Massage Mastery

From Student to Professional

Massage Mastery

From Student to Professional

Anne Williams, LMP, CHT, BFA

 Wolters Kluwer | Lippincott Williams & Wilkins
Health

Philadelphia · Baltimore · New York · London
Buenos Aires · Hong Kong · Sydney · Tokyo

Acquisitions Editor: Kelley Squazzo
Product Manager: Linda G. Francis
Senior Manufacturing Manager: Margie Orzech
Marketing Manager: Shauna Kelley
Development Editor: Tom Lochhaas
Design Coordinator: Holly McLaughlin
Photographer: Rick Giase
Production Service: SPi Global

Printed in China

Library of Congress Cataloging-in-Publication Data
Williams, Anne (Anne Eleanor)
   Massage mastery : from student to professional / Anne Williams.
      p. ; cm.
   Includes bibliographical references.
   ISBN 978-0-7817-8017-9
 I. Title.
   [DNLM: 1. Massage. WB 537]
   615.8'22—dc23
                                                                    2011035822

Care has been taken to confirm the accuracy of the information presented and to describe generally accepted practices. However, the authors, editors, and publisher are not responsible for errors or omissions or for any consequences from application of the information in this book and make no warranty, expressed or implied, with respect to the currency, completeness, or accuracy of the contents of the publication. Application of the information in a particular situation remains the professional responsibility of the practitioner.

The authors, editors, and publisher have exerted every effort to ensure that drug selection and dosage set forth in this text are in accordance with current recommendations and practice at the time of publication. However, in view of ongoing research, changes in government regulations, and the constant flow of information relating to drug therapy and drug reactions, the reader is urged to check the package insert for each drug for any change in indications and dosage and for added warnings and precautions. This is particularly important when the recommended agent is a new or infrequently employed drug.

Some drugs and medical devices presented in the publication have Food and Drug Administration (FDA) clearance for limited use in restricted research settings. It is the responsibility of the health care provider to ascertain the FDA status of each drug or device planned for use in their clinical practice.

To purchase additional copies of this book, call our customer service department at (800) 638-3030 or fax orders to (301) 223-2320. International customers should call (301) 223-2300.

Visit Lippincott Williams & Wilkins on the Internet: at LWW.com. Lippincott Williams & Wilkins customer service representatives are available from 8:30 am to 6 pm, EST.

10 9 8 7 6 5 4 3 2 1

This book is dedicated with love to my mother, Marsha Williams. Thank you for being my role model in education, for developing my passion for literature, public speaking, and life-long learning, and for your unwavering wisdom, support, encouragement, and friendship.

About the Author

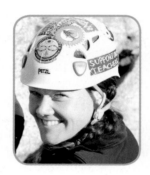

Anne Williams is a licensed massage therapist, esthetician, certified reflexologist, clinical hypnotherapist, registered counselor, aromatherapist, spa consultant, author, and educator. She is director of education for Associated Bodywork & Massage Professionals (ABMP), where she develops support materials and resources for massage students, instructors, schools, and professional members.

Before joining ABMP, she worked as a massage therapist with a special focus on healthcare massage for people recovering from car accidents. She also worked as a massage instructor for 8 years with an emphasis on curriculum development and program implementation for Ashmead College in Washington State. She has offered a number of different continuing education programs including workshops on hot stone massage, aromatherapy, spa therapies, and reflexology. In 2004, she became Ashmead's director of education and ran the education program at the Tacoma campus for 3 years.

Since she has been with ABMP, she has served on the Federation of State Massage Therapy Boards' (FSMTB) test writing committee and developed ABMP's Student Success Program and a wide range of resources for schools and instructors. She also wrote the curriculum and implemented the "Instructors on the Front Lines" massage teacher training program for ABMP and acted as project coordinator and editor for a joint book project between ABMP and Lippincott Williams & Wilkins (LWW) titled *Teaching Massage: Foundation Principles in Adult Education for Massage Program Instructors*, which was published in October 2008. She is also the author of *Spa Bodywork: A Guide for Massage Therapists*, and publishes articles for *Massage & Bodywork* magazine. When not writing or working at ABMP, Anne loves rock climbing, ice climbing, hiking, camping, trail running, biking, skiing, hanging out with friends, and anything that gets her out into Colorado's beautiful countryside.

Preface

Massage Mastery: From Student to Professional is organized into 24 chapters that cover the key areas addressed in massage programs of 500 to 1200 hours in length. It does not cover the subject of anatomy and physiology, recognizing that this important topic should probably be covered in a separate textbook. The space created by the absence of anatomy and physiology allows a broad discussion of foundation massage to be addressed with appropriate depth for a beginning student progressing to an entry-level professional. It also allows for the inclusion of new topics that are necessary to prepare today's adult learners for successful massage careers. A helpful appendix on healthcare terminology, a comprehensive massage glossary, and ancillary materials complete the package.

Organization, Structure, and Content

The textbook is broken into two parts. Part I (Theory-Focused Topics) presents program subjects that form the framework of a professional massage practice with particular focus on building "soft-skills." Effective communication, professionalism, critical thinking, maintaining a healthy therapeutic relationship with clients, and practicing good ethics are highlighted. Detailed chapters on massage effects and indications, and massage cautions and contraindications help adult learners understand the powerful reactions clients have to massage and to work safely from early in their studies. A thorough career planning a self-assessment process presented in Chapter 9 (Your Massage Career) provides adult learners with personal information to envision the future in a way that meaningfully frames their educational experiences.

Part II (Technique-Focused Topics) teaches practical skills in logical progression matching students' developing abilities. Subjects like positioning clients, modest draping, opening and closing the massage, and proper body mechanics lead to information on a variety of common massage systems including Swedish massage, seated massage, spa therapies, hydrotherapy, stone massage, reflexology, myofascial release, and deep tissue and neuromuscular therapy. For schools that introduce students to Eastern bodywork a chapter on Chinese medicine concepts that underlie Asian bodywork therapy, and a taste of techniques from tuina, shiatsu, Thai, and ayurvedic massage is helpful. Similarly, Chapter 18 (Energetic Approaches) describes key concepts in energy medicine, reiki, polarity therapy, and therapeutic touch.

Thorough Coverage of Assessment, Treatment Planning, and Documentation

Treatment planning, and documentation are essential skills that students need to practice effectively in all massage-related settings. Massage Mastery separates these issues related to wellness massage and health care massage into two in-depth chapters instead of lumping them together. In Chapter 12 (Assessment, Treatment Planning, and Documentation for Wellness Massage) students learn the basics of visual assessment, palpation assessment and session planning. They are introduced to SOAP (subjective, objective, assessment, and plan) charting and quick forms often used for recording information related to relaxation-oriented massages. Posture, range of motion, pain assessment, treatment planning, and documentation specific to healthcare massage are taught later, in Chapter 19 (Assessment, Treatment Planning, and Documentation for Healthcare Massage), when students have the foundation to absorb these sophisticated concepts.

Thorough Coverage of Massage for Clients with Specialized Needs

The final chapters of the book integrate information for adult learners ready to take on advanced skills and work with clients who have specialized needs. Chapter 22 (Musculoskeletal Injury and Massage) explores the forces that stress soft-tissue and lead to injury, the inflammatory response, and massage techniques effective for common conditions like carpal tunnel syndrome, whiplash, sprains, and strains. Chapter 23 (Massage for Chronic Pain Conditions and Selected Pathologies) explains the anatomy of pain, the impact of pain on quality of life, and describes massage for osteoarthritis, rheumatoid arthritis, fibromyalgia, headaches, cancer, and HIV/AIDS. In Chapter 24 (Massage for Special Populations), students learn how to work with athletes, mothers and babies, elderly clients, obese clients, clients living with disabilities, and the terminally ill.

Chapter Structure Designed for Today's Adult Learners

Adult learners in massage school are a dynamic group consisting of individuals from different generations, cultures, ethnicities, with different personality preferences, cognitive styles, learning patterns, and life experiences. They are often balancing multiple responsibilities including family obligations, full or part-time work, the need for social interaction, and school. Education researchers notice that specific practices can build adult motivation for learning.[1] One area that requires careful reflection is homework assignments. Researchers report that typical homework assignments can burden adult learners in ways that lead to lower motivation for learning, lower grades, and lower student retention rates.[2] Associated Bodywork & Massage Professionals (ABMP) Instructors on the Front Lines massage teacher training program recommend that teachers assign no more than 10 pages of reading per day and use a specific reading system to take notes from textbooks. Adult learners receive points when reading notes are turned in as homework.[3] In response to this research, *Massage Mastery* was structured so that each chapter is broken down into a number of specific topics. These "bite-sized" chunks of related information make perfect reading assignments for adult learners. This organization also makes it easy for teachers to match the textbook to a variety of curriculum models.

Textbook Content Designed to Address Recent Trends in Massage Education

A decade ago adult learners were often older students "dropping out" of corporate America in search of a more holistic profession. Today, approximately two-thirds of massage students are younger and choosing massage as a first profession, and this percentage is likely to get larger. This change in massage school demographics suggests that schools add material in particular subject areas to ensure their younger graduates have the skills necessary to work successfully in the massage field. *Massage Mastery* addresses these new topic areas and allows massage teachers to include instruction on building therapist emotional intelligence and understanding the psychological factors at play in a therapeutic relationship (Chapter 7), interpersonal communication skills as a precursor to professional communication (Chapter 8), and critical thinking in relationship to contraindications, client populations, and session planning (Chapters 5, 12, 19, 22, 23, and 24). In addition, Chapter 4 (The Therapeutic Nature of Massage) teaches research literacy and provides a meaningful discussion on evidenced-based massage. A feature titled, "It's True!" discussed later in this preface reinforces the value of massage research as a fundamental aspect of our technique choices. Another emerging change in the massage profession is the movement from private practice to work as an employee. *Massage Mastery* addresses this trend with an expanded section on writing resumes and cover letters, interviewing, and expectations of employers.

Textbook Features

Massage Mastery has many features that support student academic success. Chapter outlines, key words, learning objectives, and introductions help adult learners find information quickly and preview the subject of a chapter. As mentioned previously, topics inside the chapters are structured to allow for manageable reading assignments that build a student's sense of accomplishment and motivation. Every effort has been made to ensure that *Massage Mastery* is colorful and visually instructive. Tables, boxes, charts, graphs, and anatomical illustrations illuminate theoretical content. Self-assessments, proficiency checklists, and scenarios bring skill sets to life in real-world examples. Special learning features include technique boxes, concept briefs, and the Massage Fusion section at the end of chapters.

Technique Boxes

For the purposes of this textbook, a massage technique is defined as a specific procedure used to produce a particular therapeutic outcome. It can usually be applied to a variety of body areas with minor adaptations. For example, tapotement is a rapid and rhythmic percussive technique used to "drum" on the client, stimulating the muscles and improving muscle tone. Each individual massage technique is pulled out of the body of the text, illustrated with photographs, and clearly labeled. This organization of content allows students to efficiently work through step-by-step directions when learning a new skill. It also helps students understand that a particular technique is often used in a variety of massage systems or applied in integrated forms of massage. A list of techniques at the front of the textbook helps learners easily locate and practice techniques.

Concept Briefs

Concept Briefs act like note cards for adult learners when they preview or review a chapter. The purpose of these boxes is to distill relatively complex concepts into understandable bits of information that provide "anchors" for students reading through new or challenging material.

Massage Fusion Section

The Massage Fusion section at the end of chapters includes several components that assist adult learners as they integrate theory and technique.

- **Study Tips:** The Study Tips feature in the Massage Fusion section provides useful hints for how to approach information and study efficiently. In Chapter 12 (Assessment, Treatment Planning, and Documentation for Wellness Massage) the study tip is called, *Nothing Lost in Translation*. It reminds students that when they begin charting it is helpful to write out everything in long hand on a "scrap" SOAP chart in the proper sections. After the session, rewrite the SOAP chart translating the longhand into abbreviations. This insures that students collect all of the relevant information and learn proper abbreviations at the same time. While this is time-consuming at first, it is the surest way to build good skills. Soon students naturally progress to writing in an abbreviated format and charting gets faster.

- **Good to Know:** This feature provides background material that clarifies aspects of a topic to build insight or to form connections to students' personal interests or experiences. For example, the Good to Know feature in Chapter 3 (Sanitation, Hygiene, and Safety) takes a close look at allergies and explains the impact of allergies on the body's immune system. In Chapter 6 (Ethics & the Law), the Good to Know feature explains how massage therapists can get involved with legislative processes in the states where they practice massage.

- **Massage Inspiration:** This feature in the Massage Fusion pages encourages students to have fun and enjoy the process of becoming a therapist. It is particularly useful for kinesthetic learners who need to "do" in order to learn efficiently. For example, in Chapter 13 (Swedish Massage Techniques), students make a CD of their favorite songs to experience how music and the emotional state it produces affect technique application. Students play their CDs, which may contain any style of music they like, while giving a massage to classmates, friends, or family members. The goal is to incorporate the emotions of the music into the massage—even if this means departure from traditional techniques. This exercise helps students develop a flowing, connected progression of strokes. Like many Massage Inspiration activities, this can also be used as a classroom exercise.

- **It's True:** With an increased interest in the scientific basis for the benefits of massage, researchers like Tiffany Field at the Touch Research Institute have designed clinical studies that demonstrate health benefits that many massage therapists have long known. Research is showing that massage has provable benefits for the human body and should be viewed as a viable treatment for a variety of conditions including chronic pain, tension headache, fibromyalgia, and depression. It's True! highlights massage research relevant to specific chapter topics.

- **Chapter Wrap Up:** This closing feature is designed to encourage students to keep learning, even when school feels challenging. They remind students to remember how far they have come in their educational processes and relate information in a variety of chapters to one another so that students understand how various bits of massage learning fit into an integrative whole.

Online Resources

To provide support students and instructors as they use this text, a wide array of resources are offered online at http://thePoint.lww.com/Williams-Mastery.

Student Resources

Student Resources available are the following:

- Free Study Guide, with quiz questions and exercises relating to all topics discussed in the text. The Study Guide includes Learning Contracts and Rubrics for gauging progress.
- Quiz Bank
- Videos demonstrating many of the techniques found in the text
- Audio Glossary

Instructor Resources

Online resources to support instructors and massage programs are the following:

- Lesson Plans keyed to Chapter Objectives, including activities and tips for teaching the topics presented in text
- Image Bank
- PowerPoint slides
- Test Generator

A Note to Students

I am excited for you because you have chosen to embark on a challenging and very rewarding journey. Each class, each practice massage, each instructor, and each of your classmates has something to teach you that may dramatically affect how you think about your life, the human body, and the power of touch. Massage is an exciting field because it is both a science and an art. In massage school you learn that the body is both delicate and resilient. You learn that some things are easy to explain and supported by scientific research and that some things are not explained but work anyway. While massage does involve very specific procedures and detailed techniques, it is also a form of creative expression. Massage moves and flows like dance, or music, or painting. Great therapists combine the science and art of massage seamlessly in sessions that inspire many clients to make positive changes in their lives and attain a higher level of health. I hope that this textbook helps you connect information and build conceptual knowledge to inform a satisfying massage career. Massage school can be stressful at times, but if you keep your eye on your goals, stay positive, keep trying, and keep learning, very soon you will be a skilled professional massage therapist. Welcome to the massage profession!

I am grateful for the opportunity to share massage with all of the inspiring and talented therapists and students who populate our profession. I invite professionals, instructors, school administrators, and students to share with me their experiences, best practices, and suggestions. I can be reached at anne.williams20@yahoo.com.

Anne Williams,
Boulder Colorado, 2011

1. Tennant M. *Psychology and Adult Learning.* 3rd ed. London and New York: Routledge Taylor & Francis Group, 2006.
2. Wlodkowski RJ. *Enhancing Adult Motivation to Learn, Revised Edition: A Comprehensive Guide for Teaching All Adults.* San Francisco, CA: Jossey-Bass Publishers, 1999.
3. Associated Bodywork & Massage Professionals. Workshop Handout for Instructors on the Front Lines: From Handholding to Capacity Building. Information available at www.abmp.com, 2011.

User's Guide

Massage Mastery: From Student to Professional presents the theory (why) and practice (how) of massage therapy in an engaging, accessible way for today's adult and young-adult learners. Each chapter is organized into maneagable Topics, which incorporate well into any curriculum, and help you understand each component before moving on. Several key features of this title can empower your learning and help you put the topics covered into practice. We've provided this User's Guide to help you put the book's features to work for you!

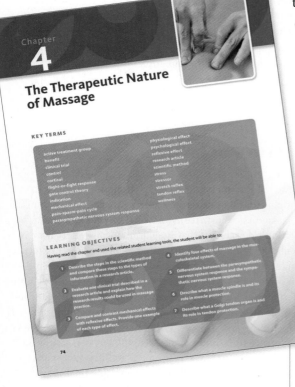

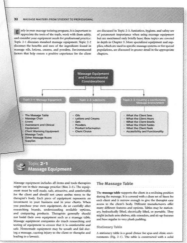

- **Chapter-opening key terms, learning objectives, and mind maps** orient you student to the material in the chapter and help you prepare for the information provided.

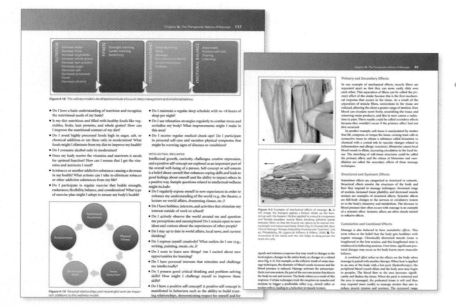

- **Unique illustrations, charts and graphs** illuminate theoretical content in a colorful and visually instructive way to help you see the topics covered and their importance in your career as a massage therapist.

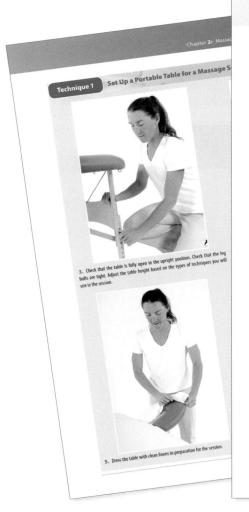

Technique 1 Set Up a Portable Table for a Massage S...

3. Check that the table is fully open in the upright position. Check that the leg bolts are tight. Adjust the table height based on the types of techniques you will use in the session.

5. Dress the table with clean linens in preparation for the session.

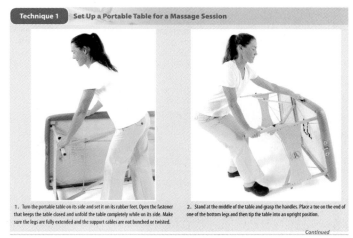

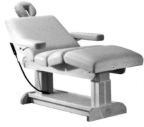

Figure 2-1 Stationary table. Image courtesy of Massage Warehouse.

Figure 2-2 Portable table. Image courtesy of Massage Warehouse.

comfortable surface for clients and allows therapists to use their body weight effectively in the delivery of certain techniques.

Massage Table Features

Manufacturers provide many options for both stationary and portable tables, allowing therapists to choose the table specifications that best meet their needs.

Frame

Massage table frames are usually made of wood, aluminum, or stainless steel. Stationary tables have heavier bases. With wood or aluminum frames, portable tables are lightweight and easy to move. Wood-framed portable tables are a little heavier than aluminum ones, but both are strong and durable. The top of the table is made of wood covered by layers of foam and fabric. Cross-braces and plastic-covered support wires provide stability. In portable tables, the four wooden or metal legs are usually constructed of two pieces that can be

Technique 1 Set Up a Portable Table for a Massage Session

1. Turn the portable table on its side and set it on its rubber feet. Open the fastener that keeps the table closed and unfold the table completely while on its side. Make sure the legs are fully extended and the support cables are not bunched or twisted.

2. Stand at the middle of the table and grasp the handles. Place a toe on the end of one of the bottom legs and then tip the table into an upright position.

Continued

- **Technique Boxes** provide step-by-step instructions illustrated by beautiful, clearly labeled photographs, giving you a clear, visual reference for each technique. A list of the techniques appears in the frontmatter.

- **Concept Briefs** placed throughout the text distill complex concepts into understandable bits of information so you can check and reinforce your learning.

Concept Brief 4-6
Flight-or-Fight Response

- The body's response to a perceived threat (run away or stay and fight)
- Mediated by the sympathetic division of the autonomic nervous system
- Causes a cascade of rapid physiological reactions to facilitate survival
- Chronic stress is a situation where persistent stressors repeatedly trigger the flight-or-fight response leading to the prolonged elevation of stress hormones, especially cortisol and epinephrine, in the bloodstream, negatively impacting health

- **Massage Fusion Section** at the end of chapters includes several components that assist you in fully integrating theory and technique:

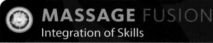

MASSAGE FUSION
Integration of Skills

STUDY TIP: there is no substitute for direct experience!

Isadora Duncan, the famous American dancer, remarked, "What one has not experienced, one will never understand in print." Massage equipment is best understood through direct experience. Students who try different bolster sizes, for example, understand that some situations require a larger bolster while others require a smaller one. Students who think about how their body feels after giving a 1-hour massage at different table heights is better able to avoid injury. Students who try the same technique with oil, cream, and powder can better understand how to make good lubricant choices. Try these ideas:

1. Place the table in a position that is too high and give massage for 30 minutes. Where does your body feel stressed? Which techniques worked well with the table high? Which techniques were difficult with the table high?

2. Place the table in a position that is too low and give massage for 30 minutes. Where does your body feel stressed? Which techniques worked well with the table low? Which techniques were difficult with the table low?

3. Lie on the massage table in the supine position using small bolsters. Feel the position of your joints and low back. Now lie on the massage table in the supine position using large bolsters. Try the same exercise in the prone position.

4. Try a massage technique using powder. Remove the powder with a dry hand towel and try the same technique with cream. Remove the cream with a hot, moist towel and try the technique with oil. Which lubricant worked best? Why?

MASSAGE INSPIRATION: Make Your Own Massage Cream

A good way to know what's in a massage cream is to make it yourself. The following natural blend provides excellent lubrication for massage strokes. A variety of natural ingredients can be found on the Internet.

Ingredients: 1 cup unrefined apricot kernel or hazelnut oil, 2 tablespoons grated beeswax, 2/3 cup distilled water, 2/3 cup aloe vera gel, 5 drops vitamin E oil.

Directions: In a double boiler, melt the apricot kernel oil and beeswax. When the beeswax melts, pour the oil mixture into a glass measuring cup and let it cool at room temperature until the edges start to turn white. Combine the water, aloe vera gel, and vitamin E in a blender at the highest speed. In a slow drizzle, pour the cooled oil and beeswax into the vortex of the blended solution while the blender is still going. Stop the blender and mix the formulation with a spatula to blend it further. Continue mixing and blending until the ingredients are completely combined. Store the product in a jar or bottle in the refrigerator.

CHAPTER WRAP-UP

The quality of your equipment and lubricants and the time and care you put into planning your massage space convey your level of professionalism to your clients. While it may seem early to start thinking about equipment needs and décor for your business, it's not too early to explore options. Try out different massage tables and different lubricants. Start to explore interior design and think about color choices and window treatments. Starting now helps ensure you will be prepared to enter the massage profession with a clear and informed plan. This also helps keep your massage career vision alive, an important motivator when the massage program gets challenging!

- **Study Tips** provide useful hints for maximizing learning benefits as well as efficient use of study time.

- **Massage Inspiration** presents activities and exercises that encourage you to have fun and enjoy the process of becoming a therapist.

- **It's True!** highlights massage research relevant to specific chapter topics.

- **Chapter Wrap Up** encourages you to keep learning! See how far you've come, and what you are now ready to learn in subsequent chapters.

Free! Online Study Guide provides the following:

- **Quizzes and Case Studies** help you enhance your understanding of the concepts
- **Learning Contracts and Rubrics** encourage you to plan and gauge your progress in the course

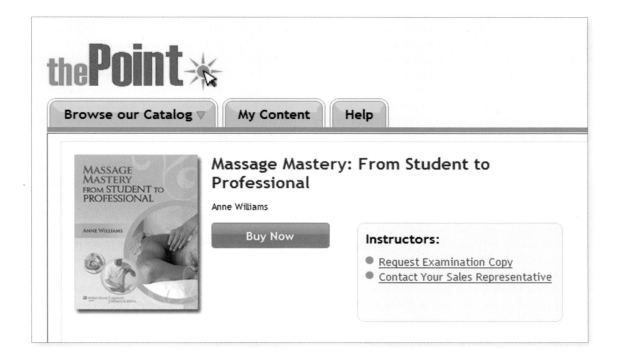

Acknowledgments

Writing and producing *Massage Mastery: From Student to Professional* has involved the contributions of many people, some who are unknown. I am thankful to all of them and would like to acknowledge those who stand out here.

During its development, *Massage Mastery: From Student to Professional* has been reviewed by a number of professionals in the massage industry, each of whom has given time and thought and provided helpful inputs. I would like to thank them for their time and contribution.

Thanks to the photographers, Rick Giase and Mel Curtis for their visual contribution to the book and for being such lovely people. Thanks to the models and also to Angie Patrick and Massage Warehouse for help with some of the images of massage equipment.

Thanks also to the amazing team at Lippincott Williams & Wilkins for their tireless enthusiasm and hard work. I would particularly like to thank Linda Francis for her understanding, great organization, and dedication to the project.

I am grateful for the insight, creativity, and vision of John Goucher who played an essential role in the formulation of the plan for this book. John will forever be one of my favorite brainstorming partners. Thank you, John. I also want to remember Pete Darcy, my first acquisitions editor, who suggested me for this project.

A huge "Thank you!" to the two people who have helped me to develop as a writer. First, Keith Shawe, whose considerate feedback of my first book helped me to learn and grow both as a writer and person. Just as important was my development editor on this project, Tom Lochhaas. Tom, I thought I was good at structuring content. You showed me just how much I still have to learn. Thank you for your insane skills as a writing coach and textbook development editor. Your insights into structure, content delivery, and style have changed me forever and influence my thinking everyday.

I am grateful for the amazing massage professionals, instructors, and administrative staff I have had the privilege of working with and learning from including Amy Klein, Amy Stark, Andrew Biel, Angie Parris-Raney, Angie Patrick, Ben Benjamin, Bill Fee, Bill Langford, Carey Rosen, Carole Osborne-Sheets, Cherie Sohnen-Moe, Cheryl Young, Chris Froelich, Christy Cael, Cliff Korn, David Christian, Debra Persinger, Deby Giske, Dennis and Gina Simpson, Elan Schacter, Felicia Brown, Gini Ohlson, Jack Elias, Jade Shutes, Jan Schwartz, Jeff Mahadeen, James Sutherlin, Jill Standard, Jesse Cormier, Kathryn Bromley, Katie Armitage, Kathy Thielen, Kim Precord, Laura Allen, Marla Gold, Marsha Elston, Marti Mornings, Mary Ann Foster, Mary O'Reilly, Mary Rose, Melanie Hayden, Melody Lickert, Meredyth Given, Nina McIntosh, Patty Glen, Ray Siderius, Rick Rosen, Rita Wynegar, Roger Patrizio, Sara Gregg, Scott Dartnall, Su Bibik, Susan Salvo, Suzanne Carroll, Til Luchau, Vickie Branch, Vicky Karr, and Victoria Robertson.

A special "thank you" to CG Funk, Darren Buford, Diana Thompson, Erin Murphy, Jenny Good, Lara Bracciante, Leslie Young, Lorine Hill, Mary Bryan, Ruth Werner, and Whitney Lowe for their great insights and influence on my thinking and work.

I extend my sincere appreciation to my parents, family, and friends for understanding when I couldn't be at events because I was working on the book, and for their unwavering support and encouragement during the time that I was writing. "Thank you" to Mom and Dad, Jill Shawe, Cindy, Larry, Jason, and Sarah Rantanen, Pam, Kurt, Joe, Gloria, and Natalie Mayer, Rick, Sharon, Jeff, and Gayle Selden, Anthony Knoll, Derek Peace, Deanna Scalf, Edana Biddle, Gretchen Pelsma, and Kim Virant.

I also want to thank my fitness trainer and friend, Burt Henry, for helping me close the computer and pick up a dumbbell. I gained 30 lb on the last book and lost 30 on this one. Thank you, Burt!

I am especially grateful to my rock climbing and adventure family who entice me away from the computer regularly, ask about progress on the book, and make my life so much fun. Thank you, Abram Herman, Jon Barr, Ronie Warner, Arthur Nisnevich, Michael Pastko, Tyler Knowles, Adele Schopf, Chris Devenney, Ryan Jaret, David Weinstein, Christy Sims, Jerilyn Sambrooke, Tiffany and Zack Shocklee, Meg Letts, Katie Mills, Eric Brown, Seth Brown, Matt Esper, Jim Erickson, and Mike Munger. Abram and Jon, I think you know you did very little to support my writing process and that more often you were a complete distraction! Both of you helped me learn to choose adventure first. The best summers of my life will forever be defined by classic trad routes in Eldo (especially Rewritten and Bastille Crack), our climbing trips to Moab and Vedauwoo, climbing in Boulder Canyon, dancing at Tahonas, hiking Colorado Fourteeners, and 32 hours in a tent on Mt. Rainier.

I want to thank everyone at Associated Bodywork & Massage Professionals (ABMP) with a special thank you to our education department team of Cindy Williams, Kathy Laskye, Taffie Lewis, Katie Mills, Kristen Coverly, Erin Merelli, and Brian Halterman. I love your ideas, dedication to massage, and enthusiasm. I look forward to coming into work everyday because of you.

I want to express my appreciation and gratitude to Bob Benson and Les Sweeney. Thank you for the most amazing job in the world and for being the best bosses and mentors I've ever known. You have given me the tools and guidance to achieve my personal best and to grow, learn, expand, and explore the possibilities. Thank you for caring as passionately as I do about massage education and for giving me so many opportunities to express that passion.

Last, but not least, I want to thank my amazing partner, Eric Brown, for helping me find the energy and determination to get this project across the finish line and for your insights, ideas, and advice. Leslie once said, "Eric Brown – big brain, bigger heart." I can't say it any better than that.

Contents

Part I
Theory-Focused Topics   1

Techniques

Theory-Focused Topics

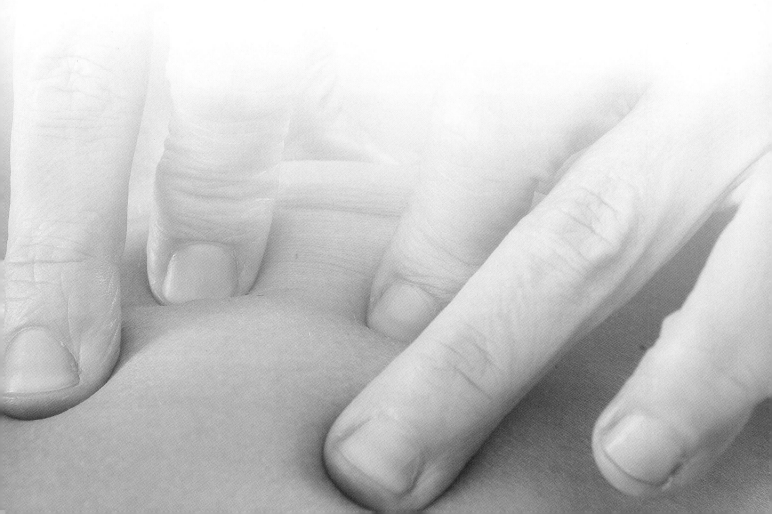

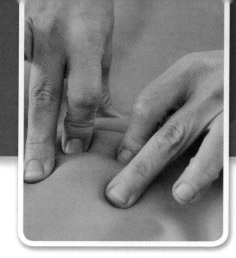

Massage from Past to Present

KEY TERMS

Andreas Vesalius

CAM therapies

Ebers Papyrus

Galen

Hippocrates

Ibn Sina

Ida Rolf

Johann Mezger

NCCAM

Per Henrik Ling

LEARNING OBJECTIVES

Having read the chapter and used the related student learning tools, the student will be able to:

1. Identify one reason why the study of history is important to contemporary massage practice.

2. Describe one ancient document that is important to our current understanding of medicine or massage.

3. Explain the contribution of one historical figure to medicine or massage.

4. Analyze the contribution of one culture to either medicine or massage and explain its relevance to a contemporary massage practice.

5. Distinguish among the terms "massage," "bodywork," "technique," "system," and "approach" in relation to the massage profession.

6. Compare and contrast the approach of conventional medicine to the body with that of alternative medicine.

7. Describe the role of the National Center for Complementary and Alternative Medicine in today's health care environment.

8. Outline one way that massage fits into today's health care system.

9. Give at least two reasons why consumers seek massage therapy today.

10. List two benefits or effects of massage that are verified by recent research.

11. List at least three different environments in which massage therapists work and describe the types of massage offered in each.

Aristotle wrote, "If you would understand anything, observe its beginning and its development." The history of massage is complex and extensive. It stretches across the globe, weaving through many different cultures and traditions. Topic 1-1 considers connections between medicine, magic, and massage in early history and how medicine evolved with contributions from the Greeks, Romans, and Arabs. The unique insights of Eastern cultures have also led to new ways of viewing the body and health. As the understanding of medicine progressed through the Renaissance and the Age of Enlightenment, ideas emerged that still influence contemporary massage. Finally, this section considers how massage developed in America, along with the influence of nurses, early physicians, and the discipline of psychology.

Topic 1-2 introduces a variety of techniques, massage systems, and ideas about how to create positive shifts in soft-tissue structures. Topic 1-3 explores the role of complementary and alternative therapies in American health care and introduces some of the research that demonstrates the benefits of massage for a wide array of conditions. We examine how the American health care system is changing to include complementary therapies like massage in treatments for many diseases and conditions formerly treated only through conventional means. This topic looks at the needs of consumers in relation to massage and discusses different environments in which massage therapists work.

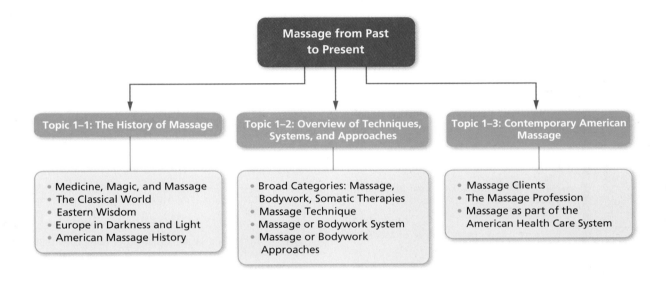

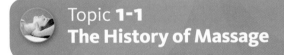

Topic **1-1**
The History of Massage

An understanding of history facilitates open-mindedness and inclusiveness, characteristics that are essential in those who practice massage. We learn that all cultures, all religions, and all peoples are connected to and "own" massage. History reminds us that as massage therapists we carry forward a tradition of working to improve the lives of others by reducing pain or bringing comfort. This chapter provides an overview of the history of massage to illuminate some of the places, people, and events that have influenced massage and bodywork (Fig. 1-1).

Medicine, Magic, and Massage

When we bump our elbow, a common reaction is to rub it until the pain decreases. A toothache prompts us to touch and hold the area that feels painful. Animals lick or rub an injured area. Massage seems to be an instinctive response to pain, and so it is likely that it was practiced all over the world long before recorded history.

In early history, medicine and magic (involving spirituality, ritual, and superstition) were closely connected. People made little distinction between the health of the spirit and the health of the body. The ancients intuitively recognized a need to address the whole individual (body, mind, and spirit), in their treatment of disease. This idea has re-emerged in the practice of alternative and complementary therapies today. The medicine man, healer, shaman, witch, priest, midwife, sorcerer, or witchdoctor worked to remove "evil" influences that caused disease. Many cultures had a practice of "anointing" another person and rubbing aromatic oil into the skin. European cave paintings from 15000 BCE show what appears to be the use of touch for healing.[1] We can learn a great deal about the roots of massage by looking at these early practices in different parts of the world.

15, 000 BCE	Early history: Medicine and magic closely linked in many cultures around the world
3500 BCE	Egypt: Evidence of civilization in Nile Valley
3000 BCE	Greece: Aegean Bronze Age–Evidence of civilization dates from 7250 BCE
2330 BCE	Egypt: Ankhmahor Tomb–Shows evidence of massage (reflexology)
1700 BCE	India: Rig Veda compiled in written form between 1700–1100 BCE from earlier tradition
1550 BCE	Egypt: Ebers Papyrus written. Found 1870s
1000 BCE	China: Classic texts compiled between 1000 BCE–221 BCE
800 BCE	Greece: 800–200 BCE medicine moves towards logical reasoning and away from magic
788 BCE	Tibet: Four Tantras compiled sometime between 786–911 BCE
753 BCE	Founding of Rome
563 BCE	India/Thailand: Jivaka Kumar Bhaccha lives 563–483. Creates Thai medicine/massage
460 BCE	Greece: Hippocrates "Father of Medicine" born. Dies 377 BCE
146 BCE	Greece/Rome: Greece physicians work in Rome after invasion of Greece in 146 BCE
129 BCE	Rome: Asclepiades born. Dies 40 BCE
30 BCE	Egypt: Death of Cleopatra. Conquest of Egypt by Rome
476 CE	Rome: Fall of Rome. Islamic nation expanding. European Dark Ages begins
529	Rome: Plato's Academy closes. Islamic physicians preserve Greek and Roman works
800	Arabia: Well developed pharmacies and extensive pharmacopeias
865 CE	Arabia: Al Razi Born. Dies 925 CE
980	Arabia: Ibn Sina Born. Dies 1037 CE
1215	Europe: First reports of witch hunts. Rise through the 1500's. Ends 1750
1275	Italy: Mondino de Liuzzi born. Writes *Anathomia* in 1315
1347	Europe/ China/ India: Bubonic Plague breaks out and over 20 million die
1400	Europe: Beginning of the Renaissance. Lasts until the 16th century
1452	Italy: Leonardo DaVinci born. Dies 1519
1514	Brussels: Andreas Vasalius born. Dies 1564
1530	Italy: Geronimo Mercuriali born. Dies 1606
1600	Europe: Translations of Greek, Roman, and Arab texts become available
1776	Sweden: Per Henrik Ling born. Dies 1839
1839	Holland: Johann Mezger born. Dies 1839
1852	America: John Harvey Kellogg born. Dies 1943
Late 1800's	Europe: Florence Nightingale includes massage in training for nurses
1897	Austria: Wilhelm Reich born. Died 1957
1950's	America: Decline of massage as public grows skeptical about its legitimacy
1960's	America: Human Potential Movement. Esalen Institute in 1962 promotes massage
1970–2012	America: Expansion of massage profession

Figure 1-1 History of massage timeline.

Ancient Egypt

In ancient Egypt, evil spirits or their poisons were believed to cause disease. The function of the priest-physician was to discover the nature of the poison and drive it from the body or destroy it. Spells, prayers to the gods, aromatic plant potions, and amulets were used. There is good evidence that massage techniques were part of Egyptian medical practice. Figure 1-2 shows a painting found in the tomb of Ankhmahor, an Egyptian priest, dated 2330 BCE. Ankhmahor's tomb contains many pictures of people undergoing medical treatment and is often called "the tomb of the physician." This image shows hands and feet being massaged with techniques very similar to those used in reflexology today.

The Egyptians documented their medical practices on a type of paper called papyrus. The **Ebers Papyrus** (1550 BCE) is a lengthy scroll that contains around 700 formulae and remedies. These entries in the papyrus demonstrate ancient Egypt's advanced understanding of human anatomy, probably related to the practice of mummification. For example, the heart is described as the center of the blood supply. Pregnancy and contraception, intestinal disorders, prevention of parasites, eye problems, dentistry, mental conditions, surgical treatments, bone setting, and skin conditions are also discussed.

Aboriginal Australia

Evidence suggests that aboriginal people have occupied the Australian mainland for over 45,000 years.[2] Our understanding of their traditional society, culture, and medical practices comes from their oral traditions and the writings of early European settlers. The aboriginals believe that life involves a network of relationships that can be traced back to the great spirit ancestors of the dreamtime.[3] Serious illness is thought to be brought about by "soul loss." Aboriginal shamans are chosen and trained to remove the influence of evil spirits and restore the well-being of the soul.[4] In one ceremony, a traditional healer conducts a healing ritual that includes sucking the sick person and spitting out a wooden object called a *yarda*, which is covered in blood. This represents the removal of evil influences. Healers also massage patients and sing over them during rituals. In *The History of Massage*, Robert Noah Calvert describes his interview with an aboriginal medicine man. Kakkib li'Dthia Warrawee'a explains that touch is vital to the aboriginal people as a means of supporting physical health and promoting relationships between the generations because the young are encouraged to massage their elders.[1]

Central and South America

The ancient Maya believed that illness had both natural and supernatural causes. Natural illness was treated with herbs, infusions, poultices, and ointments. Illness caused by supernatural causes was treated through ritual and spells.[5] The Maya had a strong spiritual connection to plants and gained a detailed knowledge of plants, their identification and use in preparations for diagnosis and treatment.

Aztec medical practices are well preserved in an advanced written language. A well-known document detailing Aztec medical practice is The Badianus Manuscript, written in 1552

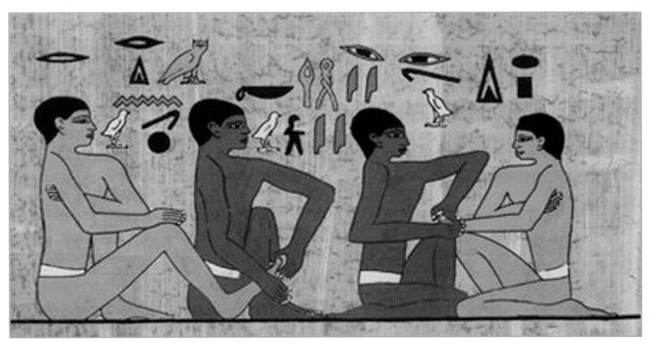

Figure 1-2 Ankhmahor's tomb.

CE by Martin de la Cruz, an Aztec physician.[6] The Aztecs understood the healing properties of plants, and 90% of the medicinal plants they identified are still in use today. For example, *Argemone grandiflora* (a relative of the opium poppy) produces a powerful analgesic known as *chicalote*, commonly used for pain in the groin. In the Aztec view, the human body was directly linked to the universe. Astronomical events likely affected body functions, and incorrect behavior could affect the function of the universe.[7] As punishment for incorrect behavior (sins), the gods sent supernatural ailments. These were treated with ritual offerings and confessions. Massage was a part of the Aztec approach to medicine and was commonly used by midwives skilled in obstetrics. Physicians also used traction and counter-traction on fractures and sprains.[9]

The *temazcal*, or sweat bath, which was a popular practice with the Maya and Aztecs, is still used in Central and South America today (Fig. 1-3). In ancient times, the baths were watched over by Temazcalteci (the grandmother of the baths), who was the goddess of medicine and medicinal herbs. The temazcal is a small, rounded mud, or stone structure with a narrow, low-ceiling entrance. It represents the womb of Temazcalteci where health, healing, introspection, and rebirth take place. Each bath is presided over by a *Temazcalera*, usually a woman, who is specially trained in diagnosis, herbs, and massage. The Temazcalera decides which herbs and techniques will be used in the treatment, along with levels of heat.[9]

Native North Americans

Native American healing methods vary depending on the specific beliefs of each nation, but many practices are common to many nations. Native Americans lived connected to the land

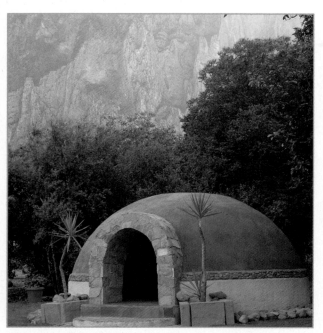

Figure 1-3 Temazcal "sweat bath." This image of a modern termazcal is used with permission from La Posada en el Potrero Chico, Camping & Lodging in Mexico (www.elpotrerochico.com).

and seasons, as many still do, so it is no surprise that they are skilled herbalists and have traditions using teas, tinctures, ointments, and salves made from local natural substances.[10] Disease is viewed as an expression of subtle forces involving the body, mind, spirit, one's relationship with the community and the environment, and lifestyle.[11] Important purification practices have been part of the practical and ritual healing traditions. The sweat lodge used for purification heats the body and exposes it to medicated steams. Smudging, a technique using smoke from a healing plant cleanses and protects the person. Some forms of smudging bring about altered states of consciousness, making the person more open to other healing techniques. Angry spirits are thought to sometimes cause disease, which might be treated in a variety of ways. Community healing rituals include chanting, singing, dancing, and praying to drive out negative energies.

Although the use of massage is not often noted in the journals of those European settlers who first wrote about Native American healing methods, James Stevenson described what are clearly massage techniques when reporting on the Navajo Indians of Arizona to the Bureau of Ethnology in 1891.[12] "Hasjelti (the medicine man) then rubbed the invalid with the horn of a mountain sheep held in the left hand, and in the right a piece of hide from between the horns of the sheep." Stevenson later explained, "On the third day the same procedures, with variations, took place. This time Hasjelti began with the limbs, and as he rubbed down each limb he threw his arms toward the eastern sky and cried 'Yo Yo!'" Many Native American practices were lost because of prohibitive laws in parts of the United States. In 1993 with the American Indian Religious Freedom Act, Native Americans gained the right to openly revive their ancient healing practices, including the use of peyote, a controlled substance.[13]

The Classical World

In ancient Greece, and later in Rome, the practice of medicine moved away from an essentially spiritual practice into the realm of science. After the fall of Rome, the knowledge gathered by the Greeks and Romans would have been lost had it not been for Arab physicians.

The Greeks

The ancient Greeks relied predominantly on the god Asclepius (or Asklepios) for healing.[14] Temples were built in his honor throughout the Mediterranean where health seekers could pray, make offerings, or conduct sacrifices to ask for his favor. His staff, bearing a single snake, identifies Asclepius in images and statues (Fig. 1-4). The snake symbolized rejuvenation and healing in many ancient Mediterranean cultures and is still used today as part of the American Medical Association crest.

From 800 BCE to 200 CE, Greek medicine moved away from magic and the divine toward observation and logical reasoning.[15] **Hippocrates** (460–377 BCE) is widely regarded as the "Father of Western Medicine" because he based his medical

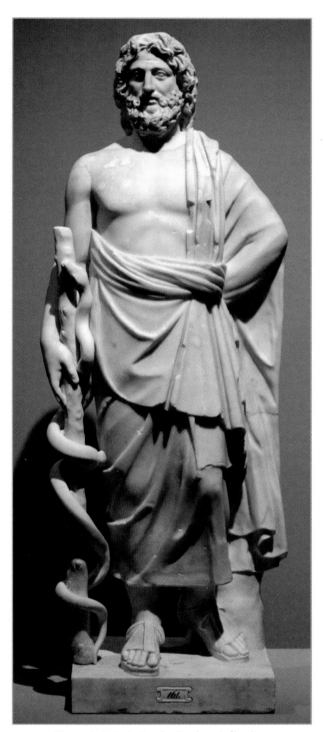

Figure 1-4 Asclepius, the Greek god of healing.

practice on observation and an extensive study of anatomy. He rejected the idea that illness was caused by evil spirits or angry gods. He believed all illness had a physical cause and a rational explanation. Hippocrates thought illness was caused when the four humors (body fluids referred to as blood, phlegm, yellow bile, and black bile) fell out of balance. To balance the humors, bloodletting or vomiting was sometimes advised. The use of the word "*anatripsis*," which means "to rub up," indicates

that Greek doctors moved away from the practice of the priest-physicians who removed evil spirits by "rubbing down" from the core of the body toward the extremities. Instead, Greek doctors massaged from the extremities toward the core of the body to support the movement of fluids.[16] This practice is still prevalent in Western massage approaches.

The Romans

In Rome, physicians were often slaves of Greek descent, taken when Rome conquered Greece in 146 BCE. Asclepiades (129–40 BCE), a Greek physician working in Rome, rejected Hippocrates' approach to medicine and believed that life was the result of "atoms" constantly on the move in the body. Hydrotherapy, exercise, and massage were important therapies for Asclepiades, who was reputed to have rubbed a dead man to life while he was on his way to the cemetery.[17] Asclepiades discovered that sleep could be induced by gentle stroking and created a device to swing the patient to promote fluid movement.[18]

Claudius Galenus of Pergamum (129–200 CE), known in English as **Galen,** was a Greek physician who built on the theories of Hippocrates. Eventually, Galen moved to Rome where he lectured, conducted experiments on animals to develop his understanding of anatomy, and wrote 22 volumes. He wrote *The Elements According to Hippocrates* to expand on the idea of the four humors. Galen accepted the benefits of massage and Asclepiades' ideas about massage and hydrotherapy and thought that muscle fibers "should be rubbed in every direction."[19] He had a major impact on medical theory and practice and was the first to demonstrate that arteries carry blood, not air as was commonly believed. He studied the brain, heart, and nervous system and demonstrated that paralysis resulted from severing the spinal column of animals. Galen's fame, ideas, and authority dominated medicine until the 16th century.

Through a desire to maintain a healthy army, the Romans developed comprehensive public health systems that included the famous Roman baths, an idea adopted from the Greeks. In the Roman Empire, public baths served an important social function as well as providing a means of exercise and hygiene. The Romans had a well-developed sense of hydrotherapy, and garrisons were often built around hot springs so that soldiers could heal their battle wounds. By the 5th century CE, there were 900 baths in Rome enjoyed by all classes of citizens. In addition to the bath itself, which housed hot pools, cold pools, steam rooms, and swimming pools, a community area often included a restaurant, library, fitness center, bar, and performance center where jugglers, musicians, and even philosophers might entertain. Massage was offered at the baths, often by skilled slave girls, who were highly regarded in Roman society.

The Arabs

In the 5th century, Rome fell and the Christian Church eventually became the new center of Europe. At roughly the same time, the Arab world was rapidly expanding geographically and melding various cultures and languages into a universal religion (Islam) and language (Arabic—Qur'an). In 529 CE, Plato's Academy in Athens closed, and its scholars sought refuge at the University of Jondishapur in Persia. After Persia became part of the Islamic world in 636 CE, the medical school at Jondishapur grew, over the course of 200 years, into the greatest center of medical teaching in the Arab world. Islamic physicians worked tirelessly to learn and preserve the works of the Greek physicians, especially Hippocrates and Galen. They also incorporated the medical knowledge of India, China, Persia, and Byzantium in their understanding. While the Islamic world advanced medical understanding, the sciences, literature, and philosophy, Europe receded deeper into the dark ages.[20]

By the 9th century, the Arabs had well-developed pharmacies with an extensive pharmacopoeia. Sienna, a clay, and new substances like camphor, nutmeg, cloves, and myrrh were used in clinical practice, and pharmacists were required to pass examinations to be licensed.

Al-Razi (also known as Rhazes, 865–925 CE) is regarded as Islam's greatest clinician. He wrote 237 books in his lifetime, many on medicine. He has been called the father of pediatrics because of his treatise *The Diseases of Children*, which distinguishes between the symptoms of smallpox and measles.

Another key figure in Islamic medicine was Abu 'Ali al-Husayn ibn 'abd Allah ibn Sina (980–1037 CE) who is most often known by his Latinized name, Avicenna. **Ibn Sina** studied and mastered medicine, philosophy, science, music, poetry, law, mathematics, physics, and statesmanship at an early age. His monumental 10th-century work, *The Canon of Medicine*, brought together and organized all existing medical knowledge including the works of Hippocrates and Galen, advances from the medical academies, and his own observations. Ibn Sina made advances in other areas that affect massage. He was the first to successfully distill essential oils (used in aromatherapy), although at the time the distillation process focused on the flower water produced, and the essential oil was an unwanted by-product.

During the 10th century, the classical texts saved by the Arabs began to find their way back into Europe and became seeds of inspiration for the Renaissance, which took hold in the 15th century. Ibn Sina's *Canon of Medicine* appeared in Europe at the end of the 12th century, became a highly regarded standard European medical reference, and was used for over 500 years.

Eastern Wisdom

Eastern manual therapy practices from China, Japan, Korea, India, Tibet, Bhutan, and Thailand have grown out of the region's rich medical history and a unique understanding of the body. In many cases, Eastern approaches to massage are an amalgamation of views from neighboring countries spread via ancient trade routes.

Ancient China

China's medical systems developed some 5,000 years ago and led to the formation of Traditional Chinese Medicine (TCM),

a comprehensive method of healing that is not only popular today but has also been shown by research studies to be effective. In *Anma: The Art of Japanese Massage*, Mochizuki points out that different components of Eastern medicine developed in different places based on the particular needs of the local people. Moxibustion, in which burning mugwort herb is applied to a small area, developed in colder regions. In the warmer flatlands, the high humidity led to a greater occurrence of muscular spasm. Cramp and spasm were treated by pressing sticks and stones directly into particular areas of the body. This practice eventually led to acupressure and acupuncture. Herbal medicine developed in western China where a wide variety of plants grew. The stretching and massaging of muscles is believed to have developed in the central region of China.[21]

Important early texts on Chinese medicine include the *Yellow Emperor's Classic of Internal Medicine*, *Essential Questions*, the *Miraculous Pivot*, and the *Book of Changes*. The content of these texts is believed to originate as early as 2500 BCE. Formally dated to the Zhou Dynasty (1000–221 BCE), these works provide the philosophical foundation on which TCM rests.

The philosophy of TCM and Eastern approaches to healing is based on the concepts of Yin and Yang, Qi, and the five elements. Yin and Yang represent relationship and connection and suggests ways to live in harmony with nature rather than attempt to subdue it. Qi (also written Chi, or Ki) is understood as life force or life energy. Qi flows along specific pathways in the body called meridians (Fig. 1-5). Eastern systems focus on promoting harmony in the flow of Qi as a means of preventing disease and promoting wellness. The five elements are wood, fire, earth, metal, and water, which correspond to qualities in nature, the seasons, and the human body.[22] Eastern healing approaches often use detailed empirical diagnostic techniques developed over thousands of years. In TCM, the information derived from the way your tongue, hair, fingernails, skin, and eyes look, as well as the smell of your breath and body and the precise feel of your pulse, is used to choose the treatment. TCM practitioners have made an art of using their senses to determine the best treatment for the patient. Chinese medical practices spread north to the Korean peninsula and Japan, where they were integrated with local customs and methods.

India

Ayurveda is both a traditional medical system and a philosophical system that offers the keys for creating harmony and balance in life. It is still practiced in India today as the primary form of medicine. In Sanskrit, "ayur" means life and "veda" means knowledge, and so the name literally means "knowledge of life" or "science of life."[23] Ayurvedic knowledge developed in India and Sri Lanka over 5,000 years ago and was written in four texts called the Vedas. The *Rig Veda*, compiled from an earlier oral history between 1700 and 1100 BCE, is the oldest of the four

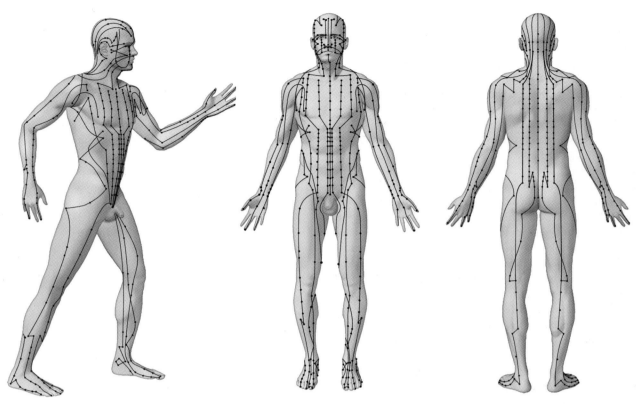

Figure 1-5 Qi flows along specific pathways in the body called meridians.

texts and outlines the main concepts in ayurveda. Ayurveda is based on the belief that everything in the universe is composed of five elements (panchamahabhutas): space (sometimes referred to as ether), air, fire, water, and earth.[24] Specific combinations of the five elements make up the three doshas (tridoshas), known individually as vata, pitta, and kapha. How the doshas combine in an individual determines body type, mental and emotional characteristics, and personality.

Abhyanga is the Sanskrit word for oil massage, which is often performed by more than one therapist. Massage strokes, oil preferences, and herbs are chosen according to the patient's dosha type or imbalance. During a treatment, marma points are usually used to restore the body to normal function, balance the body's energies, and either energize or relax the body as necessary for improved health. Marma points are energy centers in the body traditionally used with Indian massage and ayurvedic healing.[25]

In India, massage is still an important part of daily life. Mothers are commonly seen massaging their children on a blanket in the open marketplace, and women often massage each other's shoulders while chatting. Self-oiling and self-massage are also common practices.

Thailand

Thailand is situated along the great trade route between India and China, and Thai massage has roots in both ayurveda

and TCM. Jivaka Kumar Bhaccha (also known as Shivago Komparaj) lived around 536–483 BCE and is credited as the doctor of Buddha and creator of Thai medicine.[26] Thai medicine has four traditional elements: nutritional counseling, herbal medicines (both internal and external), spiritual counseling (based on Buddhist principles), and physical treatment.[27] Thai massage was also influenced by folk practices, as the farming culture needed relief from the aches and pains of hard labor in the fields. Children were trained to fill porous bags with healing herbs and press them into muscles and joints. While adults soaked in herbal baths, children would pull and stretch their limbs or knead their taut muscles. The influence of ayurveda is seen in the yogic aspects of Thai massage where "patients" are assisted in yoga positions and deep stretches. Chinese medicine introduced the idea of energetic meridian lines and acupressure points. Many of the percussive techniques and rocking movements of Thai massage are similar to Tui Na (Chinese massage).

Tibet and Bhutan

In Tibet and Bhutan, and in parts of India and Nepal, traditional Tibetan medicine is still practiced despite the invasion of Tibet by China in 1950. Tibetan medicine is based on the teachings of Buddha around 500 BCE and is known as Gso-wa Rig-pa "The Knowledge of Healing."[28] The rGyud Bzhi (Four Tantras) are comprised of 156 chapters and 5,900 verses about diseases and treatments. They are dated between

786 and 911 BCE, but the exact time of their writing is unclear. These great medical texts capture the traditions and teachings of Gso-wa Rig-pa and are still used today.[29]

In Tibetan medicine, the causes of all illness are three mental poisons described as desire, hatred, and confusion.[30] Desire is characterized by greed, attachment to objects or people, pride, and cravings resulting in disharmony of wind. Hatred, causing disharmony of energy, or bile, is characterized by anger, aggression, and aversion. Confusion, which is recognized as indecision, mental lethargy, and listlessness, causes disharmony of phlegm. The 84,000 types of disease identified in Tibetan medicine are classified as early-life, present-life, past-life, or spirit-influenced conditions.[31] Tibetan physicians interview the patient extensively and pay attention to the quality of their pulse, urine, tongue, skin, eyes, ears, and physical movement, to arrive at a diagnosis and treatment.[32] Astrological charts are sometimes used to determine the patient's predisposition to disease or the underlying cause of the disease. Treatments include herbal pharmaceuticals, moxibustion, wearing of gemstones or animal skins, burning incense, acupuncture, laxatives and emetics, mineral baths, and massage.

The Medicine Buddha is the guarding deity of Tibetan medicine and is believed to be the emanation of the historical Buddha (Fig. 1-6). The healing powers of the Medicine Buddha are invoked through visualization, speaking, hearing, or concentrating on his name (Bhaisajya guru) and prayer. Artistic depictions of the Medicine Buddha color him in the deep blue of lapis lazuli (a gem stone believed to be of divine origin). In his hand, the Medicine Buddha holds a myrobalan fruit (cherry plum), which was believed to render poison inactive.[33] Because the influence of the mind in Tibetan medicine is of primary importance, contemplation of the Medicine Buddha and his symbolism is essential to healing and harmony. Eastern approaches to massage and bodywork are described in greater detail in Chapter 17.

Concept Brief 1-1
Cultural Keys to Advances in Medicine and Massage

Egypt	Beliefs about afterlife led to understanding of anatomy
Aboriginals	Relationships to each other and to ancestors were important components of health
Maya	Advanced knowledge of plants as medicine
Aztec	Illness was punishment for bad behavior
Native Americans	Purification and ritual led to readiness of mind, body, and spirit
Greece	Moved medicine out of the realm of magic, relying instead on observation and logical reasoning
Romans	Organized related methods into systems
Arabs	Integrated many disciplines to enhance expertise
China	Philosophical foundation of yin, yang, Qi, and the five elements
India	Mindful choices in daily life promoted balance and health
Thailand	Ancient trade routes led to the integration of ayurveda, folk practices, and TCM
Tibet	A person's mindset was of prime importance in health

Europe in Darkness and Light

From the fall of Rome, through the Dark Ages, to the Renaissance, and into the Age of Enlightenment, touch and movement were a part of medicine. In the 1800s, however, medicine and massage split in separate directions, and massage as we know it today began to take shape.

The Dark Ages

At the end of the 5th century, barbarian tribes overran the Roman Empire. The Christian Church, already a powerful institution, organized resistance and eventually governed Rome.[34] The Church viewed the Roman baths and Roman technology as materialistic excess and an affront to God, and abolished them. The period known as the "Dark Ages" began and lasted into the 8th century. Across Europe, this period was characterized by low economic activity; migration of people

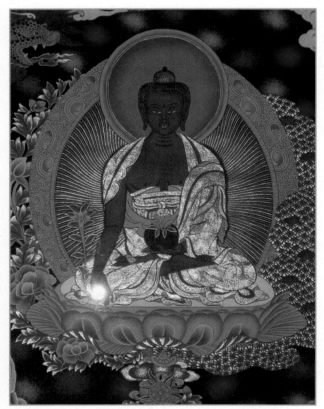

Figure 1-6 The healing powers of the Medicine Buddha in Tibetan medicine are invoked through visualization, speaking, hearing, or concentrating on his name, and prayer. Image courtesy of Vicki Harris.

into new regions; wars for control of resources; shifting politics; and a decline in art, science, literature, and medicine.

Christianity spread much more quickly in urban areas than in the countryside, and soon the word for "country dweller" (pagan) became synonymous with someone who was not a Christian.[35] Women healers had been accepted before the spread of Christianity and had developed in-depth knowledge of medicinal herbs and midwife techniques that included massage. As Christians became less tolerant of pagans' determination to maintain their own religion (some argue this was a way to increase economic power), pagans, especially women, were hunted as witches and burned at the stake.[36] Written knowledge of their practices was destroyed as heresy. Despite this persecution, the use of massage in midwifery persisted through the Middle Ages to the present day.

Women of the Church preserved massage when they created healing establishments to treat the seriously ill and dying. Although women could operate only with approval from the Church, touch and bathing practices were often used to alleviate suffering.[37]

In the 14th century, the Black Death (bubonic plague) killed an estimated third of the people in Europe (~20 million) and also broke out in China and India. Until the 1700s, the plague returned periodically and took more lives. The plague killed sinners and the pious, peasants and priests, wealthy and poor, kings and commoners alike. People began to focus more on their present life rather than the afterlife, and the Christian worldview took a serious blow.[38] Many historians feel that this shift in religious beliefs allowed the rebirth of humanistic philosophies from the Greek and Roman eras. These re-established ideas were spread further through the advent of the printing press in the 1450s.

The Renaissance

An explosion of artistic and scientific advances characterized the period spanning the 14th to 16th centuries known as the Renaissance (French for "rebirth"). The study of anatomy dramatically advanced during the Renaissance, especially in Italy where a number of authors dissected cadavers and sought to accurately describe internal organs. Prominent among these authors is Mondino de Liuzzi (1275–1326 CE), who systemized dissection and published a manual called *Anathomia* (1315), which became a medical textbook that was still used in schools three centuries after his death.[39]

Leonardo da Vinci (1452–1519 CE) was a genius who advanced architecture, anatomy, sculpting, engineering, math, music, and painting—among other fields. He is widely regarded as one of the greatest painters of all time. Leonardo learned anatomy as part of his studies in painting. He is believed to have dissected at least 30 cadavers between 1481 and 1511. He carefully studied the human skeleton and discovered that the sacrum was not uniform but composed of five fused vertebrae. He drew muscles and tendons with precision and was the first to show the fetus in the intrauterine

position. His 200 anatomical drawings were published 161 years after his death as *Treatise on Painting*.[40]

Andreas Vesalius (1514–1564 CE) wrote *On the Workings of the Human Body* in 1543, which became one of the most influential books on human anatomy. Vesalius was a Flemish anatomist, born in Brussels, who studied the medical theories of Galen at the University of Paris. Vesalius broke with common practice and handled the dissection of cadavers himself while students gathered around the table. He considered hands-on, direct observation, the only reliable source of information. Up to this time, anatomy and medicine had been taught by reading classical texts by Galen, followed by animal dissection performed by a barber-surgeon, one of two types of medical professionals at the time. Physicians were well educated and expensive. They diagnosed illness and treated wealthy individuals. Barber-surgeons were most commonly charged with looking after soldiers wounded in battle. Many set up shop to cut hair, shave beards, pull teeth, set fractures, lance boils, and let blood as needed by commoners. Physicians felt that actually conducting surgery or cutting open a cadaver was a messy, lowly task and left this task to barber-surgeons. Physicians often directed barber-surgeons in dissection while teaching other physicians about anatomy. As Galen's claims were accepted unconditionally, misinformation was passed on unchecked because physicians did not have the experience of directly interacting with the body and its structures. Vesalius' text broke from many of the anatomical models of Galen and emphasized hands-on dissection and observation in what came to be known as the "anatomical" view of the body.[41]

Geronimo Mercuriali (1530–1606 CE) was an Italian philologist and physician who studied the classical medical literature of the Greeks and Romans. Mercuriali paid special attention to classical approaches to diet, exercise, hygiene, and natural methods of healing disease. He explained principles of physical therapy and resurrected Galen's views on manual therapy. His publication of *Art of Gymnastics* (1569) is considered the first book on sports medicine.[42]

The Age of Enlightenment

Advances in the physical sciences, especially the popularity of exercise as a means of achieving health, occurred during the 17th and 18th centuries. Translations of Arab and Chinese texts provided information on new forms of exercise like yoga and martial arts. Greek and Roman ideas on gymnastics became more widely available, and books like the *Art of Gymnastics* were translated into English. Advances in chemistry and the development of drugs during this period split heath practitioners into two camps: those who favored drugs and surgery and those who favored movement as a means of preventing disease.

The Swedish Movements

A key proponent of gymnastics for health was **Per Henrik Ling** (1776–1839). While he is often credited with creating medical gymnastics, he built on the work of many other people to develop a structured movement system.

Born in the South of Sweden, Ling studied theology at both Lund University and Uppsala University and then traveled in Europe teaching languages. Ling became proficient at fencing and acted as the fencing master at Lund University in 1805. During this period, he developed rheumatism and suffered from elbow pain due to the repetitive, one-sided movements of fencing. Exercise was already popular, but Ling wanted to understand the effects of movements and their therapeutic potential. He took anatomy and physiology classes at the university to understand the body and organized the various methods used in gymnastics into a comprehensive system. Ling's medical gymnastics were classified as "active," "passive," and "active-passive."

Active movements were performed by the patient under the direction of an attendant and were basically an exercise routine. According to Calvert in *The History of Massage*, the patients stood in lines and performed lunging and isometric exercises in military fashion. With passive movements, the attendant would move and stretch the patient's body while the patient relaxed. These relaxed movements helped increase the patient's freedom of movement and lengthen muscle tissue. Passive treatment also included manipulations of soft-tissue structures that had names like "holding," "pressing," "shaking," "clapping," and "sawing." **Dr. Johann Mezger** in Holland (1839–1909) later classified these manipulations in categories with French names: effleurage (stroking), petrissage (kneading), friction (rubbing), and tapotement (tapping). Active-passive movements are now referred to as "resisted range of motion"; the patient attempted to move in a certain manner while the attendant resisted this movement. This helped to strengthen the patient's muscles.

Ling's system came to be known as "The Swedish Movements" and gained popularity across Europe and America. Mezger promoted soft-tissue manipulations and formed the earliest known association of masseurs, called the Dutch Association for Medical Gymnastics and Massage. These two individuals, building on the earlier work of many others, gave birth to what we know today as Swedish massage.

Concept Brief 1-2
Europe in Darkness and Light

The Dark Ages	The fall of Rome, the rise of Christianity, and witch hunts resulted in the loss of much traditional knowledge about midwifery, herbal wisdom, and massage; women of the church preserved massage
The Renaissance	An explosion of new ideas in science and art; the science of anatomy dramatically advanced. Mistakes of Galen corrected by Vesalius
Age of Enlightenment	Exercise a popular way to improve health; birth of Swedish massage

American Massage History

In 19th-century America, both physicians and the public embraced massage as a health-promoting practice. A number of physicians wrote books describing massage techniques and the Swedish movements. Dr. John Harvey Kellogg (1852–1943) pioneered many practices at the Battle Creek Sanitarium (the San) in Michigan. Kellogg recommended a good vegetarian diet, regular exercise, correct posture, fresh air, and proper rest. He persuaded women to discard their corsets and ignore fashion to improve their breathing. In 1895, Kellogg published *The Art of Massage, Its Physiological Effects*, and *Therapeutic Applications*, which outlined mechanical, reflexive, and metabolic effects of massage on different body systems. This text in subsequent editions has become a classic in massage, used until recently in some massage schools.

Massage in Nursing

Florence Nightingale (1820–1910), considered the pioneer of modern nursing, included massage in her training of nurses at the Florence Nightingale Training School at St. Thomas Hospital in London.[43] Her holistic and practical approach to healing encouraged nurses around the world and was an inspiration for nurses in the American Civil War. In the late 1800s and early 1900s, a number of nurses and physicians wrote books about massage for nursing. Women worked as nurses in army hospitals both at home and overseas in World Wars I and II, and massage was part of the regular duties performed by a nurse. Back massage was provided both to help patients sleep and as treatment for various conditions and recovery from surgery. Massage training remained part of the nursing curriculum until the 1950s when the expanding range of nurses' duties and time constraints forced its decline (Box 1-1).

Body–Mind Connection

In America, massage techniques became closely intertwined with the natural medicine movement and were influenced by the work of Wilhelm Reich (1897–1957).[44] Reich studied with Sigmund Freud and is often considered the founder of psychotherapeutic body therapies, sometimes called body–mind therapy or somatic therapy. In *Character Analysis* (1933), Reich theorized that unreleased psychosexual energy could produce physical blocks in muscles and organs that he defined as "body armoring." In sessions to break down "body armor," Reich used touch along with talking. He would check patients' breathing patterns and place his hand on their chest to draw their awareness to their own physical responses to the talk therapy.[45]

Skepticism and Decline

With two World Wars and the Depression behind them, in the 1950s many Americans wanted to settle behind their

BOX 1-1 What Happened to the Women?

The early history of medicine and massage is filled with male figures, making one wonder what happened to the females. Women played an important though often less publicized role in the development of massage. From the skilled slave girls in Roman times to the healing women of the church, to the midwives of the Middle Ages, to the nurses of wartime, women were often on the giving end of massage, and they still are. Associated Bodywork & Massage Professionals estimates that 80% of its members are female. Following are a few of the women who have helped to shape massage in modern times:

Louisa Despard, an Irish nurse-therapist, wrote *Text-Book of Massage and Remedial Gymnastics* (1911), which was popular in English massage up through the 1930s.

Nellie Macafee, an American nurse, published *Massage: An Elementary Text-Book for Nurses* (1920), which included in-depth information on the physiological effects of massage.

Mary McMillan, an American physical therapist, wrote *Massage and Therapeutic Exercise* (1921). McMillan became the director of physiotherapy at Harvard Medical School and founded the American Physical Therapy Association. She did a great deal to advance the understanding and value of massage.

Elizabeth Dicke, a German physiotherapist, developed connective tissue massage in the 1920s to address an impairment of circulation in her leg. Her work advanced the understanding of myofascia.

Eunice Ingham, an American physical therapist, developed reflexology and wrote *Stories the Feet Can Tell* and *Stories the Feet Have Told* in the 1930s.

Dr. Ida Rolf, an American biochemist working in the 1940s, extensively researched musculoskeletal components and founded structural integration (popularly called "Rolfing"). Her methods continue to profoundly influence massage today.

Frances Tappan, an American physical therapist, wrote numerous important books on massage, including *Massage Techniques: A Case Method Approach* (1961), and helped promote the regulated practice of massage during her lifetime.

Dr. Janet Travell, an American physician, had a special interest in musculoskeletal pain and developed a number of methods for treating and reducing muscle pain. Her extensive work on trigger points (*Trigger Point Manual*, 1968) continues to influence massage.

Dr. Tiffany Field, an American psychologist, founded the Touch Research Institute in 1992 to prove scientifically the benefits of massage.

picket fences and watch a new gadget called television. At this time, the term "massage" was often used as a cover for prostitution, and genuine therapists found that the general public was skeptical about their legitimacy. The revival of massage began in the 1960s when many young people rejected the conservative views of the 1950s and began to look for greater meaning in life.

The Human Potential Movement

The Human Potential Movement that began in the 1960s was based on the idea that humans have a large store of untapped creative and intellectual potential. To release this potential, humans needed to experience life filled with happiness, creativity, and personal development.[46] Michael Murphy and Dick Price established the Esalen Institute in 1962 in Big Sur, California, as a center for the exploration of human potential (Fig. 1-7). Spiritual practices like meditation, Buddhism, and yoga were taught in seminars side by side with massage and bodywork. Encounter groups encouraged people to explore their feelings and alternative models of communication. This movement helped to encourage the idea that massage is part of a healthy lifestyle.

In the 1970s, 1980s, and 1990s, the number of massage therapists increased dramatically as massage was increasingly accepted by the public. Massage and bodywork training programs sprang up across the country as education regulations

were established. Professional massage associations formed and developed ethical standards and practices. Today massage is flourishing, and the environment in which new therapists find themselves is dynamic, creative, and exciting. As we move to the contemporary state of American massage in Topic 1-3, it is helpful first to examine the techniques, systems, and approaches used in massage clinics, spas, and wellness centers across the country.

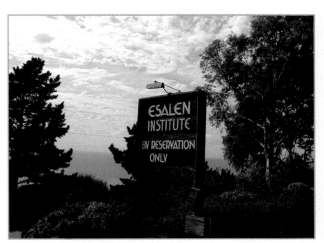

Figure 1-7 The Esalen Institute in Big Sur, California, is a center for the exploration of human potential. Photo used by permission.

Topic **1-2**
Overview of Techniques, Systems, and Approaches

Through the history of massage, new **techniques** were developed to cause physiological or psychological changes in the body. Techniques usually were later grouped together within a formalized **system** (also called a modality, form, or style). Different systems that share many similar characteristics are collectively called an "**approach**" (which might also be referred to as a modality, form, or style). These terms are often confusing, and at the time of this writing, not everyone agrees on clear-cut categories of approaches and systems. This confusion has occurred in part because people are naturally dynamic and inventive and because massage is still evolving. The story of **Ida Rolf** and structural integration is an interesting example of how terms evolve (Fig. 1-8).

Structural Integration was the name Ida Rolf gave to her revolutionary bodywork system in the mid-1900s. In 1971, Rolf founded the Rolf Institute of Structural Integration in Boulder, Colorado, to train practitioners and carry out research. Dr. Rolf died in 1979, but her instructors carried on her work. Eventually, philosophical and personal differences caused two of Rolf's senior instructors to break away from the Rolf Institute. Together they revived the Guild for Structural Integration (originally founded by Rolf) to carry on Rolf's traditions. Today the Rolf Institute and the Guild for Structural Integration teach different versions of Rolf's work. The Guild strives to teach Structural Integration as traditionally as possible, while the Rolf Institute has modified the teachings while staying true to Rolf's core ideas and concepts. The Rolf Institute owns the rights to the words "Rolfing," "Certified Rolfer," and "Rolf Movement Practitioner." The Guild, on the other hand, uses the term "Guild Structural Integration Practitioner." Thus "Structural Integration" and "Rolfing" are the same—yet different. The terminology is further complicated because new systems have been developed on Rolf's foundation. Joseph Heller ("Hellerwork") and Bill Williams ("Soma Neuromuscular Integration") both trained with Ida Rolf and used structural integration as a basis for developing their own methods.

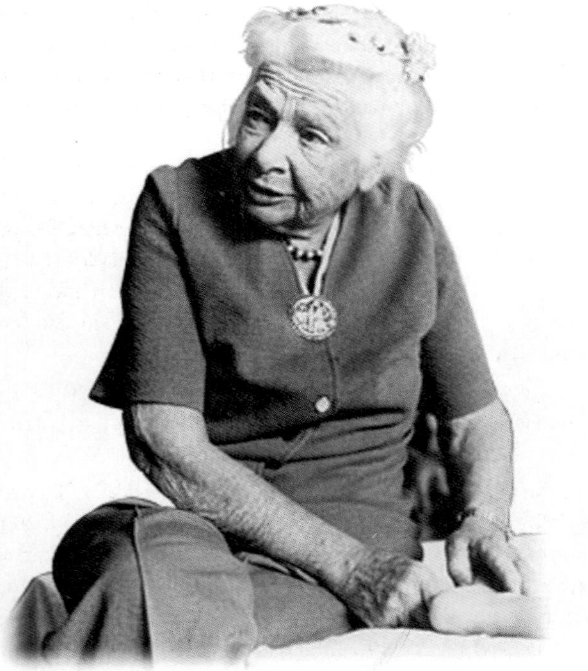

The massage and bodywork industry continues to ponder how best to define and categorize the different branches of the profession. The following section provides some useful definitions and gives an overview of some of the different systems and approaches as they exist now.

Broad Categories: Massage, Bodywork, and Somatic Therapies

Massage, bodywork, and somatic therapies are broad terms used to describe techniques and systems that promote health and wellness of the body, mind, and spirit.

Massage Defined

Massage can be defined as structured, professional, therapeutic touch. Massage techniques manually manipulate the soft-tissue structures of the body to promote health and wellness. The term "scope of practice" is used by the regulating boards of different health care professions to describe the techniques, activities, and methods licensed therapists are permitted to practice under the law. While massage definitions and scope of practice statements vary from state to state, there are some common components captured in the Massage Therapy Body of Knowledge (MTBOK) project released in May 2010 (Box 1-2). In the MTBOK, massage is defined as:

Massage therapy is a health care and wellness profession involving manipulation of soft tissue. The practice of massage therapy includes assessment, treatment planning and treatment through the manipulation of soft tissue, circulatory fluids and energy fields, affecting and benefiting all of the body systems, for therapeutic purposes including, but not limited to, enhancing health and wellbeing, providing emotional and physical relaxation, reducing stress, improving posture, facilitating circulation of blood, lymph and interstitial fluids,

Figure 1-8 Ida Rolf called her revolutionary bodywork system structural integration. Photo by David Kirk-Campbell. Used by permission.

BOX 1-2 The Massage Therapy Body of Knowledge Project

The Massage Therapy Body of Knowledge (MTBOK) project is an attempt by the massage profession to capture the essential information that defines the knowledge, skills, and attitudes required to practice massage. This baseline data is useful for setting curriculum and practice standards, and for creating greater unity across the profession. In 2007, initial meetings hosted by the American Massage Therapy Association (AMTA) led to the formation of a Stewards group comprised of representatives from the AMTA, Associated Bodywork & Massage Professionals, the Federation of State Massage Therapy Boards, the Massage Therapy Foundation, and the National Certification Board for Therapeutic Massage and Bodywork. The Stewards group funded an independent task force to gather data on the current status of the massage therapy field and to develop a general scope of practice statement for massage. In the document, they describe the competencies of an entry-level massage therapist and define the terminology specific to massage therapy. This foundational work can be used to set education standards, inform regulatory boards, and develop teacher qualifications in the future. The MTBOK was released in May 2010 and is available for review and comment until 2014 when it will be updated, expanded, and revised. You can access the MTBOK at www.mtbok.org.

balancing energy, remediating, relieving pain, repairing and preventing injury and rehabilitating. Massage therapy treatment includes a hands-on component, as well as providing information, education and non-strenuous activities for the purposes of self care and health maintenance. The hands-on component of massage therapy is accomplished by use of digits, hands, forearms, elbows, knees and feet with or without the use of emollients, liniments, heat and cold, hand-held tools or other external apparatus. It is performed in a variety of employment and practice settings.

Bodywork Defined

The term "bodywork" may include massage but also includes techniques and systems that are not massage but that may still change soft tissue. For example, Reiki is a bodywork system in which the practitioner places his or her hands on the client to "guide life force energy." Simple touch rather than massage is used because the energetic fields of the body are the focus, rather than soft tissue. Aston-Patterning includes massage but also includes movement education and exercise components. It is best described as bodywork. Assisted yoga positions could be considered a form of bodywork, as would ayurvedic bodywork in which techniques like the application of herbal pastes (udvartana) or the play of a thin stream of oil over the forehead (shirodhara) are used in combination with massage. It helps to think of bodywork as a more inclusive, broader term than massage.

Somatic Therapies Defined

The term "somatic therapies" is probably the most confusing of these three general terms because the word "*soma*" means "body" in Greek, yet many somatic therapies address the client's psychological aspects and do not use massage. "Somatic Experiencing," for example, promotes an awareness of body sensations to help people resolve and heal after traumatic events but does not involve massage. "Soma Neuromuscular Integration," in contrast, is based on the work of Ida Rolf and is very massage oriented.

Massage Technique

For the purposes of this book, a massage technique is defined as a specific procedure used to produce a particular therapeutic outcome. It can usually be applied to a variety of body areas with minor adaptations. For example, tapotement is a rapid and rhythmic percussive technique used to "drum" on the client, stimulating the muscles and improving muscle tone. This technique is most often used as part of Swedish massage (a system), but is also used in sports massage (a system) and in Russian massage (a system).

Active isolated stretching (AIS) is an advanced technique often used in sports massage and clinical massage. With this technique, the therapist asks the client to contract the muscle opposite to the particular muscle of focus (e.g., laterally flex the head to the left using the muscles on the left side). This helps the focus muscles to relax (the muscles on the right side of the neck must lengthen to allow the muscles on the left side to shorten). The therapist applies gentle pressure for 2 seconds or less to increase the stretch of the focus muscle. The key to this technique is to release the stretch before the muscles react with a protective contraction. Runners and other athletes often use AIS to protect their muscles from injury and to improve flexibility.

The word "technique" can cause some confusion in the massage profession because therapists sometimes use it when describing what generally should be called a system. Despite its name, "muscle energy technique" can be considered a system because it uses both post-isometric relaxation and reciprocal inhibition as techniques (both techniques are also used in sports and clinical massage).

Massage or Bodywork Systems

For the purposes of this book, a massage or bodywork *system* is defined as a collection of techniques organized in a complex whole. It may include a set of procedures that are carried out in a particular order to achieve a specific goal. For example, in Swedish massage, six different techniques are used in a progression from effleurage (warms the tissue), to petrissage (lifts and squeezes the tissue), to friction (compresses and broadens the tissue), to vibration (oscillates and loosens the tissue), to tapotement (stimulates and tones the tissue), to joint movements (increase joint lubrication and movement). Although many of these techniques have similar effects, each is performed to manipulate the tissue in a different way. When used together, they increase relaxation, decrease muscle tension, increase range of motion, and increase circulation (among other effects).

Tui Na is another example of a massage or bodywork system. Tui Na, or traditional Chinese massage, uses a number of techniques to promote the harmonious flow of Qi through the meridian system. Techniques include massage, acupressure to energy points, the application of herbal poultices, and the use of liniments and salves.

Massage and Bodywork Approaches

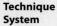 Many different massage and bodywork systems use similar techniques or procedures to achieve comparable results. Massage professionals often use the word *approach* to describe this similarity. In an earlier section, for example, different systems that evolved from the work of Ida Rolf were described, and these can all be categorized as "structural integration approaches." The next sections introduce a variety of other approaches. Since you likely have not yet been introduced to many of these techniques and approaches, it is natural to feel a little confused at first. If so, just look this section over for now, knowing that these techniques and systems will make more sense later on as most are described in greater depth in later chapters. Techniques and systems specifically designed for special populations (e.g., sports massage, pregnancy massage, etc.) are not included here but are discussed in Chapter 24.

It is important to be aware that other massage professionals may categorize these methods somewhat differently. It is best to remain flexible and curious. No doubt massage professionals will continue to discuss how techniques and approaches are defined and categorized, leading to greater clarity in the future (Fig. 1-9).

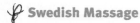

Concept Brief 1-3
Techniques, Systems, and Approaches

Technique	A specific procedure used in a particular task
System	A collection of techniques organized into a complex whole
Approach	A group of massage and bodywork systems that use similar techniques to achieve comparable results

Swedish Massage

As introduced earlier, Per Henrik Ling of Sweden formalized the gymnastics (movement therapies) of the late 1700s into a comprehensive system called "The Swedish Movements." Dr. Johann Mezger applied French terms to the specific

techniques (effleurage, petrissage, friction, vibration, and tapotement) used to manipulate soft tissue. These combined therapies gradually became known as Swedish massage. Swedish massage is sometimes called relaxation massage because it is often used specifically for stress reduction, but Swedish massage can also be used within a clinical practice. Widely recognized and popular with clients, Swedish massage is frequently the foundation of a therapist's techniques, even for those therapists who practice in different systems.

Deep-Tissue Massage

Deep-tissue massage is not really an independent system, or even a technique. It is better described as a way to approach soft-tissue structures. At any time, and during any type of massage, a therapist should be able to slow down and work more deeply when localized tension is encountered. Deep-tissue techniques aim to work the deeper fascia and muscles of the body to release adhesions and restrictions. Strokes are usually but not always applied very slowly at a depth the client can tolerate. The tissue is compressed, broadened, and stretched during the stroke and gradually softens. A therapist using deep-tissue techniques needs exceptional palpation skills because one of the keys to this type of work is "listening" to the tissue and waiting for it to "let go" and "invite the therapist in."

Many systems of massage incorporate deep-tissue techniques. For example, because friction strokes in Swedish massage can be applied lightly or deeply, Swedish and deep-tissue approaches are often integrated in one session. Some types of massage and bodywork, like Rolfing, Pfrimmer Deep Muscle Therapy, and neuromuscular therapy (NMT), predominantly use deep-tissue work.

Clinical Approaches

In general, clinical approaches are systems developed for clients who have been diagnosed with a soft-tissue condition by a physician and referred to a massage therapist for treatment. Such conditions include repetitive stress injuries (e.g., carpel tunnel syndrome), car injuries (e.g., whiplash), and sports injuries (e.g., hamstring strain). Clinical approaches use advanced musculoskeletal and postural assessment skills along with a variety of techniques to address soft-tissue pain, dysfunction, and injury. The education of clinical therapists includes an in-depth understanding of tissue injury and repair mechanisms, as well as rehabilitation protocols. The names of clinical systems include clinical massage, orthopedic massage, medical massage, health care massage, therapeutic massage, and treatment massage. Many other systems are also used to treat soft-tissue injuries, in addition to clinical approaches.

Structural Integration Approaches

This approach to massage and bodywork is based on the idea that an efficiently organized body (skeleton, joints, fascia,

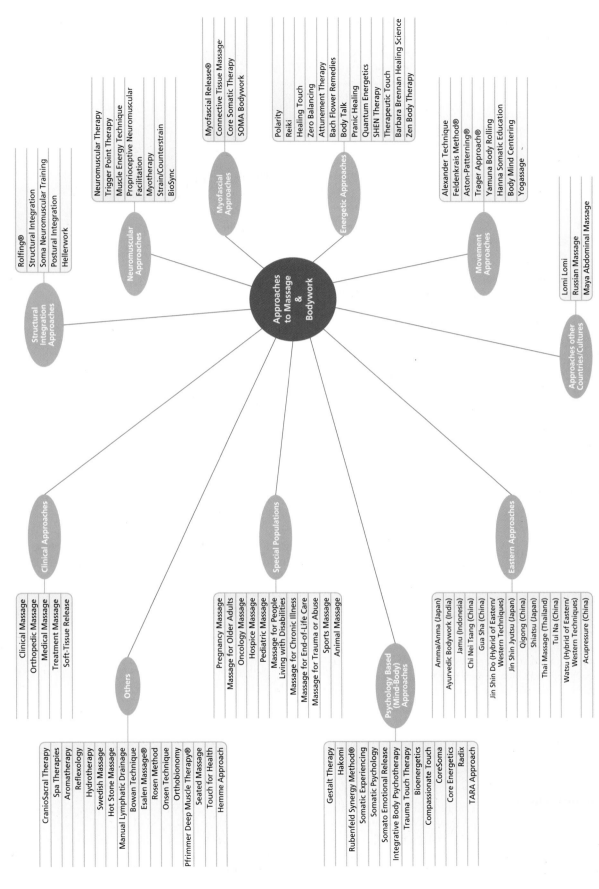

Figure 1-9 Massage and bodywork systems and approaches are likely to be defined differently by massage professionals. This chart represents one method of categorization.

muscle) functions optimally when it interacts with gravity. If habitual movements deviate from the optimal geometric movement of the skeleton in space, function changes the body's structure and the myofascial system binds the body in an altered, disorganized form. This may also lead to psychological insecurity, contributing to an overall psychosomatic dysfunction. Structural approaches aim to reorganize the body by correcting myofascial imbalance and inducing movement that is geometrically correct. Ida Rolf, who developed the underlying principles, said, "Hold structures where they are supposed to be and induce movement." Rolfing, structural integration, postural integration, soma neuromuscular integration, and Hellerwork are well-known forms of structural bodywork.

Neuromuscular Approaches

Neuromuscular approaches to the body explore the relationship between nervous system and muscular system functions to create positive reflex responses. Muscle length and kinesthetic perception are manipulated using techniques that engage the motor control center of the brain. The aim is to correct postural dysfunction and change habitual movement patterns that have led to (or have resulted from) overuse and injury. NMT, trigger point therapy, muscle energy technique (MET), and proprioceptive neuromuscular facilitation (PNF) are all examples of neuromuscular approaches. Although all of these systems re-educate or reset muscle tone and function using neuromuscular feedback loops, they accomplish this with very different techniques. Trigger point therapy and NMT use massage techniques that warm the tissue, lift it, compresses it, and stretch it, while PNF and MET use muscle contractions and assisted stretching techniques.

Myofascial Approaches

Fascia is a connective tissue that occurs throughout the body at both superficial and deep levels. Fascia is a sheet-like membranous structure that wraps muscles and organs, allowing them to slide past each other. Fascia also binds muscle fibers together and forms the walls of muscle cells; hence the term "myofascia." When fascia is in a normal, healthy state, it can move and stretch without restriction. When it is unhealthy in an area due to injury, trauma, or repetitive stress, it becomes tight, constrained, and sticky, restricting movement and causing pain. Myofascial approaches aim to release fascial restrictions to decrease pain, restore free movement to the body, and allow the body to function in an optimal state. Myofascial Release and connective tissue massage (Bindegewebmassage) are well-known myofascial approaches.

Energetic Approaches

Energetic approaches focus on energy flowing through the body and how the patterns and nature of this energy flow are affected by internal and external influences (Fig. 1-10). The general goal of many energetic approaches is to promote the uninterrupted flow of energy throughout the body and

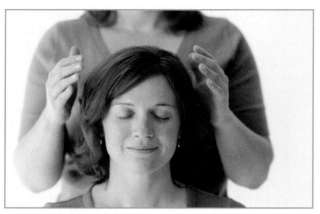

Figure 1-10 The general goal of many energetic approaches is to promote the uninterrupted flow of energy throughout the body and to help the body find emotional, spiritual, and physical balance. Image used with permission from Associated Bodywork & Massage Professionals (ABMP).

to help the body find emotional, spiritual, and physical balance. The underlying concept idea is that the connection between the human body and its external environment affects one's health. This relationship may result in either a sense of connection and belonging (a strong energetic relationship with the universe) or a sense of separation and isolation (a less than optimal energetic relationship with the universe). Polarity therapy, healing touch, Reiki, and zero balancing are well-known forms of energetic bodywork.

Although energetic bodywork is usually not associated with religion, the contemporary focus on healing with prayer (associated with many religions, including Buddhism, Christianity, Judaism, Islam, etc.) has interested many in the medical community and deserves mention. For example, Harvard Medical School sponsors a Spirituality and Healing in Medicine course that is open to researchers, physicians, psychologists, counselors, and the public. Participants study the effects of meditation, spiritual belief, and prayer on a variety of medical conditions. Such practices have been thought to have positive effects on conditions like heart surgery and some cancers. It may be that prayer elicits a relaxation response that helps to decrease the patient's stress. The reduction in stress leads to a set of physiological changes, including a decreased heart rate and decreased blood pressure, as well as an improved positive outlook. Overall, current research generally shows that spirituality can play an important role in a patient's recovery process, and courses like this promote an awareness of the importance of spirituality among health care professionals.[47]

Approaches Based on Movement

Movement approaches are based on the idea that over time, all individuals "learn" how to move in a particular way based on the person's needs and the body's reaction to the surrounding environment. In most people, habitual and often dysfunctional movement patterns become locked in the neuromuscular-myofascial system over time. Optimal function can be restored through increased self-awareness, brought about by organized movement systems (sometimes incorporating dance, yoga, or relearning specific movements). The benefits include greater kinesthetic awareness, greater flexibility, increased range of motion, better coordination and balance, decreased muscular tension, and decreased pain.

A good example of a bodywork system based on movement is Alexander Technique. F. Matthias Alexander formulated the principles of Alexander Technique between 1890 and 1900. In this system, an Alexander Technique practitioner observes the client during daily activities like walking, sitting, standing, and making gestures. The practitioner guides the client toward movement that is effortless, balanced, and free of unnecessary tension. Clients develop a better sense of their bodies in space and learn to avoid habit-forming overcompensation that leads to self-imposed tension. Dancers, singers, actors, and athletes use the principles of Alexander Technique to improve their performance. It is also used as an intervention for chronic pain conditions, repetitive stress conditions, and general health.

Another system based on movement, developed by dancer Judith Aston, is called Aston-Patterning. This system uses massage, movement training, fitness exercises, and postural awareness to promote health, reduce stress, decrease chronic tension, decrease musculoskeletal pain, and encourage effortless movement in harmony with the individual's environment. Key to Aston-Patterning is the view that the body is an asymmetrical structure that takes on three-dimensional, asymmetrical spiral patterns. Muscles and movements are retrained to facilitate long-term results and changes. Other well-known forms of bodywork based on movement include the Feldenkrais Method and the Trager Approach.

Systems from Other Countries and Cultures

Lomi Lomi and Russian massage are examples of popular forms of bodywork based on beliefs and practices in other countries or cultures. Lomi Lomi is the massage of the ancient Polynesians and Hawaiian people. Lomi Lomi is characterized by long, flowing rhythmic strokes using the forearms and hands. The practitioner moves around the massage table using hula dance movements and breathwork, which aim to increase healing energy and promote fluid techniques.

Russian massage developed in the former Soviet Union and shares many characteristics of Swedish massage. This system includes mild and moderate pressure but also deep and vigorous work. Some forms are quite forceful and use rapid friction and tapotement techniques.

Eastern Approaches

Eastern approaches to massage and bodywork are very popular today in the United States. They developed in Asian cultures in countries such as Japan, China, India, Tibet, Korea, and Indonesia. The Eastern tradition of healing is based on the concepts of yin and yang, Qi, and the five elements, as discussed earlier in this chapter. Two examples of Eastern systems are acupressure and amma.

Acupressure is a TCM bodywork technique in which pressure is applied to specific energetic points known as acupoints (or tsubos) using the thumbs, palms, fingers, or elbow. According to TCM, Qi (life energy) flows through the body along specific channels called meridians. When Qi is blocked or disrupted, it may lead to physical or emotional illness. Acupressure applies pressure to specific points to promote the uninterrupted flow of Qi. Acupuncture is closely related to acupressure but uses needles to stimulate the flow of Qi.

Amma (sometimes spelled anma) is traditional Japanese massage. Massage was introduced to Japan from China as part of TCM around the 6th century and then integrated with regional techniques into its own therapeutic form. Like many forms of Eastern bodywork, the techniques used in amma include stimulation of acupressure points along meridian channels to balance Qi. Percussive and rhythmic stroking, pressing, and stretching techniques are also used. Amma is often carried out without oils or lubricants on a fully clothed client. Some other well-known Eastern approaches to massage and bodywork include shiatsu, Thai massage, ayurvedic bodywork, Gua Sha, Jin Shin Do, Watsu, Tui na, and Jin Shin Jyutsu.

Psychological (Mind–Body) Approaches

Psychological approaches are based on the idea that emotions, beliefs, and experiences affect the body and are held as "memories" in body tissue. Over time, they can change the body's form and cause dysfunction, injury, or chronic pain. This type of bodywork seeks to draw awareness to long-held emotions and to help the body release both physical and emotional patterns, creating an opportunity for greater physical and emotional expression. Some psychologically based approaches use the body as a way of accessing the mind. The goal in this case might be to "place" the client in his or her body and process the emotions that surface with the increased level of body–spirit awareness. Gestalt, Hakomi, Rubenfeld Synergy Method, and somatic experiencing are examples of psychologically based approaches to mind–body health.

Other Important Systems

Craniosacral therapy, manual lymphatic drainage (MLD), spa therapies, reflexology, hydrotherapy, and aromatherapy are other important healing systems often used by massage therapists. These do not fit easily into the categories above but deserve a brief introduction.

Craniosacral Therapy

Developed between 1975 and 1983 by an osteopathic physician, John E. Upledger, at Michigan State University, craniosacral therapy aims to release restrictions and improve the function of the "craniosacral system." Upledger defines the craniosacral system as the membranes and cerebrospinal fluid that surround and protect the brain and spinal cord. A craniosacral therapy practitioner uses very gentle pressure to assess the craniosacral system and then follows the body's cues to release restrictions and support the body's natural ability to correct itself and find balance.

Manual Lymphatic Drainage

Emil and Estrid Vodder, Danish physical therapists, developed MLD in the 1930s. Using light, rhythmic strokes applied in a specific order and manner, MLD stimulates lymph flow and fluid movement. It is used for conditions in which fluid collects in the tissue, including inflammatory conditions, lymphedema, and circulatory disturbances.

Spa Therapies

Spa therapies aim to revitalize or relax the body and stimulate natural detoxification. Many of these therapies, like thalassotherapy (healing using seaweed, seawater, and marine environments), balneotherapy (therapeutic use of baths), and fangotherapy (the use of mud, clay, and peat for healing) have a long history of use in Europe (Fig. 1-11). Other spa therapies include hot sheet wraps, cocoons, body scrubs, and foot treatments. Some systems such as hydrotherapy, aromatherapy, and hot stone massage are often used at spas and might also be considered part of spa therapy.

Reflexology

Reflexology is a therapy based on the belief that there are points in the feet, hands, and ears that stimulate the function of different parts of the body including the glands and organs. It is most often used as a preventive therapy to soothe the nervous system, reduce stress, improve circulation, and create an optimum internal environment for balanced energy, rest, and recovery. The goal is to allow the body to draw on its natural ability to heal itself.

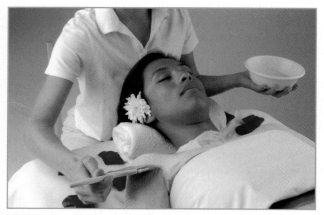

Figure 1-11 Spa therapies include fangotherapy (shown here), which is the use of mud, clay, or peat for healing. Image used with permission from Associated Bodywork & Massage Professionals (ABMP).

Hydrotherapy

Hydrotherapy uses water for healing. Traditionally water is used in one of its three forms: solid (ice), liquid (water), or vapor (steam). The environment of the body is changed by the use of water at a temperature above, close to, or below that of the body. The body's core temperature is relatively constant, even with widely varying environmental temperatures. The body produces heat when the core becomes cooled and increases heat loss when the core temperature rises. Physiological reactions occur as a result of the body's attempt to return to a constant state (homeostasis). A common physiological reaction to the application of heat is vasodilation, which cools the core and increases blood flow to the local area. A massage therapist might use a heat pack to relax chronically tight muscles before massaging the area. A common physiological reaction to cold temperatures is vasoconstriction, which reduces heat loss and decreases local edema. Another useful result of cold application is a decrease in pain due to slower nerve conduction velocity. Massage therapists therefore may use a cold pack or ice massage for an acute injury as part of the rehabilitation process. Spas often use hydrotherapy treatments in the form of Vichy showers, Swiss showers, baths, and Scotch hose treatments for general revitalization.

Aromatherapy

Aromatherapy is a holistic therapy that uses pure essential oils distilled from aromatic plants for healing. Essential oils are a complex mixture of chemical compounds that have physiological and psychological effects on the body. There are many different ways to use essential oils therapeutically. Massage therapists often consult with the client and then blend oils to be applied during massage. Many oils have gentle sedative effects and enhance the benefits of massage.

An Evolving System

Massage techniques, systems, and approaches continue to evolve, and the massage profession continues to change and grow. Associated Bodywork & Massage Professionals (ABMP) reports there are 250 types of massage and bodywork systems, with new massage approaches emerging every year. Such diversity in the massage profession may seem overwhelming for new students and may make you wonder how many systems you must master in order to give a good massage. Massage therapists do not need to know all or many different systems. The core skills massage students learn in their training programs will meet the needs of most clients. Advanced skills are usually developed later as you gain work experience in different environments, work with different client populations, or take continuing education classes.

The next topic in this chapter focuses on contemporary massage in America, different types of massage clients, different work environments, and how massage fits into the American health care system.

Topic **1-3**
Contemporary American Massage

This section considers the reasons why people seek massage and how different work environments focus on the needs of particular client groups. Topic 1-3 also discusses how massage fits into the American health care system.

Massage Clients

As we have seen, massage has been part of a healthy and flourishing lifestyle in many different cultures through history. Today, people recognize massage as an effective and pleasurable way to relieve muscle pain and stiffness, reduce stress, and feel better both physically and mentally. In addition, physicians, physical therapists, and chiropractors increasingly recognize the benefits of massage and include massage in their patients' treatment plans. In all, consumers receive 125 to 135 million massage sessions annually, making massage therapy a 7 to 10 billion dollar industry.[48]

A hospitality survey conducted for the spa industry found that spa clients focus on health, fitness, anti-aging, increased energy, and stress reduction.[49] Massage is the most frequently requested spa service, and techniques range from pampering massage integrated with luxurious enhancers like paraffin dips and aromatherapy accents to serious rehabilitative bodywork like structural integration and Aston Patterning. Many clients visit massage clinics simply for revitalization and a break from work stresses. While 27% of respondents in a survey conducted by the American Massage Therapy Association (AMTA) said they would prefer to receive massage at a spa, 30% indicated they would prefer to receive massage at home from a therapist they know, and 24% indicated they would prefer massage at the massage therapist's location.[50] The remaining 19% listed various other locations such as a chiropractor's office or physician's office.

People seek out massage for a variety of specific reasons within two general categories: wellness and health care.

Wellness Massage

Wellness massage is usually defined as massage to decrease stress, promote relaxation, and support the body's natural restorative mechanisms (Fig. 1-12). ABMP reports that 30% of people seek massage for rest and relaxation. Another 28% receive massage because they have received a gift certificate; most of these massages are likely also wellness oriented. Swedish massage is the most widely and regularly practiced massage system in America and is most often used for wellness purposes.[51] Clients seek this type of massage as a pleasurable experience that leaves them feeling refreshed and revitalized. Wellness massage is also used to reduce temporary pain from overexertion caused by activities such as weekend athletics or home repair or by unusual work stress. Wellness massage is viewed as a healthy activity to promote a balanced and functional life and is regularly promoted as such at spas, wellness centers, private practices, and massage clinics.

Health Care Massage

Health care massage (also referred to as treatment massage, rehabilitative massage, therapeutic massage, or in similar terms) is understood as massage that addresses chronic soft-tissue holding patterns that contribute to dysfunction, soft-tissue injury, or chronic pain. Health care massage is outcome based, meaning that a therapist uses critical thinking to identify the structures affected by the client's condition, the types of techniques that might cause positive changes based on reliable research, and the client's health care goals to develop a treatment plan (also called care plan). The outcomes (or results) of each session are carefully monitored to determine if adaptations to the treatment plan are needed or if the techniques used during sessions achieved anticipated results. Methods used in health care massage include advanced assessment procedures, techniques such as hydrotherapy, and some remedial exercises (e.g., resisted range of motion). Often this type of massage is provided in a health care setting such as a chiropractor's office, sports medicine clinic, or physical therapy office, and may be supervised by a physician, chiropractor, physical therapist, or athletic trainer. Sports massage for athletes is considered health care massage because the massage therapist supports the training and recovery process by including goals such as increased flexibility, increased strength, and injury prevention.

AMTA reports that 32% of Americans seek massage for medical reasons. A 2005 consumer survey revealed that massage combined with medications is most people's preferred form of pain relief. Ninety-three percent of the 1,014 adult respondents surveyed who had received massage felt that massage therapy was effective in reducing pain.[50]

Health care massage also refers to massage for clients with an illness other than soft-tissue conditions or who have experienced some physical, mental, or emotional trauma for which they are receiving medical treatment. Examples include massage in a hospital for cancer patients, massage for patients in a psychiatric ward, and massage for elderly patients in a hospice setting. In these cases, a physician or mental health professional develops an overall treatment plan for the patient that includes massage. The massage therapist is supervised to ensure that the techniques used are appropriate for the patient's overall treatment goals. Massage is often used to provide comfort, and very simple and gentle techniques are applied to nurture or calm the patient.

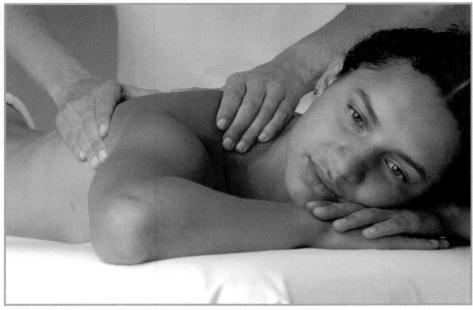

Figure 1-12 Wellness massage is massage to decrease stress, promote relaxation, and support the body's natural restorative mechanisms. Image used with permission from Associated Bodywork & Massage Professionals (ABMP).

Popularity of Massage

The popularity of massage is increasing. The total number of massage visits increased by 2 million from 2004 to 2005 in the United States, and 73% of respondents to the AMTA consumer survey reported that they would recommend massage therapy to others. About 96% of the respondents to the 2006 ABMP survey reported favorable feelings about their massage experience. While the popularity of massage is also increasing among men (up 3% in 2005 from 2004),[50] women comprise about 71% of massage clients.[51] Many corporations such as Allstate, Cisco System, FedEx, General Electric, and Hewlett-Packard have seen evidence that massage therapy increases productivity and reduces stress levels in employees. These companies and many others offer their employees massage programs through employee wellness centers, on-site massage at the office, or cost-sharing opportunities. The 18th annual list of the 100 Best Companies for Working Mothers found that 77 of these companies offered on-site massage for their empolyees.[51]

Why Some People Do Not Get Massage

ABMP's consumer survey in 2006 shows that cost and time are the two main reasons why people do not seek massage. Only 24% stated that they did not feel they needed a massage. This segment of the potential client population still views massage as a luxury. With the increased awareness of complementary and alternative medicine (CAM) among medical professionals and research showing the benefits of massage, however, these views are likely to change over time.

The Massage Profession

People generally seek massage in environments where they feel comfortable, and thus therapists choose to work in environments that attract their preferred types of clients. The job market for massage therapists is expanding as the public increasingly understands massage and values its benefits. Massage is now offered in a variety of locations ranging from private offices to chiropractic offices, gyms, hospital wards, spas, cruise ships, and many other locations.

Private Practice

Many massage therapists want to own their own business and run their practice in a leased commercial space or separate area of their home. The attractions of having your own business include flexible working hours, being able to make business decisions yourself, the satisfaction of overcoming obstacles, the opportunity for creative problem solving, and a sense of personal achievement. Drawbacks include the lack of a financial safety net, potentially longer working hours, and the duties of marketing and managing the business.

Private massage practices generally attract a specific type of client based on the type of massage offered, the facility, its visual appearance, and service prices. The therapist-owner makes these decisions. A therapist might dedicate the practice completely to relaxation services and offer Swedish massage, reflexology, aromatherapy, and certain spa body treatments. The business may focus specifically on Eastern approaches to bodywork and offer Amma, shiatsu, Thai massage, and ayurvedic bodywork. Alternatively, a therapist might form close ties with chiropractors and physical therapists in the area and offer health care massage for patients with soft-tissue injuries. Anything and everything is possible in a private practice, although not everyone is well suited to self-employment. Self-employment requires good business skills as well as good massage skills. Self-employment demands excellent time management, organizational, and communication skills. Self-employed people must also be good planners and have a positive attitude and strong determination.

Massage Clinics

In a massage clinic, a number of massage therapists often work together cooperatively, sharing a receptionist and possibly employing a manager and bookkeeper. In some cases, one person owns the business and either pays or subcontracts to the other massage therapists. When several therapists join forces to share resources, each contributes to the setup costs of the business (e.g., furniture for the reception area, massage tables, linens, washer, and dryer, etc.) and shares the cost of the lease, receptionist, phones, advertising, and other running costs. Services vary from clinic to clinic. Some clinics focus on a particular client group like pregnant woman, athletes, or people with a recent soft-tissue injury. Others might specialize in a specific modality like reflexology, NMT, or psychological body–mind approaches.

One of the benefits of working in a massage clinic is the opportunity to interact with other therapists and gain from their experience and knowledge. This can also help the business to be more successful, because one therapist might be very good at marketing while another understands insurance billing and a third retail sales. Also, therapists working in clinic often help each other by covering shifts for their colleagues when they are sick or on vacation.

Wellness Centers

Wellness centers employ many different types of health care providers. In addition to a massage therapist, the center may also employ a chiropractor, nutritionist, naturopathic doctor, physical therapist, meditation leader, counselor, fitness trainer, yoga instructor, hypnotherapist, esthetician, and life-coach among others. Wellness centers often focus on promoting health for the body, mind, and spirit. Wellness centers are now found on college campuses, in community centers, in large corporations as part of a medical clinic, in gyms, in retirement homes, and in stand-alone businesses similar to spas. As in a massage clinic, a wellness center owner may employ each therapist, or a group of different health care providers might join forces to form a partnership or association. The services offered are determined by the focus of the wellness center. For example, the center may take a broad approach to wellness and offer a variety of services, or the center might specialize in supporting clients with particular conditions such as anxiety disorders, weight management needs, or insomnia.

Spas

Like wellness centers, spas may employ a wide variety of health care professionals to offer services that address the body, mind, and spirit. Some spas focus on skin care and beauty and may offer medical cosmetic procedures such as liposuction, botox injections, laser skin treatments, and plastic surgery as well as facials and waxing. Other spas may focus on promoting healthy life choices, diet, nutrition, and exercise. Each spa is unique, but because massage is currently the most requested spa service, it is not surprising that spas are the number one employer of massage therapists.[52]

Spa work can be varied and creative, allowing therapists to offer a number of different services during the day. The day might begin with a full body massage, followed by a herbal body wrap, and then a hot stone massage, a seaweed treatment, and a foot treatment to finish. Working conditions at spas vary widely. Some spas require their staff to work long hours with little flexibility, but others try hard to work out a good schedule with therapists. Spas usually pay a flat fee to therapists for each treatment performed, regardless of the price that the client pays. Established spas tend to emphasize a structure promoting harmony and tranquility. Dress and appearance are important, as are retail sales. While many therapists resist selling products to clients, the sale of retail products is an important means of ensuring the financial success of the business. Most spas therefore require sales of retail items as part of their employment agreement. Some talented therapists work their way up in the spa industry to become spa consultants, spa department managers, and even spa directors. Others train in esthetics (skin care) to diversify their skills and practice. Many therapists now offer selected spa services such as salt-glows, body wraps, and foot treatments in their private practice without using expensive hydrotherapy equipment. These services are relaxing and provide clients with new ways to experience health and wellness.

Medical Settings

According to the American Pain Foundation, 83 million adults experience pain that is significant enough to limit their participation in daily activities. An additional 75 million people live with chronic debilitating pain.[53] When conventional medicine (drugs and/or surgery) fails, many patients seek alternative treatments for soft-tissue pain and dysfunction, such as acupuncture, physical therapy, chiropractic treatments, massage, and bodywork (Fig. 1-13).

Medical environments in which massage is offered include chiropractors' offices, hospitals, hospices, naturopathic practices, sports medicine clinics, clinical massage practices, physical therapy offices, and rehabilitation centers. The type of massage offered in medical settings varies a great deal, as do the clients. In one chiropractic office, for example, a massage therapist might provide 15-minute warm-up massages to clients. Chiropractors find it easier to adjust a client when certain muscles are soft and relaxed. A therapist providing massage in such as office is likely to find that basic Swedish and

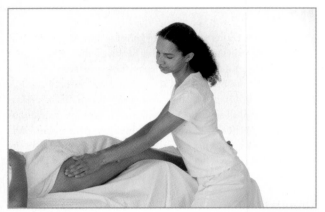

Figure 1-13 Many therapists focus on health care massage to address soft-tissue injuries and dysfunctions for such conditions as whiplash, carpal tunnel syndrome, low back pain, and many others. Image used with permission from Associated Bodywork & Massage Professionals (ABMP).

deep-tissue skills are adequate. A different chiropractor may expect the massage therapist to understand advanced massage assessment techniques and treatment massage protocols and to participate in treatment planning for clients. This requires knowledge beyond Swedish and deep-tissue techniques.

In another example, some therapists provide massage to patients and their families in hospital oncology wards. These therapists need to understand the indications and contraindications of massage in relationship to cancer, how to work around medical equipment, how to keep accurate chart notes, and how to work effectively with physicians and nurses. The techniques used may include holding strokes, guided deep breathing, gentle Swedish strokes, and some energetic approaches to calm the patient and ease pain. These basic massage techniques are not difficult to master, but the knowledge of cancer, cancer medications, and critical reasoning to make good massage-related choices for cancer patients requires deep sensitivity and understanding.

Many therapists focus on health care massage to address soft-tissue injuries and dysfunctions for such conditions as whiplash, carpal tunnel syndrome, thoracic outlet syndrome, and many others. To undertake this level of work, the therapist must have an in-depth understanding of anatomy and physiology, kinesiology, soft-tissue pathology, assessment methods, and clinical massage techniques. This type of massage might be offered in a physical therapy office, a wellness center, a sports medicine clinic, a treatment-oriented massage clinic, or a private practice. In a small number of states, health insurance plans recognize complementary medicine, and massage therapists can bill insurance companies for massage when they have a doctor's diagnosis and referral.

Cruise Ships

Some therapists like the idea of cruise ship work because it affords them the opportunity to travel and meet new people. The benefits of this type of work include free room and board

and medical insurance, which are required by maritime law. Some cruise lines also offer discounts on cruise vacations to the friends and family members of employees. Cruise ship spas most often offer wellness massage enhanced with luxurious touches that make the client feel pampered (paraffin dip for the hands, aromatherapy accents, etc.). The therapist might deal with minor sports injuries, but usually general Swedish skills suffice. One of the main difficulties for therapists working on a cruise ship is the time pressure. Often therapists move directly from one massage to the next, and a thorough health intake process is de-emphasized. Health care concerns are further complicated because a wide variety of clients with various health issues often take cruise vacations, many of whom increase their alcohol consumption during the trip. Therapists with a good understanding of contraindications for massage and critical reasoning skills are better prepared to make good decisions in this fast-paced environment. These therapists should also be in good shape and have good body mechanics. While good health and good body mechanics are always important, massage work shifts on a cruise ship are particularly demanding, lasting as long as 12 hours with back-to-back appointments. One should always research the working conditions on cruise ships carefully and compare pay rates and work hours before signing a contact.

On-Site Massage

Seated, on-site massage is currently popular in shopping malls, airports, corporate workplaces, and events like fairs and sporting events. Seated massage is often provided as a marketing tool at events to raise awareness of a massage practice at another location. Seated massage is given through the client's clothing without lubricants in 10- to 30-minute sessions. Seated massage in offices and events is a good way for new therapists to gain experience. Massage chairs can be transported almost anywhere, allowing therapists to work in a variety of locations. Clients drawn to seated massage include office workers and other busy people who want quick work on target areas. Massage students usually learn basic seated massage skills as part of their training or can take continuing education classes.

Work with Special Populations

Some massage therapists are drawn to work with a particular type of client and focus their career on those clients' special needs. Pregnancy massage, sports massage, and animal massage are some of these special populations.

Pregnancy and Infant Massage

Massage can provide relief from aches and pains related to pregnancy as long as the therapist knows how to position the client properly and use appropriate techniques. Many therapists are drawn to massage clinics where they can work with a mother before, during, and after pregnancy. The massage therapist may even become part of the labor and delivery team at a hospital or birthing center, providing

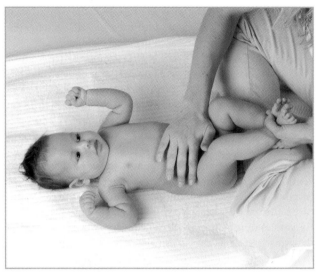

Figure 1-14 Massage can play a role in a mother's rehabilitative process after giving birth and supports the health of the infant. Image used with permission from Associated Bodywork & Massage Professionals (ABMP).

massage between contractions to help with relaxation or using specific techniques to reduce pain and pressure during contractions.

After the birth, massage often plays a role in the mother's rehabilitative process and supports the health of the infant (Fig. 1-14). Research has found that the massage of low-birth-weight infants increases their weight and decreases the length of their hospitable stay.[54] Another study showed that massage supports neurological development in infants.[4] Massage also helps to ease the discomforts of teething, colic, and emotional distress in children. A therapist might also seek additional training to become a certified doula, a person who acts as a knowledgeable companion during pregnancy, birth, labor, and the transition of the new child into the family.

Sports Massage

Athletes recognize that massage increases flexibility, supports the body's recovery process after events or training sessions, and improves performance. Some therapists, often with specialized massage training, work with professional athletes as part of the training team. Competition for such positions is often fierce, and it may be easier to find work with amateur or semiprofessional athletes in high school or college or with athletic individuals who have made physical activity a primary focus in their lives. Sports massage is mobile. Sometimes it is offered in an office setting, but it might also be offered on-site before or after an event. A recent trend is the inclusion of massage practices in gyms. In this setting, therapists work with a variety of clients, ranging from people trying to get into shape to professional athletes in peak condition. Some sports massage therapists also become trained and certified in fitness training so that they can offer a more diversified range of services.

Animal Massage

Dogs, cats, horses, and other animals respond to the calming and relaxing effects of animal massage. Performance animals like racehorses and show jumping horses benefit from massage in the same way as human athletes (e.g., better flexibility, faster recovery time, etc.). Effective animal massage requires training in animal anatomy, movement, and animal observation. Smaller animals can be massaged while they are resting on a treatment table, but larger animals such as horses usually remain standing. Some animal massage practitioners work on-site with the animal, while others have an office to which owners bring their pets.

Exploration of a Massage Career

The work environments and client types described above represent just some of the opportunities for massage therapists. Massage is a diverse field, and many graduates pursue unique occupations, defined through their own hard work, research, and interests. At the time of this writing, the 1,566 massage programs in the United States graduate approximately 70,000 massage therapists each year, and about 241,000 therapists are now working in the United States.[55] On average, therapists stay in the massage profession 7.8 years and often work in complementary occupations as massage instructors, fitness trainers, estheticians, and clinical hypnotherapists or in other forms of related bodywork. As mentioned previously, there are 250 known types of massage and bodywork, allowing therapists to continue to develop new skills throughout their careers.

AMTA and ABMP conclude that 83% of massage therapists are female, and that massage is often a second career. Therapists work an average of 15 hours a week providing massage and typically earn half of their income from their massage career. The AMTA points out that according to the U.S. Department of Labor Statistics, massage therapists earn an annual income comparable to other health care support workers.

Some massage students at the start of their training program have strong ideas about where they want to work, while others have little or no idea. Massage instructors sometimes hear students say things like, "I don't really need to know about posture and gait assessment because I'm just going to do relaxation massage," or "I'm not going to bother to learn aromatherapy because I am going into clinical massage and I won't use it." Nonetheless, the best massage therapists are always open to learning new skills and applying new knowledge in a session. For example, many clinical massage therapists do not use aromatherapy because they do not fully understand its benefits. In fact, it is very useful for helping clients relax and cope with the emotional trauma of injury. Because some essential oils have natural anti-inflammatory and pain-relieving effects when applied topically, learning aromatherapy provides new options for a therapist working with soft-tissue dysfunctions. In all cases, exploration of all options is advised. As you progress through your training program, you will learn and grow. You will be exposed to a variety of techniques, models, clients, and ideas. Students often develop an interest in a previously unknown area of massage. Some students end up doing the opposite of what they originally thought they liked. For example, a student who is determined to work with athletes and practice sports massage might be surprised to discover that he or she loves spa work. Similarly, a student planning to offer relaxation massage may discover a strength in clinical massage. At this point, it is probably best to stay flexible and enjoy learning. Planning your career ahead of graduation is a good idea, but do not let your career plan limit your learning opportunities. As we saw earlier, some of the biggest advances in the massage profession have come when people integrated existing ideas and techniques into new systems and approaches.

Massage as Part of the American Health Care System

It is helpful to understand how massage fits in today's health care system. Massage and bodywork are a type of CAM. **CAM therapies** include such diverse forms of practice as acupuncture, Tai Chi, biofeedback, chiropractic medicine, meditation, dance therapy, aromatherapy, art therapy, ayurvedic medicine, TCM, hypnosis, and many others. The term "complementary medicine" describes alternative healing practices used in conjunction with conventional medicine. In this case, a therapy like massage complements the treatment the client or patient is receiving through conventional medicine. Conventional medicine is very interested in "curing" the body by the elimination of symptoms or a particular disease-causing agent, or by intervening when the body is in an acute state of crisis (e.g., heart attack). Although physicians do make basic dietary and exercise recommendations, drugs and surgery are the most common forms of medical treatment, and a person is considered to be healthy when the body is symptom free.

The term "alternative medicine" simply means an alternative to conventional care where the focus of treatment is likely (though not always) to be more holistic. If a patient chooses not to use conventional medical intervention, or if conventional medical treatment has proven ineffective, he or she might seek out other treatment forms such as massage, acupuncture, hypnosis, or many others to reduce symptoms or improve his or her condition.

The terms "integrative medicine" and "holistic healthcare" or "holistic medicine" are often used interchangeably to refer to complementary medicine. This is something of a misuse of terminology, because the term "holistic" means an approach that focuses on the whole person, not just the disease as in conventional medicine. The physical, emotional, mental, and spiritual aspects of the individual and an individual's relationships, environment, spiritual life, diet, rest cycles, mental stimuli, and physical pressures are considered relevant, regardless of how symptoms occur. How people interact with and relate to other people and the world around them in general is a key component of health. People are considered healthy when their life is in balance. In this model, illness or pain is considered the body's way of communicating its state of imbalance and a desire for better health. People often completely change their lifestyle after the diagnosis of an illness or after a physical injury. Illness or pain becomes the motivation that facilitates rapid personal change.

The term "integrative medicine" was coined by Dr. Andrew Weil to emphasize the use of both conventional and alternative medicine to address the physical, psychological, social, and spiritual aspects of health. Integrative medicine focuses on the human capacity to heal and on a collaborative approach to patient care. A group of therapists and doctors become a health care team that "coaches" the individual to better health.

Over the last 25 years, consumer demand has forced conventional medicine to become more interested in alternative forms of medicine, and a radical shift is occurring in the health care industry. Consumer demand began in the 1980s after the Reagan administration made health care cuts that restricted the growth of CAM therapies.[56] The public was forced to pay more money out of pocket for conventional medicine, and insurance companies saw no reason to cover new groups of providers with "unproven" alternative therapies. At the same time, Americans were experiencing more stress in their lives, and musculoskeletal injuries were on the rise. Because conventional medicine offered little relief, frustrated consumers began paying for alternative therapies themselves. By 1990, 34% of Americans were spending a total of 10.3 billion dollars out of pocket for alternative health care, compared to the 12.8 billion spent out of pocket overall on hospitalization.[57] State governments took notice, and by the early 1990s, 41 states required chiropractic care to be covered by insurance policies. Washington state and Connecticut insisted that health insurance should cover all licensed alternative health care practitioners, including massage therapists. The media also did their part by promoting the benefits of CAM and profiling charismatic, self-described holistic medical doctors like Andrew Weil, Deepak Chopra, and Bernie Siegel. These highly publicized and much-published physicians are leading an integrative health care movement in which CAM and conventional medicine are practiced side by side. This integration can be seen on both a large and a small scale. For example, some hospitals have added spas to ease the discomfort of terminally ill patients and to help with pain management. Nurses often use aromatherapy and healing touch with hospital patients, and dentists use forms of meditation and guided imagery before carrying out dental procedures. Medical professionals are increasingly aware of the need to address the mind, emotions, and spirit as well as the physical aspects of the patient's condition.

In 1992, the National Institutes of Health established the Office of Alternative Medicine (OAM) to scientifically evaluate alternative therapies and to educate the public about their benefits. In 1998, OAM evolved into the **National Center for Complementary and Alternative Medicine (NCCAM)**. In 2006, NCCAM's budget topped 122.7 million to promote shared research between conventional physicians and CAM therapists and provide reliable information to the public. CAM therapies continue to progress as conventional medicine responds to public demand for integrated health care. Today, many hospitals offer some type of integrated health care program such as hospital-based massage therapy or a peaceful botanical conservatory where patients and family members can meditate. By 1997, half of America's medical schools offered courses in alternative medicine, and around 42% of Americans preferred CAM therapies to conventional medicine, spending an average total of 21.2 billion each year.[58,59]

The Spa Industry and Integrated Medicine

One of the places where integrated medicine is being practiced is in the spa industry. The 2006 International Spa Association "Spa-goer" study notes that approximately 32.2 million adults in the United States and 3.7 million adults in Canada visited a spa in 2005. The report also notes that people who regularly attend spas view the spa experience as an important part of their healthy lifestyle. These spa-goers view cosmetic services as superficial and are looking for more holistic and therapeutic benefits.[60] Destination and medical spas are particularly suited to integrative medicine approaches. Guests visit a destination spa for a weekend or longer to make significant lifestyle changes or just to relax completely. Spa programs focus on fitness, healthy diet, detoxification, and lifestyle education. Some destination spas offer classes and services geared toward spiritual as well as physical renewal. A good example is the Miraval Resort, which appointed Dr. Andrew Weil as Director of Integrative Health & Healing. Educated at Harvard, Dr. Weil has been practicing natural and preventive medicine for over 30 years. He has worked with Miraval to incorporate integrative health care into their menu of services. One result is the Life in Balance Program, in which participants explore the components of a balanced life in a 4-day program. Healthy eating, mindfulness classes, horseback riding, exercise, meditation, and bodywork are integrated so that participants feel balanced and have the resources needed for achieving greater balance when they get home.[61]

Integrative medicine is also being practiced at wellness centers that focus on alternative medical systems such as ayurveda or TCM. Naturopathic medicine, nutrition therapy, Western herbal medicine, and acupuncture all fall into this category. Dr. Deepak Chopra and Dr. David Simon founded the Chopra Center for Wellbeing in 1996 to explore the global principles of holistic healing. The Chopra Center's signature program is the Perfect Health Program. It focuses on the development of a daily routine that is balanced and encourages health and happiness. One of the primary medical systems promoted at the Chopra Center is ayurvedic medicine because of its emphasis on mindful choices to support balanced health.[62]

Some spas and massage clinics have introduced conventional medicine into their service menu. In this case, medical staff carry out a number of tests (blood tests, bone density screening, etc.) before designing a treatment program that includes massage and bodywork. Some businesses specialize in general areas such as weight loss, pain management, or pre- or postnatal care. They may also offer specific programs

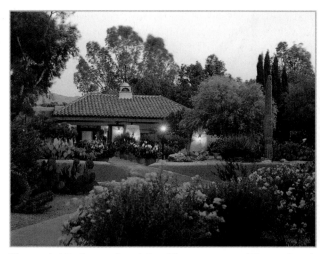

Figure 1-15 Canyon Ranch Spa. Photo courtesy of Canyon Ranch Spa, Tucson, AZ.

for particular conditions such as diabetes, high blood pressure, or chronic insomnia. The Canyon Ranch Health Resort in Tucson, Arizona, combines the well-known luxury and pampering provided by the famous Canyon Ranch Spas with a health and healing center (Fig. 1-15). Their Executive Wellness Program is a 4-day health program that includes a complete physical examination as well as lifestyle assessment. The general approach of Canyon Ranch is to encourage guests to make a long-term commitment to healthy living so as to decrease the likelihood of disease.[63]

Research and Massage

Interest in CAM therapies by conventional medicine practitioners and the public is fueled by research and clinical studies that verify its benefits. Many research studies have focused on massage. For example, recent studies sponsored by NCCAM show that massage reduces pain and improves the quality of life among cancer patients as their lives came to an end.[64] Massage also has been shown to have a positive effect on depression and quality of life in patients with advanced HIV disease.[65] Research on massage therapy indicates that massage reduces a mother's risk of premature delivery and postpartum depression.[66] It also improves sleep for babies and decreases glucose levels in diabetic children.[67] Massage reduces pain from migraine headaches and arthritis,[68] and adolescents with attention-deficit hyperactivity disorder experience reduced aggression and less hyperactivity as a result of massage.[69] Such studies have encouraged conventional medical professionals to recommend massage more often. Of the adults surveyed by the AMTA, 21% reported that they had discussed massage with their doctor, and 60% had discussed massage with other health care providers (50% physical therapist, 38% chiropractor). Two research groups of primary importance to massage therapists are the Massage Therapy Foundation and the Touch Research Institute (TRI) (Figs. 1-16 and 1-17).

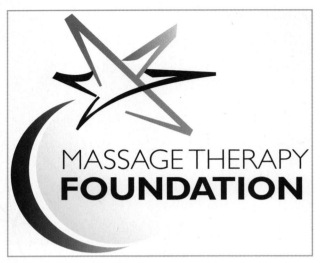

Figure 1-16 The Massage Therapy Foundation aims to advance the knowledge and practice of massage therapy by supporting scientific research, education, and community service.

Massage Therapy Foundation

The AMTA founded the Massage Therapy Foundation in 1990 to promote research into the benefits of massage, to spread knowledge to both therapists and the public, and to encourage community outreach. The Foundation receives donations from individuals and corporations and funds research projects, education and community programs, and conferences for sharing information. For example, many people have little or no access to massage in their communities, even when it might greatly improve their health and comfort. The Massage Therapy Foundation provides community service grants to community-based organizations that partner with massage therapists to provide massage in such communities. Awards between $500 and $5,000 are provided for a 12-month period to organizations that meet the Foundation's criteria.

One of the activities of the Massage Therapy Foundation of particular importance to massage students is the promotion of "research literacy," which is described by the Foundation as "the ability to find, understand, and critically evaluate research evidence that can be applied in professional practice."[70] A curriculum kit is made available to massage schools to help teach research literacy. The Foundation also has a Student Case Report Contest and a Massage Therapy Research Database that allows students, instructors, and professionals to find peer-reviewed research articles that help

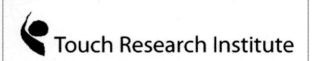

Figure 1-17 The TRI is the first center in the world that is devoted to the study of touch and its application in science and medicine. The TRI has widely researched the effects of massage on people of all ages.

validate the effectiveness of massage. Peer-reviewed research holds the most merit because these research papers are critically reviewed by well-established researchers in the particular field. The editors of peer-reviewed journals publish only those papers that have been approved by expert reviewers and thereby ensure the credibility of the research. The Massage Therapy Database also indexes relevant citations and historical references. Access to the database is free; users need only log on to the Massage Therapy Foundation website (www.massagetherapyfoundation.org) and register.

Touch Research Institute

Johnson & Johnson provided the start-up grant to found the TRI at the University of Miami School of Medicine in 1992. Tiffany Field, Ph.D., is the director of the TRI, which is the first research center in the world dedicated exclusively to exploring how touch affects health and well-being. The TRI has conducted over 100 studies on a range of conditions and age groups. For example, one TRI study showed that massage measurably decreases the pain from fibromyalgia, while another showed that massage enhances immune function. TRI researchers note that in general, decreased stress hormones mediate many of the positive effects demonstrated by the studies. The results of TRI research can be ordered directly from the TRI website (www.miami.edu/touch-research).

Concept Brief 1-4	
Health Terms in Contemporary American Health Care	
Alternative medicine	Alternative healing methods that are not traditionally practiced by medical doctors or in hospitals
Complementary medicine	Alternative healing methods used to supplement conventional medicine to address a condition or disease
Conventional medicine	Medicine that is commonly practiced at hospitals or by medical professionals using drugs and surgery as primary forms of intervention
Integrative medicine	Collaborative health care that uses a team of medical and alternative health professionals to address physical, psychological, social, and spiritual aspects of health
Holistic health care	A form of alternative medicine that seeks to address the needs of a whole person, not just symptoms or diseases

As you can see, it is an exciting time to enter the massage profession. The massage industry still has many obstacles to overcome, but gradually we are making advances. Massage is a noble profession whose history is "written" each and every day by therapists dedicated to providing the very best care to their clients.

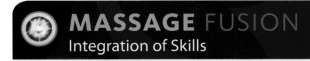

MASSAGE FUSION
Integration of Skills

STUDY TIP: Group Discussion—
What Can History Teach Us?

We all learn most effectively when we are actively involved with the information. One way to get involved is to form a study group and hold group discussions about reading assignments and class lectures. Get together with two or three other students and use the following questions as a way to explore the evolution of massage. Have one person keep notes on ideas that came up during your discussion. Photocopy these notes so that everyone in the group has a copy. Instructors can also use these questions for in-class discussions.

Introduction. If *all* we can say about history is that so-and-so did this or that on such-and-such a date, we have missed the point. While an understanding of the main people, places, and events in history is important, history is also about ideas and questions. *What did each culture know that we can use today in our massage practice?*

1. **What can the Egyptians teach us?**

   The Egyptians were very interested in the afterlife. They learned a great deal about anatomy in their efforts to preserve the body (mummification) for its journey in the afterlife. How do our current views of an afterlife affect our views of health and wellness? How might this affect the massage profession?

2. **What can the Aboriginals teach us?**

   Medicine man Kakkib li'Dthia Warrawee'a notes that massage promotes relationships between generations of people because the young are encouraged to massage their elders. Describe a relationship you have had in which nonsexual touch played a role in your bond to the other person. Some students may have had few nonsexual touching relationships—could this affect how they practice massage? Why or why not? How?

3. **What can the Aztecs teach us?**

   The Aztecs believed that the human body was directly linked to the universe and that the gods sent ailments as punishment for incorrect behavior (sins). While we might not believe that the "gods" send ailments, could "incorrect behavior" cause some forms of disease? Why or why not? How?

4. **What can Native Americans teach us?**

   Before any important activity like hunting, moving to a new location, or making a big decision, many Native Americans would purify themselves or perform a ritual. What are the benefits of such a practice? How might this understanding be applied in a massage setting?

5. **What can the Greeks teach us?**

   The Greeks introduced the idea of logical reasoning and moved medicine out of the realm of magic. Galen's ideas seemed so reasonable that they went unquestioned in medicine for 1,500 years, yet he was wrong about many things. The interesting thing to think about is how Galen's fame affected the development of medicine. Should you believe everything that you read in an accepted textbook written by a specialist or what a knowledgeable instructor tells you? If not, how will you know when you can and when you cannot believe what you read or hear?

6. **What can the Romans teach us?**

   The Romans borrowed much of their culture from the Greeks. They took what worked, organized it into an efficient system, and made the information available on a wide scale. Many therapists take existing techniques developed by other people, meld them into a new system, and teach them in continuing education classes. What is beneficial about such a practice? What are the drawbacks? How can you apply this approach in your own practice?

7. **What can the Arabs teach us?**

   Both Al-Razi and Ibn Sina wrote books on a number of topics. They both understood philosophy, science, music, poetry, law, mathematics, and physics as well as medicine. Perhaps because of their broad understanding of these areas, they were able to integrate concepts and make significant advances in their own areas of particular expertise. What skills do you already possess that will give you a broader understanding of massage? What areas, even if seemingly unrelated, might you learn from in order to improve your massage? For example, could an understanding of painting or poetry make you a better therapist?

8. **What can Eastern approaches teach us?**

   Eastern healing approaches use detailed empirical diagnostic techniques developed over thousands of years. In TCM, information about how your tongue, hair, fingernails, skin, and eyes look as well as the smell of your breath and body odor and the precise feel of your pulse is used to determine the treatment. TCM practitioners have made an art of using their senses, and current research has validated the effectiveness of TCM. Look at the person sitting next to you, and with your senses alone determine what type of massage might benefit that person (stimulating, calming, deep, light, long, short strokes, etc.). Discuss the role of observation in the practice of massage.

9. **What can ayurvedic medicine teach us?**

   Ayurveda is as much a philosophical system as a medical system. Patients must make mindful choices to balance their dosha constitution for better health. How do Americans contribute to their own health? Do they

(Continued)

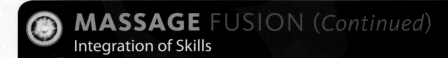

take full responsibility for their health? How might this impact a massage practice?

10. What can Tibetan medicine teach us?

The influence of the mind is of primary importance in Tibetan medicine, because the cause of illness is believed to be one of three mental poisons (desire, hatred, and confusion). Can desire, hatred, and confusion cause illness? Discuss ways in which a client's mind-set might affect the massage session.

11. What can 1950s America teach us?

In the 1950s, massage in America declined partly because the word was used as a cover for prostitution, and so the public became skeptical about its legitimacy. What current social trends fuel an interest in massage today? Currently massage is considered a legitimate health care practice, but many people still feel too shy to get a massage. How do we overcome these concerns and increase the popularity and understanding of massage in the current marketplace?

CHAPTER WRAP-UP

Having traveled from the early history of massage and medicine to massage in contemporary America, you may have noticed that ideas circle back around. In early times, people did not separate concepts of spirituality and health. Eventually, the Greek physicians developed methods of clinical observation and logical reasoning that moved healing toward the scientific methodology that we most often associate with medicine today. Now, 3,000 years later, Harvard School of Medicine "discovers" that prayer and spirituality should not be separated from health care!

Many early cultures viewed health care practices like massage as an everyday custom, and even in India today, for example, people do not view massage as a luxury. You massage your children, your parents, and your friends, and they massage you. It is considered necessary for good health.

Aboriginals practiced massage to build family relationships and as part of their connection to ancestors that had passed to the spirit world. They understood touch as a way to promote healthy relationships in the community.

In our culture, touch was de-emphasized, and people began to subconsciously protect their personal space above all else. The media often portray touch in a sexual context, leading to a deep misunderstanding of touch as something we need on a nonsexual level for good health. This misperception reached its peak in the 1950s when massage was used as a cover for prostitution and was eyed with skepticism by the general public. Americans still have much to learn about touch as part of health and family relationships. The increasing value that Americans place on massage as part of a healthy lifestyle is a good start. More and more often people are seeking opportunities to learn more about touch. This can be seen in a variety of classes for the general public focusing on topics such as massage for couples, massage to ease the pain of loved ones suffering with chronic illness in hospital beds, and massage for babies and children.

Finally, early cultures held a very holistic view of health and wellness. They understood that diet, exercise, relationships, a connection to the universe, mental attitudes, and belief systems all play a role in health and longevity. The current interest in complementary and alternative therapies brings this holistic view of the body back into focus. In fact, the American health care system is undergoing a radical shift with the reintroduction of this integrative model.

There has never been a better time to become a massage therapist, and massage therapists are in a unique position to help educate the general population about healthy, nurturing, integrative touch. You can see that you have picked a dynamic and meaningful career path that allows continual growth and life-long learning, as well as the opportunity to significantly enhance the lives of people on a daily basis.

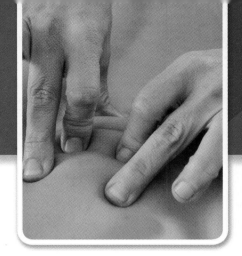

Chapter

2

Massage Equipment and Environmental Considerations

KEY TERMS

accessibility

bolster

décor

functionality

linens

lubricant

massage table

LEARNING OBJECTIVES

Having read the chapter and used the related student learning tools, the student will be able to:

1. Describe the standard equipment used to deliver a massage.

2. Compare and contrast stationary tables with portable tables.

3. Treat all massage equipment respectfully and follow safe practices that ensure comfort for both the client and the therapist.

4. Explain the use of bolsters and compare and contrast the use of larger bolsters with smaller bolsters.

5. Describe the basic ingredients in different lubricants and explain the benefits and drawbacks of each product type for use in massage.

6. List three ways you can provide clients with lubricant choices before the massage.

7. Sketch a diagram of a comfortable massage treatment space, considering design elements including décor, color, window treatments, lighting, accessibility, and functionality.

Early in your massage training program, it is important to appreciate the tools of the trade, work with them safely, and consider your equipment needs for professional practice. Topic 2-1 discusses standard massage equipment. Topic 2-2 discusses the benefits and uses of the ingredients found in massage oils, lotions, creams, and powders. Environmental factors that help ensure a positive experience for the client are discussed in Topic 2-3. Sanitation, hygiene, and safety are of paramount importance when using massage equipment but are mentioned only briefly here; these topics are covered in depth in Chapter 3. More specialized equipment and supplies, which are used in specific massage systems or for special populations, are discussed in greater detail in the appropriate chapters.

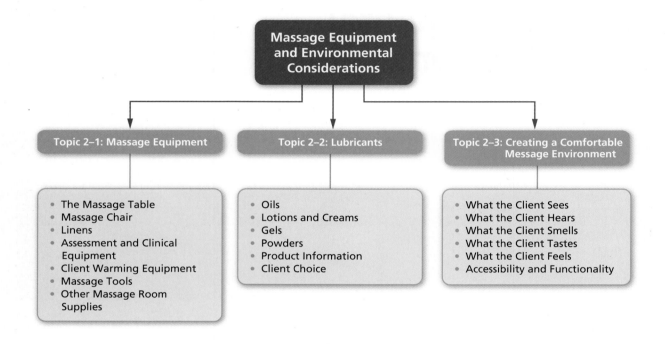

Massage Equipment and Environmental Considerations

Topic 2–1: Massage Equipment

- The Massage Table
- Massage Chair
- Linens
- Assessment and Clinical Equipment
- Client Warming Equipment
- Massage Tools
- Other Massage Room Supplies

Topic 2–2: Lubricants

- Oils
- Lotions and Creams
- Gels
- Powders
- Product Information
- Client Choice

Topic 2–3: Creating a Comfortable Message Environment

- What the Client Sees
- What the Client Hears
- What the Client Smells
- What the Client Tastes
- What the Client Feels
- Accessibility and Functionality

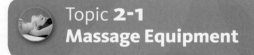

Topic 2-1
Massage Equipment

Massage equipment includes all items and tools therapists might use in their massage practice (Box 2-1). The equipment must be well made, safe, attractive, and comfortable for the client and should not cause undue stress to the therapist's body. Each piece of equipment represents an investment in your business and in your clients. When you purchase your own equipment, do so carefully after researching brands, understanding available options, and comparing products. Therapists generally should not build their own equipment such as a massage table. Massage equipment companies do much researching and testing of equipment to ensure that it is comfortable and safe. Homemade equipment may be unsafe and fail during a massage, causing injury to the client or therapist and leading to a lawsuit.

The Massage Table

The **massage table** supports the client in a reclining position during the massage. It is covered with a clean set of linen for each client and is narrow enough to give the therapist easy access to the client's body. Different manufacturers offer many different features and options. Tables may be stationary, hydraulically lifted, electrically lifted, or portable. They might include arm shelves, side extenders, and sit-up features and have regular to very plush padding.

Stationary Table

A stationary table is a good choice for spas and clinic environments (Fig. 2-1). The table is constructed with a solid

BOX 2-1 **Master Supply List**

- Massage table or mat
- Face cradle
- Massage chair (optional)
- Bolsters
  - Large
  - Small
  - Pillows
  - Other body supports
- Carrying case (optional)
- Rolling cart (optional)
- Stool
- Step stool (to get on and off table)
- Massage sheets
- Washable blankets
- Bath towels or sheets
- Hand towels
- Pillow cases
- Face cradle covers
- Bolster covers
- Heat lamp (optional)
- Table pad (optional)
- Fomentek (optional)
- Warm packs (optional)
- Client assessment equipment
- Blood pressure equipment
- Lubricants
  - Expeller-pressed oil
  - Cream
  - Gel
  - Powder
- Lotion warmer
- Forms
  - Health intake
  - SOAP forms
  - Other
- Massage tools (optional)
- References
  - Pathology reference book
  - Medical dictionary
  - Drug reference book
- Clock
- Closed storage
- Wastebasket
- Music system and music
- Cleaning and sanitation products
- Client mirror
- Disposable combs
- Container to hold personal items
- Place for clothing
- Antibacterial liquid soap
- Alcohol-based hand sanitation gel
- Vinyl gloves
- Finger cots
- Flash light
- First aid kit
- Contact lens solution
- Mouthwash
- Washer/dryer (optional)

frame that often includes built-in storage space for items like towels, lotions, oils, and cleaning products. Some newer models include features like hot towel cabinets, foot soaking tubs, and sit-up options. Most tables have some type of lift mechanism to raise or lower the table. With a manual lift, the therapist may simply turn a handle to raise or lower the table height. Hydraulic lifts use a system of pumps and motors to power the mechanical motion. Electric lift tables use motors to change the table height. The height of hydraulic and electric tables can be adjusted during the treatment, using a foot pedal, to facilitate different massage techniques or make it easy for the client to get on or off the table. Because they have heavier bases and height-adjusting equipment, stationary tables are usually much more expensive than portable tables.

Portable Tables

Portable tables are designed to fold up for easy transport to different locations (Fig. 2-2). They are ideal for therapists who visit clients' homes. Weighing from 25 to 36 lb, portable tables are lighter than stationary tables but can still support even large clients safely. Portable tables are less expensive than stationary tables and often are the first choice for students and new graduates who need flexibility. Technique 1 demonstrates how to set up a portable table and prepare it for a massage session.

Massage Mat

A massage mat (sometimes called a Shiatsu mat) is a large padded surface that rests on the floor (Fig. 2-3). The mat provides a

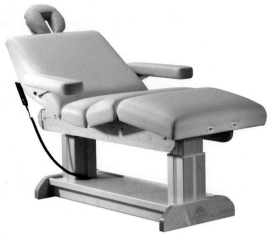

Figure 2-1 Stationary table. Image courtesy of Massage Warehouse.

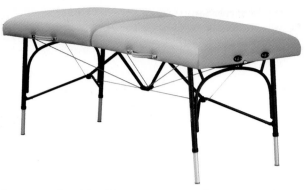

Figure 2-2 Portable table. Image courtesy of Massage Warehouse.

comfortable surface for clients and allows therapists to use their body weight effectively in the delivery of certain techniques.

Massage Table Features

Manufacturers provide many options for both stationary and portable tables, allowing therapists to choose the table specifications that best meet their needs.

Frame

Massage table frames are usually made of wood, aluminum, or stainless steel. Stationary tables have heavier bases. With wood or aluminum frames, portable tables are lightweight and easy to move. Wood-framed portable tables are a little heavier than aluminum ones, but both are strong and durable. The top of the table is made of wood covered by layers of foam and fabric. Cross-braces and plastic-covered support wires provide stability. In portable tables, the four wooden or metal legs are usually constructed of two pieces that can be

| **Technique 1** | **Set Up a Portable Table for a Massage Session** |

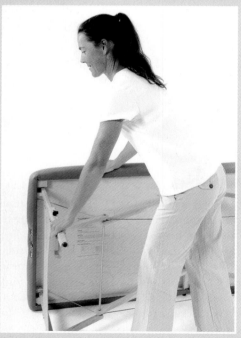

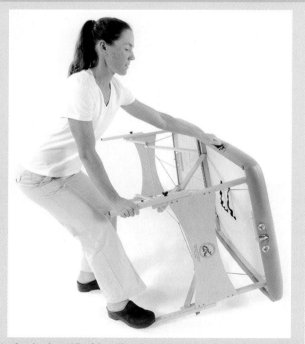

1. Turn the portable table on its side and set it on its rubber feet. Open the fastener that keeps the table closed and unfold the table completely while on its side. Make sure the legs are fully extended and the support cables are not bunched or twisted.

2. Stand at the middle of the table and grasp the handles. Place a toe on the end of one of the bottom legs and then tip the table into an upright position.

Technique 1 | **Set Up a Portable Table for a Massage Session** (Continued)

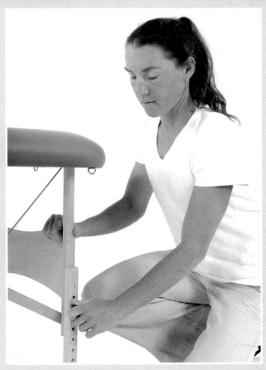

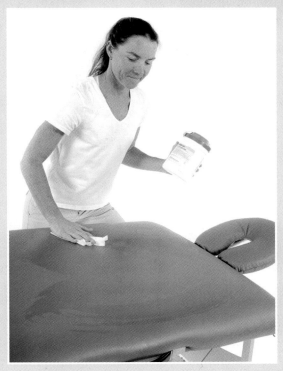

3. Check that the table is fully open in the upright position. Check that the leg bolts are tight. Adjust the table height based on the types of techniques you will use in the session.

4. Wipe the table and face cradle with an antibacterial wipe.

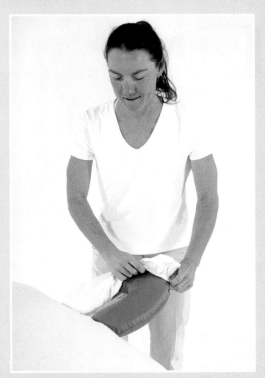

5. Dress the table with clean linens in preparation for the session.

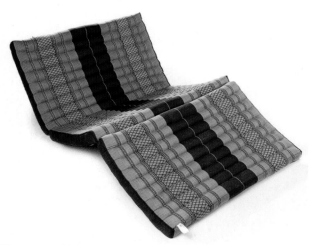

Figure 2-3 Massage mat. Image courtesy of Massage Warehouse.

bolted together at different places to change the height easily. Before each session, check the bolts on a portable table for tightness to ensure that they have not become loose due to movement during the previous session. Some tables have cutouts in the tabletop to accommodate women with larger breasts when they lie in the prone position.

Face Cradle

The face cradle (also called a face rest) is composed of a wood, metal, or heavy plastic base and a crescent-shaped foam cover attached by Velcro strips. Some face cradles are not adjustable and hold the client's head parallel to the table but do not allow for other adjustments. Adjustable face cradles allow the therapist to find the ideal position for the client's head to ensure comfort. Learning how to work with a face cradle and adjust it correctly takes time. Technique 2 demonstrates how to adjust the face cradle so that it is comfortable for the client.

Width

Massage tables range from 28 to 32 inches wide. Shorter therapists may feel more comfortable with a 28-inch table, which does not require reaching as far across the client. Taller therapists are usually comfortable with wider tables. Large clients may feel uncomfortable on a narrow table, as their arms tend to fall off the side. A short therapist using a narrow table may want to invest in arm shelves or side extenders that widen the table for larger clients.

Height

The height range of both stationary and portable tables is 22 to 36 inches. Some tables are made so that they can be

| Technique 2 | **How to Adjust a Face Cradle** |

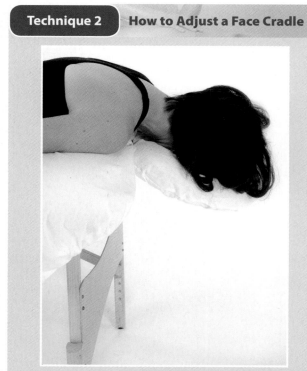

1. When you adjust a face cradle for the client, avoid placing the client's neck in too much flexion, extension, projection, or retraction. To learn proper positioning of the face cradle, it helps to first place the face cradle in a position where the client's head is too flexed as shown in this image.

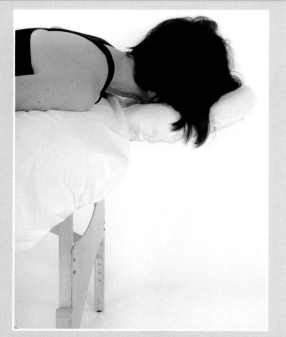

2. Now place the face cradle in a position where the client's head is too extended. After experiencing these two extreme positions, it is easier to find the correct position for the client's head.

Technique 2   **How to Adjust a Face Cradle** (Continued)

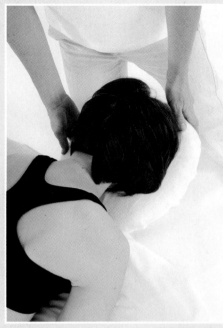

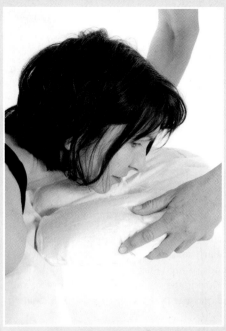

3. Find the correct position and adjust the face cradle so that the neck is open and accessible but the cradle does not put undue pressure on the sinuses or bones of the face.

4. The foam crescent can be adjusted on the base to match the size of the client's face by moving the foam sides closer or further out on the Velcro strips.

set at lower levels for use with specific modalities like Shiatsu or the Feldenkrais Method. Your height, the size of the client, and the type of massage techniques all affect the correct table height. For Swedish or relaxation massage, stand beside the massage table with your shoulders relaxed and arms at your sides. When you make a fist, your knuckles will rest on the table when it is at the appropriate height. Alternatively, use the flat of your hand or fingertips as a guide if that feels more comfortable (Fig. 2-4). If the client is larger and "sits higher" on the table, you may want to place the table a little lower than usual to compensate. If the client is very slim and "sits lower," you may raise the table a little. Some techniques are easier to deliver at a specific table height. Many therapists lower the table when providing deep-tissue techniques to be able to more easily use their body weight in the stroke. Therapists practicing Trager, craniosacral, and reflexology might set the table higher. In general, if your arms and shoulders feel sore at the end of the massage, the table may be set too high. If your lower back feels sore and stiff at the end of the massage, the table may be too low. Experiment with table height to determine what feels best for your body.

Length

Most massage tables are 70 to 73 inches long. The face cradle adds approximately 12 inches to the length, and **bolsters** shorten a client's leg length by about 6 inches. Even clients

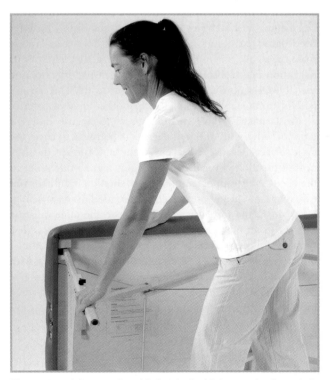

Figure 2-4 Adjusting the table height. In this image, the therapist is testing the table height with her fist. You can also test the height with the flat or your hand or fingertips.

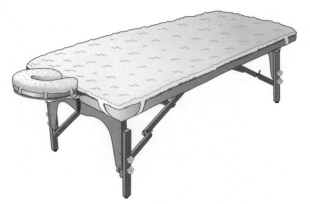

Figure 2-5 Padding on the massage table.

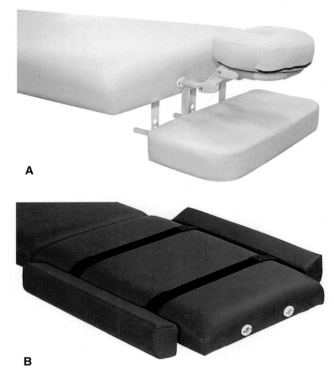

Figure 2-6 A. A front attachment often called an arm shelf is used with the client in the prone position. **B.** Side extenders provide a resting place for the arms in both the prone and supine positions for larger clients. Image courtesy of Massage Warehouse.

over 6 ft tall are comfortable on standard massage tables, although custom table lengths can be ordered for clients who are particularly tall. Ensure there is enough space in the room on both ends of the table for a chair or stool. Often you can plan time during the session to get off your feet and sit down during the massage (such as during a foot massage).

Padding and Cover

The padding on massage tables varies from a single-layer to multiple-layer systems (Fig. 2-5). Multiple-layer systems are typically more comfortable because the deeper foam layers are firm, giving support, while the upper foam layer is softer and conforms to the client's body. Padding comes in 1- to 4-inch thicknesses. Firm table padding (1½ to 2½ inches) is sometimes preferred by therapists who offer deep-tissue techniques because the client doesn't sink away from the stroke. Therapists who offer energetic bodywork or relaxation massage sometimes prefer plush padding because the table feels more comfortable and "nurturing." You can add padding to the table by using fleece or other types of covers.

Most massage table manufacturers today use different types of vinyl, with different degrees of softness, to cover the table surface. Because a sheet covers the table surface, the softness of the table cover usually does not make a difference to the client. Most important, the cover should be durable and easy to clean. Oil and creams, like those used in massage, can break down the top layer of the vinyl, so the table must be cleaned to ensure that it lasts. Wipe the table down with a suitable cleaning product between clients, and use diluted bleach solutions only if the table comes into contact with body fluids. Some therapists use antibacterial wipes to give the table a quick cleaning and prevent drying out of the vinyl top. Sanitation and cleaning products are discussed in greater detail in Chapter 3.

Accessories

A variety of massage table accessories are available from table manufacturers to increase the client's comfort and help you work efficiently without undue stress on your body.

Arm Shelf

An arm shelf can be attached to the front of the table to provide a place for clients in the prone position to rest their arms (Fig. 2-6). This is useful because it gives you easy access to the sides of the client's body. When the client is in the supine position, side extenders can be placed on each side of the table to widen the table and provide more space for the arms.

Sit-Up Feature

Some massage tables allow the therapist to place the client in a sitting position. This is a nice feature if you plan to work with pregnant clients, if you offer reflexology, or if you are also an esthetician and offer facials. A cushion is often needed to support the client's lower back because the steep angle of the upper portion of the table tends to create a gap.

Bolsters

Bolsters are used to support the client's body for complete relaxation while on the table (Fig. 2-7). These pillows and cushions come in a variety of shapes and sizes and are usually placed under the knees and neck when the client is supine and under the ankles when the client is prone. In the side-lying position, regular bed pillows are useful for supporting the client's upper body and head, and a long rounded bolster is placed under the knee and along the length of the lower leg.

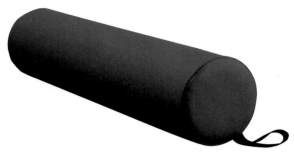

Figure 2-7 Bolsters are used to support the client's body so that she or he can relax completely without undo pressure on joints. Image courtesy of Massage Warehouse.

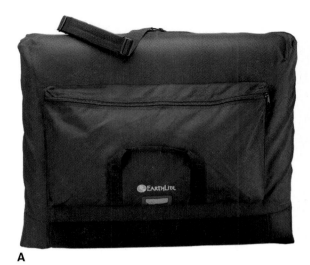

A

Several manufacturers have created elaborate body positioning systems for use with pregnant women or with any individual to position the body very specifically for massage techniques. The intention of such systems is to remove stress from the joints and position the spine and neck in a natural alignment. Pregnancy wedges can also be used to provide support for pregnant women when resting in a semi-reclined position. Supports for large-breasted women are also available. Positioning the client with bolsters is described in detail in Chapter 10.

Carrying Case and Rolling Cart

A carrying case made of tough waterproof material protects the portable massage table during transport. Straps make it easier to lift and carry the case. Cases that completely unzip on three sides are easier to put on and take off the massage table.

Rolling carts make it easy to move the table across flat surfaces and help prevent muscle stresses while transporting the table (Fig. 2-8). Although the table must still be lifted upstairs or over curbs, a cart is a valuable investment for therapists who work in many different locations.

Massage Stool

Massage stools usually have wheels so they can be rolled around the massage table (Fig. 2-9). Sitting down at appropriate points during the massage helps rest your feet. Most stools can be adjusted to different heights, and some are available with back supports. Some therapists instead sit on a Swiss exercise ball during sessions (Fig. 2-10); this can encourage good body mechanics.

Step Stool

A step stool helps clients get on and off the table. A long, flat exercise step also works well because it is wide enough to prevent missteps (Fig. 2-11).

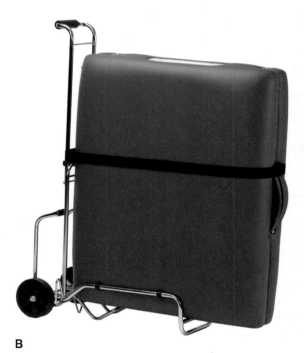

B

Figure 2-8 A. Carrying case **B.** Rolling cart. Images courtesy of Massage Warehouse.

Massage Chair

Massage chairs are used for on-site massage in offices, sporting events, fairs or community events, airports, malls, or anywhere therapists give treatments (Fig. 2-12). The client remains fully clothed in a seated position, and the chair's design provides complete support for the client to relax. Chair manufacturers have different designs with different adjustment features. Carefully research these feature differences

---

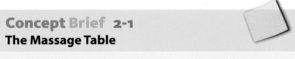

Concept Brief 2-1
The Massage Table

Massage table types	Portable/stationary/mat
Features	Frame/width/height/length/padding
Accessories	Arm shelf/sit-up/bolster/carry case/cart/ stool

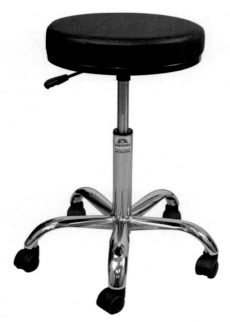

Figure 2-9 Massage stool. Image courtesy of Massage Warehouse.

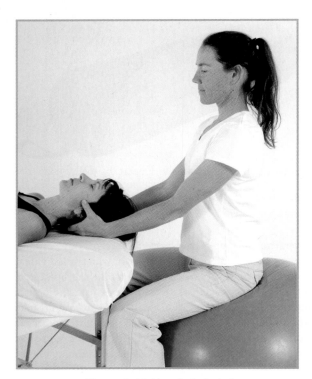

Figure 2-10 Use of a Swiss ball.

when choosing a massage chair for your practice. You will learn more about seated massage in Chapter 14. Accessories include carrying cases and disposable face cradle covers for a quick changeover between clients.

Linens

The centerpiece of a well-designed and comfortable massage room is the massage table well made up with linens. For therapists on a budget, plain sheets and a large bath towel can be used. Multitonal colors in slightly varying shades provide texture and depth. Take care to match the **linens** to the décor of the room. An upscale spa might opt for Egyptian cotton and a matching coverlet with a multitude of different throw pillows. Massage and spa suppliers provide everything from the basics to very expensive linens.

Massage Sheets

Purchase massage sheets from a massage or spa supplier or department store (twin size). Cotton, flannel, and cotton blends all work well and feel soft and comfortable. Make sure that the material is thick enough to provide sufficient coverage, avoiding thin see-through sheets that are inappropriate for draping. Make sure that sheets are small enough not to touch the ground during the session, which would create an unsanitary condition. White, cream, earth-tone, and pastel colors are easy to bleach, but darker colors tend to show oil stains. Sheets with patterns hide oil stains. Massage and spa suppliers sell laundry products that help to get oil out of

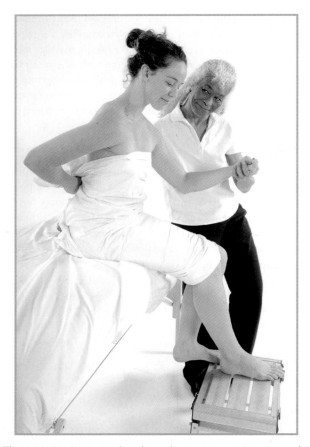

Figure 2-11 A step stool, as shown here, or an exercise step can be used to make it easier for a client to get on and off the massage table.

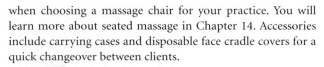

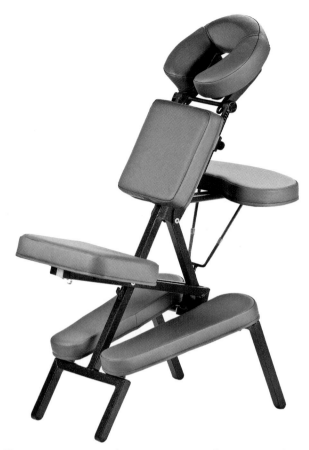

Figure 2-12 Massage chair. Image courtesy of Massage Warehouse.

often used to wrap hydrocollator packs or other hot packs to prevent burning the client. Hand towels are sometimes used as draping material, to protect the client's hair from oil, or to make a roll to support the neck. Hot moist hand towels are used to remove spa products from the client's skin or to provide a warming body steam (placed over the face, wrapped around the feet, etc.) during the session. Any towel that comes into direct contact with the client's skin or hair must be laundered between clients.

Blankets

Have washable cotton blankets on hand to help keep the client warm. Clients often experience a drop in peripheral body temperature as their blood pressure lowers during the massage. This is normal, but a chilled client cannot relax completely. Heavy blankets feel nurturing and comforting for many clients and give the client the sensation of being snug and secure. Some clients, however, find that heavy blankets feel suffocating and restrictive. Have a few options on hand to accommodate each client's needs. The blanket is always placed over the top massage sheet. If it comes into contact with the client's body (which is likely), it should be laundered between clients.

Linen Storage

Linen is washed in hot water with detergent, dried with heat, and stored in a closed container. You want to have enough linen on hand to get through 2 days of business without doing laundry if possible. The amount of linen you need varies based on the type of massage work you do. For example, if you work in a chiropractor's office, you may see 12 clients in a day for 30 minutes each. Alternately, you might offer four 90-minute sessions. A good start might be 10 sets of sheets, 10 face cradle covers, 5 bath sheets, 5 bath towels, 16 hand towels, and 2 cotton blankets. Dirty linen is stored in a closed, ventilated container, preferably outside the treatment room, until it is laundered.

massage sheets, but over time, oil usually builds up in the fabric and can smell or look dirty; plan to replace massage sheets regularly to prevent this. Disposable sheets are available from spa suppliers, but these are not as cost-effective as washable linen and impact the environment with unnecessary waste.

Face Cradle and Bolster Covers

A pillowcase can be used to cover the face cradle, provide draping material (breast drape, anterior pelvic drape, etc.), or cover bolsters. Fitted face cradle covers available from massage suppliers are better than a pillowcase because they fit the face rest snugly and do not fall off. Fitted bolster covers that enclose the entire bolster prevent cross-contamination between clients; often a bolster is not covered but placed under the bottom massage sheet. Face cradle and bolster covers that come in contact with the client's skin must be laundered and changed for each client.

Towels

Bath towels and larger bath sheets are often used over the top massage sheet to provide warmth and additional draping material. Choose lightweight ones that will not be bulky during draping. These are also easy to launder. Bath towels are

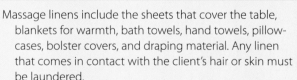

Concept Brief 2-2
Massage Linens

Massage linens include the sheets that cover the table, blankets for warmth, bath towels, hand towels, pillowcases, bolster covers, and draping material. Any linen that comes in contact with the client's hair or skin must be laundered.

Assessment and Clinical Equipment

Massage therapists working in a medical environment or offering clinical massage might need specialized equipment such as posture grids, plumb lines, and hydrotherapy equipment.

Posture Grid

A posture grid is a large, lined chart posted on a wall in the treatment room (Fig. 2-13). The client is positioned standing in front of the grid during a visual assessment. The grid helps the therapist see muscular holding patterns that affect posture (such as one shoulder higher than the other). Sometimes photos are taken in front of the grid to document progress over a series of sessions.

Plumb Line

A plumb line is a string with a weight fastened to one end (Fig. 2-13). The string is attached to the ceiling and hangs perfectly vertical. Like the posture grid, the plumb line provides a reference point for assessing a client's posture. The use of posture grids and plumb lines is discussed in Chapter 19.

Hydrotherapy Equipment

Hydrotherapy is the use of water in one of its three forms (liquid, vapor, solid) for healing. Massage therapists often use hot or cold packs to produce changes in circulation, muscle, and connective tissue that aid the healing process. For example, when a hot pack is applied to a body area, the peripheral blood vessels dilate significantly, increasing blood flow to the area. This helps to relax muscles, reduce muscular spasm, increase the extensibility of collagen, increase range of motion, and reduce pain; it is generally relaxing for the client. Different types of packs are available. Probably the most

effective hot pack is the hydrocollator pack. This pack has a canvas casing filled with silicon granules or clay particles that hold heat up to 30 minutes. The pack is submerged in water kept at 165°F in a specialized heating unit called a hydrocollator (Fig. 2-14). The pack is removed from the hydrocollator with tongs or thermal gloves and wrapped in a minimum of four to six layers of towel. Hydrotherapy principles, equipment, and techniques are discussed in Chapter 16.

Blood Pressure Equipment

Blood pressure refers to the pressure in the large arteries delivering blood to body areas other than the lungs (e.g., the brachial artery in the arm). High blood pressure may place a person at risk for stroke, heart attack, heart failure, or arterial aneurysm. Some therapists feel that it is a good idea to check the blood pressure of clients with a history of high blood pressure, first-time clients, and pregnant clients before and after a session to help ensure their safety.

Blood pressure is measured using a stethoscope and a sphygmomanometer, often referred to as a "cuff," with attached gauge. If you plan to check blood pressure, you should have small, medium, and large cuff sizes available because an ill-fitting cuff distorts the accuracy of the reading. Blood pressure and blood pressure cautions are discussed in Chapter 5.

Client Warming Equipment

There are many ways to ensure the client stays warm during the massage. Therapists use heat lamps; electric table warmers; corn, rice, or flax seed packs; hydrocollator packs; or Fomentek water bottles.

Heat Lamps

Heat lamps hung above the treatment table with a dimmer switch allow for heat adjustment. Freestanding lamps with a flexible neck are available but have large bases that take up much space in the treatment room.

Table Pads

Wool and fleece table pads provide extra softness and warmth on the massage table. Many contain electrical heating devices with adjustable heat controls to keep the client warm during the massage. Some therapists believe that electrical devices disrupt the client's electromagnetic energy field, however, and use such pads only to warm the table; they turn off the pad once the client arrives. Wool is a desirable material because it breathes and allows the body to better regulate its own temperature. The drawbacks of wool pads are that they require dry cleaning and may cause an allergic reaction in some clients. Synthetic fiber and cotton pads are also available.

Fomentek

A Fomentek is a large water bottle designed to lie flat on the treatment table (Fig. 2-15). Fill the bottle with warm, not

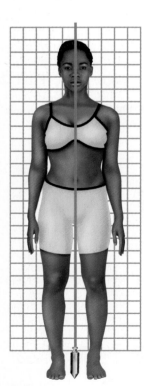
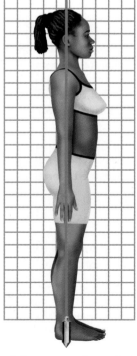

Figure 2-13 A posture grid and plumb line are two pieces of specialized assessment equipment that help therapists analyze posture and muscular holding patterns.

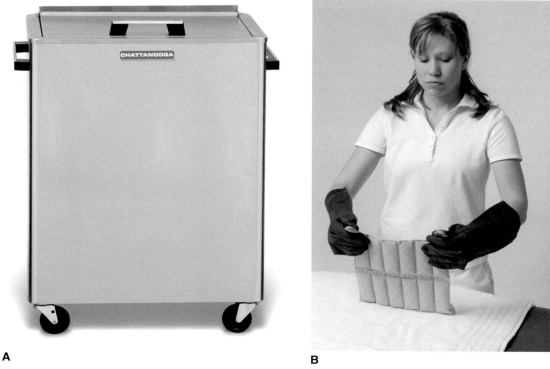

A   **B**

Figure 2-14 **A.** A hydrocollator is a specialized heating unit that heats packs. **B.** Filled with clay to 165°F.

hot, water and twist the lid on tightly. Put the bottle under a pillowcase and place it directly beneath the sheet. This provides warmth and comfort during a massage.

Warm or Hot Packs

Various types of warm and hot packs are available (Fig. 2-16). Corn, rice, or flax packs come in a variety of shapes and sizes; they are heated in a microwave. Hydrocollator packs can be used for both treatment and simply to relax tense muscles. Warm packs can be placed under the feet, on the back, on the belly, around the hands, and around the neck to keep the client warm and to draw blood to the local area. Gel face cradle inserts warm the face rest; some claim that this helps prevent sinus congestion. Some packs can be chilled in a refrigerator and used to cool a body area. For example, a cool eye pillow and neck pillow feel soothing and refreshing.

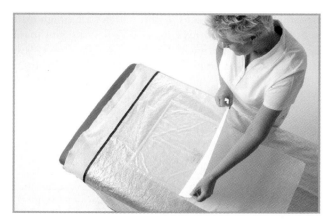

Figure 2-15 A Fomentek water bottle can be used to provide additional warmth for a client about to receive a body wrap (discussed in Chapter 15). Notice that it is always placed under a towel or sheet to insulate the client from too much heat.

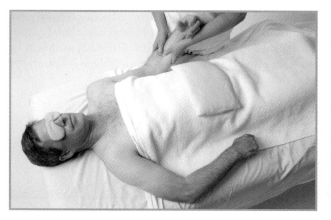

Figure 2-16 Warm packs.

Massage Tools

Some therapists use massage tools to protect themselves from stresses during certain techniques. Such tools include items with a knob used to provide pressure on a point and mechanical thumping devices that apply percussive or wave-like compressions. Many such devices are very effective and popular with clients. Before using a massage tool on a client, tell them you will use it, explain its benefits, and make sure that the client is comfortable with it. Sanitize all massage tools that come into contact with the client's skin with alcohol or an approved disinfectant (Fig. 2-17).

Other Massage Room Supplies

All massage rooms in all settings need certain basic items to be functional and efficient. These include a small reference library, clock, storage area, wastebasket, music system, and supplies for cleanliness and safety.

Reference Library

During the course of a professional practice, every therapist will need to look up a condition, medication, or other information. Available key reference books should include an up-to-date medical dictionary, drug reference, and a pathology reference book. Access to the Internet is also a plus for quickly looking up information on new drugs, pathologies, and recommendations for session protocols.

Clock

A visible clock helps you stay on schedule and adjust your treatment plan as the session progresses. Spa treatments and treatment elements requiring specific application times (body wraps, mud, or seaweed applications, etc.) are easily tracked using a digital timer.

Storage Area

A cabinet with hinged or sliding doors is best for keeping extra supplies like table cleaners, extra hand gel sanitizer, boxes of tissue, and clean linens out of sight. Soiled linens should be stored in a closed, ventilated container, preferably outside the treatment room in a separate laundry area.

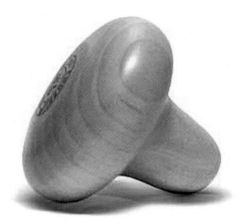

Figure 2-17 Massage tool.

Wastebasket

Wastebaskets in massage treatment rooms should have a lid opened and closed with a foot pedal to prevent hand contamination. Dispose of paper towels used for cleaning the massage table and hard surfaces, used disposable gloves, used tissues, and other items in the wastebasket. The wastebasket should be cleaned and sanitized at the end of each day.

Music System

Music often significantly impacts the client's ability to relax and enjoy the session. The music system might be as simple as a CD player or MP3/iPod system. Ensure the sound has a clean quality and that the system is in good working order (no skipping CDs, etc.).

Supplies for Cleanliness and Safety

Approved cleaning products (discussed in Chapter 3), paper towels, extra tissue boxes, gel hand sanitizer, alcohol, finger cots (vinyl finger covers to protect against the transmission of pathogens if your cuticles are rough or if your skin is broken), vinyl gloves, and a first-aid kit should be stored in the treatment room for ease of access. Also have a large, battery-operated flashlight in case of a power failure.

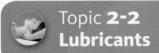

Topic 2-2
Lubricants

Lubricants are used with many massage techniques to prevent undue friction between the therapist's hands and the client's skin. While some techniques are performed on dry skin without a lubricant, most strokes feel uncomfortable to clients without some sort of lubrication. The choice of lubricant is based in part on the degree of slip and the techniques to be used in a session. For example, deep-tissue techniques work best if the client is not too slippery. With these techniques you need to slow down, sink into the tissue, and engage the deeper muscle and fascia—which is impossible if the client is too slippery. You might use very small amounts of gel or oil for deep-tissue work, or use a cream, which is absorbed rapidly and has less slip.

Sometimes the choice of lubricant depends on the client. Clients with heavy body hair may prefer massage with oil rather than cream, because cream tends to mat the hair into little balls, which can feel painful. Because hair doesn't mat into balls as easily with oil, oil provides a more comfortable massage. Some clients don't like to feel oily after a session, however, and therefore prefer cream to oil. Some clients may be allergic to certain ingredients in lubricants. It is a good idea to offer clients a few choices and let them pick what they like. As a massage student, you should work with a variety of different products to get a feel for what works for you when you apply different techniques.

In all cases, new therapists should use lubricants in moderation. Start with small amounts and add more only if your hands drag on the skin or the client reports discomfort. New massage students often use large amounts of lubricant, leaving the client greasy and dissatisfied. Clients want to feel the therapist's hands and enjoy strokes that engage the tissue. If the client is covered in a thick layer of lubricant, it is difficult to work at the appropriate depth. If too much lubricant is applied, remove the excess with a hand towel. Massage and spa suppliers offer a wide range of products for lubricating the skin. Product types include oils and butters, creams, lotions, gels, and powders.

Oils

The types of oils (also called lipids or fats) used in massage usually come from vegetable sources pressed from nuts or seeds (such as avocado oil and almond oil), but some animal fats (such as ghee, or clarified butter) may also be used. Oils are classified as "saturated," "polyunsaturated," or "monounsaturated" fats. Most oils contain some amount of all three types of fat but are classified according to the type present in the greatest amount. For massage purposes, these terms indicate something about the texture and quality of the oil and how absorbable it is. Monounsaturated and polyunsaturated fats are liquid at room temperature. Saturated fats, found mainly in animal products, are solid at room temperature and are not absorbed into the skin.

Topically applied oils soften and condition the skin, hydrate the skin, improve skin elasticity, and improve atopic dermatitis. Some oils have antiinflammatory and pain-relieving properties that make them especially useful in massage.

Whether or not topically applied oils penetrate the skin and enter the bloodstream and have internal health effects has been debated. Some research studies show that some oils, or compounds from oils, do penetrate the skin and enter the

blood circulation.[1,2] Saturated fats, like those found in regular butter and cocoa butter, are poorly absorbed but may still have benefits for the skin. Ghee, for example, is used in ayurvedic medicine to lubricate the skin, promote wound healing, and decrease inflammation. Oils tend to be slippery when first applied but can be used with deeper, slower work as they are absorbed. Because they leave a moderate-to-heavy residue on the skin, you should provide clients with disposable wet wipes and a clean hand towel so that they can wipe off after a session. Some clients prefer cream to oil because they don't like the oil residue.

It is important to use oils that are expeller pressed (also called cold-pressed or expressed) as opposed to oils (like processed cooking oils) that are refined. Refined oils are exposed to processes that damage the essential fatty acids, vitamins, minerals, and nutrients in the oil, making them less beneficial for skin health when applied topically. Mineral oil (baby oil) and petroleum products are by-products of the distillation process to produce gasoline. These oils coat the skin and are not absorbed into the skin and do not allow the skin to eliminate metabolic wastes through perspiration. When buying commercial massage oils, lotions, or gels, read the ingredients list carefully. Avoid preservatives like BHT, BHA, and EDTA; hydrogenated oils (oils that have been changed from poly or monounsaturated to saturated fats to make them more stable); lanolin, mineral oil, and petroleum; and dyes and synthetic fragrances. Natural oils are more expensive than refined oils and tend to become rancid sooner than refined oils. Purchase them in small quantities and refrigerate them between uses.

Common Oils Used in Massage

The oils described below are commonly used in massage. Some are best used in moderation or in combination with other oils because of their high cost or viscous consistency. A variety of exotic vegetable oils are available, many of which are perfectly suitable for massage. The Massage Fusion section at the end of this chapter discusses some of the components of oils in greater depth.

- **Almond oil** (*Prunus amygdalis* var. *dulcis*) is pale yellow with a light odor and medium-weight texture.
- **Apricot kernel oil** (*Prunus armeniaca*) is yellow and has a prominent odor and lightweight texture. Avoid the refined oil, which has a pale yellow color and no odor.
- **Avocado oil** (*Persea americana*) is olive green and has a strong odor and heavy texture. An avocado oil that is pale yellow in color and odorless has been refined. Avocado oil is generally expensive but is particularly useful for stretch marks, dehydrated skin, scars, and mature skin.
- **Canola oil** (*Brassica napus*) is pale yellow and has a light odor and lightweight texture. Check to ensure that the canola oil is natural, organic, and unrefined. Heavily processed canola oil is often used as an ingredient in cheaper massage and body products.

- **Cocoa butter** (*Theobroma cacao*) is pale yellow and has an odor reminiscent of chocolate (it is used to make chocolate). It is solid at room temperature but light-to-medium weight when melted and applied to the body warm or mixed with other oils. Because it contains high levels of saturated fats, it is not absorbed into the skin but forms a micro-layer on top of the skin, which is useful for preventing moisture loss in dry skin.
- **Coconut oil** (*Cocus nucifera*) is pale yellow, has a coconut odor, and is solid at room temperature but medium weight when melted. Raw coconut oil is difficult to find, and the product most often sold is refined or fractionated (to keep it liquid). Like cocoa butter, coconut oil is high in saturated fats and is not absorbed into the skin. This oil causes skin irritation in some individuals.
- **Evening primrose oil** (*Oenothera biennis*) is yellow and has little odor and a heavy, almost sticky quality. Because of its high gamma-linolenic acid content, it has been used in the treatment of conditions including eczema. This oil is often used as a spot treatment during facial massage or added to other oils to boost their healing properties for the skin.
- **Hazelnut oil** (*Corylus avellana*). Hazelnut oil is yellow and has a mild nutty odor and a lightweight texture. It is inexpensive and easy to find.
- **Hemp seed oil** (*Cannabis sativa*). Hemp seed oil is green and has a medium nutty odor and a heavy-weight texture. While it is expensive, its antiinflammatory and analgesic properties make it especially useful in massage.
- **Jojoba oil** (*Simmondsia chinensis*) is bright yellow and has a light odor and a medium-weight texture. Jojoba is a wax that is liquid and stable at room temperature. It mimics sebum, the body's natural moisturizer, and so is useful for all skin types. It is believed to regulate sebum production in oily skin when used for extended periods of time.
- **Kukui nut oil** (*Aleurites moluccana*) is pale yellow and has a sweet odor and a lightweight texture. While it is expensive, it contains high amounts of linoleic acid, alpha-linolenic acid, and vitamins A and E, which make it useful for healing sunburn, chapped skin, eczema, and psoriasis.
- **Macadamia oil** (*Macadamia integrifola*) is pale yellow and has a light odor and a lightweight texture. Like jojoba oil, it mimics sebum and is useful for all skin types.
- **Mustard seed oil** (*Brassica juncea*) is pale yellow and has a distinctive odor and a lightweight texture. It is often used in ayurvedic medicine as a heating oil for muscle stiffness and soreness. Fixed mustard seed oil should not be confused with the steam-distilled volatile essential oil of mustard seed. The volatile oil is highly toxic and avoided in aromatherapy and massage.
- **Rose hip seed oil** (*Rosa rubiginosa and other species*) is light yellow-red and has a distinctive odor and heavy, sticky texture. The CO_2 extraction (an extraction method in which CO_2 gas turns liquid under high pressure and acts like a solvent and then turns back to a gas when the pressure is removed)

is preferable to the solvent-extracted oil. It is expensive, but useful for facial massage or for use on scar tissue.

- **Safflower oil** (*Carthamus tinctorius*) is yellow and has a mild odor and lightweight texture.
- **Sesame oil** (*Sesamum inducum*) is yellow and has a distinctive toasted nutty odor and medium-weight texture. One of the primary oils used in ayurveda and often the base of taila (Indian medicated massage oils), it is considered warming and penetrating.
- **Shea butter** (*Vitellaria paradoxa—Butyrospermum parkii is the old name*) is cream colored, has a distinctive odor, and is solid at room temperature. It must be melted for use in massage. It is high in oleic acid, saturated fats, and vitamins E and A, which make it particularly healing for damaged skin and hair when applied topically.
- **Sunflower oil** (*Helianthus annuus*) is yellow and has a mild odor and medium-weight texture.

Problematic Oils

Grapeseed, corn, soybean, and peanut oils are not regularly used in massage. Grapeseed and soy oil are heavily processed and extracted with strong solvents. While corn oil can be found in an unrefined form, it is most often solvent extracted and processed. Peanut oil has a very strong smell and may cause serious allergies.

Allergic Reactions to Oils

During the health history intake, ask clients about allergies to nuts or other substances. While an allergic reaction or skin sensitivity may occur with any substance applied to the skin, nut oils and in particular peanut oil can cause mild-to-serious reactions in people with allergies to the food. Allergic reactions and strategies for dealing with them are discussed in greater detail in Chapter 5.

Concept Brief 2-3
Oils

Oils	Also called lipids or fats
Type	Vegetable or animal fats—mainly vegetable (nut and seed)
Saturated	Solid at room temperature and not absorbed by skin
Monounsaturated	Liquid at room temperature and absorbed by skin
Polyunsaturated	Liquid at room temperature and absorbed by skin
Unrefined	Cold or expeller pressed—fatty acids, nutrients, vitamins intact
Refined	Heavily processed—nutrient values for skin destroyed
Massage benefits	Soften, condition skin—benefits may be absorbed

Lotions and Creams

Lotions and creams are popular with clients because they leave the skin smooth but feel less greasy than oils. Some massage techniques work best when the therapist's hands can sink into the tissue and "grab" it instead of sliding over it. For this reason, a cream or lotion might be used instead of oil.

Lotions and creams are oil and water emulsions. An emulsion is a blend of two un-mixable substances held together by an emulsifying agent. The ingredients of some products are high quality and natural, held together by a vegetable-based emulsifier. The ingredients of other products are synthetic, heavily processed, and held together by an emulsifying wax, which is a chemical mixture of fatty alcohols and thickening agents used to bind and give body to the formulation. Creams are heavier than lotions and so provide longer-lasting slip. Lotions are absorbed rapidly but work well for certain techniques like deep-tissue techniques and for local areas like the feet and face.

Gels

Gels include natural substances like aloe vera gel or a combination of natural and artificial ingredients that create a gel-like formulation. Some massage gels are quite heavy and leave a residue on the skin as oils do. Natural gels tend to be absorbed very rapidly and leave little, if any, residue on the skin. Seaweed gels that are meant to be left on the body (some for body wraps are meant to be removed) make a good massage product. Seaweed stimulates circulation and aids the body in detoxification. Seaweed products should not be used on clients with iodine or shellfish allergies as they may cause a serious reaction.

Powders

Some therapists use baby powder (talc and fragrance), talc, cornstarch, or powered chalk to reduce friction between the hands and the client's body. Talc is usually composed of finely ground magnesium silicate, but some talc is composed of synthetic components. Some concern exists that talc may cause respiratory problems if it is inhaled. Cornstarch and powdered chalk are sometimes used, but they are drying for the skin and the therapist's hands. In ayurveda, massage powders are made from a natural ground flower like chickpea flower. These products are less drying and less irritating for the respiratory system and provide enough slip for a full range of massage techniques. Provide clients with a clean, dry hand towel to dust themselves off at the end of the session.

Product Information

Massage therapists should learn to read product labels carefully. The product label indicates the type of oil used in the lubricant, any dyes or fragrances that have been added, any ingredients that might be potential allergens for a particular client, and any undesirable fillers or chemicals. If the fixed oils included in the product are not specifically listed as expeller- or cold-pressed, they are probably refined and best avoided. The first time you try a product it's a good idea to review the complete list of the product's ingredients and look up anything you do not recognize to make sure it is acceptable for use on clients. *Milady's Skin Care and Cosmetic Ingredient Dictionary* by Natalia Michalun is a good guide to product ingredients.[3]

Botanical Extracts

Many creams, lotions, and gels include botanical (plant) extracts in their formulations to achieve a specific therapeutic goal. Botanical extracts added to a preparation are often chosen because they are antiinflammatory (German chamomile), soothing (lavender), antiseptic (tea tree), cooling (menthol found in peppermint), or pain relieving (white camphor, wintergreen, sweet birch). The concentration of the botanical extract and other components in the preparation determines the overall therapeutic value of the preparation. Sometimes an extract is added to a preparation only for marketing purposes and is present in such a low concentration that it adds very little, if any, therapeutic value to the product. Sometimes the preparation contains only an isolated chemical component of the original botanical extract. In the end, it is difficult to know how effective a product will be until you work with it and observe any benefits it provides. It is important to point out that clients may have allergies to certain botanicals or may not enjoy their aromas. Offer clients choices and be flexible.

Fragrances

Fragrances are added to enhance the smell of various formulations or to mask the smells of other ingredients. Fragrances are either natural or synthetic. Natural fragrances

---

Concept Brief 2-4
Lubricants—Slip, Absorption, Residue

Oils (unrefined)	High slip, moderate absorption, moderate residue
Oils (refined)	High slip, slow absorption, heavy residue
Massage gels	High slip, slow absorption, moderate residue
Natural gels	High slip, fast absorption, low residue
Creams	Moderate slip, moderate absorption, low residue
Lotions	Low slip, fast absorption, low residue
Baby powder/talc	Low slip, drying, low residue
Corn starch	Low slip, drying, low residue

are usually derived from natural essential oils or botanical extracts. Synthetic fragrances are usually composed of a small number of artificially synthesized compounds that may cause skin irritation or unwanted side effects such as headaches or a slightly sore throat. Avoid products that list "fragrance" or "perfume" because these are usually synthetic. Products labeled "unscented" usually contain a masking fragrance. "Fragrance-free" products contain no fragrance of any type and no masking fragrance. While many clients respond well to natural aromas, it is important always to have available a fragrance-free product for clients who are sensitive.

"Natural" Products

The term "natural" is not regulated in the cosmetic industry.[4] A company can put just about anything in a product and legally call it "natural." A product line claiming to be "all natural" usually still contains some synthetic ingredients, dyes, or preservatives. The goal is to use the best possible quality and to know the components of the products you use on clients.

Concept Brief 2-5
Ingredients to Avoid

Avoid preservatives like BHT, BHA, and EDTA and hydrogenated oils, lanolin, mineral oil, petroleum, dyes, and synthetic fragrances in massage products. Research all products carefully and give the clients choices.

Client Choice

Therapists should have a variety of products on hand to meet the needs of their clients. It works well to offer clients these choices:

- **Oil, cream, or lotion:** Briefly explain the differences and direct clients toward the type of slip that will best help them meet treatment goals. For example, if the client says, "I want really deep work" you may suggest a lotion that would ensure you won't have too much slip as you work slowly and deeply into the tissue. Alternately, if the client always gets cold easily, you might suggest an oil rather than a cream. Creams or lotions tend to feel cooling on the body whereas oil tends to warm up and stay warm.

- **Aroma or no aroma:** Many clients like the aromas of natural botanicals and essential oils. Others don't. Offer clients the choice between scented and unscented.

- **Therapeutic effect or just lubricant:** Sometimes therapists "up-sell" or use specialized products with therapeutic effects for an additional fee. For example, a therapist might offer a deep-heat massage and use a massage oil to which warming botanicals have been added to cause increased circulation and warmth to the local area. Other therapists offer these types of choices without an up-sell fee.

Pick products carefully and fully research them to ensure that they are right for your practice. Keep products, especially oils, refrigerated between uses, and follow good sanitation protocol (discussed in Chapter 3) when handling products. Remember that you yourself are the one most exposed to a product. A client may get a massage once a week using the product, but you have your hands and forearms in the product for up to 30 massages a week.

Topic 2-3
Creating a Comfortable Massage Environment

Clients' perception of the massage business is created or altered through their five senses because this is how we interpret our environment. We shape client comfort by paying attention to what the client sees, hears, smells, tastes, and feels during the session. If you own your massage business, you have control of many of the issues we are about to discuss. If you work as an employee, you will have less opportunity to determine how the environment of the business is set up. Still, by considering clients' perception and comfort issues you can make good choices in the development of your own business space or make good recommendations to your employer if it is necessary.

What the Client Sees—Décor

Every business has its own unique focus and personality. A therapist who practices relaxation massage and stress reduction is likely to operate in a different environment from a therapist who practices clinical massage. The first may choose soothing color combinations and images of natural beauty for the walls, while the second might choose a neutral color palette, medical charts, and anatomical models. To choose your own appropriate **décor**, consider the techniques you will use and the types of clients you desire. Color, window treatments, flooring, lighting, wall decorations, and extra touches are all elements of decoration.

Color

There are many ways to think about color and choose the colors that are right for your business. Therapists can learn from color psychology and color symbolism in making their decisions.

Color psychology is a field of study that evaluates the effects of colors on human behavior and emotion. Color symbolism explores the cultural significance of colors and what colors mean to different groups of people. Color psychology is appropriate for situations in which the business has no cultural overtones. For example, a therapist who delivers relaxation treatments might use a green palette because studies have demonstrated that green colors decrease tension and stress, slow breathing patterns, and in some cases decrease blood pressure.[5,6] A clinical massage therapist might note the results of a study showing weight lifters can lift more weight in rooms with a blue palette; blues seem to promote strength and physical gains.[7] A therapist working with pregnant mothers, parents, and infants would not choose a yellow palette because research shows that babies cry more frequently in yellow rooms (Fig. 2-18).[8]

Color symbolism works well when a business has cultural overtones or has a specific client group (Fig. 2-19). For example, a business focused on Eastern bodywork might choose colors with cultural significance in Asian countries. The color red might play a decisive role because in Asia, red is the color of good luck and a wedding color. It has positive, joyful overtones. A business set in a busy urban area and wanting to attract businessmen might choose a blue palette, because in Western society, blue is associated with excelling (blue ribbon), loyalty (true blue), and noble decent (blue blood). It is also associated with intelligence (bluestocking) and morality (blue laws).

Window Treatments

Window treatments are an important design feature in any room and provide privacy, light control, and style. In a massage environment, privacy is very important. Window treatments should not be so sheer that people outside can look in and see the massage session. Window treatments also control the light

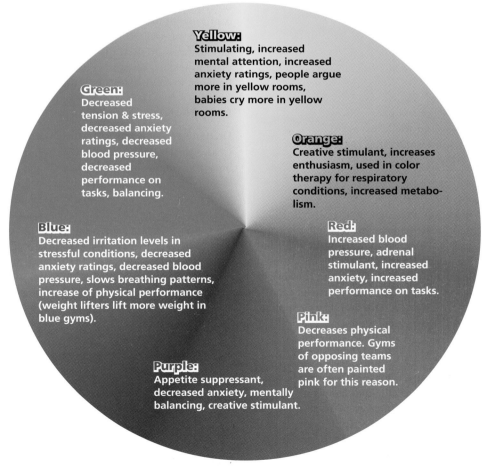

Figure 2-18 Color psychology is a field of study that evaluates the effect of color on human behavior and emotion. This color wheel shows some of the effects of color, based on research.

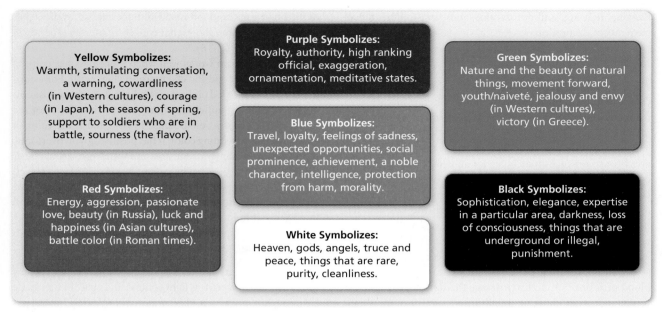

Yellow Symbolizes:
Warmth, stimulating conversation, a warning, cowardliness (in Western cultures), courage (in Japan), the season of spring, support to soldiers who are in battle, sourness (the flavor).

Purple Symbolizes:
Royalty, authority, high ranking official, exaggeration, ornamentation, meditative states.

Green Symbolizes:
Nature and the beauty of natural things, movement forward, youth/naiveté, jealousy and envy (in Western cultures), victory (in Greece).

Blue Symbolizes:
Travel, loyalty, feelings of sadness, unexpected opportunities, social prominence, achievement, a noble character, intelligence, protection from harm, morality.

Red Symbolizes:
Energy, aggression, passionate love, beauty (in Russia), luck and happiness (in Asian cultures), battle color (in Roman times).

Black Symbolizes:
Sophistication, elegance, expertise in a particular area, darkness, loss of consciousness, things that are underground or illegal, punishment.

White Symbolizes:
Heaven, gods, angels, truce and peace, things that are rare, purity, cleanliness.

Figure 2-19 Color symbolism explores the cultural significance of color and what colors mean to different groups of people.

entering the room. Natural light streaming through sparkling windows might be desirable during the client consultation or assessment. When the massage starts, softer, dimmer light is more relaxing. You can choose between semi-sheer fabrics that diffuse the light and rich opaque fabrics that shut it out completely.

Windows are often the main focal point in the treatment room. Interesting and well-planned window treatments add style and eye-catching appeal. They also absorb sounds from outside and from the room itself, helping create a quieter overall environment while conserving energy by insulating the glass.

Lighting

In the treatment room, dimmer switches work well. Lights can be made bright for cleaning or sanitizing equipment, put at a medium setting for the health intake consultation, and turned down for the massage. Several pools of soft, diffused light or diffuse natural light are more relaxing than one bright light in a corner or the room being too dark. Avoid candles because open flames are a safety hazard and they can pollute the air, especially when used in small rooms.

Wall Decorations

Wall decorations can promote the image of the business, make a soothing impression on the client, and dampen sound. In relaxation-orientated businesses, images of natural beauty are often used to help clients feel connected to the earth and nature. Clinical massage businesses benefit from medical charts and images that allow clients to see and understand the structures involved in their soft-tissue condition. Businesses specializing in Eastern bodywork may hang Asian images or

objects on the walls to evoke a sense of that culture and create continuity in the client's experience. Wall decorations can be functional as well as beautiful. For example, fabric wall hangings dampen noise, while a stylish mirror gives the client a place to freshen up at the end of the session and allows the therapist to check his body mechanics during the session.

Extra Touches

Decorative items on shelves, side tables, and windowsills help create visual interest and define the room's style. A relaxation business using an all-natural theme might display shells, non-blooming plants (to avoid allergic reactions), or interesting stones. An orthopedic business might feature anatomical models of the body. Rattan baskets, bamboo, and Japanese river stones might adorn an Eastern bodywork business. Items can be functional as well as decorative. For example, in a business focusing on ayurvedic bodywork, one therapist has different types of Indian, Nepalese, and Bhutanese bells and chimes on display. They are beautiful to look at but also sound lovely when she rings one to signal the beginning and end of the session.

What the Client Hears

The auditory environment is also important because it helps set the tone for the session and may mask outside noise. Consider the treatment room flooring. A tile or wood floor may cause echoes that are annoying or distracting. The wrong sort of music may also be disturbing and irritating to the client. Most therapists have probably heard spa or massage CDs that are downright alarming. One CD on the market features wolves howling incessantly in every song—it is difficult for a client who feels like prey to relax!

The right music can evoke strong feelings and beneficial physiological changes in the client. Research shows that music decreases anxiety, decreases systolic blood pressure, and decreases heart rate even when the person is actively stressed.[9] Music also exerts complex influences on the central nervous system and can in a short period of time change brain waves associated with an alert state to brain waves associated with a relaxed state.[10] In a single session of music therapy delivered to hospice patients with chronic pain conditions, music decreased the participants' overall levels of pain and increased their physical comfort.[11] Research also shows that the positive physiological benefits of music are increased when patients can choose their own music.[12] It is a good idea to have a variety of musical styles available and to ask clients about their musical preferences during the client consultation. Clients can also be encouraged to bring their own appropriate music for the session.

What the Client Smells

Good ventilation and fresh air are important in the massage treatment space. In the warm, closed environment of the massage room, aromas from a previous client (e.g., heavy perfume, cigarette smoke, etc.) can persist into the next session if the room is not well ventilated. Open the windows between clients if possible, or point a fan at the ceiling to circulate the air. Leafy, non-blooming foliage plants make good natural air purifiers. Because many clients have allergies to blossoms, flowers should not be used in the treatment room, despite their beauty.

Therapists must also consider their own smells and how they may impact a client. Avoid strong-smelling deodorants, perfumes, and aftershave products. Brush your teeth after meals and rinse your mouth with mouthwash between clients. Smokers should not smoke after showering in the morning until after the last session of the day. The use of a sea salt scrub on your hands can help to exfoliate skin that holds the aroma of cigarette smoke. While this might seem harsh, clients who do not smoke often find the lingering smell of cigarette smoke intolerable.

In a therapeutic setting, the good smells from natural essential oils used in aromatherapy can promote relaxation and a pleasant mood. This is important because stress is at the core of many modern diseases, and studies suggest that decreasing stress improves one's health and immunity.[13,14] Smells can evoke intense emotional reactions and can even be used to change behavioral patterns. Credible evidence shows agreeable aromas can improve our mood and sense of well being.[15] This is not surprising because olfactory receptors are directly connected to the limbic system, the oldest and most emotional part of the human brain.

In a study of how scent impacts social relationships, people in photographs were given a higher "attractiveness rating" when the test subjects were exposed to a pleasant fragrance.

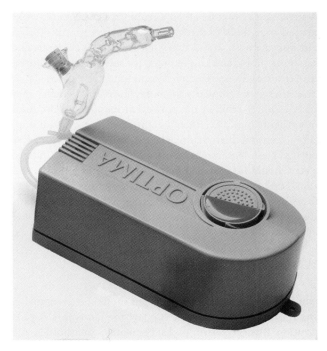

Figure 2-20 Nebulizing diffuser.

In a test of shampoos, a product initially ranked last in performance was ranked first in a second test after its aroma was adjusted.[16]

Therapists can use gentle, soft aromas to enhance the client's perception of the business and to provide an emotionally satisfying experience. For example, diffusing citrus essential oils throughout an area can purify the air, repel insects, enhance mood, and make the area smell clean and fresh. A commercial nebulizing diffuser works well to eliminate microbes and promote a clean, healthy living or working space (Fig. 2-20). Avoid the use of strong scents and even too much of a soft scent. Don't use scented carpet sprays, laundry detergent, or fabric softeners as these have synthetic ingredients that may irritate clients.

When using aromas, use products with natural rather than synthetic fragrances. Synthetic fragrances are artificial and do not come from aromatic plants, fruits, or flowers. Clients often develop adverse reactions to synthetic fragrances (headaches, sore throat, sneezing, coughing, and emotional irritation) and may come to dislike all aromas as a result. Aromatherapy and the use of pure, natural essential oils are discussed in detail in Chapter 15.

What the Client Tastes

In most cultures, food and drink have celebratory associations. Children celebrate birthdays with ice cream parties, cake is eaten at weddings, and special friends are invited over for a meal. Incorporating small food items in the session is a pleasant and smart practice. Clients can sometimes get up from a session and feel shaky and dizzy from low blood sugar.

A small snack provides an opportunity for the client to wake up and come back to the "real world" before venturing back out into the busy world. It doesn't have to be elaborate and can be as simple as a cup of green tea served from a Chinese tea set after the massage or a complimentary chocolate on Valentines Day. Similarly, a sports massage therapist may serve a sports drink at the post-event massage. In the summer, clients may leave their treatment with a colorful popsicle to remind them that massage is fun. Granola bars and a bowl of fresh fruit might be offered to clients. Fresh, filtered water should be provided before, during, and after the session. Food and drink should be simple and manageable, but focus on the intention of the offering: to welcome, to nourish on a spiritual level, and to show care, thoughtfulness, and appreciation.

What the Client Feels

Once on the massage table, the client should be enveloped in warm, soft textures. Bolsters support the joints in a relaxed position. Blankets, warm packs, Fomentek water bottles, and heat lamps help keep clients warm throughout the session. Lotion warmers heat massage oil or lotion so that it does not feel cold when applied. Never use a microwave oven to heat oil or lotion because microwaves may affect the product's therapeutic properties. Because many products break down when heated, it is recommended to use 1-oz bottles with flip or pump lids. These small bottles are filled with fresh oil or lotion at the beginning of each day so that the larger container is not exposed to heat and can remain in the refrigerator.

Some massage therapists have chronically cold hands, which can feel shocking to the client at the beginning of the session. Warm your hands as much as possible by holding them under warm water, holding a warm pack, or rubbing them briskly before the session.

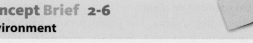

Concept Brief 2-6
Environment

Décor	Color/window treatments/wall decoration/other decorations
Color	Color psychology: how color affects human behavior
Color	Color symbolism: what colors mean to certain groups of people
Windows	Privacy/control of light/style
Lighting	Control/functional
Walls	Hangings (noise reduction)/pictures/functional (mirrors)
Floor	Noise considerations/ease of cleaning
Decoration	Theme/feelings/beauty + functional (e.g., bells)
Music	Affects physiology/variety/client choice?
Smell	Use of natural smells/adverse reactions with synthetics
Taste	Small food items/drink items/comfort/caring

Accessibility and Functionality

When designing your massage space, think about each area of the business and analyze its **accessibility** and **functionality**. Consider the entrance and reception area, dressing area, and the bathroom.

Entrance and Reception

When choosing a business location, consider its accessibility. Are doorways, hallways, and bathroom entrances wide enough to accommodate a wheelchair? Is there enough space around furniture to accommodate someone in a cast and on crutches? Does a long flight of stairs make the business prohibitive for elderly clients? Is parking convenient and user-friendly, or will clients be spending the first 10 minutes of the session looking for a space, and feeling stressed?

The reception area must be friendly, neat, and functional. Clients generally fill out paperwork in this area while waiting for their session. They might also pay for the session and book additional sessions in this area. Magazines, a retail area, tea or water, and comfortable chairs and attractive furnishings help ensure the client's comfort.

The Undressing and Dressing Space

Carefully plan the space where clients remove their clothing before the session and get dressed afterward. A screened-off area provides a sense of privacy and decreases the client's anxiety that the therapist might walk into the room unexpectedly. Place a chair and hooks behind the screen where clients can hang their clothing. A small container for personal items like keys and jewelry helps ensure clients do not misplace or forget them. A box of tissue, disposable wet wipes, and mirror are useful as well.

The Restroom

In the restroom, provide only liquid soap. Have on hand amenities that make it easy for clients to tidy up after the session. Gentle face cleanser, make-up remover, and moisturizer allow women to remove their makeup before a session or fix it up afterward. Disposable combs, bobby pins, spray gel, and hair bands come in handy, especially after a neck massage using oil. Contact lens solution, spray antiperspirant (solids or gels used by more than one person are unsanitary), and mouthwash are also appreciated.

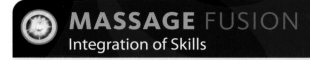

MASSAGE FUSION
Integration of Skills

STUDY TIP: there is no substitute for direct experience!

Isadora Duncan, the famous American dancer, remarked, "What one has not experienced, one will never understand in print." Massage equipment is best understood through direct experience. Students who try different bolster sizes, for example, understand that some situations require a larger bolster while others require a smaller one. Students who think about how their body feels after giving a 1-hour massage at different table heights is better able to avoid injury. Students who try the same technique with oil, cream, and powder can better understand how to make good lubricant choices. Try these ideas:

1. Place the table in a position that is too high and give massage for 30 minutes. Where does your body feel stressed? Which techniques worked well with the table high? Which techniques were difficult with the table high?

2. Place the table in a position that is too low and give massage for 30 minutes. Where does your body feel stressed? Which techniques worked well with the table low? Which techniques were difficult with the table low?

3. Lie on the massage table in the supine position using small bolsters. Feel the position of your joints and low back. Now lie on the massage table in the supine position using large bolsters. Try the same exercise in the prone position.

4. Try a massage technique using powder. Remove the powder with a dry hand towel and try the same technique with cream. Remove the cream with a hot, moist towel and try the technique with oil. Which lubricant worked best? Why?

MASSAGE INSPIRATION: Make Your Own Massage Cream

A good way to know what's in a massage cream is to make it yourself. The following natural blend provides excellent lubrication for massage strokes. A variety of natural ingredients can be found on the Internet.

Ingredients: 1 cup unrefined apricot kernel or hazelnut oil, 2 tablespoons grated beeswax, 2/3 cup distilled water, 2/3 cup aloe vera gel, 5 drops vitamin E oil.

Directions: In a double boiler, melt the apricot kernel oil and beeswax. When the beeswax melts, pour the oil mixture into a glass measuring cup and let it cool at room temperature until the edges start to turn white. Combine the water, aloe vera gel, and vitamin E in a blender at the highest speed. In a slow drizzle, pour the cooled oil and beeswax into the vortex of the blended solution while the blender is still going. Stop the blender and mix the formulation with a spatula to blend it further. Continue mixing and blending until the ingredients are completely combined. Store the product in a jar or bottle in the refrigerator.

CHAPTER WRAP-UP

The quality of your equipment and lubricants and the time and care you put into planning your massage space convey your level of professionalism to your clients. While it may seem early to start thinking about equipment needs and décor for your business, it's not too early to explore options. Try out different massage tables and different lubricants. Start to explore interior design and think about color choices and window treatments. Starting now helps ensure you will be prepared to enter the massage profession with a clear and informed plan. This also helps keep your massage career vision alive, an important motivator when the massage program gets challenging!

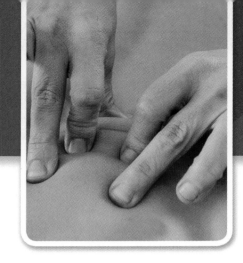

Chapter

3

Sanitation, Hygiene, and Safety

KEY TERMS

antiseptic

disease transmission

disinfectant

hygiene

infectious diseases

infectious agents

sanitation

universal precautions

LEARNING OBJECTIVES

Having read the chapter and used the related student learning tools, the student will be able to:

1. Define the word "disease" and describe three different types of diseases.

2. Define the term "infectious agent" and differentiate among bacteria, viruses, fungi, protozoa, and animal parasites.

3. Explain the specific ways in which an infectious agent can be transmitted through direct contact, indirect contact, vehicle transmission, and vector transmission.

4. Exhibit good therapist hygiene and demonstrate proper handwashing techniques in a health care setting.

5. Understand and identify health care situations in which universal precautions should be used.

6. Define the term "safe environment" and list three ways to ensure client safety in a massage business.

7. Compare and contrast the information on an accident report and incident report.

8. Describe good client screening practices and explain how they promote the therapist's safety.

Massage therapists are required by health standards and professional ethics to provide a clean, hygienic, and safe environment for their clients. Therapists adopt standard sanitation procedures to prevent the spread of **infectious disease**. Sanitation protocols include therapist **hygiene;** the **sanitation** of the treatment room, equipment, and product containers; and general cleanness of the facility. In addition, therapists must also ensure safe conditions to prevent injury to themselves or clients. Safety protocols include fire and accident prevention plus proper planning should accidents occur.

This chapter focuses on the basics of **disease transmission** and prevention; practices for good therapist hygiene; sanitation of the facility, equipment, and products; universal precautions; and safety planning. Your health as a therapist and self-care activities are described in Chapter 11.

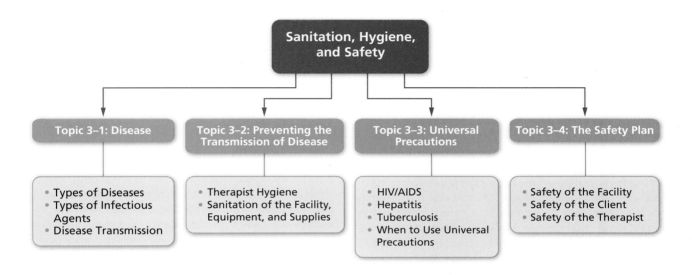

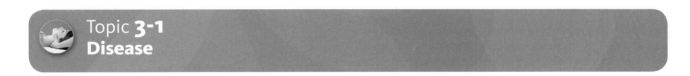

Topic **3-1**
Disease

To prevent the spread of disease, you should understand the different types of diseases, **infectious agents** (also called pathogens) and their forms, and the processes by which disease may be transmitted.

Types of Disease

A disease is an infectious or noninfectious abnormal condition that results in medically significant symptoms and often has a known cause. Diseases may cause changes in the appearance, structure, or function of cells, tissues, organs, or systems in the human body. The signs and symptoms of diseases may result from the disease process itself or the immune system's attempt to control an infectious agent. Such signs and symptoms include but are not limited to fever, nausea, an elevated white blood cell count, fatigue, and cardiovascular and metabolic changes.

The terms "acute," "subacute," and "chronic" are often used to note a disease's severity or stage. When a disease is in the acute stage, the symptoms are severe, and in some cases, the situation is more dangerous. The acute stage usually lasts a short time before the symptoms decrease and the body enters a subacute stage. A chronic disease persists for a long time or regularly recurs. Types of diseases include autoimmune, cancerous, deficiency, genetic, infectious, and metabolic diseases. Massage therapists need a basic understanding of disease to prevent the spread of infectious diseases and to rule out massage contraindications (covered in detail in Chapter 5).

Autoimmune Diseases

Autoimmune diseases occur when the immune system malfunctions and starts to treat normal body cells and tissues like an infectious agent. The immune system attacks the body, causing damage to body tissue, the abnormal growth of an organ, or changes in organ function. Although the precise causes of autoimmune diseases are unknown, researchers believe there is an inherited predisposition to develop these conditions.[1] A few types of autoimmune diseases, most notably rheumatic fever, are triggered by a bacterium or virus because part of the structure of normal cells resembles part of the structure of the infecting pathogen.[2] Examples of autoimmune diseases include rheumatoid arthritis, scleroderma, lupus, and insulin-dependent diabetes mellitus (type 1). Autoimmune diseases are not normally contagious and are not spread through person-to-person contact. Autoimmune conditions can be transferred between the mother and fetus during pregnancy, but this is rare.[3]

Cancerous Diseases

Cancer is caused by normal cells mutating and beginning to replicate uncontrollably. The abnormal cells may form masses of tissue called tumors and/or metastasize, which means spread to new areas of the body. Benign tumors rarely threaten life, do not spread to other parts of the body, and can usually be removed. Malignant tumors invade and damage nearby tissue, metastasize to new areas, and threaten life. Blood cell cancers do not form tumors but circulate through the bloodstream.

No one is certain about the precise causes of cancer, but potential trigger factors include some chemicals in processed foods, genetic predisposition, hormone levels, radiation exposure including sunburn, tobacco use, and exposure to carcinogenic chemicals in the workplace.[4] Although infection with certain viruses may increase the risk of some types of cancer as the virus interferes with the deoxyribonucleic acid (DNA) in cells, cancer itself is not contagious and does not spread from person to person, but sometimes viruses that can cause cancer, such as human papillomavirus (HPV), are contagious.

Deficiency Diseases

Deficiency diseases include all diseases caused by an insufficient supply of essential nutrients, vitamins, or minerals. For example, a prolonged lack of dietary vitamin C (ascorbic acid) may lead to scurvy. Lack of calcium and vitamin D can lead to rickets, a common childhood disease in developing countries. Deficiency diseases are not contagious and do not spread from person to person.

Genetic Diseases

Genetic diseases result from abnormalities in an individual's genetic material (chromosomes) that are either inherited from parents or triggered by external factors. Genes, or DNA, act as chemical "blueprints." They determine precisely how the body will look and function. Genes are enclosed in rod-shaped structures called chromosomes, which are contained in the cell nucleus. Every human cell has 36 chromosomes in 23 pairs, with one unit of each pair inherited from each parent at conception. A genetic disorder or disease may occur if a copying error occurs during cell division such that an abnormal version of a gene is produced or one or more chromosomes are incomplete. Sometimes the fertilized egg does not end up with a full set of chromosomes. An abnormal (mutated) gene can play a role in many illnesses including Parkinson's disease, multiple sclerosis, and Alzheimer's. Most genetic disorders are passed down from parents to children; they are not contagious.[5]

Infectious Diseases

Infectious diseases, also known as communicable diseases, are caused by an infectious agent referred to as a pathogen. Infectious diseases are spread by contact with another person or an animal, or from a mother to her fetus or infant. Disease-causing germs might be left by one person on an object like a table, doorknob, or faucet and then be picked up by another person who touches the object. Some diseases are expelled in droplets or particles when one person coughs or sneezes and are later inhaled or ingested by another person. A disease may move from host to host via an insect (called a vector) such as a mosquito, flea, lice, or tick. Good sanitation, personal hygiene, and the use of universal precautions are the best ways to decrease or prevent the spread of infectious diseases in massage settings.

Metabolic Diseases

"Metabolic diseases" is a generic term for a wide range of conditions that result from abnormal metabolic processes. A metabolic disease might be caused by an inherited enzyme abnormality, or it might be acquired as the result of the failure of an important organ like the liver. Cushing's syndrome, thyroid disorders, and Graves' disease are examples of conditions that might be classified as metabolic diseases. Metabolic diseases are generally not contagious, although conditions like hepatitis (an infectious disease that affects the liver) may lead to metabolic disorders.

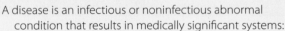

Concept Brief 3-1
Types of Diseases

A disease is an infectious or noninfectious abnormal condition that results in medically significant systems:

Autoimmune	Immune mistake—Immune system attacks self
Cancerous	Normal cells mutate and replicate uncontrollably
Deficiency	Insufficient supply of vitamins, nutrients, or minerals
Genetic	Abnormalities in genetic material lead to disease
Infectious	Communicable—spread via a pathogen
Metabolic	Abnormal metabolic processes

Types of Infectious Agents

The term pathogen comes from the Greek pathos meaning "suffering or disease" and gen meaning "producer." Therefore a pathogen is a producer of disease. The term refers to infectious organisms like bacteria, viruses, fungi, and protozoa (Fig. 3-1). Parasitic animals can also be passed from person to person or from animals to people and may cause disease.

Bacteria

Bacteria are one-cell living organisms found in every environment on earth including inside and outside the human body. They multiply independently of their host and can thrive in almost any environment including on nonliving surfaces like plastic. Most bacteria are not harmful, and many bacteria are necessary for good health. The immune system relies on probiotic bacteria (sometimes referred to as the intestinal flora), which live in the intestinal tract. Probiotic bacteria aid normal food digestion and provide immune support against certain viruses, yeasts, parasites, and pathogenic bacteria.

Pathogenic bacteria like *E. coli* (*Escherichia coli*) and *Salmonella* (*Salmonella enteritidis*) may enter the body through improperly handled food or unwashed hands (especially after toilet use) and cause food poisoning or acute diarrhea. *Staphylococcus aureus* is the species of bacteria that causes "staph" infections. It commonly lives harmlessly on the skin and hair, and around the nose. It can potentially be passed to massage clients by therapists who touch their own hair or nose and then touch a client without first decontaminating their hands. If staph gets into a cut and rapidly reproduces, it may cause serious infection and blood poisoning. *Streptococcus pneumoniae*, known informally as pneumococcus, causes pneumonia when it is inhaled into the lungs and cannot

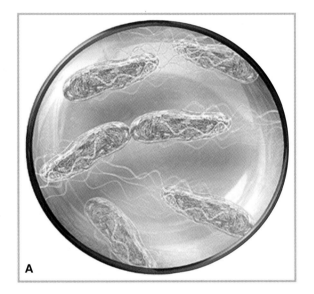

A

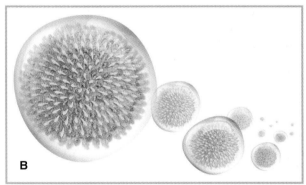

B

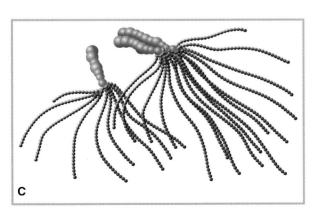

C

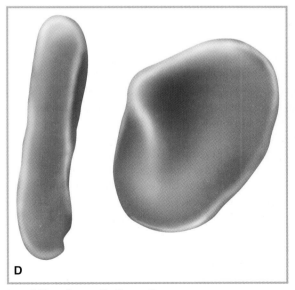

D

Figure 3-1 Infectious pathogens. **A.** *E. coli* bacteria. **B.** The influenza virus. **C.** Tinea fungus. **D.** *Plasmodium falciparum*, the protozoa responsible for the most deadly type of malaria.

be cleared. Its relative, *Streptococcus pyogenes,* causes "strep throat" among many other diseases. Pathogenic bacteria normally live on the skin and hair, in the nose, throat and lungs, or in the intestines without causing a problem. They infect the body only when its defenses are low or when a pathogenic bacterium suddenly comes into contact with vulnerable tissue.[6]

Rickettsiae and chlamydiae are smaller than bacteria but still classified as bacteria. These pathogens are parasites that must live inside cells of their hosts. In most instances, these organisms are transmitted through the bites of insects like lice, ticks, and fleas. Rickettsiae are responsible for a number of serious diseases such as typhus and Rocky Mountain spotted fever. Chlamydiae cause trachoma, an eye infection that causes blindness, the sexually transmitted diseases chlamydia and lymphogranuloma venereum, and some respiratory diseases.

Viruses

Viruses are smaller than bacteria and cannot replicate or reproduce outside a living host cell (plant, animal, or human). To grow and spread, they effectively take over the host cell, causing the cell nucleus to replicate both its own genetic material and that of the virus. The cell is usually eventually destroyed when it ruptures and the new viral particles formed are released into extracellular fluid within the body to infect more cells. Viruses mutate quickly, making them difficult to treat effectively. Some viruses lie dormant in cells until a stimulus or a decline in the host's defenses activates them. Some persistent viruses, like the human immunodeficiency virus (HIV), which causes AIDS, can enter or exit a cell without killing it.

Viruses are present in infected body fluids like blood, saliva, or droplets from the nose, mouth, or genitalia. They are transmitted person to person or animal to person. While most viruses cannot live long without a host, some, like the herpes simplex virus, can linger on surfaces for several hours and infect a person via indirect contact. This is one reason why the proper sanitation of linens and equipment in a massage environment is so important (discussed below).

Fungi

Fungi, which include molds and yeasts, comprise a large group of simple plant-like organisms that are larger and more complex than bacteria. Warm, moist environments promote the reproduction of fungi through simple cell division and the production of large numbers of spores.

A common fungus, *Candida albicans,* is present in the mouth, mucous membranes, vagina, and rectum. It can also travel through the bloodstream and affect the throat, intestines, and heart valves. *Candida* becomes dangerous when some change in the body environment allows it to grow out of control. When it grows out of control in the mouth, it is called thrush. When it grows out of control in the vagina, it is often called a yeast infection or vaginitis. In individuals with low resistance due to other diseases such as leukemia or AIDS, *Candida* can enter the bloodstream and cause a serious infection in vital organs.

A group of related fungi cause skin infections characterized by red, scaly patches known commonly as ringworm, but despite the name, the pathogen is not a worm (Fig. 3-2). Ringworm might be found on the skin (tinea corporis), scalp (tinea capitis), around the groin (tinea cruris, sometimes called jock itch), or feet (tinea pedis, most often called athlete's foot). Ringworm is highly contagious and is transmitted via skin-to-skin contact or contact with contaminated items like unwashed sheets, flooring, and combs. Therapists who practice massage barefoot can pass an undetected fungal infection to clients or pick up a fungal infection when clients walk barefoot in the same area.

Protozoa

Protozoa (from the Greek *protos* meaning "first" and *zoon* meaning "animal") are a single-cell organism regarded as the simplest form of animal life. They grow in moist environments such as fresh water, marine environments, decaying organic matter, wet grass, and mud. Protozoa cause diseases such as amoebic dysentery, which is usually contracted through contaminated water or food; African sleeping sickness, which is spread by the tsetse fly; and malaria, which is transmitted by the anopheles mosquito.

Parasitic Animals

The parasitic animals of most concern to massage therapists are mites and lice because they are spread very easily through direct contact or contact with infected sheets and clothing (Fig. 3-3). Lice and mites do not carry infectious bacteria, viruses, or fungi to the host. Instead, their wastes cause intense itching that leads the host to scratch the skin, opening it to more serious infection.

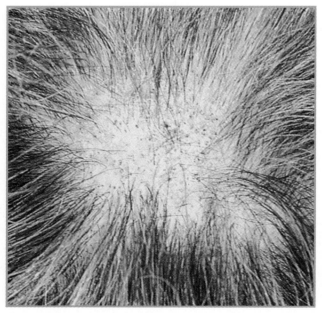

Figure 3-2 A group of related fungi cause skin infections characterized by red, scaly patches known commonly as ringworm.

Lice

Head lice (*Pediculus humanus capitis*), body lice (*Pediculus humanus*), and pubic lice (*Pthirus pubis*—often called crabs) suck the blood of the host and cause itching. Head lice often spread among grade school children and must be treated with repeated applications of special shampoos. A fine-tooth comb is passed through the hair to remove eggs. Body lice live in the seams of clothing rather than directly on the host. This type of lice is usually seen in homeless people who do not have regular access to laundering facilities. Body lice are transmitted through unwashed clothing but could be passed from clothing to massage sheets. Pubic lice are nicknamed "crabs" because of their crab-like appearance. They are usually spread through sexual contact but might also be spread to clothing or linens. While they tend to inhabit the groin area, they can live in any coarse body hair (armpits, eyebrows).

Mites

Mites (*Sarocoptes scabiei*) like warm, moist areas of the body, especially skinfolds. They burrow under the skin and live off the blood of the host. Mite infestations are often referred to as scabies. The excrement of the mite is highly irritating and leads to itchy, red allergic reactions. Like lice, mite infestations are highly contagious and spread through person-to-person contact or via clothing and linens.

If a lice or mite infestation occurs at your massage clinic (e.g., a client calls to say she just found out that she has lice), cancel all appointments until the facility can be deep cleaned. Wash any linens or cloth materials that may have come into contact with the infected person in hot water and detergent, then dry them with heat. Vacuum carpeted floors carefully and change bath mats and towels in the bathroom. Mop hard floors and wipe down all hard surfaces. Lice and mites live only about 38 hours away from the host, but care should be taken that they are not spread to an unsuspecting client.

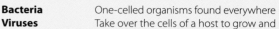

Concept Brief 3-2
Types of Infectious Agents

Bacteria	One-celled organisms found everywhere
Viruses	Take over the cells of a host to grow and spread
Fungi	Plant-like organisms (includes mold and yeast) that like warm, moist environments
Protozoa	One-celled animals that grow in moist environments
Animal parasites	Lice and mites are tiny animals that suck blood and cause itching

Disease Transmission

An infectious pathogen must breech the body's defenses to cause a disease. Some pathogens, called opportunistic pathogens, cause disease only if the host's immune system is depressed. Others, called virulent pathogens, readily cause disease when they gain entrance to the body. Pathogens are transmitted by direct contact, indirect contact, vehicle transmission, or vector transmission.

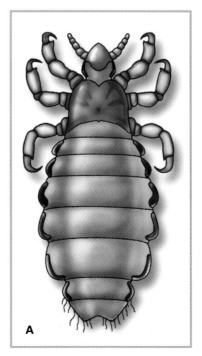

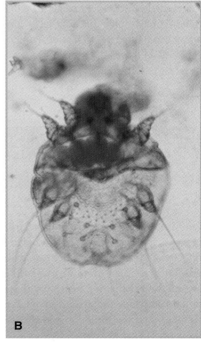

Figure 3-3 Lice and mites. **A.** *Pediculus*, the louse that causes head lice, body lice, and pubic lice. **B.** *Sarcoptes scabiei*, the mite that causes scabies.

Direct Contact

The sweat and sebum in skin provide some natural protection against the transfer of pathogens via direct contact of the skin. But if the skin is damaged by a cut, scrape, wound, burn, or even dryness that leaves the skin with microscopic breaks, the chances of infection increase.

Pathogens often reside around areas of mucous membranes such as the nose, lips, eyes, gastrointestinal tract, genitourinary tract, genital area, and anus. Lymph tissues like the tonsils, mucus, and cilia provide some protection for the mouth and respiratory system. Other mucous membranes provide less protection.

An infected person can transfer a pathogen to an uninfected person through touch, sexual contact such as kissing or intercourse, or expelling body fluid droplets by sneezing, coughing, or touching mucous membranes and then touching an uninfected person without having washed the hands.

Indirect Contact

An infected individual can transfer a pathogen to an inanimate object (known as a fomite) like a countertop, doorknob, toy, or magazine. A person might touch his or her nose or mouth and then touch the fomite, sneeze or cough on a fomite, or fail to wash hands after using the toilet and then touch a fomite. The pathogen lingers on the fomite where an uninfected person touches it.

Vehicle Transmission

Air, food, and liquid taken into the body provide a mode of transport for pathogens. This type of pathogen transmission is called vehicle transmission. Pathogens can travel in the air in droplets (usually mucous droplets such as are released by a sneeze), aerosols (very small droplets that may have evaporated from droplets on a surface), or dust particles. This is why people often get sick after flying on an airplane; because cabin air is recycled, pathogens have repeated opportunities to infect passengers.

A number of pathogens are found in food. If these pathogens are not killed during food processing, they are transmitted directly to the gastrointestinal tract. Bacteria in the intestinal flora of animals may be safe for those animals but unsafe for humans. For example, *Salmonella* is part of normal chicken intestinal flora but can cause serious illness in humans if it is not destroyed during food preparation. A food preparer may also be infected and transfer pathogens to otherwise uncontaminated food.

In the United States, drinking water is generally safe, but if a water supply is contaminated with human or animal fecal matter (e.g., sewage) it may cause serious illness. Homes and businesses with a private well should have the water tested annually to ensure its safety. Pathogenic organisms as well as harmful chemicals like lead and radioactive isotopes like radon can enter well water and cause health problems.

Vector Transmission

Vectors are insects or animals capable of transmitting diseases, including mosquitoes, flies, fleas, ticks, mites, rats, dogs, and cats. Vectors are mobile and can easily spread a disease to previously uninfected areas. The vector usually breaks the skin through a bite or sting but may also cause disease through its feces. A pathogen might be located on the outside surface of a vector and spread through physical contact with food or a surface when it lands (e.g., flies).

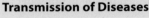

Concept Brief 3-3
Transmission of Diseases

Direct contact	Transport via person-to-person contact
Indirect contact	Infected person leaves pathogen on fomite; uninfected person later picks up pathogen from fomite
Vehicle	Transport via air, food, or liquid
Vector	Transport via insect or animal

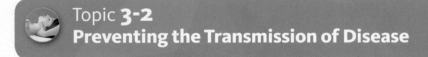

Topic 3-2
Preventing the Transmission of Disease

It is impossible to know if a client who walks into your business is infected with a pathogen. Similarly, you may be infected and not know it. Because pathogens that cause serious illness are all around us, sanitation and hygiene practices are required at all times to prevent the spread of disease. These practices include therapist hygiene; sanitation of equipment, supplies, and the building; and the use of universal precautions (discussed in Topic 3-3).

Therapist Hygiene

As health care providers, massage therapists must adhere to the highest standards of personal hygiene. This includes cleanliness of the body and hair, wearing clean, appropriate clothing, removing jewelry, proper handwashing, and attending to issues like smoking and illness.

Cleanliness of Body and Hair

Shower daily and wash your hair on work days. Avoid the use of scented antiperspirants, perfumes, colognes, aftershaves, and body care products because these may cause sensitivity or allergies in some clients. As described earlier, the hair can act as a reservoir for pathogens like *S. aureus* and must be tied back so that it does not touch the client during massage. Men should shave before each work shift or keep facial hair neatly trimmed. If you touch your own hair during a session, including facial hair, you must sanitize your hands before touching the client.

For better hygiene and client comfort, keep your nails short, natural, and filed to a smooth edge (Fig. 3-4). Long nails, nail polish, and artificial nails are breeding grounds for pathogens and may scratch a client; they are best avoided. Brush and floss your teeth before the shift and directly after eating food during breaks in the day. Because therapists and clients come into close contact during massage, it is a good idea to rinse your mouth with mouthwash before each new client.

Therapists who perspire heavily while giving massage can wear sweatbands on the forehead and wrist to prevent droplets of perspiration from falling onto the client. A clean towel can be used to absorb perspiration throughout the massage if necessary.

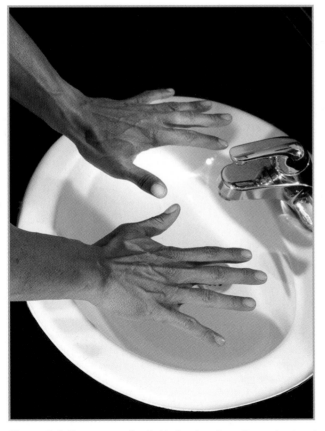

Figure 3-4 Proper care of nails. Notice that the nails are short and filed to a smooth edge and that no nail polish or jewelry is worn.

Clean and Appropriate Clothing

Launder your work uniform or clothing at the end of each working day. Short sleeves are better for massage, because long sleeves, which may touch the client's skin and become contaminated, may then contaminate the next client. While many therapists like to work barefoot, this is not advised. Your feet may harbor an undetected fungal infection, which can be spread to an unsuspecting client getting on and off the massage table. For clients with suppressed immunity, this may cause serious complications. Remove jewelry including rings, wristwatches, bracelets, and necklaces. These items contain small crevices and sharp edges that can harbor bacteria or potentially scratch a client. Small earrings that will not touch the client are fine.

Proper Handwashing

Proper sanitation of the hands is probably the single most important part of the sanitation protocol for therapists. You want to clean your nails carefully and use foaming liquid soap to thoroughly wash your hands up to your elbows. An alcohol-based hand rub is recommended for decontaminating the hands before massage, before or after certain treatment steps, and at the end of a massage. Nonalcohol-based hand rubs have not been adequately evaluated by the Centers for Disease Control and Prevention (CDC) and are therefore not recommended. In those instances where you use gloves (see the upcoming section for details), wash your hands and decontaminate them before putting gloves on and immediately after removing gloves. Decontaminate your hands with an alcohol rub before moving from a potentially contaminated body area (such as the feet) to a clean body area (such as the face) during massage. Do the same when moving from contact with an unsanitized inanimate object (e.g., a product container) to the client. As well, wash and decontaminate your hands before and after eating or using the restroom.[7] The CDC provides specific recommendations for handwashing and the use of alcohol-based hand sanitizers for health care workers, as described in Technique 3.

Therapists Who Are Smokers

The smell of cigarette smoke lingers in hair, on clothing, on skin, on the breath, on carpets, and on fabrics such as window treatments and linens. Smokers often become oblivious to the smoke odor and do not realize its impact on nonsmoking individuals. Many nonsmokers intensely dislike the smell of cigarette smoke. Some are so sensitive that they cannot tolerate the lingering smell of smoke anywhere around them. Even clients who can tolerate the smoke odor often associate it with an environment that is unclean and so may subconsciously feel uncomfortable.

Smoking should never be allowed in the treatment room, reception area, bathrooms, hallways, office area, or laundry area of a massage business. Therapists who smoke must strive to balance their personal needs with the client's needs. In the best case, a therapist would smoke before showering, washing the hair, dressing, and brushing the teeth. After showering

Technique 3   Proper Handwashing and Hand Decontamination

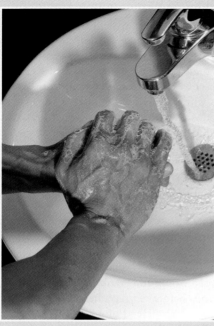

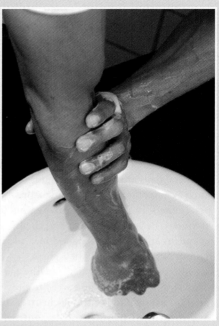

1. Clean your nails before your hands using an orange stick or a personal nailbrush that has not been used by anybody else. Wash your hands with a non-antimicrobial soap or an antimicrobial soap (liquid soap with a pump dispenser is the most sanitary—avoid bar soap) for 30 seconds using friction and lather to lift contaminants off the skin's surface.

2. Clean the area between your fingers and from your forearms up to your elbows. Rinse your arms and hands thoroughly with running water, and dry them with a disposable towel.

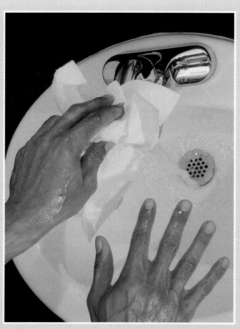

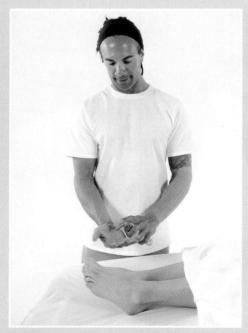

3. Use the same towel to turn off the water tap and to open any doors on the way to the treatment room.

4. Use an alcohol-based hand sanitizer at these times: (a) Directly after washing your hands and directly before touching the client. (b) Directly after washing your hands and directly before donning gloves and directly after removing gloves. (c) Directly after moving from a potentially contaminated body area (e.g., feet) and directly before working on a clean body area (e.g., face). (d) Directly after touching an unsanitized inanimate object (e.g., product container) and directly before touching the client. (e) If you accidentally touch your hair or a mucous membrane (eyes, nose) or cough or sneeze during the session. Do not retouch the client until your hands have been decontaminated with the hand sanitizer. (f) Directly after removing soiled linens from the table and directly before handling fresh linens.

and dressing, the therapist would not smoke again until after all of that day's massage sessions. A therapist who is unable to finish the day's massage sessions before having a cigarette must make every effort to minimize the impact on clients. Use a mechanic's jumpsuit to cover and protect clothing. Cover your hair with a plastic shower cap and put hand lotion on your hands before handling cigarettes (which rinses away when the hands are washed and keeps smoke odor from seeping into skin). Smoke outside at a good distance away from the massage office. After smoking, wash any areas of skin that might come into contact with smoke. You might include the use of a salt scrub on your hands to help eliminate the smell of smoke. Your face, neck, arms, and hands should all be washed. Brush your teeth and rinse with mouthwash.

Therapists Who Are Sick or Have Allergies

A therapist who is sick or may have a contagious infection must protect clients by canceling all massage appointments. The common cold is caused by a large number of different viruses and is easily transmitted through the air or by direct contact. In general, the viruses that cause colds incubate in the body for 12 hours to 5 days and then become contagious 23 hours before the onset of symptoms. The person remains contagious for about 5 days after the onset of symptoms.[8]

Therapists with allergies with symptoms similar to those of a cold are not likely to be contagious but may need to take extra precautions to prevent spreading pathogens. For example, if your eyes are itchy and watering, you must decontaminate your hands if you rub your eyes in the middle of a session. If sneezing is a problem, wear a face mask as an extra precaution. Inform clients that you suffer from allergies to prevent the impression that you are sick. If you are uncertain whether your symptoms are those of a cold or allergy, take your temperature. Allergies usually do not elevate body temperature, whereas even a low-grade cold will.

Sanitation of the Facility, Equipment, and Supplies

A clean facility has a lower risk of pathogen transmission. To provide a clean environment, pay attention to the proper use of cleaning products, sanitation of the treatment room and equipment, care of linens, proper product handling, and general housekeeping activities.

Cleaning Products

A variety of cleaning products can be used in the massage business. Use dusting aids and wood polishes on wood surfaces, and glass cleaners on windows and mirrors. Antiseptics and disinfectants are the most important types of cleaners used in a health care setting because they reduce the transmission of disease. These types of cleaners are described in detail below.

Note that cleaning products often contain ingredients that cause irritation to eyes, the skin, and the respiratory system.

Wear heavy cleaning gloves, a face mask, and eye protection when handling cleaning products, and increase the ventilation in rooms where you are cleaning by opening windows or running ceiling fans. Many cleaning products also cause damage to the environment. In recent years, there has been growing interest in natural, environmentally friendly products for cleaning. Finding suitable products is often difficult because of the unique challenges of sanitation in health care environments. Some U.S. and Canadian health care workers have formed an association called Health Care Without Harm: The Campaign for Environmentally Responsible Health Care. This group offers a kit to help health care providers "go green." The kit can be ordered through their website at http://www.noharm.org/goingGreen. At the very least, avoid heavily-scented cleaning products, and look up cleaning product dangers at the Occupational Safety and Health Administration website at http://www.osha.gov.

Antiseptics

Antiseptics are safe for use on skin, where they create an unfavorable environment for pathogen reproduction. Antiseptics are weaker than disinfectants and do not kill all pathogens but are generally appropriate for use in a massage setting so long as no blood or body fluid is present. Hand soap, iodine, hydrogen peroxide, and rubbing alcohol are commonly used antiseptics. Rubbing alcohol is often used to spray clean countertops, doorknobs, and massage equipment between clients.

Disinfectants

Disinfectants are stronger than antiseptics and should not be used on the skin. They kill or are effective against most bacteria and viruses. Disinfectants are also called germicides and bactericides. Commonly used disinfectants include bleach solutions, phenols, and quaternary ammonium compounds (quats). Disinfectants are used for deep cleaning at the end of the day, if an infectious agent may be present (e.g., if a client denied having a cold but sneezed and coughed throughout the session) or if blood or body fluids are present.

- **Bleach solution.** Bleach mixed with water in a 10% concentration is used to clean hard surfaces like countertops, equipment, and floors and to clean linens exposed to body fluids. It is noted to be effective on pathogens including *Staphylococcus*, *Streptococcus*, hepatitis, HIV, herpes, and tinea.
- **Phenols (also called cresols).** Phenols are used on hard surfaces and are effective against tuberculosis, bacteria, fungus, herpes, and the flu virus. Phenols are irritating to the skin and the respiratory system.
- **Quaternary ammonium compounds (quats).** Quats are formulated to kill pathogens on a variety of hard surfaces and are effective against *Pseudomonas*, *Staphylococcus* and *Salmonella*, certain bacteria, HIV, and the hepatitis B and C viruses.

Sterilization is the elimination of all microorganisms on and in an object through heat, chemical substances, or irradiation.

Sterilization is rarely used in massage environments but is commonly used in hospitals where moist heat (hot water or steam) or dry heat is used to sterilize medical instruments. Sterilization with an autoclave (a device using high temperature and pressure to sterilize instruments) may be used in some spa environments where estheticians use sharp implements to pierce the superficial layers of the skin when performing deep-cleaning facials that include extractions of whiteheads and blackheads.

Sanitation of the Treatment Room and Equipment

Sanitizing the treatment room and equipment involves a cleaning step that removes visible dirt and a sanitation step that removes most pathogenic organisms from inanimate objects with an antiseptic. Follow these guidelines:

- Wipe down countertops, equipment, treatment chairs and tables, the floor, and any other hard surface like doorknobs, handles, and cabinets with an antiseptic such as alcohol between clients.
- If possible, open windows and doors to ventilate the room and circulate air.
- At the end of the day, deep clean the treatment room, equipment, and hard surfaces with a disinfectant.
- Usually, a sick client is sent home without receiving a massage. After a session, if you suspect that the client was on the verge of a cold or the flu, deep clean the treatment room with a disinfectant before proceeding with the next session.
- Regularly dust window blinds, shelves, decorative items, picture frames, and lamp fixtures. Keep electronic equipment and CDs neatly organized and free from dust.
- Wash all reusable equipment such as metal or plastic bowls, spatulas, application brushes used in spa treatments, and soda coolers (used to hold hot towels) in hot soapy water, and sanitize them with alcohol between clients.

Specialized equipment like foot-soaking basins, hydrotherapy tubs, showers, and massage tools like hot stones used in stone massage must be cleaned and sanitized with a disinfectant between clients. Foot-soaking basins are of special concern especially if they have jets that might harbor bacteria:

- Wash the basic with hot, soapy water and spray it with a disinfectant.
- Allow the disinfectant to remain for 10 minutes, and then wipe the basin dry.
- If the basin has jets, flush a bleach solution through the jets to eliminate pathogens.

Follow these guidelines for cleaning a shower:

- Clean, disinfect, and dry the shower after use by each client.
- Disinfect the shower curtain and the floor outside the shower.
- Change all towels and the mat outside the shower for each client.
- Use only liquid soaps or shower gels. Bars of soap that have been used by more than one person are unsanitary and should not be left in the shower or sink.

Modern hydrotherapy tubs usually have a self-cleaning function that makes sanitizing the jets of the tub easier:

- Put a concentrated disinfectant (formulated by the manufacture of the tub) into the special holder, and then push the button.
- At the end of the cleaning cycle, dry the tub and put out fresh bath mats and towels for the next client.
- Between clients, wipe down the area around the tub, including the floor and any handrails, with an antiseptic, and deep clean the area with a disinfectant at the end of the day.

Small, one-person steam cabinets should be completely wiped with an antiseptic between clients. For larger steam rooms or steam showers, sanitize the floor and seat between clients, although the walls can be left until the end of the day. Disinfect this equipment at the end of each workday.

Proper Care of Linens

Clean linens are stored in a closed cabinet until they are brought out for use. Decontaminate your hands after touching soiled linens and before placing fresh linens on the table. Linens may include massage sheets, face cradle covers, bolster and pillow covers, uniforms, smocks, hair wraps, robes, washable slippers, blankets, draping material, and washable floor mats. Any item that comes into contact with the client's skin or hair during the session must be stored in a closed, ventilated container and washed before use with another client. Soiled linens should not be stored in the treatment room but be moved to the laundry or work area. At the end of the day, wash linens in hot water with regular detergent, dry them with heat, and return them to the closed cabinet. Handle linens soiled with body fluids with special caution as discussed in the section on universal precautions (Topic 3-3).

Proper Product Handling

Keep lubricants refrigerated between uses to prevent the breakdown of their natural oils. Transfer lubricants from larger, bulk containers to smaller bottles so that they can be heated without warming the unused product, which would break down if heated, cooled, and reheated. Some products are dispensed directly into your hand using a pump top or flip lid. Take care to decontaminate the pump container with an antiseptic both before and after each session.

If you provide spa treatments in your facility, remove spa products from their original closed containers with a sanitized spoon or spatula and place them in pre-sanitized holders for later use during the treatment. Cover the spa product with plastic wrap to avoid contamination before use. All products would become contaminated if you used your hands to remove the product or dipped into the original container during the treatment. Discard any unused spa product rather than return it to the original container. During a body treatment, proper waste disposal procedures are important. Some items used in the treatment are used only once (e.g., gauze, sponges, and plastic body wrap). Dispose these items in a closed trash can immediately after use.

TABLE 3-1   Tasks to Ensure a Clean, Sanitary, and Safe Facility

After Each Session	End of Business Day	Weekly
• Open doors and windows to ventilate room.	• Wash all bowls, implements, application brushes, trays, and other equipment with hot, soapy water and wipe with a disinfectant before storing them in closed containers.	• Clean windows, window frames, and window ledges.
• Remove soiled linen from table, face cradle, bolsters, etc.	• Wash cloth products such as massage sheets, blankets, robes, slippers, hand towels, bath towels, and shower mats in hot water with detergent and dry using heat before storing in a closed container.	• Deep clean the reception area and wipe down chairs, the beverage service, magazines, and decorative side tables.
• Wipe massage table, face cradle, and bolster with disinfectant.	• Deep clean and disinfect bathrooms.	• Wipe down shelving used to hold retail items, and dust retail items.
• Cover table, face cradle, and bolsters with fresh linens.	• Clean floors, clean and disinfect items in the reception area, clean any beverage service items, clean common areas, and disinfect items like handrails and doorknobs.	• Dust light fixtures, picture frames, the music system, shelving, and decorative items in the treatment room.
• Disinfect countertops, door handles, and any objects clients regularly touch.	• Empty and disinfect trash bins.	• Organize CDs, storage cabinets, and supplies.
• Disinfect the lubricant container.		• Check smoke detectors to ensure they are in good working order.
• If tools (hot stones, massage tools, etc.) were used during the session, wipe them with a disinfectant.		• Check and replace light bulbs both inside and outside the facility.
• If a shower or wet room has been used, disinfect and dry it.		• Water and dust plants.
• Change bath mats and towels if shower or tub has been used.		

Housekeeping Activities

The general cleanliness of the facility must be assessed and maintained on a daily basis. The reception area, retail area, office area, hallways, and bathrooms all need attention.

- Vacuum or sweep and mop floors daily.
- Wipe items such as coffee tables, beverage dispensers, toys in the reception area, doorknobs, handrails, and the reception countertops daily with an antiseptic.
- Deep clean bathrooms and empty trash bins at the end of each workday.
- Clean window ledges, retail shelving, picture frames, and light fixtures weekly.
- Fish tanks and water fountains are not advised because they may harbor pathogens and are difficult to keep clean.

Think also about the safe use of food items in the business. Home-baked products are not advised, but individually wrapped items like chocolates, granola bars, sports bars, and popsicles can be used. It's a good idea to provide filtered water from commercial dispensers. These water containers come presealed to prevent contamination. Use disposable cups for all beverages including tea, juice, or water.

Table 3-1 provides a checklist of tasks to ensure you maintain a clean, sanitary, and safe facility.

Implementation of Universal Precautions

Universal precautions is the term for the CDC policy for controlling transmission of infections carried in blood and body fluids.[9] You should practice universal precautions if a client has broken skin, if you have cuts or hangnails on your hands, or if you are exposed to a client's body fluids. Universal precautions are discussed in depth in the next topic.

Concept Brief 3-4
Preventing the Transmission of Diseases

Therapist hygiene	Clean body and hair, clean clothes, proper handwashing
Equipment	Sanitized between clients
Facility	Disinfected at the end of each business day
Products	Handled so as to prevent contamination
Linens	Laundered between clients, stored properly
Universal	Precautions understood and implemented

Topic 3-3
Universal Precautions

The purpose of universal precautions is to ensure that health care workers protect themselves from bloodborne diseases transmitted through broken skin, mucous membranes, or contact with blood and body fluid. To understand universal precautions, it is helpful to understand HIV/AIDS and hepatitis, to know when to use gloves, and to know the proper methods for cleaning up body fluids and items exposed to body fluids.

HIV/AIDS

The HIV virus causes AIDS. HIV is transmitted through body fluids including semen, vaginal secretions, and blood and can be transmitted during pregnancy from a mother to her fetus or after birth through breast milk. HIV can also be spread by drug users sharing a needle, by accidental needle pricks, and from infected blood used in a blood transfusion (rare in developed countries). There is no evidence that HIV is transmitted through saliva, sweat, tears, urine, or feces unless the fluid contains blood. There is no evidence that HIV is spread through casual contact such as sharing towels, food utensils, telephones, or swimming pools. HIV is not believed to spread by biting insects like mosquitoes or fleas.[10]

HIV is a retrovirus that can live in the infected individual for a long time before causing symptoms. The National Institute for Allergies and Infectious Diseases reports that people infected with HIV develop a flu-like illness 1 to 2 months after their initial exposure to HIV. The symptoms are often mistaken for another viral infection and clear up within a week or 2. Severe symptoms may not appear for 10 years or longer. (Children born with HIV develop symptoms around the age of 2.) During this period the HIV virus is slowly multiplying and killing immune system cells. Gradually, infected people experience periodic symptoms such as swollen glands, decreased energy, weight loss, fevers and night sweats, persistent yeast infections, short-term memory loss, persistent pelvic inflammatory disease, frequent and severe herpes outbreaks, and shingles.

An HIV infection is called AIDS when the HIV-infected person has fewer than 200 CD3+ T cells (the immune system's primary infection fighting blood cells). Uninfected adults usually have 1,000 or more CD3+ T cells. The immune system, gradually destroyed by the HIV virus, loses its ability to fight off common pathogens that usually do not cause illness in healthy individuals. In people with AIDS, these opportunistic infections can be severe and often are fatal. People with AIDS are also prone to developing various cancers, especially those caused by viruses and cancers of the immune system (lymphomas).

Massage is indicated for HIV-positive clients who do not have symptoms. In the advanced stages of AIDS, many forms of bodywork are indicated, but the most effective techniques depend on the individual client's level of health. It is very unlikely that a massage therapist would contract HIV from a client during massage, but the use of universal precautions is still required. This is especially important because an HIV-positive client must be protected from an undetected infection the therapist may have.

Concept Brief 3-5
HIV/AIDS

HIV	Human immunodeficiency virus—causes AIDS
AIDS	Acquired immunodeficiency syndrome (when HIV-infected person has fewer than 200 CD3+ T cells)
Transmission	Body fluids (semen, vaginal secretions, blood, during pregnancy from mother to baby, breast milk, needle sharing, accidental needle pricks, infected blood transfusions) Not transmitted in sweat, saliva, tears, urine, or feces, or by casual contact, food utensils, swimming pools, biting insects

Hepatitis

Several different viruses cause different forms of hepatitis, termed hepatitis A through G. These are diseases characterized by inflammation of the liver. Hepatitis A, B, and C are the most common forms.

- **Hepatitis A virus (HAV):** HAV is transmitted through contaminated food and water or by contact with feces. It usually resolves in a few weeks without medical intervention.

- **Hepatitis B virus (HBV):** HBV is spread through many of the same routes as HIV but is a hundred times more contagious than HIV. Many people who contract hepatitis B recover fully and have no long-term complications. Some individuals develop chronic hepatitis B and become carriers of the disease. These people may develop varicose veins on the stomach and esophagus, cirrhosis of the liver, and liver cancer.[11]

- **Hepatitis C:** Hepatitis C is transmitted primarily through contact with infected blood (often by drug users sharing needles). Hepatitis C spreads less commonly through sexual contact and childbirth, but these are possible routes. Of people who contract hepatitis C, 75% to 95% develop chronic long-term infections and have an increased risk for cirrhosis and liver cancer.[12]

Massage is contraindicated for individuals with acute hepatitis. Clients with chronic hepatitis can benefit from massage, but techniques should be chosen based on the individual's level of health. Universal precautions are required.

Concept Brief 3-6
Hepatitis

Hepatitis	Several diseases—inflammation of liver
Hepatitis A	Contaminated food—contact with feces—resolves in 2 to 3 weeks
Hepatitis B	Spreads via same routes as HIV—100 times more contagious
Hepatitis C	Spreads via contact with contaminated blood—chronic infection

---

Tuberculosis

Tuberculosis is not a bloodborne pathogen like HIV or hepatitis, but health care workers should be aware of this disease also. *Mycobacterium tuberculosis*, the bacteria that causes tuberculosis, usually affects the lungs but can also affect the brain, kidneys, bones, or joints. A bacterial infection, tuberculosis is spread from person to person through the air. People infected with tuberculosis may spread the disease when they cough, speak, or sneeze and other people around them breathe in the bacteria. The infection can also be transmitted through contaminated food.

Infected people in the early stages of tuberculosis often do not realize they have the disease because they do not feel sick or have symptoms. As the diseases advances, lung tissue is destroyed and replaced by connective tissue fibers. This limits the body's breathing capacity, and symptoms develop such as a persistent cough (coughing up blood in some cases), low-grade fever, loss of appetite and weight loss, and night sweats.

People with a suppressed immune system, such as those with HIV infection, cancer, diabetes, or drug or alcohol abuse are at higher risk of developing an active case of tuberculosis, and their symptoms are likely to occur more rapidly. People who travel to areas of the world where tuberculosis is common are also at higher risk for infection.

A positive tuberculin skin test (PPD) indicates that the person has a tuberculosis infection, but it does not necessarily indicate an active illness. Many people with a positive PPD have a latent infection, are healthy, and pose no risk to others. Because some of these people later develop active disease, they should be alert to changes in their health and have regular checkups. A chest x-ray, sputum culture, and other measures are used to determine if an active, contagious tuberculosis infection is present in the lungs. Antituberculosis drugs are used to cure the active disease and prevent transmission of the infection to others. Clients with an active infection are contraindicated for massage. Because of their close contact with the public, massage therapists should have a PPD skin test annually to ensure their health.

When to Use Universal Precautions

Massage therapists rarely make contact with clients' body fluids in practice, but in some situations, a therapist may be exposed to a body fluid, and therefore, be at risk for infection. A scab may rub off during a massage stroke, a blemish may erupt under the pressure of a stroke, menstrual blood may leak onto the treatment table, or a client may experience nausea during treatment and vomit in the treatment room. Universal precautions are an approach to infection control in which all blood and body fluids are treated as if infected with HIV, hepatitis, or another bloodborne pathogen. Universal precautions are guidelines for dealing with broken skin and mucous membranes, blood and other body fluids, and the cleanup of body fluids. Important components of universal precautions include:

- correctly using gloves
- properly cleaning linen soiled with blood or body fluids
- properly cleaning surfaces contaminated with blood or body fluids

Use of Gloves

Vinyl gloves are worn to protect both the client and therapist from the transmission of disease. Wear gloves at these times:

- Any time the potential exists to come into direct contact with blood or body fluid.
- If the client has broken skin such as a scratch, open cut, or blemish.
- If you have broken skin on your hands or forearms, such as a scratch, hangnail, or blemish.
- If you are likely to come into contact with mucous membranes, such as would occur with the inter-oral massage sometime used with conditions such as temporomandibular joint disorder (only in states where such work is legal and with advanced training).
- When you are cleaning linens or hard surfaces soiled with blood or body fluids.
- If the client is HIV-positive or has a condition that causes weakened immunity.
- If you are HIV-positive or a hepatitis carrier.

Wear gloves also any time you are concerned about the potential for infection or the client requests it. The correct use of gloves is shown in Technique 4.

Latex gloves break down when exposed to oil-based lubricants like those used in massage. Latex may also cause a mild to very serious allergic reaction or skin sensitivity. For this reason, vinyl gloves are recommended. Vinyl gloves do not break down when exposed to oil-based lubricants and seldom cause allergic reactions or skin sensitivity.

Proper Cleanup of Soiled Linen

Linens soiled with blood or body fluids should be handled with gloves and stored in a leakproof bag until they can be

Technique 4	**Proper Use of Gloves**

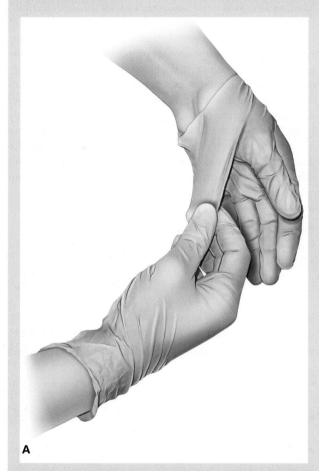

A

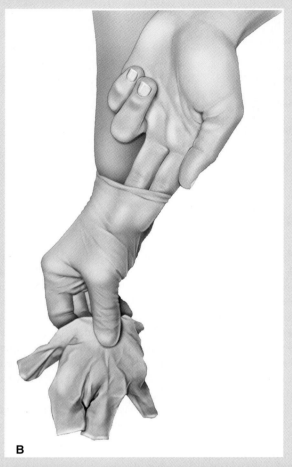

B

1. Immediately before putting on gloves, wash your hands as described in the section on therapist hygiene, and decontaminate your hands with an alcohol-based hand sanitizer. The gloves should fit snugly and not roll down your hands while giving massage. When it is time to remove the gloves, peel the first glove from the wrist to the fingers so that it is turned inside out. Any contaminants are now on the inside of the glove away from you.

2. Place the fingers of your ungloved hand inside the second glove and peel it back so that it is inside out. Make an effort not to touch the outside of the gloves with your ungloved hand. Dispose the gloves in a closed trash container, and immediately wash and decontaminate your hands with alcohol after removing the gloves.

laundered. Wash these linens separately with laundry detergent and chlorine bleach. Dry them with heat, and store then as usual in a closed cabinet.

Proper Cleanup of Blood or Body Fluids on Hard Surfaces

Add one part bleach to nine parts water (10% bleach solution) to clean hard surfaces contaminated with blood or body fluid. Wear gloves and use disposable cleaning materials such as paper towels to wipe up the spill. Dispose the cleaning materials in a closed trash container.

Because new information about communicable diseases is issued often, keep up-to-date about the most recent standards and guidelines issued by the CDC (website: www.cdc.gov).

Concept Brief 3-7
Universal Precautions

Defined	CDC guidelines for handling blood and body fluids
Approach	Treat all blood and body fluids as if infected with bloodborne pathogen
Gloves	Use with broken skin, scratches, severe blemishing, when handling linens soiled with body fluid or during cleanup of body fluids
Soiled linens	Stored leak-proof bag, laundered separately with bleach
Hard surfaces	Clean with 10% bleach solution

Topic **3-4**
The Safety Plan

Injury or harm is unlikely to happen in a safe environment. In such an environment, conditions that may cause injury have been eliminated. Procedures are adopted to increase security and plans made to efficiently handle any accidents that may occur. The safety plan should include guidelines for ensuring the safety of both clients and therapists. If you run your own practice, you have greater control over safety issues than if you work as an employee. As an employee, maintain your awareness of safety issues and alert your supervisor should you feel that the environment is not conducive to your safety or the safety of your clients.

Safety of the Facility

The facility must be accessible to a wide array of clients, including those who are unsteady on their feet and those using wheelchairs. Assess the parking area, common areas, equipment, and fire plan:

- **Parking area**: Begin an assessment of the facility in the parking area. Is the pavement smooth and even, or are cracks or an uneven surface present that may cause a client to fall? Is lighting adequate and the pathway to the front door unobstructed? If clients must climb stairs or use a wheelchair ramp, are these areas well lit and handrails provided?

- **Common areas:** All common areas such as the reception area, hallways, and bathrooms should have good lighting and nonslip flooring and be free of area rugs (which may cause a client to trip) and barriers. Bathrooms should include a lavatory at wheelchair height and handrails. Doorways should be wide enough to accommodate people with physical disabilities, and lever-style door handles used.

- **Equipment:** Regularly check massage equipment to ensure that it is in good working condition. Check bolts, hinges, and knobs for tightness before each massage session. Any exposed electrical cords should be heavy-duty and taped down around the edges of the room, behind furnishings and equipment when possible. Do not run extension cords across a doorway or in any area where therapists or clients must walk.

- **Fire plan:** Check with state authorities to ensure that proper fire and safety codes are followed. At least one fire extinguisher and smoke detector should be in clear view; more are likely needed. Check the fire extinguisher and all smoke and heat detectors monthly to ensure they are in good working order. A fire escape route should be clearly indicated in every room. The use of candles, incense, and open flames is not advised.

- **Emergency numbers:** Keep a list of emergency phone numbers by the business phone. This includes the local fire station, poison control center, police department, ambulance, and local hospital or emergency medical facility. Keep your liability insurance coverage up-to-date and display a copy on the premises.

Safety of the Client

To ensure the safety of the client, stay up-to-date with your training in CPR and first aid. A first aid kit should be kept in each treatment room along with hydrocortisone cream, which can be used to decrease any skin reactions. Never give massage without first taking a thorough health history. If you have any concern that massage is contraindicated for a particular client, err on the side of caution and ask to contact the client's health care provider or postpone the massage. Because all therapists will need to look up a health condition, medication, or other information at some point during their professional career, have available key reference books including an up-to-date medical dictionary, drug reference, and pathology reference book.

Some clients need help getting on and off the treatment table. Provide a wide step stool and offer assistance to elderly clients, pregnant clients, and clients with physical challenges. Do not leave alone a client who is unstable and may fall. Instead, assist the client to the treatment room and help with undressing if appropriate. After the session, wipe the client's feet with a paper towel to remove excess lubricant from the foot massage, which could cause a client to slip while getting off the massage table.

Alcohol, Drugs, Prescription Medications

It is a serious breach of professional ethics for the therapist to work while under the influence of an illegal drug or alcohol. This would place clients at risk of emotional harm or physical injury. These substances also interfere with logical reasoning and decision making, which might lead to making a poor treatment choice for a client. Alcohol and drugs also influence the therapist's behavior and feelings and may result in inappropriate communication or emotional outbursts. Therapists who are suffering from a hangover should cancel any massage appointments or refer their clients to another therapist.

Sometimes a therapist must take prescription medications for a condition or disorder. Each situation is unique, as is the therapist's response to the medication. Be aware that medications may alter your perception, change your behavior, or affect your physical abilities. Talk with your health care provider about possible side effects in relation to your massage duties and responsibilities. Always act in the best interests of the client. If the medication interferes with your physical or mental ability to provide a safe and beneficial massage, you may need to explore different medication options or take a break from massage until the situation improves.

Massage may also be contraindicated for clients taking a prescription or over-the-counter medication that distorts their perceptions of hot, cold, pain, or pressure, or you may have to adapt the treatment to each client's needs (see Chapter 5). Do not provide massage to a client under the influence of an illegal drug or alcohol because it would place both of you in an unsafe situation.

Accident Report

Any time that anyone at a business—including employees, the owner, clients, and visitors—is injured in an accident, causes injury to another, or causes property damage, an accident report should be written and filed. This report should provide detailed and accurate information about the accident, the people involved, injuries or property damage, and how the situation was resolved. This information must be accurate and detailed because it may be used by an insurance company to process a claim or may be evidence in a lawsuit. The accident report should include:

- The address and location in the premises where the accident occurred
- The date and time
- The name of the person filing the report and his or her job title
- The name, address, e-mail, and phone number of all individuals involved, including any witnesses
- A detailed account of what happened
- Written witness accounts of what happened when appropriate
- A description of injuries or property damage
- How the matter was resolved (e.g., the individual was sent to the emergency room, the individual refused medical treatment and went home, etc.)

If more information becomes available later, it should be documented and kept in the same file as the accident report. For example, if a client was injured by falling off a massage table and a physician diagnosed an ankle sprain the next day, record this in the file. If the accident was caused by equipment failure (e.g., the massage table suddenly buckled due to a faulty brace), file a report with the manufacturer immediately. File a copy of this letter along with any response from the manufacturer. If the manufacturer telephones to discuss the situation, document this conversation and keep it with the accident file. If a client is involved, a signed release is required before sending client information to an outside entity (e.g., insurance company, equipment manufacturer). This protects the client's privacy. A sample accident report is provided in Box 3-1.

Safety of the Therapist

While at work you may be required to lift heavy objects such as laundry, bulk spa products, or housekeeping supplies. Always use good body mechanics to prevent back injury. You will also come into contact with strong cleaning products and should wear heavy gloves, a face mask, and protective eyewear to prevent contact with your eyes, respiratory system, or skin.

When you take good care of yourself, you are less likely to suffer an injury or illness while working as a massage therapist. Proper nutrition, adequate sleep, exercise, stress reduction activities, and good body mechanics all support your health and longevity in the profession. See Chapter 11 for ways to prepare for the demands of a massage career and remain healthy and free from injury while on the job.

Client Screening

In some areas, illegitimate massage is still used as a cover for prostitution. Though most clients understand that professional massage is for wellness and good health, some people seek massage for sexual gratification. Regardless of whether your practice is based in your home or office or as a "call-out" service, careful client screening helps ensure your safety.

The screening process begins when the client calls to book an appointment or inquire about fees and services. Ask clients for their name, address, home phone number, work phone number, occupation, and how they heard about the massage business. Record all of this information in a client's new file. Ask what type of massage they are looking for (e.g., relaxation, sports, hot stone massage, etc.). Ask if this is the first massage they have received or if they regularly get massage. With clients who have had massage before, ask them to describe the results they experienced and their current expectations for massage. If their answers do not seem legitimate, be courteous but continue to question and educate them. For example, you might say, "I would like to inform you about our massage policy." This information can include the policies for a no-show client, the draping policy, and the policy on drugs and alcohol. A client who confuses massage with sexual favors may ask questions such as these: "Do you provide erotic massage?" "What will you wear during the massage?" "What do you look like?" "Can I massage myself during the massage?" or "Will you help me if I get excited?"

BOX 3-1 Sample Accident Report

Place: The accident occurred at Any Massage Clinic, 311 Any Street, Any Town, Any State, 20001, in treatment room 3.

Time: 3:20 PM

Date: Friday, December 19, 2009.

Report filed by Melody Massage, Owner and Massage Therapist.

Description: At 3:30 PM I asked my client, Susan Mills, to turn over from the supine to the prone position. When the client shifted her weight to turn over, the massage table suddenly buckled and Ms. Mills fell to the floor. Surprised, Ms. Mills jumped to her feet immediately, and I assisted her to a chair. She was shaken up and asked for a glass of water. I handed her the water and placed a blanket over her legs. After about 5 minutes she said, "I think I pulled or twisted something in my back because it's shooting pain up into my neck." I suggested calling an ambulance but Ms. Mills resisted. I suggested calling a friend who could take Ms. Mills to the emergency room or doctor and she agreed. I called Sarah Friend, who arrived after about 20 minutes. During the time that we waited for Ms. Friend to arrive, I helped Ms. Mills into her clothing. She reported that she felt stiff and was afraid to move quickly. She had moderate shooting pain up her spine into her neck intermittently with some movements. Bending over to tie her shoes was impossible, and I tied her shoes for her. She appeared to be in pain as I assisted her in walking down the hallway and out to the reception area. We agreed that she would call me after she had seen the doctor to let me know how she was doing. I helped her into the car, and she went to her doctor with her friend.

The massage tables are checked for safety every Friday at the end of massage shifts. The leg bolts of each table are checked for tightness before each session. I had personally checked the table in question on Friday, December 12, and it appeared to be in good working condition. The table was used in two previous sessions on the day of the accident. The table is the Deluxe, Super-Comfort Table model number 587; it was purchased in August of 2007 from Massage Tables R Us at 333 Any Boulevard, Any Town, Any State, 20089. The table top, vinyl, and legs are intact, but a support cable has pulled away from its fitting, allowing the table to buckle. Massage Tables R Us was contacted on 12/19/09 at 3:30 PM and alerted to the event. A representative arrived to inspect the table at 5:15 PM. The representative commented, "I have never seen a cable pull away from its fitting like this." The representative offered to replace the table at no cost based on its 10-year warranty. I asked the representative if Massage Tables R Us would agree to pay Ms. Mills' medical costs. The representative reported that his corporate office would contact me. To date, the table company has not contacted me, and I have turned the matter over to my insurance company.

People Involved:

Susan Mills: 230 Any Street, Any Town, Any State, 00091. Phone: 222-333-3333, E-Mail: smills@notarealclient.com. Client—Injured Party

Melody Massage: 653 Any Street, Any Town, Any State, 20012. Phone: 330-333-3030, E-Mail: mmassage@notarealmassagetherapist.com. Massage Therapist

Sarah Friend: 303 Any Street, Any Town, Any State, 00091. Phone 212-323-3232. E-Mail: sfriend@anyaddress.com. Friend who picked up Susan Mills.

Don Table: Representative for Massage Tables R Us at 333 Any Boulevard, Any Town, Any State, 20089. Work Phone: 333-356-3535. E-Mail: Not provided.

Additional Note Filed 12/23/09 by Melody Massage: According to a phone call from Ms. Mills, the doctor reported that Ms. Mills had strained some muscles in her back and prescribed analgesics and rest.

Additional Note filed 2/8/10 by Melody Massage: Ms. Mills submitted her medical bills and lost wages for reimbursement. A claim was filed with my liability insurance. Ms. Mills' claim was settled on 2/26/10.

Remain courteous but end the conversation and refuse the massage appointment.

All therapists should be careful about booking new clients during times when they are alone in the office. Avoid this situation whenever possible. If you cannot avoid such a situation, make arrangements with someone available to assist by telephone. Tell this person the time of the appointment and that you will call again after the intake interview. If anything feels strange during the intake interview, cancel the session and politely ask the client to leave. When the client leaves, call your backup person to say that you are safe. The backup person should be instructed to call you if you have not called by the time specified, and if you do not pick up the phone, that person should call emergency services.

Incident Report

An incident report is written whenever an unusual event occurs that creates an unsafe environment or distress for a client, therapist, or business owner. For example, a therapist might file an incident report if a client makes sexual advances during a massage session and the therapist had to end the session. The report should go directly to the business owner, who should then inform the client that he or she is no longer welcome at the clinic. Another example is a client who is unhappy with the massage and demands a refund. The therapist should document why the client was unhappy and actions taken to solve the problem. An incident report should include:

- The date, time, and place the incident occurred
- The name and title of the person filing the report
- The name, address, e-mail, and phone number of all involved individuals and any witnesses
- A detailed account of what happened
- Written witness accounts of what happened when appropriate
- How the matter was resolved (e.g., the client was informed of no longer being welcome at the clinic, the client was given a refund and referral to another therapist).

Concept Brief 3-8
Safety Overview

- Therapists should be up-to-date with CPR and first aid training. A first aid kit should be readily available. Always take a thorough health history to rule out contraindications before providing massage.
- Therapists should take care of themselves with good body mechanics, protective gloves, and masks when using cleaning products, and screening clients thoroughly.
- Accident and incident reports should be filed whenever an accident or unusual incident occurs at the business.

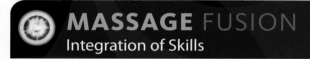

MASSAGE FUSION
Integration of Skills

STUDY TIP: Learn Health Care Terminology

Every profession develops its own language so that its professionals can communicate more efficiently and effectively. Health care terminology (also called medical terminology) is the language used by massage therapists and other health care professionals. Review the appendix at the back of this book on health care terminology now, early in your training, and develop your proficiency with the language of massage and health care. This will help you better understand the written information in textbooks and verbal information conveyed during lectures and demonstrations.

GOOD TO KNOW: Allergies

A primary function of the immune system is to differentiate "self" from "non-self" substances. The immune system tries to destroy or subdue anything identified as "non-self" as fast as possible. Allergies are an immune system response and are not caused by an infectious agent. Even substances that pose no threat to the body such as pollen, pet dander, a component in a lubricant, or other allergens (substances that causes an allergic reaction) are perceived by the immune system as a threat. Common allergies like hay fever induce mast cells (cells that play a role in wound healing and protection against pathogens) to release histamine and other chemicals that change vascular permeability. This inflammatory response leads to symptoms like runny

eyes, itching skin, swelling, a runny nose, or vomiting and diarrhea (with food allergies). In severe allergic reactions, known as anaphylaxis, mast cells release large amounts of histamine that lead to edema and sudden low blood pressure. Symptoms can include hives, redness, shortness of breath, coughing, sneezing, decreased heart rate, fainting, and shock. The rapid onset of localized swelling is called angioedema. Swelling that occurs in the tongue, larynx, or pharynx might block airflow, creating a life-threatening condition. Peanuts (and other nuts), fish and shellfish, latex, bee stings, and some foods like milk and eggs can cause severe reactions of this sort. Clients with known allergies to nuts should not receive massage with a lubricant containing ingredients from that nut (e.g., peanut oil, almond oil). Clients with a known allergy to shellfish or seafood should not receive seaweed treatments or contact products with seaweed in them. People who know they are at risk for anaphylactic reactions usually keep medication with them, such as Benadryl or injectable epinephrine (EpiPen).

IT'S TRUE!: Massage Boosts Immunity

A number of recent research studies demonstrate that regular massage improves the immune system and offers psychological benefits to patients with chronic or serious illnesses. In one study, 33 women diagnosed with stage 1 or 2 breast cancer were randomly assigned postsurgery to a massage therapy group or a control group that did

MASSAGE FUSION (*Continued*)
Integration of Skills

not receive massage. The women in the massage group received a 30-minute massage three times a week for 5 weeks. The study indicated that massage reduced overall anxiety, depression, and anger. Additional long-term effects included enhanced dopamine (a neurotransmitter and neurohormone with many important functions in the brain), serotonin (a neurotransmitter whose low levels are linked to depression), and lymphocyte numbers (important immune system cells).[13] A second similar study confirmed these findings.[14] In a study of adolescents with HIV, the massage group received two massages per week for 12 weeks. The control group participated in progressive relaxation sessions two times a week for 12 weeks. At the end of the study, those in the massage group were less depressed and less anxious and showed enhanced immune function.[15]

CHAPTER WRAP-UP

As a professional massage therapist, you are required by health standards and professional ethics to provide a clean, hygienic, safe environment for your clients. Good

sanitation skills require practice. It's easy to forget small things in the course of a busy day, but such forgetfulness may cause a client to get sick. For example, new therapists might forget to sanitize their hands before moving from foot massage to another area of the body. This client is now potentially exposed to a fungus that can take hold and grow on another area of the skin. A new therapist might forget to disinfect the oil bottle between clients. The second client is then exposed to pathogens from the first because the therapist touches the skin, touches the bottle, and then touches the new client's skin. Good sanitation practices also require you to pay attention to your every gesture. Did you touch your hair or scratch your nose as you transitioned from one body area to another? If you did, you should decontaminate your hands before you touch the client again. Be vigilant and practice thinking about sanitation as part of your massage. If you accidentally skip a sanitation step, stop and practice incorporating the step. In this way you will be ready when you are a professional to provide your clients with the best possible care.

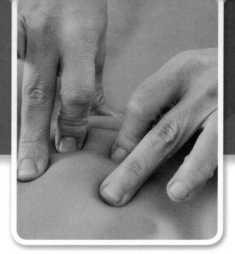

The Therapeutic Nature of Massage

KEY TERMS

active treatment group

benefit

clinical trial

control

cortisol

flight-or-fight response

gate control theory

indication

mechanical effect

pain-spasm-pain cycle

parasympathetic nervous system response

physiological effect

psychological effect

reflexive effect

research article

scientific method

stress

stressor

stretch reflex

tendon reflex

wellness

LEARNING OBJECTIVES

Having read the chapter and used the related student learning tools, the student will be able to:

1 Describe the steps in the scientific method and compare these steps to the types of information in a research article.

2 Evaluate one clinical trial described in a research article and explain how the research results could be used in massage practice.

3 Compare and contrast mechanical effects with reflexive effects. Provide one example of each type of effect.

4 Identify four effects of massage in the musculoskeletal system.

5 Differentiate between the parasympathetic nervous system response and the sympathetic nervous system response.

6 Describe what a muscle spindle is and its role in muscle protection.

7 Describe what a Golgi tendon organ is and its role in tendon protection.

8 Make a diagram of the pain-spasm-pain cycle and explain it to classmates.

9 Summarize the physiological processes that occur in the body when touch is used to reduce pain, according to gate theory.

10 Identify two effects of massage in the cardiovascular system.

11 Identify three massage indications that are particularly interesting and give reasons for the same.

12 Compare and contrast a broad definition of stress with the type of stress that triggers the flight-or-fight response.

13 Outline the role of the sympathetic nervous system in relationship to stress.

14 List three physiological reactions to the flight-or-fight response.

15 List three conditions that are caused by or exacerbated by stress.

16 In your own words describe what the concept of wellness means to you.

17 Describe the basic components of a simple wellness model.

A growing body of clinical research demonstrates that massage has proven effects and benefits for the body. Massage is indicated as a primary treatment for many conditions that affect soft tissues and is also used extensively as a support strategy for a wide variety of medical conditions. One of the key benefits of massage is that it reduces stress and helps the body rest, recover, and find balance by countering the sympathetic nervous system response to stress. Stress management is important in the movement toward wellness. This chapter explores the therapeutic nature of massage and how to use research to access massage information gathered through the scientific method in Topic 4-1. Information in research studies can inspire therapists to try new techniques or confirm their empirical findings for particular client groups. Topic 4-2 describes the changes that massage causes in each body system, in the mind, in the emotions, and in the spirit of the client. This is exciting information because it helps us understand why massage has such powerful and positive effects on clients. Topic 4-3 then explores particular conditions and client groups who experience positive changes as a result of massage. In Topic 4-4, we take a closer look at stress to better understand how massage supports stress-management processes. Wellness models are described as a way to broaden our appreciation for the role of massage in people's lives.

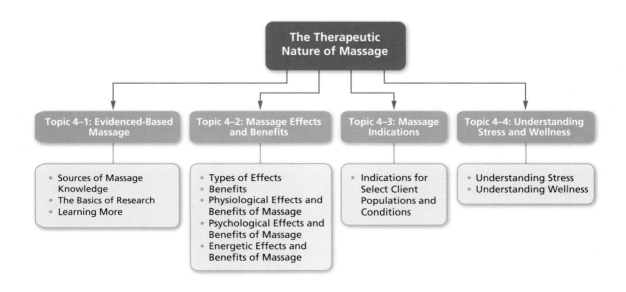

Topic 4-1
Evidence-Based Massage

Massage students and professionals should understand the theoretical basis of massage and be able to evaluate information that might affect the care of clients. The term *research literacy* has recently gained prominence in massage education. The ability to find, read, and evaluate research articles and then apply their information in massage practice supports the session planning process. Clients benefit when therapists try new techniques and approaches based on evidence of their effectiveness.

Massage knowledge began with observation, trial and error, and information passed down through the generations for hundreds of years. The recent interest in complementary and alternative medicine (CAM) therapies has spurred a move toward evidence-based massage, and now research is affirming or disproving many of our long-held beliefs. For example, Dr. John Harvey Kellogg, described in Chapter 1, first described the mechanical effects of massage. Because he stated that massage could spread cancer in patients, massage therapists treated cancer as a contraindication until very recently. Current research shows that massage does not spread cancer but in fact has many positive benefits for people living with cancer.

This topic discusses how we gain knowledge about massage and the basics of research. This understanding promotes an evidence-based massage practice where clients receive informed care.

Sources of Massage Knowledge

As massage therapists, how do we know what we know? Do we simply believe that massage is good for people and leave it at that? Do we trust textbooks and teachers and accept what they tell us without question? Do we rely on our own understanding and experience and apply that knowledge to new situations? Do we test each piece of knowledge over and over again until we are certain we can call it true? Do we use the scientific method? Massage has evolved into a defined profession through all of these valuable methods of knowing.

Tradition

The massage profession, like many others, originated in methods and knowledge passed down from one generation to the next. Some aspects of touch were natural. People instinctively placed their hands on a wounded area or an area of pain. We can speculate that through trial and error, early peoples determined which methods and techniques worked best. Different cultures developed separate beliefs and systems for creating changes in the body. Different cultures exchanged ideas first through communications carried over ancient trade routes

and later through documents that were more widely distributed. Over time, a wide body of knowledge developed. Some of this knowledge is based purely on belief, even on superstition, and some on cause-and-effect observations. Some information, passed to us in the present, still require our scrutiny and investigation. Our massage traditions are meaningful, and sometimes the body is changed by massage in positive ways that defy scientific understanding. Our goal is not to exclude something that cannot be proved with science but to question our assumptions and continue to evolve our knowledge.

Authority

Schools, teachers, textbooks, and authority figures in the profession are one way that knowledge is distilled and passed on in the massage profession. Most of this information is based on good principles and extensive experience, and students are encouraged to absorb all they can. But everyone is prone to bias, and techniques that worked well for one therapist may not necessarily work for another therapist. Although too much skepticism can hinder learning, a little skepticism in certain situations is healthy. It's a good idea to ask for proof when things don't sit right in your mind, to question how a piece of information is deemed credible if it doesn't seem credible to you, and to seek additional information to support or refute what you learn when your questions feel unanswered.

Deductive Reasoning, Inductive Reasoning, and Applied Theory

Deductive reasoning begins with a core assumption, called a premise (Fig. 4-1). The premise is applied to a specific situation to predict an outcome. For example, when you palpate a client's back, you notice that deeper muscular structures feel restricted (specific situation). Your premise is that deep friction strokes forcibly broaden and stretch muscles, breaking adhesive bonds between muscle fibers. You predict that deep friction strokes will reduce this client's adhesions, and you deduce that you should use deep friction strokes in the client's session plan.

We can reasonably suppose that when we start with a valid premise, we are likely to achieve valid results. But what if the premise is not always true? What if we base our treatment choices on an unproven assumption? In this case, we may waste time trying techniques that do not achieve a meaningful outcome for the client. Consider the example of massage therapists choosing not to work with clients diagnosed with cancer based on the premise that massage spreads cancer in the body. This was a false premise, but as a result of it people with cancer did not benefit from the therapeutic nature of massage until recently. Remember: at one point people believed the world was flat! False premises can gather so much momentum that they lodge in our psyche as if undisputable fact. It's a good idea to self-evaluate often. What do I believe? How do my beliefs shape my world and my massage practice? Are these beliefs based on sound reason? How do I know my reasoning is sound?

Inductive reasoning involves a process that is the opposite of deductive reasoning. One observes a number of outcomes from the same situation to establish a premise. This is likely how early generations gathered knowledge. For example, za therapist places a hot pack on a client's low back just to keep the client warm during a session. The therapist then notices that the muscle tissue in that area is softer and more relaxed during massage. The therapist tries a hot pack with the next client, and the next, and the next. Every time the hot pack is used, the client's muscles are softer and more relaxed. A premise has now been developed: hot packs soften and relax muscle tissue.

Applied theory is a set of principles on which a specific practice is based. Therapists with a thorough knowledge of anatomy, physiology, and kinesiology can use that knowledge to develop treatment plans and combine a variety of massage techniques for more effective sessions. Sometimes a theory from one discipline is applied to a completely different discipline. A massage therapist who is also a jazz musician, for example, might apply established theories about music composition to the development of a relaxation massage routine.

Scientific Method

The **scientific method** is a process that scientists use to
- develop an accurate representation of the world
- investigate phenomena (observable events)
- acquire new knowledge
- integrate established knowledge with new knowledge
- correct existing knowledge.

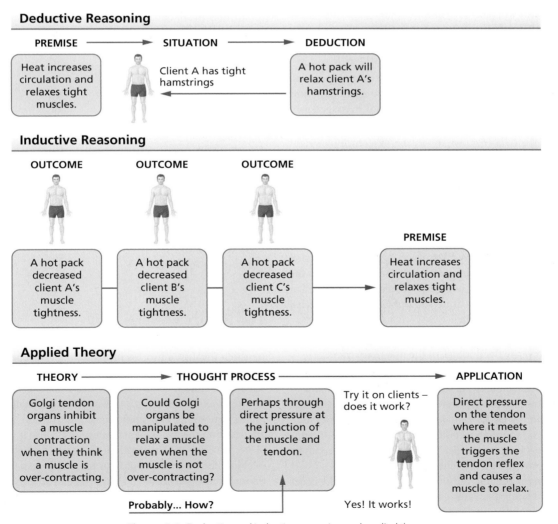

Deductive Reasoning

PREMISE → SITUATION → DEDUCTION

Heat increases circulation and relaxes tight muscles.

Client A has tight hamstrings

A hot pack will relax client A's hamstrings.

Inductive Reasoning

OUTCOME   OUTCOME   OUTCOME   PREMISE

A hot pack decreased client A's muscle tightness.

A hot pack decreased client B's muscle tightness.

A hot pack decreased client C's muscle tightness.

Heat increases circulation and relaxes tight muscles.

Applied Theory

THEORY → THOUGHT PROCESS → APPLICATION

Golgi tendon organs inhibit a muscle contraction when they think a muscle is over-contracting.

Could Golgi organs be manipulated to relax a muscle even when the muscle is not over-contracting?

Perhaps through direct pressure at the junction of the muscle and tendon.

Try it on clients – does it work?

Direct pressure on the tendon where it meets the muscle triggers the tendon reflex and causes a muscle to relax.

Probably... How?

Yes! It works!

Figure 4-1 Deductive and inductive reasoning and applied theory.

The scientific method dates back to ancient Greece. Aristotle believed that one could obtain knowledge through careful observation, and this remains an important tenet of the scientific method. The problem is that our senses and the ways we observe phenomena are unreliable, often tempered by preconceived ideas and bias, not testable, not repeatable, and often deceptive. We believe what we observe, and we observe what we believe. Our beliefs affect our observations. Scientists developed the steps of the scientific method to eliminate or minimize bias by exposing false ideas through repeated testing by different researchers. The scientific method follows these basic steps:

1. Observation of phenomenon (e.g., preterm infants seem to gain weight faster when they are massaged).

2. Formation of a hypothesis; a hypothesis is a suggested explanation for a phenomenon (e.g., massage improves weight gain in preterm infants).

3. Define a question to test the hypothesis (e.g., do massaged preterm infants gain weight faster than preterm infants who are not massaged?).

4. Design a research study to answer the question (e.g., preterm infants will receive 15 minutes of massage three times a day for 5 days, the infants' weight will be taken daily, and the weight gain of massaged infants will be compared to different preterm infants who are not massaged).

5. Conduct an experiment and collect data (e.g., how much weight did each massaged infant gain each day, how much weight did each infant who was not massaged gain each day?).

6. Analyze the data (e.g., what was the difference in weight gain each day and at the conclusion of the study in the two groups of preterm infants?).

7. Interpret the data and draw conclusions (e.g., weight gain in preterm infants who received massage was 53% higher than the weight gain of preterm infants who were not massaged).

8. Publish the methods and results in a recognized journal to share the information with other scientists (note: the example used here was adapted from a study conducted at the Touch Research Institute and published in the *Journal of Pediatric Psychology*[1]).

9. Retest: additional testing is usually conducted by other scientists to verify the findings of the first researchers.

In the PBS web publication *A Different Way to Heal*, author Jacqueline Mitchell tells the story of Dr. Stephen Rennard to illustrate how traditional knowledge passed down through the generations may be verified with the scientific method.[2] While this example does not directly involve massage, it demonstrates how long-held beliefs, like many in massage, can be tested and proven with the scientific method.

Dr. Rennard became curious about the long-held belief that chicken soup alleviates cold symptoms and wanted to see if he could prove it scientifically. In the scientific method, it is important to ask the right question. Dr. Rennard knew that chicken soup might soothe cold symptoms in a lot of different ways. It could work by promoting hydration or by providing a needed vitamin or nutrient or some unidentified therapeutic compound. He hypothesized that something in chicken soup inhibited neutrophils, the white blood cells that mediate the inflammatory response, thereby reducing upper-respiratory inflammation that causes the discomfort associated with congestion. He designed his study around this question: does chicken soup inhibit neutrophils in the upper-respiratory system?

To test his hypothesis, Dr. Rennard prepared a traditional chicken soup and tested its ability to inhibit neutrophil migration. He observed the results and recorded his findings. The statistical analysis of his data demonstrated that chicken soup significantly inhibited the neutrophils' ability to cause inflammation. Further experiments showed considerable variability in the inhibitory activity of different commercial chicken soups. Dr. Rennard published his results in the scientific journal *Chest* in 2000.[3] Other scientists are evaluating the methods and results of Dr. Rennard's research, and some may repeat Dr. Rennard's work to attempt to verify his results. Over time, the scientific community may reach a consensus on the benefits of chicken soup for cold symptoms, or others may reject Dr. Rennard's findings and test a new or revised hypnosis.

Concept Brief 4-1
The Scientific Method

Observe phenomenon
Formulate a hypothesis
Define a question to test the hypothesis
Design a research study to answer the question
Collect data
Analyze the data
Interpret the data and draw conclusions
Publish the results

The Basics of Research

Research involves a process of asking relevant questions and then seeking to answer them within the parameters of the scientific method. Claire Cassidy in *Methodological Issues in Investigations of Massage/Bodywork Therapy* states that the myriad questions that guide most research on health care are based on the fundamental questions "Does it work?" and "Does it serve?"[4] The question of "Does it work?" seeks to establish the benefits people can reasonably expect to experience from a particular massage system or technique. The second question—"Does it serve?"—reminds us that something that might work may not actually be useful. Services we provide to clients must enhance the therapeutic relationship and meet clients' needs without undue expense, discomfort, or inconvenience. If a client had to travel to a massage therapist every day for 2 months and pay $60 every session for relief of low back pain, the expense and inconvenience might make the effectiveness of the service impractical.

Cassidy outlines four domains with a list of broad questions for researchable topics (Box 4-1). Contemplating these questions can help massage therapists better understand themselves, the massage profession, and the need for more evidence-based information.

BOX 4-1 Four Fields of Research Questions: Examples of Important Researchable Topics

The questions presented here are adopted from Claire Cassidy's paper written for the Massage Therapy Foundation, *titled Methodological Issues in Investigations of Massage/ Bodywork Therapy.*

Domain 1: Sociocultural Mechanisms of Effectiveness

1. Who uses massage/bodywork therapy (MBT)?
2. What benefits do they say they receive from it?
3. What features of practice keep them coming back for more?
4. How much do they pay for care? Are they satisfied with this? What would they want to change?
5. How satisfied are they with their practitioners? The care setting?
6. For what complaints and conditions do people seek MBT?
7. What practices (types of massage/bodywork) within MBT do practitioners employ, how often, why?
8. Where do practitioners think the field is going?
9. What is the range of opinion about third-party payments, fee for service, etc.?
10. What public outreach approaches have been most effective in raising awareness in a positive way about MBT, which have not been effective?
11. What is the professionalization process in MBT?
12. What is the history of the MBT field, especially with regard to the development of particular intervention techniques and to professionalization?

Domain 2: Massage/Bodywork Therapy Practice Mechanisms of Effectiveness

1. How much time must a person experience a particular intervention to experience relief of symptoms? 15 minutes? 30 minutes? 45 or 60 minutes? Once a week, twice a month? Relief that lasts 1 day, 2 days… 2 weeks, more?
2. How does the application of an intervention by one practitioner differ from the same intervention applied by a different practitioner? How much inter-practitioner reliability is there in the delivery of care? What does "good practice" look like, feel like; how can it be measured?
3. Which MBT approaches are most effective for which conditions? Are there any popular interventions, which should actually be contraindicated?

Overlap Issues in Domains 1 and 2

1. What is the explanatory model of MBT, especially as the practices that fall under this rubric are so variable?
2. What attracts people to practice MBT, and what keeps them practicing?
3. What features of the education serve practitioners well, not so well?
4. What clinical perceptions do experienced practitioners have and how do they apply them?
5. What sorts of people respond best to particular interventions?
6. What sorts of people do best as practitioners?

Domain 3: Comparing the Effectiveness of Massage/ Bodywork Therapy to Other Medical Practices

1. For which conditions is MBT therapy as effective or more effective than the standard biomedical intervention for that condition?
2. The same question with MBT compared to other medical systems.

Overlap of Domains 1 and 3

1. What is the comparative cost-effectiveness of biomedical and MBT interventions for a particular condition?

Overlap of Domains 2 and 3: Working Toward the Level Playing Field

1. What distinctive medical insights and intervention techniques has MBT to offer biomedicine?
2. What distinctive insights and intervention has biomedicine to offer MBT?
3. How can the two medical practices combine forces so as to serve patients better?
4. The same set of questions applies to the relations of MBT with any other medical system.

Domain 4: Physiological Mechanisms of Effectiveness in Massage/Bodywork Therapy

1. What are the physiological features underlying the effectiveness of MBT practices? Of the practices that involve soft-tissue manipulation? Of those that involve bone manipulation? Of those that enter the energy fields and change them?
2. Are current observations about mechanisms accurate? Sufficient?
3. Does MBT have the same or similar effects in nonhuman animals? Why?

Different types of research yield different layers and levels of understanding. It's unusual for one study to prove a hypothesis conclusively. Usually, a body of evidence accumulates over time and over a multitude of studies until the scientific community generally agrees about a finding.[5] Case reports, a form of descriptive and observational studies, are at the low end of the evidence scale, while systematic reviews and meta-analyses are at the high end.

Observational and Descriptive Studies

Observational and descriptive studies can take a number of forms. Massage therapists are often interested in case reports and case series. In a case report, the details of each session with a patient or client are written in chart notes, the results of the sessions interpreted by the therapist, and the outcome of the sessions reported. In a case series, a number of clients or patients with the same condition are observed and described as they undergo a treatment protocol, and the results are reported. These types of observational and descriptive studies are helpful because therapists can draw on the experience of other therapists when dealing with a condition unfamiliar to them. For example, if you have never worked with a client with fibromyalgia, you might search for case reports on massage and fibromyalgia for useful treatment plan ideas. Students can participate in the student case report contest held by the Massage Therapy Foundation each year. The Foundation offers guidelines that help students develop their observation, palpation, and charting skills. For more information, search the Massage Therapy Foundation website at www.massagetherapyfoundation.org.

Correlation studies are a type of observation and descriptive study that look for relationships between variables. For example, do people with poor eyesight consistently have a head-forward posture? Do people who work at a keyboard for 6 or more hours a day commonly develop carpal tunnel syndrome? Understanding such relationships can help therapists focus on areas that need particular attention or make home-care suggestions to clients (e.g., a therapist might suggest that clients with a head-forward position have their eyes checked to rule out eye strain as a possible factor in their neck pain).

Case–control studies (also called retrospective studies, cohort studies, or case-referent studies) examine the health history (or history of exposure to a suspected risk factor) of a number of people with the same condition. They are compared to another group of people who resemble them in as many relevant respects as possible but do not have the condition. This can help to identify risk factors or exposure to a disease-causing agent. Case–control studies were used to link smoking to lung cancer.

Clinical Trials

A **clinical trial** compares a treatment like massage therapy or a medication to a placebo (inactive treatment or a medication with no active ingredients) or to another treatment or medication such as a standard treatment or care given for a particular condition. The goal is to determine the safety and effectiveness of a particular treatment. For example, a clinical trial could be designed to investigate whether massage is more effective than over-the-counter pain medications for reducing low back pain or whether slow strokes delivered to the back reduce blood pressure.

Researchers carefully choose participants for a trial. Usually participants must meet predetermined criteria so that the results are easier to measure and relevant to the study's question. In a study on low back pain, for example, the participants must all have chronic low back pain for the results to be useable. A study on slow stroke massage for blood pressure might recruit participants at age 30 to 40 with mild-to-moderate high blood pressure who are not currently taking blood pressure medications.

Next, participants are typically placed randomly into different groups by a computer program or a table of random numbers. Randomized group selection reduces the amount of bias that may occur in a study, because otherwise researchers might subconsciously or consciously place certain participants in one group or the other and unduly shift the results of the study.

One group is made up of people who receive the treatment being researched (often referred to as the **active treatment group**). The other group will receive the standard treatment (if there is one), no treatment, a placebo treatment, or a second treatment being researched as a comparison. This group is referred to as the **control**.

The specific actions in a study depend on its design, but often the health of the participants will be carefully checked and recorded at the beginning of the study, again at various points during the study, and at the end. In a study of the effectiveness of massage for low back pain versus over-the-counter pain medications, participants in both the active treatment group (receiving massage) and control group (receiving over-the-counter pain medication) likely fill out a questionnaire rating their pain levels and how the pain affects their activities each day, their mood, and their quality of life. They may fill out the same questionnaire at various times during the study and at the end. The results will be tabulated, along with changes in physiological measures taken by the researchers. For example, cortisol and substance P levels in the body might be monitored. High levels indicate high stress and higher pain, while lower levels indicate less stress and less pain. Range of motion of the back might be measured, along with blood pressure, respiration rate, and heart rate. All study data will be carefully recorded and analyzed. At the conclusion of the study, the researchers will write up their methods and findings and publish the results.

Systematic Reviews and Meta-Analyses

Systematic reviews summarize and analyze the published literature on a particular question. A meta-analysis is a type of systematic review that uses statistical methods to combine the results of several primary studies. Clearly defined methods are used to conduct systematic reviews in order to eliminate bias and faulty research processes. The published literature is reviewed, and each study is appraised to identify valid and applicable evidence. This evidence is summarized along with recommendations for changes to existing health care or new methods for treating conditions. Systematic reviews and meta-analyses are used to inform health care practices and help establish good clinical policy and treatment decision making.

Concept Brief 4-2
Research Study Types

Case report: Describes outcome from treatment of one client or patient

Case series: Describes outcomes from treatment protocol for more than one client or patient

Correlation study: Demonstrates a relationship or lack of relationship between two variables

Case–control study: Examines the health histories of similar people with and without a particular condition to identify risk factors for the condition

Clinical trial: Compares a treatment to one with a placebo (inactive treatment), to another treatment, or to standard treatment to establish safety and efficacy, using randomization and controls in study design

Systematic review: Analyzes and summarizes published literature on a particular question or treatment

Meta-analysis: Type of systematic review using defined statistical methods to combine the findings of several primary studies

---

Learning More

Massage students and professionals can benefit from searching for research on conditions they encounter in practice, especially with a condition that doesn't respond readily to the techniques they try. Although no therapist has time to spend hours a week in a library looking up research, it is fun and informative to spend an occasional afternoon learning about recent discoveries. Several key websites are helpful for students and professionals looking for research (Box 4-2). Chapter 1 described the Massage Therapy Foundation and the Touch Research Institute, both of which have websites with relevant information related to massage and research.

BOX 4-2 Student Research Resources

Massage Therapy Foundation: www.massagetherapy foundation.org
Touch Research Institute: www.miami.edu/touch-research
The National Center for Complementary and Alternative Medicine: http://nccam.nih.gov
PubMed: www.pubmed.com

The National Center for Complementary and Alternative Medicine (NCCAM) is part of the U.S. Department of Health and Human Services National Institutes of Health. According to the NCCAM website, NCCAM is dedicated to exploring complementary and alternative healing practices in the context of rigorous science; training CAM researchers; and disseminating authoritative information to the public and professionals. NCCAM supplies grants for research, research training, education, and outreach programs.

PubMed, a service of the National Library of Medicine, includes 15 million citations from peer-reviewed scientific journals. After you find a relevant abstract (described below), a librarian at your local or university library can help you find the journal where the full article is published. In many cases, PubMed also supplies links to free full-text sources for articles that can be read online.

Reading a Research Article

Research articles often use scientific language that may seem confusing, but usually you can absorb enough information to inform your massage practice. Review Appendix A at the back of the book for information about health care terminology that will be useful during your research. Research articles are usually organized the same way and contain specific sections:

- **Abstract:** The abstract summarizes the research and allows someone searching for information on a particular question to determine if the research article will be of value.

- **Introduction:** The introduction may describe the history of the question investigated and other related research findings. It likely describes why the research study is important and its objective.

- **Methods/Methodology:** This section outlines the research plan and how each step was carried out. It includes important details like the criteria for choosing participants and placing them into random groups. The way the treatment was delivered to both the active treatment group and control group is described (e.g., a 1-hour massage was delivered two times per week for 5 weeks, while the control group practiced relaxation–breathing techniques for 1 hour two times per week for 5 weeks, etc.), as are the methods for monitoring the participants' experience (questionnaires, blood pressure readings, measurement of body chemicals in urine, blood, or salvia, etc.).

- **Results/Findings:** This section analyzes the data gathered.

- **Discussion:** This section discusses the results, interprets their meaning, explains their implications, provides links to other research, and draws conclusions from the study.

- **References:** This section lists the resources and references the researchers used in designing and implementing the study.

Although reading research studies can seem daunting at first, they can help therapists stay abreast of new findings that may change our views about the body and touch. Keep three questions in mind when reading research:

1. How does this information change the way I view the body?

2. How will this information change the way I deliver a massage?

3. How will this information change my treatment planning for a particular condition?

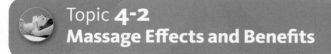

Topic 4-2
Massage Effects and Benefits

This section discusses changes that occur in the client's body and mind as a result of massage and the benefits of these for the client. This information helps you understand why some techniques are chosen over others when planning sessions for a particular client. Many of the concepts underlying certain effects of massage are quite advanced and require a thorough knowledge of anatomy and physiology which you may not yet possess at this stage of your training. Additionally, a wide variety of massage techniques produce different effects, and you likely have not yet been introduced to many of these. For now, your goal should be to absorb key principles and become inspired and committed to learning more anatomy and physiology. As your understanding of the body grows, return to this chapter and investigate the effects of massage based on your additional knowledge. As well, the upcoming chapters consider many of these concepts in more detail.

Types of Effects

An "effect" is the result or consequence of an action. When a therapist gives a client a massage (action), the client's body responds in many predictable and sometimes unpredictable ways (effects). The effects of massage are the resulting changes that occur in the body, mind, and emotions of the client. Although this topic mainly deals with positive effects and benefits for clients, in some situations massage can have negative effects for particular clients. These effects are described in Chapter 5. Massage effects are usually categorized as *mechanical effects* or *reflexive effects*, but other terms are also used and described here. Mechanical and reflexive effects are often closely related and may occur at virtually the same time.

Mechanical Effects

Mechanical effects are the direct result of the manual manipulation of the client's soft tissue (Fig. 4-2). The tissue is lifted, compressed, rubbed, pulled, and twisted during the application of strokes, and these manipulations cause changes in soft-tissue structures and cardiovascular functions. For example, when a therapist applies a gliding stroke from the ankle to the thigh, the pressure of the stroke moves the blood

> **Concept Brief 4-3**
> **Types of Massage Effects**
>
> **Mechanical:** Effects from direct manipulation of the client's tissue
> **Reflexive:** Effects from an involuntary response of the nervous system
> **Primary:** The first effect to occur in the tissue, organ, or system
> **Secondary:** Effects that occur as a result of primary effects
> **Structural:** Effects on the structures of the body
> **Systemic:** Effects on the nervous system or circulatory system, or changes to the body's chemistry and metabolism
> **Cumulative:** The buildup of effects over time
> **Combined:** Effects that occur because of two or more therapies used together
> **Physiological:** Effects that occur in the body
> **Psychological:** Effects that occur in the mind and emotions
> **Energetic:** Effects that occur in the subtle energy system

in the veins of the legs toward the heart. When a moderate-to-deep stroke is applied parallel to muscle fibers, the pressure of the stroke compresses, forcibly broadens, and separates the muscle fibers such that fibers that previously stuck together can slide over each other more easily.

Reflexive Effects

Reflexive effects involve an involuntary and rapid response of the nervous system to stimuli that results in changes to the structural or systemic condition of the body. This happens when massage techniques stimulate a sense organ in a particular area of the body. Touch receptors respond to the pressure of a stroke, while temperature receptors respond to the warmth of the therapist's hands. Other receptors monitor the length and stretch of muscle tissue, the strength of a muscle's contraction, the angle of a joint, or the body's balance during movement. This information is conveyed through the nerves to the spinal cord and brain. The brain rapidly interprets these

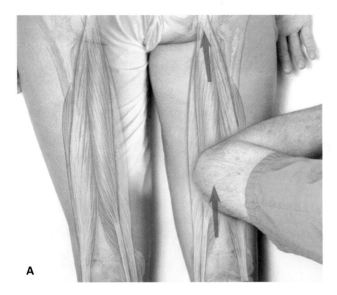

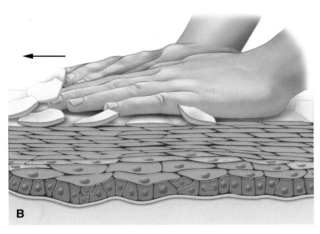

Figure 4-2 Examples of mechanical effects of massage. **A.** In this image, the therapist applies a friction stroke up the hamstrings with the forearm. Friction applied to a muscle compresses and forcibly broadens muscle fibers, breaking adhesive bonds between fibers so that the muscle can return to its normal resting length and move more freely. (From Clay JH, Pounds DM. *Basic Clinical Massage Therapy: Integrating Anatomy and Treatment.* 2nd ed. Philadelphia, PA: Lippincott Williams & Wilkins, 2008.) **B.** The movement of the hands over the skin helps to desquamate the dead skin cells.

signals and initiates a response that may result in changes in the local region, changes in the entire body, or changes in a related area (Fig. 4-3). For example, as the reflexive result of some massage techniques, the diameter of blood vessels increases and the blood pressure is reduced. Massage activates the parasympathetic nervous system, the part of the nervous system that directs the body to rest and recover. The body relaxes as a result of this response. Certain techniques trick the receptors in muscles and tendons to trigger a predictable reflex (e.g., stretch reflex or tendon reflex), leading to a reduction in muscle tension.

Primary and Secondary Effects

In one example of mechanical effects, muscle fibers are separated apart so that they can more easily slide over each other. This separation of fibers can be called the *primary* effect of the stroke because this is the first mechanical response that occurs in the tissue. As a result of the separation of muscle fibers, restrictions in the tissue are reduced, allowing the client a greater range of motion. Now blood can circulate more freely, nourishing the tissue and removing waste products, and this in turn causes a reduction in pain. These results could be called *secondary* effects because they wouldn't occur if the primary effect had not first occurred.

In another example, soft tissue is manipulated by strokes that lift, compress, or torque the tissue, causing mast cells in connective tissue to release a substance called histamine (a chemical with a central role in vascular changes related to inflammation and allergic reactions). Histamine causes local blood vessels to dilate, increasing circulation in the local tissue. The stretching of soft-tissue structures could be called the primary effect, and the release of histamine and vasodilation are called the secondary effects of these massage techniques.

Structural and Systemic Effects

Sometimes effects are categorized as structural or systemic. Structural effects involve the structures of the body and how they respond to massage techniques. Increased range of motion, increased tissue pliability, and decreased muscle tension are examples of structural effects. Systemic effects are full-body changes to the nervous or circulatory system or to the body's chemistry and metabolism. The decrease in blood pressure that often occurs with massage is an example of a systemic effect. Systemic effects are often closely related to reflexive effects.

Cumulative and Combined Effects

Massage is also believed to have *cumulative effects*. This term refers to the belief that the body gets healthier with regular massage. Chronically shortened muscle tissue is lengthened in the first session, and this lengthened state is reinforced in following sessions. Over time, significant postural changes may occur as the body learns more muscular balance.

A *combined effect* refers to the effects on the body when massage is paired with another therapy. When heat is applied to an area of the body with a hot pack (hydrotherapy), the peripheral blood vessels dilate and the body area may begin to perspire. The blood flow to the area increases significantly and flushes the tissue. When the pack is removed and the area is massaged, the preheated tissue is soft and thus may respond more readily to massage strokes that aim to reduce muscle tension and soreness. The increased range of motion, greater tissue length, and decreased pain the client experiences as a result of the session can be attributed to the combination of therapies rather than to the massage or hydrotherapy alone.

Physiological, Psychological, and Energetic Effects

Physiological effects take place in the body, while **psychological effects** occur in the mind and emotions. In following sections in this chapter, the mechanical and reflexive effects of massage are explored for the body and the mind and emotions. Some effects of massage techniques are known from research in clinical studies, others are based on a premise from applied theory, while still others are based on cause-and-effect observations documented by working massage therapists (see Topic 4-1 for more details). Energetic effects are difficult to recognize, quantify, and qualify and so are often rejected by science. This type of effect refers to changes believed to occur in the subtle energy centers inside and around the body as traditionally recognized in many Eastern bodywork practices. Energetic effects are described in more detail in a later section.

Benefits

A **benefit** is a good effect that promotes well-being, even if a specific pathology, postural dysfunction, or muscular tension pattern is not an issue. In general, massage is good for people, and people enjoy receiving massage.

The effects of massage described throughout this chapter topic demonstrate how beneficial massage can be. For the general population who are not seeking massage as part of treatment for a particular pathology, the most valuable benefits of massage are related to the parasympathetic nervous system response that allows the body to rest and recover from stress. Improved circulation, increased immunity, reduction in muscle tension, and the simple pleasure of the experience of massage are also of primary importance. In addition, massage can shift patterns in the body that might lead to dysfunction or disease. Massage can even promote the adoption of healthy lifestyle choices. For already healthy people, massage supports and ensures the maintenance of health and can become a fundamental part of a client's wellness program.

Massage as a Positive Intervention

The term "intervention" is used in medicine to denote an action or treatment intended to alter the course of a pathologic process. In massage, an intervention is a positive disruption of stressful or less than optimal repetitive patterns. While many Americans practice good healthy habits, others fall into patterns of unhealthy eating, smoking cigarettes, too much caffeine, too much alcohol, inactivity, erratic sleep schedules, and long work hours. This fast-paced life is compounded by exposure to bright lights, noise, and devices like cell phones, music systems, and computers.

These layers of responsibilities, pressures, external stimuli, and demands, are expressed in people's physical patterns. Many clients have rounded shoulders and sunken chests, for example. You may often see shallow breathing, clenched gluteal muscles, and tilted pelvises. In many work environments, people perform the same physical task over and over again, often locking dysfunctional patterns of movement into their neuromuscular myofascial memory as normal.

Massage is a positive intervention because it creates an abrupt and/or gradual shift in clients' patterns, allows them to feel and reconnect with their bodies, and reminds clients of their power to make changes. Suddenly the client is in a restful environment with quiet sounds and dim lights. This hour is just about clients. It's not about their kids, or taking the dog to the vet for a checkup, or finishing that report for the boss. This hour is the clients'. They hear their breath in their chest and pay attention to it if only for a moment. Their breathing becomes deeper and more regular. They feel the warmth of the therapist's hands and the rhythmic flow of a stroke. They are unexpectedly *in* their body—sensing its areas of tension, feeling its need for sleep, water, and uninhibited movement. The rushing has stopped, and they have this hour to take stock of their life and to think about their own needs and wants. For healthy people, massage is a reminder to remain true to their ideals and the benefits of positive lifestyle choices.

Massage is also an intervention for the body because clients often build up tension and pain from repetitive work stress that they may not recognize as tension and pain. As you work, clients are likely to feel the tenderness in their shoulders or the tension in their necks. They may question you about the sources of tension, and together you may discuss clients' work environments and repetitive motions. The next day at the office a client may sit up straighter, adjust the chair and computer screen to avoid neck strain, and stretch during breaks. Perhaps these small changes are all that is needed to prevent injury to the body.

On some level, all people are on a quest for balance, happiness, peace, calm, and ease of being in their bodies. Even the healthiest, most fit person must pay attention to stress and manage it in life. At any time, at any age, the body is capable of amazing positive transformations. Humans more than any other creature on earth have the power to change their attitudes, their habits, their minds, and their bodies. Massage is not always the launch pad for such changes, but it can be, and sometimes it is. This is evidenced by the many people focused on health and fitness who make massage a regular part of their lives.

Physiological Effects and Benefits of Massage

As noted previously, physiological effects are changes in the body as a result of massage techniques, including benefits for the client. Later discussions of specific techniques include descriptions of the particular effects of each specific stroke or method. This section looks at the broad effects of massage on cells, tissues, and body systems.

Effects and Benefits at the Cellular Level

Thousands of chemical reactions are occurring throughout the body at any given moment. You will learn more about these chemical reactions in anatomy and physiology classes, but for the purpose of this discussion, chemical reactions essentially involve the transfer of energy through the loss, addition, or substitution of atoms in the molecules of body cells. For the body to function properly, every cell relies on fluids (e.g., blood, lymph, secretions from glands, and the fluids between the spaces of cells) to deliver nutrients, hydration, oxygen, and in some cases hormones and antibodies. Cell metabolism creates waste materials that are toxic to the body if not removed by fluids. Massage is very effective at promoting fluid movement in the body, and this enhanced movement of fluid supports healthy cell function.

Effects and Benefits for the Integumentary System

The integumentary system is composed of the skin and its accessory structures, the hair, nails, sudoriferous glands, and sebaceous glands (Fig. 4-3). Sensory receptors in the skin collect information about pain, pressure, and changes in temperature, and thus the skin becomes a primary medium of communication between the client and the world. For this reason, it is difficult to separate physiological effects and psychological effects when discussing many body systems. This difficulty demonstrates the powerful connection between the mind and body.

Through the skin, people can register and interpret an overwhelming variety of sensations such as the feather-light scurry of a bug on an arm, the scratchy texture of burlap, the pleasure of descending into a warm bath, or the discomfort of sunburn. Touch helps people orient themselves in the world and informs their sense of reality. Deane Juhan writes, "By rubbing up against the world, I define myself to myself." When touching an object, people learn something about the object but also have a reaction to touching the object. Through this reaction, they learn something about themselves. Touch becomes a defining factor in the behaviors, habits, preferences, aversions, body positions, and attitudes people adopt.[6]

The importance of the skin as a means by which the therapist communicates with clients cannot be overstated. By touching the client, the therapist confirms the client's body: its position, its size, its areas of tension, its ability to

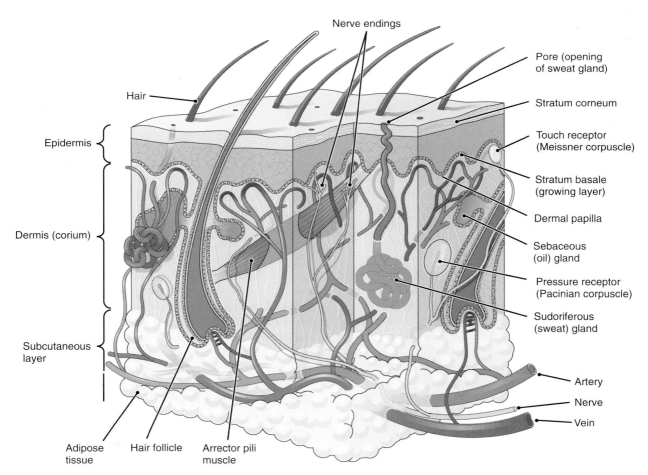

Nerve endings

Pore (opening of sweat gland)

Hair

Epidermis

Stratum corneum

Touch receptor (Meissner corpuscle)

Stratum basale (growing layer)

Dermal papilla

Dermis (corium)

Sebaceous (oil) gland

Pressure receptor (Pacinian corpuscle)

Sudoriferous (sweat) gland

Subcutaneous layer

Artery

Nerve

Vein

Adipose tissue

Hair follicle

Arrector pili muscle

Figure 4-3 Massage has many benefits for the integumentary system. It desquamates skin cells, stimulates sebaceous glands, increases scar tissue mobility, increases local circulation, and is applied with lubricants that soften and condition the skin. From Cohen BJ. Memmler's Human Body in Health and Disease, 11th ed. Philadelphia: Lippincott Williams & Wilkins, 2009.

feel pleasure or pain, and its ability to change. Through touch, clients understand their body and themselves differently.

This intimate connection between a person's sense of self and touch is illustrated in our biological development. Touch is the first sense to develop in the human embryo, becoming functional at 6 weeks. Skin and brain tissues come from the ectoderm—the same primitive cells—and the skin can thus be described as a superficial layer of the brain.[7] Touching initiates a flurry of brain activity, and the brain can precisely locate any stimulus on the body's surface. This close relationship between the nervous system and the skin allows massage therapists to trigger such important responses as the parasympathetic nervous system response through touch. Basic but significant mechanical effects also occur in the integumentary system as a result of massage:

- **Massage desquamates skin cells:** The outer layer of skin, the epidermis, is composed of epithelial cells that are constantly dying and being replaced in a natural process called exfoliation or desquamation. The movement of the therapist's hands over the surface of the skin supports this process, improving the condition and appearance of the skin.

- **Massage stimulates sebaceous glands:** The inner layer of the skin, the dermis, contains glands, blood vessels, and nerve endings. Sebaceous glands in the dermis secrete sebum, an oily lubricant that conditions the skin and hair to prevent them from drying out. Massage techniques stimulate the sebaceous glands, improving the softness, suppleness, and elasticity of the skin.

- **Massage increases scar tissue mobility:** After an injury that breaks the skin and creates a lesion, fibroblasts (fiber-producing cells) lay down crossing bands of collagen, creating scar tissue. Scar tissue is thick and strong but not as flexible as normal tissue and so may decrease tissue mobility. The application of cross-fiber friction and with-fiber friction massage to scar tissue during the remodeling and mature stages of tissue healing ensures the proper alignment of collagen fibers so that scar tissue remains mobile.[8] Some studies suggest that massage given during the healing process from burns increases the pliability of scared tissue.[9,10]

- **Massage increases local circulation to the skin:** Massage stimulates the local area and increases circulation, which brings fresh nutrients to the skin and aids in the removal of waste products. The skin is warmed by friction from the therapist's hands, which adds to client relaxation.

- **Massage lubricants skin:** The oils and creams used in massage can nourish and condition the skin, preventing the skin from drying out, aiding the skin's barrier function, and improving the appearance, texture, and elasticity of the skin.

Effects and Benefits for the Musculoskeletal System

The skeletal system is comprised of the bones and joints. Skeletal muscles attach to bones and produce movement at joints. Connective tissue in various forms weaves the body together, wrapping muscles and muscle groups, binding muscle to bone, and encapsulating the body in an interconnected mesh frame. Along with the skin, these structures are the most easily and directly manipulated by massage therapists, and massage has profound effects on how these closely related structures function.

Effects and Benefits for Connective Tissue

Connective tissue is the fibrous mesh that supports all parts of the body, as is discussed in depth in Chapter 20. For the present discussion, it is important to understand that connective tissue is found throughout the body as fascia, under the skin where it gives the body its contours (superficial fascia), in the membranes around vessels and organs, and in the walls of large arteries. As part of the deep fascial network, it wraps organs, muscle groups, and individual muscles and interweaves muscles with the denser cord-like connective tissue of tendons and ligaments. Hard, highly organized connective tissue forms cartilage and bone.

Important components of connective tissue include ground substance and collagen fibers. Ground substance is a fluid that looks something like egg whites and surrounds all the cells in the body to support cellular metabolism. Depending on where it occurs, it has a consistency ranging from a watery sol state, to a semi-fluid sol state, to a viscous gel state, to the solid crystalline structure of bone.

Collagen is a protein that forms strands, which make up the fibrous content of skin, fascia, tendons, ligaments, cartilage, bone, blood vessels, and organs. The fibers are arranged in a variety of ways depending on where they occur in the body. The proportion of collagen fibers and the state (between sol and gel) of ground substance differs depending on how the connective tissue is used. It may be fairly fluid with few collagen fibers creating a flexible network that holds skin cells in place and facilitates metabolic functions. Alternately, it may contain little fluid with large numbers of collagen fibers as in the tough, stringy material of tendons and ligaments.

Thixotropy is the phenomenon of gels becoming more fluid when they are stirred up and more solid when they are left undisturbed. The ground substance in connective tissue, especially fascia, has the unique ability to move between a more fluid sol state and a viscous gel state. Regular exercise, physical labor, stretching, proper hydration, and good nutrition promote a fluid sol state in fascia. The heat created in the tissue by movement warms and "stirs" the ground substance. On the other hand, a sedentary lifestyle, poor hydration, poor nutrition, little physical movement, and tissue trauma related to injury cause the ground substance to cool, thicken, and enter a stiffened gel state. A stiffened gel state might lead to a decrease in range of motion, patterns of tension in tissue that lead to postural imbalances, and a greater risk for injury, pain, and overall lethargy. Massage techniques that lift, twist, compress, vibrate, and stretch the tissue mechanically stir the ground substance and raise energy levels in the tissue. This leads to greater range of motion, an environment where cellular metabolism is enhanced, a decrease of fascial tension that may lead to better posture, the possibility of greater release and length in muscles (if fascia is the binding muscle the muscle cannot release properly), and less risk for injury, pain, and lethargy.

Effects and Benefits for Muscles

Skeletal muscles contract and lengthen to change the position of bones and create movement at joints (Fig. 4-4). They play a primary role in the maintenance of posture, stability of joints, and generation of heat for the body. Muscular movements are initiated by signals from nerves, a relationship characterized by the term "neuromuscular." Many of the effects of massage on muscles are actually caused by effects of massage on the nervous system. The connection between these two systems will become clearer in the following section on the nervous system. Muscle structure and function are described in greater detail in Chapter 20. The key effects and benefits of massage for the muscular system include the following:

- **Massage decreases muscle tension in hypertonic muscles.** A healthy muscle is always partially contracted because some motor units of a muscle (the nerve axon, its branches, and all the muscle fibers it supplies) remain active, even in a muscle at rest. This tone in the muscle keeps the muscle firm and is essential for maintaining posture. Too much tone in a muscle is called hypertonicity or hypertonia; when palpated, hypertonic muscles feel rigid, dense, and resistant to passive movement. Hypertonic muscles are usually chronically shortened and thus bring about muscular imbalances that cause postural adaptations that can eventually lead to painful conditions. Massage is believed to decrease hypertonicity in a number of ways. First, stimulation of the parasympathetic nervous system triggers the body to rest and

recover, generally relaxing the muscles. Relaxation massage techniques warm muscle tissue, increase circulation in tense muscles, and compress and twist the tissue to increase the pliability of muscle fibers. Certain massage techniques (e.g., Golgi tendon organ release, origin and insertion technique, muscle approximation, muscle energy techniques, etc.), which can be generally referred to as proprioceptor techniques, use sensory organs distributed in muscle and tendon (Golgi tendon organs, muscle spindles) to reset muscle length and tone. The theory and application of these techniques are discussed in depth in Chapter 21.

- **Massage reduces muscle spasms.** Muscle spasms are an involuntary, sustained contraction of a muscle often referred to in lay terms as a "cramp." A muscle may spasm due to pain in an area as an attempt to immobilize the area to prevent further injury (see the pain-spasm-pain cycle later in this chapter). Spasms may result when circulation is reduced in an area or when the body's nutritional supply is stressed such as with dehydration, perspiration, and overheating such as can occur in athletes. Stress, anxiety, or fatigue can also throw the body out of balance and cause spasms. A wide variety of massage techniques including direct pressure, agonist contraction, proprioceptor techniques, hydrotherapy, and Swedish massage are effective at reducing muscle spasms.

- **Massage reduces adhesions in muscle tissue and fascia.** Adhesions are abnormal deposits of connective tissue that form between surfaces that normally should glide over each other. Muscles are composed of parallel fibers organized into spirals, surrounded by and interwoven with fascia (thus the term myofascia). Healthy myofascia slides over itself. The myofascia strands, bundles of strands, muscles, and sheets of fascia normally do not stick together. In unhealthy tissue, collagen fibers pack together, and additional abnormal cross-links between collagen fibers are formed. Ground substance thickens and fails to adequately lubricate or nourish collagen cords. These collagen deposits are referred to as adhesions. They cause the tissue to become thicker, shorter, and less elastic. Adhesions lead to decreased blood flow, decreased range of motion, pain, and decreased function in the area. The lifting, twisting, and stretching techniques used in massage break up the adhesive bonds and make the tissue more pliable while the ground substance gets a good stirring. Strokes that compress, forcibly broaden, and stretch the tissue also break up adhesions in myofascia.

- **Massage strengthens weakened muscle tissue.** Active-resisted joint movements help to build the client's strength while taking a joint through its full range of motion to lubricate the joint structure with synovial fluid. Sometimes active-resisted techniques help to reeducate the muscle so that it can regain its normal movement pattern if it has been lost through injury or inactivity. This helps to promote greater muscular balance at the joint. In an active-resisted technique, the client carries out the movement while the therapist resists the movement, causing the client to use

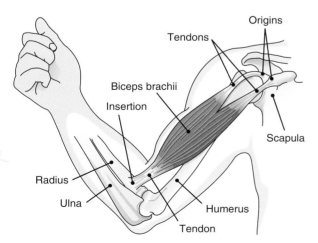

Figure 4-4 Massage has many benefits for the muscular system. It decreases tension; reduces muscle spasm; reduces adhesions; strengthens weakened muscle tissue; promotes muscular balance; increases flexibility and range of motion; decreases muscle fatigue, soreness, and recovery time; and promotes healing from soft-tissue injury. From Cohen BJ. Memmler's Human Body in Health and Disease, 11th ed. Philadelphia: Lippincott Williams & Wilkins, 2009.

stronger muscular contractions to complete the movement. Each time the client tries to carry out the movement, the therapist adds a little more resistance to build up the client's strength. For more information on active-resisted joint movements, see Topic 13-6 in Chapter 13. Other techniques that stimulate muscle spindles (sensory receptors that monitor stretch in muscle fibers) cause weak muscles to contract, thereby improving muscle tone.

- **Massage promotes muscular balance, which leads to better posture.** We know from the study of kinesiology that a muscle must relax when the opposing muscle contracts. An extension of one body area usually requires "bracing" from another body area. Contrasting muscle sensations of achiness, fluidity, soreness, pliability, stiffness, flexibility, tightness, smoothness, weakness, strength, effort, efficiency, grace, awkwardness, energy, and fatigue demonstrate the delicate balance between tension and release constantly at play in muscle and connective tissue. We also know that people develop postural habits based on a variety of factors including their type of work, attitudes, beliefs, lifestyle choices, and emotions, or in response to a period of high stress or injury. Even very distorted postures can become locked in the myofascial-neuromuscular system as "normal" and cause an ongoing situation of pain and compensation that leads to further musculoskeletal dysfunction. While we often learn individual muscles one by one, it's helpful to think of the body as one great big muscle, because the dynamic interplay of numerous muscles occurs even with the simplest gesture. A tight muscle pulls the myofascial fabric of the entire body, and even structures located at a distance to the muscle are affected. Massage and bodywork can help clients regain muscular balance by strengthening weakened muscles and lengthening chronically shortened muscles to improve posture, movement quality, and overall function.

- **Massage increases flexibility and range of motion.** At the end of a massage, clients seem to move with greater ease and with fuller motion. These inductive findings are supported by research that shows that massage increases flexibility in muscles and improves range of motion.[11,12] In one study, a group of 29 people who were assigned physiotherapy for shoulder pain were randomly divided into two groups. The first group received six treatments of massage around the shoulder area over a 2-week period. The second group did not receive massage but were placed on a waiting list for treatment. Measurements of client range of motion, pain, and functional ability were conducted before and after the 2-week treatment period by a blinded assessor (the assessor did not know a study was taking place). The group who received massage showed significant improvements in range of motion and pain reduction. They also reported improved functional ability.[13]

- **Massage decreases muscle soreness, muscle fatigue, and muscle recovery time in athletes.** A number of research studies aimed at understanding the benefits of massage for athletes demonstrated that massage decreases muscle soreness and improves muscle recovery.[14–16] In one study, 18 people were divided into two groups. One group received massage and the other served as a control group and received no massage. Study volunteers stressed their hamstring muscles with weight-lifting techniques. Two hours after the exercise, the massage group received 20 minutes of massage to the legs. At 6 hours after exercise, the groups were assessed for range of motion, intensity of soreness, and perceptions of the unpleasantness of soreness. The intensity of soreness was significantly lower in the massage group than in the control group for up to 48 hours after exercise.[17]

Another study showed that massage improved the recovery time in muscles. Thirteen male participants and seven female participants exercised their quadriceps muscles to complete fatigue using the maximum number of leg extensions they could complete at half the maximum weight they could lift. The participants then rested for 6 minutes and completed another set of their maximum number of leg extensions at half the maximum weight they could lift. The number of repetitions they could complete was documented. A few days later, the participants repeated the exercise routine but this time received 6 minutes of massage between sets. The results showed that massage after exercise fatigue significantly improved quadriceps performance compared to resting.[18]

- **Massage promotes healing from soft-tissue injury.** When soft tissue is damaged, an inflammatory and healing process begins (this process is described in detail in Chapter 22). For each stage in this process, different massage techniques have been used successfully based on the individual's needs. For example, leg edema was significantly reduced with lymphatic drainage techniques in a patient with severe distal tibiofibular fracture.[19] Scar tissue was reduced, pain was decreased, and range of motion was improved in a patient with a severe ankle injury using a variety of soft-tissue mobilization techniques.[20] The positive effects on symptom reduction and healing from a number of repetitive stress injuries like carpal tunnel syndrome, thoracic outlet syndrome, and iliotibial band friction syndrome have been documented.[21,22]

Effects and Benefits for the Skeletal System

The skeleton creates the framework of the body. Joint movement techniques focus predominantly on synovial joints, which are freely moveable and surrounded by a tough, connective tissue capsule that is further supported by ligaments and tendons. The joint capsule is filled with viscous synovial fluid, which lubricates the joint, absorbs shock, and reduces friction between moving surfaces. Hyaline cartilage (the type of cartilage that occurs at the ends of bones that form synovial joints) relies on synovial fluid for nutrients and to remove waste products. Synovial fluid moves in and out of the porous cartilage and circulates around the joint as the joint moves. As long as the joint is moved, the synovial membrane secretes synovial fluid, and the hyaline cartilage remains lubricated and creates new cells. When there is little movement at the joint, the hyaline cartilage dries out and begins to deteriorate. Joint movement techniques stimulate the production and distribution of synovial fluid.

Joints are affected by muscular imbalances that may pull the joint out of its normal alignment and lead to dysfunctional posture. Hypertonic muscles can tighten a joint, leading to decreased range of motion. Alternately, the body may compensate in another joint, leading to hypermobility of that joint (increased degree of motion) that might predispose the body to injury. Therefore, balancing the muscles around a joint may significantly improve joint health while improving overall posture. Massage, when appropriate, can decrease pain, stiffness, trigger points, edema, and spasms for conditions related to degenerative disc diseases, osteoarthritis, and temporomandibular joint (TMJ) dysfunction. The positive use of massage as part of the rehabilitation process following knee surgery and hip replacement surgery is noted in some research.[23,24]

Effects and Benefits for the Nervous and Endocrine Systems

Together, the nervous system and endocrine system synchronize all the functions of the body in an effort to maintain homeostasis. Because the nervous system is integral to the production of coordinated movement, effects on the nervous system directly impact the musculoskeletal system. Massage affects these systems on a number of levels:

- Massage activates the parasympathetic nervous system response, sending the body into rest and recovery mode.

- Massage changes the levels of chemical messengers in the body, which influence both physiological and psychological functions.

- Massage supports the biological rhythms of the body and helps the body reestablish an integrated natural tempo.

- Neuromuscular and somatic reflexive mechanisms can be manipulated by massage techniques to alter muscle tension and reeducate proprioceptors.

- Massage reduces pain through the gated mechanism of the spinal column (gate theory), by breaking the pain-spasm-pain cycle, by releasing nerves trapped by soft-tissue tension, and by reducing trigger points.

The Parasympathetic Nervous System Response

One of the most important effects of massage is activating the **parasympathetic nervous system response** that sends the body into rest and recovery mode, which is especially important because of the high levels of negative stress experienced by people as part of modern living. Negative stress triggers the body to enter fight-or-flight mode mediated by the sympathetic nervous system. Stress and its implications for health and wellness are discussed in depth in Topic 4-4.

Massage activates the parasympathetic nervous system, which balances out the sympathetic nervous system once a danger has passed, and helps the body unwind and recuperate

(Fig. 4-5). The parasympathetic nervous system slows the body's heart rate and is associated with relaxed breathing patterns. It stimulates the formation and release of urine and digestive activity so that the body can nourish and detoxify itself. This response is important for reducing all types of stress and allowing the body's chemistry to normalize.

Effects on Chemical Messengers

The body's stable internal environment (homeostasis) is achieved through carefully synchronized physiological processes (feedback reflexes or loops). This is sometimes called autoregulation. The activities of cells, tissues, and organs must be coordinated and integrated for the body to function optimally. To this end, cells must communicate with each other, sometimes over long distances.

A reflex is an involuntary response to a stimulus. If you touch a hot object, you jerk your hand away instantly—even before your conscious mind has time to register "hot." When something comes at your face very quickly, you duck and shut your eyes without thinking. Feedback reflexes or loops are occurring continually inside the body to maintain homeostasis.

Imagine you are trapped inside a room and suddenly the temperature plummets. Heat is lost from your warm skin and your body temperature starts to fall. Temperature receptors in your skin send a message along afferent pathways (afferent means "to carry to") to specific nerve cells in the brain (integrating center), alerting the brain cells to the drop in temperature. The specific cells in the brain send a response along efferent pathways (efferent means "to bear away from") to the smooth muscle around skin blood vessels, stimulating them to constrict, and to the skeletal muscles, stimulating them to contract (shiver). Blood vessels in the skin constrict, reducing heat loss, and shivering produces more heat in the body. The body's temperature normalizes. This could not happen without the work of chemical messengers.

Chemical messengers mediate the exchange of regulatory information and allow cells to communicate with one another. For example, one nerve cell releases a neurotransmitter (chemical messenger) that diffuses through the extracellular fluid to act on a second nerve cell. In some cases, a hormone-secreting gland (endocrine gland) serves as the integration center, blood serves as the efferent pathway, and a hormone instead of a neurotransmitter relays the message to target cells. The regulation of physiological functions relies on these intercellular messengers, but chemical messengers also cause feeling states such as joy, affection, depression, love, anger, hopefulness, loneliness, hunger, thirst, confidence, distrust, and attentiveness (another example of the body–mind connection). Following are some important chemical messengers:

- **Hormones:** Chemical messengers synthesized by endocrine glands in response to certain stimuli and secreted into the blood to be carried to target cells.

- **Neurotransmitters:** Chemical messengers released by neurons to communicate with another neuron or with a specific receptor in body tissue.

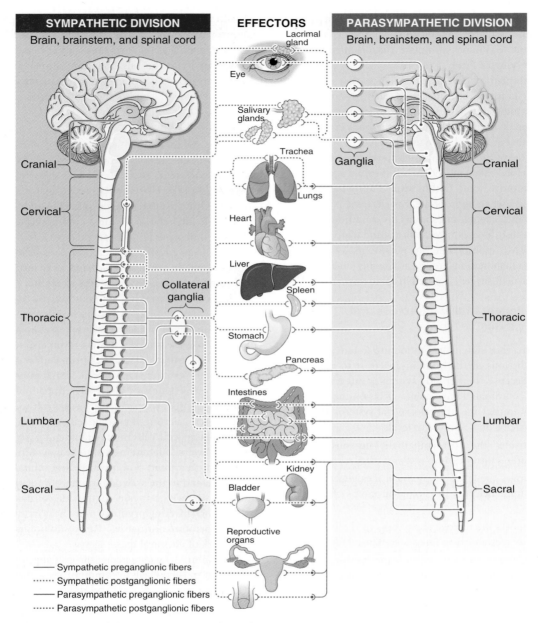

Figure 4-5 One of the most important effects of massage is activating the parasympathetic nervous system response that sends the body into rest and recovery mode. Stress triggers the body to enter the fight-or-flight mode mediated by the sympathetic nervous system. (Note: The diagram shows only one side of the body for each division.) From Cohen BJ. Memmler's Human Body in Health and Disease, 11th ed. Philadelphia: Lippincott Williams & Wilkins, 2009.

- **Neuropeptides:** A family of neurotransmitters composed of two or more amino acids that often function as chemical messengers in nonneural tissue.
- **Neurohormone:** A chemical messenger released by a neuron that travels in the bloodstream to its target cell. Sometimes these chemicals are simply called hormones, but the term "neurohormone" indicates that the substance originates in neural tissue.

Research demonstrates that massage can cause changes in the proportions of chemical messengers in the body, facilitating positive physiological and psychological changes and benefits. The following chemicals are affected by massage:

- **Cortisol:** Cortisol is a hormone produced by the adrenal glands that promotes the breakdown of proteins to form glucose to fuel muscles. It also decreases white blood cell accumulation and fibroblasts in an area of injury to reduce inflammation and has a powerful anti-allergenic action. It is one of the chemicals released during the fight-or-flight response, and when this response is triggered regularly, cortisol can remain at high levels in the body for prolonged periods of time and lead to decreased immunity, sleep disturbances, and an increase of substance P. Many studies have shown that massage reduces cortisol levels, probably due to the parasympathetic nervous system response and a balancing action on the adrenal glands.[25,26]

- **Dopamine:** Dopamine is a neurotransmitter produced in many areas of the brain, and in small amounts by the adrenal medulla. It is also a neurohormone secreted by neurons in the hypothalamus that inhibits the release of prolactin (regulation of milk production) from the anterior pituitary gland. In this capacity, it is often referred to as prolactin-inhibiting factor, prolactin-inhibiting hormone, or prolactostatin. Dopamine has many functions as a neurotransmitter in the brain and is closely related to the brain's reward system where behaviors associated with biological advantages bring a sense of gratification. For example, it is released naturally during pleasurable activities like eating and sex. Certain drugs like cocaine, nicotine, and amphetamines cause increases in dopamine levels, which may be why they cause addictions. Dopamine plays a role in motor activity, mood and sensations of well-being, sleep patterns, allocation of attention, and learning. Dopamine disorders can cause a decline in cognitive functions like memory, attention, and problem solving. Low levels are related to attention-deficit hyperactivity disorder (ADHD). Numerous studies have shown that massage increases dopamine levels and is indicated for conditions like depression, bulimia, anorexia, and ADHD and for improved cognitive function.[27–29] Increased dopamine also explains the enjoyment people experience from massage. In some cases, massage seems to balance dopamine and serotonin levels, lowering dopamine and raising serotonin.[30]

- **Endorphins, enkephalins, dynorphins:** Endorphins, enkephalins, and dynorphins are specific types of neuropeptides often referred to collectively as endorphins. Endorphins have generated interest because their receptor sites are triggered by opiates like morphine and codeine. They are released by the pituitary gland and hypothalamus and believed to act as natural painkillers and mood enhancers. During the fight-or-flight response, endorphin levels become elevated, leading to the popular term "endorphin rush" to denote the feeling of painlessness and heightened reflexes that comes with challenging or risky behavior. Studies indicate that massage, acupressure, acupuncture, thermal mud baths, thermal mineral baths, and physical therapy increase endorphin levels that decrease pain and increase positive moods in clients.[31,32]

- **Epinephrine (adrenaline):** Epinephrine and adrenaline are the same chemical substance, and the names are often used interchangeably. It is a major hormone secreted by the adrenal medulla. It is also a neurotransmitter secreted by the ends of sympathetic nerve fibers (of the sympathetic nervous system). Epinephrine plays a central role in the rush of physical and mental energy associated with the fight-or-flight response. It sharpens the senses, increases the speed

of reflexes, and boosts muscular strength. It triggers many of the responses that rapidly prepare the body for a threat. When a threat has passed, epinephrine that has not been reabsorbed produces a shaky, nauseous, pumped-up afterfeeling. In situations of chronic stress, epinephrine along with cortisol can remain at elevated levels in the body for extended periods of time, leading to overstimulation of the autonomic nervous system and adrenal exhaustion associated with fatigue and mental weariness. It is linked to conditions like high blood pressure, gastric ulcers, suppression of the immune system, and mood or personality changes. Massage has been shown to reduce epinephrine levels and quench the fight-or-flight response in patients about to undergo surgery.[33] Massage also normalizes epinephrine levels (and other chemicals) in depressed adolescent mothers.[34] It is likely that this occurs as part of the parasympathetic nervous system response to massage.

- **Growth hormone:** Growth hormone, also known as somatotrophin, is secreted by the pituitary gland and plays a central role in the reproduction and development of all body cells from embryo to adult. It stimulates connective tissue repair, growth in muscle tissue, and wound healing. Stimulation through touch is important for healthy pituitary function and may positively affect levels of growth hormone in the body.[35]

- **Norepinephrine (noradrenaline):** Norepinephrine, also called noradrenaline, is released from the adrenal medulla as a hormone and from the central nervous system and autonomic nervous system as a neurotransmitter. Like epinephrine, it plays a role in activating the body during the fight-or-flight response. Norepinephrine is closely associated with alertness, arousal, reward, and motivation in the brain and affects appetite drive and learning. It has been implicated with serotonin as a primary element in affective disorders. Affective disorders are conditions characterized by serious or prolonged disturbances of mood like depression or bipolar disorder. Research shows that massage normalizes levels of norepinephrine and proves beneficial for affective conditions like depression. It has been used in some studies as an intervention for aggressive behavioral disorders.[36]

- **Oxytocin:** Oxytocin plays an important role in pregnancy, labor and delivery, and lactation. It is also related to maternal behavior, adult bonding, feelings of affection, and calm. Increased oxytocin levels may make social contact with other people more rewarding. In one study, oxytocin levels were elevated in response to relaxation massage and decreased when sad or negative emotions were evoked. It's possible that increased levels of oxytocin during massage contribute to the feelings of being nurtured that clients often report as a result of the session.[37]

- **Serotonin:** Serotonin is a neurotransmitter found in the central nervous system. It is also found in the gastrointestinal tract and in blood platelets. It was recognized as a powerful vasoconstrictor in 1948 and later understood as an important neurotransmitter related to mood, sleep, sexuality, appetite, and other body functions. Low or abnormal levels of serotonin are associated with depression, angry or aggressive behavior, anxiety disorders, and obsessive compulsive disorder. It may also be a factor in migraine and fibromyalgia. Research indicates that massage increases or balances serotonin levels. Positive effects have been noted in relationship to depression, sexual abuse, eating disorders, pain syndromes, asthma, chronic fatigue, HIV, breast cancer, job stress, and pregnancy stress.[38]

- **Substance P:** Substance P is a neuropeptide that relays unpleasant sensory information to the brain. It is involved in several physiological activities including the vomiting reflex, changes in the cardiovascular system including vasodilation, smooth muscle contractions, and defensive behavior related to the fight-or-flight response. It is sometimes referred to as the pain transmitter because it plays a primary role in relaying sensory information related to pain. It is also involved in mental and emotional stress responses.[39] In one study, 24 people with fibromyalgia received a 30-minute massage session or relaxation therapy sessions twice a week for 5 weeks. While both groups demonstrated a decrease in anxiety and depressed mood after the first and last sessions, only the massage group had increased sleep, decreased pain, and decreased levels of substance P.[40]

Effects on Biological Rhythms

Humans have particular cycles and rhythms that help the body resist external stresses and support homeostasis. A pair of grouped cells located in the hypothalamus function as the primary pacemaker or time clock for the body, but cells in many parts of the body have their own oscillators (rhythm setters). Biological rhythms such as heart rate, respiratory rate, waking and sleeping cycles (known as circadian rhythm), digestive cycles, the urinary excretion of potassium, the menstrual cycle, body temperature changes, and the secretion of some hormones have a natural tempo. When the body is in balance, these tempos are entrained. Entrainment is defined in physics as the process whereby two oscillating systems, which have different rhythms when they function independently, assume the same rhythm. In the body, entrainment can be thought of as the harmonizing and synchronization of different rhythms so that the body finds equilibrium.

External factors provide timing cues that affect the body's entrainment. Rapid changes in environmental cues can cause biological rhythms to temporally get out of phase with each other. For example, flying into a different time zone can affect one's circadian rhythms and may lead to symptoms of fatigue, mild depression, grogginess, headache, and constipation commonly known as jet lag. Similarly, a sudden shift in work schedule, changing meal times, or exposure to bright, flashing lights, noisy environments, or loud, disruptive music can pull the body out of sync. Activities like meditation, chanting, attention to breath, positive emotional states like those experienced during religious practice, and massage are believed to help the body entrain, bringing the body's rhythms into accord.

Effects on Neuromuscular and Somatic Reflex Mechanisms

All movement relies on the close interaction and coordination of the nervous and muscular systems, denoted by the term *neuromuscular*. Motor neurons are nerve cells whose axons innervate skeletal muscle fibers (Fig. 4-6). The axon of a motor neuron divides into many branches, each of which forms a single junction with a muscle fiber. A motor neuron plus all of the muscle fibers it innervates is called a motor unit. Movement occurs when many motor units from various areas are activated in a precise order. Receptors in muscles, tendons, joints, the skin, vestibular system (sense organ in the temporal bone of the skull that provides input on balance), and the eyes send information about the body's changing position, muscle tension, muscle stretch, joint angle, load on tendons, and balance to the brain. The brain uses this information to signal muscles to better coordinate the movement. The receptors (often called proprioceptors) in muscles, tendons, and joints can be manipulated with certain massage techniques to alter muscle tension patterns and reeducate the muscle about its proper resting length in relationship to other muscles in the area. These techniques take advantage of somatic reflexes that ensure smooth movement and protect muscles and tendons from damage.

Two somatic reflexes often manipulated by massage therapists are the stretch reflex and tendon reflex. The **stretch reflex** is mediated by proprioceptors called muscle spindles that are located in the muscle belly and monitor the muscle's length (Fig. 4-7). Muscle spindles send information that helps control muscle movement by detecting the amount of stretch placed on a muscle. They protect the muscle from being overstretched and play a role in setting muscle tone.

Concept Brief 4-4
Body Chemicals and Massage

Cortisol: Stress hormone reduced by massage

Dopamine: "Feel good" neurotransmitter increased by massage

Endorphins: Natural painkiller and mood enhancer increased by massage

Epinephrine: Stress hormone/neurotransmitter reduced by massage

Growth hormone: Tissue repair hormone increased by massage

Norepinephrine: Stress hormone/neurotransmitter balanced by massage

Oxytocin: "Nurturing" hormone increased by massage

Serotonin: Mood neurotransmitter increased or balanced by massage

Substance P: Neuropeptide that transmits pain signals decreased by massage

When a muscle is stretched very rapidly or overstretched, the muscle spindles are activated and directly stimulate motor neurons causing the muscle to reflexively contract, thereby protecting the muscle from tearing. Sedentary habits, work conditions, stress, injury, and many other factors can cause muscles to lose their "memory" or their proper resting length in relationship to other muscles. Muscle spindles may become hyperactive and needlessly increase muscle tension. Techniques that reduce muscle spindle activation can help lessen hypertonicity and spasm, leading to greater muscular balance and function. One technique that manipulates muscle spindles in this way is muscle approximation. The therapist grasps the muscle with one hand close to its origin and with the other hand close to its insertion. The ends of the muscle are brought closer together, thereby lessening the stretch on the muscle spindles. This decreases their activation of motor units and reduces muscle tone or spasm.

The **tendon reflex** is mediated by proprioceptors called Golgi tendon organs that monitor muscle tension and tendon strain. Golgi tendon organs are located in tendons near where the tendon joins muscles (see Fig. 4-7). If a muscle contracts too strongly, such as when lifting a heavy load, the muscle and tendon could be damaged. When Golgi tendon organs sense that a muscle contraction is straining a tendon, they are activated and cause the inhibition of the muscle's motor units, stopping the contraction and causing the muscle to relax. One technique that manipulates Golgi tendon organs is Golgi tendon organ release. Slow, moderate, direct pressure is placed on the tendon near the junction with the muscle and held until the muscle relaxes. The pressure causes the Golgi tendon organs to react as if the tendon were being strained, activating the reflex to relax the muscle. Proprioceptors, somatic reflexes, and massage techniques that manipulate them are discussed in the upcoming chapters.

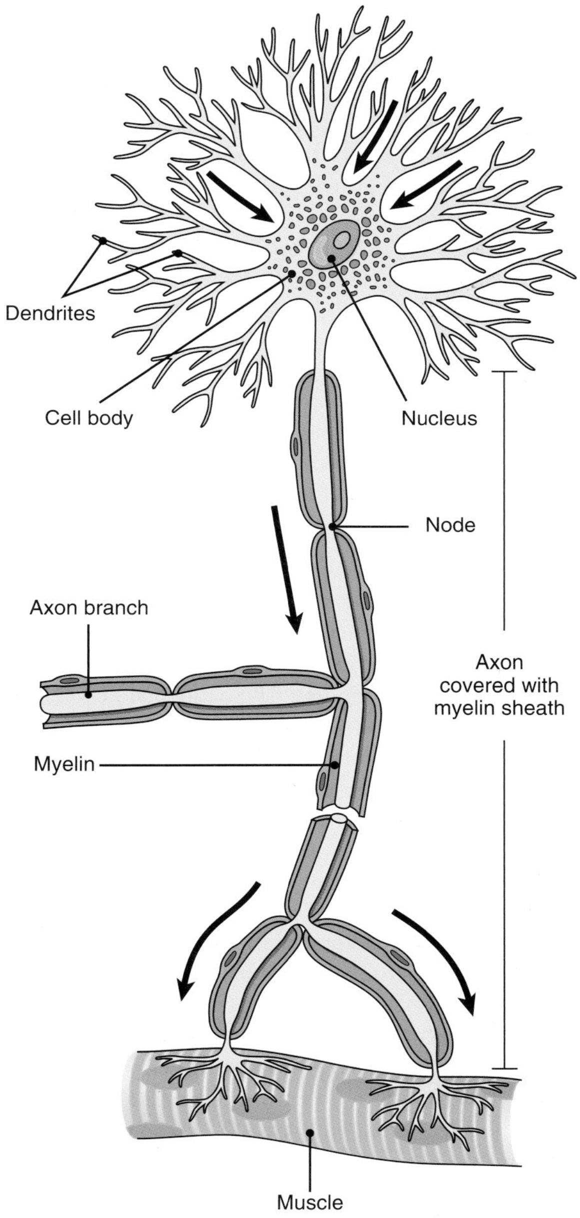

Figure 4-6 Diagram of a Motor Neuron. Motor neurons are nerve cells whose axons innervate skeletal muscle fibers. The arrows in the diagram show the direction of the nerve impulse. From Cohen BJ. Memmler's Human Body in Health and Disease, 11th ed. Philadelphia: Lippincott Williams & Wilkins, 2009.

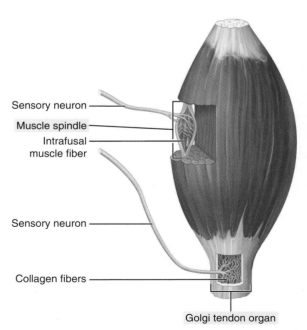

Figure 4-7 Muscle spindles send information that helps control muscle movement by detecting the amount of stretch placed on a muscle; Golgi tendon organs monitor muscle tension and tendon strain. From McConnell T, Hull K. Human Form Human Function: Essentials of Anatomy & Physiology. Philadelphia: Lippincott Williams & Wilkins, 2011.

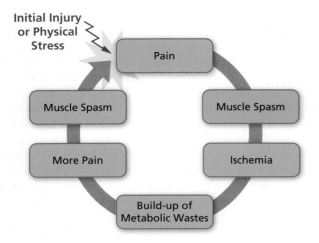

Figure 4-8 The pain-spasm-pain cycle is a persistent cycle that occurs with injury or chronic overuse in which pain triggers muscle spasms, which then lead to a series of events that cause more pain and the continuation of the cycle.

Effects on Pain

Pain receptors are widely distributed free nerve endings in skin, muscles, the periosteum of bones, joints, and arterial walls, and to a lesser extent in internal organs. The function of pain is to alert the central nervous system to damage being done to the body's tissues; thus pain also activates the fight-or-flight response and its corresponding physiological and psychological reactions. While the cause of pain signals is not certain, it is believed that the bradykinin, prostaglandins, and histamine chemicals released by damaged cells contact nerve endings and trigger the signal that indicates pain. Considerable evidence indicates that massage reduces pain, although the mechanism by which pain is reduced is not always clear. It is likely that massage breaks the pain-spasm-pain cycle, that the nervous system is "gated," and that massage frees trapped nerves and reduces trigger points.

THE PAIN-SPASM-PAIN CYCLE

The **pain-spasm-pain cycle** is a persistent cycle in which pain triggers muscle spasms, which then lead to more pain (Fig. 4-8). Imagine that you tear a muscle in your back and pain sensors alert the brain that damage has occurred in the back. Muscles in the area spasm to "splint" and "guard" the area to prevent further damage. This guarding decreases movement in the area, which prevents blood from circulating freely. The lack of circulation causes a build up of metabolic wastes in the tissue that again trigger pain receptors, resulting in more pain. More pain results in more muscle spasms, repeating the cycle. The sympathetic nervous system becomes overstimulated, while the physiological reactions of the body to the fight-or-flight response complicate the issue. Massage can break the pain-spasm-pain cycle by reducing muscle spasms, triggering the parasympathetic nervous system response to reduce sympathetic firing and increasing

circulation to the local area, which removes metabolic wastes thereby reducing pain.

GATE CONTROL THEORY

In 1965, psychologist Ronald Melzack and physiologist Patrick Wall introduced the **gate control theory** of pain management in a paper published in the Science Magazine. Melzack and Wall believed that the spinal cord had a gating mechanism whereby nerve fibers carrying somatic stimuli relating to touch, temperature, pressure, or movement can "close the gate" to dull aching pain information traveling to the brain.

Pain travels to the brain on two different types of neurons. Sharp, intense pain travels on larger, faster, myelinated A axons, while dull aching pain travels on smaller, slower, unmyelinated C axons. Like sharp pain, somatic stimuli also travel on larger, faster, myelinated A neurons. The spinal cord has a limited ability to attend to multiple sources of sensory stimuli at one time, and messages from the slower C neurons may be locked out when many sensory stimuli (like the stimuli caused by massage) are traveling to the brain. Dull, aching, or throbbing pain, the type often associated with chronic conditions, can thus be blocked by somatic stimuli like massage. This is why people instinctively hold an area that hurts and animals lick an injury. Because sharp, acute pain travels on the faster, myelinated A neurons, gate control cannot be used to reduce this type of pain. When pain is intense, these signals reach the spinal cord at the same pace as touch or pressure signals and are not locked out of the spinal cord.

NERVE ENTRAPMENT OR COMPRESSION

The peripheral nervous system consists of the nerves extending from the brain and spinal cord out to all points of the body. It transmits signals between the central nervous system and the body's periphery. The peripheral nerves can be squashed by tight muscles, tendons, ligaments, scar tissue, or fascia (nerve entrapment is the trapping of nerves by soft tissue or edema), by bones that have shifted or been pulled from their normal alignment or the development of a bony growth (nerve compression is the trapping of nerves by bone), by edema, or because of systemic conditions like pregnancy that may cause edema.

A nerve that often becomes entrapped is the median nerve as it passes through the carpal tunnel into the hand. The brachial plexus may be entrapped by structures like the scalene muscles and pectoralis minor muscle or compressed by the first rib and clavicle. The piriformis muscle can entrap the sciatic nerve, causing numbness, tingling, pain, and weakness in the affected region. Massage techniques that reduce hypertonicity in muscles, improve posture, and strengthen weakened muscles can reduce the pressure on peripheral nerves. Often the client must make lifestyle changes to ensure that body positions at work or home do not lead to a recurrence of the problem. You will learn techniques for working with common entrapment conditions in Chapter 22 and Chapter 23.

TRIGGER POINTS

Trigger points are hypersensitive spots that usually occur within a taut band of muscle or fascia (Fig. 4-9). These points cause the affected muscle to be shortened and cause a predictable pain referral pattern; when the trigger point is compressed, pain shoots down an expected path and is felt in areas distant to the point. Trigger points are related to tissue ischemia (vasoconstriction and decreased circulation) and increased metabolic processes in the local tissue brought on by many factors including stress, injury, a sedentary lifestyle, poor posture, and repetitive stress. Trigger points can mimic the pain of other conditions, such as tendonitis or osteoarthritis, and can cause continuous pain, pain when the muscle is contracted or stretched, hypertonicity in the affected muscle, muscle weakness, and dysfunctional postural adaptations.

Reducing trigger points is an important treatment goal in the rehabilitation of clients with many different conditions. Techniques include the use of heat, skin rolling, petrissage, muscle stripping, stretching, and short or long ischemic compressions. With an ischemic compression, the therapist applies direct pressure to the trigger point, causing increased ischemia. When the pressure is removed, blood rushes into the local tissue causing hyperemia. Petrissage is used to "milk" the tissue of metabolic wastes, and the area is gently stretched. Trigger point therapy is discussed in depth in Chapter 21.

Effects and Benefits for the Cardiovascular System

The heart pumps blood through arteries and veins to carry oxygen, nutrients, antibodies, and hormones to the body's cells and to remove waste products created by cellular metabolism. Good circulation is essential for proper body functions. Massage has important effects and benefits for the cardiovascular system:

- **Massage improves local circulation.** Many massage techniques produce hyperemia (increased blood flow in the local area, demonstrated by increased redness and warmth in the tissue). These changes are believed to result from a number of factors including the breakdown of muscular tension, the mechanical pressure of massage strokes on arteries, the release of vasodilators like histamine in the local area, autonomic nervous system responses caused by reflexive effects, and changes in blood viscosity.
  - When muscles are tense, they restrict blood flow in the local area, which decreases the oxygen that can reach the tissue and leads to a buildup of metabolic wastes. When muscle tension is reduced through massage, blood can circulate freely, and oxygen and nutrients are exchanged with cellular wastes more readily, improving tissue health (Fig. 4-10).
  - Massage strokes manipulate muscles and connective tissue, causing the tissue to experience pressure and torsion (stress). Histamine is a chemical released by mast cells in connective tissue when the tissue is stimulated. It is one of the chemical messengers of the inflammatory process and acts as a vasodilator, increasing circulation in the local area.

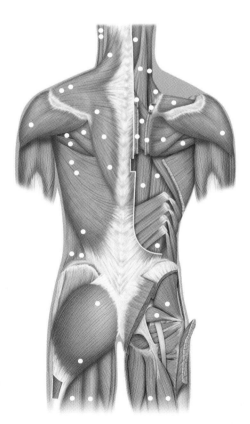

Figure 4-9 Trigger points are hypersensitive spots that usually occur within a taut band of muscle or fascia and cause a predictable pain referral pattern.

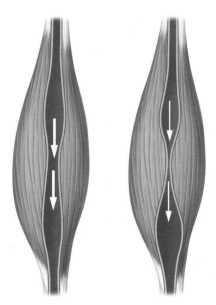

Figure 4-10 Muscle tension and circulation. Tight muscles can place pressure on blood vessels and restrict circulation to local tissue. When muscles relax, blood flow is increased and returned to normal.

- Initially massage stimulates the sympathetic nervous system and increases the heart rate, which sends blood to peripheral vessels. In a sympathetic response, the spleen, a blood reservoir, dumps extra blood into the bloodstream. These events explain why the hands and feet often become warm and flushed after application of fascial techniques in distant areas of the body.[41] As the massage progresses, the parasympathetic nervous system response is triggered (unless the techniques are purposefully stimulating, as in a sports massage), and the flushing of the hands and feet decreases as the heart rate slows; clients may report that they feel cold as the massage continues and blood is redirected to internal organs to support their processes (e.g., the digestive system becomes more active).

- Massage increases arterial blood flow mechanically because the heart acts as a pump. When massage techniques like compression, kneading, or slow deep friction are applied, they temporarily block off the flow of blood in the tissue. The blood backs up and the pressure builds. When the therapist's hands release the tissue, the blockage is removed and the blood rushes into the arteries with greater force, flushing the tissue. Light massage causes the dilation of superficial capillaries almost instantly. A 20-minute massage has been shown to decrease blood and plasma viscosity, increasing blood flow.[42] A similar result occurred in a study on Chinese Medical Massage.[43] It is theorized that this occurred because of the local release of vasodilators and because interstitial fluid was mechanically pushed from the tissue.

- **Massage supports venous return.** The arteries carry oxygenated blood to the body's tissues, and veins carry deoxygenated blood back to the heart to be re-oxygenated and recirculated. "Venous return" refers to the volume of blood returning to the heart from the veins. When a person is sitting or standing, blood returning to the heart from the lower half of the body must fight gravity. To facilitate venous return, veins have one-way valves that allow the deoxygenated blood to flow only toward the heart. Contractions of nearby skeletal muscles and the pulsing of nearby arteries help push venous blood toward the heart against the force of gravity. During massage, the techniques used to relax muscles also squeeze veins and encourage the movement of blood toward the heart. Therapists often use strokes from distal to proximal to move blood in the veins toward the heart. This decreases the accumulation of metabolic waste and stagnation of the blood and benefits the body's tissues by helping ensure adequate amounts of oxygen.[44]

- **Massage decreases blood pressure.** Massage inhibits the firing of the sympathetic nervous system, slowing the heart rate and the force of the heart's contractions.[45] This combined with vasodilation of peripheral blood vessels lowers blood pressure.[46] Numerous studies have demonstrated this effect. In a study of 30 adults with controlled hypertension, massage reduced both diastolic and systolic blood pressure.[47] In another group, a 20-minute back massage reduced systolic blood pressure.[48] Massage is likely to benefit clients with hypertension, but you should read the later cautions and contraindications chapter carefully before providing massage to these clients (Fig. 4-11).

Effects and Benefits for the Lymphatic and Immune Systems

The lymphatic system is composed of lymph, lymph vessels, lymph nodes, the spleen, and the thymus gland (Fig. 4-12). The lymphatic system filters fluids from body tissues back into the blood and transports fats from the gastrointestinal tract to the blood. It plays an important role in protecting the body from foreign substances. Massage has important effects and benefits for the lymphatic and immune systems:

- **Massage increases lymph circulation.** Protein-containing fluid (interstitial fluid) that has escaped from blood capillaries is collected from tissue spaces throughout the body by the lymph capillaries and channeled into lymphatic vessels, where it is filtered by lymph nodes before it is returned to the blood. Good lymph circulation ensures that fluids do not build up in the tissue and that the body's immune system functions properly. Movement of lymph relies on the pulse of arteries that run parallel to lymph vessels, on respiratory movements, and on the pumping action of skeletal muscles. A sedentary lifestyle, confinement to a hospital bed, pathologies, and injuries that lead to lowered mobility can seriously impair lymph circulation. Patterns of muscular tension can also reduce lymph flow. Massage techniques mechanically move the lymph fluid through the lymph vessel network in much the same way that they support venous return. Massage reduces muscle tension so that bound muscles do not restrict lymph movement.

- **Massage decreases edema.** Edema is a swelling in tissue that can have many causes. It might be caused by a chronic cardiac condition, kidney problem, or liver problem and may be a contraindication for massage. Sometimes edema is caused by an inflammatory process because of a soft-tissue injury like an ankle sprain, and certain types of massage techniques are beneficial. Very light rolling and pumping techniques are used to encourage fluid out of the swollen area in the direction of lymph flow and toward areas with many lymph nodes.

- **Massage helps manage lymphedema.** Edema caused by inadequate lymph drainage is referred to as lymphedema. Lymphedema may be caused by surgery involving lymph node removal (e.g., mastectomy), radiation therapy, the spread of cancer to lymph tissue, scarring of lymph nodes, infection, trauma, or a parasitic infestation (rare in developed countries). Manual lymphatic drainage is a specialized massage system developed by Emil Vodder, a Danish

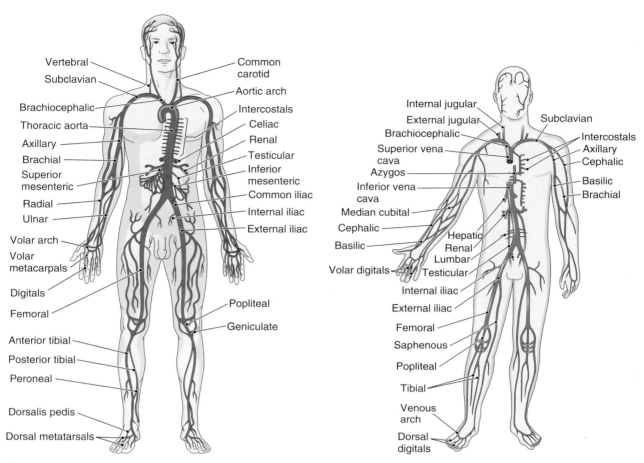

Left figure labels:
Vertebral
Subclavian
Brachiocephalic
Thoracic aorta
Axillary
Brachial
Superior mesenteric
Radial
Ulnar
Volar arch
Volar metacarpals
Digitals
Femoral
Anterior tibial
Posterior tibial
Peroneal
Dorsalis pedis
Dorsal metatarsals

Common carotid
Aortic arch
Intercostals
Celiac
Renal
Testicular
Inferior mesenteric
Common iliac
Internal iliac
External iliac
Popliteal
Geniculate

Right figure labels:
Internal jugular
External jugular
Brachiocephalic
Superior vena cava
Azygos
Inferior vena cava
Median cubital
Cephalic
Basilic
Volar digitals

Subclavian
Intercostals
Axillary
Cephalic
Basilic
Brachial
Hepatic
Renal
Lumbar
Testicular
Internal iliac
External iliac
Femoral
Saphenous
Popliteal
Tibial
Venous arch
Dorsal digitals

Figure 4-11 Massage has important effects and benefits for the cardiovascular system. It improves local circulation, supports venous return, and helps decrease blood pressure.

physical therapist. The techniques of manual lymphatic drainage include gentle stretches of the skin and focused techniques that gently pump or roll fluid along the lymph paths to lymph-collecting ducts. Lymph drainage massage is usually combined with the application of a compression bandage to limit further fluid accumulation. Many studies indicate that lymph drainage massage techniques paired with compression bandages are effective methods for managing chronic lymphedema, especially for people living with breast cancer.[49–51]

- **Massage boosts immune function.** Research on massage for people living with cancer or HIV demonstrates that massage increases the number and activity of white blood cells, improving general immune function. In one study, massage was compared to progressive muscle relaxation for women diagnosed with breast cancer. While both groups reported that they were less depressed and less anxious and had less pain from their therapy, only the massage group had increased levels of natural killer cells and lymphocytes.[52] In another study, 29 men infected with HIV received daily massage for 1 month and no massage for the second month. During the month of massage, there was a significant increase in natural killer cell numbers and activity.[53]

Effects and Benefits for the Respiratory System

During inspiration, the diaphragm contracts and moves down into the abdominal cavity (Fig. 4-13). At the same time, the external intercostal muscles contract and lift the ribs laterally, while the scalene and sternocleidomastoid muscles contract to lift the first rib, second ribs, and the sternum. The trapezius, levator scapulae, serratus anterior, abdominal muscles, pectoralis major, and pectoralis minor are accessory respiratory muscles. When any of these muscles is chronically tight and shortened, it may restrict normal breathing and disrupt breathing patterns. Massage techniques to lengthen and relax these muscles improve breathing capacity and function. Massage also improves posture, which can lead to an opening of the chest area and the structural alignment and rib cage expansion necessary for optimal lung function. When the parasympathetic nervous system responds to massage, breathing rate slows and breaths become deep and regular. Massage facilitates a client's awareness of breathing and can help establish deep, free, natural breathing patterns. These effects on the respiratory system are important for all massage clients. Other effects and benefits of massage for the respiratory system include the following:

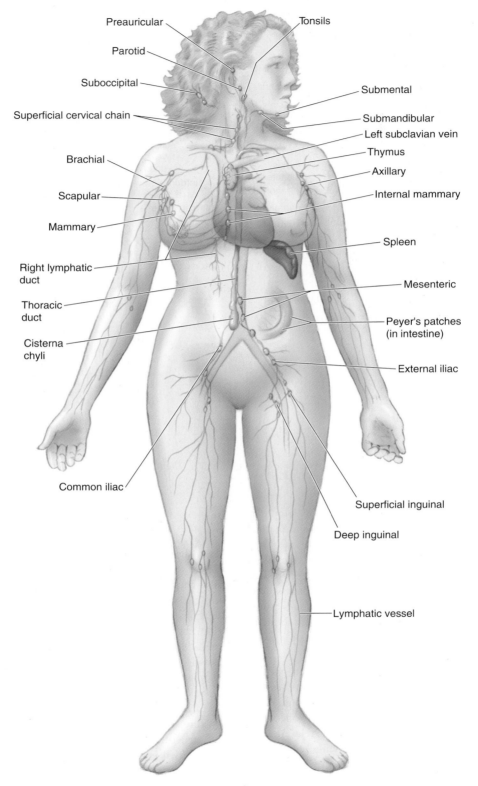

Figure 4-12 Massage has important effects and benefits for the lymphatic system. It increases lymph circulation, decreases edema, helps manage lymphedema, and boosts immune function. This image shows the location of major lymph nodes and lymph tissue. From Premkumar K. Anatomy & Physiology: The Massage Connection. Philadelphia: Lippincott Williams & Wilkins, 2004.

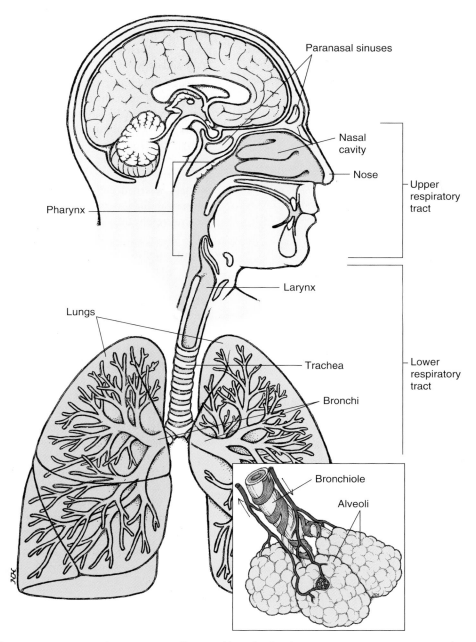

Figure 4-13 Massage has important effects and benefits for the respiratory system. It supports deep regular breathing, loosens mucus in the lungs and aids mucus expulsion, improves respiratory function, and decreases laryngeal tension. From Premkumar K. Anatomy & Physiology: The Massage Connection. Philadelphia: Lippincott Williams & Wilkins, 2004.

- **Massage loosens mucus in the lungs and aids mucus expulsion.** Tapotement techniques on the back along with vibration and shaking help to loosen mucus in the lungs and increase airway clearance for better lung function.[54] These techniques are often used to support people living with cystic fibrosis or as physical therapy for people with chronic obstructive pulmonary diseases (COPDs).[55] They may be used in combination with postural drainage techniques that place the body in different positions to facilitate mucus movement or with coughing techniques (patients are trained to cough in specific ways to best expel mucus).

- **Massage improves respiratory function.** Massage improves many indicators of respiratory function, including reduced shortness of breath and increased oxygen saturation levels, thoracic gas volume, peak flow, forced expiratory volume, and forced vital capacity.[56,57]

- **Massage decreases laryngeal tension.** Massage has been used successfully as an intervention for singers, actors, and public speakers who experience laryngeal tension as a result of overuse. Techniques focus on the muscles of the neck and shoulders. In one study, acoustic measures of the voice confirmed significant improvements in just one treatment session.[58]

Effects and Benefits for the Digestive and Urinary Systems

Many chronic gastrointestinal disorders are related to or exacerbated by chronic stress because the intestinal tract is sensitive to any changes in autonomic or endocrine function. The fight-or-flight response shuts down digestive function as the blood is redirected to the body's limbs. Massage activates the parasympathetic nervous system response, which directs the body into the rest and recovery mode. The digestive system becomes more active when the body is relaxed, and one often hears increased digestive sounds from clients during a massage session. Regular massage can be an important intervention for chronic digestive disorders. In cases of constipation, massage techniques can be used on the abdomen working from the left to the right in a circular motion with the intent to assist the movement of colon contents toward the rectum. In one study, abdominal massage improved bowl function in patients with spinal cord injury.[59]

Massage increases blood volume and filtration in the kidneys. The parasympathetic nervous system response promotes urine production, leading to increased urination after the massage.

Effects and Benefits for Pregnancy and Child Development

Pregnancy massage (also called prenatal massage) has many benefits for the mother and baby. Psychological benefits are also included in this section because positive psychological attitudes can improve the physiological health of both mother and infant.

Massage reduces pain from muscles, compensating for changes in the woman's body. Massage also improves mood and attitude, decreases anxiety about labor and delivery, and decreases labor pain. When the baby is born, touch is essential for both mother and child and affects how the child grows and develops. Massage for infants and children can influence behavior, enhance learning, improve parent–child interactions, increase restful sleep, and lead to weight gains in preterm infants. The studies presented below are just a sample of this widely researched area. Detailed information and additional research are presented in Chapter 24.

- **Massage and pregnancy.** Twenty-six pregnant women were assigned to either a massage group or a relaxation therapy group to receive 20-minute sessions twice a week for 5 weeks. The massage group reported reduced anxiety, improved mood, better sleep, and less back pain. Urinary stress hormone levels decreased in the massage therapy group, and these women had fewer complications during labor and delivery.[60]

- **Massage and labor pain.** In a study to compare the characteristics of pain during labor with and without massage, 60 women in labor were randomly assigned to a massage or control group and filled in a questionnaire at each of the three phases of cervical dilation. The massage group received massage and standard nursing care, while the control group received only standard nursing care. Massage lessened pain intensity at phases one and two of cervical dilation as compared to the control group but did not significantly change the pain experienced in phase three.[61]

- **Parent–infant interaction.** In a study evaluating whether father–infant interactions could be enhanced with massage, fathers gave their infants daily massages before bedtime for 1 month. The fathers who massaged their infants were more expressive and showed more enjoyment and warmth during interaction with their infants than the control group.[62]

- **Weight gain in preterm infants.** In a review of studies that showed that massage facilitates weight gain in preterm infants, researcher Tiffany Field noted, "Studies from several laboratories have documented a 31% to 47% greater weight gain in preterm newborns receiving massage therapy (three 15-minute sessions for 5 to 10 days) compared with standard medical treatment."[63] A study led by Field demonstrated that of 40 preterm infants receiving similar caloric intake, the infants who received massage averaged a 21% greater daily weight gain than the control infants over the period of the study.[64]

- **Massage and improved sleep.** In another study, infants and children were given massage by their parents 15 minutes before bedtime, while a control group was read bedtime stories. The massage group had fewer sleep problems and fell asleep faster than the control group.[65]

Psychological Effects and Benefits of Massage

Psychological effects are the outcome experienced mentally and emotionally by clients as a result of a massage session (Fig. 4-14). For many years, scientists viewed the body and mind as separate and did not understand how closely physiological and psychological functions were related. In 1972, Dr. Candace Pert, a neuroscientist, discovered the opiate receptor and changed how people viewed the connection between the body and mind.

Dr. Pert has spent the last two decades working to understand neuropeptides and their receptors. These "molecules of emotion" carry information that allows cells of

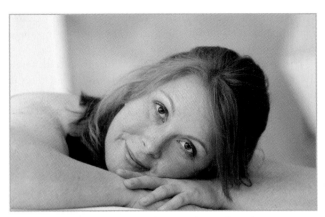

Figure 4-14 Psychological effects and benefits of massage are the outcomes experienced mentally and emotionally by clients as a result of the session. Massage reduces anxiety, depression, aggression and behavioral disorders in children and teens, improves sleep, and positively changes brain-wave patterns. Image courtesy of Associated Bodywork & Massage Professionals (ABMP).

all kinds to communicate with one another, suggesting that the brain is not just in the brain but is also in the body, being carried to all cells on neuropeptides through the bloodstream and nervous system, as discussed previously in the section on the nervous and endocrine systems. Feeling states are initiated when a neuropeptide bonds to a particular cell. Alternately, a particular feeling state can release a neuropeptide to bond with receptors on particular cells. These activities are basic to survival and create connections among our emotions, internal responses, physical patterns, and behaviors. The mind and body reflect each other. Our emotions influence our health, and our health influences our emotions.

In the previous section on the effects of massage in the nervous system, the flight-or-flight response was described as well as chemical messengers and the changes in their levels that result from a massage session. Stress creates a feeling state that is both physical and emotional. When stressed people *feel* their hearts beating, they *feel* the rush of adrenaline that heightens all their senses and reactions, they *feel* their palms sweat, they *feel* their gut tighten, and they *feel* the hairs on the back of the neck stand up. When stress is chronic or prolonged, this feeling state is dampened but persistent. Reflexes become facilitated (hair-triggered), attention becomes watchful, and behavior becomes anxious, aggressive, defensive, and urgent, even when there is no real threat. Eventually, this heightened state of constant arousal leads to physical, mental, emotional, and spiritual exhaustion. The opposite of this sympathetic state is the relaxation response initiated by the parasympathetic system during massage. During a relaxation response, the brain enters an alpha wave state. Electrical energy in the brain is expressed in a wave-like pattern when measured by an electroencephalogram (EEG). Alpha waves are a type of brain wave that demonstrate that the brain is alert in a focused, relaxed way,

rather than watchful and wary. The body and brain both rest and recover. It is not difficult then to understand the profound effect that massage can have on the mind and emotions. Therapists witness these changes daily. A client enters the treatment room keyed up, talking loudly, breathing with shallow gulps, shoulders tense, the chest caved in as if to protect internal organs, face red, and eyes darting. After the session, the client walks slower, is quiet and composed, the skin tone is warm and even, the chest is expanded and breathing deeper. Clients say things like, "I *feel* so much better," "I can face my day again," and "I needed that break." The studies referenced in the next section provide some clinical evidence that supports what we know from our observations of clients and from our own feeling states after we receive massage.

- **Massage reduces anxiety.** Some anxiety is normal, like the fear of walking down a dark ally late at night, and goes away as soon as the situation that caused it is resolved. Other types of anxiety are related to stressful situations like an upcoming wedding, major school exam, changes at work, or divorce. In certain cases, people develop chronic anxiety disorders that persist even when the person is in a relatively safe environment. Short-term situational anxiety and even anxiety-based disorders like panic disorder and posttraumatic stress disorder respond well to massage.[66–68] Massage also decreases anxiety when it is given either alone or in combination with aromatherapy for patients about to undergo different types of surgery or for people living with cancer.[69,70]

- **Massage reduces depression.** As noted previously, massage research indicates that massage changes serotonin and dopamine levels in the body, associated with decreased depression and increased well-being. A number of studies have indicated that massage is a useful support strategy for those with depression. In one study, massage was used with acupuncture and healing touch at a community mental health center to address depression in relation to trauma recovery, perceived personal safety, boundary setting, body sensations, and body shame issues. Patients reported high levels of satisfaction with these complementary therapies, and health clinicians found that complementary therapies could improve the quality of life and enhance mental health outcomes when used alongside more traditional therapies.[71]

- **Massage reduces aggression and behavioral disorders in children and teens.** In a study of 17 aggressive adolescents, 20-minute massage sessions delivered twice a week for 5 weeks lowered the adolescents' feelings of anxiety and hostility. Parents perceived their children's behavior as less aggressive during the study period.[72] Massage therapy decreased hyperactivity scores more than relaxation therapy in a study of 28 adolescents diagnosed with ADHD. Massage benefited another group of children with ADHD, who then demonstrated improved short-term mood states and better overall classroom behavior.[73,74] A study of 20 preschool children who were described as having behavior problems demonstrated that with massage sessions provided for 15 minutes twice a week for a month, the children were less active, less talkative, and more cooperative and had lower anxiety levels than the control group at the end of the study.[75]

- **Massage improves sleep.** From young children to the elderly, research shows that massage induces sleep or improves sleeping patterns in a variety of situations from preschool environments, to hospice environments, to mental health facilities, to hospitals.[76–78]

- **Massage changes brain wave patterns.** The EEG measures brainwaves of different frequencies within the brain. Electrodes are placed on specific sites on the scalp to detect and record electrical impulses within the brain. Delta brainwaves are associated with deep relaxation and deep sleep. Alpha waves are associated with an idle state of the visual cortex and calm but alert states. Beta waves are associated with an alert, processing state. In one study that demonstrated that massage changes brain wave patterns, 36 healthy adults were assigned to one of three groups. The first received moderate-pressure massage, the second received light-pressure massage, and the third received vibratory stimulation. Anxiety and stress levels decreased in all groups, but the group who received moderate-pressure massage showed the greatest decrease in stress. The moderate massage group also demonstrated an increase in delta brain wave activity and a decrease in alpha and beta brain wave activity.[79] In another study, adolescents with EEG asymmetry (the right frontal lobe of the brain being more active than the left) tended toward depression. Massage and music therapy were used for depressed adolescents with EEG asymmetry. Both massage and music significantly lessened the right frontal lobe activation, suggesting that both therapies could be used to positively alter EEG patterns.[80]

Energetic Effects and Benefits of Massage

Different therapists view energetic effects and benefits of massage in various ways. Some view energetic effects as a new way to look at and explain physiological and psychological effects. Others believe that energetic effects occur in combination with physiological or psychological effects. Eastern medical systems like traditional Chinese medicine and ayurveda have embraced the idea of energy (life force) and its role in healing for thousands of years. Western medicine has remained skeptical, perhaps because the energetic systems of the body are difficult to study, measure, and qualify. As a therapist, you will develop your own beliefs about energy in the body, if it exists, and if it functions the way that specific massage systems describe.

This section is presented as a way to examine some currently held beliefs about energy and the way that massage is believed to influence it.

In Eastern systems, health is reflected by balanced energy that flows freely throughout the body and mind. This energy is regarded as a vital life force and known as *qi* or *chi* in Chinese, *ki* in Japanese, and *prana* in Sanskrit (ayurveda). When the energy of the body is blocked or unbalanced, disease can take root or an injury is more likely to occur. Eastern bodywork systems seek to balance the body's energy and remove energy blocks.

Eastern principles underlie many of the modern energetic bodywork practices offered by Western therapists. For example, Dr. Randolf Stone, an osteopath, naturopath, and chiropractor, developed a system called polarity therapy that shares similar ideas with many Eastern practices. He believed that positive and negative electrical charges exist at every level of universal organization, including the human body. The oscillation of energy between the two oppositely charged poles could be harnessed to help balance body energy or regulate disrupted energy to improve health.

In a Reiki session, based on Chinese medicine, the beliefs about energy are a bit different. The practitioner seeks to channel vital energy from the universe to the client's energy field (the electrical energy emitted from the body that creates an invisible field around the body) to facilitate healing. Therapeutic touch, developed by Dolores Krieger, a registered nurse and PhD, along with Dora Kunz, a mystic healer, employs laying the hands on a patient to restore balance to the energy fields so that the body can heal itself. This therapy is based on the Hindu concepts of prana and chakras. Chakras are energy centers in the body that are believed to regulate psycho-physical energy to control the flow of prana and enable physical and spiritual transformation.

Interestingly, therapeutic touch has demonstrated positive results in a number of small studies for conditions including wound healing, osteoarthritis, migraine headaches, and anxiety reduction in burn patients.[81] Energetic bodywork therapists note a wide range of empirical evidence that indicates benefits for many pathologies including heart conditions, high blood pressure, and chronic pain. It is likely that as the popularity of these therapies continues to grow with the American public, researchers will strive to test these theories scientifically.[82,83]

Students often approach energetic bodywork systems with some healthy skepticism, but many believe that they can feel changes in the body from energetic bodywork techniques. While these changes might not be explainable in scientific terms, it becomes clear that something is happening. The important thing is to try energetic techniques with an open mind and remain curious. Eastern bodywork systems are discussed in detail in Chapter 17, and energetic bodywork systems are discussed in detail in Chapter 18.

Topic **4-3**
Massage Indications

Topic 4-2 explored the effects and benefits of massage on the client's body, mind, and emotions. This topic discusses client groups and conditions for which massage is indicated. It is important to distinguish between the terms *benefit* and *indication*. A benefit is a good effect that promotes well-being, even if a specific pathology, postural dysfunction, or muscular tension pattern is not an issue. In general, massage is good for people, and people enjoy receiving massage. The term **indication** is most often used in health care massage to suggest that a particular massage system or technique will

- produce a physiological or psychological effect that is likely to reduce the symptoms related to a defined condition
- help rehabilitate a particular injury
- improve function or performance
- provide comfort during serious illness or the dying process

Shared massage knowledge and research have documented the positive effects of massage for many conditions and client populations. These positive effects *indicate* massage as a treatment strategy.

Indications for Select Client Populations and Conditions

The following sections describe the indications for select client populations and specific conditions. As massage gains popularity with the public and as more research is conducted on its benefits, physicians will likely prescribe massage for these conditions more regularly. The following sections consider common client populations but cannot include all of the conditions for which massage might be used.

Note that massage is often contraindicated for conditions in an acute stage or flare-up but is indicated for the same condition in a subacute or chronic stage. Recognizing the signs and symptoms of conditions in an acute stage is important for ensuring the safety of clients. Chapter 5 explains the critical thinking process related to ruling out contraindications in depth. Chapter 12 also describes important activities to prevent adverse outcomes, such as conducting a health intake process. Massage for many of the conditions presented briefly here is described in greater detail in other chapters. The contraindications chart in Chapter 5 is useful as a quick reference guide. Massage has been documented as beneficial and indicated for all the conditions and client populations in the following sections.

Child Abuse and Child Sexual Abuse

In a study conducted at the University of Washington of 24 adult females in psychotherapy for sexual abuse that occurred when they were children, massage, body awareness exercises, and inner-body focusing were provided in eight 1-hour sessions. The participants experienced increased psychological well-being, physical well-being, and body connection.[84] Various other studies of abuse demonstrate that massage increases self-esteem while helping balance body chemicals related to stress and depression. Massage also decreases touch aversion in infants with abusive backgrounds.[85] These effects indicate massage is a means to positive therapeutic change in people recovering from abuse.

Alzheimer's Disease

In a study of massage for agitation in Alzheimer's patients, researchers concluded that the physical expressions of agitation such as pacing, wandering, and resisting were decreased after a session of slow stroke massage.[86] Expressive physical touch and verbalization improved the quality of life of patients with dementia,[87] and a French study concluded that gentle massage increased physical relaxation, improved sleep, and decreased abnormal behavior in Alzheimer's patients within 15 minutes of the session's end.[88] Massage is indicated for condition management of Alzheimer's disease.

Anxiety Disorders

A number of studies conducted in many parts of the world confirm that massage decreases anxiety and is indicated for clients with anxiety-related conditions. As noted earlier in this chapter, massage activates the parasympathetic nervous system response and moderates chemicals that are related to stress.[89–91] Massage is indicated both for condition management and for therapeutic change for people with anxiety disorders.

Athletes

A large number of studies of massage for athletes indicate that massage improves muscle recovery time after training,[92] decrease delayed-onset soreness,[93] and decrease overall muscular fatigue from exercise exertion.[94] Massage also promotes greater muscular balance and reduces muscle tension and adhesions, which can help to prevent injury. Massage is indicated for maintenance of health or for therapeutic change in athletes.

Autism

A number of studies demonstrate that massage is a useful condition management strategy for children with autism. In one study, children 3 to 6 years old with autism were assigned to massage therapy or a reading-attention control group. Parents of children in the massage therapy group were trained by massage therapists to massage their children for 15 minutes before bedtime each night. The children in the massage group showed more on-task behavior and related better socially than those in the reading-attention control group. They also experienced fewer sleep problems at home.[95] Another study demonstrated that massage helped enhance the emotional bond between parents and their autistic child.[96]

Attention Deficit Hyperactivity Disorder

Adolescents with ADHD who received massage therapy for 10 consecutive school days rated themselves as happier. Observers rated them as less fidgety following the sessions. After 2 weeks of sessions, teachers reported that these adolescents spent more time on a task and assigned them lower hyperactivity scores based on classroom behavior.[97] A second study concluded that massage benefited children and adolescents with ADHD by improving short-term mood and classroom behavior.[98] Massage is indicated for condition management of ADHD. Other undiagnosed behavioral problems in children have also improved with massage intervention.[99]

Burns

A number of studies have shown that massage is useful for therapeutic change in people recovering from burns. It decreases itching associated with healing, effectively reduces pain, improves the mobility of scared tissue, decreases depression levels, and improves skin pigmentation and vascularity.[100,101]

Cancer

Many different massage systems (acupressure, Swedish, manual lymphatic drainage, therapeutic touch, and reflexology, among others) and other complementary therapies have been widely researched to demonstrate their usefulness in condition management of cancer. Massage systems have been shown to decrease fatigue, nausea, and vomiting after chemotherapy[102,103] and decrease pain after cancer-related surgery. In general, massage is highly indicated for the management of lymphedema, enhanced coping skills and quality of life, reduced anxiety, and increased levels of lymphocytes and killer cells to improve general immunity in people living with cancer.[104–107]

Cerebral Palsy

Massage is indicated for condition management of cerebral palsy. Children with cerebral palsy who were given massage were shown to be have reduced spasticity, less rigid muscle tone, better fine and gross motor function, increased cognition, and more positive facial expressions.[108] An effort is underway to train parents to regularly massage their children with cerebral palsy. After these training programs, parents report that their children show improved muscle tone, better joint mobility, improved sleep patterns, and more regular bowel movements. In addition, the bonding between child and parents increases, and anxiety levels for parents decrease.[109,110]

Chronic Fatigue Syndrome

Not much research has investigated massage for chronic fatigue syndrome, although people with chronic fatigue tend to seek out complementary and alternative therapies including massage for condition management.[111] In one study, people living with chronic fatigue syndrome reported lower depression, lower symptom scores, and better sleep with massage. Researchers noted that cortisol and epinephrine levels were lower after massage.[112]

Chronic Obstructive Pulmonary Disease

Dyspnea is shortness of breath and distressed breathing. People with COPDs like asthma, bronchitis, and emphysema often experience bouts of dyspnea, which leads to feelings of depression and anxiety. In one study, people received acupressure for dyspnea and showed significant decreases in dyspnea and depression. Oxygen saturation levels also improved.[113] In another study, the effects of neuromuscular release therapy were assessed in relationship to pulmonary function. Thoracic gas volume, peak flow, oxygen saturation, forced expiratory volume, and forced vital capacity were measured before and after 24-weekly treatments. Eighty percent of participants had an increase in thoracic gas volumes, peak flow, and forced vital capacity, demonstrating an improvement in overall pulmonary function.[114] In a study of adults with asthma, craniosacral therapy and acupuncture improved the quality of life and reduced the amount of medication used in a particular period.[115] Thirty-two children with asthma were randomly assigned to receive relaxation therapy or massage. The younger children who received massage demonstrated improved peak flow rate and overall pulmonary function. Massage also decreased behavioral anxiety levels. Older children also experienced decreased anxiety levels but improved only in one measure of pulmonary function (forced expiratory flow, from 25% to 75%). While the reason for the greater functional benefit in younger children over older children is unknown, all children had improved airway caliber and better control of asthma as a result of the study.[116] Massage has also proved effective as part of a pulmonary rehabilitation plan for patients with emphysema. Other components of the rehabilitation plan included relaxation techniques, breathing retraining, physical exercise, and walking.[117] Massage is indicated for condition management for people with COPDs.

Constipation

Massage promotes therapeutic change for a number of client groups with chronic constipation.[118] It promotes bowel movements for people living with spinal cord injuries,[119] the elderly,[120] and people in hospice care.[121]

Depression

Topic 4-2 discussed the effect of massage on neurotransmitters, hormones, and neurohormones. Massage changes the levels of these chemicals in the body or balances the ratios of these chemicals, leading to reduced anxiety, stress, and depression. These effects indicate massage for condition management of depression.

Eating Disorders

In a study, 19 women diagnosed with anorexia nervosa were given standard treatment and massage (two times a week for 5 weeks) or just standard treatment. The massage group had lower cortisol levels after massage and reported less stress, anxiety, and body dissatisfaction. Dopamine and norepinephrine levels were increased.[122] Massage had similar results for female adolescents with bulimia.[123] These positive psychological effects support recovery from eating disorders. Massage is indicated for therapeutic change in healing from eating disorders.[124]

Elderly Clients

Massage is indicated for elderly clients for health maintenance, therapeutic changes, condition management, and comfort depending on the individual client's health. Elderly people can suffer from aches and pains as muscle and connective tissues age and the space for nerves is reduced. Because joints are worn, conditions like osteoarthritis are more common. Massage reduces pain and helps keep muscle tissue pliable, improving the range of motion. Elderly people may suffer from depression because of chemical imbalances due to aging or medications. Massage balances out the body's chemistry related to depression and can also be used to reduce some symptoms of dementia conditions such as Alzheimer's disease. Massage stimulates digestion due to the parasympathetic nervous system response, which can help in situations of lack of appetite and weight loss.

Fibromyalgia

Massage is indicated for condition management of fibromyalgia. Research demonstrates that massage decreases the anxiety and depression that often accompanies the condition, increases sleep hours, decreases substance P levels to reduce pain, decreases the number and intensity of tender points, decreases pain scores, and improves overall physical function.[125,126]

Headaches and Migraine

Massage is indicated for therapeutic change and as condition management for clients with tension headache and migraine. Massage has helped people with chronic tension headaches and migraine control the severity of their symptoms and increase their ability to cope.[127] The occurrence of chronic tension headache and the severity of pain was reduced with regular massage of the shoulders and neck muscles.[128] Trager massage (a gentle massage system based on the work of Milton Trager, MD) reduced headache intensity and medication usage, improved the quality of life for headache sufferers, and decreased the number of migraine headaches more than medication in the control group.[129]

High Blood Pressure

Swedish or relaxation massage is associated with a decrease in both systolic and diastolic blood pressure.[130] It is indicated for condition management for hypertension.[131] Some types of massage applications can temporarily increase blood pressure (sports massage, trigger point therapy), and caution is therefore required when working with clients with high blood pressure.

HIV

Massage improves immune function in children and adults infected with HIV by increasing the numbers of natural killer cells and CD4 cells and the ratio of CD4/CD8 cells. In studies, it also decreased anxiety, decreased stress, and improved coping skills for people living with HIV.[132,133] Massage is indicated for condition management and comfort care for people with HIV.

Hospitalized Patients

Massage is indicated for condition management, therapeutic change, or comfort care of hospitalized patients depending on their disease, condition, or needs. In this case, the patient's care is likely being supervised by a physician, and the massage therapist addresses specific treatment goals as part of the health care team. Therapists must often work around medical equipment like intravenous lines or monitoring devices while the client is in the hospital bed. Massage has decreased anxiety before different types of surgery or medical procedures and is useful to improve mood, decrease stress, decrease pain, and improve emotional coping skills. Massage also benefits the coping and anxiety levels of family members whose loved ones are hospitalized.[134,135]

Hospice Patients

Massage is useful for health maintenance, therapeutic change, and condition management in hospice settings. Studies indicate that massage increases the quality of life for hospice patients while decreasing a variety of physical and emotional symptoms.[136] Furthermore, massage used as a regular stress-reduction strategy for hospice caregivers promoted their better care of hospice patients.[137]

Infants

Massage is indicated for preterm infants, healthy full-term infants, and full-term infants with medical conditions for therapeutic change or condition management. Massage supports weight gain, cognitive development, and parent–child interaction and improves sleep hours.[138–140] For infants or young children who have been exposed to HIV, cocaine, or abuse, or who have medical conditions like asthma, autism, cancer, skin conditions, rheumatoid arthritis, psychiatric problems, or stress disorders, massage reduces stress hormones, lowers anxiety levels, and leads to less colic and fewer episodes of crying.[141,142]

Insomnia

Massage is indicated for therapeutic change and condition management for insomnia and irregular sleep cycles. Massage increases sleep hours for the elderly, critically ill patients, infants, and preschool children. Massage is likely to be effective for irregular sleep because it triggers the parasympathetic nervous system and encourages the body to rest.[143–145]

Irritable Bowel Syndrome

According to the National Institutes of Diabetes and Digestive and Kidney Diseases, irritable bowel syndrome (IBS) affects 20% of Americans and is directly influenced by stress.[146] Although no American studies have directly demonstrated that massage is indicated for IBS, research in China and Germany show that massage, acupressure, and abdominal massage decrease IBS symptoms.[147,148] It is likely that relaxation massage as condition management and for therapeutic change will prove beneficial for clients with IBS. As each client's experience of IBS is different, you will want to work carefully to ensure that massage does not exacerbate the condition.

Multiple Sclerosis

In one study, two massage sessions provided for 45 minutes each for 5 weeks reduced anxiety and depressed mood in people living with multiple sclerosis. Increased self-esteem, better body image, and enhanced social function were also noted.[149] In another study, reflexology improved paresthesias (sensations of tingling, prickling, or numbness in a person's skin), urinary symptoms, and spasticity in people living with multiple sclerosis. Improvement in the intensity of paresthesias remained significant at the 3-month follow-up after the study.[150] Note that massage can overstimulate or overheat clients with multiple sclerosis and cause the condition to flare up into an acute state.[151] In the subacute stage, massage is indicated for condition management of multiple sclerosis.

Overuse and Soft-Tissue Injuries

Topic 4-2 illustrated the powerful effects of massage for muscle tissue, connective tissue, and joint health. These effects indicate massage for an array of overuse and soft-tissue conditions. For example, thoracic outlet syndrome is a condition in which the brachial plexus (the nerve bundle that innervates the upper extremity) and the blood vessels running to or from the arm are impinged by the anterior and middle scalene muscles, the pectoralis minor, or the clavicle and first rib. Because tight muscles and poor posture can play a significant role in this condition, massage proves highly useful to create positive therapeutic change. An Italian study confirmed the positive results that massage therapists often note for thoracic outlet syndrome.[152] In a study to test the efficiency of massage in the treatment of carpal tunnel syndrome, 16 adults with carpal tunnel were randomly assigned either to 4 weeks of massage therapy or to a control group. The treatment included daily self-massage (clients massage themselves) and massage

with a therapist once a week. The massage group experienced improved grip strength, lower levels of pain, less anxiety, and better mood than the control group.[153] Massage is indicated for condition management and therapeutic change for a wide variety of overuse and soft-tissue injuries.

Osteoarthritis

Osteoarthritis is a wear-and-tear condition in which damage to articular cartilage in a joint causes inflammation, pain, and decreased range of motion. If the joint is inflamed and shows signs of redness, warmth, and swelling, massage is contraindicated. Typically, massage is useful to balance muscles around the affected joint and release tight muscles, tendons, and fascia, increasing the range of motion. Studies on the usefulness of massage as condition management for osteoarthritis have positive results.[154]

Pain Management

Topic 4-2 described the gate theory of pain management, the decrease of substance P that occurs as a result of massage, and the break in the pain-spasm-pain cycle brought about by massage. The following three studies on the benefits of massage for pain reduction are just a small sample of research in this area. In the first study, 262 patients with back pain were treated with 10 massage visits, 10 acupuncture visits, or self-care educational materials. The massage group scored higher on decreased symptoms and disability than either the acupuncture or self-care groups, and the massage group used less pain medication as a result.[155] In the second study, 33 people with a history of chronic headache (at least one headache per week for 6 months) received Trager massage or no treatment. The group receiving Trager massage had a significant decrease in the frequency of headaches and a 44% reduction in the use of pain medications.[156] In the third study, 19 patients and a control group of 20 patients were studied to determine the impact of massage on patients' perceptions of postoperative pain. Massage produced a significant reduction in patients' perception of pain over a 24-hour period.[157] Massage is indicated for pain management or pain reduction.

Pregnancy and Labor

A women's pregnant body undergoes extensive physical and emotional changes while she carries and delivers the baby. While pregnancy and labor are not pathologies, massage is an effective way to lessen the discomfort of some of these changes and promote greater emotional and spiritual balance. Massage is indicated for back pain and sore muscles from posture changes during the pregnancy, for stress reduction, and during labor to decrease pain and increase coping. In one study, 28 pregnant women were randomly assigned to receive massage and breath coaching from their partners during labor or to receive only breath coaching. The massage group reported significantly less pain and shorter labor, a shorter hospital stay, and less postpartum depression.[158] Prenatal depression can have negative effects on the fetus and newborn. The fetuses of depressed women have demonstrated elevated activity, delayed growth, lower birth-weight, and greater incidence of premature birth. Infants of depressed mothers have body chemistry consistent with depression, including increased cortisol levels and decreased serotonin and dopamine levels. Moderate-pressure massage has been used successfully to relieve depression and has led to a lower incidence of premature birth.[159]

Premenstrual Syndrome

In a study of massage for women with premenstrual syndrome, massage decreased the anxiety, depressed mood, pain, and water retention experienced by 24 women.[160] Another study showed that regular reflexology sessions using reflex points on the hand, feet, and ears significantly reduced the premenstrual symptoms of the women.[161] It is likely that massage can be used as condition management for premenstrual syndrome.

Skin Conditions

Some research studies indicate that regular massage improves some skin conditions such as dermatitis and eczema. In one study, children were massaged once a week by massage therapists for 8 consecutive weeks. One group was massaged with essential oils, while another received just massage. The symptoms of eczema significantly improved in both groups following the study, but there was no significant difference between the essential oil group and just massage group.[162] In a study to determine whether massage can decrease the symptoms of atopic dermatitis in young children, parents massaged their children daily for a 1-month period. The control group received standard topical care but no massage. The children who received massage improved significantly in all clinical measurements (redness, scaling, itching, etc.) during the study.[163] Massage is well known as an effective treatment to reduce scar tissue and to stimulate the sebaceous glands and desquamate dead skins cells to improve the condition, appearance, and health of the skin.

Stress

The physiological and psychological impact of chronic **stress** on people is discussed in depth in Topic 4-4. Massage can play an important role in the management of stress by activating the parasympathetic nervous system response and supporting the normalization of body chemistry related to stress. In one study, aromatherapy massage significantly reduced the anxiety levels of emergency nurses.[164] In another study to demonstrate that massage could reduce work-related stress, 26 people received chair massage for 15 minutes twice a week while a control group was asked to relax in a chair. Both groups demonstrated EEG signs of relaxation, but the massage group had increased alpha waves suggesting enhanced alertness. The massage group had increased speed and accuracy on math computations, while the scores of the control group did not change. These results show the benefit of stress-management programs for improved work performance.[165] Children with behavioral problems related to posttraumatic stress from Hurricane Andrew reported being happier and less anxious after receiving massage and had lower salivary cortisol levels than the control group.[166] Massage is indicated as condition management and for therapeutic change for stress. Conditions that are exacerbated by elevated stress levels are also likely to respond positively to massage intervention.

Substance Abuse (Recovery From)

Some evidence shows that massage can support the recovery process of substance abusers. In one study, acupressure was offered once a week for 6 weeks at a community mental health program for drug users recovering from substance abuse. The acupressure group had reduced craving and anxiety compared to the control group.[167] Massage also shows promise as an adjunct therapy to traditional medical detoxification from alcohol. Alcohol withdrawal symptoms in the early stages of detoxification were reduced when weekly massage was provided.[168] Self-massage is a viable support therapy for smoking cessation to reduce anxiety and cravings.[169]

Temporomandibular Joint Dysfunction

In one study, massage along with heat application, ultrasound, and muscle stretching decreased pain and improved jaw function in patients with TMJ dysfunction.[170]

As we can see from this small sample of massage for selected conditions, massage can act as an intervention and support wellness for the general public and for specific populations of clients.

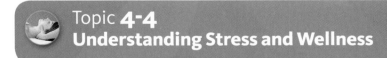

Topic **4-4**
Understanding Stress and Wellness

Wellness is a difficult word to define. It refers to all aspects of a person's life including a state of positive health, a sense of satisfaction with quality of life, and an active process of self-awareness and making choices toward a more meaningful and successful existence. Wellness programs can be adopted to help structure a person's choices that lead to well-being. An important aspect of any wellness program is stress management. This topic first explains stress and stress management and then wellness models and discusses the way massage therapists might use wellness models in their practices.

Understanding Stress

Throughout this book, stress is referred to in relationship to other massage topics. Stress is likely to influence every client you work with to some degree and can also be a factor in your health and happiness as a therapist. It is essential that every massage therapist understand stress in order to recognize the benefit of massage and the impact that massage can have on various conditions and diseases, on general health, and on a person's sense of wellness.

Stress Defined

In the broadest sense, **stress** is any event that threatens homeostasis and causes the body to adapt. With this broad meaning in mind, we understand that stress is caused by any change in external temperature, water intake, physical exertion like that during aerobic exercise, changes to diet, or even positive excitement like that experienced at a sporting event. Physiologists point out that while the reaction of the body to exposure to cold temperature is different from its reaction to fighting an infection, and different from its reaction to an event that causes anxiety and fear, in one respect all of these types of stress are the same. They all cause the secretion of cortisol by the adrenal cortex to increase. Therefore, physiologists define stress as any event that causes increased cortisol secretion.[171]

This topic focuses more specifically on stress caused by an event that triggers the **flight-or-fight response**. The flight-or-fight response is a full-body reaction mediated by the sympathetic nervous system as an inborn, automatic reflex to any perceived danger. It has protected people throughout evolutionary history by rapidly preparing the body to respond to a life-threatening event (e.g., animal attack). The problem is that the body cannot differentiate between a hypothetical threat that might be caused by something like an unpaid bill and a genuine threat where immediate action is required to survive. It is possible for the flight-or-fight response to be triggered multiple times in a day by non-life-threatening events such as sitting in traffic, being late for a job interview, worries about finances, or relationship issues. Furthermore, people are socialized to behave certain ways. You might get the full-body adrenalin rush of the flight-or-fight response when a coworker challenges you at work, but you would be unlikely to act on it. You would not run away or beat him up. Instead you suppress your physical and emotional responses with muscular, mental, and emotional tension to avoid acting in a socially unacceptable way.

Stress that triggers the flight-or-fight response can be further categorized based on its origin or duration. The cause of stress can be mental (e.g., negative speculation about the reaction of your boss to a complaint filed by a customer),

emotional (e.g., grief over the death of a loved one), or physical (e.g., pain from a soft-tissue injury can trigger the flight-or-fight response). It can be short-lived, lasting a few minutes to a few hours (e.g., you mistake your father standing in a dark room for an intruder), or chronic (e.g., you are under constant pressure at work and do your best each day to suppress it).

The regular activation of the flight-or-fight response can lead to elevated levels of stress-related chemicals like epinephrine (adrenaline) and cortisol in the bloodstream that remain for prolonged periods of time (sometimes referred to as adrenaline and cortisol poisoning). In this situation, these chemicals become destructive to the body and can lead to stress-related disorders like high blood pressure, heart diseases, ulcers, impaired immunity, and even psychological changes in personality and behavior (e.g., increased aggression or defensive behavior).

Concept Brief 4-5
Stress Defined

In the broadest sense, stress is defined as any event that threatens homeostasis and causes the body to adapt. Physiologists define stress as any event that causes increased cortisol secretion. Massage therapists are most concerned with stress caused by an event that triggers the flight-or-fight response.

The Anatomy and Chemistry of Stress

The flight-or-fight response is mediated by the sympathetic division of the autonomic nervous system, which is the automatic part of the nervous system that cannot be controlled voluntarily. It controls smooth muscle, cardiac muscle, and certain glands. It is regulated by the cerebral cortex, hypothalamus, and medulla oblongata and has sympathetic and parasympathetic divisions. The sympathetic division is the part of the nervous system that activates arousal responses during emergency situations or any state of high excitement, including nonemergency situations such as might be experienced at a sporting event or during elation or joy states. The parasympathetic division is the part of the nervous system responsible for restoring the body's resources during nonemergency states of rest (relaxation response).

The Limbic System and Stress

The limbic system consists of the hypothalamus, thalamus, hippocampus, and portions of the cerebrum. This group of structures that encircle the brainstem function in the emotional aspects of behavior related to survival. The thalamus serves as a relay station for sensory information (with the exception of smell) traveling to the cerebral cortex. It also interprets sensory impulses related to pain, temperature, light touch, and pressure. It also has some function related to processing emotion and memory. The hypothalamus is involved in homeostatic regulation of the autonomic nervous system related to body temperature, water balance, appetite, sleep, and key emotions like fear and pleasure. It receives impulses from sound, taste, and smell, and from neurons monitoring the internal environment of the body. It is the primary connection between the nervous system and endocrine system. A stressor causes a cascade of rapid physiological reactions that facilitate the flight-or-fight response.

Physiological Reactions in the Flight-or-Fight Response

When a threat is perceived by the limbic system, it stimulates the hypothalamus causing the hypothalamus to release corticotrophin-releasing hormone (CRH) into the blood stream. CRH reaches the anterior pituitary gland and causes it to secrete adrenocorticotrophic hormone (ACTH) into the blood stream. ACTH circulates to the adrenal glands and causes them to release epinephrine (adrenaline) and cortisol into the bloodstream, which then circulate throughout the body and stimulate a range of responses in different body tissues (Fig. 4-15). Research has discovered that ACTH not only stimulates the secretion of cortisol but also is a peptide related to learning and memory. We can speculate that ACTH served an evolutionary purpose in helping early humans learn to avoid danger.

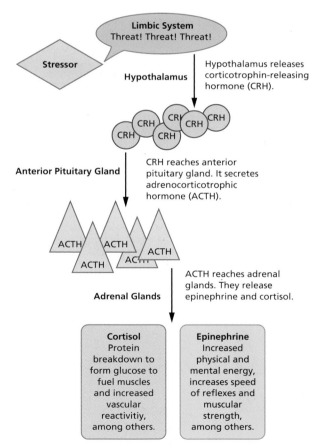

Figure 4-15 Stress causes rapid chemical changes that lead to physiological changes that facilitate the flight-or-fight response.

Cortisol is a hormone that promotes the breakdown of proteins to form glucose to fuel muscles. The action to mobilize fuels has some important implications for health. For example, a person who is sick or undergoes surgery catabolizes (breaks down) considerable amounts of body protein, while a child exposed to prolonged and severe stress experiences retarded growth. Cortisol enhances vascular reactivity, decreases white blood cell accumulation and fibroblasts in an area of injury to reduce inflammation, and has a powerful anti-allergenic action. Cortisol can also reduce the number of circulating lymphocytes in the bloodstream. It decreases both antibody production and the activity of T cells, explaining why people are more prone to colds when they are stressed.

Epinephrine plays a central role in the sensation of physical and mental energy associated with the flight-or-fight response. It sharpens the senses, increases the speed of reflexes, and boosts muscular strength. It triggers many of the responses that rapidly prepare the body for a threat, such as an increased heart rate. The flight-or-fight response produces a range of rapid changes in the body to ensure the body can respond to a threat:

- The pupils of the eyes dilate to let in more light to sharpen vision.
- The heart rate and the force of the heart's contractions both increase, and the blood pressure rises. This ensures that blood is pumped effectively to large muscle groups and to the brain so that the body can respond with maximum effort.
- The blood vessels of the skin and viscera constrict to ensure adequate blood flow for skeletal muscles, the heart, and the lungs. Blood to the hands and feet is restricted to ensure that large quantities of blood would not be lost in the event these extremities were severely injured fighting or fleeing.
- Rapid breathing occurs and the bronchioles dilate to allow for the faster movement of air in and out of the lungs.
- Blood sugar levels increase as glycogen in the liver is converted to glucose to supply the body's energy needs.
- Muscle tone increases and the body's reflexes become hair triggered for quicker responses.
- Nonessential processes such as the muscular movements of the gastrointestinal tract and digestive secretions are slowed or halted.
- Perspiration increases to cool the body, which becomes hotter due to a rise in metabolic processes.

When the body is in a state of homeostasis, the sympathetic nervous system counteracts the effects of the parasympathetic nervous system just enough to carry out normal processes requiring energy. When the body experiences chronic stress, the sympathetic system dominates the parasympathetic system, contributing to or causing many diseases and conditions (Fig. 4-16).

Concept Brief 4-6
Flight-or-Fight Response

- The body's response to a perceived threat (run away or stay and fight)
- Mediated by the sympathetic division of the autonomic nervous system
- Causes a cascade of rapid physiological reactions to facilitate survival
- Chronic stress is a situation where persistent stressors repeatedly trigger the flight-or-fight response leading to the prolonged elevation of stress hormones, especially cortisol and epinephrine, in the bloodstream, negatively impacting health

Chronic Stress and Implications for Health

Chronic stress is a situation in which persistent stressors repeatedly trigger the flight-or-fight response leading to the prolonged elevation of stress hormones, especially cortisol and epinephrine in the blood stream. These hormones, when not used in a real emergency, wear down the body's systems. For example, cortisol can cause the body to digest its own proteins, leading to decreased immunity, sleep disturbances, and an increase of substance P (related to the sensation of pain). When a threat has passed, epinephrine that has not been reabsorbed produces a shaky, nauseous, pumped up after-feeling. In situations of chronic stress, epinephrine causes over-stimulation of the autonomic nervous system and adrenal exhaustion associated with fatigue and mental weariness. These hormones are linked to conditions like high blood pressure, gastric ulcers, suppression of the immune system, and mood or personality changes.

It is possible that the weakest areas of the body, perhaps from an old injury or because of genetic predisposition, show wear and dysfunction from chronic stress first. A body under constant stress becomes more susceptible to infections and disease. People adapt quickly to challenging situations and may not recognize that symptoms such as insomnia, chronic tension headaches, or heartburn are related to stress. Massage therapists often deal with habitual tension patterns in muscles. "Bracing" physically against nonphysical, psychological threats may very well be at the root of a good deal of physical tension. One researcher speculates that in cancer the body would normally eliminate a mutant cell, but if the system is dysfunctional because of hormonal imbalances due to stress, the cell may take hold and develop into a tumor.[172]

Stressors

The term **stressor** was coined by Hans Selye, a researcher who first defined stress, and refers to any stimulus that produces

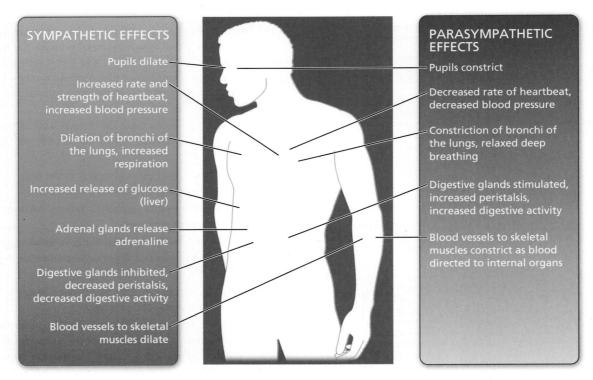

Figure 4-16 Balance of the sympathetic and parasympathetic nervous systems. When the body is in a state of homeostasis, the sympathetic nervous system counteracts the effects of the parasympathetic nervous system just enough to carry out normal processes requiring energy. When the body experiences chronic stress, the flight-or-fight response is repeatedly triggered and the sympathetic system dominates the parasympathetic system, contributing to or causing many diseases and conditions.

stress. Stressors are unique to individuals and increase or decrease in strength based on the surrounding situation. A stressor for one person may not produce stress in another. If you perceive something as a threat (whether real or imagined) and it produces the emotions of anxiety, fear, anger, or grief, it is considered a stressor. Something that you perceive as stressful today may not cause you stress tomorrow, because stressors are influenced by factors such as your mental-emotional state of mind, your physical health, the culture you grew up in, your past experiences, coping strategies, and even what you had for lunch (such as a double latte loaded with caffeine). Researchers note that stressors can often be defined as too much or too little of certain types of external stimuli. For example, extreme heat, cold, loud music, bright lights, and too much exposure to social situations or technology can

be stressors. Alternately, too much quiet and a lack of social interaction can also be stressors.[173]

STRESSOR SCALE

Psychiatrists Thomas Holmes and Richard Rahe developed a scale for rating stressors in 1967. The pair examined the medical records of approximately 7,000 patients to determine if stressful life events could cause illness.[174] The patients were asked to tally a list of life events based on a scoring system, and a strong correlation was found between these events and their illnesses. In the Holmes and Rahe Stress Scale, a specific number of "Life Change Units" are associated with each life event (Table 4-1). An adapted scale was created later to better assess the stress levels of young adults or children with different life experiences (Table 4-2). In the original scale,

TABLE 4-1   Original Holmes and Rahe Stress Scale

Life Event	Life Change Unit	Your Score (leave the space blank if you have not experienced this life event in the last year)
Death of a spouse	100	
Divorce	73	
Marital separation	65	
Imprisonment	63	
Death of a close family member	63	
Personal injury or illness	53	
Marriage	50	
Dismissal from work	47	
Marital reconciliation	45	
Retirement	45	
Change in health of a family member	44	
Pregnancy	40	
Sexual difficulties	39	
Gain a new family member	39	
Business readjustment	39	
Change in financial state	38	
Change in frequency of arguments	35	
Major mortgage	32	
Foreclosure of mortgage or loan	30	
Change in responsibilities at work	29	
Child leaving home	29	
Trouble with in-laws	29	
Outstanding personal achievement	28	
Spouse starts or stops work	26	
Begin or end school	26	
Change in living conditions	25	

(Continued)

TABLE 4-1   Original Holmes and Rahe Stress Scale *(Continued)*

Life Event	Life Change Unit	Your Score (leave the space blank if you have not experienced this life event in the last year)
Revision of personal habits	24	
Trouble with boss	23	
Change in working hours or conditions	20	
Change in residence	20	
Change in schools	20	
Change in recreation	19	
Change in church activities	19	
Change in social activities	18	
Minor mortgage or loan	17	
Change in sleeping habits	16	
Change in number of family reunions	15	
Change in eating habits	15	
Vacation	13	
Christmas	12	
Minor violation of the law	11	

the death of a spouse is extremely stressful and represents 100 life change units, while the minor violation of a law is far less stressful and represents 11 life change units. To take the assessment, people mark the life events that they have experienced in the most recent year and tabulate the associated life change units. A score of 300 or more indicates high stress and a high risk of illness. A score of 150 to 299 indicates moderate stress and a moderate risk of illness (reduced by 30% from the high rating), and a score of 149 or lower indicates lower stress and a low risk of illness. You can tabulate your personal stress score for this year by filling in the right-hand column in either the original scale or the adapted scale for younger adults and children and adding up the life change units.

Stress-Related Illnesses

If you review the glands and organs affected by the autonomic nervous system, it makes sense that stress affects every body system on some level. For example

- **Integumentary system:** Skin disorders like psoriasis and atopic dermatitis are worsened by stress. Some forms of hair loss are linked to stress. Neurodermitis is a skin disorder that causes severe itching of the skin and is likely caused by an overactive sympathetic nervous system and the subsequent imbalance in the endocrine system related to stress.

- **Musculoskeletal system:** Muscle tension is increased when the body is under stress, and this may lead to chronic tension patterns and postural imbalances. Conditions like TMJ disorder may be caused or worsened by stress.

- **Nervous system:** Anxiety is a normal response to stress, but if stress is prolonged a number of disorders can develop such as panic disorder, posttraumatic stress disorder, and social anxiety disorder. Stress also plays a role in depression and mood disorders.

- **Digestive system:** Brief bouts of stress (e.g., a presentation at work) may cause short digestive system reactions such as a stomach ache, nausea, or diarrhea. Gastritis, stomach and duodenal ulcers, colitis, and IBS are closely associated with chronic stress.

- **Urinary system:** While urinary retention (problems emptying the bladder) has many possible causes, one of them is stress. Stress can also worsen conditions including interstitial cystitis (painful bladder syndrome), in which the bladder wall becomes irritated and inflamed.

- **Reproductive system:** CRH released during the flight-or-fight response inhibits the release of gonadotrophin-releasing hormone (GnRH). GnRH is the hormone that directs reproduction and sexual behavior. Cortisol inhibits the release of luteinizing hormone, which stimulates ovulation and sperm release, and hinders the production of male and female sex hormones like testosterone, estrogen, and progesterone. Stress levels influence infertility, menstrual disorders, and sexual disorders.

- **Endocrine system:** As we discussed earlier, stress can cause imbalances in powerful hormones that help regulate many body functions. The adrenal glands can go through three different phases as they attempt to deal with chronic stress. In the first stage (adrenal adaptation), the adrenals increase the

TABLE 4-2   Adapted Holmes and Rahe Stress Scale

Life Event	Life Change Unit	Your Score (leave the space blank if you have not experienced this life event in the last year)
Getting married	101	
Unwed pregnancy	92	
Death of parent	87	
Acquiring a visible deformity	81	
Divorce of parents	77	
Fathering an unwed pregnancy	77	
Becoming involved with drugs or alcohol	76	
Jail sentence of parent for over 1 y	75	
Marital separation of parents	69	
Death of brother or sister	68	
Change in acceptance by peers	67	
Pregnancy of unwed sister	64	
Discovery of being an adopted child	63	
Marriage of parent to step parent	63	
Death of close friend	63	
Having a visible congenital deformity	62	
Serious illness requiring hospitalization	58	
Failure of a grade in school	56	
Not making an extracurricular activity	55	
Hospitalization of a parent	55	
Jail sentence of parent for over 30 d	53	
Breaking up with boyfriend or girlfriend	53	
Beginning to date	51	
Suspension from school	50	
Birth of brother or sister	50	
Increase in arguments between parents	47	
Loss of job by a parent	46	
Outstanding personal achievement	46	
Change in parent's financial status	45	
Accepted at college of choice	43	
Being a senior in high school	42	
Hospitalization of a brother or sister	41	
Increased absence of parent from home	38	
Brother or sister leaving home	37	
Addition of third adult to the family	34	
Becoming a full-fledged member of church	31	
Decrease in arguments between parents	27	
Decrease in arguments with parents	26	
Parent beginning work	26	

production of stress hormones resulting in digestive issues, jitteriness, weight gain, menstrual problems, and sleep disturbances. In the second stage (adrenal maladaption), the adrenal glands slow down resulting in fatigue, loss of sexual drive, fluid retention, and hair loss. The third stage (adrenal exhaustion) is associated with conditions like fibromyalgia, severe constipation, depression, memory loss, joint pain, and panic attacks. Thyroid disorders are also closely linked to stress.

- **Cardiovascular system:** Research indicates that stress contributes to sustained elevation of blood pressure as well as triggering or aggravating cardiovascular pathologies like coronary heart disease, angina, and ischemic cardiopathy, among others.
- **Lymphatic and immune system:** Stress makes people more susceptible to common illness and can impair the body's inflammatory response. Conditions involving excessive inflammation, like allergic, autoimmune, cardiovascular, infectious, and rheumatologic illnesses are exacerbated by stress. People experiencing chronic stress recover more slowly from a wide variety of diseases and conditions.
- **Respiratory system:** Asthma symptoms worsen under increased levels of stress.

Dr. Barbara Brown notes in *Stress and the Art of Biofeedback* that disease that results from stress is the consequence of a very complex interaction of psychological, constitutional, genetic, and environmental factors. The pattern is unique to each person.[175] As Selye noted, the body is capable of adaptation and a return to homeostasis if the stressor is removed or lessened. For instance, once the alarm stage has passed, the adrenal glands return to their normal rates of secreting hormones. If the stressor continues to be active, however, adaptation and resistance lead to a stage of exhaustion and the body becomes highly vulnerable to disease and accelerated aging. Table 4-3 lists some symptoms associated with stress, and Box 4-3 lists some common conditions related to or exacerbated by stress.

Stress Management

While it is unlikely that stress can be completely eliminated from life, people can learn how to manage stress and lead healthier lives. Stress management is often part of a wellness program (covered later). If you can learn to manage stress in your own life, you will be better prepared to support clients who are seeking to reduce stress. These basic activities can help

- **Identify stressors:** When you identify the stressors in your life, you may become more conscious of the choices you make each day that increase your stress levels. Sometimes just the awareness that a stressor is a stressor can minimize its effects.
- **Make changes:** Some stressors can be eliminated completely once they are identified. For example, if you carpool with Sally who constantly complains about your driving, the weather, her boss, and family obligations, causing you stress before work, you might simply choose not to carpool any longer. If a stressor cannot be eliminated, can it be

TABLE 4-3   Symptoms of Stress

Body Symptoms	Mental/Emotional Symptoms	Behavioral Symptoms
Chest pain	Anger	Alcohol abuse
Constipation	Anxiety	Blaming others
Diarrhea	Depression	Decreased productivity
Fatigue	Dissatisfaction	Defensive behaviors
Headache	Feelings of insecurity	Drug abuse
Heart palpitations	Forgetfulness	Emotional outbursts
High blood pressure	Guilt	Increased smoking
Jaw pain	Irritability	Overeating
Muscle aches and pain	Lack of concentration	Relationship conflicts
Perspiration	Mental confusion	Social withdrawal
Sexual dysfunction	Mental fatigue	Underrating
Shortness of breath	Mood swings	
Skin conditions	Negative thinking	
Tooth grinding	Resentment	
Upset stomach	Restlessness	
Weight gain	Sadness	
Weight loss	Worry	

BOX 4-3 Some Common Conditions and Diseases Associated with Stress

- Alcoholism
- Anxiety attacks
- Asthma
- Chronic fatigue syndrome
- Colds and flu
- Depression
- Drug abuse
- Dystonia
- Eating disorders
- Eczema
- Heart disease
- High blood pressure
- Insomnia

- Insulin resistance
- Menstrual disorders
- Migraine headache
- Panic disorder
- Peptic ulcers
- Posttraumatic stress disorder
- Postpartum depression
- Rosacea
- Teeth grinding (bruxism)
- Temporomandibular joint disorder
- Tension headache
- Urinary retention or incontinence

minimized? If you have a tight deadline at work that's causing stress, can you negotiate an extension? If you find an environmental situation stressful, can you lessen the stress you feel by taking a walk around the block?

- **Increase emotional self-awareness:** The flight-or-fight response is triggered by a perceived threat whether real or imagined. Are you blowing a stressful situation out of proportion and making yourself feel worse with negative self-talk? You can learn techniques to soothe yourself and put yourself in problem-solving mode. By paying attention to emotions and self-talk, you can reduce your stress.
- **Build physical reserves:** A healthy diet and regular exercise help protect you against stress and allow your body to cope more effectively when it is stressed. Avoid nicotine and excessive caffeine and maintain a consistent sleep schedule of no <8 hours per night.
- **Build emotional reserves:** Research shows that a supportive network of friends and family members can help manage stress and improve health.[176] You can also build your emotional reserves by being kind and gentle with yourself and giving yourself praise and encouragement.
- **Activate the parasympathetic nervous system regularly:** As you know, the parasympathetic nervous system response sends the body into rest and recovery mode. Activities like breathing exercises, yoga, meditation, positive visualization, and massage trigger the parasympathetic system. Regular participation in these activities can help combat stress.

Stress and Massage

We already know that massage activates the parasympathetic nervous system, which balances out the sympathetic nervous system once a danger has passed and helps the body to unwind and recuperate. The parasympathetic nervous system slows the heart rate and is associated with relaxed breathing patterns. It stimulates the formation and release of urine and the activity of the digestive system so that the body can nourish and detoxify itself. This response is important for reducing all types of stress and allowing the body's chemistry to normalize. Massage also helps the body normalize the levels of cortisol and epinephrine. As noted earlier, massage lowers cortisol and has a balancing action on the adrenal glands.[177,178] Massage has been shown to reduce epinephrine levels and quench the fight-or-flight response in patients about to undergo surgery.[179] It has also normalized epinephrine levels (and other chemicals) in depressed adolescent mothers.[180] Massage is a key stress-management tool that helps the body return to normal homeostasis and optimal function.

Understanding Wellness

As mentioned earlier, wellness is difficult to define precisely, although it can simply be described as a state of being comfortable, healthy, and happy while making daily choices that lead to more self-fulfillment, meaning, and success. Wellness is broad and multidimensional. For example, physical health is only one aspect of wellness. Even top athletes in the prime of their careers have difficulty finding the balance necessary for true well-being. A strong focus on physical fitness may override other important wellness components, or their training schedules may be so intense that minor or major injuries develop. Wellness is as much a state of mind and spirit as it is a state of body. It requires a balance between work time and playtime, solid interpersonal relationships, and strong emotional coping resources. Meaningful work, family activities, social interaction, and personal interests help life feel purposeful and enjoyable. Wellness requires good choices and some effort. People seeking wellness eat a healthy diet but allow themselves to splurge once in a while. They get regular sleep and take strides to manage stress, nurture relationships, pursue personal interests, and remain open and positive about life's ups and downs. Because massage is an activity that people can undertake to move toward greater wellness, it is helpful to understand wellness models. The implementation of a wellness model is also useful to massage therapists as a form of self-care.

Wellness Models

Many people use wellness models to help them focus on areas of life that feel out of balance. A wellness model is a chart, program, or document that offers basic criteria for optimum function in specific life areas and provides questions that help people explore wellness in their own lives. Sometimes, health care practitioners use a wellness model as part of their assessment and goal setting with clients. Many destination spas use a wellness concept. Clients receive a consultation that includes the development of a wellness plan for their life. The client's treatments, menu, seminars, and activities are then designed in accordance with the wellness plan.

Administering a wellness model in a private massage practice is not appropriate unless you have additional training and credentials and define the session appropriately, because otherwise you will be outside the scope of massage therapy. That focus could lead the therapist to ask information about a client's life that is not pertinent to the massage. It can also place the therapist in a situation where the client expects psychological or spiritual counseling. Some therapists find that they can introduce clients to wellness concepts without moving outside their scope of practice by providing a wellness model as a handout that clients can take home if they are interested. In other cases, a massage therapist is expected to act as part of a client's wellness team and interact with other health professionals while supporting the client's wellness goals.

Wellness components and wellness planning are described here to help you broaden your understanding of the benefits and role of massage. Massage therapists may be included in

a client's wellness plan at spas and clinics, and so must be versed in wellness concepts. This model can also be useful in your personal self-care routine, helping you maintain a long massage career.

Components of a Wellness Model

Wellness models vary somewhat, but all usually address three main areas: physical health, mental health, and spiritual health (Fig. 4-17). Figure 4-18 shows a common wellness model that promotes healthy nutrition, physical fitness, stress management, and emotional balance. As people contemplate what they need in life to feel well-being, the wellness model adapts to include areas they view as important. Figure 4-19 shows a wellness model that incorporates a focus on personal relationships and meaningful work. In Figure 4-20, the wellness model is well defined and includes social, environmental, and occupational areas of focus. It is personal and written in clients' own language to best reflect their goals and areas for focus.

It helps to consider wellness in six key areas, though many different grouping methods can be used. For example, Figure 4-20 breaks wellness down into seven areas that require awareness. These examples show that there is no one best structure for a wellness model. Each person and therefore each model will be unique. Questions are developed for each wellness area and used to inventory a person's current state of wellness. When people have insight into their state of wellness, they can set goals to improve in areas they feel motivated to change. Following are six key areas of wellness providing questions for exploration.

PHYSICAL WELLNESS

In any wellness plan, the health and fitness of the physical body are an important focus, and nutrition, exercise, sleep, and relaxation strategies might be explored. Sample questions include:

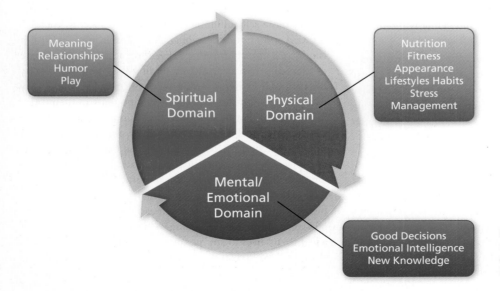

Figure 4-17 This basic wellness models include areas focused on physical, mental, and spiritual health.

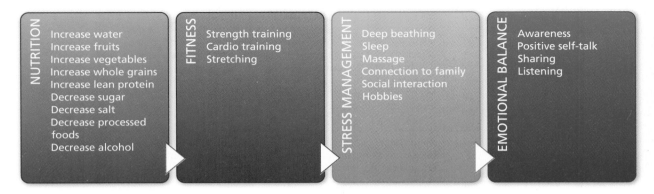

Figure 4-18 This wellness model is developed to include a focus on stress management and emotional balance.

- Do I have a basic understanding of nutrition and recognize the nutritional needs of my body?
- Is my diet nutritious and filled with healthy foods like vegetables, fruits, lean proteins, and whole grains? How can I improve the nutritional content of my diet?
- Do I avoid highly processed foods high in sugar, salt, or chemical additives or eat these only in moderation? What foods might I eliminate from my diet to improve my health?
- Do I consume alcohol only in moderation?
- Does my body receive the vitamins and nutrients it needs for optimal function? How can I ensure that I get the vitamins and nutrients I need?
- Is tobacco or another addictive substance causing a decrease in my health? What actions can I take to eliminate tobacco or other addictive substances from my life?
- Do I participate in regular exercise that builds strength, endurance, flexibility, balance, and coordination? What type of exercise plan might I adopt to ensure my body's health?

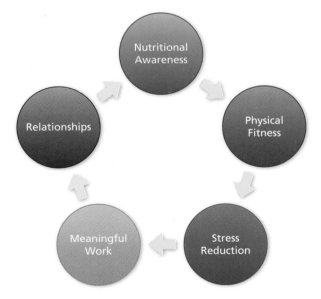

Figure 4-19 Personal relationships and meaningful work are important additions to this wellness model.

- Do I maintain a regular sleep schedule with no <8 hours of sleep per night?
- Do I use relaxation strategies regularly to combat stress and revitalize my body? What improvements might I make in this area?
- Do I receive regular medical check-ups? Do I participate in personal self-care and monitor physical symptoms that might be warning signs of diseases or conditions?

INTELLECTUAL WELLNESS

Intellectual growth, curiosity, challenges, creative expression, and a positive self-concept are explored as an important part of the overall well-being of a person. Self-concept or self-esteem is a belief about oneself that enhances coping skills and leads to good feelings about oneself and the ability to impact others in a positive way. Sample questions related to intellectual wellness might include:

- Do I regularly expose myself to new experiences in order to enhance my understanding of the world (e.g., the theatre, a lecture on world affairs, drumming classes, etc.)?
- Do I have hobbies, interests, and activities that stimulate my interest outside of work or school?
- Do I actively observe the world around me and question my perceptions and assumptions? Do I remain open to new ideas and curious about the experiences of other people?
- Do I stay up to date in world affairs, local news, and current thinking?
- Do I express myself creatively? What outlets do I use (e.g., writing, painting, music, etc.)?
- Do I want to learn new things? Am I excited about new opportunities for learning?
- Do I have personal interests that stimulate and challenge me intellectually?
- Do I possess good critical thinking and problem-solving skills? How might I challenge myself to improve these skills?
- Do I have a positive self-concept? A positive self-concept is manifested in behaviors such as the ability to build trusting relationships, demonstrating respect for oneself and for

Spiritual Aspects of Wellness	My values, purpose in life, listening to intuition, finding joy, sharing my wisdom, learning from others, my faith in mankind, living my life with courage, showing kindness to others, being responsible, being trustworthy, feeling good about the way I live and how I behave in the world.
Environmental Aspects of Wellness	My home, access to fresh air, access to clean water, noise levels, lighting, design, inspiring decorations, the environment where I work.
Intellectual Aspects of Wellness	Mind challenge, memory improvement, problem solving, decision making, imagination, life-long learning, what I know, reading, writing, communication.
Emotional Aspects of Wellness	Awareness of feelings, cultivation of serenity, joy, happiness, love, concern for others, secure relationships, willingness to express anger, willingness to say no without guilt, willingness to feel sadness, ability to change mood, ability to use emotions to meet challenges and achieve goals.
Physical Aspects of Wellness	Nutrition, fitness, blood pressure, weight, strength, endurance, coordination, vision, hearing, gracefulness, feeling good in my body, care for my appearance, regular check-ups, self-awareness.
Social Aspects of Wellness	Connection to family, time for friends, building new relationships, being an active part of my neighborhood, my larger community (state, country, planet Earth), belonging to an organization, participating in team sports, planning social events.
Occupational Aspects of Wellness	Finishing school, finding meaningful work, enjoying work friends, ongoing training, using my interests and abilities to help my community, learning new manual skills, credentials, a good income.

Figure 4-20 A complex wellness model featuring social, environmental, and occupational areas.

others, and having the confidence to take on a challenge, set goals, complete tasks, and handle disappointments. What actions can I take to develop my self-concept and build on my personal strengths?

EMOTIONAL WELLNESS

Emotional wellness involves exploring your awareness and acceptance of your feelings. One assesses one's emotions and moods to gather information for meeting important life goals and overcoming personal limitations. Sample questions for exploring emotional wellness might include:

- Can I recognize and label my emotions as they occur (e.g., being able to differentiate irritation from anger, sadness, or fear)?
- Do I feel in control of my emotions most of the time or do my emotions often come on unexpectedly and overwhelm me? Do my emotions ever seem "too big" for the situation and catch me off guard with their intensity?
- Do I recognize the relationship between self-talk and mood? Am I aware of self-talk and can I change my self-talk to feel more positive and to achieve my goals?
- Can I recognize negative moods and improve my mood through positive self-talk?

- Can I share my emotions with trusted friends and family members?
- Can I recognize and accept the feelings of other people without feeling threatened or uncomfortable most of the time?
- Can I say "no" when I need to without feeling guilty?
- Is my attitude toward life mostly positive and do I believe that I can reach my goals?

SPIRITUAL WELLNESS

Spiritual wellness refers to each person's search for meaning and purpose in life. It explores the ability to find beauty in everyday events, the ability to feel comfort and hope even when things are not going well, the ability to express compassion and caring toward others, and the ends to which we devote our time and energy. Sample questions for exploring spiritual wellness might include:

- Can I contemplate the meaning of my life and allow myself to embrace my dreams for my future?
- Am I open to the beliefs and practices of other people, and can I demonstrate tolerance and compassion for each person's unique path through life?
- Do I make time for spiritual growth and exploration? What actions might I take to explore my spiritual wellness?

- Are my beliefs and values in alignment with my daily behaviors? Where are they out of alignment? What can I do to live my ethics more fully?
- Do I take responsibility for the events in my life and contemplate the meaning and significance of these events? Do I use this understanding to create positive change in my life?
- Do I care about the welfare of other people? Do I participate in community events or activities that allow me to demonstrate my concern for the well-being of others?
- Can I talk about spiritual issues with trusted friends and family members, and do I feel comfortable explaining what I believe and why?
- Do I feel faith in mankind and in the world? Do I feel hopeful that things will get better and that I can make a difference in the world?

OCCUPATIONAL WELLNESS

Occupational wellness is concerned with finding personal satisfaction and enrichment through one's work. When people can use their talents and interests to contribute to society through work, work tends to feel more meaningful, enjoyable, and fulfilling. Sample questions for exploring occupational wellness might include:

- Do I feel challenged by and satisfied with my current work, or am I preparing now to move into an area of work that I believe will challenge and satisfy me?
- Does my work or future work align with my ethical values and personal beliefs? If not, what is the misalignment and can change occur to make this work a good fit for me?
- Can I create positive change through my work? Are my feelings and opinions respected? Can I influence decision making if this is important to me?
- Can I accurately assess my strengths and weaknesses in relationship to my work and set goals that lead to increased capacity and skill? Do I regularly strive to improve my personal performance?

- Do I believe that I have the qualities of a valuable employee and that I can obtain and secure a meaningful job?
- Am I doing what I want to with my life and career?

SOCIAL WELLNESS

The ability to build and keep supportive and satisfying relationships is an essential element of wellness. Social wellness also requires exploring how you interact with your local and even global community, because being active participants in society can enrich life and provide purpose and meaning. Sample questions for exploring social wellness might include:

- Can I adjust to new places and make new friends?
- Do I give the time and energy to old friendships and to family relationships?
- Do I value diversity and interact with people of different ages, races, cultures, and lifestyles?
- Do I maintain my values, beliefs, and ideas when interacting with other people? At the same time, do I demonstrate tolerance and openness for different beliefs and new ideas?
- Am I aware of the concerns of the different communities with which I interact (e.g., school community, work community, neighborhood community, etc.), and do I participate in problem solving or actions to build a stronger community?
- Do I feel a responsibility and commitment to the global community? How do my actions and behaviors demonstrate this commitment?

A wellness model and personal wellness inventory are used to create a wellness plan in which specific goals and action steps will lead to greater equilibrium. To create a wellness plan, clients are encouraged to identify the areas they are most motivated to change. Clients might keep track of their progress in a wellness journal or through the coaching of a healthcare professional. At predetermined dates, progress on the plan is evaluated and the plan is revised and updated.

MASSAGE FUSION
Integration of Skills

STUDY TIP: flash!

Massage is a new language. Simply look at the list of key words and terms at the beginning of this chapter and you start to realize "Hey! I'm learning a new language!" When people study a new language, they usually repeat words over and over again to memorize their meaning and

pronunciation. With massage words, repetition is key. Start with flash cards. Write the term on the front of the card and its meaning on the back. Put the cards into decks of 10 cards each. Work through the first deck by looking at the front of a card, saying the term out loud, and then giving its meaning out loud. Turn the card over. If you got it right, place it off to the side. If you got it wrong, place it on the bottom

(Continued)

MASSAGE FUSION (*Continued*)
Integration of Skills

of the deck. When you have learned the terms in one deck, move onto the next. Begin each study session by reviewing an old deck you already know and then working through one new deck of cards. The key words at the top of each chapter are an excellent place to find important words. You can also make flash decks from the health care terminology words in the tables and boxes in Appendix A, Health Care Terminology. Each time you encounter a new vocabulary word, write it directly onto a flash card. Keep building new decks of words and keep reviewing old decks to maximize your massage vocabulary. When the time comes to take your credentialing exam, you will be well prepared for study sessions and to pass with flying colors!

MASSAGE INSPIRATION

Journaling can be a powerful practice during your massage training. It allows you to keep track of the changes you are making on a mental, emotional, physical, and spiritual level. You will face challenges during your schooling—everyone does—and when you capture these in a journal you begin to see the pattern of your strength. This is exciting! Use the questions listed in the wellness model section of this chapter for a journal entry. Answer these questions now, and then answer them again toward the end of your program, and then again 6 months after graduation. You will be able

to see if you are making progress toward greater health and wellness.

CHAPTER WRAP-UP

This chapter has covered a broad area that provides a framework for your work as a massage therapist. You learned about research studies and their importance for informing your massage practice. You explored the general benefits of massage and the range of effects massage causes in the body, mind, and emotions of clients. You were presented with a large number of research studies that demonstrate that massage is indicated as a treatment strategy for many conditions, diseases, injuries, and disorders. You looked at stress and wellness in some detail. This is a lot of information. You're probably feeling like you need a stress management and wellness program just to cope! Take three deep breaths. You're through it now, and you have your entire training program to digest and integrate the materials in this chapter. In fact, as you learn about each new massage system and each new client population later in your training, and even when you graduate and have a practice of your own as a professional, you can return to the information in this chapter as a way of remembering how unique, exciting, and important the practice of massage is as a way to promote wellness and help people experience life in a meaningful and enjoyable way.

Massage Cautions and Contraindications

KEY TERMS

adaptive measures

adverse reaction

anterior triangle

area of caution

axilla area

brachial plexus

contraindication

cubital region

drug

femoral triangle

flare up

hypertension

insulin shock

medication

physician's release

popliteal region

posterior triangle

side effect

LEARNING OBJECTIVES

Having read the chapter and used the related student learning tools, the student will be able to:

1 **Indicate on a diagram of the human body where areas of superficial anatomy are unprotected and constitute an area of caution.**

2 **List the types of structures that might be superficial in areas of caution.**

3 **List three arteries, three bones, and three organs that are superficial and require caution.**

4 **Describe the borders of the anterior, posterior, and femoral triangles.**

5 **Describe massage adaptations that should be made for a client who is taking prescription non-narcotic analgesics.**

6 **Define the term contraindication and list the different types of contraindications.**

7 **List four conditions that are absolute contraindications for massage.**

8 **Compare and contrast a side effect with an adverse reaction.**

9   Define hypertension and describe when a physician's release is required to provide massage to a client with hypertension.

11   Outline the critical thinking steps a therapist can use to rule out contraindications and ensure massage is safe for a client.

10   Categorize integumentary conditions that are contraindicated or that require adaptive measures.

In his *Epidemics*, Hippocrates advises physicians, "Do good or do no harm." Over time, this advice has been distilled into the saying "First, do no harm," which is commonly quoted as part of the Hippocratic oath, which physicians take when they become doctors of medicine. Doing no harm is a long-standing guiding principle of medicine and all health care professions. This chapter aims to give you the knowledge you need to "do no harm" when you provide massage to clients.

Topic 5-1 describes the areas of the body where structures like nerves and blood vessels are superficial and could be affected by your massage strokes. You want to work with caution in these areas. Topic 5-2 explains that massage might influence a client's response to medication and a client's medication might influence the client's response to massage. Understanding these issues is important for providing a safe massage. Topic 5-3 reminds us that some effects, while beneficial for particular client groups, can be dangerous for others. Massage therapists must be vigilant and flexible in order to "do no harm" and think critically about each client's unique health history, medications, and physical condition, to adapt techniques to ensure the client's safety and enjoyment. The important concepts and principles in this chapter guide our thinking and are essential in a professional and effective practice.

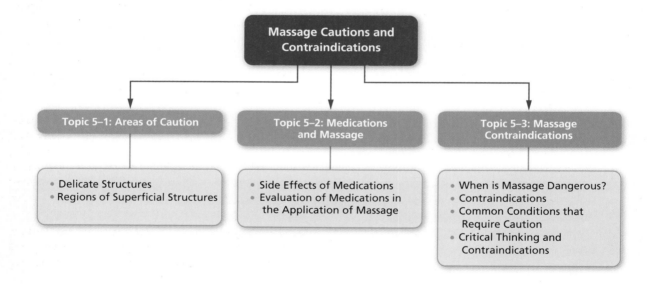

Massage Cautions and Contraindications

Topic 5–1: Areas of Caution	Topic 5–2: Medications and Massage	Topic 5–3: Massage Contraindications
• Delicate Structures • Regions of Superficial Structures	• Side Effects of Medications • Evaluation of Medications in the Application of Massage	• When is Massage Dangerous? • Contraindications • Common Conditions that Require Caution • Critical Thinking and Contraindications

Topic **5-1**
Areas of Caution

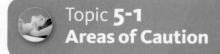

In certain areas of the body, structures like nerves, blood vessels, bones, organs, and lymph nodes are more superficial than in other areas. Care is required when working in these **areas of caution** to ensure the client's comfort and safety. The following sections discuss the types of damage that might occur to unprotected structures when strokes are too heavy or vigorous in these specific areas. A later section identifies areas where extra caution is required.

Delicate Structures

Nerves, blood vessels, bones, and organs are delicate and can be damaged if strokes are applied too forcefully or for a prolonged time in areas of caution.

- **Abnormal occurrences:** Sometimes clients have lumps or masses directly under their skin, which are often benign cysts or fatty deposits. Avoid direct pressure or heavy pressure to these abnormalities. If a mole is enlarged or irregular, alert the client and avoid massaging directly over it.
- **Blood vessels:** Arterial blood is under pressure from the heart, which acts as a pump. When an artery is closed off momentarily with a massage stroke, the pressure builds up behind the blockage. When the blockage is removed, the buildup provides an extra push to the fluid. This can be a positive mechanism that improves circulation in a local region. If arteries are blocked for too long, however, the delivery of oxygen distal to the blockage site is delayed. This can lead to feelings of discomfort, panic, and even a loss of consciousness if the blockage occurs in the anterior region of the neck. In areas of caution, arteries are superficial and thus receive the full force of a massage stroke. Avoid heavy and/or prolonged pressure over arteries in areas of caution to prevent disrupting oxygen to body tissue.
- **Veins:** Veins are weaker than arteries and have one-way valves. Light-to-moderate strokes that work from the distal areas of the body toward the heart can mechanically move venous blood toward the heart to positively support venous return. In areas of caution, veins are superficial, and heavy pressure can cause damage to a vein's fragile structure when the stroke works against the direction of blood flow in areas where the vein is not protected. This could damage the valve and potentially cause a varicose vein.
- **Bones:** In some areas, bony prominences project from the otherwise smooth contoured surface of the body. Use caution when applying strokes over these prominences because compression or forceful pressure could potentially cause discomfort, pain, pinching of soft tissue into bone, bruising of the tissue directly around the bone, or even fracture. Use special caution with clients who are frail or have bones weakened by osteoporosis.
- **Nerves:** When a nerve is compressed by a deep stroke, pinched between the fingers with a lifting stroke, or pressed up against a bony structure, pain, numbness, tingling, and discomfort can result. In some cases, clients might feel burning pain or shooting pain along the nerve path or referral path. Nerves can be irritated when a therapist applies a stroke without proper attention to the client's responses. If a client complains that a stroke causes pain, numbness, or tingling, immediately lighten the pressure or move the position of your hands or forearm to alleviate the discomfort. In areas of caution, avoid heavy pressure altogether to prevent irritation of superficial nerves.
- **Organs:** Lymph nodes are small, rounded structures located along lymph vessels and are superficial in many different areas of the body. Students and new professionals sometimes mistake lymph nodes for adhesions or trigger points and work to break them down in an effort to free the tissue. This can obviously cause damage to the structure and discomfort for the client. Heavy work or prolonged compression in areas of caution where lymph nodes are unprotected can also cause damage. Sometimes lymph nodes become enlarged when they are working to fight an infection. Avoid placing any pressure on inflamed nodes because this will cause discomfort to the client and could potentially interfere with the node's filtering and infection-fighting functions. Other organs might be unprotected in certain areas (e.g., kidneys, liver, trachea) and require caution.

Regions of Superficial Structures

The following sections describe regions of the body where delicate structures are superficial and unprotected (Fig. 5-1), including details about specific structures located in the regions of the head and face, neck, trunk, upper extremity, and lower extremity.

Concept Brief **5-1**
Area of Caution Defined

Regions of the body where delicate structures like nerves, bones, arteries, veins, and organs are superficial and unprotected.

Head and Face

The structures of the head and face that require some caution from massage therapists are shown in Figure 5-2. Most of these structures are directly accessed every time the therapist provides a face massage. Damage to any of these structures is highly unlikely unless the therapist uses heavy pressure and is not responsive to the client's feedback. The structures of the head and face that require caution include the following:

- **Blood vessels:** Both the temporal artery and facial artery contribute to blood flow in the head and face. The temporal artery arises from the external carotid artery, and its pulse is palpable superior to the zygomatic arch.
- **Bones:** The styloid process of the temporal bone is a pointed piece of bone that extends from the skull below and slightly behind the ear. It serves as an attachment point for a number of muscles associated with the tongue and larynx. This area is very tender, and even moderate pressure over this bone can cause the client pain. Because some clients also feel tenderness when pressure is placed over the mastoid process, therapists should work gently in this area when massaging the neck and face.
- **Nerves:** The trigeminal nerve carries sensations from the face, while the facial nerve controls facial expressions.

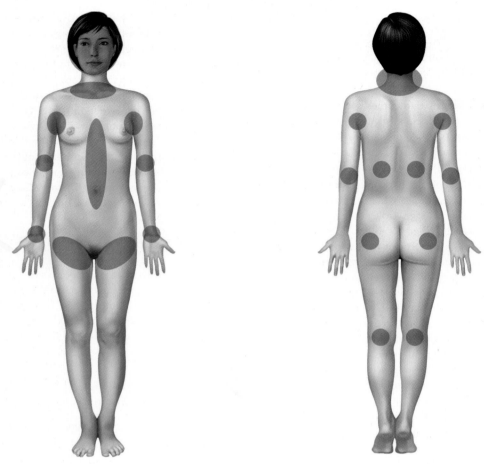

Figure 5-1 Areas of caution are regions of the body where delicate structures are superficial and unprotected.

Intense pressure with the fingers or thumb can result in discomfort, pain, irritation, or damage. Damage to the facial nerve could result in paralysis of facial muscles, or the trigeminal nerve could become irritated leading to a painful condition known as trigeminal neuralgia.

- **Organs:** The parotid glands are large salivary glands that lie on top of the lateral and posterior aspect of the mandible, just anterior to the ears. Because these glands can feel tender, only light pressure should be applied in this region of the face. Along the line of the jaw, under the chin, and alongside the ear, lymph nodes are superficial.

Concept Brief 5-2
Superficial Structures in the Head and Face

- Temporal artery
- Facial artery
- Styloid process
- Mastoid process
- Trigeminal nerve
- Facial nerve
- Parotid glands

Neck

The neck can be divided into four triangular regions; two **anterior triangles** and two **posterior triangles** (Fig. 5-3). The trachea, mandible, and sternocleidomastoid muscles on each side of the neck define the anterior triangles. These triangles contain the carotid arteries, internal jugular veins, vagus nerve, hyoid bone, trachea, and thyroid gland (Fig. 5-4). The clavicles, sternocleidomastoid muscles, and trapezius muscles define the posterior triangles of the neck. These triangles contain the external jugular vein, lymph nodes, brachial plexus, subclavian arteries, and subclavian veins (Fig. 5-5).

- **Blood vessels:** Because both the anterior and posterior triangles have many blood vessels, massage should be performed carefully in these areas. The left and right common carotid arteries, which can be palpated on either side of the trachea, divide into the left and right external and internal carotid arteries. The external carotid arteries supply the neck, esophagus, pharynx, larynx, lower jaw, and face with oxygenated blood. The internal carotid arteries supply oxygenated blood to the brain. Any prolonged compression strokes that would block off the blood flow in these arteries could cause a client to panic or lose consciousness.

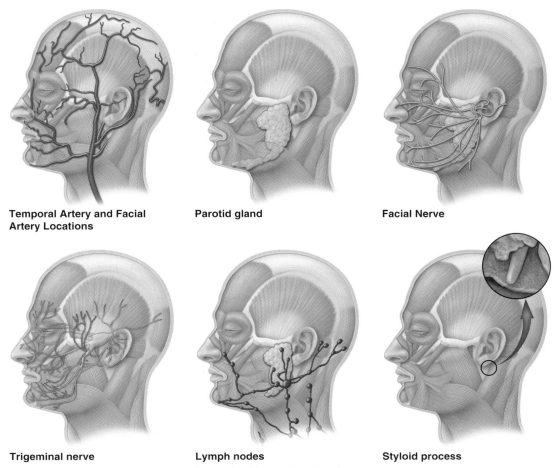

Temporal Artery and Facial Artery Locations

Parotid gland

Facial Nerve

Trigeminal nerve

Lymph nodes

Styloid process

Figure 5-2 Structures of the head and face that require caution.

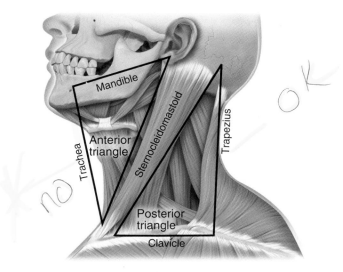

Figure 5-3 Anterior and posterior triangles of the neck. The neck can be divided into four triangular regions: two anterior triangles and two posterior triangles. The trachea, mandible, and sternocleidomastoid muscles on each side of the neck define the anterior triangles. The clavicles, sternocleidomastoid muscles, and trapezius muscles define the posterior triangles of the neck.

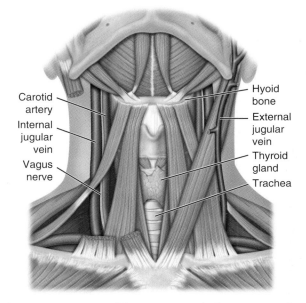

Figure 5-4 Structures of the anterior triangle that require caution.

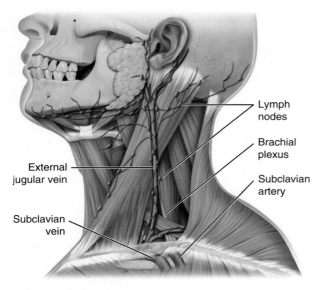

Figure 5-5 Structures of the posterior triangle that require caution.

The internal jugular veins descend from the head parallel to the common carotid arteries. The external jugular veins descend from the head on the anterior surface of the sternocleidomastoid muscles. These vessels along with the vertebral veins carry deoxygenated blood back to the heart from the head and neck. The subclavian artery and vein pass under the clavicles and carry blood to and from the upper extremities.

Later in your training program, you will likely learn techniques that address each muscle of the neck and shoulders. For example, the sternocleidomastoid muscle is lifted and stretched as the head is rotated in a "pin and stretch" technique. A therapist might apply a moderate friction stroke down the scalene muscles to the clavicle. It is important not to be fearful of working the muscles of the neck but to develop awareness of the structures that run with and through the muscles. The external jugular vein is likely to be lifted along with the sternocleidomastoid muscle. Strokes down the scalene muscles are likely to access the subclavian artery and vein just as the stroke reaches the clavicle. Pay attention to the client's reactions as you massage the structures of the neck. If veins or arteries are manipulated too forcefully, clients will experience an uncomfortable feeling that will likely be apparent in their facial expression even if they do not say anything.

- **Bones:** The hyoid bone in the anterior triangles of the neck is held in place by ligaments and serves as an attachment site for several muscles associated with movement of the tongue and larynx. Avoid direct pressure on the hyoid bone and strokes that graze the bone. The transverse processes of the spinal column can be palpated in the posterior triangle. Be aware of their position in techniques that rotate the head to one side or the other. Direct pressure on the processes can cause discomfort and potential injury.
- **Nerves:** The vagus nerve is 1 pair of 12 paired cranial nerves. It descends from the spinal cord lateral to the common

carotid arteries and is the primary parasympathetic nerve that supplies most of the viscera in the thorax and abdomen. The vagus nerves are structures that might be accessed when working in the anterior triangles of the neck. Sections of the facial nerve are accessible in the posterior triangles.

The **brachial plexus** is a network of nerves formed from nerves C5 through T1. It passes through the posterior triangle under the clavicle and over the first rib into the axilla where it divides into the five main nerves that innervate the upper extremity. Any strokes applied in the posterior triangle, which cause numbness, discomfort, or tingling down the arm, are probably compressing the brachial plexus. Lighten the stroke or change the position of your hand to alleviate discomfort.

- **Organs:** The trachea is the main air passage to the lungs and forms one border of the anterior triangles. The thyroid gland lies on the trachea in the anterior triangles. Avoid this area because strokes directly on the front of the throat or even close to the edges of the trachea can cause clients to feel as if they are being choked. Superficial lymph nodes occur in both the anterior and posterior triangles of the neck.

Concept Brief 5-3
Superficial Structures of the Neck

- **Anterior triangles**
  - Borders:
    - Trachea
    - Mandible
    - Sternocleidomastoid muscles
  - Structures:
    - Carotid artery
    - Internal jugular vein
    - Vagus nerve
    - Hyoid bone
    - Trachea
    - Thyroid gland
- **Posterior triangles**
  - Borders:
    - Clavicles
    - Sternocleidomastoid muscles
    - Trapezius muscles
  - Structures:
    - External jugular vein
    - Lymph nodes
    - Brachial plexus
    - Subclavian artery
    - Subclavian vein

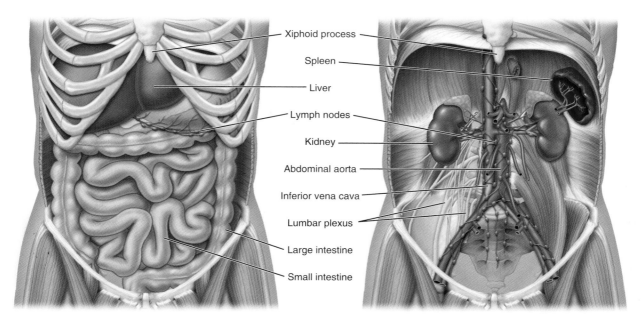

Figure 5-6 Structure of the trunk that require caution.

Trunk

The structures of the torso that require some caution are shown in Figure 5-6. These structures are accessed during massage of the upper chest, abdominal area, and back.

- **Blood vessels:** The abdominal aorta delivers blood to the abdominal and pelvic organs and divides to carry blood to the lower extremities. The inferior vena cava drains blood from the abdominal organs into the right atrium. Deep massage work in the abdominal area can access these major blood vessels and their branches. If you feel a strong pulse while doing abdominal work, change the position of your hands to avoid disrupting circulation.

- **Bones:** The xiphoid process is the inferior part of the sternum where the diaphragm and rectus abdominus muscles attach. This bone is accessed in some upper chest massage strokes that work down the sternum. Direct pressure on this bone could cause pain or a fracture. On the posterior of the body, ribs 11 and 12 are attached to the vertebrae but not to the sternum, as the other ribs are, and thus are called floating ribs. These ribs are weaker than the other ribs and more prone to bruising or fracture with application of intense tapotement, compression techniques, or heavy pressure. As noted earlier, the floating ribs are most vulnerable during seated massage. The chest plate of many massage chairs supports only the upper body, and compression strokes can cause much anterior–posterior movement in the lower thoracic and lumbar regions. Be careful of strong compressions over the floating ribs and low back in this particularly unsupported position.

- **Nerves:** The lumbar plexus is a network of nerves in the low back that supply the lower abdominal area and the anterior and medial portions of the lower extremity. Low back pain has many causes, but if a client reports that a stroke causes pain or discomfort in the lower back, abdomen, genital area, thigh, or medial and anterior aspect of the lower leg, it is possible that part of the lumbar plexus is being compressed. Change your hand position or lighten the stroke. If pain or discomfort persists, refer the client to a primary care physician because a more serious condition may be the cause.

- **Organs:** Lymph nodes along the sternum might be accessed during upper chest massage and may be tender. During abdominal massage, it is possible to access the liver, spleen, large intestine, and small intestine. This is most often beneficial because massage can help promote regular bowel movements. Sometimes a client may experience mild discomfort if the colon is full. If a client complains of pain with mild-to-moderate abdominal massage, or if you encounter areas of particular tenderness, refer the client to his or her health care provider for follow-up.

The kidneys and liver require the most caution because they are vulnerable to certain types of techniques such as heavy pressure or tapotement. The kidneys are located on the posterior wall of the abdomen against the posterior muscles of the back, just above the waistline. With the client in the prone position, striking techniques like tapotement can damage the kidneys because they are not protected by the ribs. Apply only light tapotement over the areas of the kidneys to ensure they are not bruised, irritated, or damaged.

The liver lies directly inferior to the diaphragm on the right side of the anterior body. While it is unlikely that general abdominal massage would bruise the liver, some advanced techniques like psoas massage have caused damage when the therapist did not position strokes correctly. In one psoas technique, the therapist imagines a line running from the navel to the anterior superior iliac spine and places fingers in the abdominal area at the halfway point between these two structures. This should place the therapist directly on the muscle belly of the psoas. The work can be deep and intense but very beneficial for low back issues. But if the therapist's hand is positioned too high when seeking to access the psoas on the right side, the liver could potentially be bruised. You will learn safe psoas massage techniques in later chapters.

Concept Brief 5-4
Superficial Structures of the Trunk

- Abdominal aorta
- Inferior vena cava
- Xiphoid process
- Floating ribs (ribs 11 and 12)
- Lumbar plexus
- Lymph nodes around the sternum
- Liver
- Spleen
- Large intestine
- Small intestine
- Kidney
- Liver

Upper Extremity

The areas that require caution in the upper extremity are shown in Figure 5-7. The **axilla area** is the area of the armpit, the **cubital region** is the area of the elbow, and the wrist area is directly above the hand. Major blood vessels and nerves that supply the upper extremities are superficial in these areas.

- **Blood vessels:** Remember that the names of arteries and veins change as they move from one region of the body to another. For example, the subclavian artery becomes the axillary artery when it moves through the axillary region. When it moves out of the armpit area and into the upper arm, it is called the brachial artery. In the cubital fossa, it branches into the radial artery on the lateral side of the forearm and wrist and the ulnar artery on the medial side. At the hand, it forms two arches, called the deep and superficial palmar arches that supply the hand and fingers with blood.

  The veins are more complicated. The hand and fingers drain into the digital veins, which empty into the superficial and deep palmar veins. These empty into the cephalic vein, antebrachial vein, and basilic vein, which run up the forearm. The brachial vein on entering the axillary area is called the axillary vein and then becomes the subclavian vein.

All of these blood vessels can be accessed during massage of the arms. If a client complains of discomfort or a sensation of heaviness in a limb, it may be the result of pressure on a blood vessel. Techniques that work forcefully into the axillary region are the most likely to cause discomfort, but also avoid heavy pressure on the anterior wrist and the cubital fossa.

- **Bones:** The bone structure of the elbow is comprised of the olecranon process and fossa of the ulna and epicondyles of the humerus. The depression at the posterior of the elbow is called the cubital notch. The ulnar nerve runs right through this notch, which is commonly called the "funny bone." Some types of massage techniques (e.g., cross-fiber friction on the triceps insertion) may irritate the ulnar nerve at the cubital notch. Correctly positioning the arm while strokes are applied can reduce this occurrence (e.g., place the triceps in a lengthened position).

- **Nerves:** As noted earlier, the brachial plexus is the collection of nerves that innervate the upper extremity (Fig. 5-8). Three large trunks of the brachial plexus pass under the clavicle and divide into five major nerves. The axillary nerve supplies the deltoid and teres minor muscle, the shoulder joint, and skin of the shoulder. The musculocutaneous nerve supplies the flexors of the arm, while the ulnar nerve and median nerve supply the forearm and hand. The radial nerve supplies the anterior compartment of the forearm. Damage to the median nerve or compression by the carpal tunnel (carpal tunnel syndrome) causes numbness, pain, tingling, and dysfunction in the thumb and the first two fingers and half of the third finger. Damage or compression of the ulnar nerve causes numbness, pain, tingling, or dysfunction to the little finger and the medial half of the third finger. As Figure 5-7 shows, many of these nerves are superficial and accessible in the axillary, cubital fossa, and wrist regions.

- **Organs:** Lymph nodes are superficial in both the axilla area and cubital fossa.

Concept Brief 5-5
Superficial Structures of the Upper Extremity

- Axillary artery
- Brachial artery
- Radial artery
- Ulnar artery
- Cephalic vein
- Antebrachial vein
- Basilic vein
- Brachial vein
- Axillary vein
- Subclavian vein
- Cubital notch (ulnar nerve)
- Brachial plexus
- Lymph nodes (axillary area, cubital fossa)

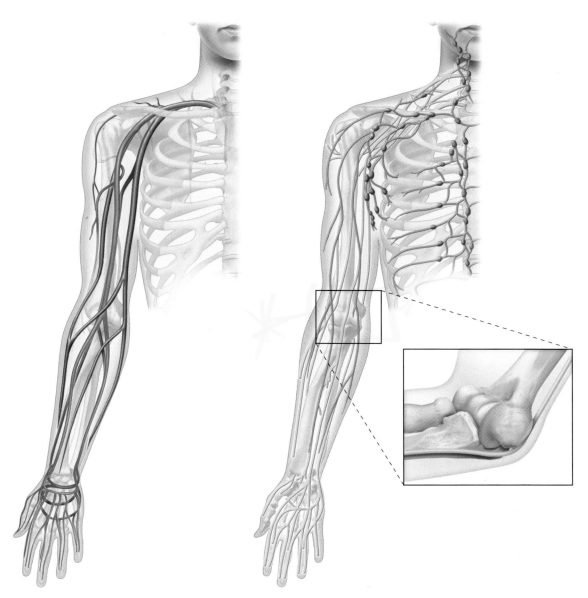

Figure 5-7 Structures of the upper extremity that require caution. The axilla area is the area of the armpit, the cubital region is the area of the elbow, and the wrist area is directly above the hand. Major blood vessels and nerves that supply the upper extremities are superficial in these areas.

Lower Extremity

The areas that require caution in the lower extremity are shown in Figure 5-9. The **femoral triangle** on the anterior body is defined by the inguinal ligament, sartorius, and adductor longus. In this area, you must be cautious of the inguinal lymph nodes, femoral artery and vein, and femoral nerve. The **popliteal region** on the posterior body is defined by the gastrocnemius, biceps femoris, and semimembranosus. The common peroneal nerve, popliteal artery and vein, and tibial nerve require caution. In addition, the great and small saphenous veins and sciatic nerve require caution in the lower extremity.

- **Blood vessels:** The abdominal aorta divides into two major arteries called the left and right common iliac arteries,

which divide into the internal and external iliac arteries that carry blood to the pelvis and lower limbs. The external iliac artery becomes the femoral artery in the thigh and then the popliteal artery in the popliteal region. The popliteal artery branches into the anterior and posterior tibial arteries. The posterior tibial artery becomes the peroneal artery, while the anterior tibial artery becomes the dorsalis pedis artery. These arteries are superficial in the femoral triangle and in the popliteal region (also called popliteal fossa). Avoid deep pressure in either of these regions.

The anterior tibial vein and the posterior tibial vein join the peroneal veins in the popliteal fossa to form the popliteal vein. In the thigh, the popliteal vein becomes the femoral vein, which becomes the external iliac vein in

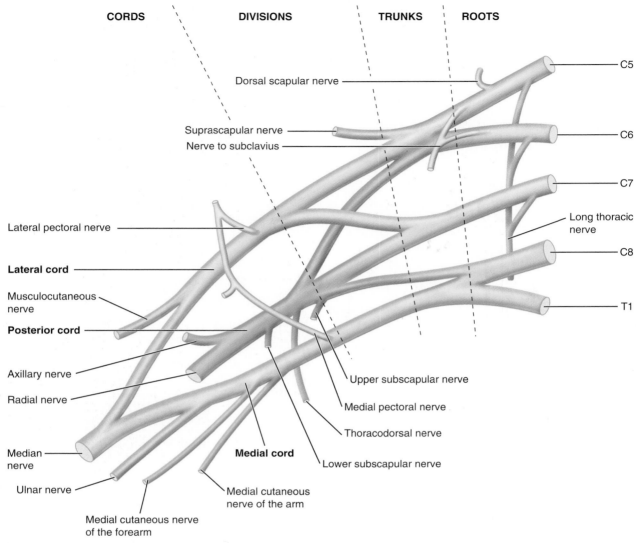

CORDS **DIVISIONS** **TRUNKS** **ROOTS**

Dorsal scapular nerve

Suprascapular nerve
Nerve to subclavius

C5

C6

C7

Long thoracic nerve

C8

T1

Lateral pectoral nerve

Lateral cord

Musculocutaneous nerve

Posterior cord

Axillary nerve

Radial nerve

Median nerve

Ulnar nerve

Medial cutaneous nerve of the forearm

Upper subscapular nerve

Medial pectoral nerve

Thoracodorsal nerve

Medial cord

Lower subscapular nerve

Medial cutaneous nerve of the arm

Figure 5-8 The brachial plexus is the collection of nerves that innervate the upper extremity. Three large trunks of the brachial plexus pass under the clavicle and divide into five major nerves.

the lower abdominal wall. The great saphenous vein is formed from the dorsal venous arch in the foot. It ascends along the medial aspect of the lower leg and thigh. The small saphenous vein is also formed from the dorsal venous arch in the foot but ascends along the lateral and posterior sides of the calf and then drains into the popliteal vein. These superficial veins, especially the great and small saphenous veins, are common sites of varicosities. Work carefully in the femoral triangle, popliteal fossa, and medial area of the leg and thigh.

- **Nerves:** In the femoral triangle, the femoral nerve is superficial. This nerve innervates the hip flexors and extensors, the skin of the medial and anterior thigh, and the medial leg and foot. On the posterior body in the gluteal and thigh region, you can access the sciatic nerve. This is the largest nerve in the body, running under the

piriformis and gluteal muscles to branch into the tibial and common peroneal nerves in the popliteal region. The nerve roots of the sciatic nerve can be compressed by a herniated disk or injured by an injection into the gluteal region, causing pain that can burn or shoot all the way down the length of the leg (called sciatica). The gluteal and piriformis muscles can become hypertonic and compress the nerve as it runs underneath them (called pseudo-sciatica). Deep pressure in the gluteal region or over the hamstrings can sometimes cause pain or irritate the sciatic nerve. Remain responsive and adjust the pressure of strokes based on the client's feedback. Avoid heavy pressure over the popliteal fossa and along the medial surface of the lower leg.

- **Organs:** Lymph nodes are superficial both in the inguinal area in the femoral triangle and in the popliteal fossa.

Anterior   **Posterior**

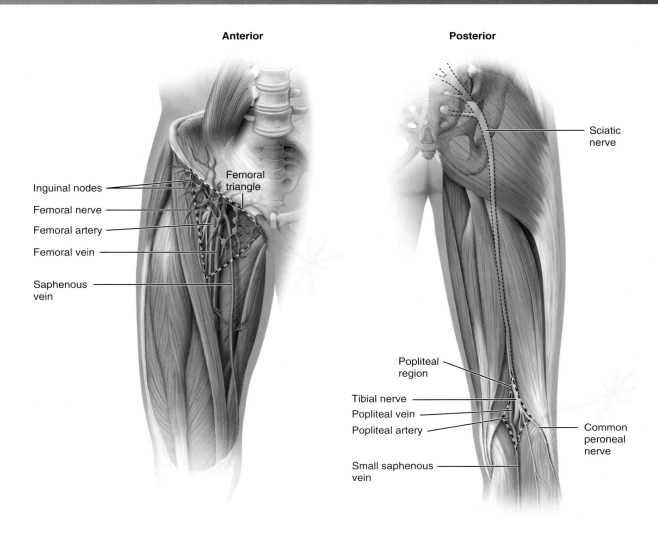

Inguinal nodes

Femoral nerve

Femoral artery

Femoral vein

Saphenous
vein

Femoral
triangle

Sciatic
nerve

Popliteal
region

Tibial nerve

Popliteal vein

Popliteal artery

Small saphenous
vein

Common
peroneal
nerve

Figure 5-9 Structures of the lower extremity that require caution. The femoral triangle on the anterior body is defined by the inguinal ligament, sartorius, and adductor longus. The popliteal region on the posterior body is defined by the gastrocnemius, biceps femoris, and semimembranosus.

Concept Brief 5-6
Superficial Structures of the Lower Extremity

- **Femoral triangle**
  - Borders:
    - Inguinal ligament
    - Sartorius
    - Adductor longus
  - Structures:
    - Inguinal lymph nodes
    - Femoral artery
    - Femoral vein
    - Femoral nerve
- **Popliteal region (also popliteal fossa)**
  - Borders:

    — Gastrocnemius
    — Biceps femoris
    — Semimembranosus
  - Structures:
    - Lymph nodes
    - Common peroneal nerve
    - Popliteal artery
    - Popliteal vein
    - Tibial nerve
    - Great saphenous vein
    - Sciatic nerve

Responsiveness is Key

Learning about the potential irritation or damage of blood vessels, nerves, bones, and organs is often distressing for students, especially when beginning to learn deep-tissue techniques. Students sometimes become so concerned with not damaging these structures that they back off from the muscles and stop engaging the tissue. Avoid this reaction if you can, and remember that clients usually speak up if something hurts. Every therapist at some point has caused a nerve to momentarily shoot pain or caused a client momentary discomfort. Stay alert, know the areas where lighter pressure is required, and pay attention to the client's breathing patterns, facial expressions, and feedback. If you make a mistake, adjust your hand or arm position, lighten your pressure, change the stroke, and proceed. Remember that you can deepen or lighten a stroke, even as a stroke progresses up or down a body area. For example, a deep-tissue stroke applied to the posterior leg might start at the ankle, drop into the gastrocnemius and soleus, and then soften to a very light stroke that just grazes the popliteal region. As you clear the popliteal region, you can then drop back into deeper pressure over the hamstrings and into the gluteals. As you reach the area medial to the greater trochanter, you might ask the client if the pressure feels appropriate, knowing that you are positioned directly over the sciatic nerve. You want to engage the tissue and provide clients with a meaningful massage experience that creates positive changes in their muscle tension patterns. So don't be afraid; instead, be responsive and adaptable.

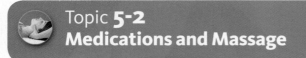

Topic 5-2
Medications and Massage

In the United States, the word **drug** usually refers to a synthesized chemical that may be prescribed by a physician to treat a particular condition, purchased over-the-counter without a prescription (e.g., cold medication, pain reliever, etc.), or categorized as illegal substances (e.g., cocaine, heroin, etc.). Alcohol and cigarettes also have active substances that classify them as drugs.

Massage should not be given to any client under the influence of alcohol or an illegal substance, but massage is often provided to clients who are taking prescription **medications**. Over-the-counter medications, including legal herbal and vitamin supplements, might also be present in a client's system during a massage. Massage therapists need to understand something about medications and how they influence a massage.

Pharmacology is the science and study of drugs, including their sources, chemistry, production, use in treating diseases, and **side effects**. Massage therapists are most interested in ways that side effects might influence the results of massage and in changes that must be made to ensure a client's safety in relationship to a particular medication.

Side Effects of Medications

A side effect is a secondary effect of a medication or therapy that goes beyond the desired effect or causes unwanted responses in addition to the therapeutic effect. Side effects occur commonly with many medicines and can range from mild sensations such as fatigue to serious problems such as hemorrhage. Each client's response to medications is unique. One may experience difficulty with side effects of a medication, while another doesn't. One may find that massage soothes the side effects of a medication, while another finds that massage increases the severity of side effects.

The common side effects of chemotherapy for cancer, for example, include nausea, vomiting, fatigue, decreased blood cell counts, hair loss, and mouth sores. These side effects occur because chemotherapy drugs used to fight cancer cells travel throughout the body and may also damage healthy tissue. A number of studies suggest that massage and acupressure are effective complementary therapies that reduce the nausea and vomiting side effects.[1,2] On the other hand, the side effects of the cancer therapy drugs Vincristine, Oncovin, and Vincasar include peripheral neuropathy, which may contraindicate massage if the symptoms are severe enough to affect a client's ability to give feedback about pressure.[3]

In some cases, clients are not aware that their symptoms are side effects. They may seek a massage because of muscle pain and not realize the pain is caused by their medications. This client may expect massage to relieve this symptom, not understanding that a symptom caused by a drug might not be lessened with massage. Therapists can help clients set realistic expectations for the massage session by researching the client's medications and alerting the client to potential side effect symptoms. Clients who recognize their side effects are more likely to discuss them with their health care provider, allowing alterations in dosages or changes in medication to be made that might alleviate some symptoms.

Elderly clients often experience greater side effects from medications than younger clients.[4] They also metabolize drugs more slowly, and drugs may build up over time in their body, causing a toxic situation. Massage increases circulation, which can move a drug through a client's system more quickly. This could support the positive effects of the drug or cause increased side effects. Additionally, therapists may encounter clients who are taking multiple medications and therefore be unable to predict side effects or the effects caused by the interaction of different drugs. In these cases, it is appropriate to call the client's physician (provided the client signed the release of information form usually completed before the client's first session). Because some physicians do not understand the broad effects of massage, you may need to describe the particular techniques you plan to use in the session.

Side effects that are extreme or place the client at serious risk are called **adverse reactions** or effects. Adverse effects can occur with an excessive dose of the drug (overdose), with an allergy to the drug, from sensitivity to the drug, or because the particular client has an intense response to the drug creating unusual symptoms. Examples of adverse effects include cardiac arrhythmias, hypertension, stroke, increased blood glucose levels, edema, breathing difficulties, rash, nausea, vomiting, abdominal cramps, diarrhea, depression, and many others. If a client exhibits unusual symptoms or a rapid increase of a symptom at any time during the session, call the client's health care provider or emergency services, depending on the severity of the reaction.

Concept Brief 5-7
Medication Terms

Pharmacology: The science and study of drugs

Prescription medication: A medication prescribed by a physician to treat a diagnosed disease or condition, or to counteract the side effects of another drug

Over-the-counter medication: A medication that can be purchased without a prescription by the general population

Side effect: A secondary effect of a medication or therapy that goes beyond the desired effect

Adverse effect: An extreme reaction to a drug that causes severe side effects or places the client in medical danger

Evaluation of Medications in the Application of Massage

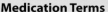

It is important to evaluate the impact of a massage on the medication or client and to adapt the treatment if needed. First, conduct a thorough health history intake (described in Chapter 12) and ask clients to list every medication they have taken in the last week, including prescription medications, over-the-counter medications, vitamins, and herbal supplements (Fig. 5-10). Vitamins and herbal supplements do not usually cause negative interactions with massage, but it is important to have all substances recorded in case an adverse reaction occurs. The substance can then be included in a physician's evaluation of the situation or in a liability claim. During the health intake interview, double-check the list with the client to ensure no medications are missing. Clients

commonly do not list over-the-counter medications like analgesics or cold medications because they don't understand that these substances also may affect their ability to respond to pressure and give feedback about the depth and comfort of a stroke. Clients similarly may forget to inform therapists of conditions like a cold or the flu, which they deem insignificant. The medication list may alert you to the client's health condition, allowing you to question the client to determine whether massage is contraindicated (such as when the client has a fever or is contagious).

Next, look up each medication the client is taking in a current drug reference book such as the *Nursing Drug Handbook*[5] or a reliable website such as drugs.com or WebMD. Ask clients to describe any side effects they experience from their medications. Often massage techniques can help the body balance or adapt to some side effects. If a client experiences drowsiness from a medication, the massage will likely increase the drowsy feelings. Applying stimulating strokes at the end of the massage can help the client wake up. If the client experiences dizziness as a side effect, you should assist the client getting on and off the massage table or when changing positions during the massage.

Reviewing medications can be time consuming. Some therapists send their clients a health history form with directions a week before their first scheduled appointment. The clients mail back the forms in a pre-addressed, stamped envelope provided by the therapist. This way the therapist has time to research any unfamiliar medications and conditions before the client arrives. It is still important to verbally review the medications list with the client as part of the health intake interview to ensure that nothing has been forgotten or overlooked.

Clients usually want some specific results from the massage, and together the client and therapist set treatment goals for the session. The client's medications or health conditions may limit some of the techniques that can be used in the session. This could potentially impede meeting certain treatment goals. It's important to discuss the limitations of massage in relationship to medications before the session begins. For example, if a client wants deep-tissue massage but you find the client has taken a full dose of an over-the-counter analgesic (pain medication) immediately before coming to the appointment, you should avoid deep-tissue work. The client's response to pain and pressure would be numbed by the analgesic, keeping the client from responding normally to the intensity of the strokes. You might overwork the client as a result and cause bruising, tissue damage, or increased pain and soreness after the massage. Similarly, you should use lighter massage techniques on a client taking anticoagulants such as Coumadin or Warfarin because these drugs prevent blood clotting by making the blood thinner, making clients on these medications prone to bruising. If you feel any doubt about performing the massage based on a client's medications or side effects, it is prudent to contact the client's health care provider, discuss the situation, and obtain a **physician's release** before proceeding.

Table 5-1 provides an overview of some common types of medication and their implications for massage. This table

Directions: Please list all the prescription medications, over-the-counter medications, herbal supplements, and vitamins you have taken this week in the space provided. Describe the reason why you take the substance and any side effects you experience as a result. This information is used by your massage therapist to ensure the safety and appropriateness of massage techniques, or to adapt the massage to better fit your individual needs. Failure to inform your massage therapist of medical conditions and medications may place you at increased risk for adverse reactions.

Name of the substance	Dosage per day	Reason for the use of this substance	Side effects?

Figure 5-10 Medications list for the health history form.

TABLE 5-1 Examples of Drugs with Implications for Massage

Drug Type	Effects	Possible Side Effects	Examples of Commercial Drugs	Massage Considerations
Antianginal medications	Increase the supply of oxygen to the heart	Dizziness, fatigue, flushing, headache, hypotension, and weakness Adverse reactions include angina, diarrhea, edema, fainting, heart failure, nausea, severe hypotension, shock, tachycardia, vomiting, and others	Apo-Atenol, Betaloc, Cardizem, Cedocard, Corgard, Detensol, Dilacor XR, Novopranol, Lopressor, Monoket, Nitrodisc, Norvasc, Noten, Timate, Tizac, and others	Dizziness at the end of the massage is common. Help the client off the massage table to prevent falling accidents. Watch for low blood pressure or increased weakness and contact the client's physician if side effects are worsened by massage
Antiarrhythmic medications	Normalize irregular heart rhythm (arrhythmia)	Anxiety, constipation, dizziness, dry mouth, fatigue, headache, hypotension, insomnia, peripheral neuropathy, tremor, and weakness Adverse reactions include angina, arrhythmias, difficulty breathing, edema, heart failure, liver toxicity, nausea, seizures, vomiting, and others	Apo-Propranolo, Apo-Quinidine, Brevibloc, Cardioquin, Detensol, Dura-tabs, Durules, LidoPen, Mexitil, Monitan, Norpace, Procainamide, Procan, Promine, Quinalan, Quinate, Rythmodan, Sctral, Tonocard, Xylocaine, and others	Consult with the client's physician to determine the most appropriate form of massage for clients on these medications. In some cases, rapid and stimulating techniques like tapotement may be contraindicated. Watch for dizziness at the conclusion of the massage. Avoid deep work and the use of hydrotherapy in cases of peripheral neuropathy
Anticoagulant medications	Reduce the ability of the blood to clot. Used in the treatment of deep-vein thrombosis, stroke, and heart disease and to prevent the movement of a blood clot	Easy bruising Adverse effects include bleeding	Bishydroxycoumarin, Coumadin, Heparin, Fragmin, Lovenox, Warfarin, and others	Heparin-based medications are delivered via injection, usually in a hospital. Avoid massaging the local injection area for 24 h. Clients on anticoagulant medications bruise easily, so avoid deep tissue, compression, deep friction, and tapotement strokes

TABLE 5-1   Examples of Drugs with Implications for Massage (*Continued*)

Drug Type	Effects	Possible Side Effects	Examples of Commercial Drugs	Massage Considerations
Anticonvulsant medications	Control seizures associated with epilepsy, or for short-term use after brain surgery or brain trauma to control seizures	Constipation, dizziness, drowsiness, dry mouth, fatigue, hair loss, headache, hypotension, indigestion, irritability, restlessness, sweating, and tremor Adverse reactions include liver toxicity, heart failure, rash, fainting, and others	Apo-Carbamazepine, Apo-diazepam, Carbatrol, Cerebyx, Depakene, Diamox, Diastat, Dilantin, Epitol, Epival, Gabitril, Keppra, Klonopin, Lamictal, Neurontin, Peganone, Topamax, Tranxene, Zarontin, and others	Use stimulating techniques at the end of the session to counteract drowsiness. Avoid scalp massage because many anticonvulsant drugs cause hair loss. Keep water available throughout the massage in the event the client's mouth gets dry. Because reaction to depth and pressure may be altered, use deep-tissue strokes with caution
Antidepressant medications	Reduce depression or the symptoms of affective disorders (disturbances in mood). May be used to treat phobias, neurodermatitis (nervous skin disorder), and other behavioral symptoms	Anorexia, blurred vision, constipation, decreased sex drive, dizziness, dry mouth, drowsiness, edema, hair loss, hypertension, insomnia, lethargy, joint pain, muscle weakness, nausea, photosensitivity, rash, sudden blood pressure drop when standing, vomiting, and others Adverse reactions include blackouts, cardiac arrest, coma, hypothyroid, palpitations, rapid heartbeat, respiratory arrest, severe hypertension, self-mutilation, seizure, speech dysfunction, suicide attempts, suicidal thoughts, and others	Alti-Moclobemide, Avantyl, Celexa, Effexor, Elavil, Lexapro, Lithium, Ludiomil, Luvox, Marplan, Norpramin, Nordil, Parnate, Paxil, Prozac, Remeron, Rhotrimine, Serzone, Sinaquan, Tofranil, Vivacil, Wellbutrin, Zoloft, Zyban, and others	Because the side effects of antidepressant medications are numerous, design the session to counteract each client's specific side effects. Watch for a sudden drop in blood pressure with standing at the end of the massage. Avoid scalp massage with clients taking lithium because this drug often thins hair and causes hair loss. Massage changes brain chemistry as noted in Chapter 4. It is unclear how these massage effects interact with antidepressant medications. Remain vigilant and report any increased side effects to the client's physician Listen carefully to clients taking these medications and watch for indications of self-mutilation (small cuts). Report any concerns to the client's physician immediately
Antidiabetic medications	Insulin and oral antidiabetic medications lower blood glucose levels. Glucagon raises blood glucose levels	Bruising or scar tissue formation at injection site, diarrhea, fatigue, flatulence, flushing, funny taste in mouth, heartburn, headache, hypoglycemia, nausea, photosensitivity, and vomiting Adverse reactions include adipose distribution changes, hypersensitivity reactions, insulin resistance, insulin shock, and others	Actos, Actraphane HM, Actrapid HM, Amaryl, Avandia, Dimelor, Diabinese, Euglucon, GlucaGen, Glucophage, Glucotrol, Glysep, Humalog, Isophane, Lantus, Lente Insulin, Novolin N, Orinase, Prandin, Precose, Starlix, Tolinase, Ultratard HM, and others	Avoid the injection site where insulin is given. If the client has developed circulatory impairments or neuropathies, avoid deep work and hydrotherapy. Massage increases the use of glucose and insulin in the body, which could lead to insulin or hypoglycemic reactions. Keep some form of sugar available such as orange juice or soda in the event of low blood sugar. If the client does not respond quickly to the sugar, call emergency services. See the section on cautions with diabetics in this chapter for more details

(Continued)

TABLE 5-1   Examples of Drugs with Implications for Massage (Continued)

Drug Type	Effects	Possible Side Effects	Examples of Commercial Drugs	Massage Considerations
Antidiarrheal medications	Decrease the peristaltic movement of the intestines and soothe the intestinal mucosa	Constipation, dizziness, drowsiness, fatigue, nausea, and vomiting Adverse reactions include abdominal distention, central nervous system depression, tachycardia, and others	Devrom, Diphenatol, Imodium, Kaodene, Kaopectate, Motofen, Pepto-Bismol, and others	Use stimulating strokes at the end of the massage to counter drowsiness. Help the client off the table if dizziness occurs. Abdominal massage is indicated for constipation, but watch for abdominal tenderness or distention, which should be referred to a physician
Antihistamines	Block histamine to combat allergic reactions	Constipation, diarrhea, dizziness, dry mouth, hypertension, hypotension, increased heart rate, loss of appetite, muscle weakness, nausea, and vomiting Adverse reactions include arrhythmias and allergic reaction.	Alavert, Allerdryl, Astelin, Benadryl, Clarinex, Dayhist, Dimetapp, Lodrane, Phenergan, Polaramine, Restall, Rynatan, Triacin, Vistaril, Zyrtec, and many others	Monitor blood pressure before and after the massage, and watch for dizziness at the end of the massage. Have water available for the client throughout the massage
Antihypertensive medications— see also vaso-dilators and diuretics	Reduce blood pressure. Used to treat hypertension	Depression, dizziness, drowsiness, fatigue, headache, hypotension, numbness and tingling in the periphery, weight gain Adverse reactions include angina, arrhythmias, bronchoconstriction, edema, liver dysfunction, and others	Accupril, Aldomet, Altace, Apo-Methyldopa, Capoten, Cardura, Catapress, Dixarit, Hylorel, Ismelin, Lotensin, Monopril, Normodyne, Presolol, Rogitine, Tenex. Zestril, and others	Stimulating strokes at the end of the massage or directly before asking a client to change positions can help combat drowsiness. Watch for low blood pressure. If numbness and tingling in the periphery is a consistent side effect, avoid deep-tissue strokes
Anti-infective medications including antibacterial, antiviral, antitubercular, and antifungal medications	To eliminate certain microorganisms or to disrupt microorganism life cycles to prevent or treat an infection	Nausea Adverse reactions include abdominal cramps, allergic reactions, arrhythmias, bleeding, confusion, diarrhea, fever, hives, hypersensitivity, hypertension, kidney dysfunction, liver dysfunction, photosensitivity, rash, seizures, vomiting, and others	Alti-Clindamycin, Amikin, Apo-Pen, Azactam, Bicillin, Cefobid, Cytovene, Declomycin, Duricef, Erygel, Etibi, Fortaz, Foscavir, Fradantin, Ilosone, Kantrex, Levaquin, Megacillin, Novo-Rhythro, Relenza, Tamiflu, Truxazole, Primaxin, Wesmycin, Vancocin, Valtrex, and many others	Anti-infective medications are prescribed for a wide variety of conditions. The types of medications and their adverse reactions are vast. Anyone on anti-infective medications has some level of immune system compromise. Avoid exposing the client to any illness and use relaxing and balancing techniques that do not overly stress the client's delicate system. It is likely that you will consult with a physician before providing massage, but still research conditions and medications carefully. You may be required to practice universal precautions in many cases

TABLE 5-1   Examples of Drugs with Implications for Massage *(Continued)*

Drug Type	Effects	Possible Side Effects	Examples of Commercial Drugs	Massage Considerations
Antilipemic medications	Lower cholesterol, triglycerides, and phospholipids levels. Used to treat athero-sclerosis and to lower the risk of the devel-opment of coronary artery disease	Constipation, fatigue, flatulence, headache, nausea, and upset stomach Adverse reactions include anemia, arrhythmias, chest pain, diarrhea, gallstones, kidney dysfunction, liver toxicity or dysfunc-tion, muscle soreness, ulcers, and others	Atromid, Colestid, Lescol, Lipitor, Lopid, Mevacor, Novo-Cholamine, Pravachol, Tricor, Zetia, Zocor, and others	Constipation is a common side effect of antilipemic medica-tions and can benefit from abdominal massage. If con-stipation is persistent and the client complains of abdominal tenderness or pain, stop the abdominal massage and refer the client to the physician
Anti-Parkinson medications	Anticholinergic anti-Par-kinson medications reduce the tremors associated with Parkinson disease Dopaminergic anti-Parkinson medica-tions improve motor function through dopamine concentra-tion and neurotrans-mission in the brain	Agitation, confu-sion, constipation, dizziness, drowsi-ness, heart palpita-tions, hypotension, insomnia, nausea, restlessness Adverse reactions include anorexia, depression, nausea, psychoses, and vomiting	Apo-Benztropine, Akineton, Alter-Dryl, Apo-Trihex, Artane, Banflex, Banophen, Benadryl, Biperiden, Lactate, Cogentin, Flexoject, Flexon, Kemadrin, Myolin, Norflex, Orphenate, Procyclid, Trihexane, Trihexane, and others Antadine, Apo-Bromocriptine, Apo-Levocarb, Carbex, Comtan, Dopar, Endantadine, Larodopa, Mirapex, Parlodel, Permax, ReQuip, Tasmar, and others	Clients may have difficulty relaxing and may exhibit restlessness or mild anxiety or nervousness. Watch for dizzi-ness at the conclusion of the massage or when changing positions. Help clients onto and off the massage table to ensure their safety
Antipsychotic medications	Reduce or control symptoms like delu-sions and hallucina-tions in conditions like schizophrenia or extreme agitation	Side effects if they occur are usually adverse and include cardiovascular dys-function, elevated body temperature, hypertension, muscle rigidity, rapid heart rate, respiratory depression or failure, seizures, and other serious reactions	Abilify, Anatensol, Apo-Thioridazine, Chlorpromanyl, Clozaril, Enanthate, Geodon, Haldol, Moban, Modecate, Navane, Loxapac, Orap, Prolixin, Risperdal, Serentil, Seroquel, Stelazine, Trilafon, Zyprexa, and others	These medications are given to treat serious mental disorders. Work with the client's physi-cian to determine the best treatment plan based on the client's individual needs. Direct supervision from a physician is important to ensure the client's and your own health and safety
Antitussive medications	Suppress coughing	Constipation, dizzi-ness, drowsiness, headache, nasal congestion Adverse reactions include arrhythmias, chills, rash, breathing difficulties, seizures, and others	Balminil, Benylin, Dayquil, Dextromethorphan, Duro-Tuss, Koffex, methylmorphine, Mucinex DM, Nyquil, Paveral, Pertussin, Tessalon, and others	Check to ensure that the client does not have a fever or a communicable disease before providing massage. If nasal congestion occurs as a side effect, you may limit the time the client spends in the prone position or avoid the prone position altogether and use the side-lying position. Watch for drowsiness and dizziness at the conclusion of the massage and help the client off the massage table if appropriate

(Continued)

TABLE 5-1   Examples of Drugs with Implications for Massage *(Continued)*

Drug Type	Effects	Possible Side Effects	Examples of Commercial Drugs	Massage Considerations
Antiulcer medications	Eradicate *Helicobacter pylori*, a bacterial infection that causes peptic ulcers Balance acid and pepsin secretions and soothe mucosal membrane in the lower esophagus, stomach, and/or small intestine	Constipation, diarrhea, dizziness, flatulence, funny taste in mouth, headache, nausea Adverse reactions include abdominal pain, back pain, electrolyte imbalance, impotence, itching, kidney stones, muscle pain, rash, vomiting, and others	Aciphex, Amoxil, AlternaGel, Biaxin, Caltrate, Cycotex, Flagyl, Maalox, Nexium, Novo-Famotidine, Pepcid, Prevacid, Prilosec, Protonix, Tagament, Rolaids, Sulcrate, Zantac, and others	Constipation is the most common side effect of antiulcer medications. Abdominal massage is indicated
Cancer medications	A variety of drugs used to combat many different forms of cancer. Chemotherapy is the use of chemical agents to stop cancer cells from growing; over 50% of people diagnosed with cancer receive chemotherapy. Other cancer drugs help people remain on their chemotherapy regime. Radiation therapy is the use of particles or waves to kill cancer cells or shrink tumors	Side effects to chemotherapy and radiation therapy are serious and include fatigue, hair loss, low red and white blood cell count, low platelet count, nausea, and vomiting. Radiation can cause dental problems, bladder, and fertility problems. In addition, clients experience high levels of stress and emotional disturbances	4dmdr, Actinomycin D, Andronate, Apo-Megestrol, Arimidex, Aromasin, Betaseron, BiCNU, Blenoxane, Busulfex, Casodex, Coladex, Colaspase, Cosmegen, Cytoxan, DepoCyt, DIC, Doxil, DTIC, Eloxatin, Emcyt, Etopophos, Euflex, Fludara, FUDR, Gemazar, Gleevec, Histerone, Ifex, Interleukin-2, Iressa, Lanvis, Leukeran, Leustatin, Matulane, Methotrexate, Mutamycin, Myleran, Nevelbine, Nilandron, Oncovin, Onxol, Paraplatin, Platinol, Prodox, Purinethol, Thioplex, Trelstar, Velban, Viadur, Zanosar, and many others	Each client living with cancer has a different experience and different needs. It is important to work directly with the client's physician to determine the best possible massage treatment plan. Working with cancer is discussed in greater detail in Chapter 23
Cardiac glycosides	Strengthen heart contraction, reduce heart rate, regulate heart rate	Dizziness, hypotension, muscle weakness, fatigue Adverse reactions include agitation, blurred vision, heart failure, hallucination, and others	Digitek, Digoxin, Lanoxicaps, Lanoxin	The condition for which the client is taking the medication is likely to influence the massage; consultation with the client's physician is recommended. Watch for dizziness at the conclusion of the massage and an abnormally low heart rate (50 or lower beats per min) during the massage
Chronic obstructive pulmonary disease medications	Reduce bronchial spasm, increase sensitivity to carbon dioxide in the brain's respiratory centers to stimulate respiration, decrease fatigue on the diaphragm.	Anxiety, cough, dizziness, dry mouth, insomnia, irritability, restlessness, and tremors Adverse reactions include anorexia, abdominal cramps,	Apo-Salvent, Accurbron, Atrovent, Bronkodyl, Choledyl, Crolom, Maxair, Norisodrine, Isuprel, Phyllocontin, and others	Anxiety and restlessness may inhibit the client's ability to relax completely. Use slow, soothing strokes and avoid strokes that stimulate the sympathetic system such as tapotement or rapid compression. Have water available

TABLE 5-1   Examples of Drugs with Implications for Massage *(Continued)*

Drug Type	Effects	Possible Side Effects	Examples of Commercial Drugs	Massage Considerations
	Decrease the release of histamine. Used to treat asthma, chronic bronchitis, and emphysema	arrhythmias, chest pain, diarrhea, joint pain, joint swelling, nausea, palpitations, rash, tachycardia, urinary dysfunction, vomiting, and others		throughout the massage in case the client's mouth becomes dry. Ensure the client is not dizzy or lightheaded at the conclusion of the massage. If dizzy, help the client from the massage table to prevent a falling accident
Decongestant medications	Constrict blood vessels in the nose and sinuses to open blocked air passages	Anxiety, dry mucus membranes in the nose, elevated blood pressure, insomnia, and restlessness Adverse reactions include allergic response, hypertension, nasal congestion, palpitations, urinary dysfunction, and others	Afrin, Bronchial Mist, Dionephrine, Pretz-D, VasoClear, and others	Clients may have difficulty relaxing at the beginning of the massage. Check the client's blood pressure before massage to ensure it is not above safe limits for massage (maximum systolic 159, diastolic 99). Refer clients who experience hypertension or other adverse reactions from decongestants to their health care provider
Diuretics—see also antihypertensive medications and vasodilators	Increase the excretion of water and electrolytes by the kidneys. Used in the treatment of hypertension	Breast soreness, drowsiness, headache, hypotension, and muscle cramps Adverse reactions include arrhythmias, confusion, dehydration, electrolyte imbalance, rash, shock, ulcers, and others	Apo-Chlorthalidone, Bumex, Demadex, Dyrenium, Edecril, Enduron, Ezide, Furocot, Inspra, Kaluril, Lozide, Metatensin, Naturetin, Renese, Spiractin, and others	Stimulating strokes used at the end of the massage or directly before changing positions can help combat drowsiness. Watch for low blood pressure. Ensure water is available directly after the massage. Apply direct pressure to muscle cramps if they occur during the session
Expectorant medications	Thin mucus so that it is easier for the body to clear it from the respiratory system. Expectorants also soothe mucus membranes. Used to treat respiratory symptoms like coughs and bronchial irritation	Drowsiness Adverse reactions include abdominal cramping, diarrhea, nausea, and vomiting	Balminil, Breonesin, Guaifenesin, Guiatuss, Robitussin, and others	People often take expectorant medications when they have a cold, flu, or acute sinusitis. Check to ensure the client does not have a fever or communicable disease before providing massage. Use stimulating strokes to combat drowsiness before changing positions or at the end of the massage to help the client wake up
Laxative medications	Draw water into the intestine to promote bowel distention and peristalsis, soften stools, and promote defecation	Abdominal cramps (mild), diarrhea, fatigue, flatulence, funny taste in mouth, irritated rectum, sore throat, and weakness Adverse reactions include abdominal cramping and distention, arrhythmias, dehydration, diarrhea, electrolyte imbalance, fecal impaction, nausea, vomiting, and others	Acilac, Citrucel, Colace, Dixidan, Dulcolax, Emulsoil, Fiber-lax, Glycerol, Hydrocil, Kondremul, Magonate, MiraLax, Visicol, and others	Have water available for the client during the massage. Gentle abdominal massage is indicated, but refer any symptoms other than mild abdominal cramps to the physician

(Continued)

TABLE 5-1   Examples of Drugs with Implications for Massage *(Continued)*

Drug Type	Effects	Possible Side Effects	Examples of Commercial Drugs	Massage Considerations
Muscle relaxants	Reduce muscle spasm, reduce muscle pain. Used to treat acute, painful muscle conditions	Constipation, diarrhea, dizziness, drowsiness, heartburn, hypotension, and nausea	Banflex, Carbacot, Carisoprodate, Dantrium, Flexeril, Flexitec, Isobamate, Myolin, Norflex Parafon Forte, Remular-S, Skelaxin, Soma, Strifon Forte, and others	Because clients likely have a reduced sensitivity to pain from the medication, avoid deep work. Watch for dizziness at the conclusion of massage or when changing positions
Narcotic analgesics	Used to reduce severe pain in acute illness, some chronic conditions, and terminal illness. May be used to reduce anxiety before anesthesia	Constipation, dizziness, drowsiness, euphoria, flushing, hypotension, pupil constriction Adverse reactions include asthma, depressed respiration, delirium, heart palpitations, and tremors	Demerol, Dolophine, Duragesic, Hydromorph Contin, Levo-Dormoran, Methadose, Morphine, Paveral, Roxanol, and others	Clients using these powerful analgesics likely have serious conditions that require massage cautions. In this case, work closely with the client's health care team to develop a comprehensive and safe treatment plan. Response to stimuli is likely reduced, and pain sensitivity may be minimal. Avoid deep techniques, and watch for a drop in blood pressure or dizziness at the conclusion of the massage or when changing positions. Monitor the client closely throughout the session and contact the physician if adverse reactions develop
Non-narcotic analgesics	Reduce pain and fever. Many also have anti-inflammatory effects	Dizziness, stomachache Adverse reactions usually do not occur with normal dosages	Salicylates: Amigesic, Aspirin, Bayer, Diflunisal, Dolobid, Empirin, Rexolate, Tricosal, Trilisate, and others Acetaminophen: Anacin, Panadol, Paracetamol, Tylenol	Because analgesics reduce the client's sensitivity to pain, avoid deep-tissue work or use caution. Some clients experience dizziness when sitting up after the massage. Use stimulating strokes at the conclusion of the massage and help the client off the massage table if the client feels lightheaded
Nonsteroidal anti-inflammatory medications	Reduce inflammation and pain	Diarrhea, dizziness, drowsiness, headache, nausea Adverse reactions include abdominal pain, bleeding, blood in the urine, bladder infection, jaundice, liver toxicity, ulcers, and vertigo	Actron, Advil, Anaprox, Ansaid, Bextra, Celebrex, Clinoril, Daypro, Feldene, Indocid, Lodine, Mobic, Motrin, Ponstan, Ralafen, Rimadyl, Tolecin, Vioxx, Voltaren, and others	Because pain sensitivity is reduced, avoid deep work or use caution. Some clients experience dizziness when sitting up after the massage. Use stimulating strokes at the conclusion of the massage to counteract drowsiness and help the client off the massage table if the client feels lightheaded
Sedative and anti-anxiety medications	Used to reduce anxiety or to induce sleep in conditions like insomnia Barbiturate sedatives depress the central nervous system and cause dependence and so are used for short periods of time only	Diarrhea, dizziness, dry mouth, drowsiness, gastric irritation, headache, hypotension, fatigue, fogginess, muscle weakness, nausea, palpitations, vertigo, and vomiting	Ambien, Amytal, Apo-Buspirone, Aquachloral, BuSpar, Buspirex, Butisol, Gen-Buspirone, Intensol, Mebaral, Nembutal, Novo-Clopate, Librium, Luminal, Paxipam, Placidyl,	Monitor blood pressure before and after the session and watch for dizziness when changing positions or getting on and off the massage table. Have water available for the client throughout the session in case of dry mouth. The effects of prescription and over-the-counter sleep aids

TABLE 5-1   Examples of Drugs with Implications for Massage *(Continued)*

Drug Type	Effects	Possible Side Effects	Examples of Commercial Drugs	Massage Considerations
		Adverse reactions include allergic reaction, amnesia, depression, drug dependence, respiratory arrest or depression, and others	Riva-Lorazepam, Seconal, Serax, Sonata, Valium, and others	often persist for 12–24 h. A client using a sedative medication could be foggy and "hung-over" on arrival for the massage. Reaction time and response to therapist questions may be slowed
Sex hormone medications	Estrogen is used in hormone replacement therapy for menopausal symptoms, or because of ovarian dysfunction or the removal of ovaries. It is also used in birth control medications. Progesterone is used to treat menopausal symptoms, for premenstrual syndrome, and in combination with estrogen for birth control	Breast swelling and tenderness, bleeding between menstrual cycles, bloating, decreased sex drive, headache, fatigue, irritability, nausea, weight gain, vomiting, and yeast infections. Adverse reactions include hypertension, blood vessel block caused by a blood clot, vein inflammation from blood clots, depression, embolism, jaundice, hyperglycemia, and others	Aygestin, Delestrogen, Depo-Estadiol, Climara, Crinone, Estratab, Estinyl, Estriol, Gesterol, Honvol, Menest, Neo-Estrone, Otho-Est, Premarin, Prempro, Prometrium, Provera, Triestrogen, and others	The main concern for massage is the development of blood clots sometimes caused by sex hormone medications. Ask the client about the presence of blood clots and look for redness, swelling, heat, and pain, especially in the legs. If blood clots are present or suspected, massage is contraindicated until a physician provides clearance
Steroids	Suppress immune responses and decrease inflammation to treat inflammatory disorders like arthritis. May also be applied topically for skin conditions	Hypertension, fluid retention, insomnia, suppressed immunity. Long-term use can lead to weakened connective tissue, muscle wasting, and decreased bone density. Adverse reactions include adrenal gland dysfunction, diabetes mellitus, impaired wound healing, osteoporosis, peptic ulcers, and others	Alphatrex, Betaderm, Compound E, Cortone, Decardron, Deltacortisone, Dexasone, Hexadrol, Hydrocortone, Inflamase Forte, Medrol, Prednisol, Propaderm, Sterapred, Winpred, and others	Massage adaptations depend somewhat on how long the client has been taking steroids. Monitor blood pressure before and after the massage because of hypertension. With long-term steroid use, avoid compression strokes because of bone density issues. Myofascial techniques could damage tissue, as could deep-tissue work. Use caution to avoid bruising the client
Thyroid medications	Reduce or increase thyroid hormones for conditions of thyroid deficiency (hypothyroidism) or thyroid excess (hyperthyroidism)	Abdominal cramps, angina, anxiety, arrhythmias, diarrhea, fever, headache, hypertension, increased body temperature, insomnia, menstrual changes, palpitations, rapid heart rate, weight loss, and others. Antithyroid drug reactions include decreased body temperature and feeling cold, diarrhea, drowsi	Armour Thyroid, Cytomel, Eltroxin, Iodotope, Levoxyl, Propyl-Thyracil, Tapazole, Thyrolar, Thyronine, Sodium Iodine, and others	Clients who have taken thyroid medications for some time and have adjusted to the medications are most likely to benefit from massage. Clients new to thyroid medications require a physician's release for massage until their reactions to the medication are established. Clients on antithyroid medications are likely to benefit from massage, but clients using radioactive iodine need a physician's release because special precautions are necessary

(Continued)

TABLE 5-1   Examples of Drugs with Implications for Massage *(Continued)*

Drug Type	Effects	Possible Side Effects	Examples of Commercial Drugs	Massage Considerations
		ness, funny taste in mouth, headache, joint and muscle pain, lymph node tenderness, nausea, vertigo, vomiting, and others Adverse reactions include blood disturbances, depression, liver dysfunction, and sensitivity reactions		
Vasodilators—see also antihypertensive medications and diuretics	Dilate veins, arteries or both, depending on the medication. Used to treat hypertension	Headache, hypotension, and fatigue Adverse reactions include angina, edema, palpitations, rash and others	Apo-Hydralazine, Apo-Gain, Apresoline, Hyperstat, Loniten, Minox, Nipride, Nitropress, Proglycem, Rogaine, and others	Negative reactions to massage are uncommon. Low blood pressure at the conclusion of the massage is unlikely but possible

serves only as a general preview, as space is not available to cover the extensive medications and side effects you might encounter in your practice. All massage therapists should have an in-depth and up-to-date drug guide and pathology guide for reference. Because drugs change and new drugs emerge frequently, you should purchase a new drug reference when you start to encounter drug names that are not covered in the reference book.

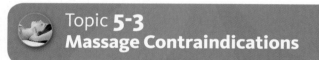

Topic 5-3
Massage Contraindications

Chapter 4 discusses the effects of massage on the client's body, mind, and emotions. These effects demonstrate the profound influence that massage can have on body systems, especially the circulatory system, nervous system, and musculoskeletal system. It should therefore be easy to understand that certain techniques could be overpowering for some clients or exacerbate a preexisting condition. While massage is usually beneficial and indicated for most clients, some client conditions make massage inadvisable; these are called **contraindications**. A contraindication is any condition that makes the application of massage unadvised or potentially dangerous to the health of the client. Before we explore specific contraindications, we'll first examine the question of when massage is dangerous.

When Is Massage Dangerous?

Massage therapy has few serious risks when appropriate cautions are followed. Investigations of insurance claims related to massage often reveal that general safety procedures were not adhered to in situations of liability. Associated Bodywork and Massage Professionals (ABMP) is the largest massage membership organization in the United States. Massage therapists receive liability insurance as part of their membership, and ABMP insurance claims can offer some useful information about massage hazards.

Burns to clients from hot stone massage resulted in the highest number of claims filed at ABMP in 2008. In some cases, burns occurred even when the stones were not placed directly on the skin but were insulated by towels. Elderly clients with thin, delicate skin should be directed to a different massage system like Swedish massage or reflexology because they are particularly prone to burning. Safety procedures for stone massage are outlined in Chapter 15.

Back injuries during seated massage comprise the second highest number of claims filed at ABMP in recent years. In many of the claims, therapists had not asked clients for a complete health history and so were not aware of preexisting conditions that contraindicated particular techniques. In one case, compression strokes, which are typical in seated massage because they are easy to apply over clothing, caused a rib fracture. The therapist was unaware that the client had osteoporosis (weakened bones) or would likely have chosen a safer technique. Safety procedures for seated massage are discussed in Chapter 14.

Rib fractures, rib bruising, and spinal injuries like herniated disks from Swedish and deep-tissue massage techniques have also occurred, though with some claims it is unclear if clients had preexisting conditions that were exacerbated by massage or whether massage actually caused the injury. In some of the claims, it is clear that therapists were working too forcefully on elderly clients or clients who were in poor physical health. It is important to remain vigilant and adjust your techniques to fit the overall health of the client.

Bruising and intense soreness occur in some clients when deep work is performed. This is why deep work is avoided if the client is on a blood-thinning medication or pain medication. Clients also experienced minor muscle strains with stretching techniques. In one case, a client sustained a serious rotator cuff injury from forceful range of motion techniques applied at the shoulder. Allergies and skin irritation caused by massage lubricant products have also occurred. ABMP notes that stroke and heart condition complications have occurred in the past but that these are very rare.

Finally, ABMP notes that a number of injuries were reported in relationship to equipment. For example, when the bolts on the table legs were not tightened down and legs fell off tables, clients fell to the floor. Clients have also fallen when getting off massage tables at the end of massages. One client fainted in a massage chair and fell out of the chair while the therapist was getting the client water.

These cautionary tales are not meant to frighten anyone, and it should be repeated that massage is a low-risk complementary and alternative therapy. Still, these claims should remind all therapists to conduct careful health history intakes, understand contraindications, use adaptive measures when the client's health indicates that adjustments are necessary, and pay attention to their judgment. If you feel doubtful about working with a client because of a physical condition, refer the client to their health care provider for a release or to a more experienced therapist. A long-standing massage motto is, "When in doubt, refer out."

Contraindications

As stated previously, a contraindication is any condition that makes the application of massage unadvised or potentially dangerous to the health of the client. Table 5-2 provides an overview of contraindicated conditions. Following are the different types of contraindications and other implications:

- **Absolute contraindication.** If the client has a condition that is an absolute contraindication, the client should not receive massage. Examples include a significant fever (100°F or higher), vomiting, a cold (unless the symptoms have been present for 5 days or longer; usually people are contagious from 24 hours before they notice symptoms to 5 days after the first symptom), an acute systemic condition (when the condition affects the entire body and not just one local region), an injury that requires medical attention, or symptoms that are intense and unexplained (e.g., intense headache pain). For example, a client with chicken pox or pink eye should not receive massage because the client is

extremely contagious and these conditions could be passed to the therapist or to other clients. Similarly, massage should not be provided to relieve headache pain in a client with a recent concussion. Not only would massage overstimulate this client, but the client needs to see a physician to rule out serious complications. Table 5-2 shows conditions that are absolute contraindications. Note that many conditions are contraindications in an acute stage, when the body is inflamed and the condition flares up, but are not contraindications in a subacute or chronic stage. Chapter 22 provides detailed explanations about the inflammatory process in Topic 22-2.

- **Local contraindication.** A condition may affect only one area of the body. Massage can be applied to the rest of the body but the local area is avoided. If a client recently had a mole removed, you would not massage over the area of reforming skin. If a client has a swollen knee, you would not massage the area distal to the swelling and the swollen area, but the area proximal to the swelling and the rest of the body can be massaged.

- **Advanced understanding.** Some therapists receive extra training and specialize in working with clients with specific conditions. Because of their experience, often through participation on a health care team, they develop an advanced understanding of the condition and know the limits of massage. These therapists can often work safely with a condition that would be a contraindication for a less experienced therapist. Novice therapists may avoid certain conditions early in their practices and then work with the same condition later as their knowledge increases with professional experience. Regardless of your level of experience, it is important to obtain a physician's release with complex conditions or clients who are taking multiple medications.

- **Physician's release.** Before providing massage to clients with certain conditions, it is prudent to obtain a physician's release. The release indicates that the physician believes that massage will not harm the client and may prove beneficial to the client's health. In some cases, physicians are champions of massage, receive massage themselves, and understand the wide range of techniques that might be employed in a session. Other physicians do not understand massage, its physiological effects, or the increased burden it can place on a weakened client's system. If possible, explain to the physician or the physician's staff the types of techniques you plan to use in the client's session and the ways these techniques might affect the client's body systems. This may help the physician make the best possible recommendations.

- **Use caution.** In many cases, the client is not contraindicated for massage but the massage must be adapted to fit the client's overall vitality and stamina. Obviously, a client who is young and in good physical condition can receive a more vigorous massage than an elderly client who is thin and frail. Sometimes the massage is shortened or certain techniques are avoided. Sometimes the way in which the client is positioned on the table is changed to accommodate a particular condition. You may be able to work with the client as you normally would but with increased vigilance. Watch for any change in the client's condition or for side effects or adverse effects that may develop. A sudden increase in pain, moderate-to-intense discomfort, agitation, nausea, headache, or excessive dizziness is a sign that the client is not responding to massage normally. If any of these symptoms occurs during a treatment, stop the session, offer the client water, and allow the client to relax. Monitor the client at all times and do not allow the client to leave until the symptoms have disappeared. If symptoms persist after the session has ended, you should consult a physician. If the symptoms increase rapidly after the session has ended, the client could be in danger and you should call emergency services.

Concept Brief 5-8
Types of Contraindications

- **Absolute:** No massage is provided
- **Local:** One area of the body is contraindicated for massage
- **Physician's release:** A physician approves the use of massage for a client
- **Advanced understanding:** A therapist with advanced training or understanding may work with a client who would otherwise be contraindicated, usually still requiring a physician's release
- **Use caution:** Massage is not contraindicated but the therapist remains vigilant

---

TABLE 5-2 Quick Contraindications Reference

Condition	C	AU	PR	LC	UC	I
Abortion (spontaneous or elective)			X	X	X	
Acne vulgaris				X		
Acromegaly			X		X	
AIDS (client condition good)			X		X	
AIDS (client condition poor)		X	X			
Allergic reaction	X					
Alzheimer					X	X
Amenorrhea					X	X
Angina pectoris			X		X	
Anemia (nutritional deficiency)						X
Anemia (non-nutritional deficiency)			X		X	
Aneurysm			X		X	
Anorexia nervosa (stable condition)						X
Ankylosing spondylitis (acute)	X					
Ankylosing spondylitis (chronic)						X
Anxiety disorders					X	X
Appendicitis	X					
Arteriosclerosis			X		X	
Asthma attack	X					
Asthma					X	X
Atherosclerosis					X	
Athlete's foot				X		
Attention-deficit hyperactivitydisorder					X	X
Avascular osteonecrosis			X	X	X	

C, absolute contraindication; AU, advanced understanding or training is required; PR, a physician's release is required; LC, local contraindication; UC, use caution and adaptive measures; I, massage is particularly indicated.

TABLE 5-2 **Quick Contraindications Reference** *(Continued)*

Condition	C	AU	PR	LC	UC	I
Baker cysts				X		
Bed sore/pressure sore				X		
Bell palsy					X	
Bipolar disorder			X		X	X
Bladder cancer			X		X	X
Boil				X		
Breast cancer			X		X	X
Bronchitis (acute)	X					
Bronchitis (chronic)						X
Bruise				X		
Bunions				X		
Burns				X		
Bursitis (acute)				X		
Bursitis (chronic)					X	
Cancer		X	X		X	
Candidiasis					X	
Cardiac arrest (history of)			X		X	
Carpal tunnel syndrome					X	
Cellulitis	X					
Cerebral palsy			X		X	X
Cervical cancer			X		X	X
Chemical dependancy (recovery from)						X
Chickenpox	X					
Cholecystitis	X					
Chronic fatigue syndrome					X	X
Cirrhosis of the liver		X	X		X	
Colitis					X	
Common cold (5 d after symptoms)					X	
Conjunctivitis/pinkeye	X					
Constipation						X
Contact dermatitis				X		
Contusion or concussion	X					
Coronary artery disease			X		X	
Crohn disease			X		X	
Cushing disease			X		X	
Cystic fibrosis			X			X
Cysts				X		
Cystitis (acute)	X					
Cystitis (chronic)					X	

C, absolute contraindication; AU, advanced understanding or training is required; PR, a physician's release is required; LC, local contraindication; UC, use caution and adaptive measures; I, massage is particularly indicated.

(Continued)

TABLE 5-2 Quick Contraindications Reference *(Continued)*

Condition	C	AU	PR	LC	UC	I
Depression					X	X
Diabetes insipidus			X		X	
Diabetes mellitus			X		X	
Disc disease (acute)				X		
Disc disease (chronic)					X	
Dislocations (acute)				X	X	
Dislocations (subacute, chronic)						X
Diverticulitis (acute)	X					
Diverticulosis (chronic)			X	X	X	
Dysmenorrhea					X	X
Eating disorders					X	X
Eczema				X		
Edema		X		X	X	
Embolism/thrombus	X	X	X			
Emphysema			X		X	X
Encephalitis	X					
Endocarditis	X					
Endometriosis					X	X
Epilepsy			X		X	
Esophageal cancer			X		X	
Fatigue					X	X
Fever	X					
Fibrocystic breast disease						X
Fibroid tumors					X	
Fibromyalgia					X	X
Flaccid muscles					X	
Folliculitis				X		
Fractures				X		
Fungal infections				X		
Ganglion cysts				X		
Gastroenteritis (acute)	X					
Gastroenteritis (chronic)					X	
Gastroesophageal reflux disease					X	
Goiter					X	
Glomerulonephritis	X					
Gout (systemic, acute)	X					
Gout (one joint, chronic)				X		
Guillain–Barré syndrome (in remission)			X		X	

C, absolute contraindication; AU, advanced understanding or training is required; PR, a physician's release is required; LC, local contraindication; UC, use caution and adaptive measures; I, massage is particularly indicated.

TABLE 5-2 Quick Contraindications Reference *(Continued)*

Condition	C	AU	PR	LC	UC	I
Graves disease			X		X	
Headache (tension)						X
Heart murmur			X		X	
Heart attack/myocardial infarction (recovery from)		X	X		X	
Heart failure		X	X		X	
Hemangioma				X		
Hematoma				X		
Hemophilia (mild)			X		X	
Hemophilia (severe)	X					
Hemorrhage	X					
Hepatitis (acute)	X					
Hepatitis (chronic)			X		X	
Hernia				X		
Herniated disk				X	X	
Herpes simplex (active symptoms)				X		
High-risk pregnancy		X	X			
HIV (non-symptomatic)			X		X	
Hives	X					
Hypercholesterolemia	X					
Hypertension			X		X	
Hyperthyroidism					X	
Hypoglycemia					X	
Hypotension					X	
Hypothyroidism					X	
Ichthyosis vulgaris						X
Impetigo	X					
Inflammation (acute)	X					
Inflammation (subacute)					X	
Inflammation (chronic)						X
Influenza	X					
Insomnia						X
Interstitial cystitis					X	
Intestinal obstruction	X					
Irritable bowel syndrome						X
Jaundice		X	X		X	
Kidney stones (acute)	X					
Kidney stones (history of)						X
Leukemia		X	X		X	
Lice	X					

C, absolute contraindication; AU, advanced understanding or training is required; PR, a physician's release is required; LC, local contraindication; UC, use caution and adaptive measures; I, massage is particularly indicated.

(Continued)

TABLE 5-2   Quick Contraindications Reference *(Continued)*

Condition	C	AU	PR	LC	UC	I
Liver cancer		X	X		X	
Lung cancer		X	X		X	
Lou Gehrig disease (ALS)		X	X		X	
Lupus (flare up or acute)	X					
Lupus (in remission)					X	
Lyme disease (acute)	X					
Lyme disease (chronic)			X		X	
Lymphangitis	X					
Lymphoma		X	X		X	
Lymphedema		X	X		X	
Marfan syndrome		X	X		X	
Meningitis	X					
Menopause						X
Metabolic syndrome			X		X	
Mites	X					
Mononucleosis	X					
Multiple sclerosis (in remission)						X
Muscle spasm						X
Muscular dystrophy			X			X
Myasthenia gravis			X			X
Myocarditis	X					
Myofascial pain syndrome						X
Myositis ossificans				X		
Neuropathy			X	X	X	
Obesity					X	
Open wounds or sores				X		
Osgood–Schlatters disease (history of)						X
Osteoarthritis (flare up)	X					
Osteoarthritis (chronic)						X
Osteoporosis					X	
Ovarian cancer			X		X	
Ovarian cysts				X		
Paget disease			X		X	
Pancreatic cancer			X		X	
Pancreatitis (acute)	X					
Pancreatitis (chronic)					X	
Paralysis		X	X		X	
Parkinson disease					X	X
Patellofemoral syndrome (chronic)						X

C, absolute contraindication; AU, advanced understanding or training is required; PR, a physician's release is required; LC, local contraindication; UC, use caution and adaptive measures; I, massage is particularly indicated.

TABLE 5-2   Quick Contraindications Reference *(Continued)*

Condition	C	AU	PR	LC	UC	I
Pelvic inflammatory disease	X					
Pericarditis	X					
Peripheral neuropathy				X	X	
Peripheral vascular disease (mild)			X		X	
Peritonitis	X					
Plantar fascitis						X
Pleurisy (nonbacterial)			X		X	
Pneumonia	X					
Polio (history of)					X	
Polycystic kidney disease			X		X	
Postural deviations						X
Pregnancy (high-risk)		X	X		X	
Preeclampsia	X					
Pregnancy (no complications)						X
Premenstrual syndrome						X
Prostatitis (chronic)					X	
Pseudo-sciatica			X			
Psoriasis				X		
Pulmonary edema	X					
Pyelonephritis	X					
Raynaud syndrome						X
Renal failure	X					
Rheumatoid arthritis (acute or flare up)	X					
Rheumatoid arthritis (chronic)					X	
Ringworm	X					
Scabies	X					
Scleroderma			X		X	
Sebaceous cyst				X		
Seizures (history of, or chronic)					X	X
Shingles/herpes zoster (acute)	X					
Shingles/herpes zoster (chronic)						X
Shin splints						X
Sickle cell disease			X		X	
Sinusitis (no fever present)					X	
Skin cancer			X	X		
Sleep disorders						X
Spinal cord injury		X	X		X	
Spondylosis			X		X	X
Sprains					X	X

C, absolute contraindication; AU, advanced understanding or training is required; PR, a physician's release is required; LC, local contraindication; UC, use caution and adaptive measures; I, massage is particularly indicated.

(Continued)

TABLE 5-2   Quick Contraindications Reference *(Continued)*

Condition	C	AU	PR	LC	UC	I
Stomach cancer			X		X	
Strains					X	X
Stroke (history of)		X	X		X	
Substance abuse (recovery from)						X
Sunburn (mild)					X	
Sunburn (moderate to severe)	X					
Surgery (postoperative)			X		X	
Temporomandibular joint disorder					X	X
Tendinitis					X	X
Tenosynovitis (acute)				X		
Tenosynovitis (subacute or chronic)						X
Thoracic outlet syndrome			X			
Thrombophlebitis/deep vein thrombosis	X					
Tonsillitis	X					
Torticollis			X			X
Tremor			X		X	
Trigeminal neuralgia				X		
Tuberculosis (no longer infective)						X
Ulcerative colitis (acute)	X					
Ulcerative colitis (chronic)			X			
Ulcers				X		
Urinary tract infection	X					
Varicose veins				X		
Warts				X		
Whiplash (acute)				X		
Whiplash (subacute, chronic)			X		X	X

C, absolute contraindication; AU, advanced understanding or training is required; PR, a physician's release is required; LC, local contraindication; UC, use caution and adaptive measures; I, massage is particularly indicated.

Common Conditions that Require Caution

While the range of conditions you might see in professional practice is vast, hypertension, integumentary issues, and diabetes are fairly common and so require special attention. Considerations for special populations such as pregnant women, infants, the elderly, people in recovery from abuse, the terminally ill, people living with a physical challenge, people living with a psychological challenge, people living with cancer, and people living with HIV/AIDS are not discussed here; cautions and contraindications for these groups are discussed in depth in later chapters.

Hypertension

Blood pressure refers to the force of blood pushing against blood vessel walls as it circulates throughout the body. A sphygmomanometer is an instrument that measures this pressure at two different moments. The systolic pressure is the peak pressure in the arteries, which occurs near the beginning of the cardiac cycle during ventricular contraction. The diastolic pressure is the lowest pressure of the resting phase of the cardiac cycle during ventricular relaxation. A blood pressure cuff measures the pressure in the arteries in millimeters of mercury, which is why the abbreviation mm Hg is used in blood pressure descriptions.

High blood pressure, called **hypertension**, is a blood pressure consistently elevated above 140 mm Hg systolic and

90 mm Hg diastolic. Usually in chart notes, physicians or nurses write this blood pressure as 140/90. The top or first number refers to the systolic pressure and the bottom number the diastolic number.

Essential hypertension is hypertension that is not due to some other pathology. Secondary hypertension is high blood pressure that is a symptom of a separate pathology such as a hormonal disorder. Malignant hypertension is a dangerous condition in which the diastolic pressure increases rapidly over the course of weeks or months and requires immediate medical attention. Most hypertension cases are essential hypertension and are caused by smoking, being overweight, a sedentary lifestyle, a salty diet, high alcohol consumption, stress, age, and genetic factors as evidenced by a family history of hypertension. Pregnancy, kidney disease, and adrenal and thyroid gland disorders are some of the causes of secondary hypertension.

Hypertension is a serious condition that causes damage to the heart and blood vessels. Left untreated, it can lead to atherosclerosis, aneurysms, stroke, heart failure, heart attack, kidney failure, and vision problems. Blood pressure parameters are:

- Normal: <120/80
- Prehypertension: 120–139/80–89
- Stage 1 hypertension: 140–159/90–99
- Stage 2 hypertension: 160 and above/100 and above

Many massage therapists feel it unnecessary to take a client's blood pressure before a massage, but because this is the best way to ensure the client's safety, blood pressure readings are becoming more common in massage clinics. Massage increases circulation and stimulates fluid movement in the body. This can be overtaxing for the heart and blood vessels if they are already under stress from high blood pressure. In some

---

Technique 5   Taking a Blood Pressure Reading

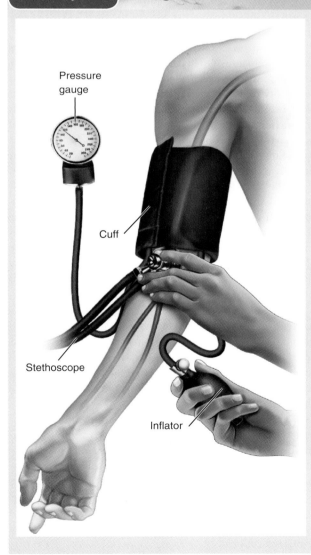

Pressure gauge

Cuff

Stethoscope

Inflator

1. A sphygmomanometer (often called sphygmometer or blood pressure cuff) is comprised of an inflatable cuff connected to an inflation bulb used to pump air into the cuff and restrict blood flow for measuring blood pressure. A gauge on the cuff indicates blood pressure in millimeters of mercury (mm Hg). It is important to use a cuff that fits the client's arm correctly; have a small, medium, and large cuff on hand. Hold the bulb in one hand and tighten and loosen the screw valve multiple times until you can manipulate it comfortably with either hand. A stethoscope is a device used to listen to internal sounds in the human body, in this case blood flow. It has earpieces and a rounded metal end often referred to as the chest piece.

2. Ask the client to remove outer layers of clothing or to roll up a sleeve to uncover the cubital fossa and the lower half of the upper arm. The client should be seated comfortably with the arm resting on a table. Deflate the bladder of the cuff by opening the screw valve and then wrap the cuff around the client's arm directly above the elbow on the lower part of the upper arm. The cuff should be snug but not too tight, and the gauge should be easy to see.

3. Palpate the radial pulse with one hand and inflate the cuff until the radial pulse disappears (because it is occluded by the cuff). Note the reading on the gauge when this occurs and quickly open the screw valve to deflate the cuff. Add 30 mm Hg to this reading. This tells you how high to inflate the cuff to take the blood pressure reading.

4. Place the earpieces of the stethoscope in your ears and the chest piece over the client's brachial artery in the cubital fossa just slightly under the bottom edge of the cuff. Tighten the screw valve so that no air escapes as you pump up the cuff. Inflate the cuff with brisk squeezes of the bulb until the pressure is 30 mm Hg above the earlier reading where the radial pulse disappears.

5. Slightly open the screw valve on the inflation bulb to slowly release the air from the cuff. Don't open it so much that all the pressure quickly releases, but don't open it so little that air doesn't escape and the cuff remains almost completely inflated. As you release the screw valve, listen carefully while watching the gauge. You are listening for a slight "blrrpp" or "prrpshh" sound. When you hear this first sound, note the reading on the gauge and continue to listen. When you hear the sound for the last time, note the reading on the gauge. The reading at the first sound is the systolic pressure and that at the second sound is the diastolic pressure. Release all the pressure from the cuff and record your findings in your chart notes (discussed in Chapter 12). If you do not get a good reading on the first arm, try again with the other arm. If you cannot take a reading on the other arm due to an IV line, edema in the limb, bruising, or some other reason, wait at least 2 minutes before trying again on the same arm. Do not take a client's blood pressure more than three times.

massage clinics, blood pressure is taken on the client's first visit. If the client's blood pressure is within normal limits, it is not taken again for a year. If the client's blood pressure is elevated, it is taken before every session. If a client is pregnant or lists hypertension on the health history form, a blood pressure is taken before every session. Note that a blood pressure reading may be temporarily elevated in clients who have recently consumed alcohol (these clients should not receive massage), smoked a cigarette, or had a large amount of caffeine.

Many massage schools do not teach students to take blood pressure readings, especially if the curriculum focuses on wellness massage. While this is understandable, it is a good skill to learn. Taking blood pressure readings is not difficult with practice and is described in Technique 5.

Some clients with hypertension take prescription medications to control their blood pressure. As long as their blood pressure falls in the range from normal to stage 1 hypertension, massage is usually not contraindicated. Deep abdominal work is contraindicated for any client with elevated blood pressure or who is taking blood pressure medications, but gentle, superficial abdominal massage for relaxation is usually fine. Also avoid very vigorous or very stimulating techniques that trigger the sympathetic nervous system. If a client's blood pressure is over 140/90, refer the client to his or her health care provider for follow-up before providing massage. This is to rule out pathologies like kidney infections and to ensure the client receives treatment for hypertension. Any client with stage 1 hypertension should obtain a physician's release before receiving massage. Any client with stage 2 hypertension is contraindicated for massage except under the supervision of a physician.

Concept Brief 5-9
Blood Pressure

Systolic pressure: Peak pressure in arteries at the beginning of cardiac cycle, with ventricular contraction

Diastolic pressure: Lowest pressure in arteries in the resting phase of cardiac cycle, with ventricular relaxation

Essential hypertension: High blood pressure not due to some other pathology

Secondary hypertension: High blood pressure as a symptom of a different pathology

Malignant hypertension: Diastolic pressure increases in a short time frame, requiring immediate medical attention

Normal range: 120/80 or lower

Prehypertension: 120–139/80–89

Stage 1 hypertension: 140–159/90–99 (physician's release required)

Stage 2 hypertension: 160 and above/100 and above (massage contraindicated without direct physician supervision)

Integumentary Conditions

Any areas of broken skin such as open wounds, scratches, blemishes, or scabs are local contraindications. Contagious skin conditions like cellulitis, impetigo, mites (scabies), and lice are absolute contraindications, and massage should not be provided. Hives is a reaction to stress or an allergy that makes the skin hot, swollen, and itchy. It is a local contraindication if it is confined to one small region, but an absolute contraindication if widespread.

With a skin condition that is contagious but confined to one small area such as boils, fungal infections including ringworm, herpes simplex, and warts, the area is locally contraindicated, but massage can be applied to other areas of the body. Separate used linens that were exposed to contagious skin conditions, especially herpes, and use bleach and hot water in the wash cycle. Sanitize your hands, wear vinyl gloves, and clean all massage equipment and the treatment room with extra care after the session.

Avoid massaging directly over areas of acne (a bacterial infection of the sebaceous glands) because massage might spread the infection to other areas of the client's skin or cause increased blemishing by massage lubricants blocking pores.

Dermatitis is a nonspecific term describing many types of skin inflammation. Often dermatitis is caused by contact with an irritating substance or allergen. Eczema is caused by hypersensitivity reactions of the skin. Psoriasis is a noncontagious skin disorder in which epithelial skin cells replicate rapidly in patches and turn itchy and scaly. If the skin of a client with any of these conditions is very inflamed, is open due to scratching, or is weepy or crusty with delicate scabs, treat the areas as a local contraindication.

If the skin is in a relatively good condition, not overly inflamed, intact, and not crusty, it may respond well to massage with a natural anti-inflammatory lubricant like hemp seed oil and skin-soothing essential oils like German chamomile and helichrysum oil (see the Aromatherapy section in Chapter 15). Do not use products with synthetic fragrances, dyes, mineral oil, lanolin, coconut oil, grapeseed oil, or cocoa butter on clients with dermatitis, eczema, or psoriasis.

Precancerous skin conditions like actinic lesions and skin cancers like basal cell carcinoma and squamous cell carcinoma are local contraindications. Malignant melanoma spreads rapidly and is treated aggressively, often with chemotherapy and radiation. Any massage for clients with malignant melanoma should take place only under the guidance of the client's physician.

Skin injuries such as burns (including moderate-to-severe sunburn), ulcers, or open wounds are local contraindications. Widespread burns and ulcerations may be an absolute contraindication, depending on their severity. The scar tissue that forms over burns, ulcers, or wounds responds well to massage in the subacute and chronic stages. Massage can improve the appearance and mobility of this type of scar tissue. Keloid scar tissue and raised moles are local contraindications.

Diabetes

Diabetes is a group of related conditions that result in elevated levels of blood sugar (hyperglycemia). About 98% of all diabetes cases are either type 1 (rarer and more serious) or type 2 diabetes (~20.8 million cases in the United States). Gestational diabetes affects about 4% of all pregnant women and accounts for around 135,000 cases each year.[6]

In type 1 diabetes, the body does not produce insulin, the hormone needed to convert sugar (glucose) into energy. It may have genetic roots, as it runs in families, or be caused by exposure to certain drugs, chemicals, or infections. It is caused by an autoimmune response in which killer T cells damage parts of the beta cells in the pancreas where insulin is created, causing a life-long deficiency. People with type 1 diabetes must take injections of insulin and monitor their blood sugar levels carefully to avoid very high levels, which can cause ketoacidosis, or very low blood sugar, which can cause **insulin shock**. Ketoacidosis is a condition in which the body metabolizes fats for fuel because the lack of insulin does not allow glucose to be used for energy in cells. The acidic waste of rapid fat metabolism changes the pH balance of the blood and can lead to shock, coma, and death.

In type 2 diabetes, the body does not produce enough insulin or target cells have fewer receptor sites for insulin than needed. While the exact cause of type 2 diabetes is unknown, it is linked to high-carbohydrate diets and is often treated with diet, exercise, and medications. Some people with type 2 diabetes have to supplement this regime with self-administered insulin. While people with type 2 diabetes do not experience ketoacidosis, they may develop a blood pH imbalance related to high blood sugar, called hyperosmolality, which can lead to shock, coma, and death.

Insulin shock, very low blood sugar, can occur in both type 1 and 2 diabetes but can be treated effectively simply by ingesting juice, milk, candy, or sugar-containing soft drinks right away to increase blood sugar levels. Over time, diabetes can lead to serious complications including cardiovascular disease, stroke, hypertension, aneurysm, edema, ulcers, gangrene, amputations, kidney disease, impaired vision, blindness, and neuropathy.

The types of massage techniques that can be used with clients who have diabetes depend on the state of the individual's health. Clients with poorly treated diabetes may have serious edema, ulcerations on their extremities, impaired circulation, and/or severe neuropathy. Very light massage or energetic techniques might be the only strokes that are appropriate for such clients. On the other hand, a client who monitors blood sugar carefully, eats a healthy diet, gets exercise, and experiences few complications may have massage as usual.

Keep in mind the fact that massage stimulates the body and uses up available glucose and insulin faster, which can lead to an imbalance, usually low blood sugar.[7] It's important to talk this over with the client, who may need to plan meal times and insulin injections to better accommodate the massage. Clients can also monitor their blood sugar immediately before massage and make the necessary adjustments by eating a small snack or injecting insulin if needed. Keep some form of sugar in your office (juice, candy, regular soft drinks) in case a client becomes hypoglycemic. If a diabetic client becomes confused, irritable, weak, or shaky or has clammy skin, stop the massage and offer the client some sugar. If the client does not respond quickly to the sugar, call emergency services immediately. It is not in the massage scope of practice to test a client's blood glucose level or inject insulin.

Massage therapists should obtain a physician's release when working with a client with advanced or poorly treated diabetes. If possible, discuss with the physician the types of strokes you would like to use in the session and their effects on the body, to obtain the best possible recommendations to ensure the client's safety.

Critical Thinking and Contraindications

Therapists may discover contraindications or situations that require caution in the client's completed health intake form and the intake interview, in their observations of the client, or from palpation findings or reactions the client has to massage treatment.

Often the client has a condition diagnosed by a physician and understands how that condition affects the body. As long as the condition is not a complete contraindication, the client and therapist can discuss session goals and plan **adaptive measures** to ensure comfort during the session. In some cases, a client's condition may be serious or complex enough to cause concern, in which case the therapist should contact the client's physician and obtain a release. Often therapists ask clients to bring a release to their first sessions. Clients who do not have a diagnosed condition but who complain of symptoms like fatigue, muscle weakness, unexplained pain or stiffness, persistent headache, or feelings of lethargy should see their physician and obtain a release before receiving massage. Undiagnosed symptoms may indicate a serious condition that might be exacerbated by massage. Following is the basic process by which therapists rule out contraindications:

1. Administer a health intake form (Chapter 12) and review the form carefully.

2. Conduct a health intake interview (Chapter 12) and ask the client to describe symptoms, general health, goals for the massage, and side effects from medications. Ensure that the client has listed all medications and conditions on the health intake form.

3. Look up unfamiliar diagnosed conditions in a pathology reference. *A Massage Therapists Guide to Pathology* by Ruth Werner is highly recommended.

4. Determine if the client's condition has flared up (moved suddenly from a chronic stage to an acute stage with intense symptoms). A condition that has flared up is more likely to be contraindicated. If the symptom level is normal for the client and the condition has not flared up, massage is more likely to be safe for the client.

5. Look up medications in a drug reference. Note the side effects of the medication and check these against the client's experience. If the client describes symptoms that are listed as adverse effects of a medication, the situation needs further discussion. A call to the client's physician is advised.

6. Conditions vary from client to client, depending on other variables in the client's life. After researching the condition and medication, and questioning the client about any side effects experienced from medications, assess the client visually. Get an overall impression of the client's physical health, level of vitality, and stamina. Don't underestimate your intuition. Even if the reference books say massage is okay, if your gut tells you "no," listen to your gut.

7. Determine if the client is contraindicated, needs a physician's release, has any area that should not receive massage, should be referred to a more experienced massage therapist, or should be referred to another health care provider. If you decide that massage is not contraindicated and that you do not need a physician's release but that adaptive measures are required, discuss your thoughts with the client. What does the client hope to achieve from massage? What type of massage does the client want? How does the client feel right now? How does the client hope to feel at the conclusion of the massage? Depending on the client's condition, you may eliminate the use of some techniques or adjust your pressure and the speed of your strokes. You may decide to avoid the use of hydrotherapy (e.g., a hot pack) and shorten the session's length (e.g., offer a 30-minute session instead of 60 or 90 minutes).

8. A client may list a few symptoms but not have a diagnosed condition or be taking medications. Question the client carefully. Perhaps a client tells you about weekly headaches believed to be from neck and shoulder tension. The client may have periods of nausea and refer to them as "nervous stomach." The nausea may occur when the client must give a presentation at work. The client also reports being unable to sleep for the last week and feeling moody and irritable. The client believes these symptoms are related to work stress and not related to any serious condition. You palpate the client's shoulders through clothing and confirm the neck and shoulders are very tense and the headaches could be the result of this tension. You have to decide if it is safe to provide massage. Probably it is. While these symptoms could be related to a more serious condition, the client has given you a logical explanation, and your shoulder and neck palpation supports the client's perception about the headaches. Your visual assessment tells you the client is in moderate physical health and has good skin coloring, and your impression of the client's overall vitality and stamina is good. You check the client's blood pressure, which is within normal parameters, and proceed with the massage but remain vigilant throughout the session.

A different client might tell you about waking up with pain in all the joints, with a pounding headache, and feeling incredible fatigue. The client can give no explanation for these symptoms. Because these symptoms came on very suddenly with no logical explanation, you refer such clients to their physician for a release and postpone the session. Remember: when in doubt, refer out.

Table 5-2 provides an overview of conditions for quick reference, but do not rely completely on such a list. Each client and each situation is different, and therapists need to learn to reason clinically so that they can make appropriate decisions for each client. Novice therapists may shy away from conditions that an experienced therapist can work with safely. An up-to-date medical dictionary, drug reference, pathology reference book, and Internet sources should be readily available for researching unfamiliar conditions and medications. If you have any doubt about the suitability of massage for a client, be cautious and postpone the treatment until you have obtained a physician's release. Contraindications for specific techniques, some soft-tissue conditions, and special populations are described in greater detail in the upcoming chapters

MASSAGE FUSION
Integration of Skills

STUDY TIP: Up to the Test!

To do well on a written test, you must know the information, but you must also have a good test-taking plan. A good plan helps prevent test anxiety and leads to better test scores. Try the PASS method to do your best on your next test:

P = Prepare: Prepare for the test by first breaking the test topics into different study sessions. Don't try to learn a whole chapter the night before the test. For example, for a test on this chapter, you might plan four study sessions.

Study one topic in each of the first three study sessions and then review all the topics together in the final study session. Write a test yourself from the chapter. By combing the chapter to make test questions, you can predict what the instructor might ask and have a good chapter review in the process.

A = Arrive early: Before leaving for school, eat a light meal but avoid sugar, which can adversely affect your thinking. Drink lots of water because people think better when they are hydrated. Get plenty of sleep the night before the test so you are well rested. Arrive early and read through

MASSAGE FUSION (*Continued*)
Integration of Skills

your notes one last time. Then put the notes aside and focus on your breathing while you clear your mind.

S = See success: Don't fall into negative thinking (e.g., "I don't know this chapter well enough and I'm sure to fail!"). Give yourself positive energy (e.g., "I studied. I'm ready. I'll do great!"). See yourself succeeding and answering every question with ease. Visualizing success helps your mind relax and focus on the test content.

S = Strategize: Proven test-taking strategies can help you score high. First, read the directions carefully. Many students assume they understand the directions and then make wrong choices based on false assumptions. Next, answer everything you know first. This warms up your brain and gives you confidence. If you're stuck, underline key words and define them in the margins of the test or on scrap paper. Thinking about key terms often unlocks the answer to a test question. Look for absolutes like *always* and *never*. Absolutes in an answer choice often signal that it's the wrong choice. Finally, when your test is returned to you corrected, look it over carefully and determine the sources of the test's information, which helps you know what to study next time. For example, if you missed two class lectures but know the textbook material well, you still might have difficulty on a test if the instructor asks questions primarily from the lecture content. You now know that attending every lecture is a must if you want a good grade in this particular class.

CHAPTER WRAP-UP

The chapter introduction discusses Hippocrates' advice "To do good or do no harm." At first you might have thought, "No problem. It's just a massage. What harm could it do?" Now the answer is crystal clear if it wasn't already. Massage causes profound changes in people's bodies. Massage causes changes in circulation, in the nervous system, in muscle tissue, in digestion, in body chemistry, in medication levels, in attitude, in mood, and even in behavior. Profound changes. Worse yet, in particular areas of the body nerves, bones, blood vessels, and organs are unprotected. This is terrifying! If massage can cause so many physiological and psychological changes, and if delicate structures are nearly everywhere, then someone could get hurt!

Students often feel overwhelmed when they first learn about areas of caution and contraindications. You may think, "I'm not a doctor. How will I know if massage is going to cause a client's medication side effects to get worse?" or "What if I hurt someone? What if someone has a heart attack or stroke because of the massage?" The honest truth is that it's unlikely a client will be hurt—but a little fear is not bad if it ensures you will be vigilant.

Topic 5-3 gave some examples of insurance claims filed with ABMP. In almost every case, these therapists made one of two errors: (1) They didn't conduct a thorough health intake process and thus didn't know about preexisting conditions that rendered some techniques dangerous, or (2) they became too relaxed. They didn't check the stones' temperature for hot stone massage. They didn't check the bolts on massage table legs. They didn't think about the overall health of the client in relationship to the treatment plan. Finally, some therapists just made downright bad choices. One gave an older woman with osteoporosis and on prescription pain medication a deep-tissue massage! We can speculate that this therapist didn't know what osteoporosis is and didn't take the time to look it up after seeing it listed on the health intake form.

A theme that runs throughout this chapter, and the skill that will protect you from adverse reactions in massage clients, is being willing to check a reference book and make inquiries. It is impossible to memorize every pathology and the effects of every drug on the market. Clients' health is also affected by their lifestyle choices, attitudes, and attention to their own health. You can't pre-learn every situation you may encounter. You have to be ready to find out about a condition or medication (or multiple conditions and medications) on the spot. Don't feel pressured to rush through this process. Take your time and look everything up in a reference book. Then trust your gut instincts. When in doubt, refer out.

Ethics and the Law

KEY TERMS

Board of Massage	kickback
certification	laws
code of ethics	licensure
confidentially	practical exam
discrimination	regulation
ethics	scope of practice
informed consent	standards of practice
jurisprudence exam	state-approved exam

LEARNING OBJECTIVES

Having read the chapter and used the related student learning tools, the student will be able to:

1 Define these terms: ethics, values, character traits, and standards of practice.

2 Discuss the role of ethics in the massage profession, and explain how ethical behavior promotes massage as a legitimate health care practice.

3 Explain at least two ethical principles, and give examples of how these principles can be upheld through the standards of practice adopted by the therapist.

4 Explain the importance of informed consent for ensuring the rights of clients.

5 Give an example of when a client can be refused a massage.

6 Outline a good draping policy and explain its relationship to ethics and standards of practice.

7 Define "scope of practice" and analyze the massage scope of practice in the state where practice is intended.

8 List two examples of how the term "certification" is used in the massage profession.

9 Research and report on the laws of the state where practice is intended.

assage is still an emerging profession, and its public acceptance depends on therapists' steadfast commitment to ethical standards and the law. This chapter investigates the evolution and purpose of ethics in Topic 6-1 and then explains how a code of ethics and standards of practice guide our behavior as massage therapists in practice (Topic 6-2). Topic 6-3 focuses on laws, massage education requirements, procedures to test competency, massage credentials, and scope of practice. Topics in this chapter are closely related to Chapter 7 and Chapter 8.

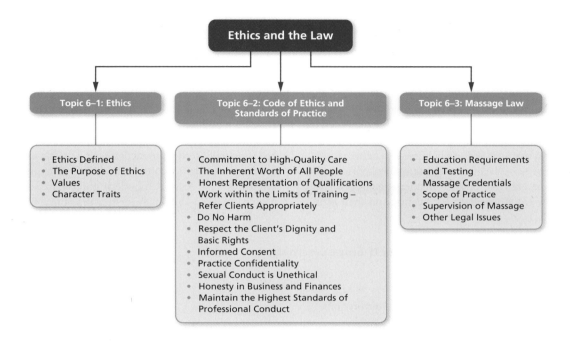

Ethics and the Law

Topic 6–1: Ethics
- Ethics Defined
- The Purpose of Ethics
- Values
- Character Traits

Topic 6–2: Code of Ethics and Standards of Practice
- Commitment to High-Quality Care
- The Inherent Worth of All People
- Honest Representation of Qualifications
- Work within the Limits of Training – Refer Clients Appropriately
- Do No Harm
- Respect the Client's Dignity and Basic Rights
- Informed Consent
- Practice Confidentiality
- Sexual Conduct is Unethical
- Honesty in Business and Finances
- Maintain the Highest Standards of Professional Conduct

Topic 6–3: Massage Law
- Education Requirements and Testing
- Massage Credentials
- Scope of Practice
- Supervision of Massage
- Other Legal Issues

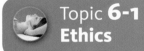

Topic **6-1**
Ethics

Massage therapists' ethics influence how they behave in professional practice and how fu lly they comply with regulations. A historical perspective helps one understand ethics. Philosophers have long sought to understand the origins of ethics, the factors that motivate humans to be moral, and the ways in which humans determine ethical values. Massage therapists need to understand basic ethical concepts and the purpose of ethics in the massage profession, as well as their personal values and character traits that influence their ethics. Sometimes situations arise in practice that create ethical dilemmas for therapists. With an understanding of and sensitivity to ethical issues, therapists can make good decisions to protect themselves, their clients, other health care providers, and the massage profession as a whole.

Ethics Defined

Ethics is a major branch of philosophy exploring values, morals, right and wrong, good and evil, and responsibility. Also called moral philosophy, ethics is a system of principles determining appropriate conduct for an individual or group. It is concerned with values and the standards by which human actions can be judged right or wrong. Ethics are different from laws, which are rules of conduct that are recognized by a community as binding or enforceable by authority. Some behaviors may be legal but not ethical. For example, it is not illegal for a therapist to date a client, but the massage community actively discourages this as unethical, because dating a client may cause the client harm. The word *ethics* is from the ancient Greek *ethikos* meaning "arising from habit." Ethics in the Western world are rooted in the Greek philosophies of Socrates, Plato, and Aristotle.

The ideas of the Greek philosophers provide useful insight into many of the ethical principles that massage therapists practice today. Philosophers speculate about factors that motivate humans to behave ethically. Is it to avoid punishment, gain praise, attain happiness, appear dignified, or fit in? Some believe that people behave ethically for self-oriented reasons. Perhaps they give to charity, for example, to feel more powerful and to be praised for their goodness. Socrates (circa 470–399 BCE) held a different, and perhaps, kinder view. He believed that humans were inherently good and behaved ethically to achieve happiness.[1] He states, "The ultimate object of human activity is happiness, and the necessary means to reach it, is virtue." He believed that people should focus on self-development, friendships, and a true sense of community to find happiness. This is good advice for massage therapists. You can develop your skills as a professional, for example, by participating in continuing education classes. At conferences and local meetings you can form meaningful friendships with other massage therapists and discuss ideas relevant to the massage profession. Some therapists are dedicated to their local community and create outreach programs to bring the benefits of massage to people who might otherwise be left out (e.g., massage for the homeless). These therapists feel more connected and use their skills to help create a better world.

Plato (circa 427–347 BCE) felt that to live a virtuous life, a person must cultivate balance in the soul.[2] People ruled by appetite or emotion are out of balance, and their actions are likely to provoke personal and social disharmony. Plato advocated rational thought before action. Insight prevents rash deeds and helps maintain harmony. Popular psychology uses the phrase "self-empowerment" for this concept. Self-empowerment is a choice a person makes to live with a sense of purpose and responsibility. What a person does, and their actions everyday, define who the person is. Actions may not define a person's best qualities, but they define who the person is in that moment. Plato advocated reflection in decision-making. One might ask oneself, "Does my behavior align with my view of who I am, or who I want to be?" Self-awareness, self-honesty, autonomy, and resilience lead to self-empowerment, a key to good ethics (Fig. 6-1).

Aristotle (circa 384–322 BCE) is considered the founder of ethics as a philosophical system. He believed that to become virtuous, a person could not simply study what virtue *is* but had to actually *do* virtuous activity.[3] In Aristotle's view, people can learn how to be good and develop their positive characteristics. Like Aristotle, modern philosophers believe that people can learn to distinguish between ethical behavior and

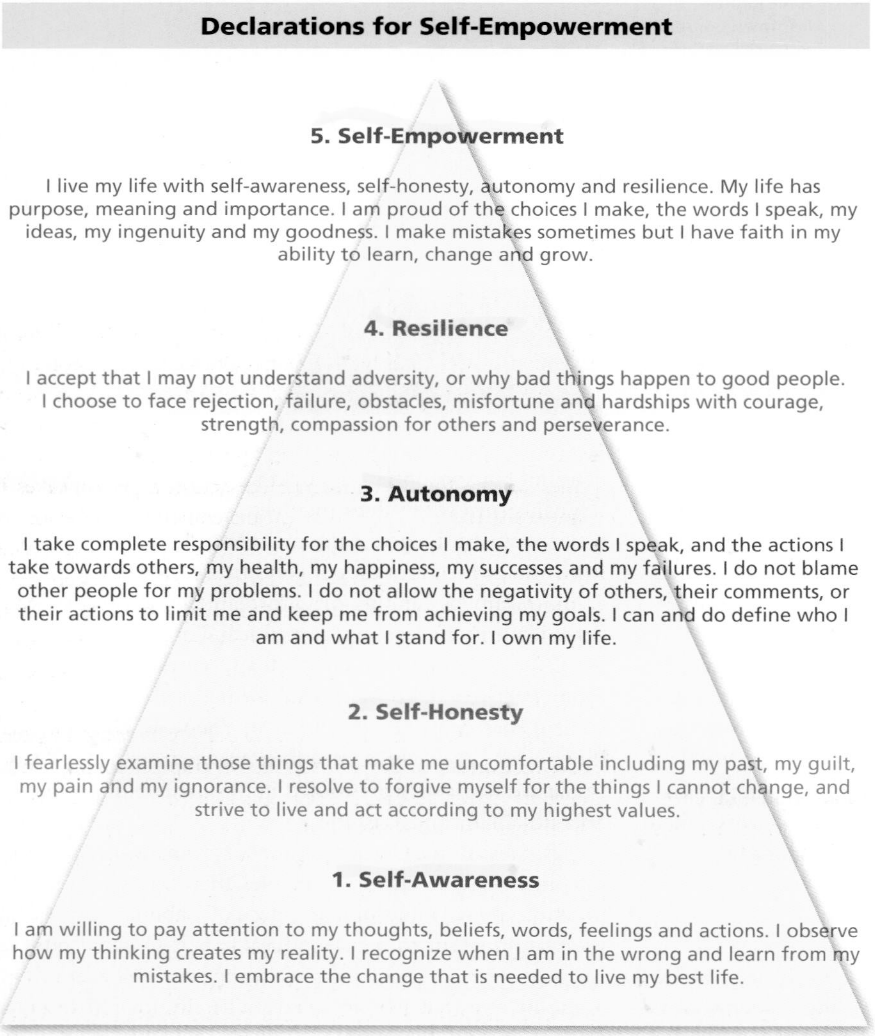

Declarations for Self-Empowerment

5. Self-Empowerment

I live my life with self-awareness, self-honesty, autonomy and resilience. My life has purpose, meaning and importance. I am proud of the choices I make, the words I speak, my ideas, my ingenuity and my goodness. I make mistakes sometimes but I have faith in my ability to learn, change and grow.

4. Resilience

I accept that I may not understand adversity, or why bad things happen to good people. I choose to face rejection, failure, obstacles, misfortune and hardships with courage, strength, compassion for others and perseverance.

3. Autonomy

I take complete responsibility for the choices I make, the words I speak, and the actions I take towards others, my health, my happiness, my successes and my failures. I do not blame other people for my problems. I do not allow the negativity of others, their comments, or their actions to limit me and keep me from achieving my goals. I can and do define who I am and what I stand for. I own my life.

2. Self-Honesty

I fearlessly examine those things that make me uncomfortable including my past, my guilt, my pain and my ignorance. I resolve to forgive myself for the things I cannot change, and strive to live and act according to my highest values.

1. Self-Awareness

I am willing to pay attention to my thoughts, beliefs, words, feelings and actions. I observe how my thinking creates my reality. I recognize when I am in the wrong and learn from my mistakes. I embrace the change that is needed to live my best life.

Figure 6-1 Declarations for self-empowerment.

unethical behavior. For this reason, massage schools include instruction in ethics and strive to impart good ethical practices to students. Students' ethical behavior includes academic integrity (no cheating or copying homework), confidentiality (not talking about classmates behind their backs), and respect for others (treating all people kindly and recognizing that all people have inherent value). The continuous practice of thoughtful, considerate actions helps prepare you for an ethical and professional practice after graduation.

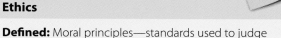

Concept Brief 6-1
Ethics

Defined: Moral principles—standards used to judge right and wrong.
Origin: Greek philosophy
Value: Creates societal structure where people can feel safe
Leading a good life may lead to greater happiness.

The Purpose of Ethics

Almost all major religions and cultures embrace some version of "The Golden Rule," a fundamental ethical principle on which the modern concept of human rights is based (Fig. 6-2). Imagine what our world would be like if most people didn't practice this basic ethical principle. Likely, the world would be in a state of complete chaos. No one could feel safe. People would spend their time protecting their possessions, family members, and selves. Ethics brings order to the world and helps create social structures that allow people to pursue happiness and feel secure. Ethics is a framework for laws that hold accountable someone who violates the rights of another.

In massage, ethical principles define appropriate therapist behaviors so that clients can feel safe. Clients are in an extremely vulnerable situation during a session. They are undressed and covered only by a flimsy drape, lying on a table in a private room with a person they may not know. How can a client who doubts the therapist's ethics relax and benefit from the session? Imagine how damaging it would be for our profession if someone took advantage of a client (e.g., sexual misconduct or business misconduct). That client would be unlikely to seek out massage again and might tell every friend and family member about the negative experience. Police might be involved and the incident could receive media attention. It only takes one event like this to convince an already hesitant potential client that massage is a risky health care choice. Every therapist thus has a duty to represent the massage profession with honesty, integrity, and respect for all people.

Ethical principles encourage excellent service and protect the rights of clients. They also provide direction in challenging or confusing situations. People come from a range of social and economic backgrounds. Some grow up with ethical role models that help them identify right and wrong, good and bad, and self-accountability from an early age. Others may not have had an ethical role model or may even have had an unethical role model. Ethical guidelines ensure that all therapists, regardless of their upbringing, have a model of professional behavior and examples of ethical norms.

People seek out touch for a variety of reasons, including some that are not legitimate. Furthermore, some clients do not recognize that some behaviors are inappropriate. Some clients know their behavior is inappropriate but want to see how far they can push the issue. Therapists with strong ethical principles are clear in their behavior and communication. They are a model of professionalism for clients who need guidance. Clients who push an inappropriate issue may find their session terminated. Ethical principles help therapists distinguish between clients who need direction and clients who seek massage for the wrong reasons.

Concept Brief 6-2
Purpose of Ethics in a Massage Practice

- Creates an environment where the client can feel safe
- Encourages excellent service
- Ensures the rights of the client
- Provides structure for therapists in challenging or confusing situations
- Provides a model for professional behavior
- Helps therapists set good boundaries for clients

Values

People's values are made up of beliefs that hold emotional worth, importance, and usefulness. Often, values are understood as a group of accepted principles or the standards of a person or group. Values can motivate a person to act in a certain way, and form the base of one's character and personality. What a person values will profoundly influence the action a person takes in a given situation. Congruence means coinciding, agreeing, or being in harmony. People who are congruent with their values feel balanced, clear-sighted, and empowered. They can make quick decisions and act decisively in a way that leaves them feeling confident and assured. But sometimes people get out of sync with their values and act in a way that goes against what they deem important. Conflicts may occur with other people who hold conflicting values. Sometimes this is caused by fear, prolonged stress, or desperation. For example, a loving spouse may burn down the family home in a rage because of a divorce. The tremendous distress of the situation causes the spouse to act against the deeply held value of protecting the family.

Usually value conflicts in a massage practice are not so extreme. Instead, they cause a therapist to get that funny, uncomfortable feeling in the pit of the stomach that signals that something is not right in the world. Therapists who learned a technique that was legal in one state but not legal in another may feel this incongruence if they used the technique where it was illegal. They may self-justify their actions

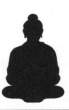

Hillel
(circa 50 BCE–10 CE)

a Jewish religious leader who lived in Jerusalem during the time of King Herod said, "What is hateful to you, do not to your fellow man."

The Dhammapada
(date unknown, between the 3rd and 5th century)

is an anthology of verses attributed to the Buddha, which states, "Every being fears punishment; every being fears death, just as you do. Therefore do not kill or cause to kill."

Confucius
(circa 551–479 BCE)

a famous Chinese thinker and philosopher, whose teachings deeply influenced East Asian life and thought said, "What you do not wish upon yourself, extend not to others."

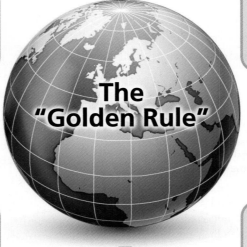

The
"Golden Rule"

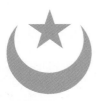

Muhammad
(circa 570–632 CE)

was a religious, political and military leader who united the tribes of the Arabian Peninsula and established Islam. He said, "Hurt on no one so that no one may hurt you."

The Mahabharata
(written sometime around 500 BCE)

is a Sanskrit epic of ancient India that has immense religious and philosophical importance to Hinduism. It says, "This is the sum of duty; do naught onto others what you would not have them do unto you."

Jesus
(circa 5 BCE–33 CE)

affirms Moses in the Gospels, Matthew 7:12, "Do unto others as you would have them do unto you."

Figure 6-2 The Golden Rule.

by thinking, "The technique is legal in California so it's stupid that it is not legal here. Besides, it made my client feel better." Perhaps such therapists value the law and have always taken pride in following the rules. Now they have acted against an important value and feel conflicted. If they spent some time thinking about their values related to this situation, they would likely not make this mistake again. They would probably find that they can use other techniques that are just as effective and thereby remain true to their values and in alignment with the ethical principles of the massage profession at the same time.

Character Traits

Character traits are inherent attributes that influence how a person responds in a given situation; they are closely interwoven with values. Plato described good character traits as

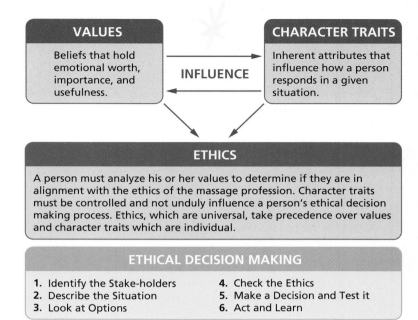

Figure 6-3 Influence of character traits and values on decision making.

wisdom, courage, moderation, justice, fortitude, generosity, self-respect, good humor, and sincerity. Four of these traits (wisdom, courage, moderation, and justice) were deemed the most important traits and hailed as the "cardinal virtues."[4] Aristotle believed that people had to seek a balance between the extremes of character traits. Too little courage leads to cowardice, while too much courage leads to rashness.[5] Both cowardice and rashness are equally disagreeable and could lead to unethical behavior. In the example described above, therapists who had too little courage (cowardice) might give in when a client requests the restricted technique, even if they had vowed never to use the technique again. A therapist who had too much courage (rashness) might have thought, "What the heck, I like the technique and I'm going to use it whether it's restricted or not." You should not be swayed by your character traits but must control your personality to maintain your ethics and professionalism.

Ethical Decision Making

In all massage practices, situations will arise that challenge therapists' ideas and requires that they make a difficult decision. As discussed in the previous sections, people's values and character traits play a role in their actions and choices (Fig. 6-3). A trained sensitivity to ethical issues, recognition of personal values and character tendencies, and a framework for making ethical choices is helpful. It is also wise to consult a mentor or supervisor for an experienced perspective. Most decision-making models follow the same general outline as shown in Box 6-1. Figure 6-4 uses this model to explore the process of a therapist trying to decide what to do about a client who requests a restricted technique, for example. Ethics, and the values that influence ethics, permeate all aspects of a massage practice, especially the professional standards of practice discussed in the next topic.

BOX 6-1 Ethical Decision Making

1. **Identify the stakeholders.** Who are the people affected by the situation or who will be affected by the decision either directly or indirectly?

2. **Describe the situation.** What are the facts? Who did what? Who said what? Where does the situation stand right now?

3. **Describe the options.** What are all the possible lines of action? What is the outcome with each option? Who benefits? Who is compromised? Which line of action provides the best outcome for the most people?

4. **Check the ethics.** Does a proposed outcome jeopardize the therapist's ethics? If yes, continue looking for another option.

5. **Make a decision and test it.** Choose a line of action but don't act. Sleep on it and spend additional time in reflection. Imagine how the situation will feel a month from now if you take the action. Imagine defending your actions to friends or family. Is it defensible?

6. **Act.** Make the decision and act on it. Reflect on your feelings and thoughts as the action takes effect. Learn from mistakes and successes to hone your decision-making skills.

1. Identify the stakeholders. Who are the people that are affected by the situation or will be affected by the decision either directly or indirectly?

The people involved are Cheryl Smith (the client) and I. My clinic owner, Dave Sanders, might also be affected.

2. Describe the situation. What are the facts? Who did what? Who said what? Where does the situation stand right now?

I used a technique that is legal in California, but not legal here, on Cheryl. I felt it would really help with her foot pain at the time but now I feel guilty. The problem is that Cheryl loved the technique and has told three of her friends and they all want to book appointments.

3. Describe the options. What are all the possible lines of action? What is the outcome with each option? Who benefits? Who is compromised? Which line of action provides the best outcome for the most people?

I think the best option is to tell Cheryl that I shouldn't have used the foot technique and explain that I can't use the technique again. She is bound to be mad because she gets angry easily. She is also going to feel embarrassed because she has three of her friends booking appointments just for that technique. Dave is sure to find out what's going on and I might lose my job.

I could tell Cheryl that she can't talk about the technique to anyone and continue to use it just with her. She will keep my secret if she gets what she wants. The problem is I would have to lie to Dave about it and I don't want to lie.

I could quit this job and go work somewhere else and start over. I like this job but I could find another one.

4. Check the ethics. Does a proposed outcome jeopardize the therapist's ethics? If yes, continue looking for another option.

If I quit my job I won't use the technique ever again unless I move back to California. If I stay I think I have to come clean and be honest. I may lose my job anyway.

5. Make a decision and test it. Choose a line of action but don't act. Sleep on it and spend additional time in reflection. Imagine how the situation will feel a month from now if the line of action is adopted. Imagine defending the line of action to friends or family. Is this an action that is defensible?

If I quit my job I let a lot of people down. What about my other clients? It's best if I come clean. After thinking about it I know I should tell the truth. I plan to tell Dave and ask him to meet with Cheryl and I. I want to offer Cheryl a free session to say I'm sorry.

6. Act. Make the decision and act on it. Reflect on your feelings and thoughts as the action takes effect. Learn from mistakes and successes to hone decision-making skills.

Dave was pretty cool about it. He supported my decision to offer Cheryl a free session and was supportive when Cheryl got mad and said she was embarrassed in front of her friends. Dave offered to give each of Cheryl's friends half-price on their first massage. Cheryl agreed but said she didn't want me as her therapist anymore. I feel really sad about upsetting Cheryl but I know I did the right thing and I won't make the same mistake again.

Figure 6-4 Ethical decision making model in action.

Topic **6-2**
Code of Ethics and Standards of Practice

A professional is an individual working within the framework of a profession. A profession is a career that requires an academic preparation to acquire a recognized body of knowledge, which is often demonstrated through standardized testing. In the massage profession, the **scope of practice** (see Topic 6-3) defines the methods and techniques a professional can use in practice. Ethics and standards further define the activities and behavior of the professional.

A **code of ethics** states a professional group's ethical principles. It suggests values by which the group abides. **Standards of practice** are professional guidelines based on ethical principles (Fig. 6-5). It is helpful to think of ethics as the principle and standards as the behavior or action that upholds the principle. For example, if the code of ethics states that "Massage therapists shall do no harm," the standards of practice might state, "Therapists will always conduct a health history intake to rule out contraindications."

Four main national massage organizations play an important role in defining the ethics and standards of practice for the massage profession. These organizations are the American Massage Therapy Association (AMTA), Associated Bodywork

TABLE 6-1   National Association Websites

http://www.abmp.com
http://www.amtamassage.org
http://www.fsmtb.org
http://www.ncbtmb.com

& Massage Professionals (ABMP), the National Certification Board for Therapeutic Massage and Bodywork (NCBTMB), and the Federation of State Massage Therapy Boards (FSMTB). Other related groups like the American Organization for Bodywork Therapies of Asia, the Feldenkrais Guild of North America, the American Polarity Therapy Association, and many others influence the code of ethics and standards of practice that define specific bodywork systems. Most states that regulate massage also have a defined code of ethics and standards of practice document developed by the board that oversees massage therapists in that state. The code of ethics and standards of practice documents for each of the different massage organizations can be found at their websites (Table 6-1).

When massage therapists join professional organizations or receive their massage credentials, they agree to abide by the massage profession's code and standards. While some variations exist between massage groups, the key principles discussed below provide insight into the standards advocated by massage professionals.

Standards of Practice Guidepost

- Commitment to High-Quality Care
- The Inherent Worth of All People
- Honest Representation of Qualifications
- Work Within the Limits of Training
- Do No Harm
- Respect for the Dignity and Rights of All People
- Practice Confidentiality
- Uphold Appropriate Sexual Boundaries
- Honesty in Business and Finances
- Maintain the Highest Standards of Professional Conduct

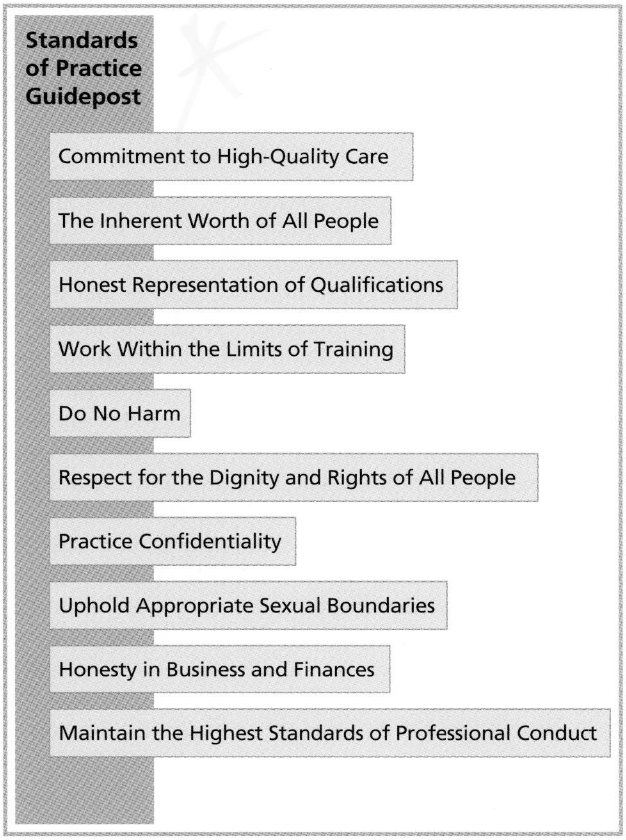

Figure 6-5 Standards of practice guidepost.

Concept Brief 6-3
Code of Ethics and Standards of Practice Defined

- A code of ethics is a document that states an individual's or group's ethical principles. It suggests values that the individual or group holds as important.
- Standards of practice are professional guidelines based on ethical principles.
- Massage organizations like AMTA, ABMP, NCBTMB and state boards of massage provide guidance to therapists on appropriate conduct.

Commitment to High-Quality Care

Ethical Principle: The Code of ethics for ABMP states, "I shall endeavor to serve the best interests of my clients at all times and to provide the highest quality service possible."

Standard of Practice: The therapist must be attentive and responsive to the client's needs in all interactions in regards to the therapeutic relationship (discussed in detail in Chapter 7). The therapist should strive for professional excellence through continuing education, feedback from peers, and regular assessments of personal strengths and goal setting.

Discussion: Commitment to high-quality service and client care is an umbrella principle that affects every aspect of the massage business. It covers the small things like phoning clients back promptly when they call for an appointment, and it covers the big things like appropriate referral of a client when your skill level does not meet the client's needs. If you start the session late, chat continually about a recent movie opening, and end the session 2 minutes early, you have demonstrated a lack of attention to quality care. If you are not responsive to the client's tissue and use deep pressure even when a client shows physical signs of discomfort, or if you fail to clean the massage table between clients and are negligent about handwashing, you are failing to provide quality care.

One way that therapists can provide high-quality care is through an ongoing program of self-improvement. This might be accomplished through continuing education classes or through self-assessment and goal setting. Some therapists form peer groups that meet throughout the year and receive input and feedback from other therapists. One national online peer group is www.massageprofessionals.com, a website dedicated to social networking for massage. Massage therapists can join various sub groups, view blogs from industry professionals, and ask questions in forums. A novice therapist might also seek out an experienced massage therapist as a mentor for support in challenging situations.

The Inherent Worth of All People

Ethical Principle: The Code of Ethics for the NCBTMB states that therapists will "refuse to unjustly discriminate against clients or health professionals." The AMTA states, "Acknowledge the inherent worth and individuality of each person by not discriminating or behaving in any prejudicial manner with clients and/or colleagues."

Standard of Practice: Treat all clients and other health care professionals fairly and with respect, regardless of personal beliefs. Strive to understand and identify discriminatory or prejudicial thoughts or actions and eliminate them.

Discussion: Different people have different values, beliefs, habits, and behaviors. In order to work with other therapists or clients effectively and capitalize on the strengths and experiences of our diverse population, we must tolerate and respect each other. We must also seek to decrease misunderstanding, prejudice, racism, and discrimination.

Prejudice is a pre-formed opinion (usually unfavorable) based on inadequate knowledge, irrational feelings, or inaccurate stereotypes. Gordon Allport describes prejudice in his classic work titled *The Nature of Prejudice* as "an aversive or hostile attitude toward a person who belongs to a group, simply because he belongs to that group, and is therefore presumed to have the objectionable qualities ascribed to the group."[6] Prejudice sometimes leads to stereotyping, in which a person adopts an oversimplified opinion or image of another group of people. It is often caused by fear that a different worldview held by another person or group challenges one's own worldview. Sometimes people believe negative stereotypes about a particular group and so come to fear that group. Prejudice can be passed from older members of a family to younger members of the family through negative storytelling.

Racism is the belief that one's ethnic stock is superior to or significantly different from another person's ethnic stock. Similar prejudices also apply to beliefs that one's sex, socioeconomic class, or generation is superior. When prejudicial or racial attitudes lead to behavior, it is called **discrimination**. Discrimination is an act based on prejudice or racism.

Prejudice and racism may survive unrecognized in people and affect their thoughts and feelings without their conscious awareness. As a health care provider, you must be sensitive to your own feelings and thoughts, and seek to better understand other groups of people. Every person who seeks massage for legitimate reasons has a right to the best possible care and a massage free from bias or judgment. Although therapists can refuse service to clients in certain situations (e.g., the client has been drinking alcohol, has a communicable disease, etc.), they cannot refuse service based on race, gender, religious or political affiliation, disability, physical build, marital status, ethnicity, sexual orientation, or social or economic status. Each of us has a responsibility to identify people, physical situations, or groups that cause us discomfort, and through reflection, strive to overcome personal fears and give excellent service to everyone.

When Is It Appropriate to Decline Service to a Client?

It is appropriate to decline service to a client when it is in the best interest of a client's health. If you do not feel that you have the experience or knowledge necessary to effectively work with a particular condition, you can and should refer the client to another therapist. Service is declined if the client has a preexisting condition that is a contraindication or because the client has consumed alcohol or illegal drugs before the session. Clients are refused service if they are seeking sexual or erotic massage, or if they break the policies of the massage business. In each of these cases, it is important to remain respectful but to explain to clients the honest facts of the situation. Communication, including difficult discussions that might occur with clients, is discussed in Chapter 8.

Sometimes a particular client may cause you to feel uncomfortable for no identifiable reason, or something about the client may trigger emotions from an earlier event in your life. You may find yourself dreading the session and emotionally exhausted as a result. Sometimes these issues can be worked through with a mentor, but sometimes the best course of action is to refer the client to another therapist. There are also situations in which a client develops an unhealthy attachment to a therapist or needs help beyond the therapist's abilities. These issues require careful reflection and a considerate and compassionate response based on the best interests of both the client and the therapist. These situations are discussed in greater depth in Chapter 7.

Honest Representation of Qualifications

Ethical Principle: The ABMP code of ethics states, "I shall practice honesty in advertising, promote my services ethically and in good taste, and practice and/or advertise only those techniques for which I have received adequate training and/ or certification."

Standard of Practice: Therapists will only provide services for which they are fully trained and hold appropriate credentials. They will not work outside of their scope of practice or use the trademarks and symbols associated with a particular system or group without honest affiliation.

Discussion: Once therapists have earned their massage credentials, they can continue to study different systems of massage. Some of these systems are very advanced and teach new skills that might be specifically suited to a certain type of injury or client group. It's important for massage therapists to honestly represent themselves. For example, many therapists learn a little bit about manual lymphatic drainage (MLD), in massage school when they work with acute soft-tissue injury. MLD stimulates lymph flow and fluid movement. It is often used for complicated conditions in which fluid collects in the tissue, including inflammatory conditions, lymphedema, and circulatory disturbances. The basic training involves around 160 hours of continuing education. Therapists who state that they are an MLD practitioner after a weekend workshop would not be representing their qualifications accurately. Similarly, certified reflexologists have completed a course of 300 hours (in addition to their massage training) and passed a written and practical exam. While massage therapists can use "reflexology techniques" in a session, they should not claim to be reflexologists unless they have been certified by a recognized reflexology organization.

Work Within the Limits of Training— Refer Clients Appropriately

Ethical Principle: The NCBTMB Code of Ethics states, "Acknowledge the limitations of and contraindications for massage and bodywork, and refer clients to appropriate health professionals." NCBTMB also states that therapists must "Accurately inform clients, other health care practitioners, and the public of the scope and limitations of their discipline."

Standard of Practice: Therapists must fully inform clients of the benefits, limits, and contraindications for massage. Therapists must carefully evaluate the needs of each client and refer the client to another health care provider if the client requires treatment beyond the therapist's capabilities or beyond the capacity of massage to benefit the client.

Discussion: Massage training hours vary widely across the country. Some courses are as short as 150 hours, while others run well over 1,000 hours. After graduation, therapists can take a variety of continuing education programs to develop their knowledge base. The typical massage therapy course length is around 500 hours, which prepares a graduate to deliver a solid "wellness" massage and work with some common pathologies like tension headaches and muscle strains. Wellness massage often uses predominantly Swedish techniques and is delivered to reduce stress and support the body's natural restorative processes. This is very valuable work and widely sought by the public.

Longer courses give graduates the understanding they need to work effectively with conditions like fibromyalgia, peripheral nerve compression syndromes, postural deviations, and whiplash. This type of training is often referred to as health care massage, treatment massage, or rehabilitative massage. Additional training hours also provide insight into appropriate and effective techniques for use with special client groups like mothers and infants, the elderly, and athletes. While therapists from both types of programs might hold the same state massage credentials, and practice under the same laws and regulations, they have different abilities. A therapist trained in a 300-hour "wellness" program may need to refer a client who was recently in a car accident to someone with more education. One should not feel inferior based on the number of hours in one's primary massage training. The point here is that all therapists, regardless of training hours, should refer a client to someone else if they have any doubt about their ability to benefit the client.

Clients sometimes share very personal information in a session. Therapists may respond to this situation by seeking to counsel the client or give advice. But even therapists who also have counseling credentials would be working outside the limits of the scope of the session and breaking this ethical principle. The session was scheduled for massage and bodywork and should focus on massage and bodywork techniques. Therapists with credentials in multiple but related disciplines form dual relationships when they seek to treat a client on multiple levels (dual relationships are described in Chapter 7, Topic 7-3). Instead, the client should be referred to a different mental health specialist.

Do No Harm

Ethical Principle: The Code of Ethics for the AMTA states that massage therapists will "accept responsibility to do no harm to the physical, mental, and emotional well-being of self, clients, and associates."

Standard of Practice: A therapist will provide massage therapy only when there is a reasonable expectation that it will be advantageous to the client. The therapist will conduct a thorough health history intake process for every client and evaluate the health history to rule out contraindications. If the client has an undiagnosed condition or describes symptoms not in keeping with those treatable by massage, the therapist must refer that client to a physician and delay the massage session until the physician determines a diagnosis or grants approval for massage. The therapist should understand the importance of ethical touch and therapeutic intent, and apply strokes with the objective to do the client good.

Discussion: If therapists have any doubt about what they feel in the tissue or the advisability of a technique for a client, they should err on the side of caution and consult with a physician or mentor. For example, a novice therapist might think that a small cyst is a trigger point and apply prolonged pressure to the area, causing tissue damage.

Therapists also do harm when they are neglectful or inattentive. While it is unlikely that these therapists intended to provide poor care, numerous cases have occurred of clients being left alone while cocooned tightly in a body wrap. In one incident, filed with an insurance company, a client became claustrophobic and panicked. The client rolled off the massage table in an effort to get out of the wrap and sustained a concussion while the therapist was in the break room having a snack. This therapist did more than make an ethically questionable choice; she was negligent, and her disregard for the client's safety led to a liability claim, insurance payout, and loss of membership in her professional massage organization.

Therapists also have an ethical responsibility to care for themselves by not overworking and by setting good personal boundaries with clients and employers (boundary setting is discussed in Chapter 7). A therapist who willingly maligns another therapist, actively seeks to steal someone else's clients, or treats another therapist disrespectfully has also broken this ethical principle.

Respect the Client's Dignity and Basic Rights

Ethical Principle: The NCBTMB states, "Respect the client's boundaries with regard to privacy, disclosure, exposure, emotional expression, beliefs, and the client's reasonable expectations of professional behavior. Practitioners will respect the client's autonomy."

Standard of Practice: Massage therapists must respect the dignity and rights of all people by providing a clean, safe, and comfortable environment, following appropriate draping policies, giving clients recourse in the event of dissatisfaction with treatment, upholding the integrity of the therapeutic relationship, and respecting the client's autonomy.

Discussion: Clients who come to a massage clinic or spa reasonably assume that proper sanitation and hygienic practices are followed. They trust that the environment is safe and that every effort is made to protect their health. In one example, a massage clinic was using the same set of sheets for two different clients by turning the sheets over between sessions to cut down on laundry. When a therapist reported this to a professional massage organization, the health department was called and the business was closed.

Draping Policies

The use of modest and appropriate draping techniques shows respect for clients' privacy and allows them to feel safe during the application of massage techniques (Fig. 6-6). The client has the right to leave on underclothing, and may choose to

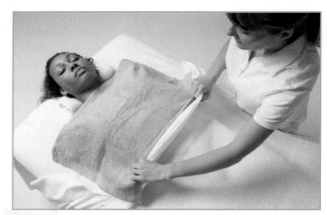

Figure 6-6 The use of modest and appropriate draping techniques demonstrates respect for the client's dignity and basic rights.

receive massage fully clothed. Only the area of the body receiving massage is uncovered. The breasts, genitals, and anus are never undraped during a session. Care is taken to use draping techniques that protect clients' modesty when they are getting on and off the massage table and when they are being turned from one position to another (e.g., supine to prone).

Recourse Policy

As part of **informed consent** (described below), the client should be apprised of the recourse policy in the event of being dissatisfied with the massage. Sometimes the client receives a refund; sometimes the client is referred to another therapist for a free session or a session at a reduced price. In all cases, clients should be empowered to have a voice in their treatment and encouraged to give honest and direct feedback about their massage experience.

Integrity of the Therapeutic Relationship

The relationship between the therapist and the client can be complex, sometimes filled with subconsciously driven emotions and expectations (discussed in Chapter 7). The responsibility for maintaining the professionalism and integrity of the therapeutic relationship falls on the therapist. Therapists demonstrate respect when they are on time for sessions, return phone calls promptly, customize sessions to meet clients' needs, and keep to an agreed schedule. Part of the therapeutic relationship involves honoring a client's right to emotional expression (e.g., emotional release) and the willingness to be present and attentive to the client's needs without counseling or giving advice.

Client Autonomy

Autonomy is defined as personal independence, self-sufficiency, self-government and the capacity to make decisions and act on them. Clients have the right to decide what happens to their own body. They can opt to discontinue treatment at any time without giving any justification for its termination. When a client says, "That hurts," the therapist has an ethical obligation to lighten the pressure. If a client says, "I don't want any work on my back today," the therapist must respect that wish even if the therapist feels the client needs the back massaged. Mental and emotional harm can be done when therapists fail to listen to the client and impose their own beliefs on a situation. For example, if a client feels shy and doesn't want to remove underclothing, the therapist has an ethical responsibility to respect the client's wishes, even if it means some difficulty and awkwardness in the application of techniques. A therapist who implies by words or attitude that the client is being a "prude" or "difficult" has broken trust with that client and potentially caused feelings of shame or embarrassment.

Working with Minors

Children and teenagers have the same rights as adults with regards to autonomy but may not have the experience necessary to assert these rights in a massage session. Always ask children, no matter how young, for the permission to touch them. The sensitivity and professionalism of the therapist is of primary importance here. Physical signals or facial expressions provide clues about the quality of the child's experience, such as a technique being uncomfortable. Young children might show they are ready for the massage to be over with their restlessness, even if the session is not complete. Teenagers may feel especially self-conscious about their bodies and require thoughtful communication that is perceptive to their developmental stage. They may choose to leave some or all of their clothing on, and these preferences may change from session to session. A parent, caretaker, or guardian should be present for all sessions with minors to provide support to the child and because of liability issues.

Informed Consent

Ethical Principle: The NCBTMB states, "Respect the client's right to treatment with informed and voluntary consent. The practitioner will obtain and record the informed consent of the client, or client's advocate, before providing treatment."

Standard of Practice: The therapist will fully inform clients of choices relating to their care and disclose policies and limitations that may affect their care. The therapist will not provide massage without obtaining the client's (or client guardian or advocate's) informed consent to the treatment.

Discussion: Informed consent is a process by which a fully informed client consents to participate in the massage treatment. It originates from the ethical (and legal) right of clients to direct what happens to their body, and from the ethical duty of the therapist to involve clients in choices related to their wellness. For clients' consent to be valid, they must be competent to make the decision to consent and that consent must be voluntary. Parents or legal guardians must provide informed consent for minors or for those unable to consent on their own due to mental or physical challenges.

The process of obtaining the client's informed consent takes place during the first health intake procedure before the client receives a massage. During this exchange, the massage therapist provides specific types of information, and the client signs a form stating that he or she understands and would like to participate in the massage treatment. Information provided to the client includes:

- A written and verbal description of massage, its limits, its benefits, indications, contraindications, and risks, along with some suggestions of alternate therapies that have benefits similar to massage.

- A written and verbal description of the massage scope of practice in the relevant state, or directions to the website where the client can read the massage scope of practice, and the contact details for reporting therapist misconduct.

- A written and verbal description of the therapist's training, credentials, and experience, and disclosure of any factors that limit the therapist's professional ability such as hearing disorders, vision impairment, or lack of experience in a particular relevant area (e.g., the client is pregnant and the therapist has never before delivered a pregnancy massage).

- A written and verbal description of business policies relating to the professional relationship between the client and therapist. This includes the fee schedule, hours of operation, returned check policy, late arrival or no-show policy, policy on draping, sanitation protocols, and expectations on the client's conduct. For example, "The client is expected to demonstrate good hygiene and not use illegal drugs or alcohol before a session."

- A written and verbal description of activities or behaviors that constitute sexual impropriety and the consequences of such behaviors (e.g., termination of the session, report to the police).

- A written and verbal description of the rights of the client including the right to terminate the session at any time, confidentiality, and the limits of confidentiality (described in greater detail in the next section).

Informed consent procedures benefit both the client and the therapist because they clarify the expectations of both parties and provide guidelines for how sessions are conducted. Informed consent establishes the framework of the therapeutic relationship. This empowers clients to feel in charge of their session and supports therapists in setting good boundaries with clients.

Sometimes the client is handed numerous documents such as a menu of services with fees and business policies, a brochure on what to expect during a massage, and a short informed consent form. You could also choose to include all the important information in one document as in the sample provided in Figure 6-7. When the client has read and understood the informed consent information, the client signs it and a copy is placed in the file.

Massage Defined
Massage can be defined as structured, professional touch. Massage techniques manually manipulate the muscles, tendons and fascia of the body to promote health and wellness. Benefits of massage include stress reduction, circulation enhancement, relief from muscular tension, soreness and pain, and increased relaxation. People may find that meditation, other bodywork systems like myofascial release, energetic bodywork and Eastern massage like Amna provide results similar to relaxation massage.

Limitations of Massage
Massage therapists do not diagnose medical diseases or musculoskeletal conditions and massage is not a substitute for medical examination and treatment. Massage therapists do not prescribe herbs or drugs including aspirin or ibuprofen, or medical treatments. They do not perform spinal adjustments and they cannot counsel clients about emotional or spiritual issues as would be provided by a mental health or spiritual leader. If you experience symptoms that lead you to believe you may have a medical condition it is recommended that you visit a medical physician for diagnosis and treatment. For detailed description of the massage scope of practice in this state please visit the Board of Massage website at www.anyboard.com.

Adverse Reactions to Massage
Massage may lead to adverse reactions in certain situations or when used with certain conditions or medications. The massage therapist will evaluate your health history intake and ask you questions to make sure it is safe for you to receive massage. In the event that the massage therapist is uncertain that massage will be of benefit to you, he or she may ask your to provide a note from your physician stating that it is safe for you to receive massage. Please provide complete details of medical conditions, and medications to your massage therapist during the health intake interview. Failure to inform the massage therapist of all medical conditions and medications may place you at increased risk for adverse reactions.

Therapist Training and Experience
All of the massage therapists working at Any Massage Clinic have completed a minimum of 500 hours of massage training from a State-approved school and passed the State licensing requirements. Therapists at Any Message Clinic specialize in Swedish massage techniques, deep tissue techniques, myofascial release techniques and hydrotherapy. Any Massage Clinic also has therapists who specialize in pregnancy massage, reflexology, spa body treatments and CranoSacral therapy. Pick up a menu of services from our receptionist to find out about these different forms of massage. We do not specialize in rehabilitative massage for soft-tissue injury. Please ask us for a copy of our preferred provider list in the event that we can't meet your particular needs.

Business Policies and Practices
You may book a thirty-minute ($40), sixty-minute ($60), or ninety-minute ($75) session. Any Massage Clinic accepts cash, personal checks and all major credit cards. We do not bill insurance companies for services. Plan to arrive ten minutes early to update your paperwork and discuss any changes to your condition with your massage therapist. The first session usually requires a longer health intake process and so clients should arrive twenty minutes early on their initial visit. Clients arriving late will be charged for the full session and the session will end promptly at the scheduled time. Clients must cancel sessions with 24 hours notice or pay for the missed session in full. Returned checks will be charged a $20 processing fee. Business hours are from 8 AM to 8PM. Walk in appointments are accepted providing therapists are available. Children and teens are welcome but an adult guardian must be present with the child or teen in the treatment room for the entire session.

Clients receive $5 off their first massage at Any Massage Clinic. Clients receive $5 towards a massage for each friend or family member they refer to the clinic who receives a session. Occasionally coupons for discounts on services are sent as part of our client newsletter. Sign up for our free newsletter with the receptionist. A tip to a therapist for exceptional service is optional but appreciated.

Figure 6-7 Example of informed consent form.

Practice Confidentiality

Ethical Principle: The AMTA Code of Ethics states, "Acknowledge the confidential nature of the professional relationship with clients and respect each client's right to privacy."

Standard of Practice: The therapist will keep client communication and information confidential within the limits of the law. The therapist will not share client information, even with other health care providers, without the client's written consent.

Discussion: Therapists are both ethically and legally obligated to keep client information confidential. Client information includes details about health conditions, documents or files relating to the client's health and status, personal information like the client's address and phone number, and information the client shares verbally with the therapist during the session. Therapists must follow the Health Insurance Portability and Accountability Act (HIPAA) laws discussed later in this chapter. Ethically, therapists must consider a number of instances where client **confidentiality** might be compromised.

Do not approach or greet a client in public unless the client greets you first. Clients may wish to keep the fact that they are receiving massage private, and approaching clients would breech their right to confidentiality. With written permission

Expectations and Rights

The client is expected to demonstrate good hygiene and not use illegal drugs or alcohol before the session (the use of drugs and alcohol make it unsafe for the client to receive massage). Clients and therapists are expected to refrain from any behavior of a sexual nature including sexual jokes, use of nicknames, or immodest conduct. Sexual behavior from the therapist towards the client is grounds for therapist termination and may lead to a formal complaint filed with the State Board of Massage. This may lead to the loss of the therapist's license. Sexual behavior from the client toward the therapist is inappropriate and will lead to the termination of the session and refusal of further service.

The client has the right to prompt, professional service in an environment that is clean, private and safe. Client information is not shared with any members of the public or other health care providers unless the client releases the information in writing. A court of law may order the client's health care records released to the court as part of a legal proceeding. Therapists are obligated to report information about the abuse of a child, elderly person or mentally or physically challenged person in the event that such information is related during the session. Therapists are obligated to report threats of self-harm or threats that the client plans to harm another person to authorities.

The client has the right to end the session at any time should they feel dissatisfied or uncomfortable with the session in any way. Clients who are dissatisfied with a therapist are encouraged to contact the manager, (manager's name), at (manager's phone number). Formal complaints can be filed with the State on the Board of Massage website at www.anyboard.com.

Your Massage Session

After you complete the health intake form you are taken to a private treatment room where the therapist will review the form with you and find out about the benefits you hope to achieve from massage. The therapist will customize the massage to meet your specific needs within the limits of his or her training, and scope of practice. The therapist will leave the room briefly while you undress and place yourself under the drape on the massage table. Only the area being massage is undraped during the session. The breasts, genitals and anus are never undraped during a session, and every effort is made to respect and protect both the client and therapist's modesty. You may leave on your underclothing if you prefer. While the therapist will ask you about the comfort of the strokes, or if you are warm enough, conversation is generally discouraged. This allows you to relax fully and enjoy the session.

Informed Consent

I, (client's name)_____

have read and understand the disclosures, policies and procedures of Any Massage Clinic and I would like to receive a massage session or request a session for my child or dependent. I understand the benefits and limits of massage and that massage may cause adverse reactions in certain situations. If I experience any discomfort during the session I will immediately inform my therapist so that he or she can modify the massage strokes. I understand that massage therapists do not diagnose diseases or conditions, prescribe medications or treatments, or perform spinal adjustments. I recognize that massage is not a substitute for medical treatment and should I need medical treatment I will seek out the appropriate health care professional (physician, psychotherapist, chiropractor, etc.). I understand that it is my responsibility to keep the massage therapist informed of changes in my child's or my dependent's health status, diagnosed medical conditions and medication changes. I understand that failure to inform the therapist of these changes may place my child, my dependent or me at greater risk of adverse reactions to massage. I release the massage therapist from any liability if I fail to disclose the appropriate health related information.

Client's Signature _____ Date _____

Therapist's Signature _____ Date _____

I authorize the therapists of Any Massage Clinic to provide massage to my child or dependent.

Name of Child or Dependent _____

Parent or Guardian Signature _____ Date _____

Figure 6-7 *(Continued)*

from the client, a therapist can discuss the client's condition and treatment goals with a mentor or supervisor. The mentor is also bound by confidentiality and cannot discuss the client's information with anyone but the primary therapist and the client.

There are limits to confidentiality that the client should be appraised of in the documents relating to informed consent. If the client discloses information relating to harming a child, elderly person, or mentally or physically challenged person, it is an ethical duty (often it is the law) to report the matter to the proper authorities. If clients threaten to harm themselves or others, this information must be reported to the authorities.

A court of law may subpoena a client's files, and those files may then be released to the public. It is important to keep honest, accurate, and organized documentation relating to client sessions. Avoid placing personal details in the file that are not necessary to treatment planning for massage therapy. For example, it is enough to note that a client's neck pain increases from work stress, but there is no need to include details of the client's conflict with his or her boss. The client release of information form shown in Figure 6-8 allows health care professionals to share details relating to the client's care.

I, (client's name) _____ ,
give my permission for (therapist's or business name) _____
to share or exchange pertinent information with (other health care professional's name)
_____ beginning on (date) _____ and ending
on (date when the agreement needs to be renewed) _____ . I understand that
this permission can be revoked at any time either verbally or in writing.

Client or Guardian Signature: _____   Date: _____

Figure 6-8 Example of client release of information form.

Concept Brief 6-4
Confidentiality

Keep confidential:

Health information and client file

Contact details

Events that occurred in massage sessions

Confidentiality limits:

Knowledge of harm to child, elderly person, person with mental or physical challenges

Threats of harm to self or others

Client misconduct as would be documented on an incident report

Client files subpoenaed by a court of law

Sexual Conduct Is Unethical

Ethical Principle: The Code of Ethics for NCBTMB states, "Refrain, under all circumstances, from initiating or engaging in any sexual conduct, sexual activities, or sexualizing behavior involving a client, even if the client attempts to sexualize the relationship."

Standard of Conduct: Therapists should understand behaviors considered sexual conduct and uphold the highest professional standards in regards to desexualizing massage. Therapists will not use sexual language, tell sexually oriented jokes, discuss their sexual experiences with clients, listen to the sexual experiences of clients, touch a client with sexual intent, allow a client to touch them with sexual intent, date a client, accept the offer of a date from a client, or allow any level of sexual impropriety from themselves or clients.

Discussion: The various levels of sexual misconduct range from lack of attention to sexual innuendo, to sexual impropriety, to sexual abuse of clients. You must always control

the atmosphere of the massage business. Allowing clients to act inappropriately is as serious as acting inappropriately yourself.

Lack of Attention to Sexual Innuendo

People often compliment each other and express their affection by positively commenting on another person's appearance. In a massage setting this can lead to mistrust. If you tell a client, "You look really good in those jeans," this may plant a seed of doubt and mistrust in a client's mind about your intentions, regardless of how long you have known each other or how innocent the comment is. Because of the intimate nature of massage, refrain from making any body comments that indicate approval or disapproval of a client's body and physical features like the eyes, mouth, or hair. Do not have magazines, pictures, or written material of a sexual nature in the work environment. Do not allow clients to make sexual jokes, and discourage clients from commenting on your personal appearance by downplaying those types of compliments with a brief "thank you" and a return to the business at hand.

Sexual Impropriety

Sexual impropriety is more serious than a general lack of attention to sexual innuendo and could lead to sexual harassment charges. Behaviors that could be labeled as sexual impropriety include:

- Any behavior that is immodest or encourages immodesty in clients. For example, a therapist who stands in the treatment room while the client undresses in view or allows clients to take a position on top of the drape exposing the genitals or breasts.
- Draping loosely or deliberately looking at a client's body while adjusting a drape. Not using draping practices or pressuring clients to take off their underclothing when they leave it on.

- Using nicknames for clients, especially those with a sexual connotation, or allowing the client to use sexual nicknames for you, like "baby," "honey," "sexy," "Romeo," or "handsome."

- Telling a client jokes or listening while a client tells jokes of a sexual nature.

- Discussing one's own sexuality within hearing of a client (it's a bad idea with co-workers as well, as it could lead to a sexual harassment claim).

- Gender-based comments or harassment, which includes verbal, nonverbal, or physical intimidation or hostility based on sex or sex-stereotyping, such as comments about another therapist's sexual orientation or criticism of a sexual orientation.

- Displaying or distributing sexually explicit drawings, pictures, or written materials (e.g., showing pictures of undraped bodies, no matter how "artistic" they are, in the reception area).

- Requests to date or acceptance of an offer to date.

- E-mailing or phoning clients or sending them notes or cards that are not specifically and exclusively related to the massage session. For example, it is acceptable to call a client the day after a session and ask how their muscles are feeling, but it is not acceptable to call a client for a conversation about personal details of events the client mentioned in the session.

Sexual Abuse

In a therapeutic relationship, the therapist develops a power advantage over the client (the power differential is discussed in Chapter 7), because the therapist is the caregiver. For this reason, any sexual misconduct, whether or not the client consents, is considered sexual abuse. The therapist is responsible and liable for sexual abuse, even if the client initiates it. Never engage in any sexual activity with a client in or out of the treatment room. This includes behavior that could reasonably be interpreted as sexual, including touching with the hands, body, mouth, or genitals the client's genitals, breasts, mouth, or anus; allowing the client to touch you; or allowing or encouraging clients to touch themselves or to masturbate during the session in your presence, or directly after the session in the treatment room. If the therapist masturbates or touches himself or herself in a sexual manner in the presence of the client, it is sexual abuse.

Sexual impropriety may lead to sexual harassment charges and the loss of massage credentials. Sexual abuse could lead to loss of massage credentials, lawsuits for personal damages, criminal charges, fines, attorney's fees, court costs, and jail time.

Honesty in Business and Finances

Ethical Principle: The Code of Ethics for NCBTMB states, "Conduct business and professional activities with honesty and integrity" and "Avoid any interest, activity or influence which might be in conflict with the practitioner's obligation to act in the best interests of the client or the profession."

Standard of Practice: The therapist must know and follow good business practices including record keeping, tax law, and compliance with regulations. Therapists will set fair fees and practice honesty in the development of marketing materials. Therapists will not accept gifts, compensation, or other benefits intended to influence a referral, decision, or treatment related to a client.

Discussion: Good business practices are covered in detail in Chapter 9. This discussion considers just a few ethical situations that arise in a massage business.

Fees

One area that needs careful consideration is the fee schedule. Set fair prices for services and charge all clients the same fees. Avoid setting fees that are dramatically reduced in an attempt to get more clients, as this practice may lead to plummeting fees in the area where the business is located and the devaluation of massage by the general public. Secure clientele through exceptional service instead. Sometimes therapists offer a sliding fee scale for clients with financial difficulty, offer an introductory massage rate (e.g., get $10 off your first massage), or offer a prepaid plan (e.g., prepay for five massages and get the fifth for $20 off). This is fine, but in all cases, fees and discounts should be clearly outlined in informational material and clarified before the start of the session.

Conflict of Interest

A conflict of interest is a conflict between a person's private interests and his or her public obligations. In a therapeutic relationship, the therapist has an obligation to provide the best possible care to the client. If therapists find themselves in a situation where they may benefit from influencing a client in a certain way, it is a conflict of interest and they should avoid the situation or step down from the therapist role. For example, a "**kickback**" in massage is any money, fee, commission, credit, gift, gratuity, thing of value, or compensation of any kind, provided for referrals of clients. If a chiropractor sends a massage therapist a thank you card containing $20 for every client the therapist sends to the chiropractor, the therapist is accepting a kickback. It is acceptable and even desirable to offer clients a list of other health care providers that you trust (often called a preferred provider list). You should refer clients to other health care providers who may benefit them, but no compensation should be exchanged. Your motives will be called into question if you receive payment for referrals. How could one be certain that the client is not being referred for the wrong reason? For example, maybe the client doesn't really need to see a chiropractor for a condition, but the therapist is thinking, "I could really use some extra money right now, and if I send five clients to the chiropractor this week it's an extra $100 bucks." Clearly this therapist has just broken this ethical principle.

Some therapists offer a referral plan where a client gets a discount for referring friends or family members to the massage therapist. This may seem a kickback but is not unethical. The difference is that the client and the friend are on an equal footing. Any health care provider develops a "power advantage" over a client because the client most often views the health care provider as more knowledgeable about health-related issues. When a massage therapist says, "I think you could really benefit from working with a chiropractor," it is likely to carry more weight than a friend saying, "You should get a session with my chiropractor, you need it!" Other conflicts of interest occur in situations of dual relationships discussed in Chapter 7.

Concept Brief 6-5
Referral Versus a Kickback

Referral: When the therapist suggests a client visit another health care provider for services outside the massage scope of practice. No compensation is exchanged.

Kickback: Any money, fee, commission, credit, gift, gratuity, thing of value, or compensation of any kind, provided for referrals of clients.

Maintain the Highest Standards of Professional Conduct

Ethical Principle: The Code of Ethics for the AMTA states that a therapist will "Conduct all business and professional activities within their scope of practice, the law of the land, and project a professional image."

Standard of Conduct: Therapists will maintain clear and honest communication with clients and make available to them, on request, their file. Refrain from the use of drugs or alcohol before or during the massage session, and present a professional image in keeping with the highest standards of the massage profession.

Discussion: This is a broad ethical principle and standard that covers such diverse areas as business, personal deportment, law, and regulations. Every massage therapist must strive to represent the massage profession in a positive way by maintaining standards of practice, working within the limits of the law, upholding good boundaries, and demonstrating the highest ethics.

Chapter 7, which explores the therapeutic relationship, discusses additional areas in which therapists must pay attention to ethics, values, standards, and decision making.

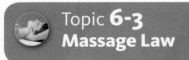

Topic 6-3
Massage Law

Laws are rules that are recognized by a community as binding and enforceable by authority. **Regulations** are directives that give official guidance about how laws should be followed. Massage laws are enacted at the local and state level with the aim to protect the safety and welfare of the public.

State or local authorities determine if a particular activity could potentially cause harm to the public. If they decide that it can, the authority seeks to limit the people who can practice that activity. A committee is formed to determine appropriate educational requirements, which are then demonstrated by a standardized test. People who meet the educational requirements and pass the test are awarded official credentials (Fig. 6-9). The scope of practice for the profession is described in state or local law and a board is appointed to ensure that professionals follow the law and don't practice the activity without proper credentials.

Each state is unique. Some states have state laws, some have local laws, and some have no laws regulating the practice of massage. It is therapists' responsibility to know and understand the local and state regulations in the state where they practice.

Education Requirements and Testing

In the states and local jurisdictions that regulate massage, massage education requirements vary widely from 100 hours up to 1,000 hours, with most states requiring students to complete 500 hours of training in order to sit for the **state-approved exam**. In regulated areas, an educational program must be accepted by the state board of education, and in some cases, by the state board of massage, for its graduates to be eligible to sit for the exam, often called "massage boards." Massage boards are designed to test massage school graduates on entry level massage concepts in the areas of anatomy and physiology, kinesiology, sanitation and hygiene, ethics, assessment, contraindications, pathology, the theory of the application of techniques, and professional standards (Box 6-2).

Some states require the student to complete a **jurisprudence exam** and/or **practical exam** in addition to the written exam. A jurisprudence exam is usually an open-book law exam that ensures knowledge of the laws relating to massage in the particular state, general massage ethics, and continuing education requirements. In a practical exam, the applicant performs massage techniques in front of a panel to

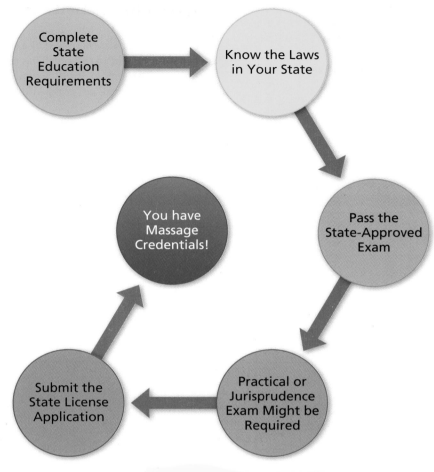

Figure 6-9 Credentialing process.

BOX 6-2 Massage Credentialing Examinations

There are three primary exams used for massage credentialing at the state level:

1. **Massage & Bodywork Licensing Examination (MBLEx):** The MBLEx was developed by the Federation of State Massage Therapy Boards on behalf of its Member Boards. It was based on a Job Task Analysis Survey and developed with contributions by over 50 content experts under the guidance of 15 testing and psychometric experts. The Job Task Analysis was validated by input from 7,646 massage, bodywork and somatic professionals and administered through Pearson VUE at test centers across the United States. To find out more about the MBLEx and utilize online practice tests visit www.fsmtb.org.

2. **National Certification Examination for Therapeutic Massage (NCETM) and National Certification Examination for Therapeutic Massage & Bodywork (NCTMB):** The two NCE exams were developed by the National Certification Board for Therapeutic Massage and Bodywork. The content areas of the two exams are similar but with variations in the percentage weights of different content areas. As the name suggests, the NCTMB contains more questions about bodywork modalities, their assessment procedures, and their application methods. To find out more about the NCE exams, visit www.ncbtmb.org.

3. **Resources for Study**: Both websites offer links for content outlines and both have downloadable handouts for applicants. Determine the test required in your state using Table 6-2 in this chapter and visit the appropriate website to gather information. A number of publishers provide textbooks with practice tests specific to these exams including Laura Allen's *Plain & Simple Guide to Therapeutic Massage and Bodywork Examinations* (Lippincott, Williams & Wilkins), Sandy Fritz's *Mosby's Massage Therapy Review* (Mosby/Elisver), Joseph Ashton's *Review for Therapeutic Massage and Bodywork Exams* (Lippincott, Williams & Wilkins), and Barbara Rice's *Outline Review of Massage Therapy* (Prentice Hall).

demonstrate competency in the application of techniques, sanitation and hygienic practices, communication with clients, and overall professionalism. Massage schools usually dedicate some portion of their program to preparing students for the state-approved exam, jurisprudence exam, practical exam, and licensing process. Education minimums and credential and licensing requirements are listed in Table 6-2.

Massage Credentials

Massage credentials are bestowed by a state or local authority to demonstrate that an individual has met the education and testing requirements to legally practice massage. The term "licensed," "registered," or "certified" may be used depending on the state.

TABLE 6-2   State Education Minimums and Massage Credentials Information is current as of January 2011

State	Required Education Hours	Competency Assessment	Designation/Title
Alabama	650	NCBTMB and state exam	License (LMT)
Alaska	0	No state regulation	NA
Arizona	700	NCBTMB exam	License (LMT)
Arkansas	500	MBLEx	License (LMT)
California	500 250	MBLEx or NCBTMB accepted as an alternative to education	Voluntary certification A. Therapist (CMT) B. Practitioner (CMP)
Colorado	500	MBLEx or NCBTMB	RMT
Connecticut	500	NCBTMB exam	License (LMT)
Delaware	300 or 500	No exam required NCBTMB exam	Certification/Massage Technician (CMT) License (LMT)
District of Columbia	500	MBLEx or NCBTMB exam	License (LMT)
Florida	500	MBLEx or NCBTMB exam	License (LMT)
Georgia	500	MBLEx or NCBTMB exam	License (LMT)
Hawaii	570	State exam	License (LMT)
Idaho	0	No state regulation	NA
Illinois	500	NCBTMB exam	License (LMT)
Indiana	0	MBLEx or NCBTMB exam	Certification (CMT)
Iowa	500	MBLEx or NCBTMB exam	License (LMT)
Kansas	0	No state regulation	NA
Kentucky	600	NCBTMB exam	License (LMT)
Louisiana	500	MBLEx or NCBTMB exam	License (LMT)
Maine	500	MBLEx or NCBTMB exam alternative to education	License (LMT)
Maryland	500 or 500 +60 College	NCBTMB or NCCAOM exam and jurisprudence exam	Registration (RMT) Certification (CMT)
Massachusetts	650	Not required	License (LMT)
Michigan	500	Pending implementation of law	Pending
Minnesota	0	No state regulation	NA
Mississippi	700	MBLEx or NCBTMB exam	License (LMT)
Missouri	500	MBLEx, NCBTMB or NCCAOM exam	License (LMT)
Montana	500	MBLEx or NCBTMB exam	License (LMT)

TABLE 6-2   State Education Minimums and Massage Credentials Information is current as of January 2011 (Continued)

State	Required Education Hours	Competency Assessment	Designation/Title
Nebraska	1,000	MBLEx or NCBTMB exam	License (LMT)
Nevada	500	NCBTMB exam	License (LMT)
New Hampshire	750	MBLEx or NCBTMB exam	License (LMT)
New Jersey	500	NCBTMB exam is accepted as an alternative to education	Certification (CMT)
New Mexico	650	MBLEx or NCBTMB exam and jurisprudence exam	License (LMT)
New York	1,000	State exam	License (LMT)
North Carolina	500	MBLEx, NCBTMB, OBTE, or NCCAOM exam	License (LMT)
North Dakota	750	NCBTMB exam	License (LMT)
Ohio	750	State exam	License (LMT)
Oklahoma	0	No state regulation	NA
Oregon	500	MBLEx or NCBTMB exam and jurisprudence, and practical exam	License (LMT)
Pennsylvania	600	MBLEx or NCBTMB exam	License (LMT)
Rhode Island	500	MBLEx or NCBTMB exam	License (LMT)
South Carolina	500	MBLEx or NCBTMB exam	License (LMT)
South Dakota	500	MBLEx or NCBTMB exam	License (LMT)
Tennessee	500	MBLEx or NCBTMB exam and jurisprudence exam	License (LMT)
Texas	500	MBLEx or NCBTMB exam	License (LMT)
Utah	600	MBLEx or NCBTMB exam and jurisprudence exam	License (LMT)
Vermont	0	No state regulation	NA
Virginia	500	NCBTMB exam	Certification (CMT)
Washington	500	MBLEx or NCBTMB exam and AIDS training and jurisprudence exam	License (LMP)
West Virginia	500	MBLEx or NCBTMB exam	License (LMT)
Wisconsin	600	MBLEx, NCCAOM, or NCBTMB exam	Certification (CMT)
Wyoming	0	No state regulation	NA

To check for legislative updates go to http://massagetherapy.com/careers/stateboards.php

Licensure

A license is a printed, state-issued document that gives a person official permission to practice massage within the limits of a scope of practice (discussed below). **Licensure** also allows qualifying therapists to use a protected title and list their massage credentials after their names. For example, Washington and New Hampshire grant licensed massage therapists (LMTs) the right to use the title "Licensed Massage Practitioner" or LMP. Most licensed states use the title "Massage Therapist", or "Licensed Massage Therapist". States that license massage therapists usually appoint a **board of massage** to supervise the profession in that area.

Registration

Maryland and Colorado "register" massage therapists and grant the title "Registered Massage Practitioner" (RMP) and "Registered Massage Therapist" (RMT). The words are different, but the legal requirements are essentially the same. People must still complete an approved training program and sit for an exam, as required with licensure. In Maryland, a therapist who has 60 hours of college credit and meets the requirements for registration can be "certified" and may use the credentials "Certified Massage Therapist" (CMT). A registered therapist can upgrade to "certified" after completing 60 hours of college credit. Maryland uses the terms "registered" and "certified" to define environments where therapists can work. RMPs cannot practice in health care settings such as hospitals, nursing homes, clinics, or doctors' offices. They can only practice in business settings such as a private business, health clubs, and spas. CMTs can work in health care settings and also in business settings, so a therapist who wants to work with hospice patients needs 60 hours of college credit in addition to massage training, even though the college credit does not need to be related to massage or health.

Certification

The term **certification** is very confusing in the massage profession because it is used in a variety of ways with different meanings.

- **Required State Certification to Practice Massage:** In Virginia, massage therapists must complete 500 hours of education and complete the state-approved exam to use the title CMT and practice massage in the state. In this case, "certification" is synonymous with licensure.
- **Voluntary Governmental Certification:** In California, massage therapists can participate in voluntary state certification by demonstrating proof of 500 hours of education and completing one of the state-approved exams. Therapists who do not voluntarily certify are subject to requirements and registration fees in different municipalities of the state. They may be able to practice massage by meeting the requirements of a particular municipality, but they cannot use the title CMT or Certified Massage Practitioner and cannot practice in a different municipality without first meeting the new municipality's requirements for practice. Certification in this case allows the therapist to work in any city in the state without the need to fulfill requirements in numerous municipalities.
- **Association Certification:** Both ABMP and the AMTA "certify" members. Members of these organizations must meet the association's requirements to join. When they have met the requirements, they are granted membership and a certificate. The designation has no legal significance at the state or national level.
- **National Certification:** The NCBTMB has a certification process that is widely recognized by the massage and bodywork community as an entry-level standard, though it is not mandated at the state or national level. Because it is called "National Certification," some students get the idea that it gives them permission to practice in any state, which is not the case. When the NCBTMB was founded, hourly minimums for education and standards for massage credentials were even more inconsistent than they are today. Many states did not regulate massage at all, and therapists had less professional recognition. The NCBTMB certification process gave therapists the opportunity to voluntarily demonstrate that they had accomplished a minimum level of competency that was clearly defined and recognized by other therapists across the country. As more and more states regulate massage, the need for this voluntary credential has decreased.

- **Continuing Education Completion:** Privately operated continuing education providers also "certify" people who have completed their courses. Because a course might be 2 hours long, 16 hours long, 250 hours long, or longer, the use of the word "certified" causes some confusion. Usually it means that the participant has been granted a certificate of completion. In this case, recognition comes only from the person running the continuing education program and holds little weight locally, at the state level, or nationally.
- **Registered or Trademarked Continuing Education Certification:** Sometimes the continuing education program is so extensive that it does hold weight on a national level and the title of those completing the program is protected. For example, Certified Rolfers complete 600 hours of continuing education in structural integration and are widely respected and recognized in the massage and bodywork community. The titles "Certified Rolfer" and "Rolf Movement Practitioner" are registered trademarks of the Rolf Institute of Structural Integration and cannot be used by anyone who has not completed their extensive program.

Concept Brief 6-6
Massage Credentials

- **License:** Official state permission to practice massage and use a protected title after meeting education and testing requirements.
- **Registration:** Registration with the state after meeting education and testing requirements.
- **Required state certification to practice:** Certification (synonymous with licensure) with the state after meeting education and testing requirements. Required to practice massage.
- **Voluntary governmental certification:** Voluntary process in which therapist meets education and testing requirements to use a protected title. Other people can provide the service but not use the title.
- **Association certification:** Granted by a professional membership organization to denote that the therapist met the requirements to be a member.
- **National certification:** A voluntary process set up by the NCBTMB to denote that the therapist has met specific entry-level requirements. No state or federal recognition.
- **Continuing education certification:** A certificate of completion from the person or group running a continuing education course. Holds little weight locally or nationally.
- **Registered or trademarked continuing education certification:** A certificate of completion from a recognized continuing education provider. It may enable the therapist to use a legally protected title (e.g., Certified Rolfer).

Scope of Practice

The term **scope of practice** is used by regulating boards of health care professions to describe the techniques, activities, and methods that are permitted to a therapist under the law. While most states define the scope of practice for massage in similar terms, small variations require therapists to carefully inspect and understand the scope of practice in the state where they practice massage. Ohio's scope of practice for massage therapy provides a good example; it states, "Massage therapy is the treatment of disorders of the human body by the manipulation of soft tissue through the systematic external application of massage techniques including touch, stroking, friction, vibration, percussion, kneading, stretching, compression, and joint movements within the normal physiologic range of motion; and adjunctive thereto, the external application of water, heat, cold, topical preparations, and mechanical devices."

Florida's definition is an example of an uncommon variation. It states that "massage means the manipulation of the soft tissues of the human body with the hand, foot, arm, or elbow, whether or not such manipulation is aided by hydrotherapy, including colonic irrigation, or thermal therapy; any electrical or mechanical device; or the application to the human body of a chemical or herbal preparation." Colonic irrigation, also called colon hydrotherapy, or colonics, involves the low-pressure injection of water into the colon for cleansing purposes using a mechanical device. It is believed to flush toxic buildup out of the colon leading to better overall health. This type of treatment is usually not included in the massage scope of practice.

Restrictions to Scope of Practice

Usually the state's definition lists some of the restrictions in the practice of massage. The Arizona definition states: "Practice of massage therapy means the application of massage therapy to any person for a fee or other consideration. Practice of massage therapy does not include the diagnosis of illness or disease, medical procedures, naturopathic manipulative medicine, osteopathic manipulative medicine, chiropractic adjustive procedures, homeopathic neuromuscular integration, electrical stimulation, ultrasound, prescription of medicines or the use of modalities for which a license to practice medicine, chiropractic, nursing, occupational therapy, athletic training, physical therapy, acupuncture or podiatry is required by law."

You may notice that three primary restrictions to massage scope of practice are universal. Massage therapists cannot *diagnose* a patient's condition, *prescribe* a medication or treatment, or *adjust a client's bones*. Some therapists fall into diagnoses accidentally and do not realize the serious ramifications of their actions. The term "diagnose" means to identify an illness or disorder through an interview, physical examination, and medical tests. For example, a client may describe to the therapist a set of symptoms that the therapist recognizes as a particular soft-tissue condition like carpal tunnel syndrome. A therapist who says, "Your condition is carpal tunnel syndrome and you need to take 1,200 mg of ibuprofen a day, wear a wrist splint, and receive treatment massage," has crossed the line and is diagnosing. Anytime therapists label a set of symptoms as a defined medical condition, they are diagnosing. Instead, the therapist should acknowledge the seriousness of the client's symptoms and suggest the client visit a physician for a diagnosis.

The term "prescribe" means to direct a patient to follow a particular course of treatment, specifically to use a particular drug at set times and in specified dosages. The therapist in the example above who advised the client to take 1,200 mg of ibuprofen a day and wear a wrist splint was prescribing. Therapists sometimes accidentally prescribe things like herbal remedies or aromatherapy cures. To say to a client, "You should drink six glasses of peppermint tea a day for your stomach condition" is prescribing.

A chiropractor is a medical professional who adjusts bones to improve structural alignment and free nerve tissue leading to better overall function. Sometimes a client's bones shift naturally during the application of a massage stroke. This is normal and should not cause alarm. But therapists are working outside their scope of practice if they try to get a bone to move. Many massage therapists develop highly refined palpation skills and sometimes can feel that a bone is not aligned normally. But if they attempt to shift the bone by using a thrusting movement, or even hold an intent to move the bone with a massage stroke, they are working out of their scope of practice. Instead the therapist should refer the client to a chiropractor.

Another area where massage therapists may venture out of their scope of practice is counseling. People seek counseling from mental health care providers to gain insight into personal or psychological problems. Clients often share personal issues with their massage therapists during sessions. This is not a scope of practice violation so long as the therapist listens compassionately but does not give advice or professional input. At other times, clients express a need for guidance or become emotional. The massage therapist must be very careful not to counsel the client or try to talk the client through the situation. If listening is not enough, the massage therapist should refer the client to a professional mental health care provider. In

---

Concept Brief 6-7
Scope of Practice

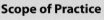

Defined	The techniques, activities, and methods permitted to massage therapists under the law.
Restrictions	Limits to the scope of practice, including: Diagnosis: The identification and naming of a condition or disease. Prescribing: Directions to take a drug or remedy at specific dosages and times. Bone adjustments: Seeking to change the position of a bone.

all cases, massage therapists must know and understand their scope of practice and its restrictions in their state.

Supervision of Massage

A board of massage is usually appointed in states that regulate massage to supervise the practice of massage by reviewing therapist applications, investigating complaints, and overseeing licensees who practice in the state. Sometimes massage is supervised by another health care board, such as the nursing board or board of chiropractic examiners. Each state board of massage has a website where massage therapists can find important information about the laws and regulations that define their scope of practice. Board members often hold meetings that are open to massage therapists and the public so that issues can be freely discussed. It is a good practice to log onto the state board of massage website and become familiar with state laws, regulations, and requirements before graduation (Table 6-3). The board of massage is likely to participate in supervising the renewal of credentials and the withdrawal of credentials.

TABLE 6-3   State Board of Massage Websites

Alabama
http://www.almtbd.state.al.us
Alaska
No state regulation
Arizona
http://massagetherapy.az.gov
Arkansas
http://www.arkansasmassagetherapy.com/
California
http://www.camtc.org/
Colorado
http://www.dora.state.co.us/massage-therapists/licensure.htm
Connecticut
http://www.dph.state.ct.us/Licensure/apps/PLIS/MassageTherapist/MSG_Endo.htm
Delaware
http://www.professionallicensing.state.de.us/boards/massagebodyworks/index.shtml
District of Columbia
http://hpla.doh.dc.gov/hpla/cwp/view,A,1195,Q,488659,hplaNav,%7C30661%7C,.asp
Florida
http://www.doh.state.fl.us/MQA/massage/ma_home.html
Georgia
http://www.sos.state.ga.us/plb/massage/
Hawaii
http://www.hawaii.gov/dcca/areas/pvl/boards/massage/
Idaho
No state regulation
Illinois
http://www.idfpr.com/DPR/apply/masst.asp
Indiana
http://www.in.gov/pla/massage.htm
Kansas
No state regulation

TABLE 6-3   State Board of Massage Websites *(Continued)*

Kentucky
http://finance.ky.gov/ourcabinet/caboff/OAS/op/massth/
Louisiana
http://lsbmt.org/
Maine
http://www.maine.gov/pfr/professionallicensing/professions/massage/index.htm
Maryland
http://www.mdmassage.org/
Massachusetts
http://www.mass.gov/?pageID=ocasubtopic&L=4&L0=Home&L1=Licensee&L2=Division+of+Professional+Licensure+Boards&L3=Board+of+Registration+of+Massage+Therapy&sid=Eoca
Michigan
http://www.michigan.gov/mdch/0,1607,7-132-27417_27529_53660—,00.html
Minnesota
No state regulation
Mississippi
http://www.msbmt.state.ms.us/msbmt/msbmt.nsf
Missouri
http://pr.mo.gov/massage.asp
Montana
http://www.massagetherapists.mt.gov/?;
Nebraska
http://www.massagetherapy.nv.gov/
Nevada
http://www.massagetherapy.nv.gov/
New Hampshire
http://www.dhhs.state.nh.us/DHHS/LRS/ELIGIBILITY/massage-license.htm
New Jersey
http://www.state.nj.us/lps/ca/medical/nursing.htm
New Mexico
http://www.rld.state.nm.us/b&c/massage/
New York
http://www.op.nysed.gov/mtlic.htm
North Carolina
http://www.bmbt.org/
North Dakota
http://www.ndboardofmassage.com/
Ohio
http://www.med.ohio.gov/MTsubwebindex.htm
Oklahoma
No state regulation

(Continued)

TABLE 6-3   State Board of Massage Websites (Continued)

Oregon
http://www.oregonmassage.org/
Pennsylvania
http://www.massagetherapy@state.pa.us
Rhode Island
http://www.health.ri.gov/hsr/professions/massage.php#Requirements
South Carolina
http://www.llr.state.sc.us/POL/MassageTherapy/
South Dakota
http://www.state.sd.us/doh/Massage/
Tennessee
http://www2.state.tn.us/health/Boards/Massage/index.htm
Texas
http://www.dshs.state.tx.us/massage/default.shtm
Utah
http://www.dopl.utah.gov/licensing/massage.html
Vermont
No state regulation
Virginia
http://www.dhp.virginia.gov/Nursing/nursing_forms.htm
Washington
https://fortress.wa.gov/doh/hpqa1/hps3/Massage_Therapy/default.htm
West Virginia
http://www.wvmassage.org/
Wisconsin
http://drl.wi.gov/prof/mass/def.htm
Wyoming
No state regulation

Renewal of Credentials

Most regulated states require a yearly fee and a specified number of continuing education hours for maintaining massage credentials. Continuing education is viewed as beneficial because it brings the therapist up to date with new advances in massage knowledge or skills and encourages therapists to diversify their practices. Usually, therapists are required to keep proof of continuing education course completion and provide it to the board of massage when requested.

Withdrawal of Massage Credentials

The board of massage can suspend or revoke a massage therapist's credentials for a number of reasons:

- The therapist obtained the license fraudulently by falsifying the license application. For example, an applicant was convicted of a crime as a teenager and failed to list the conviction and an explanation on the application.
- The therapist allowed another person or business to use the license fraudulently. In some instances, a therapist has sold the license to a business that was a front for prostitution.
- If the board receives complaints from clients that indicate a therapist is not behaving in a professional manner, or is behaving in a way that endangers the health and safety of the public, credentials may be suspended or revoked.
- The therapist is caught using a controlled substance, is convicted of a felony, is convicted of any crime relating to the

unlawful practice of massage, or is found mentally incompetent by a court of law.

- The therapist used false, deceptive, or misleading advertising to promote massage.
- The board of massage discovers that the therapist had a license revoked, suspended, or denied in another U.S. jurisdiction.
- The board receives complaints from other therapists or other health care professionals that the massage therapist is working outside the scope of practice for massage.

The board of massage may also issue fines to therapists practicing illegally or to individuals who are practicing massage without a license. Some boards list disciplinary actions on their websites so that the public and other professionals can review offences related to massage. An examination of these sites indicates that sexual impropriety and the practice of massage without legal credentials are the most common reasons for disciplinary action.

Complaints from the Public

Consumers who want to file a complaint about a massage therapist or massage business can do so via the state board of massage website. Usually the consumer fills out a form and sends it to the board. The board investigates the complaint and may take action. Consumers in states that are not regulated can contact the AMTA, ABMP, or NCBTMB and file a complaint. If the therapist is a member of one of these organizations, the complaint will come under review when the therapist attempts to renew membership. Sometimes an investigation and termination of membership occur immediately because of the nature of the complaint. If a therapist has acted illegally, the consumer is encouraged to involve local authorities as well as file complaints with the board of massage and professional organizations.

Reporting the Misconduct of a Colleague

The board of massage might also receive a complaint from another health care professional or a colleague. For example, a client might mention to a chiropractor receiving a spinal adjustment from a massage therapist during massage. The chiropractor may then alert the board of massage about the therapist working outside the massage scope of practice and endangering the health and safety of the public. The board of massage would investigate the claim, and the therapist's license might be suspended or revoked. Any knowledge of sexual misconduct or harm to a child, elderly person, or individual with mental or physical challenges should be reported immediately.

Sometimes issues are not so clearcut, and therapists must grapple with their feelings about another therapist's conduct. For example, a therapist named Susan is a heavy drinker who doesn't come to work drunk exactly but sometimes smells of alcohol. Although clients have not complained, are they perhaps concerned whether she is providing them with the best and safest care?

In another example, a therapist named John at a large massage clinic is very talented and has developed his skills through advanced continuing education courses. He regularly takes clients away from the other therapists at the clinic, and his schedule is always full. The receptionist reports hearing John making untrue claims to a client about the benefits of a particular massage technique he offers. Other therapists at the clinic become angry and get together to speak to the clinic owner and decide to file a complaint with the board of massage.

In both of these cases, careful consideration is needed before a report is filed. In the first scenario, a conversation might be enough. Maybe Susan is unaware of the fact that she comes to work smelling of alcohol. A caring, companionate dialogue might be enough to resolve the situation. In the second scenario, the other therapists need to consider their personal motivations for filing a complaint. It's hard to tell if John has really done anything wrong. Is he purposely trying to steal clients from other therapists, or does his advanced training make him especially appealing to clients? Is he purposely trying to mislead clients about the benefits of massage to get them interested, or is he making substantiated claims for a sophisticated technique that is misunderstood by the receptionist? These issues need clarification, and a discussion with the group and a mentor, perhaps the clinic owner, might be the best solution. An objective person might be better able to ascertain whether John committed ethical or legal violations that should be reported to the board of massage, or whether he simply needs coaching about his interaction with other people at the clinic.

Therapists who find that they need to file a formal complaint with the board of massage or with a professional organization should carefully and honestly document the details of the situation in writing and send it to the relevant agency. Keep a copy of the document in the event it is misplaced or goes astray. The therapist may or may not be informed about the investigative process by the board or professional organization. The information is kept confidential to protect the therapist in the event that the allegations prove unfounded.

Other Legal Issues

A therapist must understand some key legal terms and issues to practice massage in a regulated state. These issues include exemptions to the law, reciprocity, grandfathering provisions, and HIPAA regulations. Liability insurance and zoning restrictions are discussed in Chapter 9.

Exemptions to the Law

An exemption from the law is the permission not to do something that others are obliged to do. Some therapists who have met educational requirements in other forms of bodywork are exempt from complying with massage regulations in some states or municipalities. Therefore they do not need a massage license, registration, or certificate to practice. For example, reflexology is often exempt from massage law. Energetic bodywork systems like Reiki and movement systems like Feldenkrais are also often exempt. It is widely accepted that professionals who are licensed or registered to practice medicine, nursing, physical therapy, podiatry, or chiropractic can use massage as part of their practice. Athletic trainers or instructors in physical education departments at high schools, universities, and colleges can use massage with athletes without a license.

Reciprocity

Reciprocity is a right granted by regulatory bodies that have formed a mutual relationship to allow therapists to transfer their credentials from one state to another. This is sometimes allowed when one state has requirements similar to those of another state. Therapists moving from a state where they hold a license, certificate, or registration should contact the board of massage in the state where they are moving to determine if the states have a reciprocity agreement.

Grandfathering Provisions

When a state passes legislation to regulate massage, it usually includes a "grandfathering" provision in the statues that allows people who practiced massage under the old system to integrate into the new system. Therapists who do not apply for regulation under the grandfathering provision by the deadline then must meet the new state education and examination requirements.

The Health Insurance Portability and Accountability Act

The HIPAA was passed by Congress in 1996 to ensure that employees changing jobs do not lose their health care benefits, to simplify health care record keeping by requiring standardization, and to ensure patient privacy. The key part of this law for massage therapists is the privacy protection section, which requires you to maintain client files in a secure place (file or drawer in a room locked when you are not present) and not to wrongly disclose to third parties information linking an identifiable client to a particular medical treatment or condition. In other words, as discussed earlier, you must maintain client confidentiality. If you electronically submit client documents for insurance reimbursement, you must follow HIPAA standards in your submission practices and use accepted codes. ABMP estimates that only 5% of massage professionals submit files electronically for insurance reimbursement. If you work in a state where you can bill insurance companies for massage therapy, you should review HIPAA regulations carefully. Information can be found at www.hhs.gov/ocr/privacy-summary.rtf.

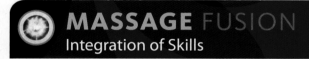

MASSAGE FUSION
Integration of Skills

STUDY TIP: Graphic Organizers

Graphic organizers are visual representations of concepts, ideas, and other information (Fig. 6-10). They can help you organize and clarify information to improve your comprehension and recall. They are especially useful for visual and kinesthetic learners. Visual learners benefit from the structure of graphic organizers, while the process of creating a graphic organizer motivates kinesthetic learners.

MASSAGE INSPIRATION: Change Minds with Massage

The AMTA and the ABMP often work with local groups to set up massage awareness events for legislators. These events allow legislators to hear from massage therapists about their concerns regarding licensing and regulation. They also get the chance to learn about the benefits of massage and experience a seated massage. Usually the hosting professional association provides a snack for the legislators and their staff. This is an excellent experience for students to learn about the logistics of an on-site seated event and have the chance to make a difference at the same time. Participants also get to meet other massage therapists who share similar interests and concerns.

GOOD TO KNOW: How do I Get Involved with Massage Issues in My State?

If you want to get involved in the legislation affecting massage in your state, the first step is to log on to the AMTA, ABMP, and FSMTB websites (see Table 6-1). Each of these groups has updated information about legislative issues in various states. Often, postings for events like massage awareness days, discussed above, are also listed. These groups send members "legislative alerts" about laws that affect massage. The alerts often provide detailed information about the issue and who to contact with your concerns. A person can also write a letter to elected representatives at the federal, state, county, or local level. The Legislative Hotline (800-363-9472) provides contact details for all elected officials.

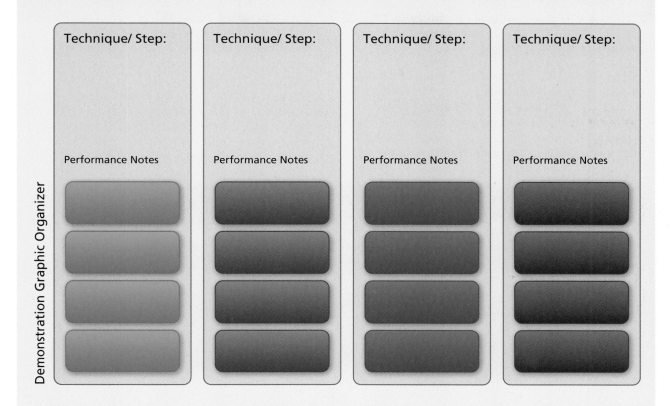

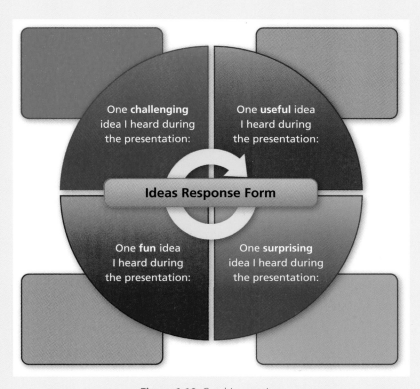

Figure 6-10 Graphic organizers.

(Continued)

MASSAGE FUSION (Continued)
Integration of Skills

CHAPTER WRAP-UP

When you signed up for massage school you probably didn't think about, or even realize, that you would be dealing with such weighty subjects as ethics, standards, and laws. You just wanted to massage people and get paid for it! Many students feel resistant to these topics because they are full of gray areas. You can't just memorize all the right answers and fill them in on a test. These topics require a therapist to think, reason, feel, assess those feelings, understand, and adapt. Each situation, each client, your reaction to each client, the client's reaction to you—everything will be different every session. Every session will require you to be aware of your feelings and behaviors, and be aware of the client's feelings and behaviors in response to the treatment. This is actually one of the more interesting aspects of massage. As you grapple with right and wrong, as you challenge yourself and question your own actions, you grow as a person and as a therapist. Embrace these topics, discuss them with classmates, and come back to this chapter regularly because at each stage of your training, new issues and ideas will stand out. Ethics, standards of practice, and laws form the foundation of your massage practice. Skills in this area are just as important as advanced massage techniques, and ultimately may have a greater impact on your client's healing process.

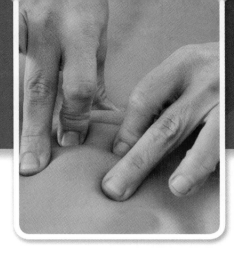

Chapter 7

The Therapeutic Relationship

KEY TERMS

armoring

bodymind connection

bodymind split

boundaries

counter-transference

dual relationships

embodiment

emotion

emotional intelligence

emotional release

physical history

power differential

psychological defenses

psychological history

therapeutic relationship

touch

transference

LEARNING OBJECTIVES

Having read the chapter and used the related student learning tools, the student will be able to:

1 Outline the importance of touch for life, development, connection, and bonding.

2 Compare and contrast ethical professional touch and unethical unprofessional touch.

3 Practice the language that might be used to manage a sexual arousal response in a client receiving massage.

4 Define these terms: power differential, trans-ference, counter-transference, and psycho-logical defense.

5 Describe the way in which armoring is used to suppress emotion.

6 Distinguish permeable, semipermeable, and impermeable boundaries.

7 Differentiate physical, mental, emotional, spiritual, and sexual boundaries.

8 List four ways to establish the boundaries of the therapeutic relationship.

9 Define the term bodymind and explain its general relevance to the practice of massage.

10 Summarize the reasons for a bodymind split and explain its general relevance to the practice of massage.

11 Categorize the components of a client's physical history and psychological history.

12 List three reasons why a client might experience emotional release during a massage.

13 Outline three principles for ensuring a safe, supportive atmosphere for the client during an emotional release.

A large body of psychology research suggests that the relationship between the therapist and the client is the single-most important predictor of therapeutic outcome,[1] even more important than the types of techniques that were used in the session.[2] One group of researchers refer to the therapeutic relationship as an alliance and define it as the "observable ability of the therapist and client to work together in a realistic, collaborative relationship based on mutual respect, liking, trust, and commitment to the work of the treatment."[3] In the massage profession, the **therapeutic relationship** is a professional partnership between a massage therapist and client in which, safe, structured touch is used to help the client achieve reasonable and clearly defined treatment goals. The work is client centered, which means that it is always provided to benefit the client and with the client's needs at the forefront.

This chapter explores five topics that illuminate factors that influence a therapeutic relationship. Topic 7-1 examines the power of touch for life and development. It compares ethical and unethical touch and establishes guidelines for managing sexual arousal responses in clients. In Topic 7-2 students learn how to work with issues including the power differential, transference, and the psychological defenses of clients. Boundaries are the subject of Topic 7-3 in which students develop an awareness of personal and client boundaries and learn to set good boundaries to establish the framework of a therapeutic relationship. In Topic 7-4 students explore concepts like the bodymind split and bodymind connection and consider how these concepts might impact the massage session. The importance of understanding client emotions is discussed in Topic 7-5, which provides guidance on managing the emotional processes of both the self and clients during a massage session.

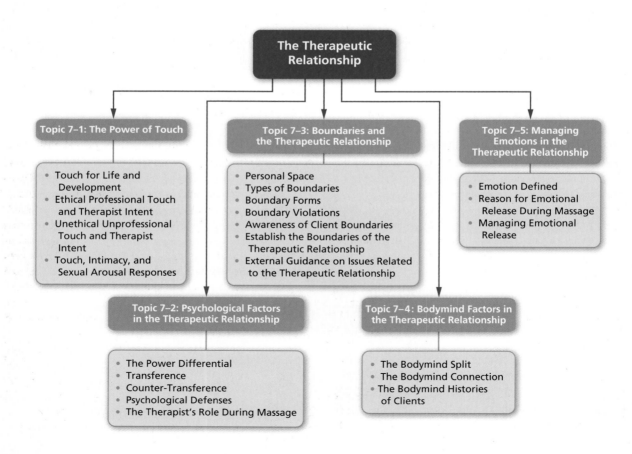

Topic **7-1**
The Power of Touch

In the *Oxford Dictionary of English*, the word **touch** has eight verb definitions and seven noun definitions. This is a loaded word! As massage therapists, we think of touch as something that is skilled, practiced, and professional. We understand that touch has power because we have already felt muscle change, witnessed the reduction of pain, and seen the reestablishment of freer movement patterns. This topic demonstrates that the power of touch goes beyond its ability to address soft-tissue tension patterns. Touch is necessary for life, for physiological and psychological development, and for connection and bonding. In a therapeutic relationship, the form of touch is important. Clients benefit from ethical, professional touch and could potentially be harmed by unethical, unprofessional touch. Because touch during massage can elicit unintentional sexual arousal responses in clients, therapists must learn how to manage these responses in a respectful manner to ensure a healthy therapeutic relationship.

Touch for Life and Development

In the early years of the 20th century, a number of physicians in America and Europe were confronting the same problem. Children placed in orphanages died – not just a few of them, but up to 99% of children in orphanages under the age of 2, according to an American study conducted in 1915 by Dr. Henry Dwight Chaplin.[4] The disease killing children in staggering numbers was called *marasmus*, the Greek word for "wasting away." The few children who did survive early orphanages were permanently damaged. They experienced retarded bone growth, low weight, suppressed immunity, poor coordination, general apathy, and decreased mental function. American orphanages followed precise rules and the children were fed properly, bathed regularly, and housed in a clean and safe environment. Why were they dying or developing physical and mental disabilities?

Investigations in both America and Europe found that childcare providers were stretched thin at orphanages. Staff only had time to feed and bathe children, change diapers, and clean the facility. There was no time for hugging, stroking, rocking, holding, or affectionate play. The children were touch deprived. They were missing an essential element for life: touch. When aides were hired to handle the children, hold them, stroke them, sing to them, and rock them, mortality rates fell to <10% and the children developed normally.

Chapter 4 discusses the effects of massage for infants and notes that massage is indicated for preterm, healthy full-term, and full-term infants with medical conditions for therapeutic change, and condition management. Massage supports weight gain, cognitive development, parent–child interaction, and improved sleep hours.[5–7] For infants or young children who have been exposed to HIV, cocaine, or abuse, or who have medical conditions like asthma, autism, cancer, skin conditions, rheumatoid arthritis, psychiatric problems, or stress disorders, massage reduced stress hormones, lowered anxiety levels, led to less colic and fewer episodes of crying.[8,9]

Clearly touch, like food, water, or shelter, is essential for normal and optimal development. While we have focused so far predominantly on infants and young children, we can speculate that clients with headache, depression, a heart condition, or back pain receive something more than a reduction in muscle tension from massage. They also receive the inherent human nourishment of being touched by another human in a respectful and nurturing way.

Concept Brief 7-1
The Power of Touch

Marasmus: Greek word for "wasting away." A condition that affected children in orphanages in the early 20th century.

Touch deprivation: The absence of touch leading to marasmus and death or severe physical disability.

Power of touch: Touch is necessary for normal and optimal growth and development and for life.

Ethical Professional Touch and Therapist Intent

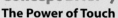

The phrase "ethical professional touch" describes all of the behaviors of the therapist toward the client, not just the actual massage techniques. Ethical, professional touch is *skilled*, *purposeful*, and *respectful* and holds *healing intent*. Touch that is *skilled* knows just which muscles are tight and require attention. Skilled touch is highly trained. It works at a depth that engages the muscle and fascia without causing undue discomfort to the client. Touch that is *purposeful* has a plan for how each area of the body will be addressed to meet clearly defined treatment goals. Strokes are applied in predictable patterns that understand the body's organization at both superficial and deep levels. Touch that is *respectful* is careful, considerate, and responsive. Each action is well thought out, and draping is smooth, snug, and modest, and the client is protected from chills or undue stress. *Healing intent* refers to the state of the therapist's mind during the session. A therapist who *intends* to benefit the client with a massage is much more likely to benefit the client than a therapist who doesn't care. Clients who experience ethical professional touch are more likely to trust the therapist and so relax completely during the session and receive the greatest benefit from the treatment.

Unethical Unprofessional Touch and Therapist Intent

Unethical, unprofessional touch is *unskilled*, *careless* touch that holds little therapeutic intent or holds *sexual intent* or *hostility*. Mistakes are easy to make in the early stages of training, and this is not viewed as unethical unprofessional touch. Still, some students are casual about learning palpation skills and demonstrate only enough effort to pass their classes. Often, these therapists get into professional practice and lose clients because their work is superficial and does not engage the muscle and fascia. This can leave a client feeling frustrated and disappointed. On the other end of the spectrum is the therapist who works too deeply and can't sense when the client's tissue is resistant. This therapist loses clients because he causes the client unnecessary pain.

Careless touch is disrespectful and includes sloppy draping, inattention to the client's comfort level, and the failure to establish and implement a clear, effective treatment plan. Carelessness is usually accompanied by a lack of therapeutic intent. The therapist's mind is on everything but the client's muscle tissue and the session. While this type of negligence is unpardonable in a professional, it is not illegal and is not likely to exert a lasting impression on the client. The client will simply schedule his or her next massage with someone else. A therapist who is sexually motivated or is hostile toward the client can cause a client emotional, physical, and spiritual damage.

Touch with Sexual Intent

Touch with sexual intent can draw out a range of emotions from slight irritation or discomfort, to feelings of fear, to feelings of anger, to feelings of shame. When a therapist has sexual feelings toward a client, she places a client in a very difficult position, even if the therapist does not act on the feelings, or express the feelings verbally. It must be assumed that the client senses the therapist's sexual intent, even if she or he cannot clearly identify what it is that feels "off." At the very least, the client probably doesn't relax completely and remains semialert and watchful during the massage. Many professional massage therapists with the highest ethics have developed romantic or sexual feelings for a client at some point during their careers. This is not abnormal or anything the therapist should feel ashamed of. It is only unethical if the therapist allows these feelings to continue to develop, fantasizes about the client during or outside of massage sessions, speaks of the feelings to the client, or makes an advance on the client. Even if the therapist feels that she can control the sexual or romantic feelings and conduct a professional session, she should probably refer the client to another therapist. Sometimes it can be as simple as suggesting that

another therapist has a range of specialized techniques that may benefit the client's condition. Oftentimes, a therapist in this situation is advised to enlist the help of a mentor or supervisor who can offer support from a more objective standpoint.

Touch with Hostile Intent

Client behaviors can sometimes lead therapists to feel frustrated, angry, or hostile. For example, a client may fail to follow self-care practices and undo all of the good work from a previous session. Some clients share personal views about religion or politics that are in conflict with the views held by the therapist, while others activate past emotions linked to personal events that bring up old disappointments or anger. All of these events, and others, lead to real feelings of annoyance and irritation.

Remain aware of feelings clients trigger. It is usually possible to release these feelings and still provide a professional and effective session, but sometimes the feelings are so strong that you could end up directing them into the client through the massage strokes. This is unhealthy for both you and clients, and clients would be better served if you referred them to another practitioner or canceled the session (Fig. 7-1).

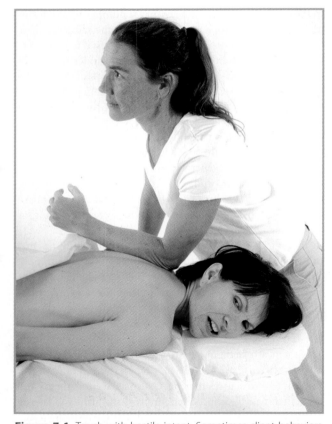

Figure 7-1 Touch with hostile intent. Sometimes client behaviors trigger feelings of frustration, irritation, or anger in therapists. If the feelings are strong and can't be dissipated before the session, it may be unhealthy for the massage to take place.

Concept Brief 7-2
Professional Versus Unprofessional Touch

- **Professional touch:** Ethical, professional touch is skilled, purposeful, and respectful, and holds healing intent. It forms the foundation of a meaningful therapeutic relationship between a massage therapist and client.
- **Unprofessional touch:** Unethical, unprofessional touch is *unskilled*, *careless* touch that holds little therapeutic intent or holds *sexual intent* or *hostility*.

Touch, Intimacy, and Sexual Arousal Responses

Massage sessions are intimate experiences in which the client and therapist share a common goal. They are moments when instantaneous transformations can take place, new insights be gained, and laughter shared. Sometimes a session shifts a client's body, and suddenly pain, experienced for years, is eliminated or greatly reduced. In some cases, massage is the first experience a client has of healthy touch that is respectful and nurturing, not sexual or violent. Sometimes clients become confused by what they feel. People usually respond to a new experience by comparing it to old experiences, whether consciously or subconsciously. It is not surprising that some clients comprehend touch as parental and nurturing and so view the therapist unconsciously as a parental figure. Other clients have only experienced caring touch as part of a romantic or sexual relationship and so comprehend touch as loving or sexual in nature.

Chapter 6 discusses sexual innuendo, sexual harassment, and sexual abuse. As a massage therapist, you must make every effort to desexualize massage and help clients understand that therapeutic touch and sexual touch are two different things. At the same time, it is also important to understand that the physical state associated with relaxation (activation of the parasympathetic nervous system) is a physiological state that is similar to sexual arousal responses, and so sexual arousal responses may occur during a massage session. A sexual arousal response does not necessarily mean that a client is interested in or seeking sexual gratification during the session. In fact, such responses may fill the client with shame and embarrassment. It is helpful to understand the reasons why these responses occur, and in some cases how to explain these responses to clients using clinical terms and a nonjudgmental tone of voice.

Understanding Sexual Arousal Responses

The sacral and lumbar nerve plexuses that carry impulses from the abdominal area, gluteal region, and lower extremities are the same nerve plexuses that carry impulses to and from the genital region. When the abdominal area, legs, or gluteal muscles are massaged, the entire region, including the genitals, may be stimulated. Men may experience a partial or full erection. Women may also become aroused, but this is less noticeable. For the purposes of this discussion, it is assumed that the client is experiencing an unwanted sexual arousal response and the client's intent is not sexual. Clients with sexual intent are discussed in the section on sexual boundaries later in this chapter.

Managing Sexual Arousal Responses

Therapists react to sexual arousal in their clients in a number of different ways. Some overreact and shame the client by terminating the session, speaking in judgmental tones, or applying overly aggressive techniques. Others respond with paralyzing fear and try to pretend the situation isn't happening. It's important to remember that this is not an abnormal response and with a few simple changes in technique the response is likely to pass and the session can continue.

1. Notice your client's face. Is it flushed and embarrassed, or is he or she deeply relaxed? Sometimes a client is so relaxed that arousal happens without full awareness. If this is the case, you might simply change techniques (see below) and not need to address the situation verbally. If the client is embarrassed, it is appropriate to be reassuring. Educate the client by saying calmly, "Sexual arousal is a normal physiological response to massage techniques and people sometimes have a sexual arousal response without having sexual intent."

2. Next, reestablish the purpose of the therapeutic relationship by saying something like, "The purpose of massage is to reduce muscle tension and pain and support relaxation. It is not my intent to cause sexual arousal. If you feel comfortable continuing with the session, I feel comfortable so long as I witness no behavior that indicates your intent is sexual."

3. Add draping material (e.g., an additional towel or blanket) to create a thicker physical barrier and to give the client a greater sense of privacy.

4. Change the massage techniques to those that are more invigorating, such as stretching, joint movements, or vigorous compression or tapotement. These types of techniques stimulate a sympathetic response from the body, and this change can help arousal pass.

5. Move away from the legs, gluteal muscles, or abdomen and focus on areas not associated with the sacral or lumbar nerve plexuses. Often it is appropriate to simply turn a male client into a prone position and work on his back, or move up to massage his neck and shoulders.

6. Some clients are unable to change inappropriate responses to massage and sexual arousal occurs repeatedly. In this case, politely but firmly end the therapeutic relationship.

7. If clients indicate by their verbal or nonverbal behavior that they want to enhance the sexual arousal state or receive sexual gratification, end the session immediately and terminate the therapeutic relationship. This issue is discussed in more depth under the section on sexual boundaries later in this chapter.

It is common to feel threatened, awkward, and embarrassed when confronted with sexual arousal responses during a session. The best way to prepare is to practice. Plan the words you would use to educate a client about sexual arousal responses and reestablish the therapeutic relationship. Practice these words out loud and even memorize them. As you practice, you may start to notice that the emotional triggers caused by these words decrease in intensity. It is also helpful to role play sexual issue scenarios with classmates. It can feel embarrassing at first, but when you get over the embarrassment you know that you are building the skills you need to manage sexual arousal responses and maintain a healthy therapeutic relationship with clients.

Concept Brief 7-3
Sexual Arousal Responses

- The abdominal area, gluteal region, lower extremities, and genitals share the same nerve plexuses. For this reason, a client may experience an unwanted sexual arousal response during the massage for these areas.
- Massage therapists can practice skills to learn how to manage sexual arousal responses in clients without causing the client embarrassment and the massage can proceed.

Topic 7-2
Psychological Factors in the Therapeutic Relationship

Topic 7-1 explored the power of touch, and you learned that touch is a profound form of nonverbal communication. Professional touch may cause a variety of feelings, thoughts, memories, and behavior in both clients and therapists. To establish and maintain a healthy therapeutic relationship, it is important that you understand something about the psychological factors that might influence a massage session. This topic explores these factors and provides some practical advice for how they might be managed effectively.

The Power Differential

In massage, a **power differential** is the authority a massage therapist is granted by a client, based on the client's perception of the massage therapist as a knowledgeable and skilled health care provider. Take a moment to contemplate your relationship with these people: parent, boss, best friend, physician, teacher, counselor, spiritual leader, or spouse. Each of these relationships involves differing levels of trust, closeness, loyalty, respect, and responsibility. It is likely that you perceive some of these people as having more authority than you in some situations. For example, if you go to your spiritual leader to discuss a personal concern, you grant him or her the power of an advanced understanding of spiritual concepts. It is easy to assume that history teachers are more knowledgeable about history than other people, or that dentists know more about teeth than other people. When clients make an appointment with a massage therapist, a power differential is at play in the relationship because the client assumes and respects the therapist's understanding of soft-tissue structures and manual techniques that reduce tension and pain. Furthermore, during the session clients share details of their personal health history and are situated at a level below the therapist, in a vulnerable reclining position, while

unclothed under a drape. The therapist by virtue of knowledge and skill in the area of massage is granted control of the situation, and so has a power advantage over the client.

Ethical massage therapists remain aware of the power differential and seek to minimize it as much as possible to ensure the mental, emotional, and physical safety of clients. When the power differential is minimized, clients are better able to:

- Take an active role in the decision-making process to determine reasonable treatment goals.
- Alert the therapist to an uncomfortable technique or voice concerns.
- Give honest feedback on the quality of strokes or the effectiveness of sessions.
- Maintain their boundaries, personal power, and responsibility for health.
- Actively practice self-care activities and other types of therapy to augment the results from massage sessions.

You can actively minimize the power differential by listening carefully to clients and responding compassionately to their needs, while representing the benefits of massage and your personal skill level realistically. You can give clients choices about the types of techniques that might be used in the session, or about which body areas will receive the most attention during the massage. If you remain attentive, you will notice when a client tenses because of discomfort and urge the client to speak up if a technique causes pain. Finally, you can encourage clients to seek out other therapists that might help them meet treatment goals and discuss self-care options that speed or enhance treatment outcomes.

If you or the client maximize the power differential, it is likely to be unhealthy for both of you. Clients who turn over all of their healing power also tend to place unreasonable amounts of responsibility for their well-being on your shoulders. Over time, they may express resentment or bitterness at their lack of progress and blame you for poor treatment. Clients without power are less able to question your decisions or voice concerns about the quality of sessions. They are less able to protect themselves in the event that you act unethically during the session. In all cases, whether the client actively gives all of the power to the therapist or not, the therapist is always responsible for what happens in a session and must constantly strive to understand and minimize the power differential.

Transference

Transference is a normal subconscious psychological phenomenon that occurs when there is a power differential. Clients try to establish the therapist in a place of importance in their personal life (Fig. 7-2). Instead of viewing the therapist as a professional who is utilized for massage, the client seeks approval, special consideration, and support from the therapist on multidimensional levels. The degree to which this occurs can vary greatly depending on the state of mind, level of self-awareness, and autonomy of the client. Some clients exhibit little or no tendency toward transference, while other cases are extreme. Often the degree to which the client is experiencing pain or coping with physical, mental, or emotional trauma can be a factor. Behaviors that signal transference include:

- Asking the therapist questions about the therapist's personal life and disclosing very personal information in early sessions.
- Regularly bringing the therapist gifts or leaving excessively large tips.

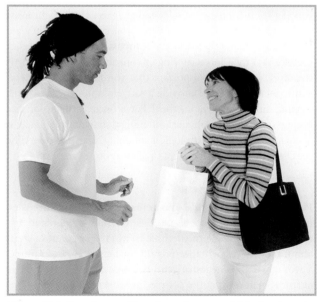

Figure 7-2 Transference: The client tries to establish the therapist in a place of importance in his or her personal life. One behavior that signals transference is the client bringing the therapist a gift or leaving an overly large tip.

- Giving the therapist too much credit for personal progress and overly praising the therapist.
- Inviting the therapist out to social engagements, asking for friendship, or seeking sexual involvement.
- Asking to set up sessions when the therapist is not on the clinic schedule, or asking for a special schedule.
- Having difficulty leaving at the end of the session and demonstrating behavior that prolongs parting, such as asking for more treatment, asking questions about the session, or starting a personal conversation.
- Seeking the therapist's support in emotional and personal issues and asking for the therapist's approval and reassurance on matters not related to massage.

In some situations, the client may experience feelings of disappointment, anger, shame, and rejection when the therapist resists allowing the therapeutic relationship to be personalized. Setting good boundaries, as discussed in the next topic, and attention to the way in which the therapeutic relationship is established are probably the best way to decrease situations of transference.

Counter-Transference

Counter-transference is the opposite of transference. In this case, the therapist tries to personalize the therapeutic relationship. Sometimes this happens if therapists perceive the client as like themselves, like someone from the past, or like another client. Subconsciously, the therapist tries to work out unresolved needs or feelings through the client. For example, therapists who perceive the client as being like themselves may believe that the client needs work on the low back, not realizing that low back issues are their own, and not the client's. The same is true if therapists perceive the client as like another client. They may apply the other client's treatment strategy to the new client and fail to understand the new client's true needs. The client may remind a therapist of a person from the past, prompting a range of emotions from strong attraction to repulsion based on the past relationship. In any case, the therapist's perception of the client is distorted, and the therapist is unable to assess the client's therapeutic needs accurately or make good decisions in treatment planning. A client's transference can set off a therapist's counter-transference leading to a confusing mix of inappropriate and unresolved needs and emotions fused into a progression of unhealthy sessions that are unlikely to be therapeutically valuable. Behaviors that signal counter-transference include:

- Any strong feelings or emotions toward the client that are excessively positive or negative.
- Physical symptoms that result from anticipation of the session or directly after the session such as elation, anxiety, nausea, exhaustion, fear, depression, or excitement.
- Feelings of anger, depression, or disappointment if the client cancels the session or fails to show up for the session.

- Seeking to prolong the session by offering extra treatment time, or starting a personal conversation at the end of the session.
- Feelings of extreme confidence ("I'm the only therapist who can help this client") or extreme insecurity ("I'm not good enough to work with this client") in relationship to an individual client.
- Encouraging the client to share personal information and sharing personal information with the client. Seeking to become involved in the client's personal life. Inviting the client to social engagements, seeking friendship, or a sexual relationship with the client.
- Taking full responsibility for the client's progress and feeling guilty or angry when the client doesn't improve or seems to receive little benefit from massage.
- Empathizing so deeply with the client that the therapist begins to manifest physical and emotional symptoms that are similar to the client's symptoms.
- Thinking obsessively about the client between sessions and putting extra effort into personal appearance on the days when the client is coming for a session.
- Feeling defensive and angry when the client asks for a change in the application of strokes or demonstrates discomfort with a technique.

Self-awareness and recognition are the first step to diffusing counter-transference. You should regularly question and investigate your feelings toward clients. While attention to boundaries can help, if you regularly find yourself feeling strong emotions toward clients, you are likely to benefit from the supervision of a mentor or even professional counseling. There is no shame in experiencing counter-transference sometimes. Problems arise when you fail to take positive actions to resolve the situation and thereby place clients at risk for emotional or physical harm.

Psychological Defenses

Psychological defense mechanisms are mental processes that enable the mind to deal with conflicts it can't resolve, and every person learns some type of psychological defense from normal experiences of life. Anxiety such as the concern that one might lose control of urges, needs, or desires resulting in shame or punishment for inappropriate behavior, or the concern that one will lose personal self-esteem and power, or the concern that one is threatened may be experienced either consciously or unconsciously. Psychological defense mechanisms are often supported by physical tension patterns that help suppress disturbing emotions, ideas, desires, and memories.

In some cases, defense mechanisms are necessary for survival, or allow a person to adapt and function in the world after an extreme trauma. Often they create imbalances that prevent people from dealing with conflicts so that they might be understood and resolved. A few primary defense

mechanisms are described here in terms of psychological dynamics that might impact the massages you give.

Suppression

Suppression is the conscious pushing down of anxiety-producing ideas, urges, desires, feelings, or memories. The item that causes anxiety is recognized on a conscious level but then actively ignored, squashed, or avoided. For example, a client reared by parents who discouraged the display of emotion might feel sadness during a particular massage technique, but view the display of emotion as unacceptable and embarrassing. The client can recognize the feeling but tenses muscles and actively dismisses the feeling in order to avoid expressing or showing the sadness through tears or sobbing.

Denial

Denial is the outright refusal to acknowledge something that has occurred or is occurring. Suppression might be used to support denial. Denial protects the mind from anxiety-producing conflicts it can't cope with. For example, alcoholics often deny that they have a problem with alcohol and insist that the situation is under control. Denial might be used to avoid the unpleasant reality that a particular lifestyle choice impedes health (e.g., smoking, lack of physical exercise, poor eating habits) or places a person at risk (e.g., participation in unprotected sex, abuse of drugs, etc.). In some cases, people have learned from caretakers that certain feelings are disgraceful. If you have been taught that showing fear or being afraid is shameful you may deny that you feel fear even when it is sensible to be fearful. As a result, you might participate in dangerous behaviors as part of your unconscious denial of fear.

In massage sessions, clients may express denial in many subtle ways. They might deny that a technique is painful, even though you can see them tense muscles and grimace. They might insist that "everything is fine," even when you can see that they are struggling to maintain emotional composure. They might reject the idea that their job is causing or contributing to their repetitive stress injury. It is important that you maintain the therapeutic relationship and provide a safe environment for clients without directly challenging them. Focus on areas of tension and keep in mind that the physical softening the client experiences is likely to facilitate a psychological softening, and that over time the client may be able to accept or allow more awareness.

Projection

Projection is the unconscious transfer of feelings, impulses, or thoughts to someone else. Projection allows people to disown or place outside of themselves what they cannot accept about themselves, whether positive or negative. For example, a woman with a negative attitude, unaware of her negative attitude, believes that the people she works with are negative. In massage sessions, clients project their unrealistic expectations (e.g., massage will change everything about my life), fears (e.g., this will just be one more therapy that doesn't work), unwanted weaknesses (e.g., I don't want to cry), and abandoned strengths (e.g., I can't heal) onto the treatment or onto the massage therapist. The massage therapist may also be projecting onto the client. This is normal but may have negative effects on the session if the therapist is unaware of it and feeds the client's projections.

One way to minimize projection is to center the sessions in reality. Ask the client questions like, "What are the results you expect from the next six sessions?" "Was last week's session like what you expected?" "How was last week's session different from what you expected?" You can also be attentive to the verbal and nonverbal signals you send clients during a session. You might make a comment like, "Well, here we go again working on this knot in your neck" and send the client the message that you have grown tired of the work and are unhappy with progress. Instead, you want to send the message that you accept the client's progress and are willing to spend as long as necessary for the condition to resolve.

People also project their moment-by-moment needs and feelings and thus decrease their level of self-awareness about their own bodies. One of the positive things that can come from regular massage is greater attention to how the body feels. When you are attentive to projection and can reflect a projection back to clients, you help them recognize their feelings and needs as welcome and acceptable. For example, clients might project their own foot pain onto you and say, "Standing on your feet all day must make your feet really tired." You reflect the possible projection by saying, "Are your feet really tired today? Do you want me to spend extra time working on your feet during the session?" In all cases of projection, you must be careful of two things. First, your response to the client must

BOX 7-1 Common Projections

- The projector believes that another person is experiencing what the projector is actually experiencing (e.g., "You look like you don't feel well" when it is the projector who doesn't feel well).
- The projector believes that the other person has characteristics that are actually characteristic of the projector (e.g., "I really admire your daredevil spirit" when the projector believes he or she doesn't have the right to be a daredevil).
- The projector believes that another person feels something the projector is afraid the other will feel (e.g., "He thinks I'm stupid" even though they have never spoken to each other).
- The projector believes that another person is "making" him or her feel emotion whether it is positive or negative (e.g., "You are making me anxious" or "You make me feel beautiful").
- The projector believes that another person feels something that the projector wants the other person to feel (e.g., "She loves me!" even though they have only been on one date).

honor the client's feelings and needs. If you said, "My feet are fine, don't project your foot issues onto me," the opportunity for self-acceptance has been eliminated. Second, you must be careful not to view all comments made by the client as projection. For example, the client says, "When you ask me to turn over it sounds a bit like you are ordering me around and then I feel less relaxed. Could you ask me more softly?" If you respond by saying, "Try not to project your issues with authority onto me," you are likely reading too much into the statement. Box 7-1 provides some examples of projections that might occur during a massage session to help you raise your awareness.

Deflection

The term *deflection* refers to ignoring or turning away from stimuli that trigger emotions in order to prevent recognition or full awareness of the material associated with the emotion. For example, clients might talk continually during a massage session to avoid paying too much attention to their feelings brought about by massage (Fig. 7-3). The client may unconsciously distract you away from a body area that is emotionally charged by

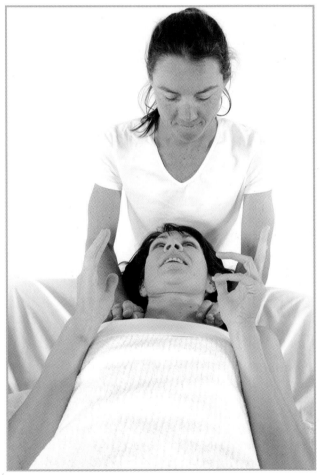

Figure 7-3 Deflection: The client in this image is talking continuously while the therapist is trying to provide massage. This might be a form of deflection where the client is trying to distract herself from the feelings triggered by massage in a particular body area.

complaining of pain or tension in another area. If an emotionally charged area is massaged, the client might try to focus on other body areas and report the sensations felt in that area to you (e.g., "When you massage my feet I feel a buzzing in my hands"). It is useful to gently ground the client in an awareness of the area where massage is occurring. You might say something as simple as, "The buzzing in your hands is interesting, but while I massage your feet, see if you can focus your awareness in this area and use your breath to release tension here."

Resistance

The term *resistance* was originally used by Sigmund Freud to refer to the blocking of memories from consciousness by patients, thereby slowing the therapeutic process. In massage, it more directly relates to the client's feeling that change, even change perceived as desirable, is threatening, resulting in an unconscious opposition to the therapeutic process. For example, Sue has been working with you to reduce tension in her shoulders and jaw. As the tension softens with progressive sessions, Sue has started to remember incidents from her childhood when she felt overwhelmed and controlled by her mother. With each session, Sue's overall discomfort and anxiety increase, and now she has fears of what might surface next. While Sue verbally affirms that she is committed to weekly massage sessions, she misses one appointment, is late for the second, cancels a third, and fails to use the warm packs on her shoulder for self-care as she agreed. You may not even be aware that Sue is starting to recall repressed memories and may think that Sue is just irresponsible.

Resistance might also surface as recurring tension. You might work with a client to free tension in a particular area, only to find that the tension is back or even increased at the next session. The client may be unconsciously reinforcing the tension pattern as a way to keep repressed items from surfacing.

Dealing with resistance is challenging, as you must be careful not to step outside your scope of practice by confronting the client. Often, acknowledging and honoring the resistance can be helpful, and you can affirm for clients that, "Tension often has a positive purpose in helping people cope with stress and anxiety. Your body may not yet be ready to release this tension. We will just keep working with this tension until your body is ready to let it go."

Armoring

Armoring is the use of physical tension to support psychological defenses such as suppression and denial. You may remember Wilhelm Reich, described in Chapter 1 as the founder of psychotherapeutic body therapies, often called bodymind therapy or somatic therapy. Reich introduced the idea of armoring in his classic text *Character Analysis* (1933).[10] Reich believed that in an effort to protect ourselves from the physical and emotional stress we disconnect from tender, venerable feelings. He called this phenomenon "body armoring," defined as when the body tightens, the muscle groups in an effort to control or minimize feelings, thereby creating physical, emotional, and mental tension patterns.

People learn how to express emotion "properly" based on the society in which they live. For example, males are not supposed to show emotions like sorrow by crying, but are allowed to show a certain amount of anger. Sorrow and crying by females, on the other hand, is generally accepted, but anger is frowned upon. In our society, sayings like "Stop crying or I'll give you something to cry about," "Keep a stiff upper lip," "You should be ashamed of yourself," and "Hold your temper" teach people to suppress emotion when necessary to avoid punishment or embarrassment.[11]

The suppression of emotion shows up in physical tension because muscular contractions can be used to block the display of emotion or suppress emotion so that it can be ignored.[12] People can develop patterns of muscular tension in relationship to repeated emotional triggers.[13] If one family member is violent and threatening toward another family member, the threatened family member may wish to strike out but suppress the impulse to strike because of fear. A pattern of physical tension in the chest and arm muscles might result from the repeated need to stifle the desire to hit. Over time, this pattern is delegated to the subconscious mind and becomes habitual. Perhaps the violent family member moves away and is no longer a threat. Tension in the chest and arm muscles is likely to remain as a chronic and unconscious expression of the repressed emotions for years or even for life.[14]

Sometimes during the health intake, during the massage, or at the end of a session, the client will share an awareness of their body or a feeling that arose during the session, and their eyes will mist over. If they don't "armor," they may welcome the tender feelings and uses their increased awareness to learn something new about themselves and their body. In the event that they do "armor," they may feel deeply uncomfortable with their tender feelings, experience them as threatening and shameful, and suppress or deny their existence. Tense muscles help numb these feelings and keep them from escaping. In Topic 7-4, you learn about the bodymind split and how it relates to armoring. Topic 7-5 explains that massage reduces

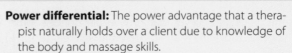

Concept Brief 7-4
Psychological Factors in the Therapeutic Relationship

Power differential: The power advantage that a therapist naturally holds over a client due to knowledge of the body and massage skills.

Transference: When a client personalizes the therapeutic relationship.

Counter-transference: When a therapist personalizes the therapeutic relationship.

Psychological defenses: Mental processes that enable the mind to deal with conflicts it can't resolve.

Armoring: The use of physical tension to support psychological defenses. Massage reduces physical tension and affects armoring. This sometimes leads to emotional release.

the muscular tension used to suppress emotion and so can lead to emotional release.

The Therapist Role During Massage

You are not expected to recognize all of the psychological defense mechanisms of clients, but by understanding the client defenses you can better recognize the dynamics at play in a massage session. The most important thing you can do for clients is provide a safe and nonjudgmental environment and encourage clients to develop their awareness of body sensations and be open to what they feel. If clients share with you that they are experiencing the surfacing of repressed items, if an emotional release occurs (discussed in an upcoming section) during a session, or if they express the desire to explore surfacing thoughts, memories, and feelings, refer them to a mental health care professional who has the training necessary for processing their experience appropriately.

Topic **7-3**
Boundaries and the Therapeutic Relationship

Boundaries are conscious and subconscious imaginary lines that mark the limits of an individual's personal space or territory. Boundaries create a separation or border between a person and other people, and between a person and the environment. People who are not aware of boundaries can cross into another person's space, causing discomfort or even harm. Part of establishing a healthy therapeutic relationship involves learning how to assert and maintain your own boundaries while respecting the boundaries of clients. This topic explores personal space, boundary types, boundary violations, boundary issues related to dual relationships, and external guidance from supervisors or mentors.

Personal Space

Personal space has been named and defined in various ways by different authors and psychologists. In this textbook, "personal space" is understood as the physical, emotional, mental, and spiritual space people "hold" around themselves. It also refers to a person's "territory" such as possessions like clothes, toiletries, car, home, furniture, books, and other personal items. Within the boundaries of personal space, an individual is free to express the rights of identity and pursue personal values. While people always maintain some personal space, in common areas a person must consider the boundaries of others and adapt to the needs of the common good.

People's family, environment, culture, relationships, and early experiences may affect their ability to set and uphold appropriate boundaries around their personal space. For example, if a person grows up in a family that does not value privacy, it is likely that this person will have more difficulty respecting the privacy of others, and asserting that others respect his or her own privacy. As a therapist, this person might have difficulty recognizing a client's need for privacy and so drape with little attention to modesty during the session.

Personal space is also defined by the things we share with other people and the things we allow other people to share with us. We tell our friends and loved ones intimate details of our lives, things we wouldn't tell a massage client. Sometimes one person encroaches on another's personal space. A therapist might sit too close to a client during the health intake interview. The client, who feels crowded, keeps inching backward, only to find that the therapist, who is not being attentive to the client's physical boundary, keeps inching forward (Fig. 7-4).

Types of Boundaries

Your boundaries are constantly in fluctuation based on the circumstances in which you find yourself. You have to decide how much to share, when to share, when not to share, when to protect yourself, and when it is safe to be vulnerable. In *The Ethics of Touch*, authors Cherie Sohnen-Moe and Ben Benjamin explain the fluctuations in boundaries by suggesting that therapists imagine a semipermeable bubble enclosing their personal space. Sometimes the bubble allows more information and energy to move in and out, and sometimes it blocks the movement of information and energy in and out.

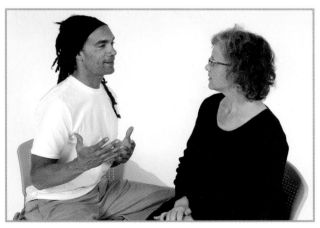

Figure 7-4 Boundaries: This therapist is not being attentive to the client's physical boundary.

Boundary types could then be described as permeable, semi-permeable, or impermeable.

Permeable Boundaries

A permeable boundary allows information, feelings, thoughts, beliefs, and energy to flow freely in and out. This type of boundary is appropriate if you are in a conversation with a close friend. It would not be suitable when conversing with a client. A therapeutic relationship is client focused, and massage sessions are delivered for the good of the client. To share very personal information with a client takes the focus off the client and places it on you. This may encourage client transference or cause irritation when the session doesn't meet the client's needs.

Semipermeable Boundaries

A semipermeable boundary is appropriate in a therapeutic relationship because it allows you to be sensitive to the needs and wants of the client, without placing yourself at risk. With a semipermeable boundary, you can work closely with a client, like and respect the client, and still say no politely when the client asks for a special session on Saturday; your day off. This type of boundary provides you with the necessary objectivity to pay attention to ethical issues while feeling empathy for a client's condition. It provides some distance so that you can question your own behavior if you begin to get too close, or too personally involved with the client. It allows you time to take a step back and reestablish the parameters of a healthy therapeutic relationship.

Impermeable Boundary

An impermeable boundary allows little information or energy to pass through and is only appropriate in limited situations, such as when a client makes an overt sexual advance. An impermeable boundary provides the distance needed to calmly state the policies of the clinic and terminate the massage session. Sometimes people's upbringing or life experiences teach them to develop a boundary that is permeable too often or in the wrong circumstances. Alternatively, people who are intolerant of other people's views, or impose their views regularly on others, are probably stuck behind a boundary that is too impermeable and doesn't allow for normal communication and interaction. An example is a therapist who refuses to work with clients who are smokers or who have a different sexual orientation. In this case, the therapist's boundary is so thick that the therapist has difficulty recognizing the boundaries of others and so fails to respect their rights, and as a result breaks an important ethical standard.

Boundary Forms

Each type of boundary (permeable, semipermeable, or impermeable) can take a different form depending on the area it relates to. Boundary forms can be categorized as physical, emotional, mental, spiritual, and sexual.

Physical Boundaries

Physical boundaries refer to the amount of space we need around us to feel comfortable as described previously. Physical boundaries can be violated if one person moves into the physical space of another with whom healthy intimacy has not been established. It should be noted that intimacy does not mean sexual interaction. It means a shared feeling of understanding, empathy, and closeness. For example, if you greet a new client with a hug, the client is likely to feel that you crossed a physical boundary and may remain alert and uncomfortable throughout the entire massage session as a result (Fig. 7-5).

Emotional Boundaries

Emotional boundaries refer to the amount of emotion we feel safe sharing, and the kinds of emotions we share with others. If David breaks up with his girlfriend, he may feel safe crying with his good friend Rob, and Rob is likely to feel safe if he cries. He is unlikely to feel safe crying with his boss or his client, and they are unlikely to feel safe if he cries. In a work environment, he would seek to contain his emotions by reinforcing his emotional boundary.

Emotional, mental, and spiritual stress, as well as physical pain, can make it difficult for people to maintain their normal emotional boundaries. These situations can wear boundaries down so that emotions seep out unexpectedly despite a person's attempts to contain them. In David's case, the most ethical decision he can make may be to cancel his sessions for the day and take care of himself. It is unethical to provide massage if a pressing personal issue will prevent you from remaining client focused and providing excellent service.

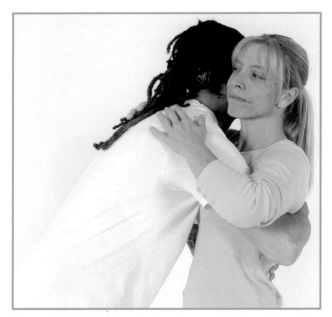

Figure 7-5 Physical boundaries: If you greet a new client with a hug, she may feel uncomfortable with the level of intimacy that you express. You have crossed her physical boundary.

Clients who are dealing with acute or chronic conditions may demonstrate poor emotional boundaries in a massage session. Clients tend to express more emotion or be more reactive because their internal resources are stretched thin. Sometimes this leads to issues of transference or counter-transference, as discussed previously. Sometimes it is appropriate to listen to the client and allow the client to "get it out." Still, you must remain aware of your emotional boundary so that you can remain objective and supportive without becoming emotional yourself, and without crossing out of your scope of practice. You must also think of the long-term effects on the therapeutic relationship. Clients may feel so embarrassed by their display of emotion that they never come back. Alternately, they may begin to look at the massage session as a chance to let their emotions run wild. In both cases, the therapeutic relationship has been compromised.

Mental Boundaries

Mental boundaries refer to the beliefs, values, and ideas we feel safe sharing with other people. People define themselves by what they believe and think. When ideas or beliefs are mocked, or rejected, a person's sense of confidence may be dampened. For example, it is unwise to discuss religious views with clients. This places both of you in a situation where you need to defend your beliefs. It's unlikely that heightened defenses lead to the best therapeutic outcome. Sometimes clients will make political or religious comments that are in opposition to your beliefs. Your mental boundary must be strong enough that you can avoid being drawn into an unhealthy or unproductive discussion. Instead, calmly direct clients back to the work of the session, perhaps by asking them to take a deep breath and let it out slowly as they focus on the muscles that are being massaged.

Spiritual Boundaries

Spiritual boundaries could also be called energetic boundaries. This type of boundary is made up of all of people's subconscious beliefs, subconscious needs, the energy the radiate out into the world, and the energy they seek to absorb from the world. This type of boundary is sometimes difficult to understand on an intellectual level, but you may be able to feel it. Some clients require a greater degree of energy output from you and may leave you feeling drained and moody. Is it possible that the client's spiritual energy is reaching out to tap into your energy? On a subconscious, energetic level, can a needy client suck energy from a therapist? Many therapists believe that some clients, referred to in massage slang as "energy vampires," can and do. In this case, seek to strengthen your spiritual, energetic boundary before each session with grounding and centering exercises (described in Chapter 11).

Sexual Boundaries

Sexual boundaries involve how and with whom we express our sexuality. Holding appropriate sexual boundaries with clients is the cornerstone of an ethical therapeutic relationship. Chapter 6 discusses the ethics and standards around sexuality and presents ethical guidelines to desexualize massage. In the section on touch, intimacy, and sexual arousal earlier in this chapter, you learned that a sexual arousal response does not necessarily mean that a client is seeking sexual gratification. Still, the steps to reestablish the therapeutic relationship described in that section were a form of strengthening sexual boundaries. For purposes of this section now, it is assumed that the client is seeking sexual gratification or seeks to enhance a sexual arousal response for the purposes of discussion.

Clients seek out massage for a variety of reasons. Some reasons are healthy ("I want to reduce my neck tension") and some are unhealthy and misguided ("I have no love in my life and if I pay for massage the therapist is obligated to love me"). There are clients whose lives are so destabilized or distorted by early experiences that they seek massage as a way to dominate or control another person, in this case the therapist. These people may have developed a skill for luring people into feeling that a special bound has developed, or that the therapist is indispensable to the client's health and wellness. Feeling important to other people is a huge ego boost, and no one is completely immune to it. When a therapist is maneuvered into feeling somehow responsible for the client, the tables turn and the client crosses the therapist's boundaries in a multitude of different ways. In some cases, sexual gratification is the aim, and part of the game for the unhealthy client is the manipulation of the therapist to act against his or her ethics. Both the client and the therapist are being damaged by this situation. The client persists and is gratified by using manipulation to find the twisted form of love and acceptance he or she is likely seeking, while the therapist faces the emotional, mental, and spiritual crisis of acting against his or her ethics and professional standards, and may lose massage credentials as a result.

Sexual boundaries are established by practicing the right degree of familiarity with clients (discussed below) by wearing clothing that does not draw attention to your body, and by paying careful attention to all other boundaries and issues. Watch for small transgressions. A client who insists on calling you "sweetheart" should be corrected politely but immediately. You might say, "My name is Carmon. It makes me uncomfortable when clients call me by nicknames. Please call me Carmon."

A client who states, "I don't know what I would do without you, you are the only good thing in my life, you are the only person I can relate to and talk to, I'm heartbroken when I'm not with you and I want to see you more often" is either giving you too much power or setting you up to be further manipulated later on. You must clarify the parameters of the therapeutic relationship politely but firmly. You might say, "Jackie, I'm a massage therapist and I can help you release muscle tension and reduce stress. It sounds like you need more support than I can offer you through massage. I am going to refer you to a really skilled counselor. He can help you develop the resources you need to feel good again."

Clients may flirt or seek to discuss a sexual issue with you (e.g., sharing with you that a spouse is not interested in sex, or sharing that the client hasn't had sex in a long time). Again, you can establish a boundary and still remain polite. You might say, "The purpose of the massage session is to provide relief from muscular tension. I'm not a counselor, and massage sessions are not designed to include counseling, so it is inappropriate for me to discuss personal issues with you. I can refer you to a skilled counselor at the end of the session."

Some clients claim, "I'm comfortable with my body, there is no need for a drape" or repeatedly expose draped areas of their bodies. They may attempt to mask a need to expose themselves as a healthy level of comfort with nudity. You must stop these small transgressions immediately to prevent an escalation of boundary violations. You might say, "Massage is a health care profession, and as such it is important that proper draping be used to protect both your modesty and mine." If you find that the client continues to undrape, you must set an even clearer boundary by saying, "I have explained that proper draping protects your modesty and mine. Our draping policy is that only the area that is being massage is exposed. The breasts, genitals, and anus are never exposed. This was explained to you during the informed consent process. If you expose any area of your body again I will terminate this session."

In some instances, a sexual arousal response turns into a desire for sexual gratification. Clients may try to hide this and touch themselves when you're not looking. They may verbalize (e.g., moaning) and try to pass it off as a general enjoyment of the massage. Watch for breathing changes, sexual movements, and muscular contractions. In some instances (though this rarely happens), the client might ask you to participate and indicate that there is a big tip involved. If you were to participate, you could be charged and convicted of prostitution. If the client demonstrates verbally or nonverbally a desire to enhance a sexual arousal response or seek sexual gratification, you should terminate the session and leave the treatment room.

A client might also hide a sexual arousal response but then masturbate on the massage table at the end of the session after you have left. You discover this only when you return to the treatment room to change the linens for the next client. Body fluids should be cleaned up according to the Universal Precautions procedures outlined in Chapter 3. Call the client or write a letter terminating the therapeutic relationship. Client sexual misconduct can take many forms, but you will notice that in most of the examples described here your response is the same:

1. Clarify the therapeutic relationship by defining the scope of practice for massage. In some cases, it is important to refer back to the informed consent process and emphasize the policies of the massage business (discussed in Chapter 6).
2. Give clients one warning that allows them to stop the inappropriate behavior.
3. Terminate the session if the client does not stop any behavior that jeopardizes the therapeutic relationship.

4. If clients ask outright for sexual gratification or if their behavior seems overtly threatening, terminate the session immediately and leave the room. Contact emergency services if you feel in danger.

The different types of boundaries described previously are interrelated and together create a therapist's professional boundary. Sometimes a therapist is very good at maintaining one type of boundary but has difficulty establishing another type. Doug has no problem setting emotional boundaries but is easy to draw into a political discussion. Erin forgets to maintain good physical boundaries and often places an arm around her clients as she walks them to the treatment room. She has no idea that a number of clients changed to another massage clinic because this physical familiarity made them uncomfortable.

From this discussion you might well be thinking, "Oh no, is every client who comes for massage going to misbehave and try to violate my boundaries? Will I spend all of my time trying to prevent clients from acting sexually in the treatment room? Perhaps massage is not for me!" In fact, clients don't misbehave very often, especially if they are introduced to the framework of sessions through a comprehensive informed consent process. Most clients seek massage for therapeutic reasons, and good screening processes (discussed in Chapter 3, Topic 3-4) can weed out those who are seeking sexual gratification. The point is that you must be aware and set boundaries so that small transgressions don't persist and become major problems.

Boundary Violations

A boundary violation occurs when one person disregards another's boundary and interferes with the other's personal space. You could cause harm to a client through simple carelessness. For example, you might say something that you view as harmless such as, "Your muscle is less dense than it used to be. It's probably because you don't work out as much." This implies a subtle judgment of the client's body and physical shape, and so may cause the client to feel a sense of shame. A therapist causes more harm through unethical boundary crossings that include asking a client on a date, or pressuring clients to take off underclothing when they want to leave it on. Clients can also cross your boundaries. The behaviors described in the section on transference explain some of the ways that clients seek to breach a therapist's boundaries. In other boundary violations, clients may not show up for an appointment without calling and alerting you first. When you ask that they pay for the missed session, they might refuse. This shows a lack of respect for your time and professional expertise.

Awareness of Client Boundaries

First, take a moment to imagine the kinds of boundary modifications a client must make to come for a first session. This may compare to the discomfort you likely felt the first time you had to disrobe in the classroom and allow another student to apply massage techniques. Clients enter a new environment, which may feel very different than the environments they usually inhabit. Business people entering a clinic filled with new age paraphernalia may feel they have landed on a new planet. Next, they meet a new person who asks them to disclose details of their health history including their stress level, their medications, their physical condition, and their goals for the massage session. These are things they probably don't often discuss with friends, let alone a stranger. Now they are taken to a private room and told to undress and lie down under a flimsy drape so that a stranger can apply techniques that are sometimes pleasurable, but sometimes slightly uncomfortable. It's amazing that clients have the courage to give massage a try!

It is important to remain aware of the client's boundaries at all times and constantly adjust your behaviors based on verbal and nonverbal input received from the client. Certain practices can help clients feel comfortable and establish their own boundaries clearly.

- **Changing levels of interaction:** During the health intake, your communication style should be friendly but matter of fact. Avoid too much familiarity with clients in this environment. Examples include touching the client unnecessarily or bringing up an emotional release that occurred in the last session. Instead, gather information efficiently and avoid probing for personal information that is not directly relevant to ruling out contraindications or making a treatment plan. Once the massage starts, the interaction level deepens naturally as the work of the session begins. When the massage ends and the client emerges to pay for the session or book another session, return to a friendly but matter-of-fact style of communication. Paying attention to the level of interactions helps clients maintain boundaries that feel comfortable.
- **Establish client boundaries:** Ask the clients questions during the intake interview and session that help clients establish their own boundaries. Questions like, "Are there any areas of your body that you would prefer I didn't massage?" or "Are there any types of massage techniques that you would prefer I didn't use?" or "Did you find that technique uncomfortable? Would you prefer I didn't use it again?" remind clients that they always retain control of their bodies. It is also important to allow clients to undress to their level of comfort. If the client remains fully clothed, work through the client's clothing.
- **Give clients a voice:** Give the clients choices and encourage them to speak up if a technique is not working or if they feel uncomfortable (Fig. 7-6). Questions like, "What type of music do you enjoy?" "Which of these massage lubricants would work best for you?" "How is the temperature? Are you too cool?" "Does this technique feel effective? Should I reduce the pressure or would you prefer more pressure?" help clients to voice concerns and give feedback on the quality of the session.

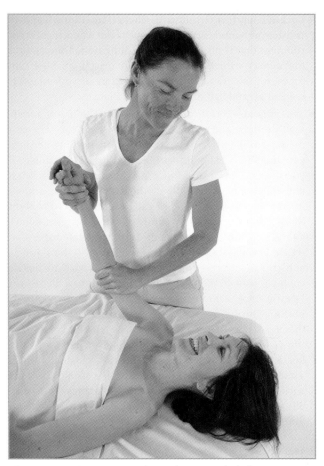

Figure 7-6 When you give clients choices and ask them questions like, "Does this technique feel effective?" you give them a voice that helps them establish their boundaries during the session.

- **Alert clients to their rights:** Clients have the right to terminate the session at any time and should be reminded of this during the informed consent process. Ask for honest feedback at the end of the session to empower your clients. It can be as simple as, "What types of techniques would you like to experience during the next session?" "Were you comfortable with the pressure and flow of the massage?" "What changes can I make in the next session to better meet your needs?" If a client expresses dissatisfaction or asks for a technique that is out of your skill set or scope of practice, willingly refer the client to another therapist.

Establish the Boundaries of the Therapeutic Relationship

Professional boundaries form the foundation of the therapeutic relationship and are communicated to clients during the initial intake interview as part of the informed consent procedure. Some boundaries are communicated through subtle signals that establish the professionalism of the business on a nonverbal level.

- **Location and environment:** Clients are more likely to respect the boundaries of a therapist who works in an environment that is professional. Avoid the use of decorations that convey seductiveness or that are overtly spiritual. Opt for clean, safe, functionality. Post a copy of your massage credentials and liability insurance in plain view.

- **Therapist dress code and deportment:** The use of a massage uniform and name tag sends perhaps the strongest message to clients. It creates subconscious distance between you and the client and identifies you as a professional. If you do not wear a uniform, your dress should be modest and functional. Avoid any clothing that projects sexuality, reveals too much skin, or calls attention to your body. Refrain from using swear words or slang during sessions, and practice instead the use of calm, moderate tones that soothe and relax. Clients should receive only ethical touch, and you must prevent situations where sexual or hostile energy is transferred to the client through massage strokes (see the next section for details). Also watch your body position during the application of techniques. Sometimes therapists start to lean on the massage table and place portions of their bodies on clients without being aware of it. For example, a female therapist might accidentally touch a client with her breasts as she performs a stroke down the back. A male therapist might accidentally lean his genitals against the side of a client while delivering a stroke. If unintentional contact takes place, apologize and pay closer attention to your body position in the future.

- **The informed consent process:** During the initial intake interview, clients are informed of the policies and practices of the massage business. They are also alerted to client and therapist behaviors that are considered unethical and that may lead to actions such as termination of the massage session. Clear informed consent materials are important because they define the role of the therapist, the limits of the therapist's role, and the role of the client. When clients sign an informed consent form, they agree to abide by the policies of the massage business, and so the form becomes a logical and apparent boundary.

- **Scheduling:** Time defines a massage session, and an efficient schedule demonstrates respect for both the client and therapist. Clients arrive at a specific time for a session that lasts a specific amount of time and ends at a specific time. Boundaries are violated when clients fail to show up on time but still expect the full time allotted to their session, or when they request that you work past the time when the session should end.

- **Payment of a fee:** The payment of a fee by the client creates a professional boundary. It demonstrates that the relationship is business and service oriented and not social. Boundaries are violated when you give a certain client a special fee, or when a client fails to pay a fee for the massage.

- **Self-disclosure:** In a therapeutic relationship, it is appropriate to share with clients the amount of training hours you've had, continuing education training that has led to the practice of advanced massage techniques, and your years in practice. It is not appropriate to share personal information such as the particulars of a divorce, your discontent with the massage business manager, or a crush you have on an acquaintance. In some cases, it is appropriate to share some personal information, if it will benefit the therapeutic process. For example, a client who is frustrated with the slowness of the healing process after a car accident may benefit from your experience of healing from a car accident. In this case, you express empathy and demonstrate that healing can occur over time.

Concept Brief 7-5
Boundaries

Defined: An imaginary border that marks the limits of an individual's personal space.

Personal space: The physical, emotional, mental, and spiritual space a person holds around self, including possessions and personal items.

Fluctuations: Normal changes in a person's boundaries to allow adaptation to a variety of different situations and people.

Types: Permeable, semipermeable, impermeable.

Forms: Physical, emotional, mental, spiritual, sexual

Violations: When one person disregards another's boundary and interferes with the other's personal space

---

Boundaries and Dual Relationships

A **dual relationship** is defined as a situation in which more than one relationship with a client is present. In cases of dual relationships, the therapeutic relationship is compromised by a secondary relationship that stretches beyond the massage session. Anytime you provide massage to a friend, family member, business associate, love interest, teacher, or employer, a dual relationship exists. If you form, or allow to form, a friendship, romantic connection, business association, or other relationship with an established client, you have created a dual relationship. From the previous discussion, we know that an ethical therapeutic relationship should be client centered and you should focus entirely on the needs of the client. Clients must be able to focus on their own healing process during the session and not be distracted by your needs. When a dual relationship is present, it is much more difficult to keep the session client centered, and conflicts of interest, boundary violations, the potential for poor treatment planning, and a range of emotions from disappointment, to sadness, to rage may occur for both you and the client.

Dual Relationships with Friends, Family, and Other Professionals

There is some debate as to whether dual relationships are permissible in some situations or should be completely avoided. Many massage therapists say that dual relationships of any type are never permissible. In this mindset, you would never provide a massage to a friend, family member, work colleague, or social acquaintance, ever. Other professionals say that dual relationships are permissible under certain circumstances but need careful attention. For instance, a friend or family member might seek massage. You might set appropriate boundaries and clearly differentiate between the therapeutic relationship and the friendship or family relationship, and the dual relationship might work. The question becomes: Are you able to separate the relationships consistently, or will the boundaries of the relationships get blurred leading to possible conflicts and negative consequences? In all cases, you must take full responsibility for understanding the risks, communicating the risks to the friend-client, and maintaining the parameters of the different relationships. For example, you might have just broken up with your girlfriend or boyfriend the night before a massage session with a friend. In a normal therapeutic relationship, you would never dream of sharing your emotions about the split. But if you are not careful, the boundaries between a friend and client may be blurred and you may tell your friend-client all about the breakup during the massage. Clearly, this massage is not client centered, and the therapeutic relationship and your ethics are compromised.

You are likely to find it more difficult to set good boundaries with friends and family members. What will you do if your friend fails to show up for a session? Will you charge a friend the full price of the session as you do with other no-show clients? Your friend may feel dismay after receiving the bill because you are friends—aren't you? What happens when you are at a family gathering and Aunt Sue, who is also a regular massage client, begs to have her shoulders massaged and wants to talk about the aches and pains she is feeling since the last session. Aunt Sue now expects family time to also be her client time. It is easy to see that the potential for conflict and boundary violations is immense.

In some cases, social acquaintances become clients. You may belong to a nonmassage-related group or club. When club members find out that you are a massage therapist, they may seek massage. Allowing a stranger to provide massage can feel very threatening for many people. Because an acquaintance feels safer, they may want to become your clients. Again, you must navigate the parameters of the two relationships carefully, but in this situation there is less risk of difficulty than with friends and family members. While you should never bring up massage sessions with the client at club meetings (which is a breach of confidentially), or bring up club business during massage sessions, the lower level of intimacy experienced with an acquaintance makes setting and maintaining boundaries easier.

It sometimes happens that you run into a client outside the massage clinic (e.g., at a movie, grocery store, community gathering, etc). Don't walk up and greet the client. Allow the client to identify that a relationship exists or not, as he or she deems appropriate. If you are pulled into a conversation with the client, separate the dual relationships by talking only about nonmassage-related topics. Keep the massage work with the client separate from the social event.

You might barter services with another health care professional leading to a potentially confusing situation for both of you. Now both of you act in some sessions as the therapist and hold responsibility for the therapeutic relationship, and in some sessions you are the client. You must both pay careful attention to roles and feel comfortable reversing roles regularly.

Dual Relationships that are Prohibited

In some cases, dual relationships are completely prohibited as a breach of professional ethics. When the therapeutic relationship is the first relationship formed with another person, all secondary relationships should be avoided. As discussed previously, clients readily give power to massage therapists in massage settings, and issues of transference and counter-transference are common. To engage in a social or sexual relationship with clients puts those clients at risk mentally and emotionally and may lead to other poor treatment planning choices. This is not to say that massage therapists are not human. Massage can feel like a lonely profession sometimes, and client interaction may be the only human contact a therapist makes in a day. It is normal to want to make connections with other humans, and the client is right there and often longing to connect as well. Attraction may lead to friendship and the desire for outside contact, which may in turn lead to a sexual or romantic relationship. In this situation, you would more likely spend massage sessions focused on exploring the client as a possible friend or romantic partner and meeting your personal needs for connection. The therapeutic relationship would be compromised, and the possibility for client abuse and exploitation is increased.

Avoid starting secondary relationships. If this is impossible, end the therapeutic relationship before pursuing the secondary relationship. The client can be referred to another therapist, preferably in a different massage clinic. It is best if both parties wait a period of time before pursuing a personal relationship (National Certification Board for Therapeutic Massage and Bodywork mandates 6 months). This allows issues related to the power differential, transference, and counter-transference to subside.

As you can see, the issues related to dual relationships are not always black and white. Gray areas depend a lot on your maturity level, willingness to communicate honestly, attention to ethics, and general self-awareness. In all cases, dual relationships require careful thought on your part and a dedication to act in the best interests of the therapeutic relationship and individual client.

Concept Brief 7-6
Dual Relationships

- A dual relationship is a situation in which more than one relationship with a client is present.
- Some dual relationships are never permissible, while others require careful attention and heightened awareness to preserve boundaries and the therapeutic relationship.

External Guidance on Issues Related to the Therapeutic Relationship

Massage therapists are constantly dealing with a variety of ethical and professional issues that often stem from complex psychological causes. Added to this, massage can often feel like a lonely profession where the only contact a therapist has during the course of a day is clients. The need to uphold the therapeutic relationship does not allow for the development of friendships. Supervisors, mentors, and peer groups can help you at any stage of your career deal with ethical issues, feel supported, and develop friendships.

Supervisors

Supervisors are people who oversee massage therapists. Supervision is a formal arrangement, and often the supervisor is the therapist's boss. Supervisors may help you set goals for performance improvement, monitor your relationships with clients, coach you to overcome any personal limitations that may affect client relations, or give feedback on treatment plans for clients. For example, a supervisor might role play boundary setting with clients to coach a shy therapist in verbalizing boundaries. A supervisor might review client health history forms (with client consent) to ensure that you have not missed a possible contraindication to massage. Good supervisors are a lot like mentors, discussed below. They create an open, respectful, and supportive environment so that you can share your concerns and grow as a professional.

Mentors

Mentors are experienced massage therapists who provide insight for newer therapists into ethical, professional, and technique issues. Mentorship is less formal than supervision, but the mentor still plays an active role in helping you grow as a professional. A mentor might give you insight into dealing with difficult clients or provide teaching stories that help you see different ways of handling client misconduct. You can discuss with the mentor issues of transference, counter-transference, and boundary violations and get feedback based on personal experience. A mentor can also help in treatment planning with clients, as long as the client gives consent. The mentor is held to the same confidentiality as you are regarding client records.

Peer Groups

A peer group may form as a regular gathering of massage professionals to discuss issues related to massage. Peer groups decrease the isolation many therapists feel because they provide a social outlet that still serves as a professional growth activity. A group of peers can offer a multitude of different perspectives on issues you face in the course of a workday. While the client's identity and identifying factors must not be disclosed, peers can usually discuss treatment options, new methods, and client-related dilemmas without breaking the client's confidentiality.

As you progress through massage school, you will develop your professional boundaries. A good first step is awareness. Pay attention to how permeable your boundaries are with different people and in different situations. Assess if your boundary is too permeable, not permeable enough, or just right for the situation. It is also helpful to label boundaries as physical, emotional, mental, spiritual, and sexual, and pay attention to them. Are your boundaries weaker in one of these areas? Why? Finally, watch out for boundary violations and practice speaking up if another student violates your boundaries when you act as the client in a massage exchange. Always treat student-clients or practice-clients as if they are real clients when you perform practice massages, and think about how you assert your boundaries and show respect for theirs. This awareness will help you maintain strong and appropriate boundaries with clients when you graduate and become a professional.

Topic 7-4
Bodymind Factors in a Therapeutic Relationship

The term *bodymind* describes both a philosophical or scientific viewpoint and the personal experience of connection or disconnection felt by an individual. Prominent viewpoints (philosophical, political, societal, religious, etc.) have influenced the way that people experience their bodies throughout history. Early people accepted the intimate links between the body and mind without question. The Greeks and then subsequent philosophers and scientists explored the body and mind as separate entities, leading society to accept and experience a disconnection between the body and mind that still influences the way that people feel today. Massage and many other complementary and alternative therapies embrace the philosophy that the body-mind cannot be separated and use the term "bodymind" to refer to the interconnected workings of the body, mind, and spirit of a person and ways in which those parts mirror and influence each other. How people view themselves, move through space, feel about the world around them, enter and interact with that world, experience emotion, learn, behave, and take action are expressions of their degree of bodymind connection.

This topic explores the bodymind split and its ramifications on health, the science behind a new recognition of the bodymind connection, and the bodymind histories of clients. While massage naturally facilitates bodymind connection, a therapist aware of bodymind concepts is better able to create a therapeutic relationship that reinforces a positive client state leading to greater health and wellness.

The Bodymind Split

The **bodymind split** is the view that the body and mind are separate and that one does not directly reflect the other. With this unconscious philosophical attitude, people suppress the urges and impulses of the body forcefully in order to elevate the mind. It's not difficult to see how this split occurred when we consider that the ancient Greeks developed a high regard for the intellect and reason and investigated the nature of the mind separately from that of the body.[15] We can speculate that the ability to write language and thereby divorce a person's thoughts from the physical body further supported the elevation of the mind above the body. Some religions view the body as inherently sinful and teach that it must be purified and transcended through higher thinking and control of bodily drives. For example, in the Middle Ages, the Catholic Church promoted practices that deprived and tortured the body as a way to atone for sins.

This view of the body and mind as split reached its height in the Western world in Victorian times (1837–1901). During this historical period, people upheld a precisely defined and rigid set of manners to overcome what was considered the "animal impulses" of the body. Human sexuality and normal body functions were associated with immorality, and the sounds and smells of the body were forcefully repressed. Clothing was layered and restrictive. High necklines, long skirts, long sleeves, and corseting hid the body from view and required shallow breathing and stiff postures. Women who acknowledged their sexual urges were diagnosed as mentally ill, and homosexuality was punishable by death.

Some researchers believe that the legacy of the bodymind split can be recognized in postural holding patterns, sensations of disconnection from the body, psychological disorders, and many physical conditions. The bodymind split has led us to learn and then train future generations to suppress emotion, often viewing it as "bad," and so it is not processed in a healthy way. In fact, there is substantial evidence to show that emotions that are not expressed get stuck in the body and become part of a person's physical tension patterns.[16] We can see this in the way that clients continue to participate in repetitive motions, forcing themselves to work, often ignoring the pain they feel until it is so severe that they must stop. Often they don't stop but seek instead to mask the pain with analgesics (again, suppressing the feelings and needs of the body).

The shifting of our understanding from a belief in a bodymind split to a belief in an inseparable bodymind is a slow process, because beliefs often operate outside of conscious thought. They are so ingrained that we don't recognize the way they limit us or influence our lives. For example, consider that medicine and psychiatry are practiced as separate sciences despite the weighty amount of research that shows that emotions, attitudes, and beliefs (the mind) play a major role in a person's health and the ability to survive many serious illnesses of the body. In mainstream medicine, psychiatry, and alternative therapies, new research is helping to shift our understanding and adjust our thinking for the benefit of clients and patients.

The Bodymind Connection

Massage embraces the philosophy that the interconnected workings of the body, mind, and spirit of a person, and the ways in which they mirror and influence each other, demonstrate an inseparable **bodymind connection**. Science is also shifting to a philosophy of a connected bodymind because of research evidence. In fact, the bodymind connection was first "officially" recognized in research that led to the discovery of stress and in the mid-1900s when psychiatrists noticed that psychiatric patients demonstrated immune changes in relationship to depression, delirium, dementia, and schizophrenia. In studies to verify these findings, psychiatric subjects showed decreased lymphocyte numbers and poor antibody response to vaccinations compared with nonpsychiatric subjects. The disordered states of the patients' minds were reflected in the disordered states of their immune systems.[17–19]

Research related to the emerging field of psychoneuroimmunology (psycho = mind + neuro = nervous system + immuno = immune system + logy = study of) explains that certain molecules in the body carry information that allow cells from many different body systems to communicate with one another across long distances. It shows that the view of the brain as a control center that only sends information via a hard-wired, one-nerve-to-the-next-system is incomplete. The hard-wired system is valid and important for many functions, but operating right alongside it is a brain system that closely resembles the endocrine system and more dynamically links the body's different systems together.[20–22]

Concept Brief 7-7
Bodymind Concepts

Bodymind: Refers to the whole person; body, mind, and spirit and how those parts relate.

Bodymind split: The unconscious belief that the body and mind do not reflect each other.

Bodymind connection: The recognition that the body and mind mirror each other and are intimately connected.

Psychoneuroimmunology: The study of the links between the psyche, nervous system, endocrine system, and immunity.

Information Molecules

Information molecules are the molecules in the body that allow different body systems such as the nervous system, endocrine system, digestive system, and immune system to chemically communicate with one another to influence function. Information molecules fall into two categories:

1. **Receptors:** Receptors are protein-binding sites found on a cell membrane or found inside the cell. Many different types of receptors might be found on a cell surface. As researcher Candace Pert explains, "If you were to assign a different color to each of the receptors that scientists have identified, the average cell surface would appear as a multicolored mosaic of at least seventy different hues—50,000 of one type of receptor, 10,000 of another, 100,000 of a third, and so forth."[16]

2. **Ligands:** Ligands (from the Latin *ligare*, meaning "that which binds") is the term used to describe the chemical keys that unlock cells by binding with receptors. Ligands are divided into three chemical types—neurotransmitters, steroids, and peptides—and are either natural or artificial substances (e.g., drugs) that bind selectively with particular receptor sites.

Binding occurs when the fluids that surround cells carry ligands to specific receptors. When the right ligand bumps into the right receptor, the vibrational binding that is produced unlocks the cell so that information from the ligand can enter and cause cellular level activities that can lead to changes in physical activity, changes in mood, and changes in behavior.

Massage therapists notice that emotions and memories may surface when particular areas of the body are manipulated with techniques. For example, in one session a client started to sob when her neck was massaged. The therapist stopped working but the client encouraged her to continue. After the session, she told the therapist that the work on her neck caused her to remember an incident where she was mugged and her attacker placed his hands on her neck cutting off her air supply. The client speculated that her neck had carried the suppressed trauma from that event for years

and that massage had somehow released it. This event can be explained by the physical softening of body armor but is further clarified by the findings of psychoneuroimmunologists who believe that memories are stored throughout the body as changes in the structure of receptors at the cellular level. In this new model of a fully integrated bodymind, the body *is* the unconscious mind and stores memories, repressed emotion, traumas, and joys. It is no wonder that clients may experience a range of emotions from sobbing, to irritation, to anger, to joy, to elation, to uncontrollable laughing during sessions. So when you provide massage to a client, you're not just manipulating soft tissue, you're also manipulating the entire person, body, mind, and spirit, and potentially causing changes to ligands and receptors at a cellular level (Fig. 7-7).

The Bodymind, Emotion, and Health

Much research has been conducted on the role of emotions in the development and progression of diseases, especially cancer. People in touch with their emotions and who expressed emotion had faster recovery rates from cancer than those who suppressed or denied emotion.[23] People who expressed emotion, even emotions perceived as negative like anger, had better survival rates in relationship to cancer than those who repressed emotion.[24]

Psychoneuroimmunologists believe that emotional expression is related to a specific flow of peptide–ligands in the body. Suppression of emotion leads to a massive disturbance of this peptide–ligand flow, altering, on a cellular level, the delicate bodymind network and weakening immunity. For example, viruses may use the same receptor sites as ligands to enter into a cell. The virus will find it less easy to enter a cell if the particular ligand for that cell is available to bind. The reovirus, the cause of the common cold, uses the receptor for norepinephrine to enter cells. Norepinephrine is abundant in upbeat, positive, and joyful mind states. In all probability, when people are in positive moods, they are less susceptible to colds because

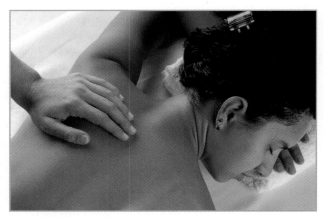

Figure 7-7 When you provide massage to a client, you're not just manipulating soft tissue, you're also manipulating the entire person, body, mind, and spirit! Photo courtesy of Associated Bodywork & Massage Professionals (ABMP).

norepinephrine receptor sites are blocked to the reovirus by norepinephrine.

This information helps us understand why some research suggests that massage boosts immunity. Massage creates a safe environment where long-buried memories can surface through the power of touch into conscious awareness. It also facilitates a state of enjoyment that likely shifts the peptide–ligand flow in the body balancing the body's chemical information system. Massage helps people find their way back into their bodies and experience life from an embodied prospective.

The Bodymind Histories of Clients

We know from the previous section that massage embraces the view that the mind and body are closely connected and reflect each other. What happens in the mind causes changes in the body. What happens in the body causes changes in the mind. Each client comes to a massage session with a bodymind history made up of everything that has happened to the client physically and everything that has happened to the client psychologically. Clients' sense of "me-ness" determines how they respond to you as a therapist, to your massage techniques, to the changes in their soft tissue, to the feelings and thoughts that arise in response to touch, and to life after the session. The massage you provide the client today becomes part of the client's ever-evolving bodymind history (Fig. 7-8).

The Client's Physical History

To better understand the **physical history** of clients, take a moment to explore your own physical body. How do you stand, for example? Are your shoulders rolled back or forward, does one foot turn out or in, does your chin tilt to one side or jut out? How did you get this way? How did you learn to stand with your jaw clenched? How did you learn to dance gracefully around the room? What are all the factors that played a role in creating the person you are today in terms of your movement patterns, muscular tension patterns, range of motion, use of space, and more than that, the way you feel inside your body and about your body?

A client's physical history is based on many factors including genetics, nutrition, age, fitness level, past diseases, conditions, or injuries, and current diseases, conditions, or injuries. As a massage therapist, it is important to be aware of these factors in your dealings with clients. This increased sensitivity can help you adapt techniques or remain responsive to the client's needs during the session.

Genetics

Genetics is the biological science that deals with the way in which living organisms inherit traits from their parents. Humans receive their physical characteristics from their parents; even tension patterns in muscle may show an arrangement in the offspring that is similar to that in a parent. Physical traits are modified due to environmental factors.

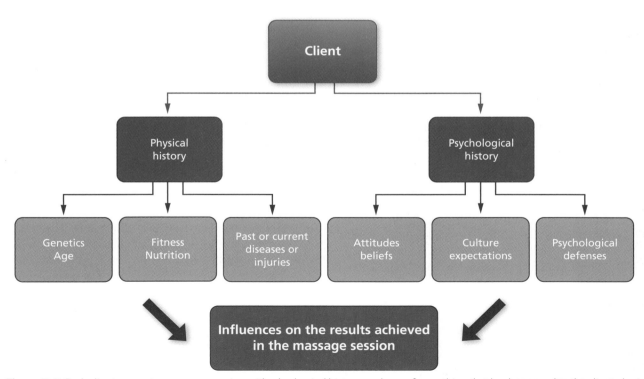

Figure 7-8 Each client comes to a massage session with a bodymind history made up of everything that has happened to the client physically and everything that has happened to the client psychologically. The massage you provide the client today becomes part of the client's ever-evolving bodymind history.

Many diseases and conditions are genetically based, caused by abnormalities in a person's genetic material.

Nutrition

Our bodies need fuel for proper growth, energy, heath, injury recovery, and optimal function. Most people are aware that some diseases are caused by a lack of essential vitamins, minerals, proteins, or nutrients in the diet. Usually people think of malnutrition as only affecting people who don't have enough to eat, but it can also occur from eating the wrong foods. Without proper nutrition, a client might be more prone to injury, bruise easily, heal more slowly from injuries, and experience fluctuations in energy levels and possibly mood swings and behavioral changes.

Age

The age of the client may directly influence the massage session in a number of ways. Children and young adults are likely to heal more rapidly from an injury than a middle-aged person, but may have less personal autonomy. A child or young person may have been taught to be suspicious of strangers. Allowing someone unknown to apply massage may feel uncomfortable, and yet children may not understand why they feel uncomfortable. An elderly person is more likely to be taking multiple medications, suffer from a chronic condition or disease, experience dehydration, or suffer from disrupted sleep patterns. Many elderly people are alone because of the death of spouses and friends. The physical and interpersonal contact with the massage therapist may cause strong emotions to surface.

Fitness Level

Regular physical activity strengthens muscles and bones, increases flexibility, strengthens the heart, aids circulation, relieves stress, and improves sleep and energy. Clients who are physically active may heal more quickly from an injury, tolerate deeper massage techniques more readily, and feel more positively about their bodies. Physical people also tend to demonstrate better posture and better muscular balance. Clients in poor physical condition tend to require more adaptive measures from therapists. It is easier to "overwork" unfit clients with too much massage because the increase in circulation places an increased load on their cardiovascular systems. You may notice that the physical histories of clients are often present in the way they view themselves during the session. Discomfort when certain body areas are touched (e.g., the abdominal area) might be related to clients' feelings about their fitness level and body shape.

Past Diseases, Conditions, or Injuries

The past diseases, conditions, and injuries clients have experienced are likely to influence their bodymind sense of self even after the injury has healed. A physical tension pattern may have developed when they compensated for the injury with other body areas. This new pattern may be placing the body under stress, and yet they may not be aware that they

are still compensating for the old injury. In one example, a client broke his tibia 2 years before his massage session and was seeking massage because he still had pain in his lower leg. While watching him walk, the therapist detected a subtle limp, a movement pattern the client learned in order to compensate for the leg's weakness while it healed. His leg was fully healed, but every time he took a step his brain instructed his body to produce the faulty movement pattern, even though the compensation was no longer necessary. His brain was quick to adapt and learn a new protective movement pattern, but it was slower to shed that pattern when it was no longer needed.

Clients may feel venerable from memories of a past disease or condition and believe that their body is susceptible to catching the disease again, or that the condition or injury might recur. In response to feeling venerable, they might subconsciously avoid certain situations, treat a particular body area with more care, feel uncomfortable when the area is touched, or use muscular tension to wall the area off in an effort to protect it. Sometimes such strategies are necessary, but often they place new stresses on the bodymind of the client and operate at a level below conscious awareness.

Current Diseases, Conditions, or Injuries

Clients with current diseases, conditions, or injuries are likely to be coping with symptoms that impact their lives and the lives of their families and friends. One symptom that you are likely to encounter regularly is pain. Research on chronic pain indicates that the brain leans to be more pain sensitive. While another person might describe a particular body sensation as "uncomfortable," a person living with chronic pain is likely to describe it as "painful." So as time progresses, more and more body sensations are perceived as painful, and the client may fall into a pattern of closely analyzing the pain and doing everything possible to manage it, or avoid it.

Sometimes a massage therapist encounters clients who have exhausted every resource by visiting a variety of health care specialists in an effort to manage their disease or condition. Massage and other alternative therapies become a last resort, and the session is charged with the client's feelings of desperation and fear of failure. In all cases, a current disease, condition, or injury is not just a set of symptoms that cause physical discomfort. They cause deep feelings and fears to surface that may trigger a client's psychological defenses (described earlier in Topic 7-2). Working with chronic pain conditions is discussed at length in Chapter 23.

The Client's Psychological History

The **psychological history** of clients is based on their attitudes, beliefs, expectations, and cultural influences. Psychological defense mechanisms they have adopted and the way in which they use "body armor" to control their emotion will directly influence some aspects of the session.

Attitudes, Beliefs, Expectations, and Suggestions

Attitudes (a view of something), beliefs (ideas held as true), and expectations (what a person thinks will happen) can play a powerful role in health and well-being. When people have a sense of control over their lives, believe they have the capacity to make choices to cope with problems, express optimism about outcomes, and demonstrate enthusiasm for life, they are healthier or survive terminal illnesses longer.[25–27]

Attitudes toward life lead to changes in physiological function. People who smile often have autonomic nervous systems that are less reactive to stress, while facial expressions of happiness increase blood flow to the brain and stimulate changes in neuropeptide levels, improving immunity.[28,29] An open attitude to change can increase resistance to illness.[30] On the other hand, chronic cynicism can increase the risk for atherosclerosis and heart disease, while an attitude of helplessness decreases the body's resistance to disease.[31,32]

Beliefs can be very powerful, as seen in the placebo effect (when people believe a medication is real when in fact it is an inactive substance like a sugar pill). If people believe that the medication will be beneficial and have strong faith in a positive outcome, they often experience the effects of the drug without the drug.[33] Beliefs affect clients on the musculoskeletal level because they become attached to particular postural habits and movement patterns. If clients sit hunched over their computer screen every day for 3 years, they may come to believe that this is the way that they sit naturally. When you suggest that they would feel less neck, shoulder, and back pain if they sat upright, they report that this new upright posture "feels uncomfortable" and resist. Even though you point out that hunching causes repetitive strain to muscles and may damage the spine, they maintain that their sitting posture is okay because it feels normal.

A client's expectations for massage will influence the outcome of the session. The suggestions a therapist makes to clients can sometimes shift their attitudes, beliefs, and expectations in either positive or negative ways. For example, physicians began to notice that some people who underwent surgery emerged with fixed ideas about their prognosis that were different from the expectations they exhibited before the surgery. Research showed that patients could subconsciously hear what physicians said while they were under anesthesia and that the effects of the physician's comments had profound consequences. Physicians began to receive training to monitor their comments during surgery.[34]

Massage therapists should also monitor the suggestions they make to clients, just as physicians do. Therapists sometimes make unmonitored statements like, "I just spent twenty minutes on your shoulders and they are still so tight I doubt you will have much relief from your headache." Without meaning to, the therapist in this case just suggested that the client will still have a headache after the session. This can promote the client's previously held expectation of pain. If on the other hand, the therapist says, "I just spent twenty minutes on your shoulders and the tissue is much better now. I bet your headache will feel a lot better now that the tension is gone," this provides a foundation for the best possible outcome for the client.

Cultural Influences

Culture is the system of values, beliefs, history, and pattern of behavior shared by a particular group of people. People's culture is learned from their family and others and is manifested in art, science, moral systems, consumption of consumer goods, and lifestyle. Your perception of the world around you, your concept of time and space, the way you think, your language, the way you hold your body and the gestures you make, your values, your behaviors, your decision-making, and the types of people you form relationships with are all influenced by your culture.

Culture directly impacts the shape of the body and the way people feel about their appearance. For example, research suggests that exposure to mass media depicting the ideal body type as very thin has led to body image disturbances in women and an increase in eating disorders.[35,36] Men are not exempt from body image disturbances caused by cultural norms. One study noted that men from a range of cultural groups (Whites, Blacks, Hispanics, Asians, and Middle Eastern) engage in extreme body change strategies to increase muscle size and decrease body fat to achieve a lean body ideal.[37] The emphasis of American culture on youth and beauty has led to the increasing popularity of cosmetic medical treatments over recent decades.[38]

The goal for health care providers is to be aware of the beliefs and values held by people of different cultures about health care and touch to facilitate cross-cultural understanding. While it is not possible to understand every nuance of every culture, it is important to learn as much as possible about the cultures represented in your community. In their online training program for health care professions, Laurine Charles and Beth Kennedy describe cultural competence as;[39]

- An awareness of one's own cultural values
- Sensitivity to and acceptance of the influence of a person's culture on health and wellness
- A willingness to understand another's perspective and an awareness that people of different cultures have different ways of communicating, behaving, and problem solving
- A commitment to the life-long pursuit of understanding different cultures and developing skills to improve cultural competence
- The ability to provide care that is meaningful and fits with the cultural beliefs and lifestyle of the patient
- A balance between an individual's autonomy and freedom to practice personal beliefs versus the right of a community to be protected from harm

By understanding your own cultural background and differences in other groups, you are more likely to provide care that fits the needs of the individual.

Psychological Defense Mechanisms

In Topic 7-2 in this chapter, you learned that psychological defense mechanisms are mental processes that enable the mind to deal with conflicts it can't resolve, and every person learns some type of psychological defense from normal experiences of life. The way in which a client uses psychological defenses impacts the results achieved during the session and is part of the client's psychological history. Review Topic 7-2 for more information on working with the psychological defenses of clients.

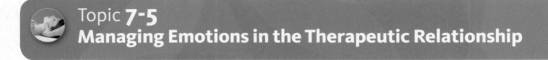

Topic 7-5
Managing Emotions in the Therapeutic Relationship

Massage directly affects the bodymind and overall health of the client through the power of touch. As explained in Topic 7-1, touch is a unique form of nourishment that is essential to life. When touch is therapeutically structured, as in a massage session, physical tensions are softened and the chemical information system of the body is affected as discussed in Topic 7-4. These changes at both the structural and chemical level can lead to the surfacing of emotions in clients. Massage therapists must learn to manage these emotional releases in a way that supports bodymind learning for clients and maintains the integrity of the therapeutic relationship.

Emotion Defined

Robert Plutchik, a well-know researcher based at the Albert Einstein College of Medicine, is considered an authority on emotion. He notes that more than 90 definitions of **emotion** were proposed during the 20th century and that "emotion is one of the most confused (and still open) chapters in the history of psychology."[40] When looking at the word emotion, Plutchik notes that three aspects of emotions can be distinguished:

- Emotions are private, subjective feelings that arise spontaneously rather than through conscious effort.
- Emotions are a state of psychological arousal accompanied by detectable physiological responses.
- Emotions are sensations that spur us to actions so that mental and physical equilibrium is maintained or reestablished.

Some psychologists and researchers make distinctions between emotions, moods, temperament, and drive states:

- Emotions are transient (temporary and short in duration) and usually have a cause.
- Moods are an overall feeling or mental state, often without a perceived cause, which can last for several days.
- Temperament refers to genetically based characteristics and aspects of personality that we are born with that endure into adulthood. For example, infants that are anxious and nervous tend to be anxious and nervous as adults.
- Drive states are based on the idea that all living organisms have physiological needs that must be satisfied for survival or to maintain homeostasis. Disruption of homeostasis causes a state of psychological arousal (drive), which impels the organism to take action to reduce the drive and return to homeostasis. If you are hungry or thirsty, you take action to find food and water.

Emotions help us to determine what to pay attention to, what to care about, what to remember, and what to forget.[41,42] Emotions could be described as "bodymind truth." They help people connect to what has meaning, what is really happening, what requires attention, and where letting go can occur. So when **emotional release** happens in a massage session, it can be viewed as a natural process in which a healthy shift of the client's bodymind leads to greater equilibrium.

Reasons for Emotional Release During Massage

Emotional release in the practice of massage is defined as the sudden or gradual rise of feeling in the client and the expression of that feeling before, during, or after the massage session. Clients might experience a variety of emotions during a session, and the stories shared here are meant to serve as examples and not to represent the spectrum of what might occur (Fig. 7-9).

The Fullness of Life

Massage can evoke tender, open feelings that are not based on sadness but rather on the recognition of the fullness and uniqueness of life. Massage allows a space for inner exploration, in which people can reconnect with themselves and embrace their challenges and triumphs. Every person struggles at some point, and it is how we deal with these struggles, learn from them, and grow that defines who we are and where we can go. Massage facilitates an embracing of self, an acceptance of self, and a clarity about self that may lead to feelings of peacefulness or to important life decisions for self-transformation. As the therapist, you might see the client's face soften and the eyes turn misty. Gentle tears may escape from the sides of the eyes and the client may take deep breaths. Sometimes the chest will contract and clients will hold their breath as a type of physical defense reaction to the internal

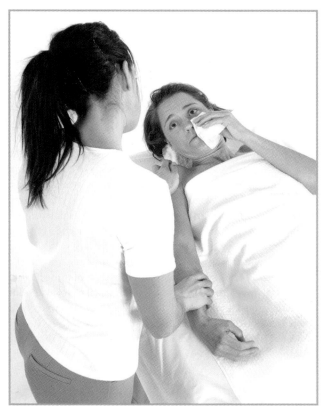

Figure 7-9 Emotional release is the sudden or gradual rise of feeling in the client and the expression of that feeling before, during, or after the massage session.

openness that is experienced. If client take a breath and allow the chest to expand naturally, this initial defense is lessened, allowing them to enter fully into their internal space.

Embodiment

The term **embodiment** refers to the subjective sensation of having and using a body. Each of us has the sensation of being in our bodies, and that sensation has shaped the way we view and explore the world around us, interact with people, develop habits, think, feel, and behave. Think of your childhood experience of embodiment where you reveled in the slick, heavy goop of mud, gave your full attention to the feeling of the rain on your hands, and buried your nose in the warm, familiar smell of your pet dog, cat, or horse. To be fully embodied is to be fully aware of the body and what it senses and experiences.

Disembodiment refers to the sensation, often unconscious, of being disconnected from the experiences of the body, or alienated from the body. People who gain weight may see a photo of themselves and get a shock. They say things like, "I didn't know I was so heavy!" or "I can't believe this is me!" People also get a shock when a therapist points out a physical holding pattern such as hunched shoulders in a mirror. Clients don't view themselves in their own mind as hunched and fail to recognize the physical sensation of hunching.

Disembodiment can happen to anyone and is part of the legacy of the bodymind split that is passed from one generation to the next. The nature of modern life is disembodying. People might spend time in online chat rooms, where they are divorced from their physical presence and the physical presence of the people they are socializing with. A hectic schedule doesn't allow much time to contemplate the sensations or experiences of the body. We are also exposed to multiple stimuli like bright lights, cell phones, noisy environments, and electronics that cause disruptions to entrainment (the natural osculating rhythms of the body discussed in Chapter 4), leading to disembodiment.

Massage brings people back into their body, and suddenly they are connected with their body's sensations and needs. This can stir deep emotions, because on both a conscious and unconscious level we want to feel our bodily sensations and embrace the physical aspects of ourselves. A sensation of grief might be felt as clients recognize their disassociation from their body and experience the sense of dismay this produces. In one example, a professional athlete had an emotional release related to embodiment. He was suddenly gasping for breath and struggling to hold back tears. In a few moments, he gave in and tears ran down his cheeks as he began to sob. When his emotions had cleared, he told the therapist, "My body told me to back off. That I'm driving it too hard and that I never recognize how hard it tries for me, and it's true, I don't recognize how hard it tries. I'm always angry with my body for its pains and limitations. I just want it to be superhuman, and it never will be. My body told me that it is breaking down and if I don't back off now, I won't play the rest of the season."

It is not rare for clients to report that their bodies "spoke" to them during a session. In the case of the professional athlete, the message was clear and uncompromising, but it allowed him to make different choices in his training schedule and play without injury for the season.

Remembering Repressed Memories

As discussed in Topic 7-4, researcher Candace Pert's theory is that repressed emotions, and the memories that surround them, become stored in body tissue on a biochemical level in the structure and function of ligands and receptors.[16] Massage manipulates the tissue where these memories may be biochemically stored. The changes in biochemical levels caused by massage allow repressed emotion and memory to surface into consciousness, where they are re-experienced by the client. For example, Donna is an accomplished horse rider and schedules monthly appointments with Joe to keep her muscles supple for riding and because she has intermittent bouts with low back pain. During one session, Joe used a technique that placed downward pressure on Donna's sacrum while Donna was in the prone position. Joe saw Donna suddenly tense her back muscles and immediately released the pressure, thinking that it caused her pain. Donna lifted her reddened face out of the face cradle and said, "No, it's okay. Put your hands back where they were." Joe again applied the technique to Donna's sacrum and saw Donna begin to shake with tears. "Should I stop?" Joe asked gently and Donna replied, "No, keep going and let me work through this." "Okay" Joe said, "I'll keep working here until you tell me to stop." Finally, Donna lifted her head and said, "I just remembered a time when I was a kid and I was thrown off my horse Sunny and onto my back. I think I've been holding the fear and pain from that fall in my back for a long time. When you started to work on that spot, it came flooding back, but I think it wanted to leave my body today and it feels like it is gone now. I feel so much better."

In some situations, the memories that surface may be frightening for the client, or so loaded that they seem completely overwhelming. Clients may worry that they will lose control of their life if they have to try to process their feelings about things they have long repressed. They might strive to re-suppress the emotions by layering new physical tension on top of the old physical tension. They might even feel angry with you and blame you for what they are feeling. Memories brought back to consciousness during a massage may not present themselves fully during the session. As the hours and days progress after the session, the client might have dreams related to the memories or have bits and pieces of memory emerge at various times.

Clients may distrust the memories that surface during and after a session. They may wish to avoid the internal conflicts these memories produce and so disavow their memories and further disassociate from their bodies. All of the psychological defense mechanisms discussed in Topic 7-2 might be used to close the body off to the opening that occurred during massage.

Freeing Emotion Held by Physical Tension

A related explanation is that physical tension is used to repress and numb emotion, as discussed in the section on armoring earlier in this chapter. As the physical tension in a client's body is reduced and softened, emotions held in by tension patterns are freed. Often the client doesn't have a specific memory that goes with the emotion, perhaps because different emotions have been building up over time.

In one example, a client experienced high levels of stress and pressure each day in her job as a stockbroker. The emotional roller coaster of her work left her elated one moment and defeated the next. During the massage, she suddenly turned angry and became highly critical of the massage therapist. She ordered the therapist to "Stop massaging my legs that way! I hate that! Where did you learn to massage anyway? Massage my back!" The therapist complied, only to hear the client say, "I wish you would work deeper...No! Not that deep." The massage therapist wisely stopped the massage and said, "It seems like my style of massage is not working for you. I'm going to end the session and I'll only charge you for the first thirty minutes when it seemed like you were enjoying the techniques. If you will get dressed, I'll meet you up at the front

reception area." The therapist was then surprised when the client burst into tears and began sobbing. When the client's emotion calmed, the therapist asked gently, "Are you okay? What just happened?" The client told her, "I suddenly felt this buildup of pressure like I was going to snap, and it made me so angry. I realized with one part of myself that I was being unfair to you but I couldn't stop myself. I just wanted to ease the pressure before I exploded."

In this case, the client was able to move from her experience of the emotion into self-awareness fairly quickly. It is also possible, however, for clients to remain in the emotion, or travel through a variety of conflicting or related emotions, without self-awareness and leave the session angry, confused, exhausted by emotions, depressed, or feeling isolated. As a therapist, you have to honor the client's experience but not allow the client to cross professional boundaries. When the therapist in the example above sets a boundary for the client, this action shifted the client into greater awareness. It disrupted an unhealthy pattern of using criticism to deal with personal anger and allowed the client to understand what made her critical and to deal with it in a new way. If the client had remained unaware and continued to be critical, the therapist's best choice was to end the session.

Laughing Fits and Euphoria

Some clients release pent up tensions with laughing fits or intense sensations of euphoria (Fig. 7-10). The therapist might notice the client smiling, and then some giggles might escape, and then laughter might erupt. The client might laugh so hard that the massage is disrupted and the therapist has to stop and wait for the laughing to subside. Euphoria causes a heady, expansive feeling akin to joy, and the client might become talkative, boisterous, and "high." While these types of emotional releases seem easier to deal with than sobbing, anger, or fear, they are just as complex. In some cases, they are defense mechanisms clients use to distract themselves or the therapist. In other cases, they are real feelings created by massage that may transition into other, less comfortable feelings later. Laughter may be followed by tears, or euphoria may transition into feelings of disappointment or even depression.

Managing Emotional Release

When emotional release occurs during a massage session, therapists must manage two processes. First, therapist must manage their response to the client's emotional expression while maintaining appropriate boundaries; second, they must manage the process of maintaining a safe, supportive atmosphere for the client.

Self-Management During a Client's Emotional Release

While the factors related to the expression of emotion by clients may be complex, the actual process of managing

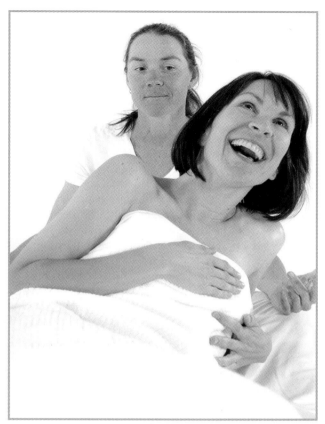

Figure 7-10 Laughing fits and sensations of intense euphoria may be an emotional release where the client lets go of pent up tensions. These types of emotional releases are just as complex as sobbing, anger, or fear.

emotional release is really very simple. Perhaps the toughest part is managing the personal emotions the client's release may trigger in you.

Based on your bodymind history (discussed in Topic 7-4), you are likely to feel something in response to the client's release. Perhaps you were raised in a family where emotion was discouraged, and witnessing another person's emotions frightens you or causes you to withdraw. Maybe the client's tears remind you of your own sadness over a recent event, and you suddenly feel overwhelmed by grief. Maybe you take on the emotions of other people and if the client gets angry you find yourself responding with anger. While all of these responses are normal, they may prevent you from holding good boundaries while providing appropriate support for the client. One of the skills you can develop to improve your ability to manage occurrences of emotional release is emotional intelligence.

Emotional Intelligence Skills

In 1990, psychologists John Mayer and Peter Salovey introduced an exciting concept in psychology in *Emotional Intelligence: Imagination, Cognition, and Personality*.[43] In those days, the IQ (intelligence quotient) test was the primary standard for assessing intelligence, but researchers were starting

to question if there weren't other measures that indicated a person would be successful in life. In 1995, Daniel Goleman wrote the bestseller *Emotional Intelligence: Why it Can Matter More Than IQ* and popularized a new definition of what it means to be smart.[44]

Emotional intelligence is often considered a subset of social intelligence. Social intelligence is the ability to understand and manage people, and the ability to understand and manage oneself.[45,46] As a subset, emotional intelligence is concerned with the "ability to monitor one's own and other's feelings and emotions, to discriminate among them and to use this information to guide one's thinking and actions."[43] Massage therapists need good emotional intelligence skills when relating to clients (Fig. 7-11). Emotional intelligence skills can be broken down into four key areas:

- Perception of emotion in self and others
- Use of emotion to facilitate thinking
- Understanding emotion in self and others
- Management of emotion in self

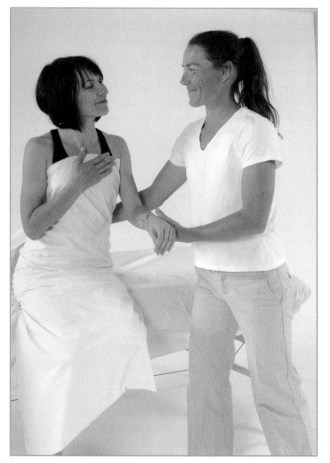

Figure 7-11 Emotional intelligence skills include perception of emotion in self and others, use of emotion to facilitate thinking, understanding emotion in self and others, and management of emotions in self.

PERCEPTION OF EMOTION IN SELF AND OTHERS

Progressive schools with emotional intelligence curriculums teach early elementary students to recognize and label emotion. What is "angry" and in what way is it different from "annoyed," for example. This learning is then applied to oneself, "I'm feeling something. What is it? Is this anger? Is this fear? I think its anger—I feel angry!" These first steps in self-awareness may be undone by socialization at home, as we have discussed earlier in this chapter (e.g., males are not supposed to show emotions like sorrow by crying, but are allowed to show a certain amount of anger, etc.). For many people, and massage therapists are no exception, life socialization has dampened self-awareness. Perhaps we can label our inner states, but often this identification occurs along with a lot of self-judgment such as, "Pull yourself together because you're losing control!" or "You're feeling sad again, stop it!" or "I shouldn't get so mad about this, calm down, get over it." It is likely that we are using the same defense mechanisms as our clients.

Emotional intelligence training systems seek to revitalize people's self-awareness to improve their perception of emotions without judgment. It's not that emotions are allowed to run rampant or that emotive displays are encouraged. Rather, people are taught a healthy process for using emotion in a way that leads to greater life success. This means you can manage your emotional process as needed to reach your goals and communicate with other people more successfully.

To understand, use, or manage emotions, you must first be able to perceive them in yourself and others. Think about the emotions that might arise during an assigned massage exchange. Perhaps one particular classmate, Susan, always causes you stress. As Susan approaches, you tap into the physical sensations you experience and describe them to yourself. "Here comes Susan for her massage. I feel tightness in my stomach. I feel pressure right behind my eyes, and there is tension in my shoulders. My breathing has gotten shallow and my palms are sweaty." Now label the sensations as an emotion if possible: "These sensations tell me I'm feeling anxious." Now, avoid the urge to evaluate this feeling by labeling it as good or bad. Instead, stay with the feeling and allow yourself to continue to watch your physiological reactions and thought processes throughout the session. If you practice this exercise regularly you will develop your understanding of your own emotions and know instantly what you are feeling moment by moment.

The ability to identify what others are feeling is equally important to emotional intelligence and requires attention to multiple external cues. You will build this skill in Chapter 8 when you learn new techniques for communication. One simple method for raising your awareness of the emotions of others is to practice on your classmates. Before class each day pay attention to one or two classmates. What is their body language like? What are their facial expressions conveying? How are they holding their shoulders? What is the tone of their voice when they speak? What emotions do you suspect they feel? By developing the ability to identify emotions and moods in classmates now, you will be ready to apply this skill in massage sessions.

USE OF EMOTION TO FACILITATE THINKING

People who use emotion to facilitate thinking know how to focus their emotions to improve their attention and motivation. They communicate honestly and assertively, and use their high-level awareness of feelings to help them make good ethical decisions or to solve problems. For example, if a client has an emotional release and becomes angry and aggressive, a therapist with high emotional intelligence skills can constantly monitor both self and client to set appropriate boundaries. The therapist recognizes feeling nervous about the degree of anger expressed by the client. Instead of disregarding or judging this nervous feeling and using defense mechanisms to suppress it, the therapist pays attention to it and uses it when responding to the client. The therapist honestly tells the client, "It's normal to have emotions come up during a session, and the fact that you are expressing anger is okay. I need to let you know that I am feeling some nervousness right now because your anger seems to be escalating. I don't want you to shut down your feelings but can you continue to allow your anger to be freed from your body without shouting at me?"

UNDERSTANDING EMOTION IN SELF AND OTHERS

People with high emotional intelligence understand what causes their own emotions and can empathize with others who are processing an emotional state without judgment. Part of this skill is the ability to pay attention to the changes an emotional state undergoes (in self and others) as the emotion progresses and transforms, eventually resolving into a state of calm. It is also important to understand what trigged an emotion and its historical context in your own emotional process. It is not necessary to know what triggered an emotion or its historical context of your client. For example, during an emotional release by a client, a particular therapist with high emotional intelligence was watching her own process while also monitoring the client. Because she had done the work necessary to feel comfortable with her own emotions, this therapist treated the emotions of the client as normal and natural. It is important to convey that emotions are not dangerous and that the process of going through an emotional release is positive, even while it feels uncomfortable.

To feel comfortable with your own emotions, you may want to write a journal entry about some basic emotional questions. Review the emotional behaviors described in Box 7-2. Now imagine a client having an emotional release and exhibiting these behaviors. How does each different emotional behavior make you feel, and how will you handle the situation? Ask yourself these questions:

- What physical sensations do I experience when I imagine a client displaying this emotional behavior?

- What thoughts do I think I'll have when I imagine a client displaying this emotional behavior?

- Which emotions might I experience if a client displays this emotional behavior?

- Do I have any memories that come up from my past when I imagine a client displaying this emotional behavior? (e.g., does it remind you of the time your mom went through a brief period of depression after the death of your grandfather, or does it remind you of the way your father expressed anger?)

- What is my degree of comfort with this particular emotion? Very comfortable, somewhat comfortable, uncomfortable, very uncomfortable.
- How can I improve my level of comfort with this emotion?

MANAGEMENT OF EMOTION IN SELF

The goal in the management of emotion is to control emotional expression when necessary by employing strategies to soothe oneself (Fig. 7-12). At the same time, it is important to stay with feelings and not suppress them through physical or mental tension. Emotion rapidly becomes calm when positive self-talk and self-understanding are used effectively. High emotional intelligence leads to better problem solving and conflict resolution. To understand this, let's use an example of two students in massage school. Both fail an anatomy exam. Student A thinks one of two things: "I am so stupid. I'm never going to get through massage school. I should just quit now before I waste any more money on tuition!" or "The teacher never covered this material! If she had taught the class better, I would never have failed!" Clearly neither of these modes of thinking will lead to calm or to personal success. Student B thinks differently: "I failed! Take three breaths and feel this feeling. What do I feel? I feel disappointed in myself. I went into class knowing I didn't study hard enough. I need to meet with the teacher and find out if there is some way I can improve my grade. I'll study extra hard this weekend to catch up in the class. I won't make this mistake again." Student B's thinking and feeling model is likely to serve this student well after graduating and meeting the challenges of a professional practice.

BOX 7-2 Emotional Behaviors

Emotional behaviors that could occur during an emotional release include:
- Anger
- Anxiety
- Childlike behaviors
- Complaining
- Criticizing
- Cynicism
- Euphoria
- Fear
- Fidgeting
- Freezing and withdrawal
- Hysteria
- Irritation
- Laughing fit
- Restlessness
- Sadness
- Screaming
- Sobbing
- Talkativeness
- Tearfulness
- Terror

During an emotional release, therapists with high emotional intelligence can monitor their own process while remaining attentive to the client. A therapist may think, "I'm

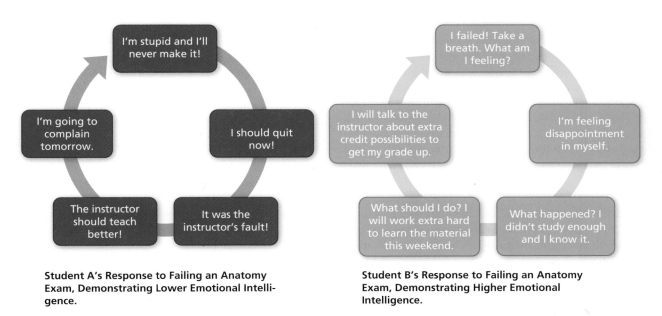

Student A's Response to Failing an Anatomy Exam, Demonstrating Lower Emotional Intelligence.

Student B's Response to Failing an Anatomy Exam, Demonstrating Higher Emotional Intelligence.

Figure 7-12 Two students in massage school fail an anatomy exam. Student A's emotional intelligence is not as developed as Student B's. As a result, Student A's thinking process doesn't lead him or her to solutions and new behaviors that might support success. Student B's process allows him or her to learn and grow from failing the exam.

feeling like I want to cry with my client because this client reminds me of my mother and I can't bear to see my mother upset. This is not my mother. Refocus on the client and remember this is not about you right now. Breath. Focus. You can handle this. Pay attention to the client. Good."

By developing our awareness of what we feel, what others feel, how emotions influence thinking, and how we can manage the emotional processes of ourselves and stay focused on the client, we can improve our therapeutic relationships and experience greater comfort and confidence when an emotional release happens.

Ensure a Safe, Supportive Atmosphere for the Client

It is important to point out that emotional release happens, but it doesn't happen that often. In most sessions, clients simply feel open, refreshed, and relaxed by their massages. While any client could have an unexpected emotional release, those who are coping with pathologies that limit their activities of daily life, working through substance abuse issues, dealing with depression, the death of a loved one or divorce, or living with a chronic pain condition are more likely to have strong emotions surface.

If you are actively working to develop your communication skills, as discussed in Chapter 8, and if you are willing to build your emotional intelligence by developing greater awareness of yourself and your own emotional triggers, as well as attentiveness to the feelings of others, you will likely handle a client's emotional release effectively. The process is simple because emotional release only happens when the client's bodymind is ready. Box 7-3 provides concise guidelines for managing emotional release.

Emotional Release Principles

Your goal as a therapist is to create an environment where clients feel safe, supported, and honored, where emotional expression is viewed as normal, natural, and acceptable, where you communicate nonverbally your fearless permission to clients that it is okay to speak up, feel sensations, and experience their body in a way that frees them from emotional, mental, and physical tension. These ten principles support the emotional processes of clients in a way that is appropriate in a massage session.

Principle 1: Acknowledgement and Normalcy

Physical changes will alert you to a client's emotional release. Watch for increased physical tension, changes in facial expression, breath holding or irregular breathing, misty eyes, tears, or overt signs of emotion like sobbing or prolonged laughter. When you perceive an emotional release, acknowledge it and immediately communicate that emotional expression is normal, productive, and acceptable. For example, you might say, "Mary, I can see that you are experiencing some feelings around this work I am doing on your neck. It's normal to have feelings emerge as tension is softened in muscles. By allowing

BOX 7-3 Guidelines for Managing a Client's Emotional Release

1. Acknowledge the emotional release and affirm it as normal, natural, and productive.
2. Remain present and responsive to the client's needs (e.g., provide a tissue or a sip of water if requested). Maintain contact with the client's body.
3. Suggest slow, deep breathing and give the clients time to process what they are feeling, thinking, and remembering. Listen supportively if they share what they are feeling, but do not ask probing questions.
4. As the emotion begins to dissipate, ground the client in the area that triggered the release by placing your hands on that area.
5. Honor the event as productive and meaningful.
6. Proceed with the massage if it is sensible, or refer the client to a mental health care practitioner.
7. Provide privacy if the client is still feeling vulnerable or emotional at the end of the session.
8. Maintain the boundaries of the therapeutic relationship and avoid behaviors that are damaging or would take you outside your scope of practice.

your emotions to surface and move out of your body, you help to free tension on many different levels. Emotions are signs that we are making good progress."

In some cases, clients are not aware that what they are feeling is an emotional release. For example, they may get restless and irritable. Again, acknowledge what you are witnessing in a nonjudgmental tone and affirm it as normal. You might say, "Bob, just a minute ago you were relaxed and chatting happily about your daughter. Now, your muscles are building tension and you're bouncing your leg up and down. It is not uncommon for massage to trigger feelings like restlessness and even irritability. What are you feeling when I work on your hands? You don't have to share the feelings with me if you don't want to, but just recognizing them yourself can help them move freely out of your body."

Principle 2: Presence, Responsiveness, and Contact

During an emotional release remain present and responsive to the client's needs without losing physical contact with the client's body. Depending on the intensity of the emotional release you may need to stop the massage to allow the client to focus on surfacing emotions. Explain what you are doing by saying something like this: "Mary, I'm going to stop the massage for a moment so you can pay attention to what you are feeling. I'm right here with you." Don't remove your hands from the client as this could cause feeling rejected or abandoned. Instead, place your hands in a holding position on one hand or a foot, lightly on the belly, shoulders, or under the neck. Don't place a hand on the head or forehead or stroke the hair as this can feel parental and may increase the power differential while the client is already vulnerable. Sometimes a client will want to change positions on the massage table, such as to move from the prone position to wipe the face with a tissue. Help the client change position and offer a tissue or glass of water (also see Principle 4).

Principle 3: Connect with Breath

Suggest that a client takes slow, deep breaths. If the client is trying to stifle sobbing by gasping and holding the breath, say that it is okay and perfectly normal to cry, and encourage the release of the chest muscles so that breathing can normalize. You might say something like, "Bob, don't feel like you have to hold back your feelings. It's okay and normal to express emotion in massage. Try to take a deep breath and release your chest. That's good. Keep breathing. I'm right here with you." Sometimes clients are put off and distressed by any suggestions by the therapist. If your gut feeling is keep your mouth shut, then pay attention to that feeling and give clients some time to normalize their breathing on their own.

Principle 4: Give the Client Time

The body processes and releases emotions naturally when it is given the time and space it needs. If the client is actively processing an emotion and you are maintaining contact, all you may need to say is, "I'm here—you're doing good" or "I'm listening." In fact, when clients are moving forward in their emotional processing, you don't want to interrupt them with too much verbalization. On the other hand, clients might try to rush through the process and say things like, "Okay, okay, I'm okay and you don't have to wait for me." In this case, communicate to clients that there is no rush and that they can take the time they need to fully experience the thoughts, memories, and feelings that have surfaced. Let them know that this process is productive and may support the positive results of massage. You might say something like, "Mary, take all the time necessary to allow this process to progress in the way that is right for your body because what you are feeling, and thinking right now may be just what your body needs to move forward in releasing muscle tension and pain."

Don't offer a sip of water or a box of tissue too early in the client's process. Clients might interpret this as a sign that you are impatient with their emotions and want them to finish up so the massage can continue. But if the client sits up and asks for water or a tissue, provide it.

Principle 5: Allow Sharing or Allow Privacy

Affirm for clients that they can share with you what they are experiencing or not as they choose. Let them know that if they find they would like to describe their experience later or during a future session you are available. You might say, "Bob, it is often productive to talk about what you are feeling and if you sense that this would be helpful I am here to listen. If you don't feel like you want to share this now, that's okay to. If you should decide later that you want to talk about it, I can listen in an upcoming session."

Never probe clients for personal information or make them feel that they must share with you. If they start to share, keep your responses attentive, encouraging, and short, along the lines of, "I understand," "I'm listening," and "That makes sense." Avoid any tendency to try to solve the client's problems by offering advice, equalizing, psychoanalyzing (analyzing and interpreting the information), giving inappropriate reassurance, or expressing sympathy. These communication blockers are discussed in depth in Chapter 8.

Principle 6: Ground the Client and Honor the Event

If emotions are allowed to flow freely without interruption from the client, they will naturally dissipate and the client will most often enter a calm, open, and peaceful state. Ground the client by helping a return to the here and now, while honoring the event as productive and meaningful. To do this, you might say something like, "Mary, it seems like your emotions are dissipating and that you are feeling calm inside your body. Continue to follow your breath and bring your attention to your shoulders and neck (or to the area where the release was triggered). Notice that they feel softer and stronger. Emotional release always happens when the body is ready, and you allowed yourself to go with it. I think this experience will mean a lot to your body going forward." Notice that this sentence contains a positive suggestion that facilitates the best possible outcome for the client's muscles as an after-effect of the release.

Principle 7: Proceed or Refer

An emotional release may take as little as 5 minutes or may take up the entire session. If the client enters a calm space, you can suggest that the massage continues. If the client is willing and wants to proceed with the massage, finish the session as you normally would. If the client chooses not to proceed with the massage, respect this and reschedule. It is appropriate to charge the client the fee for the session. By expecting a fee for the time spent, you establish the boundaries of the therapeutic relationship, and confirm to the client that emotional release is a normal occurrence in a massage session. If you suddenly get embarrassed and say, "You don't have to pay me for this session," you may give an impression like this: "This never happens and this was really weird."

In some cases, you may decide that the session can't proceed because the client has acted outside the bounds of the therapeutic relationship during the release (e.g., a client becomes violent and starts hitting the wall—this is highly unlikely but possible). In such cases, or if the clients say they are overwhelmed or frightened by what they are feeling, remembering, or thinking, refer them to a counselor, other mental health professional, or a therapist who specializes in somatic or bodymind-oriented bodywork.

Clients may say that they learned a great deal from the awareness produced by the emotional release. They may anticipate emotional release in future session, and even come to view emotional release as a sign that the session was successful. They may feel disappointed if massage does not lead to an emotional release, or they might store up emotions to release during the massage, such that every massage turns into an emotion-processing session. This is an unhealthy pattern for the client to enter with a massage therapist. Again, refer this client to a trained mental health specialist.

Principle 8: Manage the End of the Session

If a client has experienced an emotional release during the session, the end of the session and the departure of the client from the clinic can feel uncomfortable if these moments are not managed effectively. This can be challenging when the emotional release happens late in the session. What will you do if Mary is crying on your massage table and David, your next client, is waiting in the reception area? It can feel very stressful because your tendency may be to take care of Mary and neglect David. Remember that emotional processes are normal and that you affirm for clients that emotional release is normal when you maintain the boundaries of the session. You might say to Mary, "Mary, our session time is over. I can see that you are still feeling some emotions surface. You were able to free a great deal of tension during this session and so you may continue to have emotions surface. If you like, I can refer you to an excellent counselor in the area who can support this process. I feel like this was really positive and that we made excellent progress today. I'm going to leave the room now so that you can get dressed, but I will come back in 5 minutes and process your payment here so that you can have some privacy." Process the payment in the privacy of the treatment room and escort Mary to the door as you normally would. Avoid giving Mary encouragement or further discussing the emotional release in the reception area where other people might hear the exchange. The minute you enter public space behave with warmth but avoid showing Mary undue attention that might alert others to an emotional episode and so compromise Mary's privacy.

Principle 9: Avoid Behaviors that Are Damaging

In Chapter 8, a number of communication blockers are discussed in depth. These communication blockers include making judgments or judgmental statements, problem solving for other people, equalizing or the use of balancing statements to naturalize something that feels negative, psychoanalyzing, inappropriate reassurance, and sympathy. Such behaviors are damaging when they are used to manage an emotional release and should be avoided. Review those communication blockers regularly and seek to eliminate them from your communication methods. Also refrain from advising clients or offering suggestions for next steps. Don't analyze an emotional release and assume you know why it occurred. For example, the therapist would cross and line and potentially cause emotional damage by saying to Mary, "I've been watching you over the last four sessions and I think your neck tension is all about your issues with authority. It always gets worse when you've had a disagreement with your boss. You should tell your boss how you feel or find another job." Remember that there is a power differential created by the therapist's role as a health care provider and Mary is in an especially vulnerable space. By analyzing and offering advice, the therapist would be distracting Mary from what she is feeling in her body and disempowering her by assuming Mary can't figure it out for herself.

Principle 10: Stay in Your Scope of Practice

If a client has an emotional release, you remain inside your scope of practice by offering support but refraining from offering your opinions, analysis, or advice. Counseling is outside your scope of practice and requires special training and a separate license. Even if you have credentials as a counselor or mental health care specialist, you should not practice these skills within a massage session. You would form dual relationships with clients if you worked with them on multiple levels. It would be better for the client to see you either as a mental health care provider or as a massage therapist, but not as both. Review Chapter 6 to revisit these concepts.

In all the previous examples, the therapists confirmed that emotional release is normal and productive. They explained emotional release within the framework of massage as something that might occur when physical tension is softened. They remained supportive and willing to listen but they did not try to deepen the emotional release, direct the emotional release, or intellectually process it. To participate in any of these activities is to step outside your scope of practice and face possible censure from the Board of Massage in your state.

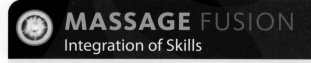

MASSAGE FUSION
Integration of Skills

STUDY TIP: Personalize to Familiarize

Heady concepts like those discussed in this chapter make the most sense when you explore how they operate and manifest in your own life. While an ongoing exploration of these concepts is recommended, it can be helpful to focus on one concept at a time and then move onto the next concept. Write these terms on pieces of heavy paper (one term on each piece of paper): power differential, transference, counter-transference, suppression, dual relationships, bodymind split, bodymind connection, armoring, embodiment, and emotional intelligence. Carry one piece of paper with you and take the paper out regularly. Every time you

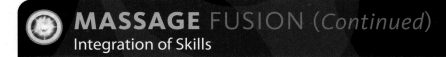

MASSAGE FUSION (*Continued*)
Integration of Skills

take out the paper, contemplate the term and think about it in relationship to your own life. Write down any thoughts, memories, ideas, or feelings that come up. When you have filled both sides of the paper with your notes, move onto the next paper. Once you have worked through all of the papers you will "own" these concepts because they will be familiar to you on a personal level.

MASSAGE INSPIRATION: My Touch History

It can be helpful to write a touch history of your life to identify the power of touch in your own life and to think about how it might influence the way you interact with clients and provide massage. Answer these questions in a journal:

1. When I was growing up, affection in my family was expressed _____.
2. In the culture in which I was raised, emotions and touch were viewed as _____.
3. When I think of nonsexual touch, I think of _____.
4. When I touch people in ways that are not related to massage, I feel _____.
5. When I touch people in ways related to massage, I feel _____.
6. When I am touched during a massage, I sometimes feel _____.

7. When I contemplate the answers I have given to these questions, it makes me think about _____ and feel _____.
8. These thoughts and feelings could affect the massage I give because _____.

CHAPTER WRAP-UP

One of the most wonderful things about going through a massage training program is the opportunity it offers for self-growth and personal transformation. This chapter has introduced you to psychological dynamics that are constantly at play in relationships with other people. If you are willing to explore these concepts in your own life and pay attention to yourself, your actions, and your reactions, these concepts can help you understand yourself better, not only as a therapist but also as a human. The depth to which you embrace and integrate this understanding mirrors the depth to which you will be able to create meaningful therapeutic relationships with clients. You are likely to find that your greater comprehension of boundaries, emotions, psychological defenses, touch as human nourishment, and the bodymind connection not only enhances the relationships you build with clients but your interpersonal relationships with friends, family, and loved ones as well.

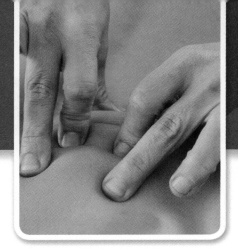

Chapter
8

Professional Communication

KEY TERMS

active communication
assertive relating
conflict resolution

filter
personal space
reflecting

LEARNING OBJECTIVES

Having read the chapter and used the related student learning tools, the student will be able to

1. Explain the concept of personal space and recognize verbal and physical space violations in daily interpersonal interactions.

2. Distinguish among submissive, assertive, and aggressive relating behaviors in daily interpersonal interactions.

3. Analyze different learning styles and mental processing differences, and recognize these differences in others.

4. List three communication blockers and describe how they obstruct open communication.

5. Categorize the components of active communication and describe the basic concepts of awareness, active listening, and the delivery of a message.

6. Describe three points in a massage session at which client and therapist communication plays a vital role for achieving treatment goals.

7. Appraise the benefits of using an assertive communication model with clients.

8. Describe three strategies for reaching a fair and equitable resolution to a conflict.

Communication skills include the ability to listen to and understand another person and the capability to convey ideas and information in both spoken and written language. These skills affect every aspect of your massage training and professional practice. Students must be able to communicate effectively with instructors and fellow classmates to get the most from their massage training program. As professionals, therapists must convey their values and business approach to potential clients and encourage those clients to feel welcome and safe. During a health intake interview, the client's safety and satisfaction with the session both rely in part on the ability of the therapist to gather meaningful information and mold it into an effective treatment plan. Therapists must also be able to share their boundaries, policies, regulations, and business practices with clients in a way that is assertive yet therapeutic. When talking with other health care professionals, therapists also want to use appropriate health care terminology and express their knowledge and understanding of the body.

This chapter introduces basic communication concepts and skills (Topic 8-1), communication blockers (Topic 8-2), active communication skills (Topic 8-3), and conflict resolution (Topic 8-4). This chapter is closely related to Chapter 6 and Chapter 7 because establishing the therapeutic relationship and maintaining professional boundaries involves the ability to communicate effectively. Equally important, written communication is discussed in depth in Chapters 12 and 19 in the sections on documentation and charting.

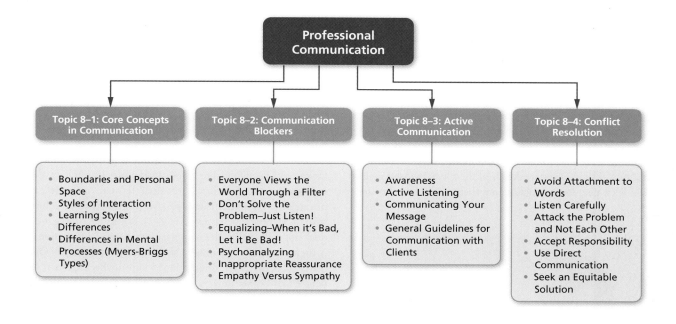

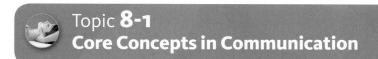

Topic 8-1
Core Concepts in Communication

Successful human relationships are built on meaningful communication. People must be able to listen to others, formulate an appropriate response, and articulate their own ideas in a clear manner. Sharing one's thoughts and feelings with a trusted friend is an opportunity for self-discovery and development. Problems are "talked through" and the "air is cleared" with a good conversation. Open, honest, sensitive, and caring communication nurtures relationships and helps people grow in self-confidence and autonomy. People with strong communication skills exert a transformative influence on the people and situations around them. They can revitalize another person's sense of self or infuse a work team with positive energy. They create an environment where everyone's ideas can thrive. On the other hand, poor communication with family, friends, clients, or colleagues erodes self-esteem and can be devastating.[1]

Some people believe that communication skills are like hair color: you're either born with them or you're not. In fact, people learn their communication skills from important adults like parents and teachers, influential friends, early romantic partners, and even people in the media. Anything learned can be unlearned, relearned, or developed. Therefore, all people can improve their communication skills and experience more self-confidence, pleasure, and understanding in their relationships with others.

Boundaries and Personal Space

In Chapter 7 you learned about boundaries and personal space. A quick review here might be helpful. Boundaries involve conscious and subconscious imaginary lines that mark the limits of an individual's personal space or territory. Boundaries create a border between a person and other people, and between a person and the environment. Boundaries can take different forms and may be physical, emotional, mental, spiritual, or sexual in nature. Because different situations call for different types of boundaries, boundaries are constantly in fluctuation.

Personal space is the physical, emotional, mental, and spiritual space people hold around themselves. It also refers to a person's "territory," including possessions such as clothes, toiletries, car, home, furniture, books, and other personal items. Most people have experienced an occasion when their boundaries were crossed and their personal space violated. Someone might stand too close to another person during a work conversation (Fig. 8-1). The person who feels crowded keeps backing up only to find the other person inching forward. It's also uncomfortable when new acquaintances ask very personal questions or share intimate details of their lives without invitation—such people are violating another's space but also their

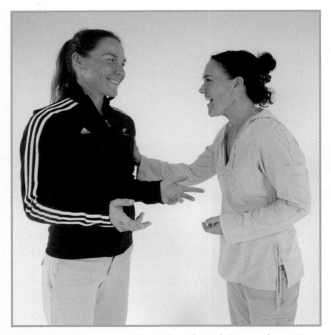

Figure 8-1 People need about three feet of distance from others to feel comfortable. We allow people we know and trust much closer physically and share with them details of our personal life. When acquaintances stand too close, make unnecessary physical contact, or share personal information usually reserved for close friends or family, it creates discomfort.

own space. They are asking about or sharing information that is usually reserved for a close friend or family member.

One of the first steps to good communication in both personal and professional settings is an awareness of boundaries and personal space. Good communicators understand how to maintain their own space without aggression and how to assert themselves without violating the boundaries of others. They are always conscious of the reactions of those they are talking with, and adjust their behavior based on nonverbal cues they observe. For example, a person aware of physical boundaries would not continue to inch forward when the other person is inching back but would recognize the backward step as a signal of being too close.

Styles of Interaction

People learn methods for relating to other people from early caregivers like parents and teachers. They also demonstrate preferences for how they learn new information, generate energy, and order their world. An awareness of these different styles helps therapists understand differences in their clients, adapt their communication style, and practice tolerance for others.

Relating Styles

Many psychologists have described the attributes of people who build strong, healthy relationships, influence their communities or work environments in a positive way, express their creativity, and live life to the fullest. In popular psychology, these multifaceted characteristics are often termed "assertive" and placed on a continuum with passive (nonassertive or submissive) or aggressive behaviors (Fig. 8-2). While this simple model does not fully reflect the complexity of human interactions, it is useful for understanding basic communication styles. Often behavior patterns are unquestioned and unchecked, such that people may behave in ways that do not lead to desired outcomes. Positive behaviors that lead to better communication can be learned, however, and negative behaviors can be unlearned simply through awareness and a desire to make changes.

PASSIVE (NONASSERTIVE/SUBMISSIVE) RELATING

People who adopt passive ways of relating allow others to frequently impose on their personal space. They hold back their true feelings and mold themselves into what they believe other people find lovable. They bend to the opinions of others rather than stating their honest needs and desires, or they state their needs and desires so indecisively that they are ignored. Passive people avoid conflict and seek approval from others by being agreeable and selfless. Someone who related to the world through passive behavior may find pleasure in always being the "nice" person. In fact, these passive people frequently offer to do so much for friends and family that they either are taken advantage of or cause friends and family to feel uncomfortable.

There are many advantages to passive ways of relating. Passive behavior involves never assuming a leadership role, and thereby avoiding any responsibility for outcomes. Passive people often use their "niceness" to control and manipulate other people while always appearing to be good. In extreme cases of passive relating, some people may become helpless

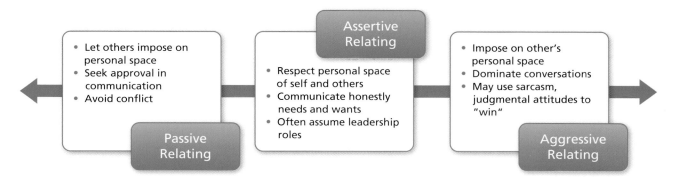

Figure 8-2 Relating styles can be viewed on a continuum from passive to assertive to aggressive. Psychologists notice that assertive communicators build healthy relationships and influence their communities and work environments in a positive way.

and depend on others to care for or protect them. People with passive behavior patterns may suddenly shift to very aggressive relating behavior and have angry outbursts that leave them feeling guilty and submissive again. These outbursts result from built-up tension from the constant need to repress their emotions in order to maintain a selfless persona.

ASSERTIVE RELATING

Assertive people are self-aware and self-confident without being egotistical, respecting themselves while respecting the rights and feelings of other people. They can communicate their ideas, values, opinions, and feelings in a manner that is appropriate and direct, without encroaching on other people. In fact, they encourage others to share, and they look for outcomes that serve everyone's needs. They set goals and follow through with plans. They know who they are, where they are going, and how they plan to get there. They communicate this to the people around them and often have leadership roles because they are not afraid to take responsibility for projects or plans. They learn from their mistakes and are willing to be wrong or unpopular sometimes. They can laugh at their foibles and find humor in otherwise trying situations. People who use assertive behavior to relate never seek to dominate others, even those with opposing plans or ideas. Instead, they strive to communicate clearly, listen carefully, make good decisions, remain flexible, adapt as needed, and maintain their values and humanity. Use the questions in Box 8-1 to determine how you yourself relate to others.

Aggressive Relating

People who relate to others with aggressive behaviors are determined to "win" at any cost. They often fall into sarcasm, judgmental attitudes, or cynicism as a way to communicate superiority. They express their needs and ideas without regard for others and in such a way that the rights and beliefs of others may be violated. Aggressive relating includes dominating conversations and arguing with other people's ideas. Because aggressiveness seems historically to have had some benefits, aggressive relating is often promoted as "successful" behavior in the media and the business community. Aggressive people

control their own lives and some part of the lives of others around them. They make sure their material and physical needs are met, and in the business world their competitive spirit and determination often land them in management roles. On the other hand, aggressive people are generally ruled by some degree of fear: fear that things will get out of their control, fear that their weaknesses will be uncovered, and fear of failure. They meet aggression with more aggression of their own or by sabotaging people in submissive roles. People who use aggression as their primary relating style often find no one is on their side when the tables are turned. While they may dominate a relationship, they rarely experience the joy and satisfaction of intimacy between equals.

Most people relate with a particular style most of the time, but the types described above are much less absolute and fixed in real life. For example, Diego may be friendly, outspoken, honest, and very supportive of his massage classmates until in a class discussion he can't stand to be wrong and bullies others until they agree he is right. In that example, Diego changes to aggressive relating behaviors. In contrast, Mila is goal oriented and self-confident in the massage clinic but becomes soft-spoken, nervous, and self-depreciating around chiropractors who share the same office space. When she is with people she views as authority figures, she reverts to the submissive relating behaviors she used around her father growing up.

BOX 8-1 **How Do You Relate?**

Take a moment to think about your primary relating style and where you fall on the continuum of passive and aggressive relating behaviors. How have these behaviors benefited you? How have they held you back? Think about situations that have caused you to radically shift your style of relating. Why did the shift occur? Where do your relating styles come from? Through contemplation and self-vigilance, you can develop your awareness of your relating style and then make the best possible choices about how to relate to your friends, family, classmates, and future clients.

Sometimes it is appropriate to aggressively defend one's personal space, while at other times it is appropriate to give way. The goal is to be aware of how you relate to others, identify the relating styles of others, improve your relationships, have a good experience in interactions, and not lose your personal space or violate the space of another. These skills serve all people well in life. In a profession like massage therapy, where the client and therapist work closely together, they are important for behaving in a manner that best supports the therapeutic relationship.

Learning Styles Differences

People take in and process information in a variety of different ways (Fig. 8-3). Some people are visual and like to see information, others are auditory and like to hear information, while still others are kinesthetic and like to work through information. Massage therapists must understand how to engage these three types of learners to ensure that all clients feel safe and comfortable. Visual learners like charts, diagrams, and written directions. These clients are drawn to a well-crafted brochure full of pictures that show the clinic's services. They would rather see a picture of the particular muscle causing their neck pain than hear the therapist describe it. This type of learner notices details of the environment and may be soothed or aggravated by how the treatment room looks upon entering. This type of learner has little patience with much talking during the health intake process, but is likely to look over the clinic's forms carefully to absorb policies and procedures.

Auditory learners process information by hearing it. They do much better with spoken directions and are likely to tuck away the clinic's brochure without looking at it. With a particular pain, they prefer the therapist to explain the muscle and why it is causing pain; a picture is unnecessary. They are less likely to read the clinic's forms carefully and may sign the informed consent form without looking at it. For these learners, the therapist must take the time to verbally review policies and procedures. While the visual environment has less influence on their ability to relax, music often is very important. The wrong music or volume easily distracts auditory learners.

Kinesthetic learners do best with information they can touch or experience through their senses. These learners would respond well to finding out about the clinic's services by attending an open house event where they can try things out. They understand a painful muscle best if the therapist palpates the length of the muscle and moves the muscle slowly through its actions. In this way, they experience the muscle and differentiate it from other muscles in the same area. These clients benefit from a multilayered presentation of the clinic's information. They may be drawn to a lovely image on the brochure or to the fine texture of the paper in the clinic's forms. They may listen carefully at first but then grow impatient with the initial health intake interview. Provide this type of client a cup of warm herbal tea during the interview or offer a foot soak as described in Chapter 10 in the topic Opening and Closing the Massage. Every sensual element of the treatment influences these learners, who may absorb more of the clinic's important information and develop greater rapport with a therapist who can engage all their senses.

These differences in how people learn information and communicate can sometimes cause a misunderstanding.

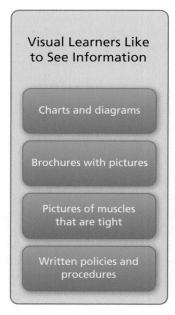

Visual Learners Like to See Information

- Charts and diagrams
- Brochures with pictures
- Pictures of muscles that are tight
- Written policies and procedures

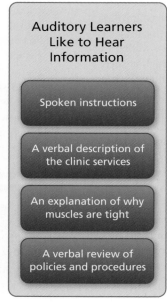

Auditory Learners Like to Hear Information

- Spoken instructions
- A verbal description of the clinic services
- An explanation of why muscles are tight
- A verbal review of policies and procedures

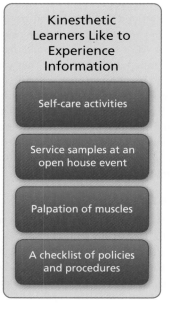

Kinesthetic Learners Like to Experience Information

- Self-care activities
- Service samples at an open house event
- Palpation of muscles
- A checklist of policies and procedures

Figure 8-3 People take in and process information in a variety of different learning styles. Professional massage therapists must understand how to engage different types of learners to ensure that all clients feel safe and comfortable. Make sure to use a variety of methods to communicate with your clients.

A person who communicates information in a particular learning style may become frustrated if another person with a different learning style doesn't get the message. For example, Larry, the receptionist, gives Carole the directions to the massage office three times over her cell phone but Carole still seems confused. Larry gets frustrated and passes the phone to Haya, a massage therapist standing close by, and says, "She can't figure out how to get here!" Haya says to Carole, "Can I get your email address? I'll send you a link to a map to the clinic." Haya sends Carole a link to a map and Carole has no problems finding the office. Larry is an auditory learner and has no problems taking directions over the phone. Carole is a visual learner and has difficulty with audio directions.

During interpersonal exchanges, it is helpful to keep learning style differences in mind. If a friend, loved one, or colleague seems to be missing your point, you may need to shift how you are conveying the information to better match the other's learning style. With new clients, it is best to cover information in as many ways as possible. For example, you might verbally describe the clinic's policies and practices but also hand out a brochure. You might verbally describe where the restrooms are located but also show the client in a tour of the facility. When you work with clients over time, you are likely to learn their preferences for taking in information and can then adjust their sessions to meet their learning styles.

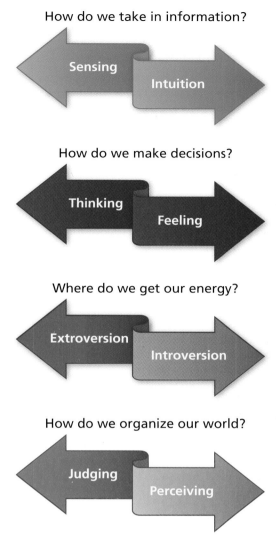

Figure 8-4 Myers–Briggs personality types: People differ in the way they get energy, take in information, make decisions, and organize the world. Understanding people's personality preferences aids communication. More information about this system is available at http://www.myersbriggs.org/.

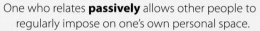

Concept Brief 8-1
Styles of Interaction and Learning

One who relates **passively** allows other people to regularly impose on one's own personal space.

One who relates **assertively** maintains one's own personal space while respecting the personal space of others.

One who relates **aggressively** regularly imposes on the personal space of others.

Visual learner likes to "see" information and relies on pictures and written words.

Auditory learner likes to "hear" information and relies on discussion and hearing words.

Kinesthetic learner likes to "work through" information and relies on doing activities.

Differences in Mental Processes (Myers–Briggs Types)

Katharine Cook Briggs and her daughter Isabel Briggs Myers developed a personality test that identifies four primary ways in which people vary (Fig. 8-4): People get energy, take in information, make decisions, and organize their worlds differently. They called these differences "preferences" to indicate that all people have access to different ways of relating but that everyone tends to be stronger in one of the four areas. This tendency is often compared to being right- or

left-handed. We all use both our hands, but most of us use one dominant hand in many activities.

Sensing and Intution

The first group of preferences relate to how people take in data (perceive). People who prefer *sensing* like tangible information that is clearly defined and has a basis in reality "right now." They like facts, details, and information with a proven, viable source. They are less likely to enjoy speculative data or spending too long looking at possibilities that are related to a distant future. On the other end of the spectrum is someone who prefers *intuition* or more abstract information. Intuitive people like to imagine all possibilities and look at the big picture. They enjoy speculating about how information fits into both related and unrelated models. They are able to connect one set of data to another in broad imaginative leaps but are less likely to enjoy examining every detail.

Thinking and Feeling

The second group of preferences describes how people make decisions (form judgments). People who prefer *thinking* like to make decisions in a logical, objective way that focuses on goals to be achieved and tasks to be accomplished. They may ignore the impact of tasks on people in an effort to reach their goals. On the other end of the spectrum are people who prefer *feeling* and like to make decisions based on finding harmony for all people. This personality type is concerned with the impact of a decision on everyone who might be affected. They might find it difficult to complete tasks or reach goals if they can't ensure that everyone will be happy with an outcome.

Extroversion and Introversion

The third group of preferences describes the place from which people draw their energy. People who prefer *extroversion* draw energy from the outside world of people and activity. They can work all day in a busy office, go out for dinner after work with friends, and still feel talkative and excited when they get home. The more they are out in the world and participating in activities, the more energy they feel. This type may have difficulty with downtime and feel restless and irritable when alone. On the other end of the spectrum are people who prefer *introversion* and draw their energy from a quiet inner world of thoughts and ideas. They are very comfortable in a solitary setting and like to work on projects alone. People who draw their energy from introversion are easily exhausted by too much activity in the outside world and need a period of rest and quiet to recharge.

Judging and Perceiving

The fourth group of preferences describes how people prefer to arrange their world (self-management). People who prefer *judging* like a well-planned, neat, organized, and well-managed environment. They make to-do lists, shopping lists, and lists of goals and stick to a planned schedule. They may have difficulty letting go of outcomes and allowing projects to flow in an unfixed time frame. On the other end of the spectrum are people who prefer *perceiving* and like to go with the flow, driven by their curiosity. They have more difficulty accomplishing a predetermined goal or working with a timeline and due dates. They want to see where the world will take them and are often happy to drift.

Conflicts Among Different Preferences

It is easy to see how conflicts in communication can occur between people on different ends of the spectrum in their mental processes. Imagine a strongly *sensing* massage student who has a strongly *intuitive* massage teacher. The student wants information delivered in a logical progression with clearly defined goals and objectives, while the teacher feels that classes work best when people share their ideas and discuss the material in any order. The student wants detailed facts while the teacher delivers large concepts.

Now imagine massage business partners where one partner is *thinking* and the other is *feeling* when they make decisions. When a big decision comes up, the *thinking* partner wants to look at business goals and make decision based on them. The *feeling* partner frustrates the *thinking* partner because he or she wants to consider staff members, colleagues, and long-term clients in the decision-making process. One partner wants to achieve goals, while the other wants to achieve harmony.

If two massage students are trying to plan study sessions, they could experience conflicts if one is *extroverted* and the other is *introverted*. The *extroverted* person wants to plan a study party with lots of classmates and have study games with prizes, while the *introverted* student suggests a quiet session at home. One student will learn best with excitement, while the other will learn best with quiet.

Finally, imagine a *judging* massage therapist and a *perceiving* client. The therapist has a clear plan for the session and wants to do a thorough assessment before starting the massage. The client arrives 2 minutes late and isn't interested in a thorough assessment but just wants to get on the table and get started. The therapist wants to meet treatment goals, while the client wants to enjoy the session.

The important thing to remember is that people are different and it is vitally important to be tolerant. When you find yourself irritated by a friend, partner, family member, colleague, instructor, classmate, or client, take a moment to identify the other's style of relating. It is likely that the person's preferences and learning and relating style are different from yours and that the person simply perceives information and orders his or her world differently from you.

Topic 8-2
Communication Blockers

Several ways of thinking and responding can get in the way of good communication. These communication blockers remind us that "just listening" and "just speaking" are not as easy as they might seem. By becoming more aware of communication blockers, however, people can adjust their communication styles to better facilitate open and honest sharing. Table 8-1 provides an overview of communication blockers.

TABLE 8-1   **Overview of Communication Blockers**

Filters	A view of the world based on one's past experiences, culture, and upbringing. Causes people to attach to certain ideas that influence how they listen to others.
Judgment	The need to quickly determine if something is good or bad, right or wrong, thereby impeding an exploration of the subject.
Inappropriate problem solving	When one person tries to solve others' problems instead of allowing them to talk through their own solutions.
Equalizing	Attempting to balance something negative with a positive, thereby blocking the speaker's need to express feelings.
Psychoanalyzing	The tendency to "diagnose" the speaker's psychological state, thereby blocking the speaker's free expression.
Inappropriate reassurance	Reassurance stops the speaker from exploring the issue fully and reaching better self-understanding.
Sympathy	The listener expresses pity for the pain of others, causing them to feel a need to defend themselves. Not to be confused with empathy, with which the listener understands the speaker's point of view and can feel and reflect the other's feelings.
Aggressive relating	Communication is blocked because a person who relates aggressively dominates the conversation and has difficulty hearing the views of others.
Submissive relating	Communication is blocked because people who relate submissively allow others to impose on their personal space and do not state their true needs to others.
Learning styles differences	Communication is blocked because the speaker and listener take in and process information differently.
Mental processes differences	Communication is blocked because the speaker and listener have different ways of interacting with and managing the world.

Everyone Views the World Through a Filter

All of us have individual needs, values, beliefs, attitudes, assumptions, and experiences that become a **filter** for how we view the world, listen to others, communicate ideas, or feel in certain situations (Fig. 8-5). Words that excite little emotional response from one person may be charged with particular meaning for another. Situations that make one person uncomfortable cause another to shrug with indifference.

Sometimes we meet people who share many of our values, beliefs, and attitudes, or have experiences that are similar and

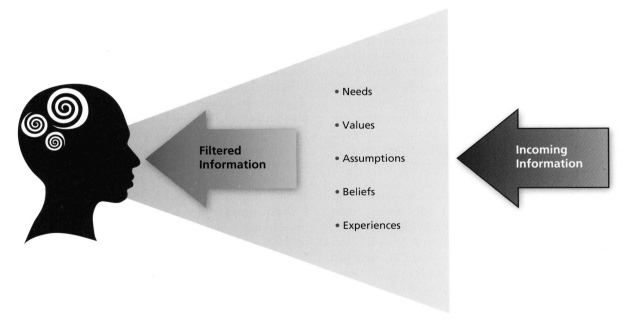

• Needs

• Values

• Assumptions

• Beliefs

• Experiences

Figure 8-5 All of us have individual needs, values, beliefs, attitudes, assumptions, and experiences that become a filter for how we view the world, listen to others, communicate ideas, or feel in certain situations.

communication flows freely. These people have filters colored in a similar hue to our own. At other times, we may find that the ideas we try to communicate cause resistance, distrust, or even anger in another person because the filters are different. For example, the word "alcoholic" carries a particular charge in our society, but each individual still reacts differently. If my mother was an alcoholic and my childhood was disrupted by her behaviors, then I'm likely to feel more emotion in a discussion of alcoholism than another student who has no experience with alcoholism.

To minimize the impact of filters on communication, you can raise your awareness of your own filters and pay attention to the filters you notice in others. Notice the words that cause an emotional change when you hear them. Explore your attitudes. Does a particular situation cause you to become angry or defensive? Why? Seek to better understand the dynamics at play behind an exchange of ideas and information. Simply by remaining alert and listening actively (discussed later), you can minimize the impact of your filters on communication.

Judgment

It is often difficult for people to converse without taking a side on issues being discussed. This need to approve or disapprove, agree or disagree, becomes a barrier to the exchange of ideas. Imagine three massage therapists at a massage clinic having a conversation on their lunch break. One says, "Energetic bodywork is really cool. I went to a workshop this weekend, and the instructor completely released the client's muscle tension by using only holding positions with his hands." The other two therapists immediately make judgments about what they just heard. The second one says, "You're wrong—everyone knows that energetic bodywork is a load of bull." The third says, "I agree that energetic bodywork is effective, but I don't believe it can reduce muscle tension as well as Swedish massage."

The two listeners reacted to the communication of the first by viewing it from their own perspectives and evaluating it as right or wrong, good or bad. This may be a natural tendency, but it sets people up to misunderstand each other, become defensive, and conflict. What if the listeners did not judge the statement as right or wrong, good or bad? What if the second person said, "Really? I haven't heard that. Tell me more about what you know." In this case they potentially could have a real conversation, and all three might learn something new.

"Should" and "Ought"

Some people fall into the habit of defining everything in terms of "should" and "ought." They block communication by promoting their own ideas as the only right thing to do. Phrases like "You should take better care of yourself," "You really ought to do something about that," and "If I were you I wouldn't let her talk to me that way" imply that the speaker is clearly right and the other person does not have the intelligence or fortitude to figure it out. Avoid using words and phrases like "should," "ought," and "if I were you," especially in your role as a massage therapist. Such words increase the

power differential with clients (discussed in Chapter 7) and can lead a client to feel shame or embarrassment. For example, saying, "Your tissue is completely dehydrated—you really ought to take care of yourself and drink more water" sounds moralizing. Just say, "Your tissue feels a bit dehydrated today. Drinking more water after the session will help your body release tension more completely."

The more aware you are of communication, the easier it is to remove unhelpful moralizing statements from your language. When you recognize them in the language of others, you can choose not to react.

Avoid Labels

People also have a natural tendency to label each other, which leads to less understanding. A man in a group might say, "I wish our clinic would do more to conserve energy and recycle. I'm really worried about global warming, and I'm afraid that polar bears will become extinct in my lifetime." Others in the group evaluate his statement from their own perspective (filter). One of them thinks, "I never knew Dmitri was such a left-wing radical." Another says, "Dmitri, you're a big softy, but don't worry, the polar bears will be fine." These two people both just missed an opportunity to know Dimitri better. Instead of asking him more about his concerns and thoughts about how the clinic could conserve energy to help reduce global warming, they labeled him. Instead of seeing, hearing, and honoring him as a complex individual, they reduced him to a "left-wing radical" and a "softy." When people fall into labeling, they often miss the point of the communication and get stuck on the label and how they view it (good or bad, right or wrong). Even labels with positive connotations (hard worker, beauty, intellectual, etc.) can cause fixation and not allow people to be understood as their perfect, imperfect, dynamic, boring, smart, uninformed, multifaceted selves. With labels, people are convinced that they know someone else and lose the opportunity for greater depth of understanding.

Extreme forms of labeling include stereotyping, bigotry, and prejudice, and racism, sexism, and ageism. We would like to think that these do not occur in the massage profession, but they do. In one example, a therapist was very physically fit and ate a vegan diet. He labeled anyone who was not physically fit or vegan as "lazy," "carnivore," "fat," and "undisciplined." His tendency to apply negative labels influenced his interactions with clients, and he was blind to the fact that he behaved unethically as a result. While talking with his supervisor about a client, he commented, "There is no way this person's knee problems are going away without some serious weight loss. Massage is pointless until she gets her act together, goes on a diet, and starts to exercise." How could this therapist do good client-centered work? What about upholding ethical standards like "Do no harm" and "Value the inherent worth of all people"? When did it become his role to decide what is best for clients? In a client-centered therapeutic relationship, clients decide how to best facilitate their own health, and massage is one of many ways to approach wellness. If you find yourself labeling someone, imagine for a moment that the person is a client. How could this label affect your treatment decisions and your ability to provide the client with the best possible care? By developing an understanding of these principles now, you prepare yourself to work with and honor the wide array of clients you will encounter in practice.

Don't Solve the Problem—Just Listen!

Only rarely do people want someone else to solve their problems for them. Usually, people just want someone else to listen while they talk through their problems to arrive at a solution. Problem-solvers block communication and may send others a message that they don't have the experience, knowledge, or understanding to work it out on their own. For example, Erin, a massage therapist, tells Deepti, the clinic owner, "I had a client the other day who asked me out on a date. I told him it was not appropriate for a massage therapist to date her client. He said he understood, and then said he would like to date me and find a different massage therapist. When I told him no, I didn't want a date, and that I would have to end the session if he kept talking about it, he apologized, said he understood my position and wouldn't mention it again. We finished the session without incident. He's a really nice person, and I think he'll respect my feelings and not mention it again, but he called yesterday to book another appointment and I'm not sure what to do." At this point, Erin is about to tell Deepti what she views as her options, but Deepti thinks she has already solved the problem herself. She says, "I'll tell you what to do! You call that jerk up and tell him he's no longer welcome in the clinic! You tell him if you ever see him again, you'll get a restraining order. Oh! Guys like that make me so mad! In fact I'm going to call him right now and cancel all his appointments!" Erin is now in the uncomfortable position of having to defend the client to Deepti and to calm Deepti down. When did the conversation become about Deepti and the types of men she doesn't like? Deepti didn't give Erin the chance to work it out for herself, and now Erin wishes she hadn't told Deepti about the client. Instead of rushing in to "solve" Erin's problem, Deepti could have promoted conversation and sharing by simply saying, "What do you plan to do?"

Equalizing—When It's Bad, Let It Be Bad!

Sometimes things happen to people that seem unfair. People who equalize always try to see the bright side of a situation to balance out anything negative with a positive. While there is nothing wrong with cultivating a positive attitude to life's ups and downs, this can block communication when it doesn't allow the person who is feeling bad to process his or her emotions (Fig. 8-6). For example, a young man visits a massage therapist two years after recovering from a serious car accident. During the health intake interview, he opens up and talks about his concern that he will never be able to race road bikes again. His neck and shoulders still give him problems

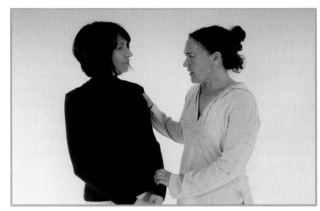

Figure 8-6 It's not always best to "look on the bright side" of a situation, as doing so can block communication when a person who is feeling down needs to process emotions. When it's bad, let it be bad.

caused by the neck injury he sustained in the car accident, and when he rides they ache so badly he has to stop. The therapist shakes his head in sympathy and says, "Yeah, but at least you can walk. You must feel glad about that."

People often work through emotionally painful things by talking with friends, grieving, and eventually finding a way to either change or accept the situation and adapt. People find their own way through grief. The therapist in this case needed only to hear and understand the biker's concerns. He could have said something as simple as, "Oh man, that's tough! How many minutes can you ride before the pain flares up?"

Psychoanalyzing

Popular psychology and self-help books lead some people to fall into pseudo-psychoanalysis, which blocks honest and open communication. Someone psychoanalyzing generally breaks into conversations to say things like "You seem really defensive right now, so take a deep breath—you need to breathe!" or "Your lateness was a sign of your hostility toward your client—perhaps you should take some anger management classes" or "It sounds like you were projecting your feelings onto the client. No wonder it went badly." A person with this habit tends to judge others' behavior as good or bad, right or wrong, and tries to diagnose their "psychological" shortcomings, thereby falling into judging and labeling.

Inappropriate Reassurance

Sometimes, people feel downhearted about some aspect of themselves or their lives because they haven't lived up to their own expectations. It is natural to want to reassure a friend, loved one, or client but sometimes reassurance becomes a communication blocker. For example, Kathy failed her anatomy exam and was sharing her feelings with Ichiro. She said, "I've just been so lazy and uncommitted, it's no wonder I failed that test!" Ichiro replied, "You're not lazy and not uncommitted—that test was really hard and you are perfect just the way you are." Kathy was exploring her feelings, but Ichiro sidetracked her. She had a moment of personal honesty and had recognized that she had been lazy and uncommitted to her studies. What she really needed was to feel those feelings and then seek to understand why she had been lazy and uncommitted. Ichiro reassured her, but now she doesn't feel better because she is no closer to solving the problem. Ichiro could have simply said, "Why do you feel you have been lazy and uncommitted?" This would have given Kathy a chance to explore the situation freely.

Empathy Versus Sympathy

Empathy is the ability to identify with and understand another person's feelings and difficulties. People who are empathetic for others can "live in their skin," "stand in their shoes," "see through their eyes," and "feel their emotions." Empathic people are nonjudgmental, open-minded, and understanding because they can see the situation from the other person's point of view and comprehend how the situation impacts that person's life. They say things like, "Wow, I can see why you are so upset about that, I would be upset too." Sympathy, on the other hand, can be a communication blocker when one person expresses pity or sorrow for the pain or distress of someone else. It puts the sympathizer in a more powerful position and weakens the other's position, because the sympathizer can think and say, "Oh, poor, poor you! I'm so glad my partner doesn't treat me that way" or "I feel so sorry for you! That must be so humiliating!" Receiving sympathy usually makes people feel uncomfortable and defensive. Instead of being able to simply feel and express their emotions, they are now in the position of defending their life.

In addition to the communication blockers described above, relating styles, learning styles, and mental processes can also cause communication to break down. If someone has a strongly aggressive relating style, others will grow weary of feeling unheard and may shut off communication with that person. We must remember that people take in information and order their worlds differently. Awareness and patience are vital. Great communicators overcome these differences in style and find ways to relate to most people.

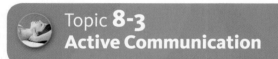

Topic 8-3
Active Communication

Active communication requires three primary skills: awareness, active listening, and the ability to communicate your message. With these skills, communication becomes more interesting and more informative. Each of these primary skills involves smaller, more specific skills. In a professional massage practice, all of these skills are integrated to communicate effectively and professionally with clients (Fig. 8-7).

Awareness

Is someone sharing too much and not allowing others in the group to express their ideas? Is someone sharing too little and not contributing because of anxiety or resentment? Is the environment conducive to a comfortable exchange? Active communication requires give and take as well as attentiveness to both one's own needs and other people's needs. In a shared conversation, people monitor their input and pay attention to

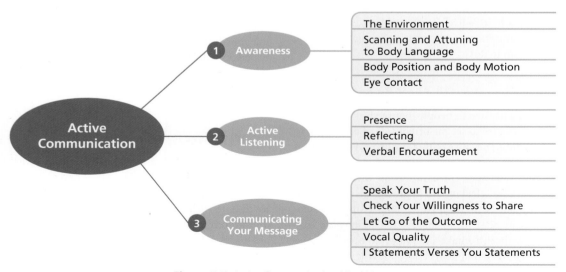

Figure 8-7 Active Communication Mind Map.

body language, the environment, and moment-by-moment changes in interpersonal dynamics.

The Environment

The environment where conversation takes place can facilitate a successful exchange or impede it. Environmental distractions should be eliminated or kept to a minimum. If you are trying to hold an important conversation with a friend or family member, you would turn off the TV, music system, and telephones, and close doors to eliminate noise from other rooms. Newspapers, notebooks, magazines, and other reading materials would be put aside. In a massage office, large pieces of furniture, like a desk, create a physical barrier that may prevent free and easy sharing. If you talk to a client in an office, come out from behind the desk and sit on the same side of the desk as the client to minimize this distraction. Attempt to sit at the same height as your client. One person sitting higher than the other creates a subconscious power differential that makes it more difficult to feel open and equal. Sit at a comfortable distance from the other person. Friends and family members may sit close together, but in most other instances three feet of distance is appropriate.[2] As a matter of confidentiality, all conversations with clients that pertain to their health or status should be conducted in a private space. When the environment is free of distractions, people can better gather and convey their thoughts and listen to the thoughts of others.

Scanning and Being Attuned to Body Language

Scanning involves placing yourself in an objective state and using your senses to take in emotional, physical, and instinctive information about yourself, others, and the environment. Some people scan naturally. These people can walk into a party and know who feels anxious, who feels left out, who is having a great time, and who feels bored, simply by looking around the room. Part of the skill of scanning is tuning into nonverbal communication such as body language (Fig. 8-8).

Body language is thought to be the earliest form of human communication, used long before spoken or written language developed.[3] Most people have some skill at reading body language, although they may not be aware of it. A listener's attentiveness to a speaker's body language can reinforce that what the speaker is saying is true, can alert the listener to an inconsistency between what the speaker says and truly feels, or can tell the listener that the speaker is not verbalizing something important.

Imagine that you are conducting a health intake interview with an elderly client who was dropped at your office by a protective daughter. You ask the client if he is taking over-the-counter pain medications for his shoulder issues. He hesitates and crosses his arms over his chest, averts his eyes, and says, "No." Something is up. What he's saying does not completely coincide with his body language. You decide to question him further about pain medications and find out that his daughter gets upset when he uses them regularly. You reassure him that his daughter will not see his health history forms, and he uncrosses his arms, looks you in the eye, and says, "Then yes.

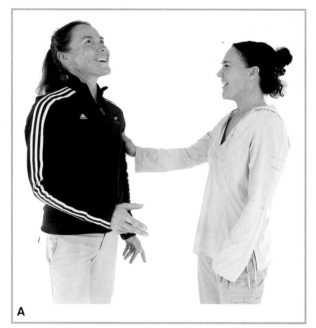

A

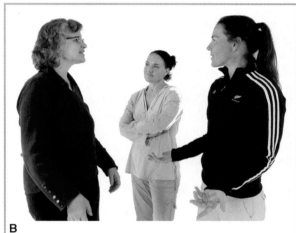

B

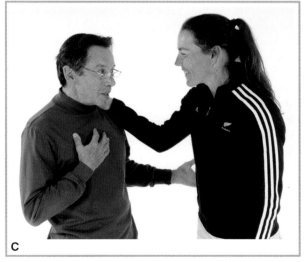

C

Figure 8-8 Each person comes into a situation feeling a certain way. Being attuned to body language gives us clues about how a person is feeling.

I have taken pain medication today." Your attunement to body language helped you realize that the situation needed further investigation that could protect this client from receiving techniques that are too deep for his tissue.

Body language includes vocal cues like the pace and volume of words, facial expressions, body positions, and gestures. A person who speaks slowly, mumbles, or uses a low pitch and volume may be feeling sad. A person who speaks quickly and in a higher pitch is more likely to be excited or enthusiastic about something. Abrupt speech indicates that the speaker may feel defensive. Tense, rapid, loud speech indicates anger. Facial expressions are many and varied but certain patterns hold generally. A flushed face and misty eyes often indicate the person is experiencing a deep emotion. Annoyance or anger is generally expressed with narrowed eyes, tense features, and a flushed face. Widened eyes, a relaxed jaw, and soft, open mouth indicate receptiveness, enjoyment, affection, or enthusiasm.

Often a person's fleeting facial expressions tell others that the person is not openly expressing true feelings. For example, a person might listen to her colleague in a meeting with a fixed smile on her mouth and then roll her eyes without realizing it, thereby expressing her true annoyance or impatience with the topic. People who are angry may hold their body in a tense, highly alert posture, while people who are feeling sad cave in the chest and tend to look down more often. People can improve their scanning and skill for reading body language by paying attention to their own reactions to situations as well as the reactions of others. When others are having an argument, watchers often hold their bodies in alert positions, tighten their stomachs, and tense their faces. They are reading and mirroring the body language of the people in conflict.

Body Position and Body Motion

Being aware of body language helps you hold your body in a position that encourages another to share and that helps the other take a position that encourages listening. An open body position invites a person to reveal information, while a closed body position discourages interaction. In an open body position, you face the other squarely while sitting at the same height. You lean forward slightly and uncross your arms and legs. When listening, your body movements respond to what the other is saying. You might nod your head to show understanding or lean forward at certain moments to indicate anticipation. These positions and movements tell the other that you are comfortable and interested in hearing the information.

In a closed body position, the listener turns the body slightly so that the chest and abdomen are shifted away from the talker. A closed body position indicates weariness about sharing or a lack of confidence. Slumping in one's seat or leaning the body backward is another sign of disinterest or discouragement. When conversations get heated, people often fold their arms over their chests. This is a defensive position that physically closes off the listener and speaker. Distracted or disinterested listeners move their body in a way that is out

of sync with the speaker's body. They might flip a pen in their hands, crack their knuckles, search for something in a bag, fiddle with an object on a table, cross and uncross their legs, or shift their weight often.

In *People Skills: How to Assert Yourself, Listen to Others and Resolve Conflicts,* Robert Bolton shares a story about Allen Ivey and John Hinkle, who trained six students in good listening behaviors. The students began a class taught by a visiting professor in non-listening body positions, slumped in their chairs and with crossed arms and legs. The visiting professor read his lecture from note cards and did not use gestures or interact with students. When signaled, the students assumed good listening positions, nodded at the instructor's comments, and actively listened. The instructor then began to use gestures within a half a minute of the change, his speaking speed increased, and he began looking directly at the students. The lecture improved, and soon a lively discussion was taking place.[4]

During conversations, classroom lectures, and discussions, think about your body position and body movements. Seek to place yourself in the best position to encourage the other person and exchange the best possible quality of information. If you practice often enough, good body positioning will become second nature and you will naturally use good body positioning when talking with clients as a professional massage therapist.

Eye Contact

The eyes help one understand the feeling and intent of another's message because they are continually gathering nonverbal data consciously and subconsciously. Facial expressions, hand gestures, and breathing patterns help convey the speaker's feelings behind the words. Good eye contact can be difficult to achieve, especially with new acquaintances or colleagues, because eye contact creates an instant intimacy that sometimes feels uncomfortable. With good eye contact, you gaze at the other person's face, might look down briefly to follow a hand gesture, and then come back to the face. Avoid staring intently or blankly, or keeping your eyes down or averted. A lack of eye contact can feel hostile, indifferent, or submissive.

Active Listening

Active listening involves encouraging the sharing of information, gathering the information conveyed by another person, interpreting and understanding the information, reflecting the information back to the sharer, and remembering what is said. Passive listening refers to a state where you are awake and your ears are working properly but you are not fully involved in what the speaker is communicating. Table 8-2 contrasts active and passive listening. Many psychologists comment that our society tends to teach people to be non-listeners.[5] This begins at home when parents give non-listening messages or model non-listening behaviors. When a parent comes home wanting to discuss something that happened at work, the other parent may model non-listening by continuing to watch TV and giving only half-hearted

TABLE 8-2   Active Versus Passive Listening

Active Listening	Passive Listening
• Willing to listen (being "present")	• Distracted, not fully present
• Attuned to body language cues	• Misses body language cues
• Open body position	• Closed or slumped body position
• Body motions in sync with speaker	• Body motions out sync with speaker
• Good eye contact	• Inconsistent or little eye contact
• Removes or diminishes environmental distractions	• Distracted by things in the environment
• Uses short verbal interjections to encourage speaker	• Interrupts the speaker or asks questions that take the speaker off track
• Reflects thoughts and feelings of the speaker back to the speaker	• Does not reflect thoughts and feelings of the speaker back to the speaker
• Is aware of communication blockers and seeks to avoid them	• Regularly uses communication blockers without awareness

responses. Non-listening is also taught at school where too much lecture time in early classrooms teach young students to tune out while the teacher is talking. Schools rarely teach how to listen and communicate with other people, even though we all need these skills to succeed. Furthermore, because the world is noisy and distracting, people have learned to tune out anything that does not actively excite their interest. Good listening skills are imperative to gather knowledge from classroom lectures, participate in class discussions, build strong relationships with friends and loved ones, and facilitate a safe and professional massage practice.

Presence

Some people find it easy to be present with other people, tune out everything else around them, and focus only on the person who is talking. This focused attitude builds trust and openness so that deeper and more meaningful communication can take place. Sometimes people are not willing to listen to someone else or listen only half-heartedly because they are weary of what is being said or because they would rather give their attention to something else. Sometimes people automatically feel guarded or on the attack when a particular person approaches. The first skill to cultivate in active listening is "presence," the ability to deliberately focus on the listener to the exclusion of all else. Pay attention to your ability to tune into other people and notice if you feel guarded, on the attack, bored, weary, or any other emotion while they speak. Simply by being more aware, you will have more control over your listening attitude. Jen tells the story of how she learned presence with her husband. "I would come home each night from work complaining about my boss or coworkers, and I couldn't understand why he was always so withdrawn. One day he blurted out, 'You're always in a bad mood. You never stop to ask how my day is, and you complain all night about your job. If you hate it that much, get a new job. I don't feel like we have anything real to say to each other.' I thought hard about what he said, and I started practicing 'losing my mood'

at the door. I would take three deep breaths and enter the door as positive, fun Jen. Then I would ask about his day and really listen. Gradually he shared more and more information about his day, and then I could talk about my problems with my boss and he would give me good feedback. It was an easy change to make, and it changed the dynamic of our relationship, just that one little thing."

Practice presence with a friend or loved one and with your classmates at school when you perform massage exchanges. If you can learn to hone your presence now, you will be more prepared to interact with clients in an effective manner later.

Reflecting

Earlier we discussed how people develop a view of the world based on their past experiences and upbringing. This perspective is a filter through which information must pass before the person accepts or rejects it. This is one reason that communication often goes astray. Speakers give information through their filters, and listeners hear it through their own filters. Somewhere between the two filters the pure content of the information can be lost. Reflecting is a method that can be used to overcome the confusion caused by these filters.

Reflecting is a listening skill with which the listener gathers information conveyed by the speaker and then summarizes the information in a brief phrase back to the speaker. This technique ensures that the listener really understands what the speaker means, while confirming for the speaker that the listener has understood the message. The first key to good reflecting is to keep the summary brief and reflect only the essential message, free of details and descriptive phrases. A reflective summary should also be stated in the listener's own words, not the words of the speaker. This demonstrates that the listener understands the information well enough to paraphrase it. If Mariana is discussing a career option with Francisco, she might say, "I don't know how I feel about working on a cruise ship. I always saw myself working in a hospice with elderly people, and that still really appeals to me. Then again, I want to travel, and this might be one way to do it. But Dana said she did so many massages everyday when she worked on a cruise ship that she was too exhausted to see anything on her day off, so maybe that's not the way to travel. Then again, she was able to get a free cruise vacation for her mother. I'm feeling really confused and I need to decide soon." Francisco might reflect back to Mariana, "I think you're saying that you really want to travel but you're not sure this is the right massage job for you." If Mariana says "Yes," "That's right," or "Exactly," Francisco knows he's on target. If Francisco is off target, on the other hand, Mariana is likely to say, "No, not really, it's more like…" and can then clear up the misunderstanding. One of the chief benefits of reflecting is that misunderstandings are cleared up immediately. Reflective statements also help speakers view their own thoughts through another person's filter. This sometimes gives speakers a more objective viewpoint from which to contemplate their own ideas. Francisco may have helped Mariana to see that her career goals and travel goals are very separate.

Reflecting also helps speakers better understand their feelings. A listener pays attention to the speaker's words but also to body language and facial expression. The listener "reads" the speaker's emotion and reflects that emotion to the speaker. For example, Mariana might say to Francisco, "I'm so sad I didn't take that job at the hospital when it was offered to me. It was such a fantastic opportunity, but I was too worried about commuting in traffic. Now Sarah has that job, and she says it will become a full-time position next year. It makes me want to cry, it really does." As Mariana says this, Francisco notices that her fists are clenched and her face is flushed. Her movements are agitated, but she doesn't look as if she is going to cry. Francisco reflects to Mariana, "You don't seem sad. Is that what you're really feeling or is it something else?" Mariana stomps her foot, "You're right, I'm mad! How could I be so stupid?" Now Mariana is closer to understanding how she really feels, processing those feelings and moving toward a resolution.

Verbal Encouragement

Verbal encouragement includes questions a listener asks, sounds made while listening, and even attentive silence. A loved one, friend, or client often needs encouragement in order to feel safe sharing feelings and experiences. Something about what speakers want to share may show in their body language and facial expressions. Speakers with great news might beam or grin. Speakers who are angry might have a flushed face and tense expression. Speakers who are feeling downhearted may drag their feet and hunch their shoulders. It's important to read the person's body language and use verbal encouragement that is free of judgment, reassurance, or advice. Regardless of the situation, people usually just want to be heard and understood. When the listener makes a judgment, offers reassurance, or offers unwanted advice, this causes the speaker to withdraw instead of opening up and sharing feelings. For example, the verbal opener, "What happened to you? You look like someone ran over your dog!" sounds cynical, while "Look on the bright side, by tomorrow

you'll feel better" attempts to be reassuring but really just shuts off the chance for the other to process emotions. Greeting a friend with "What did you do now?!" or "Don't tell me you're depressed again!" is unlikely to inspire trust and sharing. Instead, a listener can demonstrate interest in the other person with an open body position and an invitation to talk. For example, say, "You look like things are not going so well, do you want to tell me about it?" or "You're beaming! What are you so excited about? Tell me!" Both of these examples describe the other person's body language as a way to open the conversation without making judgments.

Once the speaker begins sharing, the listener may demonstrate interest by periods of attentive silence or by brief verbal interjections that demonstrate understanding. You can listen without agreeing with the speaker, while still encouraging the other to talk. For example, verbal interjections like "Really?" or "Go on" or "And then?" or "I'm listening" provide space for the speaker to keep exploring ideas. Sometimes you may agree and briefly interject phrases such as "That makes sense" or "Yes, I understand why you would think that" to encourage the speaker and build trust that there is mutual understanding. Avoid lengthy questions or questions that require the speaker to jump ahead in the narrative. Such interjections tend to take speakers off track and prevent communicating their story in their own way.

Box 8-2 provides a checklist of good listening skills.

Communicating Your Message

Just as good listening skills are important, so too are good speaking skills. All people can benefit from learning how to speak their truth directly with good body language and vocal control. As a professional massage therapist, you can use these interpersonal skills to better communicate your policies and regulations to clients, to establish solid therapeutic boundaries, and to use appropriate self-disclosure as discussed in Chapter 6.

Speak the Truth

As noted previously, people are always communicating their true feelings with their body, even when their words

BOX 8-2 Good Listening Checklist

✓ I am present and willing to listen.
✓ I eliminate or minimize distractions.
✓ I am attuned to the speaker's body language.
✓ My body position is open and receptive.
✓ My body motions are in sync with the speaker.
✓ My eye contact is consistent.
✓ I use short verbal interjections to encourage the speaker.
✓ I reflect the meaning of the communication back to the speaker when appropriate.
✓ I reflect the speaker's feelings back when appropriate.
✓ I am aware of communication blockers and avoid them.

say something different. There are numerous reasons why people don't always "tell it like it is." Some are afraid they won't get what they want, others feel ashamed to express their true needs and desires, while others don't want to deal with messy emotions. Sometimes a person believes that the other can't handle the truth and so tries to skirt or avoid the issue. Oftentimes, differences in personality, filters, or learning styles cause misunderstandings, and the speaker fears the listener's feelings will be hurt or their friendship jeopardized. Although occasionally it may be better to conceal the truth, learning to speak directly and honestly is an important step toward assertive relating.

It is important to build your awareness of when you don't speak your truth and to identify why not. As you're speaking, step outside yourself and listen to what you're saying. If you can, pause and redirect your communication to make it more truthful. This can be as simple as saying, "Wait, I'm not being as honest as I want to be because I don't want to hurt your feelings. The truth is…" Sometimes you may find that you are not ready to speak your truth, and you carry on an entire conversation skirting the issue, telling small untruths, or lying outright. Again, think about what you said, why you said it, and how it all turned out, and then vow to be more honest in the future.

Check Your Willingness to Share

To share, a person must feel willing and able to relate something to someone else. Notice the way your body feels as you contemplate sharing your message and the attitude you hold toward the listener. Are your arms crossed over your chest? Are your face and eyes averted? Do you feel mistrust, hostility, or weariness toward the listener? These signs clearly tell you that you don't feel ready to share the message. If your body is in an open position and you are making eye contact with the listener, you more likely feel ready to share.

Let Go of the Outcome

Notice if you are fixed on the direction you think the conversation should take. Starting a conversation with a predetermined outcome in mind usually prevents free and open communication. With predetermined outcomes, a person is more likely to get emotionally attached and defensive if the conversation goes astray, or this predetermination prevents the possibility of a better outcome that the person might not have thought of. It helps to hold a wish for an open and positive outcome in your mind. Say to yourself, "I am going to communicate directly and honestly and trust that a fair and positive outcome results from this conversation."

Vocal Quality

When speaking, think about what your tone of voice says about how you think and feel. Do you state your message directly, enunciating the words in a clear tone, or do you speak very slowly or rapidly, mumble, or loudly and aggressively? As you relate your message, choose your words and tone appropriately, and watch for submissive or aggressive relating behaviors. It's also important to monitor how much you say before allowing the other to contribute to the conversation. When you pay attention to your communication methods, you can identify areas of weakness and develop new skills.

I-Statements Versus You-Statements

I-statements are messages that share how a person feels about something. Such messages help the listener comprehend how the situation impacts the speaker. They also provide an opportunity for both to understand the consequences of the situation and to explore new possibilities. Here is an example of an I-statement: "When I'm told my draping is bad but not given an explanation, it makes me feel angry and mistrustful [sharing one's feelings and stating the impact]. It causes me to doubt our ability to work well together [stating the consequences]. I would prefer it if I was told one way to make my draping skills better [stating the ideal behavior]."

You-statements use shaming, blaming, judgmental, or hurtful language in an attempt to "win" the situation. They don't address how the person feels, the impact of the situation, or opportunities for better ways of relating. Following is a you-statement: "You're telling me my draping skills are bad when it was you who couldn't figure out a side-lying drape last week!" Clearly, this conversation is not going to be very productive and neither student's draping skills will improve. This conversation will lead to more hurtful words and a further breakdown of trust and respect.

The use of I-statements requires self-awareness and a willingness to control one's attachment to words and one's emotions. It takes some practice to remain objective and prevent an impulsive emotional reaction. All I-statements follow the same format: When _____ occurs I feel _____. This results in _____. Instead I prefer _____.

General Guidelines for Communication with Clients

All the core communication skills described so far in this chapter are involved in therapists' interactions with their clients. Clients respond to therapists who treat them as

Concept Brief 8-2
Communicating Your Message

Feel willing to share

Speak your truth

Use I-statements

Assert yourself

State your expectations

Provide a rationale

Describe the consequences

Identify obstacles

Clarify the future

equals, speak to them honestly, and include them in the planning process.

Therapists must also practice being responsive to clients' needs. For example, it is not professional to make a client wait for 2 days before returning a phone call. Return phone calls within 24 hours. Therapists regularly require 24 hours' notice from clients to cancel an appointment. They must show the same respect for clients and give them 24 hours' notice when rescheduling is needed.

Therapists should never use profanity or slang words when speaking with clients and should strive for good English language. Eliminate the "yep," "nope," "like," "kinda," "ya-know," and "yeah-sure" from your professional interactions. Although you use medical terminology with peers and other health care providers, always be careful to speak in everyday words to clients. For example, the client is unlikely to know what the cubital fossa is. Instead, use the phrase "inner elbow" when talking to the client.

Key Areas of Client Communication

Communication plays a primary role in 10 areas of working with clients. Each is described below as an overview of the types of therapist–client communication that take place throughout the total massage experience, even though you may not yet understand the intricacies of each stage in the complete client interaction. Appropriate aspects of communication at various times are discussed further in later chapters detailing these different stages.

1. **Introduction to the Massage Business:** Some potential clients will learn about your massage business from friends or family members. Others see your marketing information on a web site, brochure, or display ad. Some may hear you speak at a health food store or health fair or meet you at an event on your premises such as an open house. In all cases, strive to communicate your philosophy of health and wellness clearly and define the parameters of your skills and areas of expertise.

2. **The Booking Phone Call:** When you speak to a new client the first time, you are performing three major tasks. You inform clients about policies like your draping policy, no-show policy, and required paperwork. You are also screening clients to ensure they are seeking massage for legitimate reasons. Finally, encourage clients to ask questions so that you can allay any fears or apprehensions about the massage.

3. **Introductions:** Before the intake interview and massage session, introduce yourself and share your credentials with the client. At this time, the client forms a first impression and consciously or subconsciously evaluates your appearance, manner of speech, level of knowledge, and capability. Explain your intake forms to the client in a clear, concise manner.

4. **Intake Interview:** After the client has completed the intake forms, you discuss this information together to make a plan for the session. You use several communication skills for a successful intake experience. You need to describe the benefits and limitations of massage as well as appropriate policies, procedures, rules, and regulations. Through your communication style, you establish rapport with the client. Rapport is mutual trust and understanding. If you have not established your credibility and trustworthiness, the client may not relax completely and experience the full benefit of the session.

   While talking over the completed health intake form, ask the client appropriate health questions to ensure that it is safe for the client to receive massage. You need to know what questions to ask and how to ask them in such a way that the client is encouraged to share additional relevant information. Finally, discuss with the client the goals for the session and together make a treatment plan.

5. **Monitor the Client's Experience:** During the massage, ask the client for feedback about the techniques being used, the client's comfort with the room temperature and draping procedures, and how muscles are responding to the massage strokes. Articulate these questions clearly, interpret the client's answers, remain responsive to the client's needs, and adapt appropriately.

6. **Receive Feedback:** After the session, ask the client for honest feedback, receive the feedback objectively, and plan to make appropriate adaptations in your techniques or session enhancers.

7. **Maintain Boundaries:** Before, during, and after the session, maintain well-defined boundaries and communicate these to clients as the need arises. In certain instances, you may need to confront a client, resolve a misunderstanding, and create a plan to improve your therapist–client relationship in the future.

8. **Follow Up:** When you follow up with clients to check on the results they experienced, ask good, leading questions. Use the information you receive to adapt future sessions to better meet clients' needs.

9. **Documentation:** Communication skills include properly documenting every session and keeping up-to-date records. This written information includes vital details about the techniques used and the client's response.

10. **Confidentiality and Privacy:** Therapists must practice confidentiality with all client information and always protect the client's privacy. These policies should also be communicated to clients.

Assertive Communication with Clients

Assertive people communicate their ideas, values, opinions, and feelings in an appropriate, direct manner, without encroaching on other people. Communicating assertively (rather than passively or aggressively) is an important skill, especially when working with clients. Assertive communication is clear, direct, and honest and carries a minimum of emotional overtones. In contrast, submissive communication involves hints of inadequacy, an inability to cope, and low self-esteem. Submissive speakers depreciate themselves and minimize ownership or responsibility. Aggressive communication has antagonistic, defensive, and hostile overtones. It suggests deep-seated fears and a strong attachment to ideas. Compare the following examples:

- **Assertive communicator:** "Afternoon appointments start promptly at 1:00 PM and end exactly at 2:00. I'm afraid you missed some of your appointment time."
- **Submissive communicator:** "Oh no, you're late! I'm really sorry but I have to end the appointment at 2:00 because I will get in trouble if I don't. I hope that's okay with you."
- **Aggressive communicator:** "You're late again and my other clients will manage to be on time so I won't be able to give you the entire hour."

Clear, assertive communication leads to fewer misunderstandings, hurt feelings, or angry responses. When dealing with minor conflicts, use the following process for assertive communication:

1. **State your expectations:** Let the client (or other person) know what you expect without using language that makes him feel judged or shamed. If a client refuses to fill in a health history form and says that you do not need to know this personal health information to perform a massage, you might say assertively, "The policy at Sundance Massage Clinic is that we conduct a through health history intake process before we provide a massage to a client." Remember to avoid judging language. A therapist with an aggressive communication style might say, in contrast, "If you're going to be a client here, you must behave properly and fill out the form like everyone else. You are wasting your massage time by making a fuss." That would likely inflame the client and lead to further difficulties.

2. **Provide a rationale:** People like to know the reasons for things and why they should meet someone else's expectations. You might say assertively, "It's important to conduct a through health intake process to rule out conditions or medications that might make massage unsafe for you to receive. The purpose is to ensure our clients' safety and comfort." Again, your tone should be unemotional and factual. In contrast, a passive communicator might say, "Fill out the form real fast and I'll give you an extra five minutes of massage to make up for it." Now this client will expect an extra 5 minutes of massage every session. This therapist has let the client know that policies can be violated.

3. **Describe consequences:** Sometimes you must describe the consequences of a behavior, in order to establish how sessions will run in the future. Assertively, you might say, "I cannot provide a massage unless the health form is finished accurately and completely." In contrast, an aggressive communicator might inflame the client by stating, "If you want a massage, you have to finish the form just like everyone else."

4. **Identify obstacles:** Sometimes clients (and other people) have obstacles that make it difficult for them to meet the expectations of others. As an assertive communicator, ask clients if there are obstacles and invite them to share their views. You might say, "Can you explain why you would prefer not to fill in the health history form?" It may be as simple as the client saying. "I don't really mind filling out the form, but I forgot my glasses and I can't read a word of it." In this case, the solution is easy: you can read the form to the client and fill in the answers. More complex issues often require some negotiation between you and the client.

5. **Clarify the future:** It is a good idea to summarize the conversation and confirm the plan. You might say, "I think I understand you now. You will fill in the form if I will read it to you?" The client agrees, and you can now proceed with the massage session with no hard feelings between you.

Concept Brief 8-3
Communication with Clients

Treat clients as equals
Be honest, clear and direct
Include clients in planning for sessions
Respond to clients' needs in a timely manner
Avoid slang and profanity
Speak in everyday words

General Guidelines for Communication with Health Care Providers

Chapter 1 described the increasing public interest in complementary and alternative medicine (CAM). This has led to a more integrated health care system in which health care professionals are forming alliances to better support clients in achieving wellness goals. Physicians, naturopathic doctors, herbalists, midwives, physical therapists, chiropractors, traditional Chinese medicine (TCM) practitioners, acupuncturists, nutritional experts, fitness trainers, and counselors are just some of the other health care professionals with whom a massage therapist might interact.

When communicating with other health care professionals, use proper health care terminology and avoid profanity and slang. While you might say "inner elbow" with clients, use the anatomically appropriate term "cubital fossa" with health care professionals. Appendix A introduces health care–related terminology. Embrace this terminology early in your training program and use it when speaking with classmates and instructors. By building and strengthening this vocabulary, you are preparing not only for better grades but for a professional career.

Understanding the work of different health care professionals enhances your ability to communicate effectively. If you meet a TCM doctor and do not know anything about TCM, it may be difficult to strike up a meaningful conversation. On the other hand, if you do know something about TCM, you can ask relevant questions and make comparisons to the results achieved by massage. As a professional massage therapist, you will develop a referral list of other health care professionals who might benefit your clients. For example, you would not counsel a client experiencing depression because this is out of your scope of practice. You could, however, refer the client to a psychotherapist or counselor for help. Similarly, you would want that psychotherapist or counselor to refer clients to you for massage. It is therefore important to help other health care professionals understand massage and its benefits. Some therapists provide a free massage to health care professionals they want to work with, so that they experience the benefits of massage firsthand. You might also join a local wellness organization, take part in health fairs, or volunteer to provide massage to local hospital staff once a month. All of these activities help you build your connections and your knowledge to better support your clients.

Students sometimes feel uncomfortable when they start practicing active communication skills, especially when beginning to interact with clients. A heightened awareness of body position requires some concentration at first. Learning to interject reflective summaries may also feel disjointed and forced at first. But if you persist in learning and use these skills now, they will feel natural and easy by the time you begin work with clients and meet other health care providers.

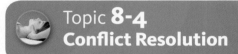

Topic 8-4
Conflict Resolution

Even with good communication skills, conflicts sometimes occur. Rarely is either person "right" or "wrong" in a conflict. The tension usually results from personality differences, value clashes, divergent views of a situation, fears over personal objectives and interests, misinformation, or misunderstandings. The different ways that people deal with conflict may lead to even more strain. Some people do nothing, hoping the problem goes away, or they give in and accept changes made by someone else until the tension builds again, leading to more conflict. One person might simply avoid another, or ask a higher authority to handle the problem. Some people fight and argue aggressively. When people's views are opposing, they tend to attach strongly to words and fix themselves in their dominant relating style. People with an aggressive relating style become loud, angry, and threatening, make personal attacks, and are determined to win at any cost. People with a submissive relating style fall back on sabotaging techniques and are unlikely to openly attack their opposition unless cornered. Instead they gather other people around them to support their cause and use gossip and sometimes slander to manipulate a win. None of these actions results in an equitable resolution. In contrast, an assertive person remains open and listens during a conflict. While some of the other person's words might trigger a reaction, assertive people monitor their own thinking and do not attach to the words. They take responsibility for their part in the conflict and participate in a fair **conflict resolution** process.

Avoid Attachment to Words

While others are sharing their views, notice if you begin to attach to words and react emotionally. Practice self-control, and use your heightened level of self-awareness to gain greater clarity. Inga accused Emma of stealing her clients while she was sick. She said, "The moment I'm down, you sneak in and try to steal my clients. You're completely unethical, and you shouldn't be allowed to work here! You make me sick!" Emma listened to Inga and was aware of wanting to attach to the words "stealing" and "unethical" and the tendency to fight back by saying something mean about Inga's skill level. Instead, she took a deep breath and said in a calm, even tone, "Inga, I can see that you are very upset with me [acknowledging and reflecting Inga's feelings]. I think it's because I worked on Mr. Smith while you were out sick, and he scheduled with me again this week. Is that right? Is that why you're upset?" In this way, Emma refused to respond to Inga's attack but instead asked Inga to focus on the specific problem (Mr. Smith). Watching your own thinking helps you remain objective and avoid responding with a counterattack.

Sometimes one or both conflicting parties are very upset and use threatening, mean-spirited language. In this situation, it is unlikely that the conversation can be productive. It's then okay to say, "This conversation feels threatening. I really want to hear what you have to say, and I really want to work this out, but I think we should discuss this when we both calm down."

Listen Carefully

During a conflict, it is important to listen carefully and allow the other person to finish talking. Using a reflective summary to make sure you understand the other's message helps the other person feel heard. Use a phrase like this: "What I heard you say is…." A person who feels understood is more likely to calm down and listen to other viewpoints. If the other interrupts your reflective summary, it's okay to say in a calm and nonjudgmental tone, "Excuse me, I would like to finish my thought. I want to hear what you have to say, but I was responding to your last statement and I haven't had a chance to finish."

Attack the Problem and Not Each Other

Because conflict is emotional, people often attack each other instead of the problem. In the example above, Inga made a personal attack on Emma by calling her unethical and a thief. Emma redirected the conversation by clearly identifying the problem and stating it objectively. Stay focused on the problem and avoid calling a person names or making a personal attack during a conflict. With self-control, you keep your personal integrity and professionalism intact.

Accept Responsibility

Both parties likely played some role in creating any conflict. When people accept responsibility for their portion of the problem, it is easier to reach a fair resolution. In the example above, Emma knew that Mr. Smith had booked an appointment with her 3 days before Inga found out. Emma could have called Inga earlier to explain the situation. Instead, Inga came to work and found that the hour usually reserved for Mr. Smith was open and that his name was on Emma's schedule. Emma might have said, "Inga, I should have called you the moment I knew that Mr. Smith was on my schedule and discussed it with you." In that way Emma would have demonstrated that she was willing to accept responsibility for her part of the misunderstanding.

Use Direct Communication

When making a point, use I-statements to prevent the defensiveness people feel when you-statements are used. Sometimes in conflicts, people enlist the help of others rather than deal with the conflict directly. They might complain or gossip about the person with whom they have a conflict. Sometimes when this happens, the other person doesn't even know there is a problem. Part of professional communication is the willingness to resolve your own grievances without involving other people.

If this is impossible, you may ask a mediator, such as a mentor, instructor, or clinic owner, to help resolve the issue fairly.

Seek an Equitable Solution

To resolve the conflict, both people should consider how they will act and relate to each other in the future. When people strive to find an equitable solution, one where everyone wins, relationships generally improve in the future. If one person has an upper hand, however, or if one person likes the outcome while the other feels browbeaten, more conflict will likely occur in the future.

Conflict may develop quickly, or tensions may grow over time into a problem. A conflict resolution worksheet helps a person prepare to resolve the conflict through conversation or mediation. Review the worksheet shown in Table 8-3. This worksheet is also useful for preventing conflicts, as it helps a person understand and address tensions that might be percolating under the surface.

Concept Brief 8-4
Conflict Resolution

- **To resolve conflicts:**
  o Avoid attaching to words
  o Avoid making personal attacks
  o Listen carefully and reflect on what you hear
  o Accept some responsibility for the misunderstanding
  o Seek an equitable solution to the problem

TABLE 8-3   Preparation for Conflict Resolution

Directions: On a clean sheet of paper answer these questions in as much depth as possible. At the end of this exercise, you should have a much clearer view of the situation.

My Perspective	Their Perspective
What is the conflict from my point of view?	What do I believe is the conflict from the other's point of view?
How have I contributed to the current situation and conflict?	How do I believe that the other has contributed to the current situation and conflict?
How is this situation currently impacting me?	How is this situation currently impacting the other?
What drives me in this conflict? What motivates the choices I am making and the actions I am taking?	What do I believe drives the other in this conflict? What motivates his or her choices and actions?
What am I feeling as I contemplate this situation?	What do I believe the other feels when contemplating this situation?
What do this situation and my behaviors say about me as a person? How would I do things differently if I could do it again?	What do this situation and the other's actions say about him or her as a person? What might the other have done differently?
What are other people saying about this conflict and how does that affect my actions?	What do I believe people are saying to the other about this situation and how might that affect his or her actions?
Where do we share common ground? What are the issues or points we agree on?	
How would I like this situation to be resolved? Does this solution benefit both of us?	
What do I want to accomplish by having a conversation with this person?	

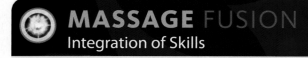

MASSAGE FUSION
Integration of Skills

STUDY TIP: Once a Day

Because this chapter introduced a variety of communication skills, you may feel uncertain about how to integrate these new skills in your daily life. Here's an idea. Write each skill on an index card with its name on one side (e.g., I-Statements) and a description on the other. Pull one card from this deck each morning. Keep the card in your pocket and take it out periodically throughout the day to read the description. Focus on bringing that skill into your communication that day. At the end of the day, reflect on how using that skill changed your communication with friends, family, instructors, and classmates. Tomorrow, pick another card. Continue to cycle through the cards until you feel that you "own" all of the skills and can use them effortlessly.

MASSAGE INSPIRATION:
Open and Close

In Topic 8-3, an open body position and active listening attitude are compared with a closed body position and passive listening attitude. Research has shown the changes that can occur in an instructor when students simply change from a closed body position to an open body position. Pay attention to your body position and those of your classmates. Try to get them to open up their positions and actively listen to lectures and demonstrations. You will likely find that your instructors deliver material more effectively and dynamically and that you get more out of their lectures and demonstrations.

IT'S TRUE! good communication improves perception of care

A study published in *Medical Care* reported that physicians who understood body language, facial expression, and voice tone cues and were aware of their own body language and what it conveyed received higher trust and perception of care ratings from patients. Researchers noted that physicians with these nonverbal communication skills more effectively built physician–patient relationships that enhanced the patient's perception of their treatment. This study suggests that training in communication could improve the quality of medical care and prove to be cost effective.[6] These studies have ramifications for all health care providers because they demonstrate the value of communication for building client loyalty and facilitating positive treatment outcomes.

CHAPTER WRAP-UP

This chapter explains core concepts of good communication and outlines how communication is used with clients and other health care providers. Communication skills can be mastered through self-awareness, practice, and a desire to improve. The massage classroom is a perfect setting for trying new communication skills, making mistakes, receiving feedback, and learning.

Some students wander blindly through their massage education, failing to see the amazing opportunity to build communication skills during their training. Everyday in your classrooms you interact with instructors and classmates. In student clinic you interact with members of the public as clients, and indeed they are clients who expect excellent service. Pay attention to your conversations, how they progress, and how they make you feel. Do you get the result you want from exchanges of ideas? Do you feel good after a conversation? Too often, people blame a failed communication on someone else. But think about how communication would improve if every person thought this way: "If I'm misunderstood, it is my responsibility. It is possible that I'm not forming my message in a way that best matches the other person's learning style and mental processing preferences. If I don't understand, I'm not paying attention to all of their verbal and nonverbal cues." That is a powerful thought. You are in control of what you communicate, how you communicate, and what you understand. You are in control of how people react and interact with you. And you can change or improve your skills anytime you want.

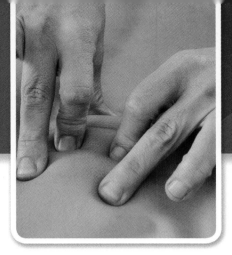

Your Massage Career

KEY TERMS

advertising

business plan

continuing education

cover letter

employee

expenses

independent contractor

marketing

promotion

publicity

resume

revenue

self-employed

target market

LEARNING OBJECTIVES

Having read the chapter and used the related student learning tools, the student will be able to:

1. Use self-assessment activities to investigate career-planning choices.

2. Differentiate among the terms employee, self-employed, and independent contractor.

3. Describe three strategies for identifying potential employers.

4. Write the first draft of a chronological resume.

5. Write the first draft of a cover letter.

6. List three areas that might be discussed during the negotiation of an employment package.

7. Discuss common expectations of employers of massage therapists.

8. Outline the components of a business plan.

9. Analyze the factors to consider when choosing a business name and location

10. Compare and contrast businesses that are structured as sole proprietorships with businesses that are limited liability companies.

11. Explain the concept of marketing and provide three examples of business promotions.

12. Explain the information that would be found on a balance sheet, cash flow statement, and profit and loss statement.

13. Predict the start-up costs for a massage business.

14. Outline a simple record keeping system for a sole proprietorship.

Each person enters the massage profession for a different reason. Some are seeking meaningful work where they can help other people feel better. Others want a flexible schedule, to meet new people, skills that can travel with them wherever they go, or interesting part-time work they can balance with family life or another parallel career. All of these reasons are valid and should be kept in mind as you plan your massage career. In Topic 9-1, we look at some of your career options and you develop a written plan to follow when you graduate from massage school. Topic 9-2 explains the process for getting your first massage job including how to write a resume and cover letter, how to build your interviewing skills, and thoughts about negotiating the employment package. Starting a private practice is the subject of Topic 9-3, which explores the basics of starting a business and writing a business plan.

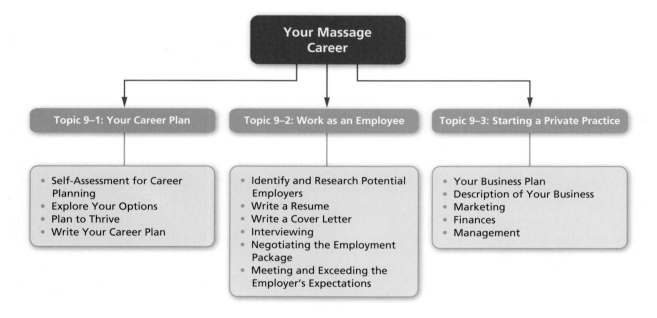

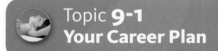

Topic **9-1**
Your Career Plan

Career planning is a lifelong process that takes place as people grow and change through new experiences. A career in massage allows for constant growth because you can work in a variety of different environments, specialize in knowledge related to particular populations of clients, and learn a multitude of massage systems that approach the body and healing from new perspectives. Many therapists also gain knowledge and credentials in related fields like fitness trainer, esthetics, yoga instructor, nursing, and physical therapy to practice alongside massage. The career-planning process can be broken into a three-step procedure that involves a self-assessment step, an exploration of the options, and a written plan.

Self-Assessment for Career Planning

Self-assessment is the process of gathering information about yourself in order to make good career decisions. There are numerous ways to conduct a self-assessment for career planning and many free tools available on the Internet to help in the self-assessment process. It is helpful to evaluate these key areas:

- A **value assessment** helps you determine what things are most important to you. For example, is job security more important than autonomy? Is helping others more important than a high salary?

- A **personality and skill assessment** helps you explore your personal qualities, motivation level, needs, attitudes, and skills. Different careers in massage fit better with different personality types. In some cases, particular skill sets are required to work with special populations, specific pathologies, or in a health care versus wellness environment.

- **Visualization** helps you identify your hopes, dreams, and possibilities regarding your career in massage therapy and how your career fits into your life.

The information you discover from self-assessment provides you with valuable insight when you write a career plan. For example, if you find that you have many of the characteristics of an entrepreneur, you may be well suited to private practice. If your value assessment reveals that you like working on a team, you may want to seek work in a busy clinic where you are surrounded by other therapists and have much contact with the public. Remember that you can develop interests, values, and skills you don't have now. If a particular career path requires some personal development and is important to you, then make the changes you need to reach your goals. The self-assessment exercises in Box 9-1 can help you gather key data about yourself as you write your career plan.

BOX 9-1 Self-Assessment Activities for Career Planning

ACTIVITY 1: VALUE ASSESSMENT

Review the list of values associated with career planning and place a 1, 2, or 3 in the space provided. 1 = things I value highly, 2 = things I value, 3 = things I don't value very much

Score	Personal Values	Description
	Help my community	I want to participate in career activities that contribute to improving the community I live in.
	Help people	I want to participate in career activities that contribute to improving the quality of people's lives.
	Contact	I want to participate in career activities where I have high levels of contact with other therapists and with the public on a day-to-day basis.
	Work alone	I want to participate in career activities where I have limited day-to-day contact with other therapists and members of the public.
	Team	I want to participate in career activities where I work with a team of people to achieve common goals.
	Autonomy	I want to participate in career activities where I plan my own schedule, make my own business decisions, decide my own policies, and personally determine the success or failure of my business based on my own actions.
	Influence	I want to participate in career activities where I can influence the attitudes or opinions of others.
	Knowledge and mastery	I want to participate in career activities where I can master knowledge of the body, work in situations where attention to detail and accuracy are very important, and be an expert in the field.
	Creativity	I want to participate in career activities where I can create new programs, organizational structures, and materials or express myself artistically.
	Management	I want to participate in career activities where I am directly responsible for the work of others and for the financial viability and operations of a business.
	Supervision	I want to participate in career activities where I am responsible for my own work and am not directly responsible for the financial viability and operations of a business. I want to work in a situation where I have regular guidance from a mentor or supervisor.
	Change and variety	I want to work in a career environment where work activities frequently change.
	Stability	I want to work in a career environment where my duties and routine are predictable.
	Security	I want to work in a career environment where I can be assured of receiving satisfactory compensation.
	Risk	I want to work in a career environment where I determine my own salary based on my willingness to commit to activities that bring in income. I can tolerate risk and uncertainty.
	Recognition	I want to participate in career activities where I can be publicly recognized for the high quality of my work.
	Money	I want to participate in career activities that will lead to the achievement of high monetary gain for my work.
	Physical challenge	I want to participate in career activities that use my physical capabilities to the fullest measure.
	Physical comfort	I want to participate in career activities that are not physically challenging.
	Time	I want to be able to work according to my own schedule.

(Continued)

BOX 9-1 Self-Assessment Activities for Career Planning (Continued)

Identify your top five values and consider them when you write your career plan.

ACTIVITY 2: PERSONALITY AND SKILL CHARACTERISTICS OF AN ENTREPRENEUR

One of the key choices that graduating massage therapists must make is whether to be an entrepreneur or to work as an employee. An entrepreneur is a person who owns his or her own company, enterprise, or venture and assumes significant accountability for the risks and outcomes. Numerous studies have been conducted to determine the personality characteristics of people who are successfully self-employed or own their own businesses. In his book, *The Young Entrepreneur's Guide to Starting and Running a Business,*[1] Steve Mariotti lists many of the following characteristics of an entrepreneur. Additional characteristics that are particularly important for a massage entrepreneur have also been included. Place a check by the traits you think you have already, and an X by the traits you think you can develop. In a journal or on a separate piece of paper, answer the questions that are asked under each trait. Don't be discouraged if you find you possess few of the traits listed here. Entrepreneurship is not a good fit for many massage therapists, but these therapists often find success and happiness working as employees. The point is to discover where you can best find personal success right now. Remember, you will continue to grow as you gain life experience and may be ready for entrepreneurship later in your career, even if you aren't ready for it now.

- **Characteristic No. 1: Adaptability**—Are you able to cope with new situations and find creative solutions to problems? Are you flexible and look at opportunities and challenges from a number of different perspectives? Describe one situation where you demonstrated adaptability to overcome an obstacle.
- **Characteristic No. 2: Competitiveness**—Are you willing to compete with and test yourself against others? Describe one event in your life where you drew on your competitive instincts to achieve your goals.
- **Characteristic No. 3: Confidence**—Do you believe that you can do what you set out to do? Explain the ways you demonstrate confidence in your life now and describe how you developed your current level of confidence. How might you gain more confidence?
- **Characteristic No. 4: Discipline**—Are you able to stay focused and stick to a schedule and deadlines? Describe a time in your life when you had to be disciplined to reach an important goal.
- **Characteristic No. 5: Drive**—Are you willing and able to work hard to achieve your goals? People with drive demonstrate high levels of motivation, energy, and initiative and have good physical health. Describe an event where you needed to sustain your drive over a period of time to achieve an important goal. How did you maintain your energy and motivation?

- **Characteristic No. 6: Honesty**—Are you committed to telling people the truth even when it causes discomfort? When you make a promise do you stand by your word? Do you deal with all people fairly? Describe a time when you had to be honest with someone even though it was difficult.
- **Characteristic No. 7: Organization**—Are you able to plan and structure your life in a logical manner? Are you able to place tasks in an order to structure the completion of a project? Are you able to differentiate between priorities so that you finish important tasks first? Describe a situation where you had to organize and follow through on tasks to complete a project.
- **Characteristic No. 8: Perseverance**—Are you able to keep your goals in sight even when obstacles present challenges? Do you refuse to quit and keep working at a goal or project even if you have encountered difficulties or failures? Describe an event where you had to persevere even when you were faced with obstacles.
- **Characteristic No. 9: Persuasiveness**—Do you have a knack for convincing people to see your point of view? Are you able to get people interested in your ideas? Describe an event where you had to win people to your side to achieve your goals.
- **Characteristic No. 10: Risk Taking**—Are you willing to expose yourself to possible losses to try a new venture? Explain a time in your life when you took a risk and succeeded. Explain a time in your life when you took a risk and failed. What did you learn from these experiences that might help you in your massage career?
- **Characteristic No. 11: Thinking Ability**—Are you able to analyze problems and come up with possible solutions? Can you look at projects from multiple perspectives to generate creative ideas? Do you readily see ways to overcome obstacles or rework processes to be more efficient? Explain a time when you had to think creatively, analytically, or critically to solve a problem or complete a project.
- **Characteristic No. 12: Human Relationships**—Are you able to listen to other people and understand their points of view? Can you empathize with people to comprehend what they are feeling and why they are behaving in a certain way? Do you strive to reach a fair resolution when you have a conflict with another person? Describe a time in your life when you had to let go of your own point of view to reach a resolution in a conflict with another. What did you learn from the experience?
- **Characteristic No. 13: Communication**—Are you able to verbally express your ideas and point of view? Do you share your thoughts, ideas, and opinions openly with others? Do you possess a strong health care vocabulary and do you feel comfortable conversing about massage and the body? Do you have basic writing skills? Describe your

level of communication skills and give one example of a time you have to communicate in a written format.

- **Characteristic No. 14: Vision**—Are you able to see the end result of your goals while you are working to achieve them? Describe a time where you had to hold a vision of a goal in your mind while you worked toward that goal. Did fears and doubts cloud your vision? What was the outcome?
- **Characteristic No. 15: Technical Skills**—Are your draping skills, hands-on massage skills, and body mechanics solid? Are you able to observe new techniques and integrate them with your existing hands-on skills? Do you constantly strive to improve your hands-on skills? Describe your current technical skill level and list three areas where you are actively striving for improvement.

ACTIVITY 3: WHICH DO YOU LIKE BETTER?

In each column pick the activity you would most like to do in each and every line of the table by placing an X by that activity. At the end, total the number of X marks in each column.

I would rather have 15 regular clients that I see one time a week than lots of one-visit clients.	I would rather see lots of one-visit clients than see the same clients over and over again.
I would like to develop detailed treatment plans for each client and set long-term and short-term goals for progress.	I don't feel that detailed treatment plans are necessary. I like to get on with the massage and release muscle tension.
I like SOAP charting and use SOAP documents to track the progress of my clients over time.	I like simple charting systems that don't require me to track the progress of clients over time.
I like to analyze a client's posture, range of motion, and movement patterns to plan my treatments.	I like to add creative flourishes like the use of aromatherapy and special music to help my clients relax.
I like to research pathologies to find out more about them. I am not afraid to work with clients who have diagnosed pathologies and conditions.	I don't particularly like to work with clients who have diagnosed pathologies. I would rather focus on stress reduction because stress causes or exacerbates many diseases.
Musculoskeletal injuries fascinate me. I like to use massage to facilitate healing and to support rehabilitation.	I want to explore my creativity by planning treatments that please the senses and promote mental, spiritual, emotional, and physical wellness.
I want to work with a team that includes athletic coaches, physicians, nurses, physical therapists, and chiropractors.	I want to work with a team that includes skin care specialists, cosmetologists, dermatologists, yoga instructors, and spiritual coaches.
Total	Total

If you have more X marks in the first column, you may particularly like to work in a health care setting like a hospitable, sports medicine clinic, chiropractor office, hospice, or athletic center. If you have more X marks in the second column, you may particularly like to work at a spa, salon, wellness center, resort, or retreat.

ACTIVITY 4: VISUALIZE YOUR IDEAL LIFE

Visualizing the life you want can help you choose activities and behaviors that lead to the attainment of your goals and dreams. Life visualization includes your living environment, relationships, finances, spirituality, health and wellness, social life, and personal development as well as career. Find a quiet place and collect your thoughts about your future in a journal or on sheets of paper. Don't question whether your desires about your life are realistic; just get them down on paper and grant yourself permission to dream big. During visualization exercises people often have doubts and fears surface. Dedicate one area of your journal to list your fears and doubts about the future. When you acknowledge fears and doubts, they immediately lose some

of their power, and you will be better able to plan strategies for overcoming obstacles if they are clearly identified. Use these questions to structure your visualization process:

1. In your perfect life where do you live (e.g., I live in Boulder, Colorado) and what is your living environment like (e.g., I live in a beautiful three-bedroom, modern home with hardwood floors and large windows that look out at the mountains)?

2. In your perfect life what are your relationships like? How do you want to interact with your parents, siblings, spouse, partner, children, coworkers, and friends? How do your relationships support your personal goals and give pleasure and meaning to your life?

3. In your perfect life how much money do you make and how do you use your money to achieve the lifestyle you want, contribute to the wellness of the world, and feel secure about your financial future?

4. In your perfect life how do you connect to your spiritual beliefs and practice those beliefs in the world? How do your beliefs influence the choices you make and the ways

(Continued)

BOX 9-1 Self-Assessment Activities for Career Planning *(Continued)*

you interact with other people? How do you nurture and care for the mental, emotional, and spiritual aspects of yourself?

5. In your perfect life what do you look like? What is your fitness level and eating habits? What do you do to maintain your health and wellness and how do you feel about participating in these activities?

6. In your perfect life what do you do for fun? What sort of friends do you have and what sort of interests and activities do you pursue for recreation?

7. In your perfect life what activities do you undertake to develop as a person? What makes you curious, excited, and motivated? How do you foster your mental, emotional, spiritual, and physical growth?

8. In your perfect life what is your career like? What is the environment like? What kind of people do you work with? What are your daily tasks and responsibilities? How do you feel about your job? What is your financial status? How does your job feed your other goals and desires?

9. In your perfect life what do you care about and what do you focus on?

10. Describe how you feel when you think about this life. What feels good? What feels scary? What feels possible? What feels impossible? Now describe three things you can do everyday, right now, to achieve the life you want.

Use the information you uncovered in your visualization when writing your career plan.

Explore Your Options

As you have progressed through massage school and learned more about the massage profession, it is likely that some of your ideas about where you want to work have changed. As you plan your massage career, evaluate all of your options with an exploration of massage environments, specialization opportunities, and employee versus self-employment preferences.

Massage Environments

In Chapter 1, you were introduced to a variety of environments where massage is practiced. If you completed Topic 9-3 in that chapter, you should have a strong idea about whether health care massage–oriented tasks or wellness massage–oriented tasks are more appealing to you. Box 9-2 outlines massage environments, but it will take some investigation into the nature of each individual business to determine if it provides health care or wellness massages, or both. For example, it is easy to assume that spas want a therapist to offer wellness massage, when in fact some have a very strong treatment focus and require the documentation, treatment planning, and health care skills you might normally see in a medical setting. Review Box 9-2 and pick the top three massage environments that interest you.

Specialization

Massage therapists often specialize by learning and offering a specific massage or bodywork system or by studying additional knowledge and treatment protocols for a particular pathology or special population. You have probably already been introduced to popular massage and bodywork systems as part of your entry-level training. For example, many students aspire to work at big resort spas and offer body treatments like salt glows and body wraps in addition to massage. Others hope to land a job with a sports team and work with athletes.

Maybe pain reduction is your objective and you want to work in a medical setting with clients who are living with chronic pain conditions. If specialization is part of your career plan, you need to carefully evaluate your skill levels. You may need additional training above the entry level to achieve your goals.

BOX 9-2 Common Environments Where Massage Is Practiced

Chiropractor office

Cruise ship

Day spa

Fitness center

Gym

Hospice

Hospital

Massage clinic

Naturopathic practice

Nursing homes

Onsite massage (corporations, dance studios, health food stores, etc.)

Pain management center

Physical therapy office

Physician's office

Private practice

Racetrack (animal massage)

Rehabilitation center

Resort spa

Salon

Sports medicine clinic

Veterinarian office (animal massage)

Wellness center

BOX 9-3 **Client Types**

Animals

Athletes

Children

Clients recovering from musculoskeletal injury

General public

Infants

Men

People living with cancer

People living with chronic pain conditions

People living with HIV/AIDS

Physically challenged

Pregnant women

Psychologically challenged

Survivors of abuse

The elderly

The terminally ill

Women

Specialization can make you more marketable to an employer or to a client population. Alternately, in some cases, employers or clients won't know enough about a particular system of bodywork to seek it out. If you plan to specialize, include these areas in your career plan. Box 9-3 can help you identify specific client groups that you may want to target. Over 250 different systems of massage and bodywork have been identified. Many of these systems were outlined in Chapter 1. If you plan to learn a specialized massage system, review Figure 1-9 in Chapter 1, determine if you will need continuing education, and include this information in your career plan.

Continuing Education

Continuing education is education you pursue after you have completed your entry-level training and received your massage credentials. It is often called "CE" in massage publications or on the Internet. While it might seem strange to think about getting more education when you haven't even graduated yet, you want to factor continuing education into your career-planning process. In fact, if you want to work with certain client groups or specialize your work to focus on a particular pathology or condition, you may need continuing education shortly after graduation in order to meet your career goals. Most states where massage is regulated require massage therapists to complete a specified number of continuing education hours to maintain their massage credentials. Continuing education is beneficial because it brings therapists up to date with new advances in massage knowledge or skills and encourages therapists to diversify their practices, as discussed previously. As part of your career plan, it can be helpful to include continuing education activities that will help you grow and develop as a person and as a professional.

Employment Options

Probably, the biggest decision you have to make about your career is if you are going to be an **employee**, **self-employed**, an **independent contractor**, or a combination of these.

- **Employee:** An employee is hired by another person or company to perform particular duties for a set fee. The employer is required by law to withhold income taxes, withhold and pay social security and Medicare taxes, and pay unemployment tax on wages paid to an employee. As an employee, you agree to abide by the rules and processes of your employer. You may have to follow a specific dress code, work a fixed schedule, and perform other duties in addition to massage such as laundry and answering phones. In many instances, employers pay an hourly rate for the hours you are on a shift and an additional fee for every massage you perform during your shift. The responsibility for **marketing** and **promotion**, abiding by state and local business ordinances, organizing and tracking inventory of retail items, and all other activities for running and managing the business fall largely on the shoulders of the employer.

- **Self-Employed**: Self-employed people work for themselves and are not employed by someone else. In this case, you set your own schedule and dress code but must also secure your own clients through marketing and promotional activities. You are responsible for keeping your own tax records and for reporting and paying taxes to the Internal Revenue Service (IRS), and for abiding by any rules that regulate businesses in your local area.

- **Independent Contractor**: An independent contractor is a self-employed person who contracts with another business to provide specific services. This is a common arrangement in the massage profession where a massage business owner contracts with massage therapists instead of hiring them as employees. The difference between employees and independent contractors is subtle. An employer has the right to direct the means and methods an employee uses to accomplish a job. A person hiring an independent contractor has the right to control only the result of the work and not the means and methods of accomplishing the job. Still, in many instances, the contract is written in such a way that the independent contractor must follow a dress code, keep to a specific schedule, and perform other duties in addition to massage, just as an employee would. Independent contractors may be responsible for securing a specific number of client sessions per week, or they might share the responsibilities for marketing and promotion with the business owner. Independent contractors must keep their own tax records and report and pay taxes to the IRS.

Each situation has pros and cons that require careful examination. In addition, your personality may predispose you toward one particular employment model, as demonstrated in Activity 2 in Box 9-1. If you found in Activity 2 that you don't have many of the characteristics of people who are successful when self-employed, you should not be discouraged.

If self-employment is an important goal, you can develop the skills and attributes you need to be successful, although developing personality traits that are not natural to you may take some work.

Many therapists don't make a choice about whether to be an employee, self-employed, or independent contractor; they do it all. This is an excellent career strategy, especially when you are trying to build a clientele. For example, Elena has diversified her practice to ensure that she always has clients. On Mondays, Elena has two corporate office accounts where she offers seated massage to employees. She sees the first in the morning from 9:30 AM to 12:00 PM and the second after lunch from 1:30 PM to 4:00 PM On Tuesdays, Wednesdays, and Fridays, she works shifts at a nearby spa as an employee. On Thursdays, she is working to build her private practice and massages friends, family, and clients she has met through her seated practice. She acts as an independent contractor at a massage clinic, specializing in car accident treatment and rehabilitation every other Saturday, and takes Sundays off.

Activities for Further Exploration

As you can see, you have a lot of choices to make when planning your massage career. If you feel confusion or if you want to make certain that your plan is good, you can pursue some specific activities that may provide you with invaluable information:

- **Job shadowing** is learning about a job by walking through the workday as an unpaid "shadow" to a competent worker. You witness firsthand the massage work environment, client interactions, and skill sets required for the particular job. Some schools set up job shadowing opportunities for students. If your school doesn't do this, you can call local massage businesses and ask if they would allow you to job shadow. You might also provide massage to the working massage therapists on staff for feedback.
- **Internships** are school-sanctioned, supervised programs where students get hands-on, career-related experience that supplements classroom academic experiences to enhance a student's education. For example, at one school students can apply for a spa, sports, or hospital internship. Students chosen for the spa internship work at a local spa to gain classroom credit 1 day a week. Students in the sports internship work with a professional football team, and students in the hospital internship work in the oncology ward of a hospital providing massage to patients, family of patients, and nurses.
- **Volunteer opportunities** are often organized by schools to help students understand the value of community outreach and to give students insight into potential career paths. A school might take students to a nursing home as part of the learning activities in a module on geriatric massage. Alternately, students might provide massage to pregnant women at a birthing center, or experience seated massage in a corporate environment. Often volunteer opportunities are not required and students have an option as to whether they participate. These activities can provide you with invaluable insight into work environments and also help you round out your massage resume.
- **Online Forums** provide opportunities to ask questions of seasoned massage professionals over the Internet. Associated Bodywork & Massage Professionals (ABMP) powers a website for massage professionals and students (www.massageprofessionals.com) that allows you to take part in online forums and discussion groups. Log on, join groups that interest you, and ask massage professionals to give you input on career paths in massage.

Plan to Thrive

If you ask professional therapists what was the one thing that most surprised them when they began their career in massage, they may tell you that massage can be a bit lonely. While you are working with other people, it is not appropriate to chat about personal interests or the latest movie release to clients. Sessions are often very quiet, and the focus is on the client and the client's changing muscle tissue. Time between sessions is usually spent changing table linens, sanitizing the space for the next client, and completing chart notes, leaving little time for friendly conversation with other therapists. Many therapists build a thriving practice by cultivating relationships with mentors and with other professionals. These activities develop knowledge, provide useful feedback and guidance, and help prevent burnout by creating a social outlet that balances the solitude of a massage practice.

Mentors

A mentor is a more experienced person who provides guidance as you establish your career and grow as a massage therapist. Mentoring can be a formal relationship established by your school or by the business that employs you. Informal mentoring often occurs spontaneously between two people who share common interests but have different levels of experience. The older or more experienced person naturally falls into the role of directing and encouraging the younger or less experienced person. For example, the manager who employs you might take an interest in developing your skills, or an established massage therapist might steer you toward treatment choices where you can work with people who have pathologies or conditions. Massage therapists in private practice might seek out a mentor who is an established business owner in a noncompeting area. Finding a mentor is a good idea because it gives you someone to contact if you encounter challenges in your career. This trusted person might also help you celebrate new learning and the development of new skills.

Possible mentors are all around you. Is there a person you work with or have met who you admire and respect because of his or her insight and knowledge? Does this person have experience he or she would be willing to share? Approach the person and ask if he or she would consider being your mentor. Let him or her know about your interests and what you hope to learn. Ask that the relationship have some structure such as a weekly phone call to discuss issues and challenges you faced during the week, or a monthly lunch meeting to talk over your career development. You can also find online mentors through your professional membership organization (ABMP or American Massage Therapy Association [AMTA]).

Professional Networks

Professional networking is the development and cultivation of friendships and acquaintances that can help you build your business. Professional networks give you access to the insights and knowledge of other people, put you in contact with people who might offer career advancement or business opportunities, and provide an outlet for pleasant social interaction. As part of your professional networks, you might belong to a local massage group that meets every other month to discuss massage profession trends and happenings in the region. This group can provide knowledge, advice, and information on massage-related topics. If you start your own business (Topic 9-3), you might also join a small business group where you meet other owners and managers of small businesses who provide information, experience, and recommendations that can help you better manage the business aspects of your practice. General networking groups in your area can put you into contact with people from diverse backgrounds who may become clients when they get to know you and find out more about massage. Online social tools like Facebook, Twitter, and massageprofessionals.com, among others, provide a virtual networking option.

Preventing Burnout

Massage is a physically and mentally demanding profession in which you give your energy and focus to helping other people feel better in their bodies. If you don't plan ways to nurture and care for yourself while you are nurturing and caring for others, you may experience burnout. Burnout is a state of emotional, mental, and physical fatigue caused by prolonged job-related stress. The signs and symptoms of burnout include mental, emotional, and physical exhaustion, loss of interest in your job, the inability to care about your job performance, and feelings of hopelessness, irritation, resentment, cynicism, and unhappiness. If you start to show up late for sessions or dread working on your next client, you may be headed toward burnout.

Burnout happens in every profession but is most prevalent in employees who feel underpaid, underappreciated, or criticized for things beyond their control. If managers set unrealistic goals for you in terms of the number of sessions you must provide in a workday, or if you must work under rules that are particularly restrictive, you may be at higher risk for burnout. Boredom can also be a factor if you are asked to provide the same massage routine over and over again despite the needs of the individual client. If your work never changes and you never feel challenged to learn and grow, you may feel bored and dissatisfied. Health care professionals, including massage therapists, often find themselves in contact with some of the more tragic aspects of human experience, like people living with chronic pain or serious injury, or work with the terminally ill. This type of work can expose you to prolonged emotional stress that may lead to burnout.

If you notice that you start to experience the symptoms of burnout, take some time to identify the reasons. It can be useful to take a few days off to rest and evaluate the situation. Once you identify the problem, brainstorm solutions with mentors or people from your networks. The recommendations and activities described in Chapter 11 can help you prevent burnout in your massage career.

Write Your Career Plan

A written career plan helps you focus your activities to achieve specific goals related to your career. Plans can be written for 1 year, 3 years, 5 years, or longer. While there are many different models for career planning, the following is specifically related to massage. A sample plan is provided in Figure 9-1.

- **Goal:** Describe your primary career goal for the year ahead.
- **Employment Status:** Describe the employment status you prefer. Do you want to be self-employed, work as an employee, work as an independent contractor, or a combination of these? List activities that will help you prepare for your chosen employment status.
- **Work Environments:** Describe your top three preferred work environments and list activities that will help you prepare to obtain a job in such an environment or create such an environment for a private practice.
- **Target Clients:** List the top three client types you would like to work with, and describe ways you can reach out to these client groups and educate them about the benefits of massage. A description of target clients is provided in Topic 9-3 in the section on marketing.
- **Specialized Skills and Knowledge:** Describe any areas where you would like to specialize, and list any additional training you need in order to offer a specialized massage system or work with a particular group of clients.
- **Mentors and Professional Networks:** List people or groups you would like to meet or develop relationships with to grow yourself and your business.
- **Plan for Self-Care and Personal Growth:** Describe activities you will undertake to care for yourself and grow as a person over the course of a year.

Once you have written a career plan, post it where you can see it regularly and keep track of your progress. It is a useful exercise to reevaluate and rewrite a career plan annually.

Name: Mary Massage
Career Plan Time Frame: 1 Year, January 2010 to January 2011

Goal: To work as an employee of a busy massage clinic where I can interact with a health care team and develop my massage skills with supervision from experienced professionals.

Employment Status: I want to work as an employee for the first year in order to observe business management procedures and so that I can interact with experienced professionals who can help me continue to improve my massage skills after school.

Tasks
- [ ] Identify potential employers
- [ ] Write a resume
- [ ] Write a cover letter
- [ ] Obtain interviews
- [ ] Practice interviewing
- [ ] Negotiate an employment package

Work Environment: I want to work in a busy rehabilitation clinic or wellness center. It would be ideal if there were different types of health care professionals employed at the business so that I can make connections and learn more about related professions. I want to identify a mentor or supervisor who is willing to help me continue to develop my health care massage skills.

Tasks
- [ ] Research local area businesses to identify work environments that meet my needs.
- [ ] Request the opportunity to job shadow to make contacts and to test my feelings about the environment and people.

Target Clients: I am interested in working with clients who have sustained a musculoskeletal injury or who want condition management for a soft-tissue pathology like fibromyalgia. I want to develop treatment plans and utilize my assessment skills to choose the best techniques to help clients make progress.

Tasks
- [ ] There is a local support group for people living with fibromyalgia that meets monthly. I will call the group facilitator and ask if I can sit in on a meeting to learn more about fibromyalgia.

Specialized Skills and Knowledge: I feel good about my assessment, treatment planning, and documentation skills. I would like to take the advanced neuromuscular class offered by the school when I graduate to further develop my treatment massage skills.

Tasks
- [ ] Save the money needed to take the advanced neuromuscular workshop.
- [ ] Buy one new book on fibromyalgia and read it.

Mentors and Professional Networks: I plan to ask Elaine Murphy to act as my mentor during my first year in massage. She was an amazing teacher and I felt that we formed a respectful relationship. I want to find a local massage group to join and also start a network with my classmates and the alumni from my school.

Tasks
- [ ] Ask Elaine Murphy to act as a mentor
- [ ] Contact ABMP and AMTA and ask if they know of local massage groups I can join.
- [ ] Ask school to conduct a mailing to alumni for me as I launch my own professional network.

Plan for Self-Care and Personal Growth: I am going to treat myself to a spa treatment and spa massage to celebrate graduation from massage school. I am going to continue to focus on practicing good body mechanics when I give massage and enroll in a series of yoga classes when school is out.

Tasks
- [ ] Research yoga classes offered in the area.
- [ ] Eat a nutritious diet
- [ ] Commit to my exercise plan
- [ ] Focus on body mechanics

Figure 9-1 A written career plan like the sample shown here helps you focus your activities to achieve specific goals related to your career.

Topic **9-2**
Work as an Employee

There are plenty of opportunities if you want to work as an employee in a variety of environments, such as spas, clinics, medical settings, and fitness clubs. The benefits include a dependable income, a regular schedule, freedom from the responsibilities of running a business, and having taxes automatically withheld from your paycheck. The drawbacks are that you make less per hour for the massages you provide than you would in private practice (though this must be balanced against the fact that you have no overhead costs), you must meet employer expectations, and you are likely to be required to perform duties in addition to massage, such as laundry and answering the phone. To get your first massage job, you will need to identify and research potential employers, write a **resume**, write a **cover letter**, be interviewed, get a job offer, and negotiate your employment package. Once you are working, you will want to meet or exceed your employer's expectations to potentially move to a higher position as you gain experience.

Identify and Research Potential Employers

A search on the Internet is probably the easiest way to develop a list of potential employers in your area, though both ABMP and AMTA offer job search boards for their members. Employers often send job announcements to schools to be posted on the school job board. Develop a list of at least 10 potential employers, and then use the Internet or make a phone call to the business to gather basic information. Ask

- Are they currently hiring massage therapists?
- What is the pay rate for entry-level massage therapists?
- Do they offer an employee benefit package (e.g., will they pay your liability insurance, will they pay for continuing education, and do they provide paid vacations and sick days)?
- What are the hours of operation and how long are massage shifts?
- What type of clientele does the business attract and what types of massage do they provide?
- What is the name and spelling of the person in charge of hiring massage therapists?
- What is the job application procedure?

It's a good idea to travel the route from your house to the business and back to determine how much commute time is involved. You might also want to visit the business as a client to get a feel for the environment and the general working conditions. Narrow your list down to your top five best options, and prepare a resume and cover letter. Follow the job application procedure for each business, or, if there isn't a specified procedure, send a resume and cover letter to the person in charge of hiring massage therapists.

Write a Resume

A resume is a summary of your background, experience, education, training, and skills. Employers use it to determine if you have the experience necessary to fill an open position. A well-written resume is a first step to securing a job interview. Effective resumes are:

- **Brief and concise**: Keep your resume to one page if possible, or two pages at the most. If your resume is long or difficult to read, the employer may skip some parts or put it aside entirely.
- **Positive**: A resume should emphasize positive elements in your record and use action verbs such as "planned," "organized," "collected," "initiated," "assessed," and so on to show employers what you have accomplished.
- **Relevant**: Write your information in the resume in such a way as to make it meaningful to the employer and pertinent to the specific position.
- **Readable**: Take care to present your information neatly, so that it is easy to gather information at a glance. Pay attention to the font and the font size you use, to the balance of information on the page, and especially to spelling and correct punctuation. Avoid abbreviations of words or incomplete sentences.
- **Honest**: Don't fabricate any of the information on your resume, and make sure that the dates for previous experience are correct. If an employer finds out that part of your resume was fabricated, you are likely to be dismissed.

The sample chronological resume in Figure 9-2 is easy to write and is appropriate for entry-level positions as it illustrates both your education and experience. There are, however, many different types of resume formats you might use. An online search for "resume formats" or "resume services" provides a variety of examples and resources. A chronological resume includes:

- **Contact Information**: List your name, address, phone numbers, and e-mail address. Avoid the use of nicknames and surnames like "Senior," "Junior," or "II," and spell out all the words in the address (e.g., "Street" and "Avenue").
- **Career or Job Objective**: An objective tells potential employers what sort of work you are hoping to do. Be specific about the type of job you want, and be sure to tailor your objective to the specific position or employer.

Jane Anybody

214 Any Street #202
Any Town, Any State   98000
(303) 222-3232
janeanybody@internet.com

OBJECTIVE: To obtain a position as a massage therapist at a leading spa where I can use my skills in massage, body treatments, aromatherapy, and reflexology.

EDUCATION: Massage Diploma, June 2005
Any Massage College, Any Town, Any State
800 Hours, Combined GPA 3.66

Spa Certificate, June 2005
Any Massage College, Any Town, Any State
200 Hours, Combined GPA 3.66

Reflexology Certification, October 2005
Any School of Reflexology, Any Town, Any State
300 Hours

Aromatherapy Certification, January 2006
Any School of Aromatherapy, Any Town, Any State
300 Hours

EXPERIENCE: Student Massage Clinic Coordinator, January 2005–June 2005
Any Massage College, Any Town, Any State

As part of the work-study program, I answered phones, assisted clients, and managed client files. I implemented a new policy for tracking client files that is now being used at the school's three campuses.

Walk for Breast Cancer Massage Coordinator, May 5, 2005
Any Massage College, Any Town, Any State
Initiated and coordinated an onsite massage event at the Walk for Breast Cancer Event in Any Town, Any State. As the event coordinator for Any Massage College, I met with event planners, organized the site where massage would be provided, coordinated volunteer massage therapists, and managed the flow of clients at the event.

ASSOCIATIONS: American Massage Therapy Association (AMTA)
Associated Bodywork and Massage Professionals (ABMP)
National Association of Holistic Aromatherapy (NAHA)

REFERENCES: References are available on request.

Figure 9-2 The sample chronological resume shown here is easy to write and appropriate for entry-level positions as it illustrates both your education and experience.

- **Education**: Include the name and location of the institution and the date of your degree, diploma, or certificate. List your most recent education experience first and include your grade point average if it is higher than 3.0. Describe your main area of study (e.g., massage and spa, or health care massage), list the hours of training you underwent, and mention any academic honors or awards you received. If you have taken continuing education in addition to your entry-level training, list the courses after your main educational experience.
- **Work Experience**: Include any relevant work experience in reverse chronological order with the most recent job first. List the title of the position, name of the organization, location of the work (town and state), dates of employment, and a description of your work responsibilities. If the experience is not an actual job, list it under the heading "Experience" as in the sample resume.
- **Other Information**: Depending on the specific job for which you are applying, you may choose to include leadership experience in volunteer organizations, special certifications or accreditations, membership in professional organizations, special accomplishments, computer skills, or foreign languages.
- **References**: Do not include your references on the bottom of your resume. Instead note, "References are available on request." Ask people if they are willing to serve as references before you give their names to potential employers.

Once you have completed a draft of your resume, share it with your instructor or mentor for feedback. Many people contact professional resume writers to help them create a professional-looking resume. Again, the Internet is the best source for locating resume writers.

Write a Cover Letter

A cover letter introduces you to employers and arouses their interest so that they read your resume and ask to interview you for the job (Fig. 9-3). Write each letter to address the specific employer and the specific job using paragraphs (avoid bulleted lists) and a conversational yet formal tone. Cover letters have three sections:

- **Section One—Opening**: In the opening section of your cover letter, briefly state the job you are applying for and how you learned about it. If you have any personal contacts with the company, mention them in this section. State your general qualifications for the job.
- **Section Two—Body**: In the body of the letter expand upon your qualifications and describe why you are a good fit for the specific position. For example, if you are applying for a spa job and the spa is well known for aromatherapy treatments, highlight your aromatherapy training and experience. If you are applying for a job at a hospice, highlight the fact that you took part in a hospital internship and worked with terminally ill patients. Pick out the most relevant qualifications listed in your resume and discuss them in detail to demonstrate your particular suitability for the job.
- **Section Three—Conclusion**: To conclude the letter, request an interview (or some other response, as appropriate) and include the times when you can be reached. Thank the reader for his or her time and consideration.

Follow up with a phone call a few days latter to ensure that the package has been received and to speak to the person who hires massage therapists, if possible. This initial discussion is important. It provides you with the opportunity to outline your credentials, special skills, and knowledge, which will hopefully lead to a request by the employer for an interview.

Interviewing

In an interview, the employer will appraise your suitability for a specific position and for the company as a whole. Your self-confidence, the way in which you express yourself, your level of professional dress, and the validity and content of your answers to questions will influence the employer's evaluation. The interview is also a time for you to gather information about the company's policies and determine if this is a job that matches your personal career goals.

When you set up the interview with the employer, be sure to inquire if you will be asked to provide a sample of your work. If the answer is no, dress as professionally as possible and even consider wearing a business suit. If the answer is yes, wear professional massage attire such as black pants and shoes and a short-sleeved polo shirt so that you can deliver a massage. The hands-on massage segment of the interview should last no longer than 30 minutes unless the employer is paying you for the massage. An experienced employer can determine your skill level very quickly based on your quality of touch, professional communication, and draping skills.

One way to prepare for an interview is to role-play with a friend or classmate so that you can practice answering standard interview questions (Box 9-4). Ask your friend to honestly evaluate your strengths and weaknesses, and practice until you can answer questions fluidly, concisely, and without hesitation. During the role-playing session, assess the manner of your speech and your body language. For example, if you speak too quickly, you may seem high-strung and chatty. If you speak with too little volume, you may seem to lack confidence. Eye contact is extremely important during an interview as averting the eyes might be interpreted as a lack of self-confidence or as dishonesty. Smiling too much looks unnatural, but a tight mouth could be read as disapproval or as a judgmental personality. Crossed arms convey defensiveness, while a slouched position sends a message that you might be lazy or disinterested. Avoid gesturing too much with your hands, which can be distracting, and do not touch your hair or face during the interview.

200 Any Street, Suite 300
Any Town, Any State 98000
janeanybody@internet.com

February 5, 2006

Mr. Eric Sanders
Recruiting Coordinator
Express Spa
Any Town, Any State 79000

Dear Mr. Sanders:

Your advertisement for massage therapists in the January issue of *Spa Spectrum Newsletter* caught my attention. I was drawn to the advertisement by my strong interest in aromatherapy and reflexology, areas where Express Spa has a well-known focus.

Although I have only recently finished my education in massage, spa body treatments, aromatherapy, and reflexology, I have had the opportunity to work in a high-pressure, customer service oriented team environment as the student massage clinic coordinator for Any Massage College. I am seeking a career with a recognized and respected spa that will allow me to integrate my understanding of wellness and relaxation while building my practical skills in aromatherapy and reflexology.

I would very much like to meet with you to discuss your open positions for massage therapists. If you wish to arrange an interview, please contact me at the above e-mail or by telephone at (303) 222-3232.

Thank you for your time and consideration.

Sincerely,

Jane Anybody

Jane Anybody

Figure 9-3 A cover letter like the sample shown here introduces you to employers and arouses their interest so that they read your resume and ask to interview you for the job.

BOX 9-4 **Examples of Standard Interview Questions**

1. Describe the experience and skills you possess that directly relate to this particular position.
2. What is it about working at this company that particularly interests you?
3. What is your primary weakness? Note: Some feel that it is best to identify a weak area honestly but then focus on a plan for self-improvement (e.g., "I have a tendency to be overly sensitive when criticized. I'm working on listening closely to constructive criticism, not becoming defensive, and then working to make positive changes."). Others feel that it is best to mention something that will be perceived as a strength (e.g., "I'm something of a perfectionist" or "I'm a bit of a work-alcoholic."). There is no one correct answer to this question, and the best advice is probably to answer truthfully.
4. What is your primary strength?
5. What do you hope to be doing 5 years from now?
6. What is your greatest accomplishment?
7. Why should we hire you?
8. Describe a problem or conflict you have had in a previous job or at school and explain how you solved it.

An interview provides you with an opportunity to find out more about the employer and to decide if the business is a good fit for you. Decide on questions you would like to ask during your interview, and practice politely interjecting them during different points in your interview. Some sample questions are provided in Box 9-5.

Show up 10 to 15 minutes early to your interview and treat everyone cordially, including the receptionist or assistant. When introductions are made, offer to shake hands and make it a firm handshake while looking the employer in the eye and smiling. Remember the employer's name and use it when speaking to him or her during the interview. Do not smoke directly before the interview or chew gum or drink a beverage during the interview. Bring an extra copy of your resume, a copy of your school credentials or transcripts, and

BOX 9-5 **Examples of Good Questions to Ask During the Interview**

1. What are the company's challenges and current goals?
2. Is a detailed written job description available for this position?
3. Are there opportunities for advancement?
4. To whom would I report?
5. Why is this position open?

a reference sheet. At the conclusion of the interview, express your appreciation for the interviewer's time and show enthusiasm for the job.

Negotiating the Employment Package

When a job offer is made, discuss the employment package, schedule, dress code, training procedure, and additional duties. Some employers require therapists to participate in training on businesses policies, procedures, and/or special treatments (e.g., a spa may want to train you to provide salt glows in a particular series of steps). Some employers pay for therapists to train, while others don't. Your employer might require you to perform a number of additional housekeeping activities like cleaning the restroom, sanitizing wet-room equipment, or doing the laundry, while others have support staff who handle such duties. Be sure to understand the expectations of the employer before accepting the job. Table 9-1 outlines some questions you may want to ask to clarify the employment package. While you should always behave in a calm, professional, and flexible manner, you should also ask for what you need in terms of scheduling and the employment package. It never hurts to ask about opportunities for advancement, especially if you have skills or credentials in addition to your massage certificate or license. Once these items have been discussed, consider the job in relationship to your specific needs and career goals. Sometimes a job is an ideal fit, and sometimes it is not an ideal fit but provides a stepping-stone toward your ultimate career goal.

Meeting and Exceeding the Employers' Expectations

Employers will expect you to meet certain expectations to maintain your position. If you exceed employer's expectations, you may be able to earn better wages, take on additional responsibilities, or work your way up to a higher position. Employer expectations fall into two general areas. First, you will be expected to have the knowledge and demonstrate the skills of an entry-level massage therapist:

- Knowledge of anatomy and physiology, especially the muscular system and individual muscles.
- Knowledge of the benefits and effects of massage techniques and of cautions, contraindications, and standard adaptations made for special populations.
- A basic understanding of common pathologies and chronic pain conditions.
- Knowledge of assessment, treatment planning, documentation, and record keeping procedures.
- Exceptional draping skills.
- Exceptional Swedish massage skills, deep tissue, and other massage and bodywork techniques based on the services provided by the business.

TABLE 9-1   Evaluation of the Employment Package

Compensation	How will you be compensated for your work? Will you receive an hourly fee and commission on massages that you perform, or will you receive a flat rate per massage, or a flat hourly fee regardless of the number of massages you provide on a shift?
Scheduling	Who will determine your work schedule, and how are schedule changes made when necessary? How will your shifts be covered if you become sick or have a personal emergency?
Extra duties	Will you be expected to perform housekeeping duties between appointments? Who does the laundry? Who cleans the bathrooms, retail area, reception area, and showers?
Staff meetings	Will you be compensated for time spent in staff meetings? Are staff meetings mandatory? When and how often are they scheduled?
Dress code	What is the dress code? Are uniforms provided or are you expected to purchase your uniform?
Inappropriate client behavior	How does the business define inappropriate client behavior? If you are uncomfortable working with a particular client, will you be required to work with him or her? When is a client refused service and who informs the client that he or she is being refused service?
Performance reviews/wage increases	Are there annual staff performance evaluations, and are wage increases tied to the outcome of the evaluations? Are bonuses given on overall performance or on meeting certain company goals (highest retail sales for the month, etc.)?
Training	How will you learn how the business operates? When will you be expected to train? Will you be compensated for training time or costs? Does the company contribute to outside training such as continuing education workshops to help you maintain your massage credentials?
Professional exchanges	Are you allowed to trade services with other professionals at the business? Are you required to pay for the linens, use of the room, and supplies when participating in trades?
Discounts	Do you receive discounts on services or products provided by the business? Can you get discounts for family members for massages?
Retail sales	Will you be expected to sell retail products? How will you be compensated for retail sales? Are there quotas for sales of retail product? What happens if you do not reach your quota for a particular month?
Health plan	Does the company provide a medical insurance plan or life insurance?
Liability insurance	Does the company provide liability insurance to cover clients who may be injured in a treatment, or are you required to provide your own liability insurance? (Review the company policy carefully if you are told it covers you. Often clients sue both the business and the individual therapist. In this case you will not be covered if you don't hold your own policy.)
Termination of employment	What is the procedure for termination of employment? Where can you work after you terminate employment? Some companies have noncompete clauses in their contracts that may prevent you from working in a certain radius of the business or working for a direct competitor.

- Exceptional client communication skills and customer service.

Second, employers will expect you to demonstrate the characteristics of a good employee and health care professional at all times:

- **Professionalism:** You dress appropriately, refrain from using slang and swear words, behave in a calm and collected manner even when dealing with difficult clients, and perform your duties without complaint. If you have a grievance with a client, coworker, or your supervisor, you follow the company's grievance procedure or speak privately and assertively with the other person avoiding gossip and unnecessary conflict.

- **Ethics:** You demonstrate high ethics at all times and set good boundaries for clients while maintaining client confidentiality. Your intent is to do no harm and to do good, and to never place the client in mental, emotional, or physical danger.

- **Dependability:** You show up on time and can be counted on to perform the duties assigned to you.

- **Responsibility:** In the event you are sick or unable to work a shift, you notify your employer promptly and try to find someone to cover your shift. If appropriate, you contact your clients to cancel appointments.

- **Initiative:** You look around and see what needs to be done and do it. You don't wait for someone to ask or assign you duties. You demonstrate a willingness to take on new tasks and responsibilities.

- **Curiosity:** You demonstrate a desire to learn new information and skills. You ask questions and show interest in your job, clients, and the skill sets of other therapists.

- **Positive Attitude:** You show up ready and willing to work while demonstrating a high regard for your job, clients, coworkers, and employer. You encourage others to be positive or to deal with conflicts in a productive manner.

- **Motivated:** You strive to do your job to the best of your ability at all times.

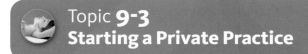

Topic **9-3**
Starting a Private Practice

In Topic 9-1, you assessed your values and skills and wrote a career plan to carry you through your first year as a massage therapist. This topic provides an overview of issues that concern therapists who start a private practice or work as independent contractors. Because the process of running a business is complex, view this chapter as an introduction to these topics and use it to structure further research. This topic does not cover aspects of running a business that includes hiring and managing other massage therapists, but it describes each of the sections of a business plan so that you can write a basic business plan and use it as a map for running your business.

Your Business Plan

The Small Business Administration (SBA) describes a **business plan** as a written guide to starting and running a business. A business plan helps you identify areas that need your attention as a business owner and helps you plan useful business activities to ensure your success. While few massage therapists need to seek a loan from a bank to start their businesses, a loan officer would expect to see a business plan, as will shareholders should you set up your business as a corporation (described below). Because each massage business is unique, the business plan helps you answer these key questions:

- What services does my business provide and what needs do my services meet?

- Who are the potential clients for my services and why will they purchase them from me?

- How will I reach potential clients?

- Where will I get the financial resources to start my business and keep it running?

Business plans can take many forms, but the SBA suggests that you break your plan into four areas:

- **A Description of the Business:** In this section, you determine your business name, location, and the way in which your business will be structured. You describe your business mission, vision, services, and fees.

- **Marketing:** The marketing section describes your business identity and helps you recognize your potential clients,

their special needs, and how you intend to meet those needs. It also examines the competition and your strengths and weaknesses in regard to the competition. In the marketing section, you explain how you intend to alert clients to your presence, services, and value, and convince them to visit your business.

- **Finances:** In the finances section, you describe how you intend to start the business financially and keep it running while you build a client base. You analyze the costs associated with starting and running the business and set goals for client sessions in order to make a profit.

- **Management:** The management section explains how the business runs, including licenses, regulations, and insurance needs; hours of operation; policies and procedures; staff roles and job descriptions (if applicable); and how services are provided.

Each of these areas is described in greater detail in the following sections. Box 9-6 provides an overview of the components of a basic business plan.

Description of the Business

Describing your business requires you to make important choices that influence your ability to attract and retain clients and meet your business goals. You must choose a business name, a business location, and a structure. Furthermore, you write a mission and vision statement to guide your business activities and outline your services and fees.

Your Business Name

Choosing the right business name is an important part of your public image. You want to find a name that is distinctive and memorable, is easy to pronounce and spell, suggests the services you offer, and separates you from the competition. A search on the Internet will tell you if names you like are currently being used by other massage businesses in your area or nationally by massage chains. You might also check for availability of the web domain name (or an easy variation of it) before making a choice so that the name you choose can also be the name of your Web site, making it easier for clients to find your business.

BOX 9-6 Your Business Plan

As you work through the pages of this topic, start to think about and fill in the sections of your basic business plan as outlined below. If you use your business plan to approach a bank for a loan or to entice stockholders for a corporation, you may want to enlist the help of an accountant to prepare the correct financial statements.

SECTION 1: DESCRIPTION OF THE BUSINESS

a. Business name

b. Business location

c. Business structure

d. Business mission and vision

e. Services and fees (describe the services you provide and the benefits of these services for clients, as well as the fee you charge for each service)

SECTION 2: MARKETING

a. Business identity

b. Target market

c. Competition

d. Advertising, promotion, and publicity plan

SECTION 3: FINANCES

a. Balance sheet

b. Cash flow statement

c. Profit and loss statement

SECTION 4: MANAGEMENT

a. Licenses, permits, and insurance

b. Operating procedures

c. Policies

d. Personnel

Sometimes therapists make the mistake of naming their businesses using words from a foreign language. While these names are often distinctive, clients may not know what they mean or how to pronounce them, and so avoid the business as a result. Another mistake is naming your business after a type of technique that clients may not be familiar with. The name "Center for Neuromuscular Therapy" may aptly describe your services but might mystify someone who just wants a regular massage. In fact, most clients won't know that neuromuscular therapy is a form of massage therapy.

Sometimes clients perceive a business as too "new-agey" because of its name. Will the general public be attracted to a business called "New Spirit Place of Touch"? Alternately, you might name your business to attract a particular clientele such as "Massage for Pregnancy and Children," but remember you are now limiting your potential for sessions because your client pool just got smaller. To choose a name, brainstorm ideas and share them with the types of people you want to attract to your business.

Location

The location of your business influences whether or not potential clients feel comfortable visiting you in the first place, whether they return, and whether they recommend you to friends and family. Think carefully about these issues when choosing a location:

- **Proximity to Clients:** Is drive-by and pedestrian traffic heavy enough that your sign alone generates new clients? Are you located in an area where clients feel safe walking to and from their cars? If you are focusing on a special population, are other services for that population located nearby? For example, if you specialize in pregnancy massage, you are likely to get more business if you are located next to a midwifery business or birthing center than if you are located next to an auto mechanics shop or sporting goods store.

- **Ease of Access:** How easy is it to find parking and are parking areas safe and well lit? How far will clients have to walk to reach your front door? Will a steep stairway and no elevator prohibit some client groups from accessing your business (e.g., the elderly and injured clients)?

- **Practicality:** Sometimes a space is located in a busy high-traffic area, with great parking and easy access, but is simply too expensive to be practical. You have to balance the need to attract clients against the possibility to make a profit. For example, you might rent space in a busy shopping mall boutique for $3,000 a month (rent in such a space could be much higher). You would then need to provide a minimum of 60 massages a month at $50 each just to cover rent. It's unlikely you could be profitable in such an expensive space unless you were sharing costs with other therapists.

- **Functionality of the Space:** The space has to be functional so you can greet clients, process their payment, provide an assessment, and deliver a massage without undue noise or loss of client privacy. For example, will clients need to walk down an outside hallway to use the restroom? How will they manage if they should have to use the restroom in the middle of a session?

- **Zoning and Signage Restrictions:** In some situations a business space may not be zoned for massage (see information on zoning in the section on management). In others, signage restrictions (where you can or cannot place signs advertising your business) are so extreme that it will be impossible for you to alert drive-by or pedestrian traffic to your location. Before you rent or lease a space, understand the zoning and signage restrictions and consider how these restrictions might impact your business.

- **Public Image:** The businesses around you can reflect favorably or unfavorably on your business. If you are located next to an upscale coffee shop, bookstore, or fitness center, that will reflect more favorably on your business than if you are located next to a video store, pawnshop, and nightclub. Consider the surrounding business and the types of clients they attract when choosing your location.

- **Home-Based Businesses:** Many therapists choose to offer massage from a home-based business because it is convenient and cost-effective, allows household tasks to be accomplished between sessions, and provides more time for family. If you offer massage from your home, you must consider noise levels (are children playing noisily in another room or outside?), pet issues (are clients allergic to your cat or dog? will your pet make noise, or sniff around the client making her uncomfortable?), cleanliness (any area of the house the client might see or use must be spotlessly clean), and family boundary issues (is your spouse lounging on the sofa in a bathrobe when the client enters or exits?). Many clients feel unsafe going to a therapist's home unless they already know the therapist's work. This may decrease the number of sessions you can fill in a workweek. In addition, zoning regulations might prohibit the use of a home for a business, or special permits might be required.

- **Shared Space:** Many therapists share space with other therapists or with chiropractors, naturopathic doctors, or other health care providers. This can be a cost-effective option with other benefits such as onsite referrals from other health care providers and wellness of health care goal planning for clients as a team (with the client's informed consent).

Business Structure

As a massage therapist, you might structure your business in a number of different ways based on your goals and whether you intend to partner with other people.

- **Sole Proprietorship:** Most massage therapists who are starting private practices structure their businesses as sole proprietorships. The business can be operated under your own name or under a business name, and your business profit or loss is reported on Schedule C of your individual tax return. All you need to set up a sole proprietorship is a business license issued by the city or county where your business operates. The drawback to sole proprietorships is that you are personally liable in the event that someone sues your business, and a lawsuit involves your personal assets, like your home (see the section on insurance).

- **Independent Contractor:** As a sole proprietor, you may form a contract with another business to provide your skills as a massage therapist without becoming an employee. In this type of arrangement you act as an independent contractor. You receive a fee based on the completion of a task, in this case, a massage. Independent contractors are often required to provide their own equipment and supplies. The business owner will not withhold your taxes, and you are expected to keep track of your profit and loss and report it on your individual tax forms.

- **Partnership:** If you go into business with another massage therapist, you might want to structure your business as a partnership. It's a good idea to have an attorney write up a partnership agreement that defines the parameters of the relationship to avoid confusion and conflict as the business grows. As in a sole proprietorship you will need a business

license from the city or county where the business operates, and each partner reports his or her own income on a standard income tax form. While you must share decision making with your partner, you are also able to share expenses and rely on each other's skills and strengths. The drawback to a partnership is that you are liable for all of the business debts if your partner dies, and if your business is sued you can be held liable for actions of your partner.

- **Limited Liability Company (LLC):** Two or more massage therapists might decide to form a LLC. An LLC protects your personal assets in the event of a suit brought against the business. Each member of the LLC claims profits and losses on their personal tax forms. The drawback to an LLC is that it requires you to file articles of organization with the secretary of state and to establish an operating agreement to help define profit sharing and ownership responsibilities. In the event that a member dies or files bankruptcy, the LLC is automatically dissolved. Check with your local state office about the rules regarding an LLC in your area, as these can vary state to state.

- **Corporations:** You might also structure your business as a corporation where shareholders hold stock in the company and a board of directors oversees operations. This is the most complicated type of business structure and usually requires the involvement of an attorney.

Concept Brief 9-1
Business Structure

Sole Proprietorship: A business owned and operated by one individual.

Independent Contractor: A person or business that performs services for another person or business under an agreement. An independent contractor is not subject to the other person's or business's control in regard to the manner and means of performing the service.

Partnership: A business in which two people enter into a contract to supply part of the capital and labor for a business and agree how profits and losses will be shared.

LLC: A business structure in which shareholders of the company have a limited liability in regard to the company's actions.

Corporation: A legal entity created under the authority of the laws of a state consisting of a person or group of people who become shareholders. The business is considered separate and distinct from that of its members.

Business Mission and Vision

A mission statement describes what your business aims to accomplish, the people it helps, and the problems it solves. Your mission statement should align with your values (see Box 9-1, Activity 1), be short enough that you can memorize it easily, and be powerful enough to make you feel inspired. Sample mission statements include:

- To provide massage customized to individual clients to improve the quality of people's lives.
- To decrease the pain and discomfort of fibromyalgia through state-of-the-art therapeutic massage techniques.
- To create a safe and supportive environment where people with mental health challenges can receive the benefits of therapeutic touch.
- To provide therapeutic services promoting physical, mental, emotional, and spiritual health and wellness.

A vision statement is a vivid idealized description of a desired outcome. It might describe how the world will be better when your business achieves it mission, or it might describe what success looks like to you. Sample vision statements include:

- (Name of business) is the recognized leader in helping people improve the quality of their lives through massage therapy.
- People living with fibromyalgia lead normal and productive lives.
- (Name of business) is regarded as the center of excellence in the provision of touch therapies to anyone with mental health challenges.
- Alternative wellness therapies are valued and used by people everywhere to maintain healthy and happy lives.

Services

Many massage therapists think of themselves as providing one service—massage. It can be useful to think of all of the different types of massage you offer as separate services to help clients better identify what they need and want from a session. In your descriptions of services, you want to identify the benefit of the service for the user, and when appropriate, the specific client for whom the service is intended. Massage therapy is not the only service you might offer. You might branch out and learn esthetics to offer skin-care services. You might be a fitness trainer and offer other health-enhancing opportunities. The sale of retail products could be considered a service, as could classes you teach or presentations you provide to community groups. Your services can be written out in a brochure often called a "menu of services" as shown in Figure 9-4. Your services should be posted on your Web site and in your office.

RETAIL SALES

The sales of retail products is a service that some therapists choose to provide clients. Chapter 6 describes the ethical considerations a therapist must make when offering retail items because there is a power differential that makes the sale of retail items to clients unethical in some circumstances. Before offering retail items to clients, review that chapter's section on Code of Ethics and Standards of Practice to make an informed choice about this practice.

If you choose to sell retail items, the retail area should be visually exciting and positioned in such a way that clients see it when they walk through the door. To keep returning clients interested, you may want to change the color, décor, and some of the products seasonally for fall, winter, spring, and summer promotions. Important retail selling times are Valentine's Day, Mother's Day, Father's Day, Christmas, and New Year. The retail area must be spotlessly clean and well organized. It's a good idea to choose products related to the effects of massage (e.g., a bath product that relaxes tense muscles) or to general stress reduction. Wholesale product lines for retail can be purchased from both massage and spa suppliers (search the Internet for "massage retail items" or "spa retail supplies"). Usually you must pay for the items in your retail area in advance, so this cost must be factored into your start-up budget.

You need some sort of system for tracking retail inventory. Those retail items that sell best should be highlighted. Retail items that sit and collect dust should be cleared in a special promotion and discontinued to make space for other more viable products. Computerized inventory tracking systems can be purchased for larger businesses. A smaller business may want to set up a simple system such as a running list of items that are sold, the employee who initiated the sale, and the client who purchased the product. A physical inventory should be conducted on a regular basis to check written records against stock. Items commonly sold for retail in massage businesses are outlined in Box 9-7.

Fees

Market-based pricing is the most common means of setting fees in the massage profession. If everyone in your area charges $60 per hour of massage, then so do you. The most common pricing error is setting fees too low. Some mistakenly believe that the lower price will entice clients away from other therapists, but the opposite occurs. Clients wonder if there is something wrong with your massage or if you can't attract business, and so avoid you. Once clients pay a low fee for massages, they are unlikely to pay a higher fee. It's a better strategy to charge the average market fee for massage and set yourself apart from the competition in other ways. An exception to this rule is prepaid package plans and special promotions that last a limited amount of time and are geared to bring in new business (discussed in the section on marketing).

Value-based pricing is determined by what a service is worth to a buyer. You may offer associated services that make the value of your massage higher than the value in the marketplace. For example, you might have an upscale spa facility with complimentary sauna and mineral salts soaking pool. If every client has free access to these facilities when they come for a massage, your massage is probably worth more than the going rate in the market. Similarly, if you offer a type of massage that clients can't get anywhere else, you can charge more per hour than you would for regular Swedish massage.

Cost-based pricing is used to set fees for items like retail products. You buy the products for wholesale and then mark

Your Body in Balance ~

YOUR MASSAGE BUSINESS

Menu of Services ~ Massage Therapy

At Your Massage Business our goal is to help our clients make good choices for healthier lives. Each service is designed to meet the needs of the individual client.

222 Any Street, Suite 300 Any Town, AS 00990

222-333-4444

www.ymb.com

Hours
Mon-Fri – 10-8
Sat & Sun – 12-5

Classic Swedish Massage: 1 Hour $60
This revitalizing full-body massage is customized to meet your needs. Swedish massage promotes circulation, improves skin condition, reduces muscular tension, supports good posture, and eases stress.

Spa Massage: 1 Hour $70
Aromatherapy touches such as a sweet sage facial steam, therapeutic aromatic massage oil and aroma mist are combined with traditional Swedish massage for a complete full-body indulgence.

Deep Tissue Massage: 1 Hour $70
A combination of Swedish and deep tissue techniques release tight, painful muscles and leave the body feeling balanced and relaxed. Your massage therapist will target areas where you want focused attention.

Hot Stone Massage: 90 Minutes $130
Hot stones are placed on points of tension and used in the therapist's hands to relax the body as the heat penetrates deeply into muscle tissue. This is a one-of-a-kind, must-try treatment for the massage enthusiast. Hot stone massage makes a great gift! Ask your therapist about gift certificates.

Pregnancy Massage: 1 Hour $60
Our Swedish classic tailored to the specific needs of the mom-to-be. Our special pregnancy pillows make this a comfortable and relaxing experience.

Onsite Seated Massage for Your Employees: Fees Negotiable
Research shows that massage improves the health and productivity of office workers. Your Massage Business brings the massage to your office where your employees can enjoy 15–30 minute sessions on break or during lunch. Find out more by speaking with your therapist.

Benefits of Massage Presentation: Free
At Your Massage Business we enjoy the opportunity to educate people about the benefits of massage for conditions like low back pain, over-use injuries, sport performance, fibromyalgia, and more. Talk to your therapist about arranging a 30 minute presentation at your office, natural foods store, support group, club, or other organization.

Figure 9-4 Think of all of the different types of massage you offer as separate services to help clients better identify what they need and want from a session. List your services in a type of brochure called a menu of services.

them up between 50% and 90% for retail resale. For example, if you pay $3 per unit of a bath soaking product, you would charge between $4.50 and $6.00 for the product.

PAYMENT PROCESSING
You want to think about the ways you process payments from clients and accept as many forms of payment as possible. In a

few states, such as Washington and Ohio, you may be able to bill insurance companies for massage.

While there is a setup and processing fee for to credit card sales, most people expect to be able to use a credit and debit card system when buying something as expensive as massage. Not offering this service to clients will likely impact your business and decrease the number of sessions you can fill in a week.

BOX 9-7 Retail Items Commonly Sold in Massage Businesses

Aromatherapy diffusers	Essential oils	Loofah mitts
Bath cushions	Exfoliation gloves	Natural baby care
Bath oils	Flower remedies	Natural hair-care products
Bath salts	Foot masks	Peppermint foot lotion
Bath soaks	Foot soaking aids	Sea sponges
Body lotion	Gift baskets	Shower gels
Body scrubs	Hand lotion	Soap
Books	Herb-filled dream pillows	Sore muscle balm
Candles	Herb sachets for bath	Spa bath-robes
Essential oil blends	Lip balms	T-shirts

Talk to your bank about setting up a merchant account to provide credit card processing. ABMP offers credit card processing as part of its member benefits package to massage therapists.

TIPS

Tips are payments that clients make of their own volition. While many therapists expect clients to tip, tipping is optional and clients have the right to choose how much they tip. If tips from clients exceed $20 per month, they are considered taxable wages and you must track the amount you make in tips and include it in your income records. IRS Publication 1244 (Federal Requirements for Reporting Tips) provides useful guidelines and information about tips.

Concept Brief 9-2
Fees and Tips

Market-based pricing: When you charge what everyone else in the market charges for a similar service.

Value-based pricing: When additional services or special services are valued by the buyer and therefore worth more than common market value.

Cost-based pricing: When wholesale products are marked up and resold for 50% to 90% more than their wholesale cost.

Tips: Additional payments clients make of their own volition.

Marketing

The term *marketing* refers to all of the things you do to attract new clients and retain existing clients. You want to consider your business identity, target markets, competition, advertising choices, promotional programs, ways to generate publicity, and a plan for building client loyalty when developing a marketing plan.

Business Identity

Your business identity is based on the message you want to communicate to clients and how clients perceive you as a result. Starbucks, Apple Computers, and Target are examples of companies that have powerful business identities. One important way to establish your business identity is through the design and use of a logo. You want your logo to reflect your values and be easy to associate with your services. It should stand out and have a style that can persist through years of change, new massage trends, and the growth of your business (e.g., you add a new service like skin care to your service menu). Hire a graphic artist to help you create a professional and meaningful logo, and then use your logo on all of your printed materials, on the uniform you wear to provide massage, on your Web site, and on your business sign. It becomes a unifying element for all things that relate to your business and helps clients remember who you are and what you stand for (Fig. 9-5).

You want to make sure to have a highly visible sign with your business name and logo placed in at least one location on your premises where drive-by and pedestrian traffic can see it. Some massage therapists use printed words on windows or doors to provide additional detail about services. For example, you might have a large sign with your name and logo over your doorway and the words "Swedish Massage," "Sports Massage," "Injury Rehabilitation Massage," and "Aromatherapy" printed on your doorway.

Your business cards, Web site, brochures, promotional materials, signs, newsletters, and everything else you print or publish provide a means to reinforce your mission and vision

YOUR MASSAGE BUSINESS
A Life in Balance

Figure 9-5 You want your logo to reflect your values and be easy to associate with your services.

for clients. All of these items should feature your logo and use a consistent color scheme and font style. Plan to have these items professionally designed and ready when you start your business.

- **Business Cards**: Your business information (business logo, business name, your name and position, phone number, address, e-mail, Web site, and a summary of services) is printed on heavy card stock about the size of a credit card. Pass out business cards to all of your friends, family, and acquaintances so that they can contact you for a massage (Fig. 9-6). Business cards can also be used for appointment reminders (write the client's next appointment date and time on the back of your business card) or for easy promotions (write "$10 off your next massage" and give it to clients to use as a coupon for their next visit).

- **Web site**: It is important to have a web presence so that potential clients can find you easily; most people have abandoned the Yellow Pages and head straight for the Internet when they want information. Websites are useful tools to communicate a wide array of information to clients and potential clients. Pages might include general information about your business (location, hours of operation, and phone number), your services and fees, policies (no show policy, termination of session policy, informed consent, etc.), a description of what to expect during a massage session, and even research articles that discuss the proven benefits of massage. Professional membership organizations like ABMP offer Web site hosting for members. You can often use simple programs to create your own Web site that looks professional and is attractive and functional.

- **Brochures**: You want to have one brochure that acts as an overview for your business. It should include your logo, business name, address, phone number, e-mail address, and Web site. Use it to explain to clients each of the services you provide and your fees. Include a basic description of your policies and a biographical sketch that outlines your credentials, training, and experience. This overview brochure might be supplemented with a Menu of Services that gives greater detail about each treatment and its benefits. You might also provide clients with a number of different informational brochures to give them in-depth information about a special service. For example, brochures on sports massage, reflexology, pregnancy massage, and health care massage explain to clients the benefits and techniques associated with each type of massage system.

- **Gift Certificates:** Make gift certificates available for purchase so that clients can buy friends and family massages when they visit for their own sessions.

Target Market

Target market is a term that refers to the specific group of customers that a business aims to attract. Target markets are identified as people with needs and/or wants that can be met with the products or services of the business. Massage therapists usually seek to capture the general public (anyone who wants a massage and is not contraindicated), plus particular target markets that interest the individual therapist. Possible target groups can be broken down into broad categories such as men, women, teens, and children, and into special populations such as athletes, pregnant women, the elderly, people living with cancer, people living with fibromyalgia, and others. Sometimes massage therapists target groups that have specific goals like individuals starting a self-improvement program, dieters, or people looking for a spiritual experience.

Demographic Indicators

Much can be learned about how to attract and retain target markets by paying attention to demographic indicators and lifestyle indicators of each market. Demographic indicators include age, income level, occupation, gender, geographic location, and education level. Lifestyle indicators include philosophical beliefs, social customs, health care needs, specialty activities, and personal priorities. For example, client A is a female (gender) with a bachelor's degree (educational level), who earns an income of $40,000 a year as a schoolteacher (occupation). She is also a yoga enthusiast (specialty activity) who practices Buddhism and organic gardening (philosophical beliefs). She has fibromyalgia (health care need) and is a single parent of a small child (personal priority). This client would most probably be attracted to your business if you had a spa featuring a well-known yoga instructor with meditation classes and on-site childcare. She will want linens made from organic fibers, natural, unprocessed massage lubricants, and music with a spiritual feeling. Client B is a 60-year-old male (age and gender) who works as an executive in a financial firm (educational level, income, and occupation). He recognizes that stress is affecting his health (health care need) and is focusing on staying fit and healthy as he ages (personal priority). He considers himself an atheist (philosophical belief) and doesn't like advertising that makes unsupported or unscientific claims. Client B is more likely to attend your business if you own an upscale massage clinic offering treatments targeting men. He is likely to be put off by any mention of treatments that are of a spiritual nature and or by new age decor in the treatment room.

As you plan your business, think about the target markets that interest you and try to understand these markets by investigating the relevant health care needs, specialty focus,

---

YOUR MASSAGE BUSINESS

A Life in Balance

Melody Massage ~ Massage Therapist

222 Any Steet, Suite 300
Any Town, AS. 00990
222-333-4444

www.ymb.com

Figure 9-6 A business card provides your contact details so people can reach you to set up a massage appointment.

concerns, and goals of each group. Next, assess the skills and services you provide, your business identity, the decor of your facility, and all the other aspects of your business in relationship to these groups. Make sure that your business will appeal to the clients you want to attract, and that your services will meet their particular needs.

Competition

The primary goal of marketing is to clearly communicate your advantages over the competition to the general public and your target markets. To do this, you must analyze your competitor's strengths and weaknesses. Use the sample competitor analysis form shown in Figure 9-7 or make up your own form to record your findings.

First, use the Internet to locate every massage business within a 25-mile radius of your business and gather general data including their name, address, phone number, and Web site. Use their Web site to find out about their services, fees, the client markets they target, and their areas of expertise (e.g., spa therapies, sports massage, injury rehabilitation, pregnancy massage, energetic bodywork, and Eastern bodywork). Pick out the five businesses you consider to be your primary competitors and call them to set up a massage appointment (massages used for competitive analysis can be deducted on your tax return). Pay attention to phone etiquette. How fast was your call answered or returned? Did you immediately get a live person or did you have to leave a message? Was the receptionist friendly and helpful? Visit

---

Competitor Name: Serenity Massage

Address: 222 Any Steet, Any Town, Any State, 00090

Phone: 222-333-7777   **Website:** www.serenitymassagenow.com

Services	Fees
Swedish Massage	1 hr. $60, 90 min $80
Deep Tissue	1 hr. $70, 90 min $90
Sports Massage	1 hr. $70, 90 min $90
Pregnancy Massage	1 hr. $70, 90 min $90
Hot Stone Massage	1 hr. $80, 90 min $100
Salt Glow	1 hr. $80
Herbal Body Wrap	1 hr. $80

Target Clients:

General public, weekend athletes, pregnant women, people who want a basic spa experience but don't want to go to a fancy spa.

Onsite Visit Experience:

When I called to make an appointment a receptionist answered after one ring and was able to provide me with a massage that day. It was hard to find the parking lot the receptionist described and I had to pay for parking on the street. Signage was poor. There is just one small sign above the door and the color scheme (purple and beige) gets lost against the other colors of the building. The reception area was pleasant, comfortable and clean and the intake paperwork was straightforward and quick to fill out. My therapist met me on time and was friendly but professional. He provided a standard Swedish massage that was good but not exceptional. My overall experience was good, especially booking the appointment, but not anything out of the ordinary.

Analysis of Stengths and Weaknesses:

Serenity Massage is stronger than my business in booking appointments and in spa therapies. Because a receptionist is available to answer the phone I was able to get an appointment arranged with one phone call. My business cannot afford a receptionist at this time so I must make every effort to return calls promptly. While Serenity Massage only offers two spa treatments, these services round out their menu and allow clients to try something new once in a while. My strength is that I offer reflexology. I need to spend time to develop good client education materials about reflexology and promote this special service to the general public.

Figure 9-7 A competitor analysis form helps you analyze your competitor's strengths and weaknesses.

their establishment as if you are a client and pay attention to their signage, location, ease of access, attention to cleanliness, and decor. Pretend to be a curious client and ask a lot of questions. How many clients does your therapist see each week? Is it easy to get appointments or is the clinic always busy? What type of clients does the clinic attract? Finally, pay attention to the quality of intake procedures and paperwork, to the quality of the massage itself, and to the ease with which payment is processed. Identify your competitor's strengths and weaknesses in relationship to your own strengths and weaknesses. If you find a competitor has a clear advantage over you, you want to undertake activities to correct this imbalance if possible. If you find you have a clear advantage over a competitor, highlight this strength in your marketing materials.

Promotion

Promotional activities increase your visibility in the marketplace and attract the attention of potential clients. These activities might include holding an open house, providing a free workshop, sponsoring an event to benefit the community, renting a booth at a community event or health expo, sending out informational newsletters, offering free foot treatments at a local walkathon, and mailing flyers to current and potential clients that include a special offer or personalized gift item. Important methods of promotion include client education, client referral programs, health care provider referral programs, and special offers.

CLIENT EDUCATION

Educating people about the benefits of massage supports the growth of your client base. Your client education plan may include activities such as speaking at meetings of support groups for specific conditions (e.g., fibromyalgia, cancer, and HIV/AIDS), or to particular groups like a women's group, runners group, business networking group, or others. Presentations at fitness clubs, health food stores, sporting events, community events, and coffee shops raise the awareness of the general public to the benefits of massage. You want to focus your efforts on your target market because these are the groups that interest you, and it is likely that you have developed special services just for them. For example, if pregnant women are your target market, to alert them to your practice you might create a flyer offering discounted pregnancy massage on Monday evenings (your slow day). The flyer can also note the proven benefits of massage to decrease pregnancy aches and pains, support the labor and delivery process, and promote healthy birth size in infants. Post the flyer where pregnant women are most likely to see it (Lamaze classes, fitness centers, health food stores, obstetrician's offices, midwifery centers, maternity clothes shops, etc.) and partner with Lamaze teachers to provide free informational presentations about the benefits of massage for pregnancy to their classes.

Newsletters are another effective way to maintain contact with clients between sessions and educate them about different styles and systems of massage. Newsletters might also alert clients to an open-house event, introduce a promotion, and provide a coupon for $10 off the client's next massage. E-newsletters have become popular in the last few years because no printing or mailing of published materials is necessary and so costs are low and there is less impact on the environment. Make sure to gather your clients' e-mail address on your intake forms and then use any of a number of web-based e-newsletter generators (search the Internet for "e-newsletter generator") to send clients information. Be sure to provide a link so that clients can choose not to receive your newsletters if they prefer.

Open-house events educate clients about your business and entice them into your business so that they are comfortable with their surroundings. This makes it more likely that they will visit you for a massage. An open-house event usually includes refreshments, sample services (e.g., free foot soak and seated massage), a presentation on the different types of massage the business offers, and even displays that allow attendees to feel, smell, and try out spa or retail products. It's important to have a receptionist ready to book appointments on the spot instead of waiting for the client to call in after the event.

CLIENT REFERRAL PROGRAMS

A client referral program enlists your regular clients as sales agents for you as a way to get a reduced rate on massage. Provide clients with referral cards (Fig. 9-8) and have them write their names on the cards. Clients hand out the cards to friends and family members and encourage them to visit you for a massage. The friend or family member gives you the card when they show up for a massage and receive a reduced introductory rate. You keep the card on file and give the discount to the referring client when he or she comes in for a session.

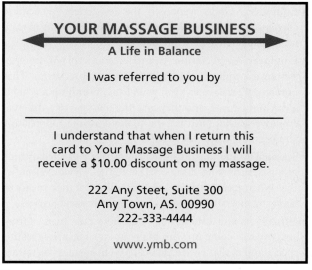

Figure 9-8 A client referral program enlists your regular clients as sales agents for you as a way to get a reduced rate on massage. Give your clients referral cards like the sample shown here that are returned to you and kept on file.

HEALTH CARE REFERRAL PROGRAMS

As part of your practice you will develop a referral list of other health care professionals. This group of physicians, naturopathic doctors, traditional Chinese medicine practitioners, acupuncturists, movement teachers, chiropractors, physical therapists, mental health specialists, nutritional advisors, fitness trainers, yoga instructors, and others will be ready to support your clients with services other than massage when they are needed. You can ask the health professionals on your referral list to direct clients/patients to you when they need massage. Building solid health care alliances takes time but builds important relationships in your community that will feed your business for years to come. It is helpful to write a letter to the health care provider introducing yourself, set up a brief meeting, and offer the other health care provider a free 30-minute massage. This way the health care provider can feel the quality of your work and better understand the benefits of massage for clients/patients.

SPECIAL OFFERS

Special offers are promotions that provide discounts on services when users meet specific criteria or for a particular amount of time. Ideas for special offers to bring in new massage clients or to increase repeat business include:

- **Massage Club**: Clients join a "massage club" where the price for one massage is automatically charged to their credit cards once a month. After they have enjoyed the once-a-month massages any additional massages they book during that month are provided at a discounted rate (e.g., $10 or $20 off).
- **Prepaid Cards**: Clients pay up front for a certain number of massages and receive a reduced rate on each massage as a result.
- **Punch Cards**: Clients receive a punch card on their first visit to your business. Every time they get a massage, you punch the card. When they have the necessary number of punches (e.g., 5, 10, or 15), they turn in the card for a heavily discounted massage or for a free massage.
- **Coupons**: Include coupons in the newsletters you send to clients to generate repeat visits, or pass them out in your immediate area to generate new client visits.
- **Employee Appreciation**: Approach local corporations or businesses with an idea for employee appreciation. They purchase 12 massages from you (1 per month for a year) at a discounted rate, and they give the massage to a different employee each month as a way to demonstrate appreciation and promote employee health.
- **Seasonal Promotions**: Pick a holiday usually associated with gift giving like Christmas, Mother's Day, Father's Day, or Valentine's Day. When clients purchase a gift certificate for their friends or family members, they get a discount on their own massages.
- **Others**: As you can see, special offers take many forms, and you can come up with many unique ideas for creating special offers that entice clients to your business or reward regular clients for their loyalty.

Advertising

Advertising is different from promotion in that it requires direct payment in order to gain public notice. The most common types of advertising used by health care professionals are classified ads, display ads, phone book ads, and Web site ads. Identify where to place the advertisements and then contact the publication for a media kit. The kit will contain the rates for different ads, deadlines for placing ads, and art development information. Statistics show that an advertisement needs to be seen at least three times before it is noticed. It may need to be seen at least seven times before the reader decides to take action. Ads seem to work best when they contain a strong visual image and clearly define the benefits and incentives of a service. Because advertising can be expensive, other methods of marketing a massage business may be preferred.

Publicity

Publicity is media exposure that usually arises from an event held by the business. Publicity might arise from an interview, news coverage of participation in a community event, or a feature story about the business or a particular service. For example, a local magazine might have a "tips for better living" section. Try sending in a press release outlining the benefits of one of your services for stress reduction. If the magazine is interested in this "new" approach to stress reduction, they will contact you about the service and may write a story about it including your comments and contact details in the story. Research the media outlets in your area. Identify those that target the same client markets as your business or that focus on health-related topics, and regularly send them press releases.

WRITING A PRESS RELEASE

A press release draws the attention of a media representative to a newsworthy event (Fig. 9-9). It is generally one page in length and lists the business name, address, phone number, and contact person in the top left-hand corner of the page. The release date (usually "For Immediate Release") is placed in the top right-hand corner of the page. A headline is placed in the middle of the page in bold capital letters. The body of the release contains short, concise paragraphs with the most important information described at the top. The final paragraph indicates the action the reader is meant to take as a result of the story (book an appointment, attend the event, conduct an interview, etc.). A press release is sent out each time the business participates in a community event, offers a free information workshop, donates their services in support of a charitable cause, introduces a new treatment, or provides an important service to a particular client group (e.g., free fitness checkup on Mondays for seniors).

Building Client Loyalty

Most massage therapists truly care about their clients and enjoy building a strong relationship as a partner in good health. This natural tendency of therapists to relate positively to their clients is the foundation of good customer relations and helps build client loyalty. You must also keep good client records, use high-quality products, make realistic claims for your services, provide a safe, comfortable, and sanitary environment, be prompt and reliable, refer to other health professionals when appropriate, and treat clients warmly and respectfully, even when clients are perceived as "difficult."

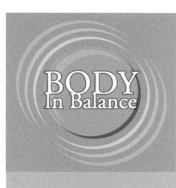

For Immediate Release

REDUCE WORK-RELATED STRESS WITH REFLEXOLOGY

Take off your shoes and relax! That's how easy it is to reduce work week stress at the Body in Balance massage clinic and spa. The clinic has designed a selection of unique foot spa treatments that target foot pain and stress through reflexology.

Reflexology is a holistic treatment that works on the theory that points on the feet, hands, and ears correspond to all areas of the body. Through stimulation of these points, the body is able to rest, relax, and recover from the pressures of everyday life.

Body in Balance offers a full menu of massage, body treatments, aromatherapy services, and reflexology. Melissa Massage, the owner, is an American Board Certified Reflexologist. She personally designed each of the seven reflexology foot spa treatments offered at the spa.

Athletes will enjoy the Pain-Away Treatment, which uses therapeutic Moor mud from Austria. This special healing mud has been used in Europe to treat joint pain and inflammation. Also popular is the Sedona Clay Ritual, which utilizes the powerful red clays of Sedona, Arizona, together with juniper and sage essential oils.

Melissa notes that "anyone bashful about getting undressed for a spa treatment should try reflexology. Reflexology is a great way to unwind from a stressful work week, and it's literally as easy as taking off your shoes."

To contact a Body in Balance and find out more about reflexology and foot spa treatments, call 255-555-5252.

Contact:
Melissa Massage

400 Any Street #1
Any Town, Any State
10000

Ph: 255-555-5252
Fax: 252-222-5555

info@bodyinbalance.com
www.bodyinbalance.com

Massage
Aromatherapy
Body Treatments
Reflexology

A balanced
body is achieved
when time is made
for self-care

Figure 9-9 A press release draws the attention of a media representative to a newsworthy event.

It is a good idea to set up procedures to maintain contact with clients between scheduled sessions and to acknowledge special dates. These activities might include checkup calls the day after the massage, a birthday card with a discounted or free massage on the client's birthday, newsletters with coupons, anniversary cards on the anniversary of the client's first massage appointment at your business with a coupon for a discounted massage, and thank you notes for referrals. An annual open-house event for clients and their guests is a nice way to thank clients for their loyalty. The event might include hors d'oeuvre, seated massage, paraffin dips, a gift of bath salts, and a free massage as a door prize.

Your Marketing Plan

It is helpful to write a marketing plan that gives details on daily, weekly, and monthly marketing activities. Time moves fast and opportunities to promote the business will come and go if a clear schedule is not maintained. Even a small business with a correspondingly small marketing budget should plan to spend 6 to 8 hours a week on short-term or long-term marketing activities. First think about seasonal promotions, and then do a search on the Internet to discover community events coming up in your area. Plan an open-house event or set up at a street fair. Make sure that clients know who you are, what you do, and where they can find you.

Concept Brief 9-3
Marketing

Marketing: All the things you do to attract and retain clients.

Target Market: The group of specific clients that your business aims to attract.

Promotion: Marketing activities that increase your business visibility and attract the attention of potential clients.

Advertising: Paid means to gain public notice.

Publicity: Media exposure arising from an event related to your business.

Finances

Your business finances include financial statements needed for a business plan, record keeping to track start-up and operating costs, bookkeeping systems that help you predict income, **expenses**, and taxes, as well as considerations for personal financial management.

Concept Brief 9-4
Terms Related to Finances

Balance sheet: A document that shows your assets, liabilities, and equity.

Cash flow statement: A document that shows your income and expenses for a fixed period of time.

Profit and loss statement: A document that shows how your business performed for a certain period of time.

Start-up costs: All of the expenses related to starting a business.

Operating costs: All of the expenses related to running a business.

Revenue: All of the monies that come into a business through clients' payments for services.

Expenses: All of the monies that go out of a business related to start-up or operational costs.

Net income: The money from revenue that is left over after expenses have been deducted.

Net loss: The amount owed when expenses exceed revenue during a certain period of time.

Financial Statements for Business Plans

When you write up your business plan, especially if you intend to submit it to a bank as part of a loan application, you will need to prepare a balance sheet, cash flow statement, and profit and loss statement. If the business is new, you will not have the financial history necessary to organize these documents. In this case, you must be prepared to demonstrate your earning power and the ability to support your new business with your personal income from wages at a job.

- **Balance Sheet:** This document demonstrates the current status of your business or personal financial situation at a given point in time (usually at the end of a quarter or year). It shows what you own (assets), what you owe (liabilities), and what your business is worth (owner's equity). Assets include cash on hand, money in checking and savings accounts, money that is owed you or your business, prepaid expenses like the deposit on your rental space or prepaid utility bills, equipment you own like your massage table and computer, and the building if you own it. Liabilities include outstanding bills yet to be paid to suppliers, wages you owe but have not paid to contractors or employees, payments you owe on a loan, or taxes you owe but have not paid. Your equity is the difference between your assets and your liabilities.

- **Cash Flow Statement:** This type of statement is prepared weekly as part of your normal bookkeeping procedures. You list **revenue** from sessions, sales of retail product, sales of gift certificates, and sales of other services against expenses like rent, utilities, office supplies, and laundry expenses. A cash flow statement helps you make good choices about purchases and upgrades to your business, and helps you track your net income or net loss week to week.

- **Profit and Loss Statement (also called Income Statement):** This statement shows how your business performed during a certain period of time (usually reported monthly, quarterly, and/or annually). It documents the total amount of money that came into your business (revenue), the money spent to operate the business (expenses), and what was left over (net income). If your expenses exceeded your revenue, you show a net loss.

While these documents may seem daunting, they are not difficult to compile. Search the Internet for "balance sheet sample," "cash flow statement sample," and "profit and loss statement sample" to view examples of these documents and then compile these documents for your business.

Financial Record Keeping

Good financial record keeping provides you with financial data that helps you operate your business more efficiently to increase your profitability. Accurate records are essential for the preparation of financial statements like those described in the previous section and ensure that you don't pay more than you really owe in taxes. The first step in setting up an ongoing system is to get baseline information for your business. This involves estimating your start-up costs and operating costs.

START-UP COSTS

All of the expenses related to setting up businesses are called start-up costs. Estimate your start-up costs by listing all the equipment, furnishings, supplies, and decor you need to outfit your business. These items were discussed in depth in Chapter 2. Factor in the cost to develop marketing materials and your Web site, as well as all licensing, permit, and insurance fees. Include security deposits on rental property and utility setup fees. If you plan to have a gift shop, also include the cost to purchase wholesale items that you sell to clients when you open your doors. Be as accurate as possible in your estimates or err on the side of estimating too high.

OPERATING COSTS

Some expenses such as the purchase of a massage table and music system are only made one time and are listed as part of your start-up costs. Other items are consumables and will run out at some point (e.g., liquid soap for bathrooms and massage lubricant) or need to be replaced as they wear out (e.g., linens, terry robes, and table pads). In addition, you will have regular costs related to laundry, utilities, the phone, and rent. These expenses are your operating costs. Get a monthly calendar and think about the year ahead. For each month list expenses you know you must pay, like rent and utilities. If you have annual fees related to licenses, insurance renewal, or mandatory continuing education, pencil these in for the months they are due. Try to predict when supplies and marketing materials will need to be ordered or reprinted, and add them in. Look at your marketing plan and factor in costs to advertise, promote, or publicize your business. For example, if you plan to set up a booth at a street fair, how much will the booth cost to rent? You want to know, with as much detail and precision as possible, what it will cost you to run your business each month. The first year you write your operations projection you are likely to miss some costs. If you keep good records, you will be able to refine the operations projection over time.

ESTIMATING INCOME

ABMP notes that therapist salaries range from $10,000 to $60,000 a year. This vast difference in salaries demonstrates the diverse nature of massage businesses. Many therapists practice massage part-time and may provide as few as three sessions a week. For others, massage is a full-time job, and they provide 20 to 25 sessions per week. It is very rare for therapists to provide 40 hours of massage per week because massage is such a physically demanding profession. Your income will likely be influenced by a number of other factors including the market rate for massage in the area where you practice, your ability to attract and keep clients, the number of sessions you are willing to provide each week, and your ability to manage expenses. Once you set your fees, you can do a simple calculation to estimate your gross income (before taxes and expenses are deducted) and net income (after taxes and expenses are deducted), as shown in Figure 9-10. This basic example does not account for massage offered at special rates, for weeks when the therapist does not provide 20 sessions, or for variations in expenses.

RECORD KEEPING SYSTEMS

Many types of established record keeping systems are described in financial management books and used in small business software packages. Small business software packages are recommended because they are easy to learn and have a reporting function that compiles all of the data you have entered in different worksheets into useful reports that help you track the financial health of your business. Some massage therapists choose to hire a bookkeeper or an accountant to manage their finances. This is a useful practice especially if you have little interest in learning a software package or

	Gross Income		Expenses		Income After Tax Deductable Expenses	Taxes	Net Income
WEEKLY	20 massages per week at $60 per massage	$1200	Rent ($700)	$337.50	$862.50	$215.62 (25%)	$646.88
MONTHLY	4 x $1200 a week for massage	$4800	Utilities ($250) Supplies ($150)	$1350	$3450.00	$862.50	$2587.50
YEARLY	12 months of 20 massages per week	$57,600	Marketing ($250)	$16,200	$41,400	$10,350	$31,050.00

Figure 9-10 Once you set your fees, you can do a simple calculation to estimate your gross (income before taxes and expenses are deducted) and net (income after taxes and expenses are deducted) income.

learning to keep records yourself. Record keeping for sole proprietorships can be very simple.

1. **Business Checking Account:** Open a separate business checking account for your massage practice. If you need to make cash purchases, write a check for petty cash from this account. Deposit all the income you make for any of the services you provide into this account. Have credit card income automatically transferred to this business account. Pay all of your expenses, including the salary you pay yourself, from this account. If you pay some bills with a personal credit card, pay the amount back to the credit card with a business check. Don't pay for business expenses with cash or a personal check if you can avoid it. This way there is accurate documentation of all of the financial transactions your business makes that you can reconcile with your other business records.

2. **Record Transactions:** Set up a ledger (financial record book) to record all of your financial transactions (money coming in and money going out). You can keep a handwritten ledger in a simple columnar book from an office supply store, set up a simple spreadsheet on your computer, or use a ledger as part of a financial software package. People often separate income from expenses and write these two different categories of transactions on separate pages of the columnar book (Fig. 9-11). You want as much information about each transaction as possible. For example, if a client pays for a session and also purchases a gift certificate, note these separately in the ledger. Record the client's name, method of payment (cash, check, visa, etc.), the check number if the client paid with a check, amount of payment, description of the service (e.g., 1 hour Swedish massage, or 30-minute foot treatment), and date.

3. **Keep Receipts:** Keep every receipt associated with purchases and expenses for your business and store them in the same order as they are recorded in your ledger. If you lose a receipt or didn't get a receipt for an expense, record the transaction in your ledger and make a note that you are missing the receipt. Reconcile your receipts with your checkbook and credit card statement at the end of every month.

4. **Keep Records:** Most business-related records must be kept for 6 years. Some records, like those related to property purchases, should be kept forever. If you are in doubt, keep the record. Store your records in a safe place such as a safety deposit box at your bank or in a fireproof filing cabinet. Items that should be kept for 6 years include receipts, bank statements, copies of tax returns, ledger sheets, check, cash, and credit card payments, balance sheets, cash flow statements, profit and loss statements, lists of inventory, equipment and furnishings, and automobile mileage logs if you do outcall services.

Taxes

The taxes you pay will depend somewhat on the way your business is structured (e.g., do you have employees?) and the types of services you offer (do you sell retail products? are clients charged sales tax on massage in your state?). Tax laws change regularly, so it is a good idea to review IRS Publication 334 (Tax Guide for Small Businesses) each year to stay informed about current tax regulations. As a small business, you may be required to pay income tax, self-employment tax, employment tax, and sales tax.

- **Income Tax:** Income tax is the federal and state taxes you pay on your business profits. The amount of your business profit is determined by subtracting deductible expenses from your revenue as discussed in the bookkeeping section (Box 9-8). The percentage of tax you pay depends on how much you made during the year. Because state taxes vary, check with your local department of revenue for

Date	Description	Income	Expenses	Balance
1/6/10	1 hr. Sw. Massage with Sue Smith – check #1123	$60		$60
1/6/10	90 min Sw. Massage with Dave Johnson – cash + $10 tip	$90		$150
1/6/10	1 hr. sports massage with Jenny Good – Visa + $5 tip	$75		$225
1/6/10	30 minute infant massage with Amy Morgan – Visa	$35		$260
1/6/10	90 min Stone Massage with Jane Murphy – cash + $10 tip	$120		$380
1/6/10	Utility Bill – paid check #2345		$60	$320
1/6/10	Liability insurance renewal		$199	$121

Figure 9-11 Set up a ledger (financial record book) like the sample shown here to record all of your financial transactions (money coming in and money going out).

BOX 9-8 **Examples of Business Expenses that Can Be Deducted from Taxes**

Accounting fees

Advertising costs

Business personal property insurance

Cleaning services

Continuing education (including travel and expenses at the workshop/seminar)

Costs to purchase a uniform

Depreciation on equipment purchases

Health insurance

Interest on loans

Laundry services

Legal services (attorney, business consultant, etc.)

License fees

Mileage for outcall services or business related travel

Office supplies

Postage and shipping

Postage and shipping costs

Practice supplies (e.g., massage lubricant and supplies for the bathroom)

Printed business materials costs

Profession related magazines

Professional conferences, conventions, and national meetings

Professional liability insurance (including general liability and product liability)

Promotion costs

Reference books

Rent or lease

Repairs on office equipment

Service charges (bank fees and credit card processing fees)

Telephone and Internet fees

information. Usually, small businesses pay estimated taxes to the IRS on a quarterly basis. To find out more about paying quarterly taxes, download IRS Publication 505 (Tax Withholding and Estimated Tax) from the IRS Web site.

- **Self-Employment Tax:** If you work as an employee, your employer withholds social security and Medicare taxes from your wages. Self-employment tax is social security and Medicare taxes you withhold for yourself.

- **Employment Tax:** If you hire employees, you are required to withhold federal income taxes, social security tax, and Medicare taxes from their wages and pay these taxes to the IRS for employees. In addition, you must pay a matching amount of social security and Medicare tax on behalf of each employee to the IRS. If your business hires employees,

download IRS Publication 15 and 15A (Employer's Tax Guide, and Employer's Supplemental Tax Guide) for more information from the IRS Web site.

- **Sales Tax:** Sales tax is a state or local tax based on a percentage of the selling price of products or services that the buyer must pay. The seller simply collects this tax from the buyer and passes it on to the state or local government. In most states and in many cities you must collect sales tax if you sell retail products to clients. In some areas sales tax is collected on the massage itself. You must obtain a sales tax permit (see the management section); contact your local department of revenue and taxation for information about sales tax rates and submission in your area.

Personal Finance Management

Personal finance management is an important area to research as a small business owner. Many books are available at your local bookstore or library that can help you sort through these issues. It can also be useful to contact a financial advisor to help you set up systems to manage your personal finances effectively. This section provides an overview of areas to consider as part of business planning.

- **Contingency Planning:** Contingency planning is planning for an unforeseen emergency. As a small business owner, you must plan ahead for events like an injury that could prevent you from providing massage to the usual number of clients each week, or a downturn in the economy that causes people to cut back on the number of massages they receive. As discussed earlier, you will pay yourself a salary each month from your business account. Try to pay yourself less than your business income and put at least 10% of your income into a savings account each month. Contingency planners suggest that you save 6 months of salary and business expenses to ensure that you can maintain your life and business in the event of an emergency.

- **Your Will:** You should write a will if you have money or possessions that you want to distribute according to some plan. Wills provide clear, legal instructors regarding your intentions and ensure that your family members are protected. While you can download will-generation programs, most small business resources suggest that you contact a lawyer to create your will.

- **Retirement Accounts:** Retirement accounts ensure you have money to live on when you retire and provide a tax advantage for small business owners. Four self-employed retirement plan options are commonly used by small business owners. These are the individual 401K, SEP IRA, Defined Benefit Plan, and IRA. The plan you choose depends on your income and the type of tax protection you need. Visit your local bookstore or your bank to find out more about these types of accounts, and start a retirement fund early in your business.

Management

To manage your business successfully, you will need to be aware of regulations in your area including necessary licenses and permits. You should have insurance to protect your business and should have policies and procedure that help you and your clients understand each other's expectations.

Licenses and Permits

In Chapter 6, you learned about the process to attain and maintain your massage credentials, including education requirements, state testing and licensure, registration or certification, and scope of practice. You may also need to obtain other licenses and permits at the local, county, state, or federal level to operate legally.

- **Business License:** In most cities or counties, you are required to get a business license that grants you the privilege of legally operating a business within a certain city and/or county jurisdiction. Contact the city hall and/or county government offices to obtain the application paperwork. Complete the application and file it in person with the appropriate government office (the application will provide the location). Fees range from $30 to $150. Business licenses are usually renewed annually.

- **Sales Tax Permit (also called seller's permit or sales tax license):** In most states, a sales tax license or permit is required if you sell products to clients. In a few states, sales tax is collected on the massage itself. You collect sales tax from clients when you sell them products (or provide massages) and then report and pay the sales tax to the state or county monthly, quarterly, or biannually. Contact your State Franchise Tax Board to obtain this permit.

- **Zoning Permit:** Don't sign a lease or rental contract on a property until you first check that the space is properly zoned for a massage business. Some cities require all new businesses to get a zoning compliance permit before they open. Contact the local planning department or the zoning board in your area for information.

- **Home Occupation Permit:** In some areas, the local government requires a home occupation permit if you practice massage out of your home. You may also need approval to run a home-based massage business from your local homeowners association. Contact the city hall or zoning board in your area for information.

- **Registration of a Business Name:** If you are a sole proprietor, the legal name of your business is your full name. If your business is a partnership, the legal name is the name given in your partnership agreement or the last names of the partners. For LLCs and corporations, the legal name of the business is one that is registered with the state government. If you want to conduct business under a different name (e.g., Mary Smith wants to conduct business as Soothing Massage Company), then you may have to file a "fictitious name" (also called assumed name, trade name, or DBA name, which is short for "doing business as") registration form with the country clerk's office or with the state government.

- **Employer Identification Number (EIN):** If you are a business that hires employees or if you are a corporation, you are required to obtain an EIN (also known as a Federal Tax Identification Number), which is used to identify your business at the federal level. To obtain an EIN, fill out Form SS-4, available from the IRS. You can apply online at www.irs.gov in the section for businesses.

If you are uncertain which agency in your city or state to contact for specific questions about business licenses and permits, the SBA (www.sba.gov), and your local chamber of commerce can help.

Insurance

People obtain different types of insurance to protect themselves in the event of a liability suit, personal loss because of fire, flood, or theft, or loss of income due to health care bills, injury, or illness. Assess what type(s) of insurance you need to protect yourself and your business.

- **Professional Liability Insurance:** This type of insurance protects you in the event that a client is injured by your treatment or your treatment causes complications in conjunction with another pathology. Many states require proof of professional liability insurance in order to obtain your massage license. It is very important to hold this type of insurance if you are practicing massage on the public.

- **General Liability Insurance:** This type of insurance is often nicknamed "slip and fall" protection because it covers you in the event that a client is injured (e.g., slips and falls walking up your stairs), or that the client's property is damaged (e.g., a lamppost on your property falls on the client's car).

- **Product Liability Insurance:** If you sell products to clients or use products like lotions, oils, and creams in your practice, this insurance protects you if the client has an allergic reaction or injury caused by the product.

- **Business Personal Property Insurance:** In the event of flood, fire, or theft, this insurance covers your losses (depending on how the policy is written). Sometimes therapists think that their homeowner's policy will cover the loss of their business property if the business is home based, but usually this is not the case.

- **Health Insurance:** Health care required by illnesses and injuries are covered to some degree by health insurance. Self-employed people can obtain health insurance through the National Association for the Self-Employed (NASE). Find information on the NASE Web site at www.nase.org.

- **Disability Insurance:** If you are unable to work because of an injury or illness, disability insurance ensures that you still have income from which to pay your bills and live. Insurance companies that provide life insurance usually offer disability insurance, or you can search "disability insurance + self-employed" to compare rates on the Internet.

Professional massage membership organizations like ABMP and (AMTA) provide professional liability, general liability, and product liability insurance as part of membership. Both organizations provide business personal property insurance for a small additional fee. Compare and contrast the policies carefully to make sure you get the right coverage for your business.

Business Policies and Procedures

Your business policies and procedures are the ways you deal with specific situations. They explain to clients what clients can expect from you and your business, and what you expect from clients receiving massage. Polices and procedures are shared with clients as part of the informed consent process as discussed in Chapter 6 and shown in a sample in Figure 6-6 in that chapter. Please review that figure and keep these areas in mind:

- **Hours of Operation:** Some businesses are *by appointment only*. The advantage is that you don't have to be on the premises during standard business hours. You are only at the business if you have an appointment. The disadvantage is that you miss the chance to increase client sessions with walk-in business. *By appointment only* works well for home-based businesses and businesses that don't have pedestrian or drive-by traffic.

- **Phone Etiquette:** One important aspect of good customer relations is phone etiquette. There is nothing more frustrating for a client in pain than not being able to reach a massage therapist promptly. Think hard about how you will manage your phone and be available to clients. Sometimes a group of therapists will share the expense of a receptionist to ensure that clients always reach a live voice when they book appointments. At the very least, you want to inform clients that you will be checking voicemail and returning calls every 90 minutes (usually massage sessions last no longer than 90 minutes).

- **Fees and Payment Options:** You want to clearly describe your fees for different services and payment options, as shown in Figure 6-6. If you offer standard discounts (e.g., $5 off your first massage), publish them and offer them to every client without exception.

- **Scheduling:** You want to establish clear no-show, late arrival, or late cancelation policies for clients. Once these policies are set, it is important to maintain these business boundaries even with friends or family members. Figure 6-6 shows standard policies and wording often adopted by therapists for no-shows, late arrivals, and late cancelations.

- **Client Rights:** Clients have legal rights to service, confidentiality, and control of their bodies. These rights are discussed in depth in Chapter 6 and described in Figure 6-6.

- **Therapist/Business Rights:** As a therapist or business owner, you also have rights and can refuse service to clients who don't demonstrate good hygiene, use illegal drugs or alcohol before the session, may be contraindicated, or behave in a sexual or immodest way, as demonstrated in Figure 6-6.

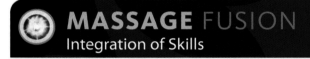

MASSAGE FUSION
Integration of Skills

STUDY TIP: Space Out for the Big Test

As you near graduation, it is likely that you will start preparing to sit for one of the three primary licensing exams if you plan to practice in a regulated state. Information for the Massage & Bodywork Licensing Exam (MBLEx) can be found at www.fsmtb.org. Information for the two exams offered by the National Certification Board of Therapeutic Massage & Bodywork can be found at www.ncbtmb.org. Often students cram for these exams shortly before their exam dates. Research studies have shown that people retain more information when they study 7 hours over 4 days (spaced practice) instead of 7 hours in 1 day (massed practice). Studying for short periods of time prevents boredom, improves concentration, and helps reduce fatigue. Spaced practice also works well for students who have jobs and family obligations. For example, Anisa goes to massage school during the day and works as a food server at night. In class, she writes her lecture notes directly onto flash cards. She carries the flash cards with her each night on her shift. When her tables are slow or while she waits for the kitchen, she pulls a flash card out of her apron and reads and repeats the information it contains. Anisa is able to memorize 6-7 flash cards each shift. Plan ahead at least 4 weeks before your licensing exam so that you can space your study sessions and refresh the information from your education slowly over a period of time.Text flush

GOOD TO KNOW: Helpful Business Resources

- Resume Writing: www.resumeedge.com, www.career-perfect.com, www.professional-resumes.com, www.resumeservices.com, wwwlresumelines.com.

- Small Business Resources: SBA at www.sba.gov, Inc. A Daily Resource for Entrepreneurs at www.inc.com, Small Business Service Bureau at www.sbsb.com.

- Books:
  o *The 250 Job Interview Questions You'll Most Likely Be Asked* by Peter Veruki. Adams Media, 4th Edition, 1999.
  o *One Year to a Successful Massage Therapy Practice* by Laura Allen. Lippincott, Williams & Wilkins, Baltimore, MD. 2009.
  o *Business Mastery: A Guide for Creating a Fulfilling, Thriving Business and Keeping it Successful,* 3rd Edition by Cherie Sohnen-Moe. Sohnen-Moe Associates, Inc. Tucson, AZ. 1997.

(Continued)

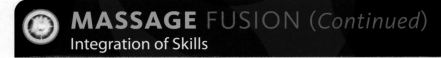

MASSAGE FUSION (*Continued*)
Integration of Skills

CHAPTER WRAP-UP

In this chapter you have begun to put together a concrete plan for your massage career after you graduate. You read about all of the practical things you will need to think about and do, like writing a resume and constructing a start-up budget. Career planning can bring up some uncomfortable feelings in massage students, especially when they try to balance their excitement with their fears about starting a new career. Some students share that they feel guilty charging money for massage. They feel that they entered the profession of massage to help people, not to make lots of money! How can I reconcile my desire to be helpful with a desire to be paid fairly for the service I provide? Others are concerned about all the regulations for self-employed people. What happens if I do my taxes incorrectly or don't put aside enough sales tax for when the bill comes due? These are real and reasonable concerns and everyone feels some uncertainty when starting any type of new venture. The best advice is to talk through your concerns while you dedicate yourself to careful planning. Discuss your worries with teachers, classmates, established professional massage therapists, family members, and friends. At the same time, cultivate your excitement for all the possibilities that are before you. This passion will help you face the challenges that arise with spirit and determination so that you can meet your goals and build the massage career of your dreams.

Technique-Focused Topics

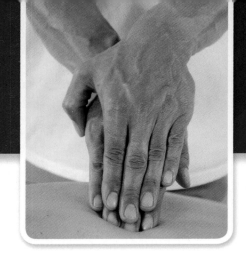

Foundation Skills for Therapeutic Massage

KEY TERMS

diaphragmatic breathing

draping

closing the massage

opening the massage

positioning

pursed-lip breathing

resting and holding strokes

wellness massage

LEARNING OBJECTIVES

Having read the chapter and used the related student learning tools, the student will be able to:

1 Outline the events that are likely to occur in a client interview and explain the importance of each.

2 Compare bolstering in a supine position to bolstering in a prone position.

3 State three reasons why draping is used in massage sessions.

4 Differentiate among simple draping, range-of-motion draping, and spa draping.

5 List three benefits of using breathwork in a massage session.

6 Describe two methods for using breathwork in a massage session.

7 Explain the importance of a well-planned opening and closing to the massage client.

8 Outline one method for opening a massage and one method for closing a massage.

A massage session is comprised of a variety of skills, often happening simultaneously and on many levels. You have already learned how to set up and organize massage equipment for the session. You have also learned how to practice good hygiene and sanitation. Knowledge of ethical issues provides a framework to think about therapeutic touch on a deeper level. This chapter teaches foundation massage skills, many that you will likely use in every session. Topic 10-1 helps you understand the sequence of skills you commonly use in a relaxation-oriented massage. The purpose of this topic is to give you the big picture so that you know where you're going and the skills you need to practice to get there. Topic 10-2 takes you step by step through the process of using bolsters to support clients in various body arrangements that give you access to different body areas during the session. The ability to undrape different body areas while maintaining the client's modesty is a key foundation skill taught in Topic 10-3, while opening and closing a massage effectively are discussed in Topic 10-4. Topic 10-4 also looks at the use of breath during a massage because breathwork can be a powerful aid for releasing areas of tension and pain. Understanding and mastering the techniques presented in this chapter will prepare you for the coming chapters on assessment and Swedish massage.

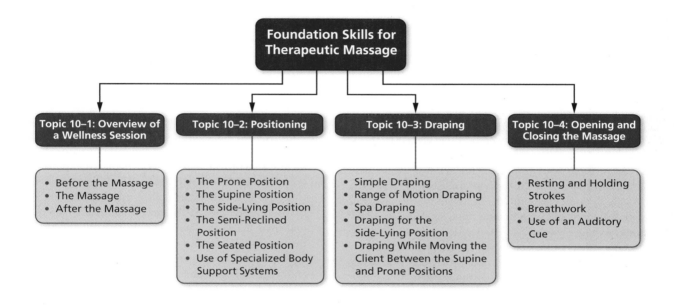

Foundation Skills for Therapeutic Massage

Topic 10–1: Overview of a Wellness Session

- Before the Massage
- The Massage
- After the Massage

Topic 10–2: Positioning

- The Prone Position
- The Supine Position
- The Side-Lying Position
- The Semi-Reclined Position
- The Seated Position
- Use of Specialized Body Support Systems

Topic 10–3: Draping

- Simple Draping
- Range of Motion Draping
- Spa Draping
- Draping for the Side-Lying Position
- Draping While Moving the Client Between the Supine and Prone Positions

Topic 10–4: Opening and Closing the Massage

- Resting and Holding Strokes
- Breathwork
- Use of an Auditory Cue

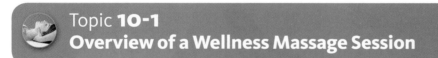

Topic **10-1**
Overview of a Wellness Massage Session

Massage theory and technique are sometimes taught in isolation, especially in the early portions of a massage training program. Students focus on one skill at a time and then put them all together into an organized whole. By previewing the big picture, however, students can better understand where and how different skills are used during the session. Previous chapters have explained differences between wellness massage and health care massage. The public seeks **wellness massage** to decrease stress, promote relaxation, support the body's natural restorative mechanisms, and have an enjoyable experience that leaves the body feeling refreshed and revitalized. Wellness massage is also used to reduce temporary pain from overexertion caused by activities such as weekend athletics or by unusual work stress. This type of massage is generally viewed as a healthy activity to promote a balanced, functional life and is regularly promoted at spas, wellness centers, private practices, and massage clinics. This topic examines the sequence of events that occur in a wellness massage. Note that the sequence of events in a health care massage (also called treatment or rehabilitative massage) is typically somewhat different. Usually a health care massage requires more in-depth assessment of the client and more detailed treatment planning. Later chapters discuss these skills.

Before the Massage

When a client arrives for the first massage appointment, make every effort to make the person feel welcome. Orient the client to the new environment. As discussed in Chapter 6 the new client is making numerous boundary adjustments to participate in the massage session and is likely to feel some nervousness or discomfort as a result.

The Greeting

As the client walks through the door, you or the receptionist should be on hand with a warm greeting. Step out from behind the reception desk to shake the client's hand and smile while making eye contact. Hand the client a clipboard with the required paperwork (usually a health history form and documents relating to informed consent), and explain each document. Show the client to a seat in the reception area and perhaps offer a cup of herbal tea. The client fills out the paperwork and hands it in to you.

The Tour

With paperwork in hand, you escort the client into the treatment area. Point out where the bathroom is located and any amenities like a steam room or sauna the client might use on the next visit. Let the client know if a shower is available before or after the massage. Show the client into the treatment room and explain where to undress and hang clothing. It's a good idea to remind clients to remove jewelry before the session, because lubricants can cause jewelry to look tarnished and delicate pieces may be damaged during massage strokes. Use a small dish to hold personal items so that jewelry is not lost or forgotten.

The Interview

The client interview, a complex and important process, is discussed in detail in Chapter 12. The overview here is to describe where and how an interview occurs in the progression of a wellness massage. Offer the client a seat, and sit down facing the client. The initial intake interview should accomplish a number of tasks:

1. **Policies and procedures:** Review your practice's policies and procedures and information relating to informed consent, including the scope of practice for massage and the limitations of massage. This process is discussed in Chapter 6. Ensure that the client has signed the informed consent form.

2. **Rule out contraindications:** Review the client's completed health history form. In some cases, you may need more information from the client about a particular condition to rule out contraindications. When you feel you understand the client's medical picture and that massage is not contraindicated, treatment planning begins. Health history form samples are provided in Chapter 12 along with complete directions for how to use the forms. Contraindications are discussed in depth in Chapter 5.

3. **Client expectations:** Ask the client to share his or her expectations for the session. "What results do you want to achieve?" It's sometimes helpful to ask, "When you leave here today after your session, what do you want your body to feel like?" In a relaxation session, it is common for clients to want to feel more relaxed or to have less tension in a particular area. First-time clients may not know what to expect and may be anxious. They may have seen a picture of massage or read about the benefits of massage in a magazine. Perhaps a friend described a positive massage experience. A client who has received only one previous massage is likely to expect this massage to be exactly the same as the first. In this case, the client may wonder what's going on when you use a different style or techniques. In each of these circumstances, you can set the client up for a good experience by explaining that there are many different types of massage and then describing some of the techniques you plan to use and their effects.

   While concerns about the therapist's gender have diminished as people become more educated about massage, some clients want to choose the gender of their therapist and may be surprised if this was not discussed during the booking phone call. In our culture, many men and women tend to feel more comfortable with a female therapist. Many women may feel less self-conscious about how their bodies look to other women. Some women have concerns about potential sexual misconduct by a man based on some past experience, while others may worry that their male partners will feel uneasy if they receive massage from a man. Some men feel anxious about receiving an enjoyable experience from a man's touch. Cultural and religious beliefs can also influence clients. While these stigmas can frustrate male therapists, this situation continues to improve as people embrace massage as a regular health care practice. As discussed in Chapter 6 all clients have the right to determine what happens to their body. If the client asks for a therapist of a specific gender, this request must be honored. Sometimes a client's expectations for massage are not reasonable, however. In this case, outline for the client what is realistic and what is beyond the scope of massage.

4. **Determine treatment goals:** With the client's input, determine specific treatment goals for the session. This can be fairly simple, as in the following example, or fairly complex. In a wellness massage, treatment goals are based on the client's expectations and often help you focus on areas that need the most attention during the session. For example, the goals for a session might be to decrease bilateral neck tension, decrease upper back tension, and decrease foot soreness. You then know that you will be massaging this client's back, neck, and feet. Will the client want other areas massaged? In a health care massage, in which the therapist is working with a specific condition or soft-tissue injury, treatment goals are determined differently. That treatment planning process is discussed in depth in Chapter 19.

5. **Plan the massage:** Sometimes clients only want selected areas massaged, or they may want a full-body massage with extra focus in certain areas. Clarify the plan before the session starts. You might say something like, "I'm going to start on your back to focus on your upper back tension and your shoulders. These tense areas are probably contributing to your neck pain. Would you like me to work on the back of your legs? Yes? Okay, then I will massage your legs before I turn you over and focus on your neck. Would you like me to massage your arms and the front of your legs? Great. How about your abdominal muscles? No? Okay, I will finish with a good twenty minutes on your sore feet." This is a good time also to ask clients about their music preferences and preferences for lubricants. When all these things have been decided, the session can begin.

Transition to Massage

Before you leave the treatment room, show the client the massage table and explain the position you would like the client to take on the table after undressing. Because clients may feel very nervous about how much clothing they need to remove, it's important to reassure them. You might say something like this: "Undress to your level of comfort. Some clients choose to remove all their clothing, which is fine, and others prefer to leave on some of their underclothing, which is also fine. You will always be draped during the session, and I will only undrape the area where I am working. This is to keep you warm but also to preserve modesty." This is also a good time to check if the client needs to use the restroom before undressing. Unless the client needs assistance getting on the massage table, leave the room while the client undresses. Because some clients feel nervous that the therapist may walk back in while they are partially undressed, it helps to say that you will knock and wait to hear they are ready before you enter.

Prepare Yourself for the Massage

Usually clients need no more than 5 minutes to undress and situate themselves on the massage table. Use this time to warm up your hands and to ground and center your energy for the session. These techniques are discussed in detail in Chapter 11. Use the restroom if you need to, and wash your hands carefully directly before returning to the treatment room.

The Massage

Knock and wait for the client's response. Enter the treatment room and greet the client again. If the client is in the prone position and cannot see what you are doing, explain your actions or movements (e.g., "I'm just going to start the music and turn on this space heater so you don't get cold."). A client who doesn't know what you are doing may become nervous when hearing you moving about the room.

1. **Bolster:** Decontaminate your hands and use bolsters to support the client's position on the table (discussed in Topic 10-2).
2. **Check in:** Ask the client about the room temperature and turn on a heater or add a blanket over the drape if the client is cold. Warm packs might be placed on the client at this time (discussed in Chapter 16).
3. **Open the massage:** There are a number of ways to open a massage. You might choose to use a breathing exercise like those described in Topic 10-4. You might apply a resting and holding stroke or perhaps add a creative flourish like ringing a small chime to mark the start of the session.
4. **Follow the treatment plan:** Once the massage starts, follow the plan you discussed with the client. If you discover an area of particular tension that needs massage but was not part of the original treatment plan, talk with the client about this. It's as easy as saying something like, "Carole, I've found an area on your low back where the tissue is very bound up. I would like to spend some extra time working on this area. We didn't discuss this earlier, but would you mind if I cut some time off the massage of your legs to work longer on your low back?" Carole will answer yes or no or may ask a question. This negotiation helps minimize the power differential and encourages clients to make decisions about their own body, as discussed in Chapter 6. Make sure to address each area where the client wants work.

   Sometimes new massage therapists frustrate clients by not getting to important areas in a timely manner. In one case, the client reported to the clinic manager that she specifically requested 30 minutes of work on her back and 30 minutes on her neck. She told the therapist she didn't want any other areas massaged. The therapist massaged the client's legs, feet, and arms and spent only 15 minutes on her back and 5 minutes on her neck. The manager questioned the new therapist and found that she felt uncomfortable with neck massage and was avoiding it. In school, she had learned a full-body massage routine, and that was what she was most comfortable doing. Ethically, this therapist should have explained her limitations up front and referred the client to another therapist until she had the skills needed to meet the client's needs.
5. **Close the Massage:** The massage can be closed in a number of ways, as discussed in Topic 10-4. Many therapists match their massage opening to their massage closing. For example, if they opened with a breathing exercise, they close with a breathing exercise.

After the Massage

Your actions following the massage help ensure the client has had a good experience:

1. **Transition out of the massage:** After **closing the massage**, remove the bolsters and ask the client to get dressed. Provide disposable wet wipes and a dry hand towel for the client to clean up. Sometimes therapists give clients

suggestions for activities they can use at home to improve the condition of their muscle tissue, such as stretches or self-massage. If you intend to give home care, ask the client to dress and remain in the treatment room. This way you can demonstrate the stretches or massage techniques privately. If not giving home care, ask the client to meet you at the reception desk after dressing.

2. **Collect the fee:** Back in the reception area, collect the fee for the massage and offer the client water. Clients appreciate bottled water they can take with them. Ask if the client would like to book another session. Some therapists choose to collect the fee and schedule additional sessions before the massage. This way, clients can be on their way as soon as the session ends. Both methods are fine.

3. **Book a session:** Book the session and give the client an appointment card with the date and time.

4. **Say goodbye:** You might remind clients to pay attention to how their body feels as a result of the massage. Phrase this in "goodbye language" to avoid opening a new conversation that would be better in the privacy of the treatment room. Say something like, "Remember to keep track of how your body feels so we can discuss it when I see you at your next session." Shake the client's hand warmly as you walk toward the door. This behavior helps the client transition out of the massage session and back into the real world. It also helps to maintain the boundaries of the therapeutic relationship, as discussed in Chapter 7.

5. **Chart notes:** Complete your chart notes and documentation for the session, and file the client's record neatly. Documentation is discussed in Chapter 12.

6. **Change the room:** Clean, disinfect, and sanitize the treatment room as needed to prepare it and the massage table for the next session, as discussed in Chapter 3.

7. **Self-care:** You might now perform any regular self-care activities like stretching or eating a snack before the next client arrives, as discussed in detail in Chapter 11.

As you can see, the massage session involves interpersonal skills like professional communication, ethics, and boundary setting and practical skills like draping and bolstering along with the actual massage techniques. The theory that underlies all of these skills is of primary importance. Without an understanding of the physiological effects of massage techniques, you wouldn't know which methods to use to address a client's neck tension. Without an understanding of the structures of the neck, you wouldn't know where to apply techniques. Each skill is important, and these different types of skills combine together in accomplished massage professional.

Concept Brief 10-1
Overview of a Wellness Session

- **Before the massage,** use your skills to greet the client, give a tour of the facility, and take the client through the intake process and interview.

- **During the massage,** use your skills to manage bolstering, positioning, draping, **opening the massage**, applying massage techniques, adapting the treatment plan with the client's permission, and closing the massage.

- **After the massage,** use your skills to collect the massage fee, book another session, transition the client back into the world, chart the session, clean the treatment room, and prepare for the next session, while also taking care of yourself.

Topic 10-2 Positioning

Clients take different positions on a massage table or chair. **Positioning** allows access to specific areas of the body. Bolsters are foam supports placed under the neck, knees, ankles, abdominal area, or upper chest or along the side of the body to decrease stress on joints and provide soft surfaces to support the client. Pillows and folded or rolled towels are also used to support a client comfortably in a given position. To maintain sanitation and hygiene, bolsters and pillows are placed under the bottom massage sheet or enclosed in a cloth cover that is laundered between clients. Bolsters are always removed before a client changes position (e.g., rolls from supine to prone) and at the end of the massage before the client gets off the table. This is for safety. If a client tried to

change position with a bolster in place, it could restrict movement and cause a muscle strain or the client to feel off balance.

The five positions commonly used in massage are the prone position, supine position, side-lying position, semireclined position, and seated position. Techniques for bolstering in these positions are shown in Technique 6.

The Prone Position

In the prone position a client is face down lying on the abdominal muscles. The face is situated in a face cradle to maintain the cervical spine in a neutral position. A bolster is placed under the ankles to reduce stress on the ankles, knees, and low back. If the client feels pressure on the low back because of this position, a pillow can be placed under the abdomen and pelvis to reduce the discomfort. For clients with large breasts who may feel discomfort in a prone position, a rolled towel under the upper chest elevates the client's upper body and reduces pressure on the chest. After such bolstering, the face cradle will likely need adjustment.

The prone position allows access to the back and lateral areas of the trunk, posterior neck, posterior arms, posterior legs, gluteal muscles, and feet. Some clients are most comfortable in this position because they feel more protected with their genitals and breasts beneath them. On the other hand, a client in a face cradle can't see the therapist, which sometimes makes new clients nervous. Be sure to describe what you are doing at times when you are not applying strokes or are away from the table. In one case, a male therapist started the massage of a new female client in the prone position. He left the table to remove the top cover from a bolster by unzipping the cover. When she heard the zipping sound, the client jumped off the table wrapped in her sheet, gathered her clothes, and rushed from the room. She told the manager that the therapist had unzipped his pants. She had been so nervous about the possibility of sexual misconduct that she wildly misinterpreted the sound she heard—a situation that could have been prevented if the therapist had said what he was doing.

Some clients don't like using a face cradle. It can feel claustrophobic and put pressure on the sinus cavity. When the client is face down, gravity drains fluids into the sinus cavity, causing congestion. The face cradle complicates the problem by restricting circulation to the face and head. If the client already suffers from allergies or chronic sinus problems, this can be very uncomfortable. In this case, you can adapt the prone position by moving the client toward the end of the massage table so that the head rests on a pillow instead of in the face cradle. Remind clients to turn their head regularly to keep the neck from becoming fixed and tight.

In the last stages of pregnancy, women are usually uncomfortable in the prone position. Use a side-lying or semireclined position instead.

The Supine Position

In the supine position, the client is face up lying on the spine. A bolster is placed under the knees to relieve tension on the knees and low back, and a small pillow or rolled hand towel is placed under the cervical spine to support the neck. Sometimes a bolster is also placed under the ankles to elevate the feet, assisting blood circulation to the heart and further reducing pressure on the back.

The supine position allows access to the face, neck, upper chest, abdominal area, anterior arms, hands, anterior legs, and feet. In this position, the client can observe the massage therapist if desired. Ceiling lights or sunlight through a window may bother the client. Ensure that the table is positioned to prevent direct light on the client's face. An eye pillow can be

placed over the eyes to dampen the light if necessary. A pillow may be placed under the head of a client who suffers from congestion to help gravity drain fluid from the sinus cavity. Many therapists start their clients in the prone position and switch to the supine position for the second half of the treatment. This way, congestion from the prone position has time to drain before the end of the session. The client leaves the massage with less facial puffiness and greater mental clarity.

The supine position is contraindicated in the last few months of pregnancy because the fetus is directly on top of the abdominal aorta and inferior vena cava, dangerously restricting the woman's circulation. Pregnant clients are often massaged in the side-lying and semireclined positions.

The Side-Lying Position

In the side-lying position (also called the lateral recumbent position), the client lies on one side. A bolster or pillow is placed under the knee and ankle of the upper leg so that the client can roll forward slightly and rest against the bolster or pillow. A second pillow is placed under the neck and head, and a third pillow is placed in front of the chest with the uppermost arm resting on it.

The side-lying position allows access to the back, neck, shoulder, gluteal muscles, abdominal muscles, anterior and posterior legs, arms, hands, and feet. It is an ideal position for clients with certain shoulder conditions because it allows anterior and posterior access to the shoulder structures at the same time and provides an unobstructed path for range-of-motion techniques. This position also allows access to the psoas muscle, an important hip flexor involved in many low back conditions. Clients who dislike the face cradle, who are uncomfortable in the supine and prone positions because of a back problem, who have large bellies, who have large breasts, or who are pregnant may prefer the side-lying position. Additional detail for positioning pregnant women is provided in Chapter 24.

Draping can be more difficult in the side-lying position and requires practice. As well, some massage techniques are not as effective in this position; for example, it is not as easy to use your body weight for deep tissue techniques on the back, and you must adapt your body mechanics to prevent stress on your joints.

The Semireclined Position

In a semireclined position, the client is lying on the back with the upper body elevated to a semisitting position. Pillows or special wedges are placed under the back, neck, head, and sometimes under each arm, and a bolster is placed under the knees. Some clients prefer only a slight elevation of their upper body and others prefer to sit almost upright. This position allows access to the face, head, neck, upper chest, abdominal area, arms, hands, anterior legs, and feet. The semireclined position is most often used in the later stages of pregnancy but can also be used for a client with allergies, a chronic sinus condition, congestion from the prone position, or a headache. As in the supine position, the client can see the therapist and may dislike direct light on the face. This is a good position to use for pregnancy massage because the client can spend some time on her back without the fetus weighing directly on the abdominal aorta and inferior vena cava.

The Seated Position

In the seated position, the client sits in a regular chair or a massage chair with the upper body supported. In a regular chair, pillows on the massage table or a face cradle or special desktop face cradle support the upper body. In a massage chair, the chair's structure supports the client's chest and face. The seated position is often used for on-site work on a fully clothed client who receives a 10- to 30-minute session, such as in an office or at a sporting event. Other clients may have a physical issue that makes the other positions uncomfortable. For clients who are too modest to remove their clothing, the seated position allows for effective compression techniques, tapotement, and kneading through clothing. The seated position does restrict your work in some ways. Access to the legs and feet is possible but requires unwieldy positioning that can stress your body. Abdominal work and work on some areas of the gluteal muscles and posterior legs is impossible or particularly awkward. Techniques that require a massage lubricant usually are applied only to the arms and hands or to the feet. Seated massage techniques are discussed in depth in Chapter 14.

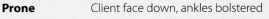

Concept Brief 10-2
Client Positioning

Prone	Client face down, ankles bolstered
Supine	Client face up, knees bolstered, neck supported
Side-lying	Client on side, knee and ankle bolstered, head and neck supported, pillow in front of chest
Semireclined	Face up, upper body elevated to half-sitting position, knees bolstered
Seated	Regular chair: upper body supported with pillows
	Massage chair: supports client's body

Use of Specialized Body Support Systems

Specialized support systems use foam forms that match the body's contours. Typically many pieces are included to fill in every gap where a client might need support. Velcro strips keep these pieces in place during massage. These systems are particularly useful with pregnant clients, larger clients, or clients with large breasts or abdomens.

Technique 6	**Using Bolsters**

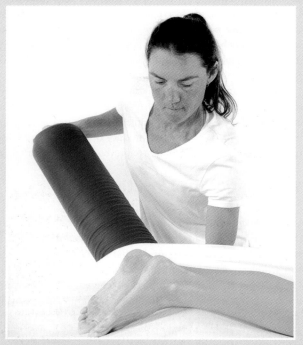

1. Prone Position. To bolster the client in the prone position, reach under the bottom sheet with the hand closest to the bottom end of the table and lift the client's ankles. Place the bolster under the bottom sheet and position it under the ankles.

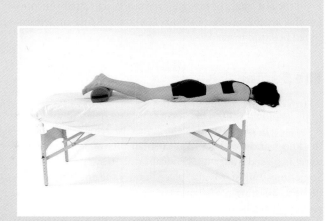

2. Prone Position. This image shows the placement of the bolster without the top massage sheet to more clearly show the correct position. Sometimes clients feel more comfortable if a pillow is placed under the abdominal area when they are in the prone position. If this is requested, ask the client to raise the abdomen and slide a pillow under the bottom sheet. The client adjusts the pillow or body position to feel comfortable.

Technique 6	**Using Bolsters** (Continued)

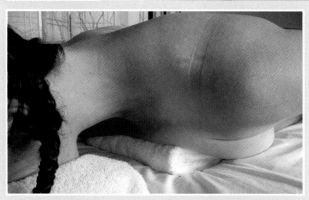

3. Prone Position. To position a rolled towel under the upper chest, ask the client to raise the head and shoulders, and place the towel under the upper chest. Have the client adjust the towel as needed for greatest comfort. Be sure to check the position of the face cradle.

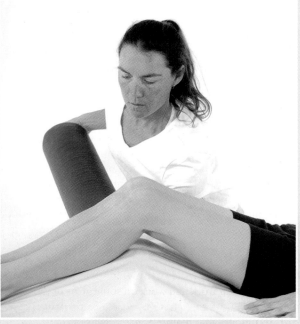

4. Supine Position. Reach under the bottom sheet with the hand closest to the bottom of the table and lift the client's knees. Place the bolster under the bottom sheet and position it under the knees.

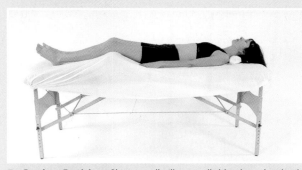

5. Supine Position. Place a small pillow or rolled hand towel under the client's neck.

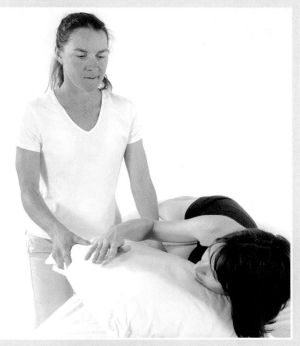

6. Side-Lying Position. Ask the client to lie on the side. Place a bolster or pillow lengthways under the bottom massage sheet so that the ankle, leg, knee, and length of the thigh are supported. Place a pillow under the client's head and neck. The same pillow can be used to support the arm.

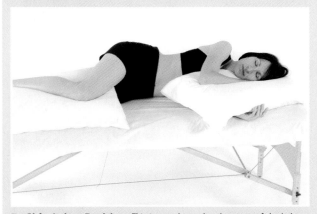

7. Side-Lying Position. This image shows the placement of the bolsters and the client's body without the top massage sheet and from a different angle to more clearly show the correct position. If you are bolstering for pregnancy massage in the side-lying position, use a larger bolster to bring the client's leg to a height even with the hip. This client is comfortable with just a pillow.

Continued

Technique 6   **Using Bolsters** (Continued)

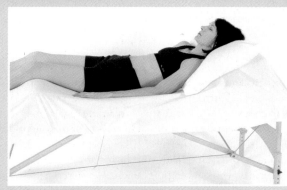

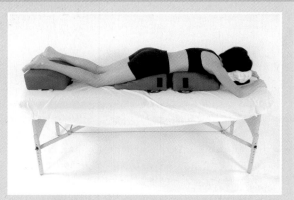

8. Semireclined Position. Preposition a wedge under the bottom massage sheet or ask the client to sit up and place a wedge. Use pillows to support the neck and head. Place a bolster under the bottom massage sheet to support the client's knees. Place additional pillows under the client's upper body if needed. This client is comfortable resting at a low angle. Some clients prefer to rest higher on the pillows.

9. Body Support Systems. This image shows the use of a specialized body support system in the prone position. Usually the wedges and bolsters are placed under the massage sheet. They are outside the massage sheet in this image for clarity.

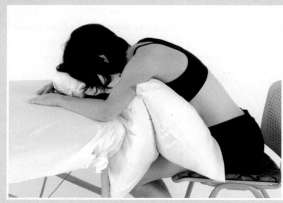

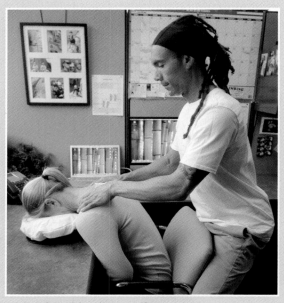

10. Seated Position without a Massage Chair. Place a chair close to the massage table, and position two or three pillows under the client's upper body and head so that the client feels supported.

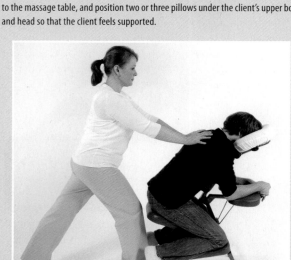

11. Seated Position in an Office. In an office, a desktop face cradle might be used to support the client's chest and head.

12. Seated Position Using a Massage Chair. Adjust a massage chair so that the chest support, face cradle, armrest, and leg supports fit the size of the client. Make sure the joints are open and the client looks comfortable. You will learn more about positioning clients in massage chairs in Chapter 14.

Topic **10-3**
Draping

A sheet, towel, blanket, or a combination of these always covers the client during massage. Even if the client leaves on underclothing or is dressed in clothing such as a sports bra and shorts, draping is used. **Draping** establishes professional boundaries, preserves the modesty of both the client and therapist, and ensures that the client stays warm during the massage. In some states or municipalities, draping is required by law. Even where draping is not regulated, professional ethics and massage standards require using draping to promote the client's and therapist's safety.

Cotton sheets, jersey sheets, flannel sheets, bath towels, pillowcases, hand towels, and blankets are common draping materials. A flat sheet covered by a cotton blanket or large bath towel works well for the main drape. Some therapists use just a towel, but towels feel scratchy to some clients, and because towels are smaller, it is easier to accidentally expose a client. Jersey and flannel sheets feel warm and snug, but these fabrics stick together and require more practice for efficient draping. Hand towels and pillowcases can be used for certain drapes such as a breast drape, anterior pelvic drape, or gluteal drape.

The only area exposed at any time is the area receiving massage techniques. Except for the head, all other areas remain covered by the drape. The breasts, genitals, and anus are never exposed. Sometimes clients become warm and move their arms or feet from under the drape. This is fine as long as the client doesn't expose large body areas or the breasts, genitals, or anus. New therapists sometimes make the mistake of fluffing the sheet to straighten it. This pulls the sheet away from the client's body and may expose all or some of the body to the therapist. In the massage classroom, fluffing the sheet may expose the client's body to the entire class of students. New therapists also might pull down on the bottom of the sheet to straighten it, and if the client is not holding the top of the sheet, this action could expose the breasts. Pulling the sheet up too high when a client's arm is undraped can also expose the breast.

When students first learn draping techniques, mistakes happen frequently. Most massage schools therefore first teach draping with clients fully clothed, and then with clients wearing underclothing. As draping skills improve, eventually draping is done without underclothing, and mistakes are rare, although even in professional practice a mistake can happen. If it does, handle the situation calmly, apologize to the client, ensure that the client feels safe continuing with the session, and proceed.

Draping should be smooth, neat, snug, and efficient. The drape should be tight enough to prevent being easily dislodged by a stroke. Learn to undrape an area with a series of precise, competent movements; avoid fussing with the drape. Some students tend to tuck the drape in multiple places, roll the drape up, anchor it here and adjust it there. This can be frustrating for a client who just wants to get on with the massage. There are many different ways to drape and undrape body areas. Since some schools have preferred methods for draping, always check with your instructor.

Three types of draping will be described here. The first, "simple draping," is used when range-of-motion techniques will not be applied to the shoulder or hip joints. Range-of-motion draping is tighter than simple draping. When a limb is moved, the drape must be circled around the proximal portion of the limb and sometimes held taut by the client. Otherwise, movement may cause the drape to fall away from the body, exposing the breasts or genitals. Spa draping is used during spa treatments and specific types of massage like abhyanga (Indian massage) or stone massage. Choose the most appropriate draping method for the techniques you plan to use in the session and to provide the most coverage of the client at all times. Techniques 7 to 11 demonstrate these different draping methods.

Usually you leave the room when the client gets on the massage table under the drape. In some instances, a client may need assistance on and off the massage table because of a physical condition or because the table is set high to accommodate the massage therapist. Many clients can manage by themselves with a wide step stool situated beside the table before and after the session. If your table has a lift feature, move it to the low position before the massage and again at the conclusion. Even with a step stool or lift feature, an unstable client may need assistance. Specialized draping techniques are then needed to ensure the client's modesty. These techniques are also effective in the massage classroom where student clients get on and off massage tables in a room full of other students. These methods are shown in Technique 12.

Concept Brief **10-3**
Draping

- Draping is always used to establish professional boundaries, protect the modesty of the client and therapist, and ensure the client's warmth, comfort, and safety.
- Therapists should drape using precise, efficient steps to create a smooth, neat drape that is snug and safe. Avoid excessive rolling, tucking, folding, or adjusting of the drape.

Technique 7   **Simple Draping**

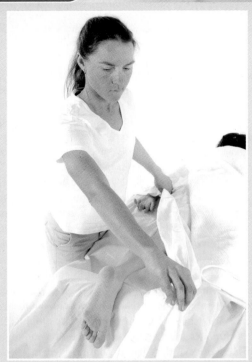

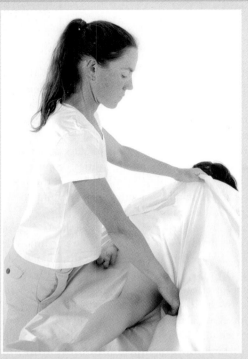

1. Posterior Leg. To undrape the posterior leg using a simple drape, gather the drape at the greater trochanter and at the ankle. Fold the bottom end of the drape at an angle across the opposite leg while holding the drape at the greater trochanter as a pivot point.

2. Posterior Leg. With your lower hand, grasp the fold of the drape and tuck it under the opposite thigh. Fold the top section of the drape across the back, leaving the gluteals and posterior leg exposed.

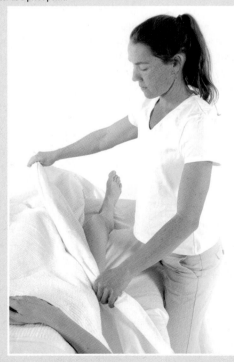

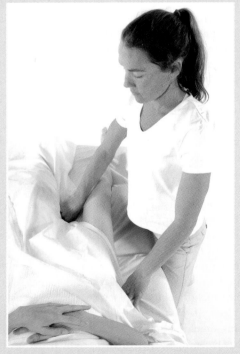

3. Anterior Leg. To undrape the anterior leg using a simple drape, gather the drape at the anterior superior iliac spine (ASIS) and at the ankle. Fold the bottom section of the drape at an angle across the opposite leg using your upper hand to hold the drape at the ASIS as a pivot point.

4. Anterior Leg. With your lower hand, grasp the fold of the drape and tuck it under the opposite thigh. Fold the top section of the drape across the abdomen, leaving the anterior leg exposed.

Technique 7   **Simple Draping** (Continued)

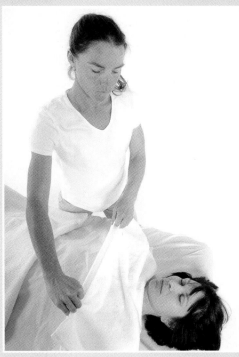

5. Breast Drape. For a simple breast drape, align the top edge of the main drape with the bottom edge of the hand towel or pillow case that will be used for the breast drape.

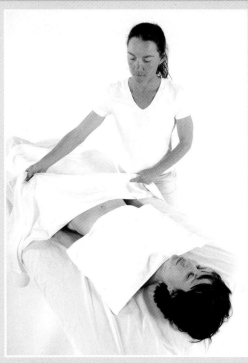

6. Breast Drape. As you pull the main drape down, the breast drape takes its place.

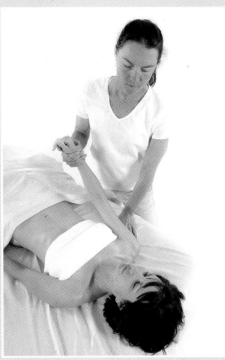

7. Breast Drape. Fold the edges of the drape neatly to give you access to the upper chest and abdominal region. Lift the client's arms and tuck the drape under the arms for more security.

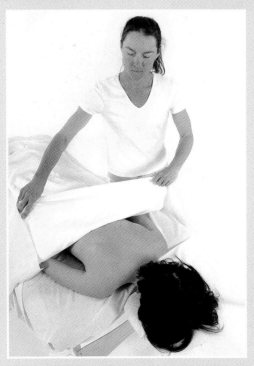

8. Back Drape. Expose the back by folding the drape down to the gluteal cleft. The gluteal muscles can be exposed by folding back the drape into a V-shape.

Continued

Technique 7 | **Simple Draping** (Continued)

9. Arm Drape. To expose the arm, lift the arm by the wrist and hold the drape tight beside the breast as you circle the arm around the drape and place it on top of the drape. If the drape is not held at the breast, the drape may be pulled up too high and expose the client.

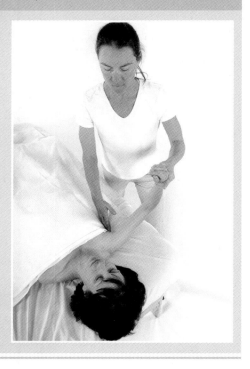

Technique 8 | **Range-of-Motion Draping**

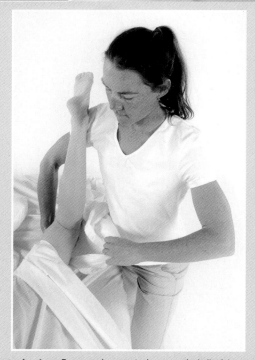

1. Posterior Leg. To expose the posterior leg, move the bulk of the towel out of the way and undrape the leg, placing the sheet between the legs. Lift the leg with your hand directly above the knee, and pull the sheet under the leg.

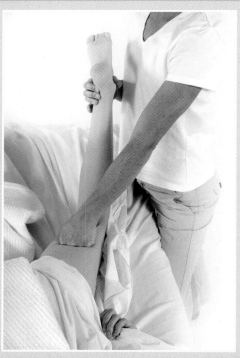

2. Posterior Leg. The client can grasp the edge of the sheet and hold it tight to prevent exposure during range-of-motion techniques.

| **Technique 8** | **Range-of-Motion Draping** (Continued) |

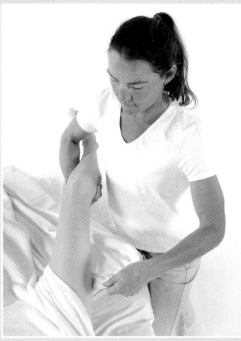

3. Anterior Leg. To expose the anterior leg, move the bulk of the towel out of the way and undrape the leg, placing the sheet between the legs. Lift the leg at the knee with one hand while pulling the sheet under the leg with the other.

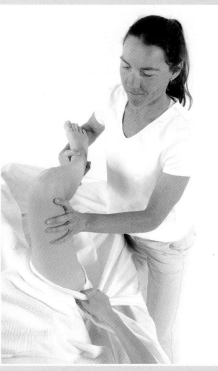

4. Anterior Leg. The client can grasp the edge of the sheet and hold it tight to prevent exposure during range-of-motion techniques.

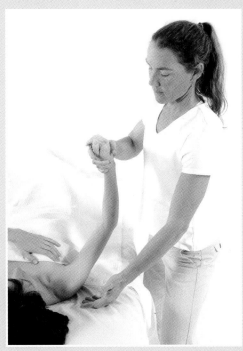

5. Arms. When performing range of motion on the arms, a client can anchor the drape across the breasts or chest with one hand to prevent exposure.

Technique 9 **Spa Draping**

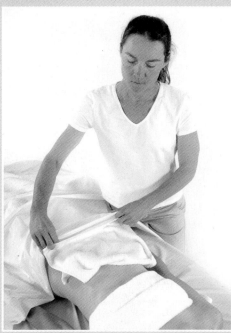

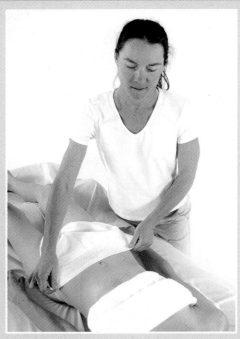

1. Anterior Pelvic Drape. An anterior pelvic drape is used when a spa product is being applied to the body or during certain types of massage. After the breast drape is in place, continue to pull the main drape down until the abdomen is uncovered. Align the fold of the main drape with the bottom edge of the hand towel or pillow case that will be used for the pelvic drape. As you pull the main drape down, the pelvic drape takes its place.

2. Anterior Pelvic Drape. Tuck the bottom section of the pelvic drape between the legs, leaving a safe distance between your tucking hand and the genitals, and adjust the top of the drape to ensure the client's modesty is protected.

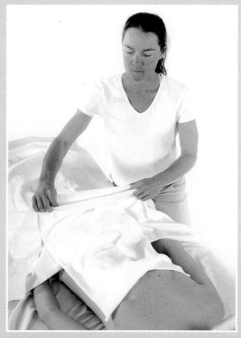

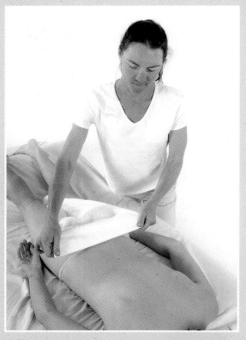

3. Gluteal Drape. A gluteal drape is used when a spa product is being applied to the body or during certain types of massage. Uncover the back and fold the drape down to the gluteal cleft. Grasp the folded edge of the main drape and the bottom edge of the hand towel or pillow case that will be used for the gluteal drape.

4. Gluteal Drape. As you pull the main drape down to expose the gluteals, the hand towel or pillow case replaces it. Tuck the bottom of the gluteal drape between the legs, leaving a safe distance between your tucking hand and the genitals, and adjust the top edge to ensure the client's modesty is protected.

Technique 10 | **Draping for the Side-Lying Position**

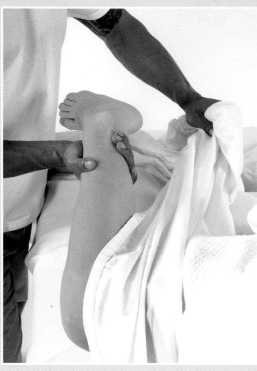

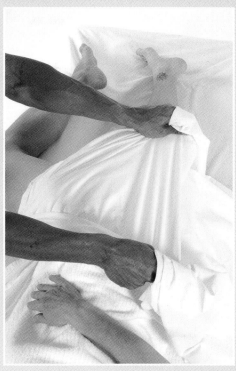

1. Legs. To undrape the legs, gather the sheet between the legs and pass the sheet between the legs.

2. Legs. Circle the remainder of the sheet over the pelvis to ensure the gluteals are covered. A towel can be placed over the pelvic area for extra protection.

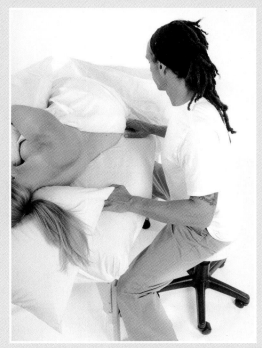

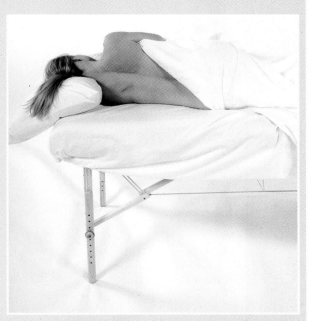

3. Back. To undrape the back, ensure that the top arm is positioned over the drape to anchor it. Fold the sheet back to expose the back, and anchor the sheet by tucking it under the hip. A pillow can be placed in front of the client to provide comfort and to anchor the drape at the front.

4. Back. This image provides another angle to view the back drape in the side-lying position.

| Technique 11 | **Draping While Moving the Client between the Supine and Prone Positions** |

Remove any bolsters, and place the client's arms under the sheet. Pull the sheeting up to the neck so that there is extra drape at the top of the table. Make the sheet into a tent, and anchor the side of the sheet by holding it with your body. Tap the client on the far shoulder to indicate the direction the client should turn. The client should always turn toward you so that your body prevents the client from rolling off the table. As the client turns, hold up the sheet in the tent to provide space for the client to roll over.

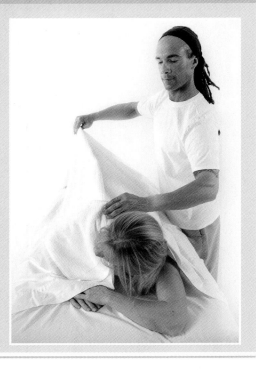

| Technique 12 | **Assisting a Client On and Off the Massage Table** |

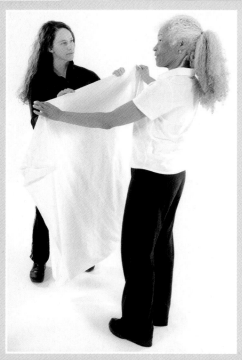

1. Getting On the Table. To help a client onto the massage table, offer the dressed client a sheet folded neatly in half, with the edges pointing up. Demonstrate how the client should position the sheet under the armpits with the opening overlapping at the front.

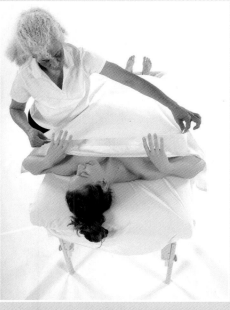

2. Getting On the Table. Leave the room so the client can undress and wrap the sheet. Return when the client is ready. Stabilize the client while using the step stool to get onto the table in a seated position. From the seated position, the client moves into a prone position. Then pull each side of the wrapped sheet out from under the client. Unfold the sheet so that it covers the client completely. You may now place a blanket or bath towel over the sheet to provide warmth.

Technique 12	**Assisting a Client On and Off the Massage Table** (Continued)

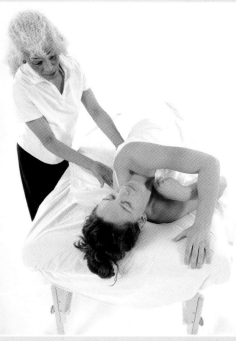

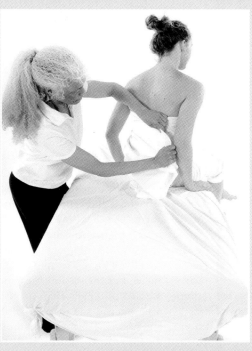

3. Getting Off the Table. To help the client off the massage table, first turn the client into the supine position. Have the client hold the top section of the drape. Pull the drape down straight, and then fold the bottom end up to the client's armpits. Tuck the drape around the body.

4. Getting Off the Table. Assist the client to a seated position, wrapping the edges of the drape around the client to conceal the gluteals.

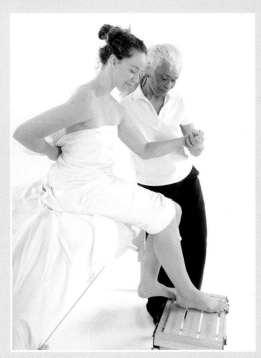

5. Getting Off the Table. Help the client off the table while anchoring the drape at the back. Ask the client to pull the drape around the body while moving off the step stool. Leave the room so that the client can dress.

Topic 10-4
Opening and Closing the Massage

Consider the following examples of how two different massage therapists open and close their sessions.

Steve pays attention to how he opens and closes his massages. He likes to use resting and holding strokes and breathwork (described below). To open the massage, he places his hands on the client with clear intent and allows the client to accept and become use to his touch. He asks the client to take three deep breaths and release all body tension with each exhalation. Steve's touch is assured and firm. The client feels a therapist who is energetically balanced and focused and who has a plan. The client relaxes before Steve even undrapes a body area, confident that Steve knows what he is doing. The opening is a simple moment, and yet it can affect clients' trust level and willingness to allow their body to let go and relax. At the end of the session, Steve finishes the massage, redrapes the client, and places his hands in the same position as when he opened the massage, this time with the client supine. Steve asks the client to breathe deeply for three breaths and to slowly wake up with each exhalation. The exhalation of each breath brings the client gently back to the real world and leaves the client feeling peaceful.

Jay doesn't worry much about how he starts and finishes his massages. When he enters the treatment room, he fusses with the drape, leaves the client to look around for the massage lubricant, and then struggles to place the bolster under the client's knees. The client's body tenses to ward off the irritating sensations of all this disjointed activity. Jay undrapes the client's leg and starts massaging, but the client remains watchful for the first 20 minutes of the session. Once Jay settles into the massage, he has good massage techniques, and the client eventually relaxes deeply when Jay works on the posterior legs and back. The client is calmly drifting when Jay abruptly replaces the drape and says, "Okay, time's up, and I'll meet you up front in the reception area when you're dressed." He pulls out the bolster and leaves the room. The client gets up quickly from the massage table and gets dressed. The client has less muscle tension but feels oddly irritated.

The opening and closing of the massage are important moments because they "frame" the entire massage experience. The **opening of a massage** is a formal moment that recognizes the importance of what is coming. Massage is an opportunity for the body to change in a positive way, to release long-held tension, to rest, to recover, and to have a healthy experience of touch. In many ways, a massage starts the minute a therapist enters the treatment room and approaches the client. Even if the client is in a prone position and cannot see the therapist, root hair receptors in the skin will recognize changes in air movement and heat. This may trigger instinctive survival responses that cause the client naturally to be tense during the initial contact.

It is better to look at the client, offer a verbal greeting, and approach slowly with therapeutic intent. Don't look around for bolsters or massage lubricant. Have everything ready before the client enters the treatment room so that your entrance into the room can be calm and relaxed.

The **closing of the massage** should leave a client feeling complete, peaceful, and balanced. You want the client to know the massage is ending before it actually ends and to start to return to normal waking consciousness smoothly without being jarred awake. Avoid abrupt closings that leave a client feeling rushed or disturbed.

Therapists use a variety of techniques to formally open and close the massage, including resting and holding strokes, breathwork, and auditory cues.

Resting and Holding Strokes

In **resting and holding strokes,** the hands are placed, without lubricant, on the client with the intent to greet the client and allow time to become accustomed to the unfamiliar touch. You might match your inhalations and exhalations to those of the client during a resting stroke, to feel in sync with the client's rhythms. Tension in the client's body, the client's temperature and breathing patterns, and the quality of the tissue under your hands all convey an impression, which may affect how you proceed with the session. Technique 13 describes the process of applying a resting stroke.

Breathwork

Breathwork in massage is an important skill. A breathing exercise such as the diaphragmatic breathing technique described in Technique 14, the pursed-lipped breathing technique described in Technique 15, or simply asking the client to take three deep breaths can help clients drop into their body, center themselves energetically, and consciously release unnecessary muscle tension. The use of breathwork to open the session or during the session also aids venous and lymph return, reduces pain, and can help a client deal with the discomfort of a particular technique. Breathwork also helps you tune into the client's breathing rhythms and thereby pace the massage to the client. Many people breathe with a disturbed pattern that can disrupt the delicate balance of carbon dioxide and oxygen in the blood. Proper breathing during a session revitalizes the body by ensuring the correct levels of oxygen and carbon dioxide in the body. The use of breathwork in a session helps clients become more aware of their breathing patterns and can lead to better breathing on a regular basis.

Technique 13   Resting or Holding Strokes

You may use numerous resting/holding hand positions. This image shows a resting/ holding stroke with the hands positioned on C7 and the sacrum. To apply the stroke, approach the client and stand at the side of the massage table. Place your feet shoulder-width apart, and bend your knees slightly. Check the position of your back and shoulders: they should be straight, upright, and relaxed. Avoid hunching your shoulders or shifting one hip to the side. Your weight should be between your feet. As you hold the stroke, develop an overall impression of the client's current physical, mental, and emotional state. Let this impression guide the massage. For example, if the client is visibly relaxed, you might move into deeper, more focused work sooner than if the client begins the session feeling stressed. Other resting/holding hand positions you might try include one hand on the upper back and one hand on the head, hands on the shoulders either supine or prone, and one hand on the abdominal area and one hand on the head in the supine position.

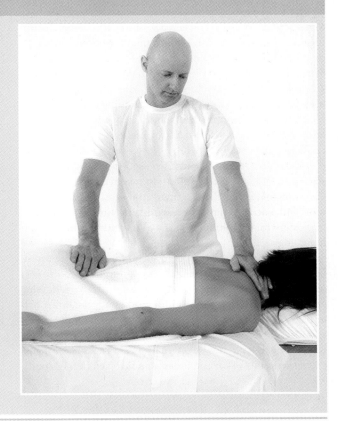

Informal Breath Assessment

Chapter 12 discusses client assessment, treatment planning, and documentation. For the purposes of this chapter, informal breath assessment is briefly introduced.

All massage assessment begins the moment the client walks through the door, and sometimes *before* the client walks through the door. For example, a client who gets out of the car slowly, with head fixed and wincing with pain, provides some indication for the focus of the massage session (probably on the upper back, shoulders, upper chest, and especially the neck). The same is true with breathing. Watch how the client breathes while filling out paperwork, talking to the receptionist, and walking to the treatment room. Breathing patterns vary a great deal, but in a normal breathing pattern, often referred to as diaphragm breathing, the abdominal area expands first on the inhalation, followed shortly by expansion laterally through the ribs and finally a mild lifting of the upper chest. Other typical patterns include apical breathing, often called upper-chest breathing. The upper chest lifts with the inhalation, but the lateral movement of the ribs and expansion of the abdominal area are minimal. Paradoxical breathing is a breathing pattern in which the lateral movement of the ribs and the upper chest compensates for abdominal holding. The abdominal area is held tight, and no expansion occurs with inhalation. This often happens in people who must maintain a fixed posture in their work, such as ballet dancers and military personnel.

Breathing can also be informally assessed while the client is on the massage table, at any time during the massage. A resting or holding stroke used to open the massage provides a perfect opportunity to track the client's movement of air and notice where breathing may be limited.

Students in the early stages of their massage training may wonder, "What am I supposed to do with this information? I can see that there is something happening on the right side, because the muscles in the neck on the right side get tenser than the muscle on the left side when the client inhales—but what does this mean? How should I change my massage to help the client?" Early in your massage training, you don't need to know what an usual breathing pattern means or how to change your massage to address it. You just need to notice it and experience it. When you see such a pattern, place your hands on the structures on either side of neck and feel what happens when the client inhales. Do your hands confirm what your eyes noticed? Where else do you see tension? How rhythmic is the client's breathing? Where does the air flow as it moves into the client's body? Where does the air stop? Continue to palpate and observe. Trust that as your skills progress, you will soon learn how to base the client's treatment plan on your observations and palpation findings to best support the client.

Opening and Closing the Massage with Breathwork

Many therapists begin and end a session with a short breathing exercise such as the diaphragmatic breathing exercise or pursed-lip exercise described in Techniques 14 and 15. These exercises support treatment goals while providing an opportunity to develop clients' awareness of how they breathe. Therapists must walk a careful line here. Too much focus on a breathing pattern can disrupt the client's relaxation experience and may cause resentment. Some clients resist breathwork because they just want to "get on with the massage." Breathing exercises used in wellness massage should be brief and to the point. In health care massage sessions involving specific treatment massage work, you have more latitude and may spend significant time assessing and working with breathing patterns as a means to meet treatment goals.

The diaphragmatic breathing technique and the pursed-lip breathing technique are brief enough to be used in every session, as desired by the client, and can help clients develop greater breath awareness and help change poor breathing patterns. These exercises set the client up to breathe more evenly and deeply throughout the session, enhancing relaxation, supporting lymph flow and venous return, and ensuring proper amounts of carbon dioxide and oxygen in the blood.

Diaphragmatic Breathing

Diaphragmatic breathing is used with the client in a supine position both to assess the client's breathing pattern and to educate the client about proper breathing. It works well to use this technique at the beginning of a session. Communication skills are key because you will "coach" the client into a functional breathing pattern. Focus on ensuring that the client's breaths are slow, rhythmic, and relaxed. Keep the exercise short enough that the client does not become concerned about losing time from the massage. The process of coaching a client through diaphragmatic breathing is shown in Technique 14.

Pursed-Lip Breathing

Pursed-lip breathing tones and strengthens the diaphragm and helps to reeducate the client's kinesthetic sense of breath. When the client exhales with lips "pursed" (imagine the lips closing around a straw), this creates resistance for the diaphragm. The diaphragm contracts on the inhalation and relaxes on the exhalation. Pursed-lip breathing keeps the diaphragm working at the same time that it is relaxing. Use this technique at the opening or closing of the massage session with the client in a supine position or sitting up in a chair. As with diaphragmatic breathing, communication skills are important as you coach the client through pursed-lip breathing. This process is described in Technique 15.

Technique 14 **Diaphragmatic Breathing**

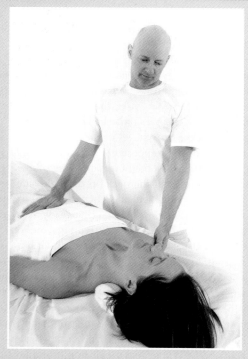

1. Place your hand on the client's abdominal area and ask the client to lift your hand with each inhalation up to three times.

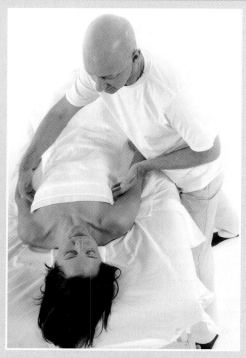

2. Place one hand on each side of the ribs and ask the client to move your hands outward with each inhalation up to three times.

Technique 14 **Diaphragmatic Breathing** (Continued)

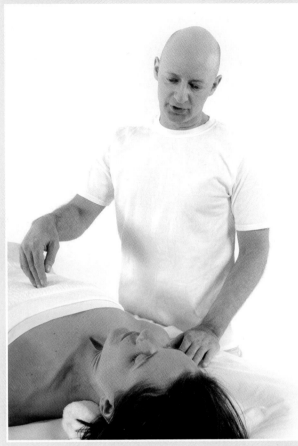

3. Place the fingers of one hand on the lower section of the sternum and ask the client to lift your hand with each inhalation up to three times.

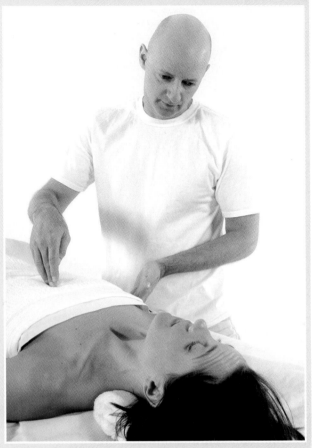

4. Have the client put the breaths together by cueing your hands. Ask the client to inhale, first filling up the abdominal area, then laterally expanding the ribs, and then allowing the chest to rise. Touch each area in order as the client inhales and pace the client on a full, even breath. As the client exhales, it can be effective to gently massage any areas of the upper neck that look tense, such as the shoulders, which may tend to pull forward or up during breathing. Repeat the cueing and coordinated breathing up to three times.

Breathwork throughout the Massage

Breathwork is important throughout the massage and can be used in a variety of circumstances. Sometimes you may notice that a client is taking a breath, holding it without conscious awareness, and then letting it out suddenly. Some clients regularly hold their breath without realizing it. You might say, "As I massage, try to focus on the even inward and outward movement of your breath. Try to make each breath full and complete. This will help regulate your breathing pattern and help relax your muscles." Clients then become aware of their breathing. Clients typically focus on breathing for a short time and then forget about it, but they are likely to breathe more regularly throughout the remainder of the session.

You can also match your own breathing to the client's to help pace the massage to the client's natural body rhythms. Alternatively, focus on your own breathing to add intention to a stroke or to ensure that your movements flow in harmony with breathing. In this case you are likely to exhale as strokes move away from your body and inhale as strokes come back. Your breathing pattern can also cue a client to breathe more regularly. For example, if you take an audible inward breath at the start of the stroke, you may find that the client joins in. As you exhale during the application of the stroke, the client might again follow along.

Technique 15   **Pursed-Lip Breathing**

Place your hand on your client's abdominal area, and instruct the client to raise your hand with each inhalation by breathing in through the nose on a slow 2- to 4-second count.

Demonstrate the pursed-lip position of the mouth for the client, and instruct the client to exhale through the lips on a slow 4- to 8-second count. The client should exhale through the lips as slowly as possible. Practice the technique a few times. Clients who are interested in improving their breathing and toning the diaphragm can practice pursed-lip breathing 20 to 40 times twice a day at home.

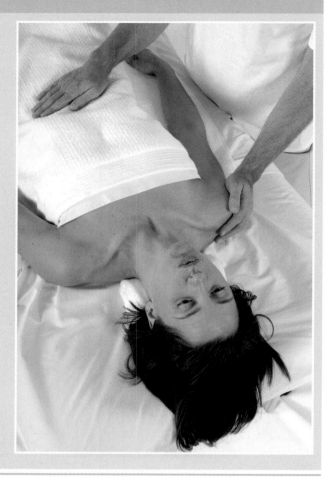

Clients can be encouraged to release bound muscle tissue with their breathing. As a muscle is lengthened, as you move from the origin of a muscle to its insertion during a stroke, or as you move from distal body areas to proximal body areas, encourage the client to take a full breath and then exhale as the stroke is performed. Your directions to the client should be simple: "Please take a full breath, and now release it." If an area is particularly painful or tense, the client can use breathing to release the area or decrease the pain. For example, if you are applying a stoke on the back and as you approach the rhomboid muscles the client tenses and you feel increased muscle tension, you can say to the client, "I'm going to drop into this bound tissue. Take a full breath and feel as if you are using your breath to lift up my forearm. Good. Take another deep breath and feel the tension dissipate as you release the breath. Good!"

In certain stretching techniques, like active isolated stretching and postisometric relaxation (described in later chapters), the use of breath is fundamental to the technique. Potentially painful methods like trigger point therapy require a client to breathe through the technique to better tolerate the discomfort.

Concept Brief 10-4
Use of Breath in a Massage Session

Benefits	Releases overall body tension
	Decreases muscular holding patterns
	Supports venous return and lymph flow
	Decreases pain
	Allows client to deal effectively with discomfort of some techniques
	Revitalizes the body
	Increases breath and body awareness
	Normalizes blood pH
	Educates clients about functional breath
	Helps pace massage to the client's rhythms
Techniques	Diaphragmatic breathing, pursed-lip breathing, breath instructions from therapist during strokes

Use of an Auditory Cue

An auditory cue, such as the ringing of a chime, can be used to signal the beginning and ending of the massage session. This opening might be paired with resting and holding strokes, an aromatherapy inhalation (described in Chapter 15), or a breathing exercise. This form of massage opening and closing creates a sense of ritual and lends the session a more spiritual formality. Over time, an auditory cue may become linked in the client's mind with relaxation, causing an instantaneous relaxation response.

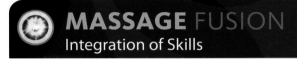

MASSAGE FUSION
Integration of Skills

STUDY TIP: Party! That's Right. Party!

Students sometimes feel like their social lives are curtailed by the need to study. One way to study and also have some social time is to hold a study party. To be productive, the party should have clear learning objectives and planned activities. For example, the schedule might be planned like this:

- 1 to 2 PM—Anatomy review—led by Steve
- 2 to 2:30 PM—Muscles of back flash card circle—led by Ellen
- 2:30 to 3:00 PM—Food! Everyone brings one dish for a potluck
- 3:00 to 4:00 PM—Draping Olympics (see explanation below)
- 4:00 to 10:00 PM—Watch a movie and more food!

MASSAGE INSPIRATION: Bring It On!

Many very talented massage therapists never fully master draping and positioning skills. A therapist may get the client bolstered in a side-lying position, but instead of this being an elegant series of carefully practiced steps, the client is asked to move this way and that to accommodate the therapist. Poor draping is epidemic in massage. Even though the client's modesty is preserved, unpracticed draping styles often involve tucking, rolling, retucking, adjusting, and more rolling—a messy, unpleasant experience for the client. Think of each draping skill, in each position or on each body area, as a series of steps to be performed like a dance routine, and plan your every movement around the massage table. Plan where to preset bolsters before the session. Plan each drape so that it is graceful and involves the fewest steps to ensure that the drape is snug enough that later adjustments are not necessary. This requires careful thought and lots of practice. One way to make this process fun is to hold a positioning and draping "Olympics." Ask your instructor to set a date and arrange for three judges. Make a set of large cards with the numbers 1 to 10 for each judge. It works well to organize each drape and each position into "events" such as the supine positioning event and gluteal draping event. Three different competitions can take place at once (each competition needs one judge). Arrange for prizes and generate some enthusiasm! You can learn a lot by practicing for your event and by watching your competition perform. If your instructor does not have time for this in the class schedule, this is a fun activity for a study party.

IT'S TRUE: Diaphragmatic Breathing Exercises Support Different Client Groups

Several research studies on diaphragmatic breathing exercises demonstrate that this technique can help a diverse group of clients meet health care goals, as long as the technique is practiced regularly. In one study, asthmatic adults who practiced diaphragmatic breathing exercises experienced a significant reduction in the medication they used to treat asthma and a lower intensity of their symptoms. This reduction in symptoms led to increased physical activity, which improved their overall health. Unfortunately, most participants decreased their practice of diaphragmatic breathing after the study and relapsed into previous medication levels and sedentary habits.[1] Another study showed that diaphragmatic breathing lowered blood pressure as long as it was practiced regularly.[2] Patients with anxiety disorders and panic attacks found that the diaphragmatic breathing exercise helped them experience less fear, fewer cognitive symptoms, and fewer catastrophic thoughts during an attack, and the technique sometimes served as an intervention to prevent an attack.[3] Finally, patients suffering from chronic low back pain improved significantly with breath therapy (a variety of techniques were taught including pursed-lip breathing and diaphragmatic breathing). This study reports that "changes in standard low back pain, measures of pain and disability were comparable to those resulting from high-quality, extended physical therapy." Again, the regular practice of these methods was important for continued benefit.[4]

(Continued)

⊙ MASSAGE FUSION *(Continued)*
Integration of Skills

CHAPTER WRAP-UP

The topics in this chapter illustrate the diverse skills needed by a professional massage therapist to manage a client before, during, and after a session. These skills involve four primary areas: knowledge, organization and client management, communication, and hands-on skills. The section on use of breathwork shows how important the knowledge of anatomy and physiology is for a massage practice. If you read your anatomy and physiology textbook, you will better understand the implications of breathing exercises, their benefits, and why they work.

Topic 10-1 shows the importance of organization and client management. Getting a client in and out the door involves many steps along with giving them an exceptional bodywork experience in between. An organized therapist who is skilled in client management can better plan and implement a meaningful opening and closing of the massage that add to the client's experience and help build client loyalty.

Therapists often emphasize learning advanced soft-tissue skills and fail to fully appreciate skills that seem less technical, such as positioning and draping. While it is desirable to master a range of therapeutic techniques, the foundation skills of positioning and draping lead to an uninterrupted client experience and allow the client to relax completely and enjoy the session. Underlying all of these skills is the ability to communicate effectively when explaining paperwork to clients, directing them to the treatment room, describing the benefits of a technique, giving direction during the session, and coaching the client through an activity like diaphragmatic breathing. Lack of skills in any of these areas can directly impact the therapist's ability to attract and retain clients and make a good living from massage.

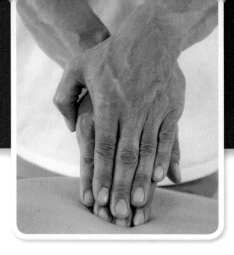

Body Mechanics and Self-Care

KEY TERMS

body mechanics
centered
flexibility
grounded
posture

repetitive stress
self-care
stamina
strength
structural alignment

LEARNING OBJECTIVES

Having read the chapter and used the related student learning tools, the student will be able to:

1 Explain four ways to prepare for the demands of a massage career using basic health-improving activities (nutrition, sleep, fitness, and stress reduction).

2 Analyze the principles of body mechanics and apply them in body positions used during massage (standing, sitting, bending, lifting, etc.).

3 Explain the concept of repetitive stress and describe how poor body mechanics contributes to repetitive stress-related conditions.

4 List three examples of jobsite pressures that can increase the number of injuries massage therapists experience.

5 Identify three self-care activities you can use on the job to promote a long, satisfying, healthy career in the massage profession.

Massage therapy is a physically challenging career that involves many body stresses. Topic 11-1 provides general information about ways you can improve your health now and prepare for the demands of a massage therapy career. Topic 11-2 explains the principles of good body mechanics and techniques for achieving depth and pressure without being injured. Topic 11-3 provides strategies for **self-care** while on the job. Chapters that discuss special populations (e.g., pregnancy massage) or particular techniques (e.g., seated massage) include additional recommendations for body mechanics.

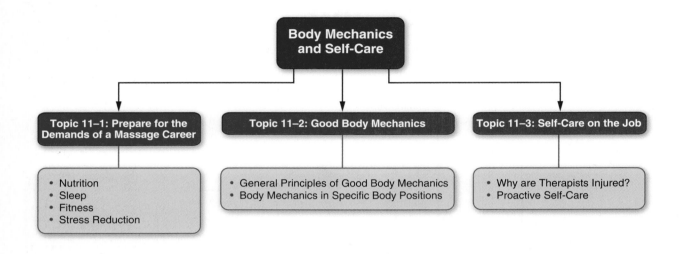

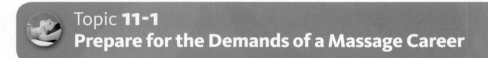

Topic 11-1
Prepare for the Demands of a Massage Career

Massage is like an athletic sport. It takes strength, stamina, flexibility, balance, coordination, and overall physical fitness to deliver an effective massage, even a relaxation massage! Massage therapists may become models of healthy living for their clients and to have credibility must practice good self-care. It is more difficult to convince clients to adopt meaningful self-care activities if you are out of shape and unhealthy. This doesn't mean that you must have <15% body fat and arms like a bodybuilder to be successful in massage. The goal is to support your body with good nutrition, rest, exercise, and stress-reduction activities, all of which reduce your risk of injury.

Nutrition

A person's nutritional requirements are unique and influenced by genetics, body type, lifestyle, cultural background, medical history, and current health. A nutritionist or naturopathic doctor can help you understand the role that food plays in your life and what types of foods and supplements are particularly important for your good health, if you have special needs or are particularly curious. Many books and articles discuss diet and specific diet plans, and these may prove helpful, but sensible eating does not need to be complicated. It involves only a few simple guidelines (Table 11-1).

Eat Regular Meals of Moderate Portions

Skipping meals and eating at odd times can lead to a greater hunger that causes overeating or low blood sugar. Symptoms of low blood sugar include shakiness, fatigue, headache, difficulty concentrating, and irritability. These symptoms signal that the body needs food. Aim to eat smaller meals every 2 to 3 hours throughout the day to best cope with the demands of a busy massage schedule. Pack healthy snacks you can eat between clients to maintain your body's energy levels, but avoid eating to the point of discomfort. The right-sized portion is one that satisfies hunger but leaves the body feeling alert and energized rather than heavy and sleepy.

Eat a Predominance of Fruits and Vegetables

Fruits and vegetables are packed with vitamins, minerals, antioxidants, and other phytochemicals (plant chemicals) that promote healthy body function, boost immunity, and protect against many diseases. For example, dark green leafy

TABLE 11-1   Healthy Foods to Include in a Nutritious Diet

Food	Basic Composition	Serving Size
Apples	Carbohydrate	½–1 small fruit
Artichokes	Carbohydrate/protein	1 medium leaves and heart
Asparagus	Carbohydrate	1 cup
Avocado	Fat	½ or less
Banana	Carbohydrate	1 small banana or ½ banana
Beans	Carbohydrate/fat/protein	¼–½ cup
Beets	Carbohydrate	½–1 cup
Blueberries	Carbohydrate	½–1 cup
Bok choy	Carbohydrate	2 cups
Boysenberries	Carbohydrate	½–1 cup
Bran	Carbohydrate	½ cup
Bread (whole grain)	Carbohydrate	1 slice
Broccoli	Carbohydrate/protein	1 cup
Brussels sprouts	Carbohydrate	1 cup
Cabbage	Carbohydrate	1 cup
Cantaloupe	Carbohydrate	¼–½ cantaloupe
Carrots	Carbohydrate	½–1 cup
Cauliflower	Carbohydrate/protein	1 cup chopped
Celery	Carbohydrate	1–2 cups
Cereal (whole grain)	Carbohydrate/fat/protein	½–1 cup
Cheese (nonfat)	Protein	1 oz
Cherries	Carbohydrate	½–1 cup
Chicken (skinless white meat)	Protein	3 oz (about ½ chicken breast)
Citrus fruits	Carbohydrate	½–1 small fruit
Collard greens	Carbohydrate/protein	1–2 cups
Corn	Carbohydrate	½–1 cup
Cottage cheese (low fat or nonfat)	Fat/protein	½–1 cup
Cream cheese (nonfat)	Protein	1–2 tsp
Cucumbers	Carbohydrate	1–2 cups
Eggs (whites—no yolk)	Protein	1–3 egg whites
Eggplant	Carbohydrate	1–2 cups
Fish	Fat/protein	3 oz
Flax seed	Fat	1 tsp
Garlic	Carbohydrate	1 clove
Granola	Carbohydrate	½–1 cup
Grapes	Carbohydrate	½–1 cup
Hummus	Carbohydrate/fat/protein	2 tsp
Juice (fresh squeezed)	Carbohydrate	½ cup
Kale	Carbohydrate/protein	1–2 cups
Kiwifruit	Carbohydrate	1 fruit
Lettuce (green, red leaf, romaine)	Carbohydrate	2 cups
Mangoes	Carbohydrate	1 fruit
Milk (nonfat, 1%, soy)	Carbohydrate/fat/protein	1 cup

(Continued)

TABLE 11-1   Healthy Foods to Include in a Nutritious Diet *(Continued)*

Food	Basic Composition	Serving Size
Melon (honeydew)	Carbohydrate	¼–½ melon
Mushrooms	Carbohydrate	½–1 cup
Mustard	Carbohydrate	2 tsp
Nectarines	Carbohydrate	1 fruit
Nuts (raw)	Carbohydrate/fat/protein	1 tsp
Oatmeal	Carbohydrate/fat/protein	½–1 cup
Olive oil	Fat	1 tsp
Olives	Fat	10 small or 5 large olives
Onions	Carbohydrate	½–1 cup
Pancakes (buckwheat)	Carbohydrate/protein	1 pancake (moderate size)
Papayas	Carbohydrate	½ fruit
Peaches	Carbohydrate	1 fruit
Pears	Carbohydrate	1 fruit
Peas	Carbohydrate/protein	½–1 cup
Peppers	Carbohydrate	½–1 cup
Pineapple	Carbohydrate	½–1 cup cubes
Plums	Carbohydrate	1–2 fruits
Prunes	Carbohydrate	3
Radishes	Carbohydrate	½–1 cup
Raisins	Carbohydrate	1 tsp
Raspberries	Carbohydrate	½–1 cup
Rice (brown or wild)	Carbohydrate	½ cup cooked
Ricotta cheese (nonfat)	Protein	½–1 cup
Salsa (fresh)	Carbohydrate	½ cup
Seeds (pumpkin, sunflower, etc.)	Carbohydrate/fat/protein	1 tsp
Spinach	Carbohydrate/protein	2 cups
Squash	Carbohydrate/protein	1 cup
Squid	Protein	3 oz
Strawberries	Carbohydrate	½–1 cup
String beans	Carbohydrate/protein	1 cup
Sweet potatoes	Carbohydrate	1 cup
Tea (green, black, herbal)	NA	NA
Tempeh	Carbohydrate/protein	½ cup
Tofu	Carbohydrate/protein	½–1 cup cubes
Tomatoes	Carbohydrate	1 cup
Tomato sauce	Carbohydrate	½–1 cup
Tortillas (whole wheat)	Carbohydrate/fat/protein	1 tortilla
Turkey breast	Protein	3 oz
Vegetable juice (fresh squeezed)	Carbohydrate/protein	1 cup
Veggie burger	Carbohydrate/fat/protein	1 patty
Vinegar	NA	NA
Watermelon	Carbohydrate	2 cups cubes
Yogurt (low fat, no sugar)	Carbohydrate/fat/protein	1 cup

vegetables like broccoli and green leaf lettuce are high in fiber and antioxidants. Fiber supports intestinal health, and antioxidants neutralize free radicals. A healthy diet contains five to nine servings of fruits and vegetables a day.[1]

Eat Whole Grains Instead of Processed Grains

Whole grains like wheat bread, brown rice, and oatmeal help stabilize blood sugar levels and provide a source of fiber, vitamins, minerals, and energy. Eating whole grains has been shown to reduce the risks of heart disease, stroke, cancer, diabetes, and obesity.[2] Use whole grain foods instead of refined foods like white bread, processed cereals, and regular pasta. Those carbohydrates cause blood sugar to rise quickly, causing a surge of insulin, which leads to increased fat storage, unstable blood sugar levels, mood swings, and overeating.[3] Eat 6 to 11 whole grain servings a day (1 slice of bread, ½ cup oatmeal or brown rice, etc.).

Include High-Protein Foods in Three Meals

Foods that are high in protein help control hunger and promote balanced energy levels. Protein is needed to help maintain and replace body tissue and is required for making hemoglobin in red blood cells. Muscles, organs, and many hormones are composed of protein, which is also needed to produce antibodies in the immune system. Protein-rich foods include tofu, nuts and seeds, fish, poultry, lean meat, eggs, yogurt, cheese, cottage cheese, and beans. Most adults need two to three servings of protein each day. A serving is approximately 3 to 4 oz of fish or lean meat; ½ cup of cooked beans, lentils, or legumes; one egg; or 2 tsp of peanut butter. Hard-boiled egg whites are a convenient good source of protein and make healthy snacks between clients.

Eat Healthy Fats in Moderation

Healthy fats such as the mono- or polyunsaturated fats found in olive oil, flax seed oil, fish, pumpkin seeds, and nuts improve the condition of hair, skin, and nails and also help the body absorb vital nutrients from other foods. The consumption of healthy fats in moderation helps prevent diseases, including diabetes, heart disease, and cancer, as well as obesity, muscle pain, and inflammation. These fats have a positive effect on cholesterol levels, blood pressure, and blood clotting.[4–6] Some components of healthy fats such as omega-3 fatty acids are necessary for proper brain growth and function. To add healthy fat in your diet, use olive oil and vinegar instead of processed salad dressing, and include avocados, nuts, and olives to liven up salads. Opt for a small handful of nuts or seeds in place of unhealthy chips, cookies, or snack cakes. Aim for one to three small servings of fats each day (about 10 to 15 nuts, 1 tsp of olive oil, ¼ avocado, etc.).

Avoid saturated fats, hydrogenated oils, and trans fats in products like margarine, shortening, snack foods, processed cooking oils, and frozen desserts. Read the ingredients on products, and avoid those with hydrogenated or partially hydrogenated oils. These unhealthy oils are implicated in high cholesterol levels, heart disease, and weight gain.[7]

Limit Sugar and Salt Intake

Sugar can be safely consumed in moderation (~2 tsp of added sugar in an otherwise healthy diet each day). What concerns physicians and researchers is added sugar in large amounts, such as in many processed foods and sugary drinks or as added to cereals or other foods. According to the United States Department of Agriculture (USDA), the United States is the world's largest consumer of sweeteners, including high-fructose corn syrup.[8] High sugar intake leads to weight gain and tends to replace more nutritious food over time. The best way to cut down on sugar is to enjoy naturally sweet and nutritious foods like fruit.

Diets high in salt (sodium) contribute to high blood pressure in some people. High blood pressure puts a person at greater risk for heart disease, stroke, and other medical problems. Avoid adding salt to foods but instead flavor them with herbs and spices. Herbs and spices like rosemary, thyme, fennel, tarragon, and sweet marjoram add fragrance and flavor and also contain compounds that promote good digestion and health.

Drink Water

The average adult human is 55% to 65% water. Approximately 2.5 L (about 4.25 pints) of water is consumed and lost per day in a healthy adult.[9] Water provides a medium for chemical reactions in the body and helps to dissolve minerals and other nutrients to make them accessible to the body. Blood is about 55–60% water. Water also supports healthy body weight maintenance,[10] waste elimination,[11] and heat regulation.[12] Mild dehydration can cause daytime fatigue and decrease short-term memory and concentration.[13] Water lessens the burden on the kidneys and liver by flushing waste products. It also plays a role in the lubrication and function of joints. In general, a healthy adult should consume 6 to 11 glasses of water each day.

Take a Daily Multivitamin

The body needs small amounts of vitamins everyday for normal functioning. Deficiencies stress the body and can lead to diseases like scurvy or rickets when deprivation is severe. Researchers now believe that many vitamins play a role in preventing conditions like heart disease, cancer, osteoporosis, and other chronic diseases.[14] Vitamin A, for example, supports good vision, stimulates the production of white blood cells, plays a role in remodeling bone, and regulates cell growth. Folic acid (a B vitamin) deficiency is linked to birth defects such as spina bifida and anencephaly. Vitamin C plays an important role in controlling infections and preventing colds, neutralizing free radicals, producing collagen, and maintaining healthy teeth, bones, and blood vessels.[15] It is unhealthy to take some vitamins in doses above the recommended daily allowance. A once-daily multivitamin ensures that a person gets enough vitamins to support normal function.

Concept Brief 11-1
Nutrition

Eat regular meals	Eat a moderate amount every 2 to 3 hours
Fruits and vegetables	Eat 5 to 9 servings daily
Whole grains	Replace processed grains (6 to 11 servings daily)
Protein	Eat 2 to 3 servings daily
Fats	Mono- or polyunsaturated (1 to 3 three small servings)
Sugar and salt	Only in moderation—salt implicated in high blood pressure
Water	Drink 6 to 11 glasses daily
Multivitamin	Important to ensure minimum vitamin requirements

Sleep

The proper amount of sleep, 7 to 9 hours a day for most adults, is essential for good health. Sleeping 6 hours or less triples a person's risk for a car accident.[16] Because sleep is cumulative, missing sleep builds up a sleep debt that must eventually be replaced. Even minor sleep deprivation can cause irritability, reduced concentration, memory impairments, and poor hand–eye coordination.[17] Prolonged sleep deprivation leads to increased stress, burnout, frequent moodiness, and aggressive behavior. It may also be related to a greater incidence of high blood pressure, heart disease, and lowered immunity.[18]

To ensure a good night's sleep, stick to a schedule. Go to bed at the same time each night, and wake up at the same time each morning. Avoid exercise close to bedtime, and engage in relaxing activities like taking a warm bath or reading. While alcohol can make a person feel sleepy, it interferes with natural sleep cycles and should be avoided close to bedtime. The effects of caffeine last as long as 6 hours and may affect a person's ability to sleep when consumed in the late afternoon and at night.

Over 40 million Americans experience sleep disorders, including sleep apnea, insomnia, restless leg syndrome, and narcolepsy.[19] While everyone lies awake unable to sleep at times, persistent problems with sleep indicate a need for a consultation with a physician. Sleep specialists recommend getting out of bed and moving to another room if you can't sleep. Watch TV, listen to music, or read until you feel tired. Napping can help to decrease a sleep deficit and improve one's concentration and mood in the afternoon. Studies show that a 20-minute power nap in the afternoon is more beneficial than an additional 20 minutes of sleep in the morning. Experts recommend a nap of 15 to 60 minutes but no longer, because longer naps disrupt one's sleep schedule and may lead to a sleepless night. Even closing the eyes for 5 minutes or meditation has restorative benefits.[20]

Fitness

The human body has great potential for increased health in its musculoskeletal and cardiovascular system. This potential can be tapped and optimized at any stage of life through a conditioning program. Different conditioning programs affect posture, flexibility, and strength in different ways. Posture, flexibility, and strength are key components of good body mechanics and overall physical fitness.

Posture and Body Awareness

Posture involves how people hold or carry their bodies while standing and moving. People often think of "posture" as a static position, but in fact people are always moving, adjusting, shifting, adapting, and balancing, even when they are "still." The ways in which body parts relate to each other and align are important, because gravity constantly exerts pressure that pulls body parts down. Ideally, a person stands and moves in a position of easy balance that requires a minimum amount of effort to achieve maximum mobility and function. Over time, however, people develop habitual movement patterns that increase stresses on bones, joints, and muscles, leading to inefficient movement and painful soft-tissue conditions. Figure 11-1 describes and illustrates the characteristics of good posture and gives criteria for vertical and horizontal symmetry.

Given the physical nature of massage work, massage therapists must be aware of their posture and strive to improve it if needed. First, stand before a mirror and observe for symmetry or lack of symmetry in your body while standing, sitting, walking, bending, and lifting. Notice how fluid movements are, and look for common postural holding patterns that can lead to dysfunction. Notice if your head is pushed forward. Notice if your shoulders are rounded or if your lower back is more arched than it should be. Are your knees locked in a hyperextended position?

Now bring your body into a neutral position. Place your feet shoulder-width apart and bend your knees slightly. Imagine the weight of your body dropping straight down between your legs. Pull your abdominal muscles in toward your spine, and lift your ribcage. Point the top of your head toward the ceiling to elongate your neck, and open your shoulders to expand the upper chest. Allow your arms to drop naturally at your sides. This corrected position may at first feel very strange because habitual movement patterns become fixed in the neuromuscular-myofascial system as "normal."

Remember that posture is dynamic and adaptive, not static and fixed. Therapists cannot force themselves or their clients into left/right or horizontal/vertical symmetry. Simply trying to "sit up straight" or "stand up straight" misses the point and moves the body into a reactive correction likely to be as problematic as the original posture. Instead, seek to develop greater awareness of how your body is moving and where the body is stuck. Be watchful for common habits that lead to

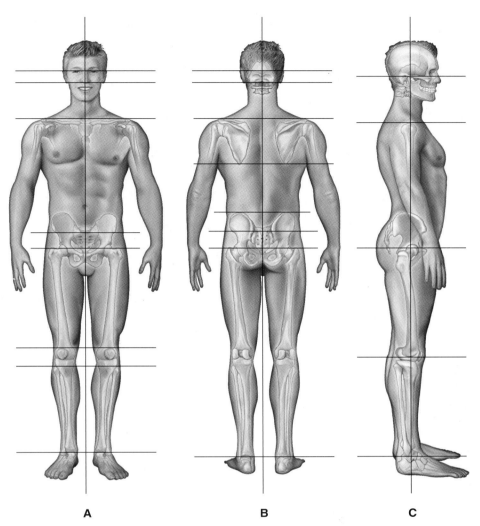

A B C

Figure 11-1 Characteristics of good posture. **A.** A person with good posture looks symmetrical and moves gracefully. The nose, chin, sternum, spine, and navel align vertically down the center of the body. Bilaterally from the anterior view, the eyes, ears, shoulders (acromion process), pelvic girdle, anterior superior iliac spine, fingertips, knees (patella), and outer anklebones (lateral malleoli) align on the same horizontal level. **B.** Bilaterally from the posterior view, the ears, shoulders, superior angle of the scapulae, pelvic girdle, posterior superior iliac spine, fingertips, and lateral malleoli align on the same horizontal level. **C.** When viewed from the side (lateral aspect), an imaginary vertical line runs through the center of the ear, the center of the shoulder joint (glenohumeral joint), the bodies of the lumbar vertebrae (the vertebrae in the lower back), the center of the greater trochanter of the femur, the center of the knee joint (tibiofemoral joint), and the ankle joint (talocrural joint).

faulty posture, strengthen the core muscles that support good posture, and work toward greater overall muscular balance. These are discussed in the following sections.

Eliminate Common Habits That Lead to Bad Posture

Even the simplest movement made in a weak or unsupported position can lead to injury. A person opening a window or tying a shoelace with the body in an awkward position can injure a disc or strain a ligament. A common bad habit that leads to postural weakness is slouching. People slouch in front of the computer, in front of the TV, and while standing in

line. Continual slouching compresses the sacrum and places the lower back in a prolonged stretch, weakening ligaments. Over time, this displaces the discs in the lower back (lumbar region) while placing the upper spine (thoracic region) in a chronically bent position, causing pain.

When standing, many people lock their knees and arch the back or roll their shoulders forward and thrust out the chin. High-heeled shoes affect the body's center of gravity and place the body in a weakened position that strains the back. Never wear high heels during massage or bodywork sessions. Avoid carrying a heavy purse or bag on one side of your body or sitting on a wallet in a back pocket. When seated, place your feet on the floor and do not cross your legs. Don't regularly grip a phone receiver between your neck and shoulder.

Imagine the spinal muscles and abdominal muscles moving toward the spine and wrapping around the body like a thick but flexible support as you assume a neutral position. Imagine the top of your head lifting up toward the sky, your ribcage lifting, your chest expanding, and your arms balanced and free. Do a mental check of your posture regularly, and ask yourself, "Is this a supported position from which I can move efficiently, fluidly, and without the fear of injury?"

Strengthen Core Muscles That Support Good Posture

As you progress through your massage training program, you learn in-depth information about specific muscles that stabilize posture. For now, it is enough to focus generally on the muscles known in popular fitness literature as "the core." Think of the core as the three muscle regions located between the pelvis and the base of the ribcage: the abdominals, the pelvic muscles, and the lower back muscles. The exercises

outlined in Figure 11-2 strengthen these muscle groups and support good posture. Do not continue any of these exercises if they cause you pain.

Work Toward Greater Overall Muscular Balance

Assessing and working with muscular imbalances involve complex skills you learn gradually over time. To improve your posture and general health, become aware of your body and contemplate how it feels. Stand in a neutral position and think about how your feet feel. Think about each toe, the ball of the foot, the heel. Do you feel pain or tension? Move your sense of awareness up your lower legs and to the knees. How do your knees feel? How do your calves feel? Do you feel any pain or tension? Continue up the legs to your hips and gluteal muscles. Tighten the gluteals and then relax them. Was there any unconscious "gripping" of the gluteals? Contemplate your lower back and spine. Are there areas of tension and pain? Contemplate the abdominal muscles and the ribcage and then the upper chest and shoulders. Contemplate your neck, jaw, forehead, ears, eyes, and scalp. Identify any areas of tension and pain, and think about how

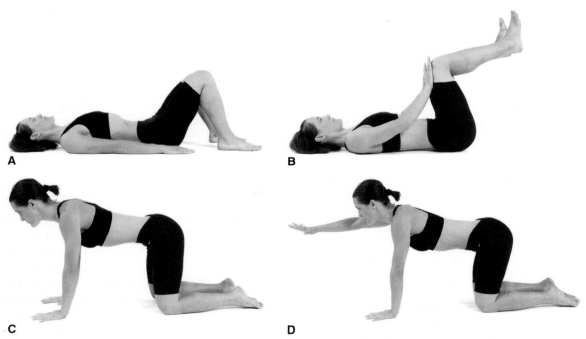

Figure 11-2 Strengthen the core for good posture. **A.** The "abdominal squeeze" exercise. Lie on your back with knees bent and your feet flat on the floor. Imagine pulling your navel in toward the spine while tilting your pubic bone toward your navel. Your shoulders are down and chest lifted. **B.** With knees bent, lift both legs up during an inhalation, and place a hand on each knee (keep your shoulders and head on the floor). Use your hands to push your knees forward, and with your knees resist the force during an exhalation on a slow count of 6 seconds. Return to the starting position and repeat the exercise six times. **C.** The "quadruped" exercise. Start the exercise on hands and knees with your hands directly below your shoulders and your neck and head in a straight line with your spine (don't drop your head forward or lift your chin up—your eyes are looking at the ground). Imagine pulling your navel in toward your spine and inhale. **D.** Exhale and lift one arm off the floor, and reach forward with the arm straight at shoulder height. Hold this position for three breaths, and repeat on the opposite side.

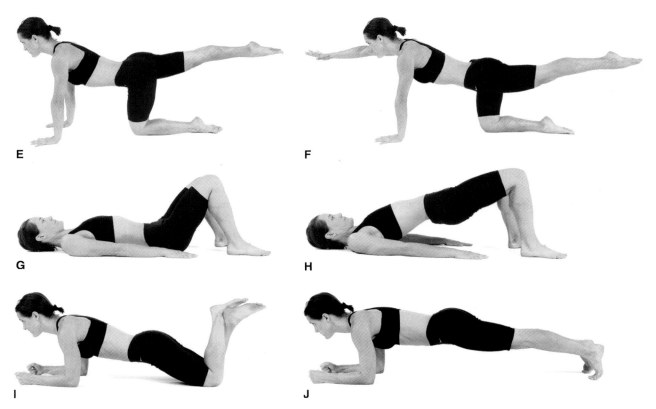

Figure 11-2 *(Continued)* **E.** Now imagine pulling your navel in toward your spine and inhale. Exhale and lift one leg off the floor, and reach it straight out from the hip. Hold this position for three breaths, keeping your abdominals pulled toward your spine. Repeat with the other leg. **F.** As core strength builds, try raising one arm and the opposite leg at the same time while keeping your abdominal muscles pulled toward your spine. Repeat with the other arm and leg. **G.** The "bridge" exercise. Start the exercise on your back with your navel pulled toward your spine. The knees are bent, your feet flat on the floor. **H.** Inhale and press your feet into the floor, and lift your pelvis on the exhalation while squeezing your buttocks together. Hold for three breaths. As your pelvis is lowered, think about your spine coming back to the floor one vertebra at a time. Repeat the exercise up to six times. **I.** The "modified plank" exercise. Starting on hands and knees, place your elbows and forearms on the floor in front of your body, a little more than shoulder-width apart. Cross your bent legs at the ankle, and pull your navel toward your spine with your head in a neutral position in alignment with your spine. Hold this position for a count of six and relax. Repeat three to six times. **J.** As you gain strength move to a regular plank position.

your body is held during the course of the day. Identify positions that provide the muscles, joints, ligaments, and tendons with better support, and use stretching exercises to help release tension.

If you struggle with posture, coordination, or balance, consider scheduling a session with a practitioner of Alexander technique, Aston patterning, or Feldenkrais method or another movement specialist. These classes help improve your body awareness, posture, and ease of movement and at the same time provide information useful for massage training.

Practicing tai chi is another valuable way to improve posture, fluidity, balance, and body awareness. Tai chi is a form of martial arts that seeks to relax and soften the musculature. It is often used as a mind–body relaxation exercise consisting of intricate sequences performed in a slow, relaxed manner over a 30-minute period.

Flexibility

Flexibility is the range of motion available at a given joint or series of joints. The elasticity of the muscles that cross the joint and the connective tissue in the region both affect the quality and suppleness of the joint's movement. Muscles have an optimum length that allows for the best possible strength and function. It is important to keep the muscles in balance. Muscles that are excessively short and tight or excessively long and weak can alter the position of a joint and predispose a therapist to injury. Flexibility can be improved through stretching and through certain movement systems such as yoga.

Stretching

Stretching aims to move a joint through its full range of motion, thereby lengthening the muscles, tendons (contractile structures), ligaments, and joint capsule (noncontractile structures). While stretching increases the elasticity of both contractile and non-contractile structures, contractile tissue is more elastic and so responds better to stretching.[21] Stretch when the body is warm to improve your flexibility. If your body is cold, stretch carefully to avoid injury to a muscle. Never bounce during a stretch or stretch so far as to cause pain, as these activate the stretch reflex and may lead to more tension in the muscle. Anytime muscle fibers are stretched too far or too fast, to prevent injury a nerve reflex sends a message to the muscles to contract. The result is increased muscle tension rather than relaxation. Bouncing up and down in a stretch can cause microscopic tearing of muscle fibers. This can lead to the formation of scar tissue and additional loss of elasticity. Later chapters describe advanced forms of stretching that aid in the rehabilitation process, such as active isolated stretching, postisometric relaxation, and proprioceptive neuromuscular facilitation.

Stretching can be performed throughout the day to ease tension and relax the body. You can stretch in the morning just after waking, after sitting or standing in one position, after watching TV or reading a book, before and after physical activity, after a long drive in the car, or anytime your body feels stiff. Massage therapists should practice good self-care by stretching before and after massage sessions. During massage, tension builds in the hands, forearms, upper arms, back, neck, chest, and legs. Pay particular attention to form and posture during stretching so as to achieve the maximum benefit without injury. Take a stretching class at a local gym, or consult a fitness trainer to learn the best techniques for stretching. Books and videos also provide detailed advice. The stretches shown in Figure 11-3 are a basic self-care practice for therapists before and after a day of massage.

(Text continued on page 315)

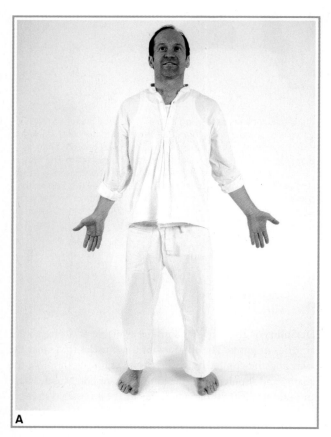

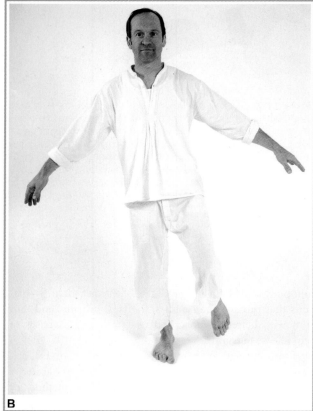

Figure 11-3 Stretching for self-care. Note that the man in these photos is a yoga instructor who is very flexible. Work at your own pace and with your own flexibility. It is normal to feel some tension and mild discomfort, but avoid any positions that cause pain. Ease into each of the stretches outlined here by moving your body to a point where you experience mild tension. Now think about relaxing your muscles, and take a deep breath into the area that feels tension for a count of 10 to 15 seconds until the tension decreases. Repeat the stretch and move a little further into the stretch until you feel tension again. Breathe into the area that feels tension again, and hold it for a count of 10 to 15 seconds. If the tension does not release, or if the stretch feels painful, ease off. **A.** Begin the sequence with your feet shoulder-width apart and knees slightly bent. Pull your abdominal muscles in toward the spine, elevate your ribcage, lift the top of your head toward the ceiling, and open and expand your upper chest. Breathe and feel the breath expanding your abdominal area. Sense your body and identify areas of stiffness or tension. **B.** Shake your arms and hands as they hang at your sides, and allow the shaking to progress up your arms to your shoulders. Stop shaking your arms and shoulders, and balance on one leg so that you can shake the other to loosen it. Grasp the top of a chair for balance if necessary. Repeat the shaking on the second leg. With both feet on the ground and knees slightly bent, swing your hips gently from side to side.

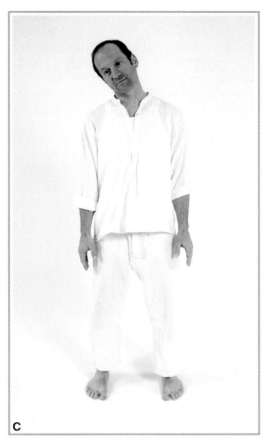

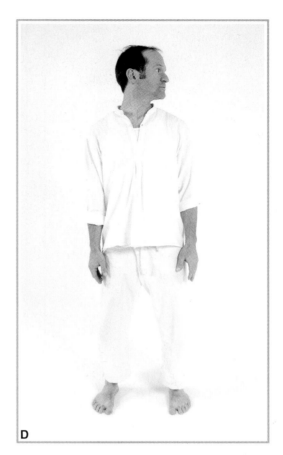

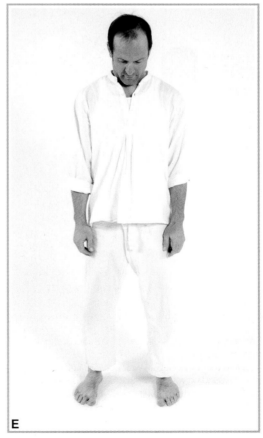

Figure 11-3 *(Continued)* **C.** Standing in a neutral position with your abdominals pulled toward your spine, take your right ear to your right shoulder to stretch the lateral flexors of the neck (don't allow your head to rotate). Repeat this stretch on the left side. Stretch the lateral flexors on each side three times. **D.** Lift the top of your head toward the ceiling to elongate your neck, and rotate your head to the right by turning your chin to your right shoulder (don't allow your head to laterally flex). Look over your shoulder so that your eyes are looking straight out from your face. Repeat this stretch on the left side. **E.** Elongate your neck by lifting your head toward the ceiling, and drop your chin forward until you feel a stretch in the posterior neck. Ensure that your body is still in a good neutral position, and bring your chin up toward the ceiling until you feel a stretch in the anterior neck.

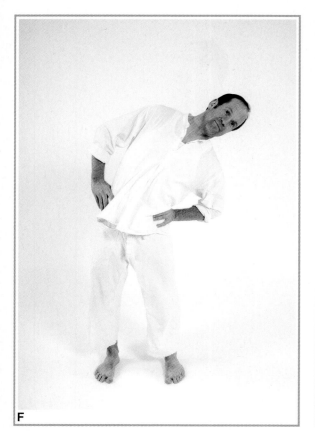

F

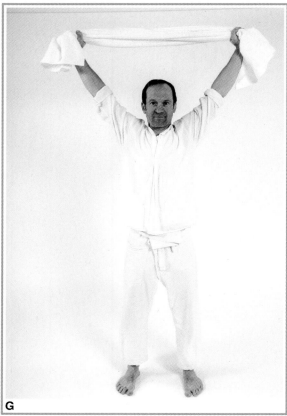

G

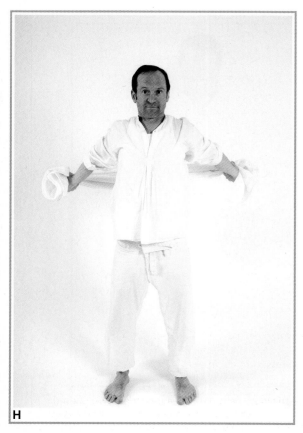

H

Figure 11-3 *(Continued)* **F.** Stand in a neutral position with your hands on your hips. Pull your abdominal muscles toward your spine and inhale. Exhale and bend at the waist to one side. Maintain the stretch for 10 to 15 seconds, and come back to the starting position slowly. Repeat the stretch on the other side. **G.** This stretch opens up the upper chest and shoulders. If you have had a previous shoulder injury, proceed slowly and discontinue this stretch if it causes pain. Stand in a neutral position, and hold a towel at both ends in front of your body. Exhale and lift the towel straight out and up, then over your head. Avoid arching your back. Move slowly and maintain a supported body position with your knees slightly bent. **H.** Continue to move the towel behind your back until it is parallel to your lower back. Stop and hold the stretch at any place in the movement where you feel tension. Use breathing to help release tension and keep your body supple.

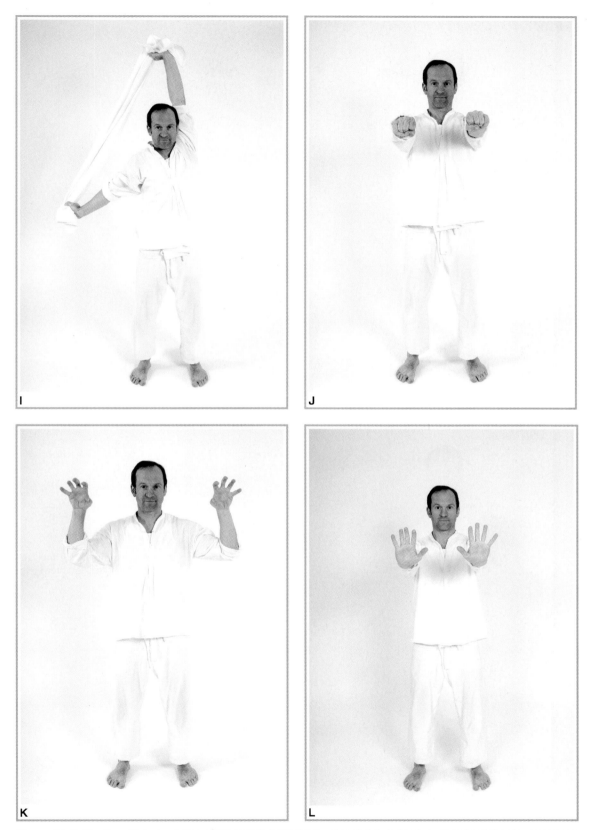

Figure 11-3 *(Continued)* **I.** In a variation of this stretch, bring the towel to slightly behind your head and then lower one arm or the other to further stretch the upper chest. **J.** Make your hands into fists and squeeze them for 5 seconds. **K.** Bend fingers at the knuckles so that they look like claws for 5 seconds. **L.** Straighten and separate your fingers for 10 seconds. Repeat this sequence three times. This warms up your hands and prepares them to apply massage techniques.

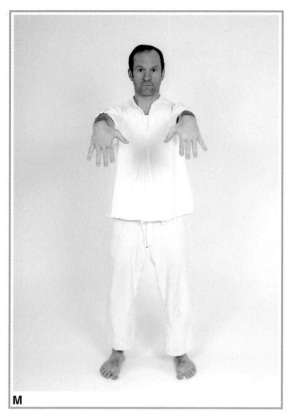

M

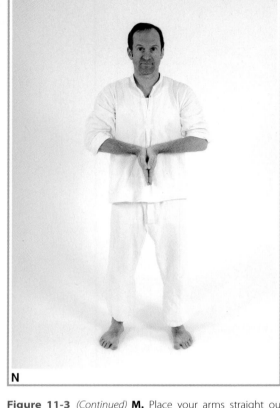

N

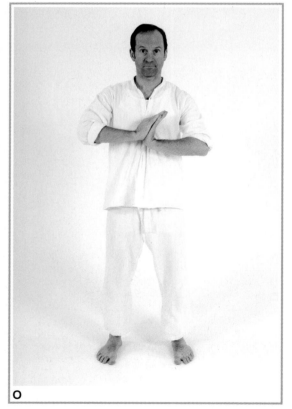

O

Figure 11-3 *(Continued)* **M.** Place your arms straight out from your shoulders, and bend your wrists so that your fingers reach toward the ceiling or slightly back toward your shoulders. Keep your arms straight out from your shoulders but bend your wrists so that your fingers point toward your feet. Repeat this sequence three times, holding each position for 10 to 15 seconds. **N.** Place your hands in a "prayer position" in front of your body, and rotate them down toward the floor until you feel a stretch. Hold the position for 10 to 15 seconds, and repeat the stretch three times. **O.** From the prayer position, push the fingers of one hand over to stretch the fingers of the other hand in extension. Repeat on both sides three times.

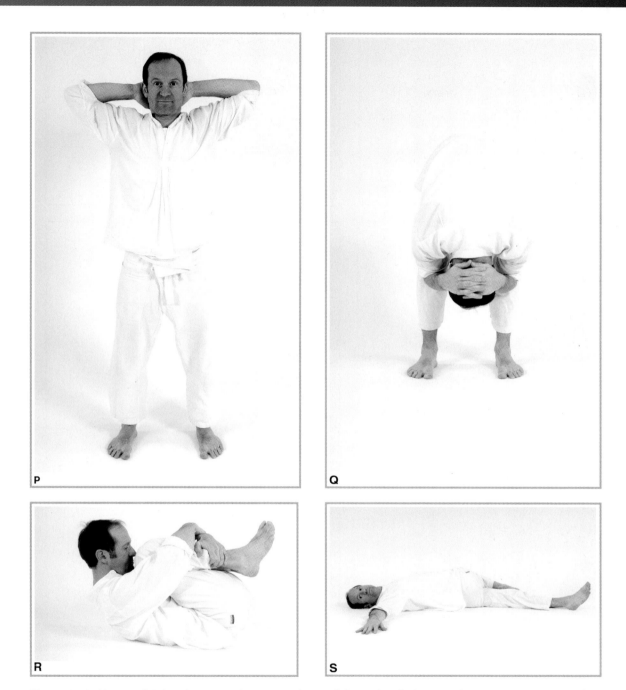

Figure 11-3 *(Continued)* **P.** Stand in a neutral position with your abdominals pulled in toward your spine, your ribcage lifted, and your head lifted so that your neck is elongated. Interlace your fingers behind your head so that your elbows point out to each side. Exhale while imagining that your elbows are being pulled together behind your head. Hold this position while breathing into the tension for a count of 10. **Q.** Bring your elbows together in front of your head while curling down and placing your elbows on your knees; breathe into your upper back to expand it. **R.** Sit on a soft surface and grasp your knees with your arms, hugging your bent knees close to your chest. Gently roll forward down your spine, keeping your head tucked so that your chin rests on your chest. Roll back into the starting position, and repeat 6 to 11 times. **S.** Lie flat on your back on a soft surface and stretch your arms over your head and point your toes out. Bring one knee up into a bent position and use your hands to push your knee to one side. Breathe into your lower back area where you feel the tension for 10 seconds. Repeat the stretch on the opposite side.

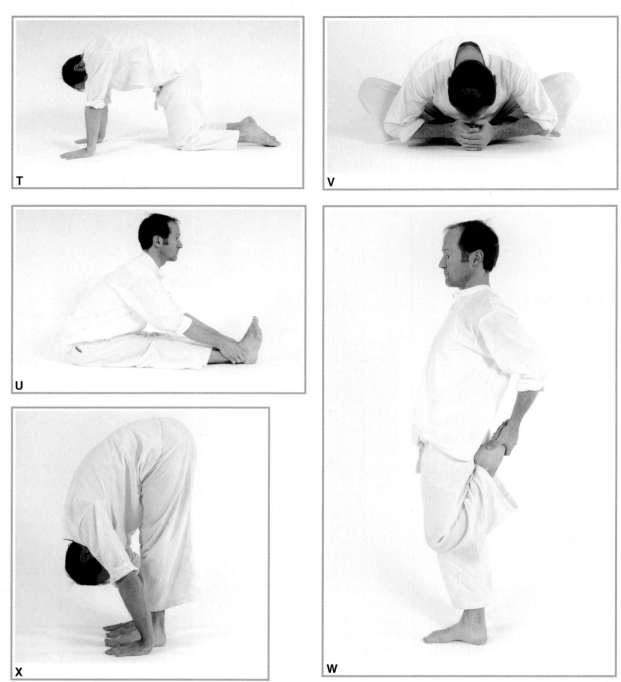

Figure 11-3 *(Continued)* **T.** Starting on your hands and knees, arch your back on an exhalation and hold it for 10 seconds while breathing into the position. Now round your back and breathe into this position for 10 seconds. Repeat the arching and rounding three times. **U.** During these stretches, you may feel tension in your lower back, hamstrings, and groin area. Sit with your legs straight out and your back straight. Inhale and pull your abdominal muscles toward your spine. Exhale and bend from the hips so that your upper body is over your legs. Grasp your ankles or feet with your hands, and breathe into areas of tension. Repeat this stretch three times. **V.** Bring the soles of your feet together while holding onto your feet. Bend forward from the hips and press your knees down with your forearms. Breathe into areas of tension for 10 seconds, and repeat the stretch three times. **W.** Stand facing a wall, and place one hand on the wall for balance. Reach your other hand behind your back to grasp the opposite foot. Pull your heel toward the gluteal muscles so that you feel a stretch in the quadriceps muscles. This stretch may be challenging if you have knee problems; proceed slowly and cautiously. Discontinue any stretches that cause pain. **X.** To complete the stretching routine, stand up in a neutral position and slowly roll forward down the spine until the trunk hangs between your legs. Keep your knees slightly bent. Roll back up the spine and shake out the muscles.

Yoga

Yoga originated in Hindu philosophy in India as a family of spiritual practices. Yoga is sometimes viewed in the West purely as exercise, but ideally it should not be separated completely from spiritual practice. It is helpful to view yoga as a living tradition and a way to physical health, spiritual balance, and vibrant mindfulness. Yoga classes might combine physical exercises, breathing exercises, and meditation or may focus only on yoga positions and breathing (e.g., Hatha yoga). Yoga postures (*asanas* or *asans*) are specific body positions that help stretch the body, promote the free flow of energy through the body, and calm the mind. A number of good yoga videos are available, and classes are popular and offered in many locations. Yoga is challenging, so it's good to take it slowly at first and discontinue any exercise that causes pain. Many therapists find that the dedicated practice of yoga leads to better overall strength, flexibility, calmness of mind, and good health.

Stamina and Strength

Good body mechanics, discussed in Topic 11-2, involves using the body effectively so that maximum physical effort is never exerted. By increasing your stamina and strength, you increase your work capacity and decrease the risk of injury.

Exercises That Increase Stamina

Regular moderate aerobic exercise helps reduce high blood pressure, diabetes, heart disease, obesity, and other health-related conditions.[22] Even easy activities like gardening, performing the stretching sequence or core exercises described previously, taking the stairs instead of the elevator, doing housework, or parking further away from work can improve one's overall health. However, while moderate exercise of this sort is important for everyone's health, massage therapists also need **stamina** to deliver a consistently good massage to five or more clients during a full day of work.

Walking is an excellent way to improve one's cardiovascular health and stamina because it's free, doesn't require expensive equipment, and holds little risk of injury. Fitness experts say that simply walking 15 minutes a day can make improvements in health, but the ideal is a brisk walk of 30 to 60 minutes.[23] Dancing is another good stamina builder for massage therapists. Vigorous dancing (30 to 40 minutes, three or four times a week) improves the condition of the cardiovascular system and develops coordination. The side-to-side movements of dance also strengthen weight-bearing bones and can help to prevent the slow loss of bone mass.[24] Team sports like football, basketball, and soccer allow participants to socialize while they exercise. Rollerblading, jogging, skating, skiing, and tennis also improve cardiovascular health, although some of these activities involve an increased risk of an injury that could reduce a therapist's ability to work.

Exercises That Increase Strength

Strength training is a form of active exercise in which a muscular contraction is resisted by an outside force (e.g., gravity, free weights, or resistance bands). Strength training improves muscle tone and the density of bones, ligaments, and tendons to help stabilize joints. It increases the ratio of muscle mass to fat, improving one's calorie-burning metabolic potential. A variety of videos and books describe strength-training programs and provide instructions for how to carry out specific exercises. The ideal approach is to hire a fitness trainer to develop a strength-training program that takes into account one's individual fitness level, specific goals, body type, and interests. This is ideal because good movement patterns use a full range of motion and require proper form and posture. A fitness trainer can demonstrate proper form and give feedback as you practice each exercise.

Figure 11-4 demonstrates some general areas for focus that help build general strength. Before practicing any strength-conditioning exercise, warm up with 10 minutes of gentle stretching or movement. Use weights that feel light when you start a program to prevent undue stiffness and soreness. Work with more challenging weights after achieving a moderate level of fitness.

Stress Reduction

Traffic jams, bills to pay, relationship problems, health concerns, eating on the run, work pressures, and other demands trigger the body's flight-or-fight response and may lead to physical symptoms like headaches, teeth grinding, fatigue, insomnia, muscular aches, anxiety, depression, mood swings, forgetfulness, poor concentration, and a negative attitude. Unrelieved stress clearly takes both a mental and physical toll and often contributes to serious conditions including severe anxiety attacks and clinical depression.[25]

Therapists must carefully monitor their own stress level and take steps to avoid burnout. When interacting with a client, a therapist who thinks things such as "You think your stress level is high?", "I'm sick of listening to people complain about their muscle tension all day long!", or "If you could feel the adhesion in my rhomboids you would give *me* the massage!" is overly stressed. Therapists must take care of themselves to be in the right frame of mind and body to provide the best care to their clients.

To reduce stress, one of the first steps is to become aware of your own stressors and your body's emotional and physical reactions to these stressors. Each person is different. A situation that causes extreme stress for one may have little effect on another, because a wide variety of factors influence how people respond to an event.[26] Memories, associations, expectations, thought processes, and body sensations contribute to the nervous system's reaction. Consider an example of someone experiencing road rage, when another driver's actions cause intense anger and physical symptoms such as a "knotted" stomach and dry mouth. Because the body is wired to survive at all costs, it treats a threat like THREAT!

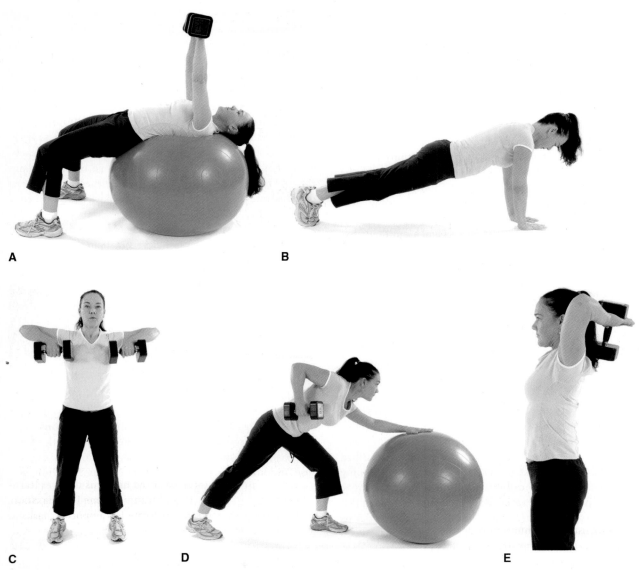

Figure 11-4 Strength-training exercises can be used to build the muscles of the chest, shoulders, back, triceps, biceps, quadriceps, hamstrings, calves, and abdominal muscles. Numerous exercises can work to build strength in each of these areas. Massage therapists often focus on upper body strength because we tend to use our arms a great deal during sessions. The abdominal muscles that make up our core are also important because they support good posture and body mechanics. Exercises for the core were outlined in Figure 11-2. **A.** Chest exercises. Exercises like a dumbbell bench press performed in this image on an exercise ball, inclined dumbbell press, dumbbell flyes, and barbell bench press build the pectoral muscles. **B.** Pushups are a great way to work the chest, triceps, and anterior deltoid muscles. **C.** Shoulder exercises. Exercises like upright rows shown in this image, seated dumbbell press, standing barbell press, side raises, and bent-over raises build strength in the deltoids. Other muscles, such as the trapezius, are often recruited to support these movements. **D.** Back exercises. Dumbbell rows shown in this image on an exercise ball, wide-grip pull-downs, reverse-grip pull-downs, and dumbbell pullovers work the latissimus dorsi muscles and other muscles of the back. **E.** Triceps exercises. Dumbbell extensions shown in this image, close-grip push-downs, bench dips, and lying dumbbell extensions work the triceps muscles.

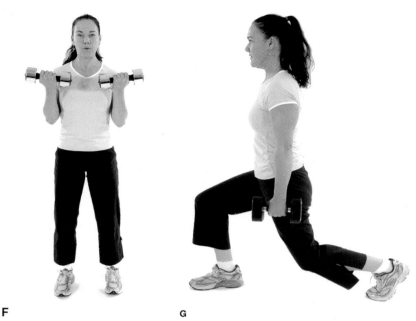

F   G

Figure 11-4 *(Continued)* **F.** Biceps exercises. Dumbbell curls that build strength in the biceps muscles are shown in this image. They might also be performed seated, standing with a barbell, or on an incline. **G.** Lower body exercises. A number of different exercises are useful for building strength in the quadriceps, hamstrings, and calves. Lunges, shown in this image, are a staple exercise for building lower body strength.

and danger like DANGER![27] But people can become aware of this and learn to moderate their emotional and physical reactions so that a minor threat, like an annoying driver, is treated as a minor threat—not as a life-and-death situation. Spend some time listing the things in your life that you find stressful. When you know your stressors, you can use some of these stress-reducing behaviors:

1. **Breathe:** When an event triggers a stress reaction, focus on your breathing. Take slow, deep breaths, and pay attention to your breathing pattern until the reaction subsides.

2. **Relaxation techniques:** Practice relaxation techniques (described below) to reduce muscle tension and build body awareness.

3. **Build reserves:** Build up physical and emotional reserves with a nutritious diet, regular exercise, and regular sleep. Develop supportive friendships and participate in social events to give life greater emotional and spiritual meaning.

4. **Delegate:** When feeling stressed, alert a loved one or friend to your feelings and delegate some responsibilities at work or home. For instance, if you are the one who always does the shopping and prepares the food, it can relieve some of your stress if your partner picks up these responsibilities for a week. The key is to be able to recognize stress and ask for help.

5. **Reschedule:** It may be necessary to reorganize your schedule to maintain a more balanced life. This involves learning to say no to others and planning time for relaxation. Prioritize your tasks and delegate less important tasks to other people, or simply eliminate them altogether if they are not really important.

6. **Write it down:** Writing down the events of the day in a journal helps put things in perspective. This exercise also supports a proactive thought process that leads to better organization and problem solving.

7. **Seek professional help:** If your stress noticeably affects your health, causes feelings of desperation (e.g., a desire to run away, quit school, leave a relationship that is fundamentally sound, or quit a job), or leads to anxiety attacks, regular tearfulness, or depression, it is time to seek professional help. Mental health professionals can help you better identify your stressors, the history behind them that gives them power, and ways to overcome them and manage your life with less stress in the future.

Relaxation Strategies

Two simple, effective methods for decreasing stress are progressive relaxation and meditation. Both involve deep, slow breathing patterns that help the body unwind and balance.

Progressive Relaxation

To practice progressive relaxation, lie in a comfortable position without crossing your arms or legs, and focus on your breathing to create a slow, deep breathing pattern. Inhale through your nose while counting to 10 and expanding your abdomen. Hold the breath for 1 second, and exhale through your nose through a count of 10. Inhale and exhale in this pattern five times.

Beginning with your head, tense your facial muscles as tightly as possible and count to five. Release the muscles completely, and sense the muscles feeling heavy and still. Work down your entire body, tensing muscle groups and then relaxing them. After the head, move to the neck, chest, arms and hands, abdomen, back, thighs and gluteals, lower legs, and feet. After relaxing each set of muscles, scan the body for any areas of remaining tension and ask those areas to relax completely. Repeat the slow breathing exercise. Gently move the body to come out of its deeply relaxed state. Try using progressive relaxation directly before bed or as a pick-me-up in the late afternoon.

Meditation

Meditation has been used for thousands of years in Eastern cultures as a way to quiet the mind and reach heightened states of consciousness. It is widely accepted as a way to promote mental clarity and relax. Sit upright on the floor with legs crossed, or sit upright on a straight-backed chair with both feet flat on the floor. Close your eyes and focus on slowly inhaling and exhaling. If you have an idea or thought, simply label it as "thinking" and return your focus to breathing. It's helpful to think of thoughts as just thoughts, removing the power they sometimes hold over us. In a meditation session, a thought such as "I am selfish" might surface. If you dismiss it as "just thinking," some of its power will dissipate as you return to focusing on your breath. This type of meditation works well in the morning as a means of getting the day off to a good start. You can also use it anytime to relax, though it may cause disturbed sleep if used directly before bed.

Mindfulness during simple and regular activities is a type of meditation. It involves an increased awareness of your immediate environment and immediate experience. For example, while taking a bath, focus on the sensation of the water, the sound the water makes as it moves in the tub, the dampness in the air from steam, the smell of the water, and the color of the water. If you begin to think about some worry, a task that needs completion, what's going to happen tomorrow, or what happened during the day, focus attention again on a sensory contemplation of the water. This disrupts stressful thoughts, leads to greater relaxation, and helps promote an appreciation of simple pleasures. Stress and its effect on the human body have been discussed in detail in Chapter 4.

Concept Brief 11-2
Prepare for the Demands of a Massage Career

Nutrition	Bring nutritious foods into the diet, and cut back on sugar and salt
Sleep	Develop a consistent sleep schedule of 7 to 9 hours
Fitness	Focus on posture, flexibility, strength, and stamina
Stress reduction	Participate in stress-reduction activities daily

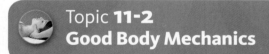

Topic 11-2
Good Body Mechanics

Extensive use is made of the forearms, wrists, hands, fingers, and thumbs in massage. Incorrect placement of the feet, repeatedly bending over the table, hyperextending the knees, or overusing the hands during a massage can lead to foot, ankle, knee, wrist, thumb, and low back injuries. A therapist who understands the principles of good **body mechanics** and is aware of proper ways to stand, sit, bend, and lift is likely to be more self-aware during a session and avoid movements that lead to injury or burnout.

General Principles of Good Body Mechanics

Body mechanics is the use of proper body movements to prevent and correct posture problems and injuries, reduce stress, and enhance physical capability. Massage therapists must pay attention to centering and grounding, structural alignment, technique variety, and the proper use of body weight and breath to prevent repetitive stress when giving a massage.

Centering and Grounding

People who are **centered** and **grounded** have a physical, emotional, and mental sense of who they are, where they are, what they stand for, where their personal boundaries lie, and how they are connected to the earth and the people on it. Contrast this with someone who is not centered and grounded. This person may speak too loudly, share too much personal information with an acquaintance, gossip, change subjects often during conversations, or have difficulty finishing a complete thought. The person may seem constantly enveloped in personal chaos, unfocused, rushed, and irritable.

Centering and grounding are skills that massage therapists can cultivate to improve the client's perception of the massage and to ensure their own health. Clients are drawn to centered, grounded therapists because they deliver a quiet, focused, intuitive massage. Clients often arrive for appointments in an uncentered and ungrounded frame of mind and can transmit this state to a therapist who is also uncentered and ungrounded. This negative, frenetic state may cause the therapist to feel ill, emotionally exhausted, or stressed at the end of the session. Alternatively, a centered, grounded therapist can calm an uncentered and ungrounded client so that both leave the session feeling good.

Centering and grounding have important physical implications in addition to the mental and emotional benefits. A person who is centered and grounded has found a point of perfect balance where movement feels effortless. Physical actions like those of the arms and legs radiate from a strong, stable, solid core. Think of this core as the abdominal and pelvic area, where the body's vital metabolic functions take place (abdominal area), and the large and powerful gluteal muscles, quadriceps, and hamstrings attach (pelvic area). The muscles of the iliopsoas connect the upper body to the lower body and form the powerful lever that flexes the thigh or the trunk. Like a horseback rider balancing the body above and between the stirrups, a centered and grounded therapist balances the core above and between the legs and can deliver a variety of techniques with effortless grace. Techniques 16 and 17 provide exercises for experiencing centering and grounding.

Technique 16   Centering

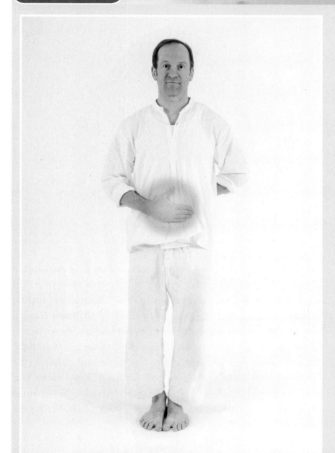

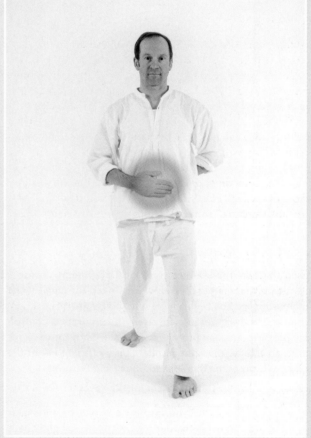

1. To experience and develop a centered state of being, stand in a neutral posture with your feet shoulder-width apart, knees slightly bent, ribcage elevated, and abdominals pulled toward your spine. Lift your head toward the sky to elongate your neck, open and expand your upper chest, and let your arms hang freely at your sides. Place one hand on your abdomen directly under your navel and the other parallel to it, directly on the small of your back. Visualize the area between your hands as a radiant ball of energy.

2. Imagine that there are bits of disconnected energy all over your body, and imagine gathering these errant bits of energy and moving them to your spinal column, where they flow down the spinal column into your core energy that you are visualizing as the area between your hands. View your core energy not only as the source of your physical strength but also as the source of mental clarity, self-confidence, and emotional peacefulness. Lift one foot up and feel your core energy stabilize your body as the weight shifts. Move this foot out from your body so that one foot is in front of the other. Imagine your core energy balancing directly above and between your legs. Shift your weight to the front leg and then to the back leg, visualizing your core energy directly above and between your legs at all times.

Continued

Technique 16	**Centering** (Continued)

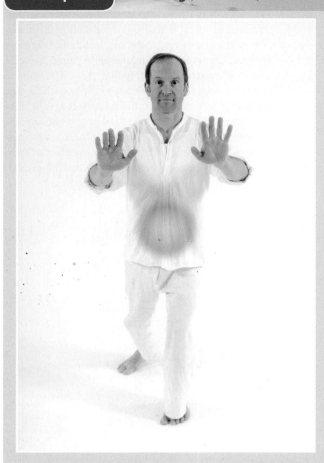

3. Lift your hands up in front of your body and begin to circle them out from your body, around and back toward your body. As your hands circle out, shift your weight to your front leg, and as your hands circle back, shift your weight to your back leg. Add breathing to the movement, exhaling as your weight shifts to the front leg and inhaling as your weight shifts to the back leg. At all times, visualize your core energy anchoring your body's core directly above and between your legs. As you develop your center, your breath and body will work together and the movement will feel balanced, graceful, smooth, and effortless.

Structural Alignment

When the body has proper **structural alignment** during a massage, physical stress is evenly distributed throughout the body and does not build up in one body area (Fig. 11-5). When the body is misaligned, strength, endurance, control, and pressure are compromised, and the body must work harder to achieve the same results. This inefficient use of the body predisposes the therapist to injury and burnout.

Alignment of the Feet, Knees, and Hips

Regardless of the stance you take for a stroke, balance your weight above and between your legs, with knees slightly bent and hips even. In some stances, your back leg may bear most of your weight and be almost straight, but it should never be locked or hyperextended. Your feet and hips should face the direction of the stroke (the feet can turn out slightly). Do not turn your feet out at extreme angles; although that may seem stable, that foot position limits your ability to mobilize your body quickly and places undue stress on the knees.

Alignment of the Back, Neck, and Head

Pull your abdominal muscles back toward your spine, and avoid twisting at the waist during a stroke. Instead, line your body up directly behind your hands so that it is positioned behind the work instead of on top of it. In this case, your feet and the hips will face the same direction. Your chest should remain expanded and open, with your head lifted toward the ceiling to elongate your neck. Avoid looking down at the stroke or tilting your head during the massage. These habits can cause you to hunch over the table and collapse the chest so that your shoulders roll forward. Keep your face and mouth relaxed, with lips slightly parted. This ensures that you do not unconsciously clench your teeth during the session.

Alignment of the Shoulders, Arms, Wrists, Fingers, and Thumbs

Think of the shoulders as sitting directly on top of the ribcage in a relaxed position. The shoulders sometimes migrate up around the ears during the course of a massage due to tension. Pay attention to your shoulder position and keep your chest expanded to ensure your shoulders don't roll forward. Breathe into the shoulders and jostle them occasionally to keep them loose.

Your arms change position based on the technique you are using. In a lengthened position, hold your arm at an

Technique 17 | Grounding

1. To experience and develop a grounded state of being, stand in a neutral posture with your feet shoulder-width apart, knees slightly bent, ribcage elevated, and abdominals pulled toward your spine. Lift your head toward the ceiling to elongate your neck, open and expand your upper chest, and let your arms hang freely at your sides. Feel the earth with your feet. Do this with your imagination; there is no need to remove your shoes or go outside. Imagine your body as a tree. Your feet are roots that reach deep into the soil to pull nutrients and moisture from the earth. Your torso is the trunk, and your arms and hands are the branches. Visualize your feet (roots) pulling energy up from the soil, conducting it through the core of your body (trunk) and out through your hands (branches and leaves). Lift your hands over your head and imagine that the energy splits and runs up each arm, exits your hands, and circles back to the earth. Move around the room and continue to imagine energy flowing up from the earth through your body. The tree visualization can help you feel connected and grounded to the earth before a massage session.

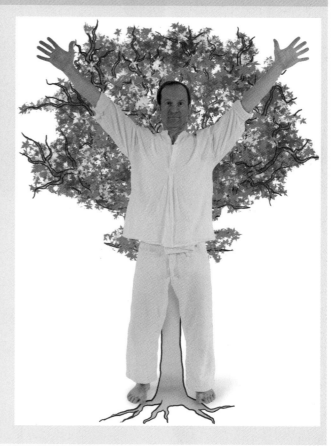

angle of approximately 45 degrees to the body, but do not hyperextend the elbow. If your forearm is used to apply the stroke, the arm is bent at a 90-degree angle but is still held approximately at an angle of 45 degrees to the body. The further your arms get from your body, the weaker they become and the greater risk of injury to the back (e.g., reaching across the client and attempting to use deep pressure or lift a body area). If you lean directly over the top of a stroke, you may expose the glenohumeral joint to undue stress. In most cases, it is better to apply pressure from an angle.

Your wrists should remain relaxed and straight whenever possible. Some strokes require the wrist to flex and extend with the movement in the stroke (e.g., petrissage), but when you apply pressure with your thumbs, palms, or fists, minimize the angle of your wrist. Hyperextension or hyperflexion of the wrists while applying pressure may lead to repetitive stress injuries like carpal tunnel syndrome (CTS). Also avoid abducting or adducting the wrist while applying pressure because this misalignment places undue stress on the wrist and may lead to injury.

Your fingers and thumbs should also be straight but not hyperextended. With direct pressure techniques, brace your thumb with the fingers of your closed hand, or reinforce one thumb with the other. Don't use your fingers for direct pressure techniques, except for the application of mild pressure such as on the face; use your elbow, reinforced thumb, or forearm instead.

Use of Body Weight

During a massage, many techniques require applying pressure to compress the tissue. Using muscular strength to apply this pressure would overstress the body and make the session exhausting. Instead, learn to use your body weight effectively to provide the pressure necessary for certain massage strokes. Keep the work close to your body (e.g., don't let your arms get too far out from your body), and keep your body properly aligned. Lean on the client to drop your body weight into the client's tissue (Fig. 11-6).

Often therapists use an asymmetrical stance (described in detail below) with one foot in front of the other and most of the body weight on the back foot. The heel of the back foot is aligned with the glenohumeral joint, and pressure is increased as the therapist widens the stance and leans into the client. Often the arm on the opposite side to the back foot in the

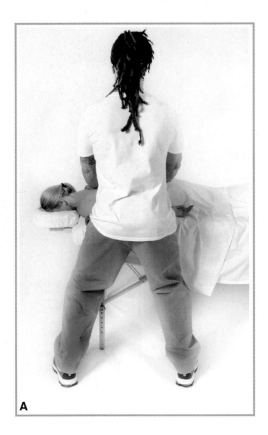

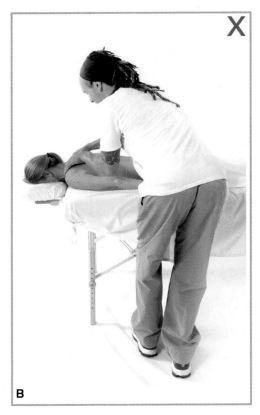

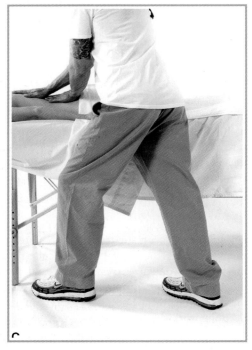

Figure 11-5 Proper structural alignment versus misalignment. **A.** Proper alignment. **B.** Misalignment. **C.** Proper alignment of the feet, knees, and hips.

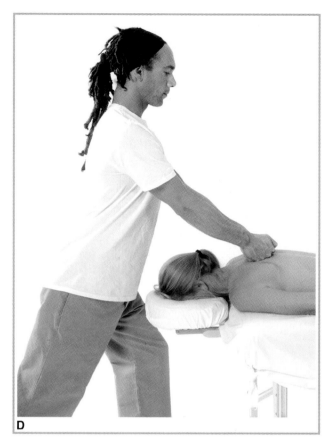
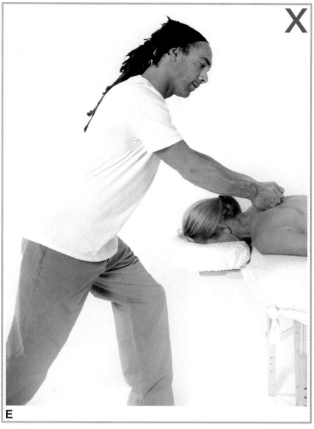

Figure 11-5 *(Continued)* **D.** Proper alignment of the back, neck, and head; shoulders, arms, and wrist. **E.** Misalignment of the back, neck, and head; shoulders, arms, and wrist.

stance is used to apply the pressure. Sometimes the therapist's body faces up or down the length of the client's body and the weight-bearing foot and arm are on the same side of the body. The danger with that position is that the therapist may overstress the glenohumeral joint by standing directly over the top of the stroke. Do not lean on the client to the extent that you cannot react quickly to the client's needs. For example, if a client tenses muscles because the pressure is too deep, you must be in a position to immediately lighten the pressure.

Use of Breath

Chapter 10 discusses the use of breathwork in a massage session in relationship to the client's needs. Breath use also benefits the therapist. Sometimes therapists hold their breath unconsciously during a session. This causes tension to build in the body and lets the chest collapse, leading to misalignment of body structures. Take full, deep, even, rhythmic breaths throughout the massage session. Proper breathing provides oxygen to the muscles and body, helps you stay relaxed and centered, helps with the correct body alignment, and sends a cue that encourages the client to also breathe deeply during the session. With good body mechanics, exhale when applying a stroke that moves away from your body and inhale with strokes that come back toward your body.

Movement and Variety

Some therapists develop a habit of stabilizing their body against the massage table. They may hyperextend their knees, lean their thighs on the table, hunch and half-sit on the table, hitch a hip onto the table, or lock themselves into one stance or position. Ideally, the whole body should be used when applying a stroke. The strength of the lower body conducts physical energy to the upper body and hands. The dynamic interaction of the body as it moves with proper alignment contributes to the intention and fluidity of the stroke. Fixed positions make it more difficult for the therapist to remain responsive to changes in the client's tissue and adapt techniques efficiently.

Keep your body in motion and move around the massage table to keep your body motion fluid. For example, when massaging the back, apply some strokes from the side of the client, some strokes from the head down the back, and some strokes from the pelvis up the back. Constantly adjust the position of your feet in relation to the client as the stroke moves up or down a body area. Use a variety of different tools to prevent

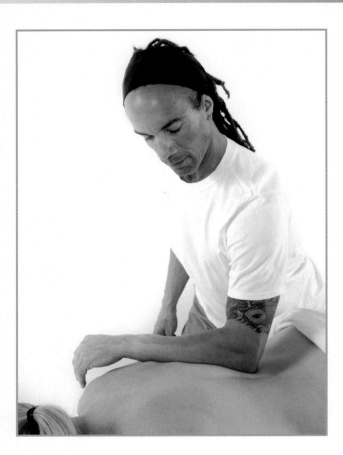

Figure 11-6 Proper use of body weight. Keep the work close to your body, and drop your body weight into the client's tissue by leaning on the client. Avoiding using unnecessary muscular strength to apply pressure.

hand fatigue. After applying a stroke that uses the hands (e.g., petrissage), apply a stroke with the forearm (e.g., a gliding stroke) to give your hands a rest. Find places in the routine where you can apply a stroke from a seated position. Often you can sit during the foot massage and during the neck and face massage. Some therapists also sit for sections of the back, leg, and arm massage.

Many therapists resist using massage tools like knobs to apply direct pressure techniques. These therapists feel that it is too difficult to adequately palpate the changes that are occurring in the client's body. However, if you find that your fingers or thumb is experiencing regular fatigue, you might experiment with massage tools to decrease the stress on your body. Many find that over time they can palpate through the tool and that it becomes an extension of their hands.

Body Mechanics in Specific Body Positions

During a session, therapists use a wide variety of movements and postures: standing, sitting, bending, and stretching, as well as pulling and lifting body parts, applying compressive strokes to an area, and working deeply into tissue. When performing these movements and postures from a properly supported position, you have less risk of injury and conserve body energy. Students often take these specific body positions, hold them rigidly, and "fix" themselves to a spot in a particular stance. Think of stances as fluid. You might start a stroke in a stance but then move your feet and body as the stroke progresses. Avoid situations where you feel you need to plant your feet and remain in a particular posture.

Standing

Therapists use two primary standing positions during massage (Fig. 11-7). In the symmetrical stance, the feet are placed shoulder-width apart with the toes pointing forward. The knees are slightly bent and directly above the feet. The back is straight and the pelvis is balanced so that it can easily shift side to side without restriction. The shoulders are relaxed, and the chest is open and expanded. The head is not laterally flexed or rotated. A symmetrical stance is appropriate when the work is directly in front of you, such as when doing petrissage or tapotement on the legs or back. You can move up and down a body area by sidestepping, and can allow your hips to sway gently with the movement of the stroke. This keeps your pelvis loose and fluid and helps keep the stroke rhythmic and energized.

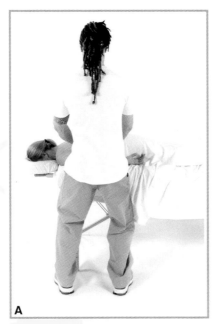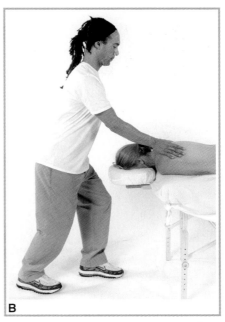

Figure 11-7 Standing. **A.** A symmetrical stance is appropriate when the work is directly in front of you, such as when doing petrissage or tapotement on the legs or back. **B.** The asymmetrical stance is ideally suited to strokes that travel the length of a body area, like gliding strokes and some vibration strokes.

In an asymmetrical stance, one foot is placed in front of the other about shoulder-width apart. The stance may be wider when you perform deeper work or need more stability for a sustained compression stroke. The front knee is flexed and the front foot points in the direction of the stroke. The back leg is straight with the knee slightly flexed and the foot slightly rotated laterally. The hips face the same direction as the front foot (in the direction of the stroke), with the weight predominantly on the back leg. The back is straight so that an imaginary line runs from the heel through the glenohumeral joint and through the ear. In this position you can lunge deeply, pushing off the back foot, thereby increasing the pressure of a particular stroke. This stance is ideally suited to strokes that travel the length of a body area, like gliding strokes and some vibration strokes.

Sitting

At certain points in a massage, you may choose to sit while applying techniques. This removes pressure from the feet and conserves your energy. In a seated position, the knees are spread wide and the feet are firmly on the floor. The back is straight with the chest open and expanded; the shoulders are open and relaxed. The head is straight. Avoid looking down at the client with your head dropped forward. Instead, look down occasionally only with your eyes to check your hand position and the client's reaction to a stroke, but then bring your head back up again. A rolling stool allows you to adjust your position easily in relation to the stroke. Some strokes are easier to perform when you

are closer to the massage table. With other techniques, you might roll out from the table and lean back to traction an area or complete the stroke. Some therapists sit on a Swiss exercise ball because it is easy to roll out of the way, and the ball also encourages good body mechanics. To balance on the ball, the abdominals must be pulled toward the spine, the back must be straight, and the feet must be flat on the floor (Fig. 11-8).

In some situations sitting may result in poor body mechanics, especially when using the wrong types of strokes. A therapist who is not standing may have to use muscular strength in the arms instead of body weight when sitting. It is also easy to abduct or adduct the wrists when applying some strokes from a seated position. Pay attention to these tendencies, and stand if the stroke feels awkward in a seated position.

Bending

As much as possible, avoid bending because it places your body in a weakened position and places undue stress on your lower back. Instead, lunge deeper into an asymmetric stance, or squat in a symmetric stance to lower your body without bending. Many therapists begin to hunch over the massage table as their careers progress. They may fail to lift body parts (during range-of-motion techniques) with their legs, instead relying on the strength of their back and arms. Some forget to keep their hips and feet pointing in the same direction and so twist and bend during strokes. These unsupported positions soon lead to lower back pain, tension in the upper back and shoulders, and neck pain.

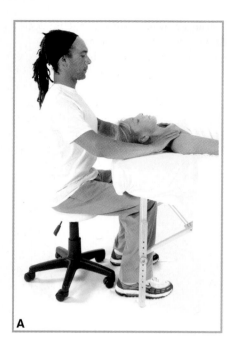

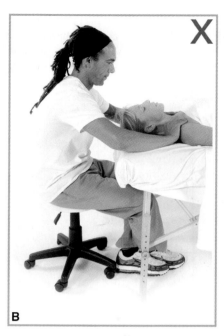

Figure 11-8 Sitting. **A.** In a seated position, the knees are spread wide and the feet are firmly on the floor. The back is straight with the chest open and expanded; the shoulders are open and relaxed. The head is straight. **B.** Avoid rounding the back and hunching over the table or crossing your legs or ankles.

Lifting, Stretching, and the Application of Range-of-Motion Techniques

Techniques that include lifting, stretching, jostling, and moving body parts require special attention to body mechanics. Make a conscious effort to initiate such techniques only from a position in which your body is in proper structural alignment. To lift a limb, sink lower into a lunge position and grip it firmly, holding it close to your body (Fig. 11-9). By holding the limb close to your body, you avoid using muscular strength in your arms and back to move the limb. Use your legs to lift the limb and bring your body up out of the deep lunge keeping your back straight. In most circumstances, you stand on the same side of the table as the limb being moved. To traction a limb, lean back with your back leg bearing the weight of your body, keeping your knee flexed. Your front leg straightens and balances your body but bears little weight. Your back should be straight and your upper chest should remain expanded and open. Avoid hunching your shoulders and looking down at the limb.

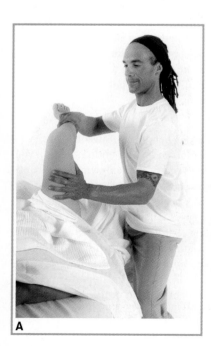

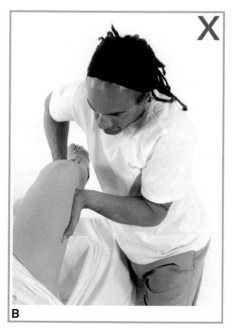

Figure 11-9 Lifting a limb. **A.** To lift a limb properly, sink lower into a lunge position and grip the limb firmly, holding it close to your body and think about keeping your back aligned, shoulders relaxed, and wrists aligned. **B.** Avoid hunching over the limb, bending too far at the hips, or hyperextending the wrists.

When pushing a limb into a stretch, stay behind the limb and lunge forward keeping your back straight, front knee flexed, and shoulders open. In this situation, weight shifts from your back leg to the front leg during the movement. Avoid twisting at the waist or standing on tiptoe to move the limb. Always keep your feet flat on the floor and your hips and feet pointing in the direction that the limb is moving.

When you pull a body area toward you, bend both knees with your weight first on your front leg. Shift the weight to your back leg as your arms pull the body area. While jostling an area, allow your own body to sway with the rhythm of the jostling. This helps to keep your body soft and fluid and also keeps the stroke rhythmic. Finally, if a large client's limbs are too heavy for you to lift them safely, do not perform range-of-motion techniques if possible. If range of motion is required to meet treatment goals, you may need to consider referring the client to another therapist.

Sustained Compression

When a sustained compression (direct pressure) is applied to specific points to achieve treatment goals, therapists often overstress their thumbs and fingers. Whenever possible, use the elbow or forearm to apply sustained compression techniques. Place your body in an asymmetric stance and drop into the client's tissue with your forearm. Lean rather than push on the tissue. Move onto the edge of your elbow when you have identified the tissue you wish to compress. Drop into the tissue as the client exhales but do not lean so much that you can't quickly reduce the pressure if the client experiences discomfort. Do not apply the pressure from directly above the point of contact. Instead, apply pressure from a slight angle to reduce the stress on your glenohumeral joint.

In some body areas, or for some specific techniques, the thumbs or fingers are used to apply sustained compression. In this case, reinforce the thumbs by holding the fingers in a fist directly behind the thumb, or place your second thumb directly on top of the first. Reinforce a finger with a second finger on top to apply the pressure, or use a knuckle instead of a finger. Avoid hyperextension of your thumb or fingers, and limit the amount of sustained compression in any one session to minimize the stress on your body (Fig. 11-10).

Concept Brief 11-3
Principles of Good Body Mechanics

Centering	Find an emotional, mental, and physical center
Grounding	Find a relaxed and connected state of being
Structural alignment	Align joints to distribute stress evenly
Use of body weight	Lean your weight on the client, avoid using arm strength
Use of breath	Focus on deep, even breathing to pace the massage
Movement and variety	Keep the body in motion, use a variety of techniques

---

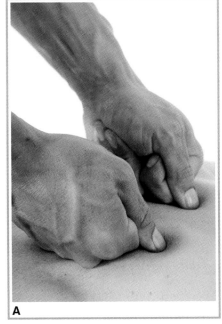

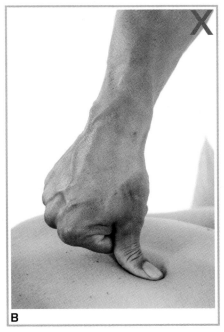

Figure 11-10 Sustained compression. Avoid overstressing your thumbs and fingers during application of sustained compression techniques. **A.** Correct position of the thumbs. **B.** A position that would overstress the thumb.

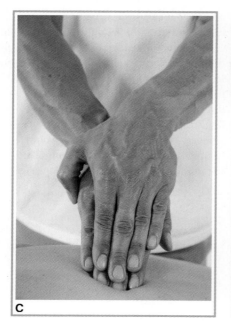

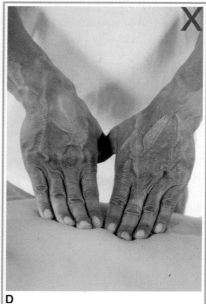

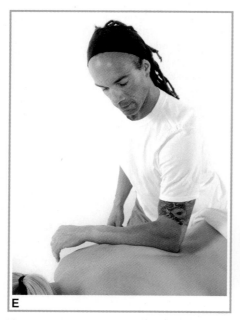

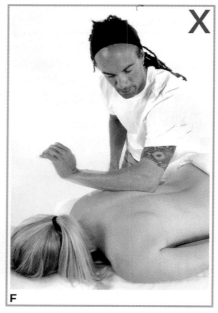

Figure 11-10 *(Continued)* **C.** Correct position of the fingers. **D.** A position that would overstress the fingers. **E.** Correct position of the elbow. **F.** A position that would overstress the body while using the elbow.

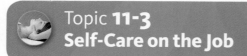

Topic **11-3**
Self-Care on the Job

A full-time massage career is demanding, and without good on-the-job **self-care**, therapists are more likely to develop repetitive stress injuries or burnout and leave the massage profession. Topic 11-1 explored ways you can prepare now for the challenges of a massage career by improving your overall health. Topic 11-2 discussed the principles of good body mechanics. This topic looks closely at repetitive stress and reasons why therapists are injured. You will learn strategies to take care of yourself while on the job. The goal is to work longer, deliver higher-quality work, prevent injury, increase income potential, and have a long and healthy massage career.

Why Are Therapists Injured?

Therapists are injured because of poor body mechanics and/or repetitive movements that overstress one area of the body. Sometimes job pressures cause therapists to continue working when they are tired. When exhausted, a therapist is more susceptible to injury and burnout.

Repetitive Stress

Therapists perform the same or similar massage techniques over and over again during a day, week, month, and year. Your joints, muscles, tendons, ligaments, and nerves may experience stresses from this repetitive movement, especially if you hold your body in a less-than-optimal position during the activity. Repeated small trauma might lead to pain, loss of function, or a specific **repetitive stress** injury like CTS, tendonitis, or thoracic outlet syndrome (TOS). (Repetitive stress injuries are also called repetitive motion disorders, overuse syndromes, cumulative trauma disorders, and other similar names.)

When abnormal tension is placed on soft tissue, especially over a period of time, it leads to tissue damage (e.g., microscopic tearing of muscle fibers) and inflammation. Chemicals released as mediators of inflammation irritate nerve endings, causing more pain and muscle guarding. This in turn causes hypertonic muscles and ischemia (lack of blood flow and low oxygen to the tissue), which increases the chemical toxicity in the tissue. A therapist who ignores the pain of a soft-tissue condition and continues to practice massage unchecked may experience permanent damage to the body.[28] The following sections describe common repetitive stress injuries and how they can affect therapists (Fig. 11-11).

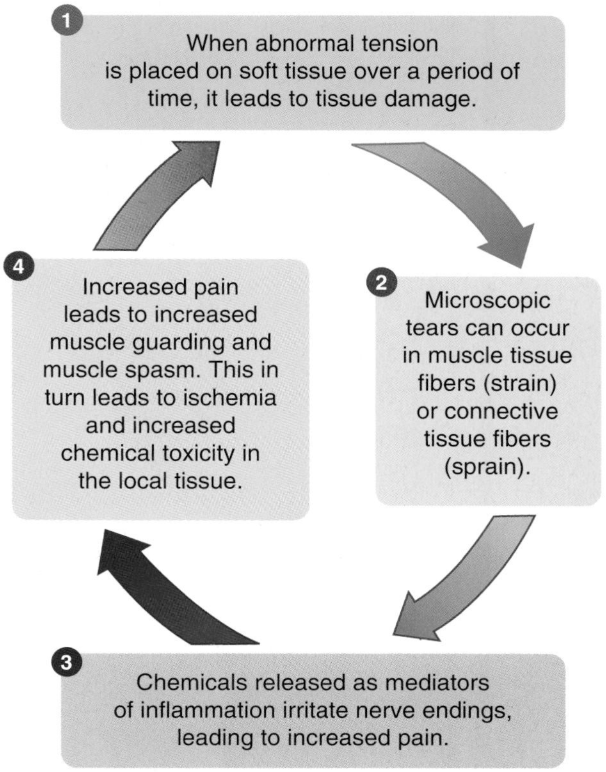

Carpal Tunnel Syndrome

CTS is a repetitive stress injury that may occur in massage therapists who regularly apply massage strokes with hyperflexed wrists or who overuse the hands (Fig. 11-12). In this condition, the median nerve is pinched by surrounding structures as it passes through the tunnel created by the carpal bones and the flexor retinaculum (also called the transverse carpal ligament). The flexor retinaculum is a strong fibrous band that spans the carpal bones forming a tunnel through which the flexor tendons and median nerve pass (the flexor tendons attach muscles originating around the elbow and forearm to the fingers). Usually the carpal tunnel provides enough space for the median nerve to pass through unhampered, but when the area is under stress, the flexor tendons thicken, the flexor retinaculum thickens, irritation causes inflammation, and inflammation causes edema (fluid retention), and this combined situation puts pressure on the nerve.[29] The median nerve provides sensation for the thumb, index finger, middle finger, and half of the ring finger. When the nerve is squeezed, numbness, weakness, burning sensations, shooting pain, and/or tingling result. Without proper attention, permanent nerve

① When abnormal tension is placed on soft tissue over a period of time, it leads to tissue damage.

② Microscopic tears can occur in muscle tissue fibers (strain) or connective tissue fibers (sprain).

③ Chemicals released as mediators of inflammation irritate nerve endings, leading to increased pain.

④ Increased pain leads to increased muscle guarding and muscle spasm. This in turn leads to ischemia and increased chemical toxicity in the local tissue.

Figure 11-11 Your joints, muscles, tendons, ligaments, and nerves may experience stresses from this repetitive movement, especially if you hold your body in a less-than-optimal position during the activity.

damage can occur. CTS is also caused by factors other than repetitive stress. For example, edema caused by pregnancy, menopause, or obesity can fill space in the carpal tunnel, as can a subluxation (when a bone loses its proper juxtaposition with neighboring bones) of the capitate bone (a centrally placed carpal bone). Other conditions in the neck, shoulder, arm, wrist, and hand can also cause symptoms that mimic those of CTS.

A number of treatment options exist for diagnosed CTS. The therapist must rest the hands and wrists and may be advised to wear a splint to keep the wrist in a neutral position. Vitamin B6 and B2 treatments might be used, as these vitamins have reduced symptoms of CTS in clinical trials.[30] A physician might prescribe diuretics or corticosteroids to reduce edema and decrease pain, or recommend surgery to remove scar tissue from the flexor retinaculum.

Tendonitis, Tenosynovitis, Tendinosis

A tendon is a tough, semiflexible band of connective tissue that connects muscle to bone. Some tendons have synovial sheaths that reduce friction where the tendon travels over a bone or through a fibrous tunnel. When an area is overused or suffers trauma, small tears can occur in the tendon, leading to irritation and inflammation. Sometimes the tendon sheath becomes inflamed (tenosynovitis), and sometimes a

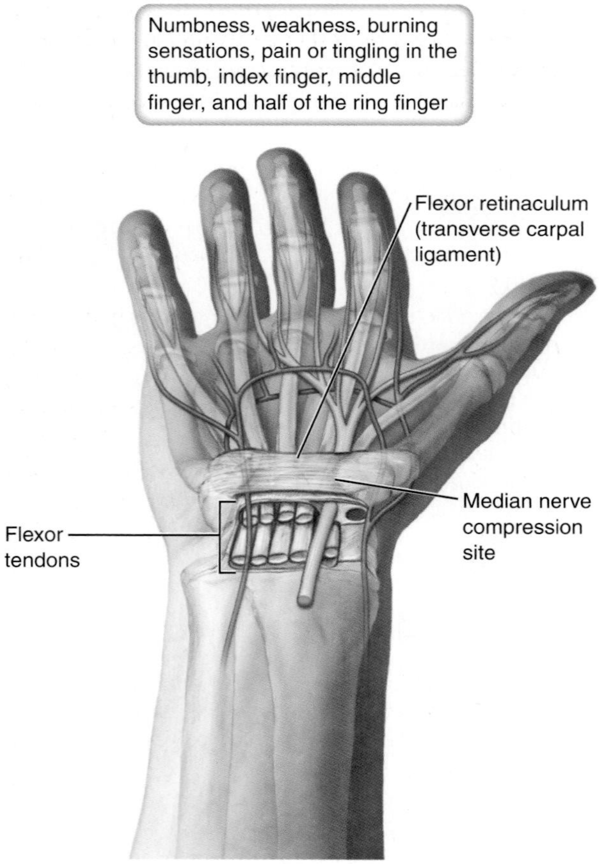

Numbness, weakness, burning sensations, pain or tingling in the thumb, index finger, middle finger, and half of the ring finger

Flexor retinaculum (transverse carpal ligament)

Flexor tendons

Median nerve compression site

Figure 11-12 In CTS, the median nerve is pinched by surrounding structures as it passes through the tunnel created by the carpal bones and the flexor retinaculum (also called the transverse carpal ligament).

significant accumulation of disorganized scar tissue occurs without inflammation that reduces strength and function (tendinosis). Massage therapists may be prone to rotator cuff tendonitis, lateral epicondylitis, and medial epicondylitis.

A group of four muscles and their tendons (supraspinatus, infraspinatus, teres minor, and subscapularis) wrap around the front, back, and top of the glenohumeral joint—referred to collectively as the "rotator cuff." Inflammation of any of these tendons is called rotator cuff tendonitis (Fig. 11-13). Although most often caused by sports that involve throwing (e.g., baseball) or swimming, it can occur in therapists who regularly lean directly over the arm while doing deep work, thereby stressing the glenohumeral joint.

Lateral epicondylitis, commonly called tennis elbow because it often affects tennis players, is a tendonitis that causes pain and tenderness in the region of the lateral epicondyle. It results from injury or irritation to the common extensor tendon caused by repeated twisting motions of the forearm and wrist, as well as excessive lifting and gripping with the hand. Medial epicondylitis, often called golfer's elbow because it affects golfers although less commonly than tennis elbow, is tendonitis that causes pain and tenderness in the region of the medial epicondyle. It results from injury or irritation to the tendons of the pronator teres and/or the common flexor tendon brought about by repeated pronation of the forearm and wrist flexion.

The treatment for tendonitis includes rest, massage, and physical therapy. During the healing process, collagen fibers (scar tissue) are deposited in a haphazard pattern. As this scar tissue matures, weight-bearing activities and stretching cause it to align along the lines of physical tension so that it heals correctly. If the area has too little activity during the scar

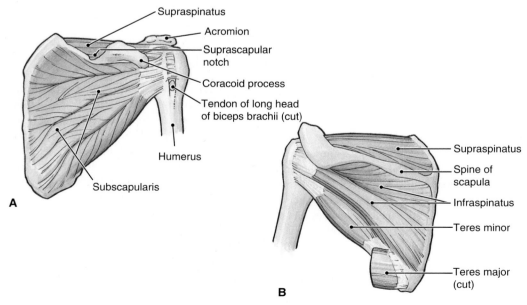

Supraspinatus

Acromion

Suprascapular notch

Coracoid process

Tendon of long head of biceps brachii (cut)

Humerus

Subscapularis

A

Supraspinatus

Spine of scapula

Infraspinatus

Teres minor

Teres major (cut)

B

Figure 11-13 Inflammation of any of the tendons of supraspinatus, infraspinatus, teres minor, or subscapularis is called rotator cuff tendonitis **A.** Anterior view. **B.** Posterior view.

tissue maturation phase, the area is permanently weakened (tendinosis). However, if the area is overworked, the problem may flare up and return to an acute state of inflammation, leading to excessive scar tissue formation.

Thoracic Outlet Syndrome

The brachial plexus is a bundle of nerves arising from the cervical spine that supplies the arm with sensation. The subclavian vein and subclavian artery run parallel to the brachial plexus as it travels under the clavicle and pectoralis minor muscle to supply the arm with blood. (The vein and artery names change as these structures travel down the arm; in the axillary region, as the structures pass under the pectoralis minor, they are called the axillary vein and artery.) TOS is a collective name for several conditions caused by the compression of these structures anywhere between the base of the neck and the axilla (Fig. 11-14). A therapist who slouches and rolls the shoulders forward while performing massage may cause the space between the clavicle and first rib to decrease, thereby compressing the brachial plexus and the subclavian vein and artery. Similarly, a therapist who constantly looks down at the client while laterally flexing the neck to one side may develop tension and tender points in the scalene muscles. The brachial plexus and subclavian artery pass between the anterior and middle scalene muscles where they can be compressed if these muscles are tight. In a therapist who regularly collapses the chest while working, the pectoralis minor muscle might compress these structures if it becomes chronically tight.

Symptoms of TOS include a feeling of fullness in the lower limb from compromised circulation. Compression of the brachial plexus results in numbness, loss of motor control, weakness, tingling, or shooting pain. The treatment for TOS depends on its specific cause and the region where compression occurs. While many other TOS-related conditions and various contributing factors also play a role in this condition, the TOS conditions described above are those most often related to poor body mechanics.

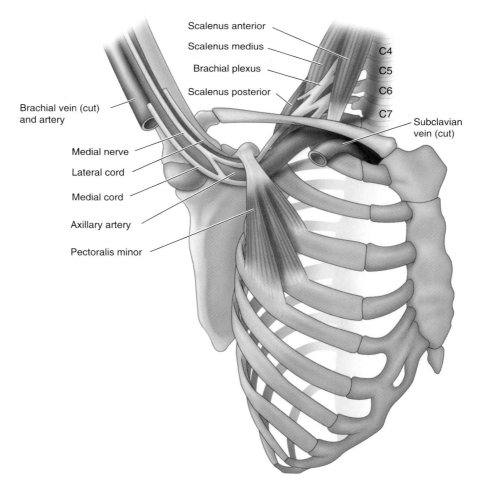

Figure 11-14 TOS is a collective name for several conditions caused by the compression of brachial plexus, subclavian vein, and subclavian artery anywhere between the base of the neck and the axilla.

Torticollis

Torticollis (also called wryneck) is caused by a severe spasm on one side, usually of the sternocleidomastoid muscle. This unilateral spasm locks the head in a rotated, flexed position. Simply sleeping in the wrong position or poor body mechanics may cause it, or it might be caused by congenital abnormalities or central nervous system problems. Therapists who continually look to one side during sessions or carry equipment (e.g., a massage table or chair) to on-site work with the strap over the same shoulder may be prone to torticollis. Stretching the neck before and after massage sessions, applying warm packs to the shoulders and neck, and paying attention to body mechanics help prevent torticollis.

Lower Back Pain

Lower back pain results when muscle fibers are torn (strain), when connective tissue fibers are torn (sprain), or when disc problems put pressure on the spinal cord or spinal nerve roots. Even mild postural deviations like mild lordosis (exaggerated curve of the lumbar spine), mild kyphosis (exaggerated curve of the thoracic spine), or mild scoliosis (an abnormal horizontal curve of the spine) cause some muscles to be overly tense and others to be weakened. This can predispose a therapist to strains and sprains that cause inflammation, pain, and loss of function. Therapists who regularly hyperextend their knees, slouch, bend over the table, twist the spine, or lift the client's limbs from an unsupported position while giving a massage have increased problems associated with these postural deviations, which might lead beyond sprains and strains to a more complicated disc condition.

Intervertebral discs are situated between spinal vertebrae to cushion and separate the vertebrae. A disc has two parts: a tough connective tissue exterior called the annulus fibrosus, and a soft, gelatinous center called the nucleus pulposus. With aging, the annulus fibrosus begins to degenerate and the nucleus pulposus becomes thinner and dryer. Numerous types of disc problems may develop. In one scenario potentially affecting massage therapists, poor posture, poor body mechanics that place repetitive stress on an area of the spine or a sudden trauma (simultaneous lifting and twisting from an unsupported position) may cause a disc to bulge, placing pressure on the spinal cord or on nerve roots (Fig. 11-15). The pressure and pain may change with different body positions, but pain, inflammation, loss of function, and nerve damage can result. Therapists can protect their backs with good body mechanics on the job and good posture in everyday life.

Piriformis Syndrome

The piriformis is a muscle that originates on the anterior sacrum and inserts on the greater trochanter of the femur to laterally rotate the thigh; it abducts and medially rotates the thigh if the thigh is flexed. The sciatic nerve, which is the largest nerve in the body, supplies sensation to the leg and foot. It originates in the lower back at L5–S2 and travels between the piriformis and the superior gemellus (another muscle that laterally rotates the thigh) before branching into the tibial nerve and common peroneal nerve at the popliteal fossa. A tight piriformis may compress the sciatic nerve, resulting in numbness, a burning sensation, sharp and shooting pain, tingling, and loss of function (Fig. 11-16). In some

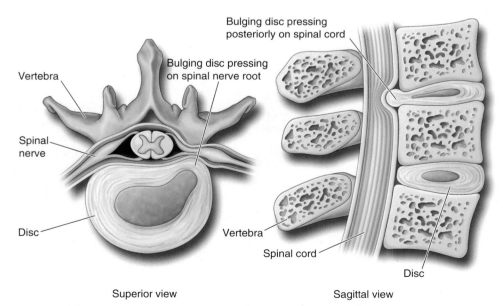

Figure 11-15 Numerous types of disc problems may develop. In one scenario potentially affecting massage therapists, poor posture, poor body mechanics that place repetitive stress on an area of the spine, or a sudden trauma may cause a disc to bulge, placing pressure on the spinal cord or on nerve roots.

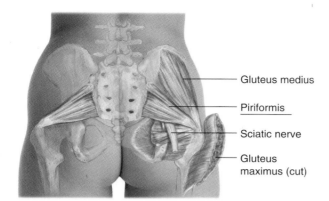

Figure 11-16 A tight piriformis may compress the sciatic nerve, resulting in the piriformis syndrome with numbness, a burning sensation, sharp and shooting pain, tingling, and loss of function.

individuals the sciatic nerve travels directly through the fibers of the piriformis, which might predispose them to piriformis syndrome. Standing with the weight on one leg or laterally rotating the thigh while giving massage can lead to piriformis syndrome. The piriformis is released and softened with massage, stretching, and good body mechanics.

Pressure on the Job

Sometimes job pressures cause therapists to continue working when they are tired. When exhausted, a therapist is more susceptible to injury and burnout. Job pressures may increase because of too many clients, too little time between massages, and too few days off.

Too Many Clients

In massage school, many students perform four to six massages a week. In a busy massage clinic, this number could increase to 30 massages a week. New graduates with a sudden full schedule may be at a greater risk for an injury. This can also happen to professionals who have worked several years at a certain level and then change jobs and suddenly have more clients.

To prevent injury, it is best to increase the number of massages you perform slowly and steadily over the course of a few weeks. Although new massage professionals may feel they can't request this courtesy from a new employer, it is in the employer's interest to ensure the health of employees. Discuss the matter openly and try to develop a plan such as starting with 8 massages in week 1, 12 massages in week 2, 16 massages in week 3, and so on until reaching the desired number of clients.

Therapists in some chiropractic offices may be prone to injury due to a large number of clients per day. Clients often see a massage therapist for a brief session directly before receiving an adjustment from the chiropractor. The massage helps warm up the client's muscles to reduce muscular tension pulling on bones, making it easier to shift the bones back into a proper alignment. Therapists in this work setting often do intense physical work with time constraints. They may overuse their hands with lifting motions like petrissage that quickly warm tissue, or overuse their thumbs in friction

or compression techniques to break up adhesions. Often the minute they finish with one client, the next is on the way. If this situation is prolonged, the therapist is at risk for injury. The goal is to be proactive and develop a sensible plan that can be negotiated with the chiropractor. For example, two therapists can tag team, trading off so that each has a brief rest before working again. Therapists should never feel powerless but must strive to protect themselves. Don't remain in a situation that could lead to injury, burnout, or a loss of spirit. Plenty of jobs are available, and a therapist who feels good is more likely to give a good massage and develop a loyal clientele.

Too Little Time Between Massages

After completing a massage session, you must wash your hands, change the table linen, disinfect some areas of the treatment room (e.g., wipe door knobs with a disinfectant), and finish chart notes. You may also process the client's payment and schedule another session. If you do not schedule enough time between massages to complete these tasks and take a short break, each successive massage gets more and more stressful. You may end the day emotionally and physically exhausted.

While a tight schedule may maximize income, one's ability to do exceptional work decreases over time, and as a result client loyalty declines. Remember that if you are injured because your body does not have enough time to recuperate between sessions, you may lose all income until the injury heals.

New graduates may want to start off with a 30-minute break between clients until they develop a system for making the transition between one client and the next. Soon you will likely feel comfortable with 20 minutes between clients. Therapists should never have <15 minutes between clients unless a support person carries out most of the changeover duties (e.g., changing table linen, processing payments, and booking clients).

Too Few Days Off

In the excitement of getting their career up and running, some new therapists may take more than one massage job and end up working, for example, five mornings at a chiropractic office and four evenings at a spa. Even if you pace yourself in each work environment and practice good body mechanics, over time this schedule is sure to be wearing. Strive to find a balance between making money and having a good life. If possible, plan to take 2 days off from massage every week to give your body adequate rest. In the beginning, while still building up your strength and stamina, try to work only 2 or 3 days in a row and then have a day off. Although it is always nice to have 2 days off in a row, a staggered schedule helps prevent injury and fatigue.

Many longtime professionals teach massage, write books and articles about massage, perform a variety of different massage systems, or pair massage with other related and complementary careers (e.g., fitness trainers, yoga instructors, doulas, and estheticians). This job strategy protects the body from repetitive stress while providing income from a variety of massage-related sources.

Transporting Equipment

On-site work requires transporting a massage table or massage chair to different job locations. Lifting and carrying equipment, moving it in and out of a car, and bending and twisting to set it up and take it down can take a toll on the therapist's body. Be sure to purchase equipment specifically designed for travel. Get a lightweight massage table or chair with a strong carrying case and a rolling cart. Don't place the strap over the same shoulder each time you move the equipment, but alternate shoulders to distribute the stress. Pay attention to your body mechanics and lift equipment using your legs while holding it close to your body. Avoid bending at the waist and twisting.

It would be a wise choice not to work in locations that require hauling equipment up long flights of stairs or providing massage in cramped spaces. Clients sometimes have dogs, cats, children, or an unclean environment that disrupts the massage and makes it difficult to feel grounded and centered during a session. Avoid giving massage in situations that don't feel conducive to good work, because these situations often lead to emotional irritation and fatigue.

Proactive Self-Care

All massage therapists should consciously control the environment where they work to ensure they promote good body mechanics. Take proactive steps to organize the treatment space, adjust equipment, and plan self-care activities that ensure your health and wellness. Furthermore, pay attention to signs and signals from your body that indicate fatigue or bad postural habits.

Organize the Massage Environment

Sometimes a therapist gets lazy and fails to pay attention to the work environment. For example, a therapist might follow another therapist's session and not adjust the table height. Working with the massage table at the optimum height is important for good body mechanics. If the table is too low, you may bend at the waist and lean over the table rather than widen your stance and lunge lower. If the table is too high, you may allow your shoulders to hunch and use too much muscular strength instead of your body weight in the strokes. The floor under the massage table should be smooth and unobstructed. If you must maneuver around extension cords, loose area rugs, or uneven floorboards, you are more likely may be caught off balance and sustain an injury.

Some treatment rooms are so small that there is not sufficient space to perform massage using good body mechanics. You may be forced to deliver a foot or neck massage from the side of the table instead of its top or bottom. Move any unnecessary furniture to create as much space as possible. Place music systems and supplies like tissue boxes and gel hand sanitizer on a wall shelf to tidy the floor. Pay attention to any adapted postures and strive to practice good structural alignment despite the limited space.

Good ventilation, a place to sit during portions of the session, and enjoyable, inspiring music create a greater sense of comfort and enjoyment for therapists during a session. Air out the treatment room by opening windows and doors between clients, or leave a window slightly open so that fresh air circulates through the room. Keep a glass or bottle of water on hand to sip from during a session.

Plan Self-Care Activities

Plan ahead for your day by packing healthy snacks to eat between clients. Arrive early and warm up with stretches, especially for the hands, arms, neck, and shoulders. Therapists who ease into the day tend to feel more grounded and centered than those who show up late and must rush. After each massage, it is a good idea to rinse your hands in cold water and/or ice your wrists and forearms. Cold temperatures decrease inflammation and fluid buildup in the local tissue. Immediately before the next massage, make sure your hands are warm again by running them under warm water or holding a warm pack.

At the end of the day, stretch your muscles out and use warm applications to decrease muscular tension. You might take a warm bath or shower, soak in a hot tub, or use warm packs. Warm and hot applications increase the blood flow to local tissue, which softens muscles, reduces muscular spasm, increases the extensibility of collagen, "melts" the superficial fascia, increases the range of motion in joints, reduces pain, and is generally relaxing.

Ideally, have massage exchanges with colleagues once a week. Therapists who receive regular massage are more likely to remain free from injury and address repetitive stresses before a major problem results. A therapist who receives regular massage may feel emotionally and mentally supported. It's difficult to give, give, give if your own body feels stiff and sore.

Listen to Your Body

Everyday, before and after every massage shift, assess your body and pay attention to your feelings, sensations, thoughts, and emotions. Ask yourself, "Am I mentally, emotionally, and physically ready to give massage today?" We all have days when we don't feel like working or have difficulty getting up and running. But you don't have to be chomping at the bit and jumping up and down to be ready. Instead, through self-awareness, make small adjustments in your plans to avoid injury. Perhaps you find that you feel sore and achy from taking on an extra two massages for a sick colleague yesterday. You may need to do additional stretching before the first massage to feel loose. You might also need to set good personal boundaries if you are pressured often to pick up more extra massages. Saying no to an employer can feel scary, but your first priority must be your own health. If your body is still feeling the effects of extra massage sessions, it's not a good idea to stress it for a 2nd day in a row.

What Does Pain Mean?

Remember that pain is not normal. Pain happens for a reason. If your body is in pain, something is wrong. A tight muscle, a bone, or fluid from inflammation is probably putting pressure on a nerve. Perhaps you are overusing one technique, resulting in microscopic tears in the muscles of the hands or forearms causing inflammation and irritation. Perhaps you have adopted a less-than-optimal position while using deep tissue techniques and are stressing your joints. Too many therapists ignore pain and adopt an attitude of "I can work through the pain and it will eventually go away." Pain is not likely to go away; pain is likely to get worse. But if you acknowledge the pain from the beginning, when it is just a minor twinge or a sensation of fatigue, you can act to identify and eliminate the cause.

During a session, if you become aware of pain, immediately assess your body position and technique. Sometimes only a small adjustment is needed to fix the problem. Areas of the body that are commonly affected by poor body mechanics or overuse are discussed in following sections.

PAIN OR TENSION IN THE NECK AND SHOULDERS

If you feel pain or tension in your neck or shoulders, you are likely laterally flexing your head and neck during sessions or looking down at the client for prolonged periods of time. Check to make sure that you are applying deeper pressure by leaning on the client and dropping into the tissue rather than using the strength of your arm muscles. Apply pressure from a slight angle, not from directly on top of the area.

PAIN OR TENSION IN THE HANDS, THUMBS, AND FINGERS

Pain or tension in your hands, thumbs, and fingers indicates that you are probably overusing your hands during a session. Strive to alternate strokes applied with the hands with strokes applied using your forearm or fists. Check to ensure that static compression or friction strokes applied with your thumbs are not causing the thumbs to hyperextend. Always reinforce the thumb and fingers during compression strokes, or use a knuckle or your elbow instead. Rinse your hands in cold water for 5 to 10 minutes directly after the session, and ice your wrists regularly.

PAIN OR TENSION IN THE LOWER BACK AND GLUTEALS

Pain or tension in the lower back indicates that you are bending at the waist for prolonged periods during the session, twisting your spine unnecessarily, or lifting the client's limbs from an unsupported position and not using your legs for the lift. The gluteals can feel painful if you unconsciously clench them to stabilize your body core. This means that you need to pay more attention to the position of your feet and hips during the session.

PAIN OR TENSION IN THE KNEES

Keep your knees slightly flexed and pointed in the same direction as your hips and feet. Twisting your upper body during a stroke can cause undue stress on your knees. If your knees hurt, you are likely hyperextending them and possibly leaning your thighs against the massage table. Pay attention to the position of your knees and try to keep them flexed and fluid.

PAIN OR TENSION IN THE ANKLES AND FEET

The most common cause of foot and ankle pain is poor-fitting shoes.[31] People often wear shoes that are one or two sizes too small for their feet. This usually occurs because people try on new shoes while sitting down (nonweight bearing), lace the shoes tightly around their feet, and then stand up and walk around. The shoes hold the foot in a cramped position such that the bones cannot lengthen out into a strong arch. Over time, this may lead to foot pain and may contribute to knee, hip, and lower back conditions. It's a good idea to try on shoes in the afternoon when the feet are at their largest due to normal swelling. Remember also that because your feet widen with age, you should expect your shoe size to increase over the years.[32]

Use this quick foot size test to determine if your shoes are too small for your feet.[33] Sit on a chair with your bare feet shoulder-width apart. Ask a colleague to place pieces of cardboard under each of your feet, and then stand up. The other person then traces around each of your feet onto the pieces of cardboard. Because your weight is on your feet and you are barefoot, the tracings will indicate the true foot size to which shoes should be fitted. Then cut out your foot impressions and try to slip them into your shoes. If the cardboard impressions do not fit into your shoes, the shoes are too small. Ideally, discard any shoes that do not fit the cardboard impressions. Note that when you first wear shoes that fit your cardboard impressions, the shoes may feel too large because it takes some time for the foot to relax back into its natural lengthened position.

Concept Brief 11-4
Proactive Self-Care

Always adjust the table to the proper height

Ensure that the space around the massage table is clear

Keep the treatment room ventilated

Drink water during the session

Eat healthy snacks

Stretch before and after the session

Ground and center before the session

Rinse hands in cold water directly after a session; ice regularly

Use warm applications to reduce muscle tension

Pay attention to pain, and make adjustments immediately

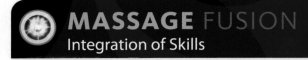

MASSAGE FUSION
Integration of Skills

STUDY TIP: Exercise and Study

Many students have full schedules that make it difficult to balance the demands of a job, school assignments, family, and self-care activities. If possible, study while exercising. Write information on flash cards and strive to memorize five to seven flash cards during a fitness session. This works particularly well for kinesthetic students (students who like to "do" rather than see or hear information), because body movements become memory cues that help one identify information placed into long-term memory.

MASSAGE INSPIRATION: Roll the Tape!

It can be difficult to pay attention to your body mechanics while also learning new techniques and strokes. When your body falls into poor postural habits, those habits start to feel normal and may become difficult to change. One way to develop more self-awareness is to ask a friend or classmate to videotape you while you deliver a massage. This way you can see how you hold your body during each technique. Identify two areas that need improvement, and focus on those areas. Repeat the video process latter to see where you have made progress and where you still need further improvement. Therapists who pay careful attention to body mechanics while in massage school usually carry good habits with them into professional practice.

IT'S TRUE! STRESS REDUCTION IS IMPORTANT FOR GOOD HEALTH AND INJURY PREVENTION

Your instructors will tell you, and you in turn will tell your clients: "Reduce stress to improve your health." One important body chemical closely connected to stress and health is cortisol. Cortisol is a corticosteroid hormone produced by the adrenal cortex. It helps regulate glucose metabolism, the immune system, the body's response to stress, and inflammatory responses. Because cortisol profoundly reduces the inflammatory response when administered in large doses,[34] cortisone and other similar drugs, cortisol's synthetic counterparts, are used to treat allergies, arthritis, soft-tissue injuries, and other inflammatory conditions.[35] Cortisol secretion increases in response to physical and psychological triggering of the fight-or-flight response (stress). In life-or-death situations this is a good thing, but daily chronic stress can lead to "cortisol poisoning" causing increasingly noticeable negative side effects.[36] Chronic high levels of cortisol may impair cognitive performance,[37] lead to blood sugar imbalances, decrease bone density,[38] increase blood pressure,[39] lower immunity, and increase abdominal fat storage.[40] Prolonged episodes of elevated cortisol also systematically weaken all types of connective tissue, increasing the risk for soft-tissue injury, reinjury, and pain.[29] Consider this in terms of body mechanics and self-care. A therapist who is overstressed is likely to have higher levels of cortisol in the body. This cortisol weakens connective tissue, which is already under pressure from repetitive motions used during massage, increasing the likelihood of injury. The point to remember is that although it's easy to disregard and ignore stress, stress-reduction activities are very, very important for self-care. Try to understand stress and take action to participate in stress-reduction activities everyday.

GOOD TO KNOW: Use of the Term "Energy"

Students sometimes feel uncomfortable with some of the metaphors used in massage. The word "energy" is used a good deal. The term is often used to describe how intangible information is passed between a client and a therapist, or between the therapist and the world. Using the word "energy" attempts to make complicated and sometimes unexplained phenomena understandable. Physical manifestations of energy, such as electricity, can be measured by physiological tests like electroencephalography, electrocardiography, and lie detector tests that measure galvanic skin responses. These tests show that the body *is* primarily driven by different forms of energy, but can humans pass intangible forms of energy-based information back and forth, or pick up "energetic" patterns from others? Many therapists believe that they can and do. Many therapists believe that a silent, energy-based form of communication continually occurs between client and therapist in a massage session, whether we are aware of it or not. Some therapists also use the word "energy" to explain subtle, elusive happenings that sometimes occur in sessions. Sometimes unexplainable changes may take place in the client's or therapist's body. If you have not yet experienced anything like this, you may be skeptical of such uses of the word "energy." Skepticism is healthy and leads to further inquiry and hopefully a deeper understanding. You are encouraged to share your feelings with teachers and classmates. Remember that you don't

MASSAGE FUSION (Continued)
Integration of Skills

have to believe everything you hear. You don't have to believe in these forms of "energy" to be a good therapist. Instead, be open to new ideas and reserve judgment until you have gathered enough information to make a decision.

CHAPTER WRAP-UP

People drawn to work in a health care profession are often very good at taking care of other people but sometimes not as good at taking care of themselves. Good self-care is essential because massage really is an athletic sport. You have to treat yourself like an athlete. Eat good, nutritious food, get rest, drink water, stretch, build strength, build stamina, and relax regularly. Then enjoy the benefits of working in a field where you are on your feet and moving everyday. When you know and practice good body mechanics, you get a great workout from performing a massage but don't feel overworked. Because massage is very centering and invigorating, if you avoid stressing your body by paying attention to your posture and movement, at the end of the workday you can feel more invigorated than when you began. Take time now, while still a student, to teach your body good habits. Slow down when you learn techniques so that you can figure out how to position your body to avoid stress. This will become a good habit that can sustain you through a long and fulfilling career.

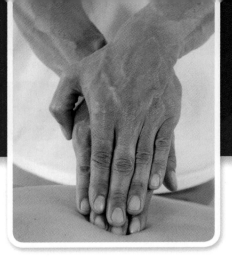

Chapter 12

Assessment, Treatment Planning, and Documentation for Wellness Massage

KEY TERMS

abbreviations

assessment

bony landmarks

customized wellness session

documentation

health intake form

health intake interview

objective data

palpation

session planning

standardized wellness session

subjective data

wellness chart

LEARNING OBJECTIVES

Having read the chapter and used the related student learning tools, the student will be able to:

1. Explain the concept of assessment and explain its role in a massage session.

2. Discuss the purpose of session planning and describe one method for getting the client involved in the process.

3. Compare and contrast subjective and objective data.

4. Provide three examples of information to include on a health intake form and explain the relevance of each.

5. Summarize the information that is explained to the client as part of the informed consent process.

6. Evaluate the goals of a health intake interview and defend the value of a thorough interview process.

7. List the objectives of palpation assessment.

8. Describe the skills a massage therapist must develop to palpate effectively.

9 Compare methods for palpating muscle tissue with methods for palpating skin and superficial fascia.

10 Identify the reasons why massage therapists document sessions.

11 Interpret the acronym *SOAP*.

12 Give examples of the types of information that are recorded in each section of a SOAP chart.

A ssessment, session planning, and documentation are interrelated skills that, when mastered by a massage therapist, ensure the client's safety and comfort and the choice of effective and appropriate techniques. Topic 12-1 describes subjective and objective data and how to collect it before, during, and after massage sessions. Palpation is an essential skill discussed in depth in Topic 12-2. Using these guidelines, you are likely to pay greater attention to what you feel in soft tissue and begin to differentiate tissue textures and types. Topic 12-3 explores session planning for both a standardized wellness massage and a custom wellness massage. Topic 12-4 describes how to record data on either a SOAP chart or wellness form. The skills discussed in this chapter form the foundation for more advanced assessment, session planning, and documentation methods described in Chapter 19.

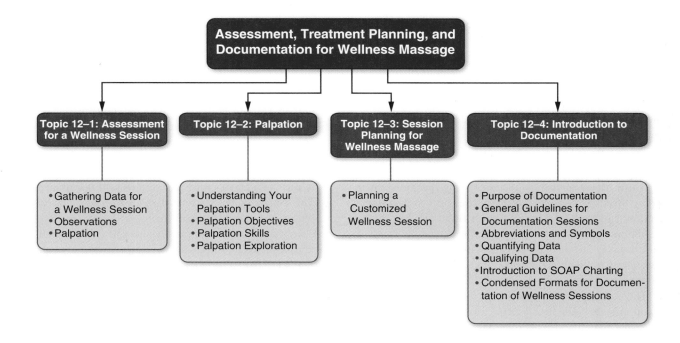

Topic **12-1**
Assessment for a Wellness Session

Assessment is a process of collecting information about a client, interpreting the information to better understand the client's condition, and then making safe and effective treatment decisions based on this understanding. Presession and postsession assessments can be compared to document changes in the body brought about by the massage session. Assessment skills help therapists know when massage is contraindicated for a client, when adaptations to the session are required, or when the client should be referred to another healthcare provider. An assessment is not the same as a medical diagnosis (Box 12-1).

BOX 12-1 Assessment Versus Diagnosis

A massage **assessment** is the evaluation of the client's signs and symptoms to rule out contraindications and choose effective techniques. **Diagnosis** is the medical evaluation of the client's signs and symptoms, plus the use of special tests, to identify an illness or condition. A diagnosis is provided only by a medical professional whose scope of practice includes procedures that lead to the identification and naming of an illness or condition.

Gathering Data for a Wellness Session

Much of the information the client writes on the health history form or tells you verbally during the health intake interview or during the massage is **subjective data**. The term *subjective* means information based on opinions or feelings rather than on observable facts. Subjective information includes the client's complaints or symptoms and usually the reason for seeking massage. In a wellness session, the client's symptoms are likely to be mild, or the client is interested in using massage as a stress reduction strategy. For this reason, the assessment in a wellness session is much less in-depth than an assessment conducted for a healthcare massage (Chapter 19).

An overview of a wellness session was provided in Chapter 10. Review that section if needed to understand where within the scope of the entire session intake and other forms are used and the health intake interview occurs.

The Health Intake Form

A **health intake form** is a document that clients complete before their first session that provides personal contact information, current health conditions, medications, past health conditions, and health-related goals. The primary purpose of the form is to rule out contraindications, indicate when adaptations to treatment might be required, and help the therapist determine appropriate session objectives.

The design of the form depends on the type of massage that is provided. The health intake form for wellness massage is usually more condensed than an intake form for healthcare massage. In a wellness massage, the focus is most often relaxation, but you still need to rule out contraindications and determine the client's preferences to provide an enjoyable session. A healthcare massage requires greater insight because to ensure that treatment goals address the client's functional limitations (limitations to activities of daily living like lifting grandchildren, cleaning the house, and working at a computer), and that improvements can be monitored to influence treatment choices in subsequent sessions. The client is asked to list and prioritize current health concerns, how these concerns impact the client's daily activities, and the severity of symptoms.

Therapists who often work with special populations, or in specific environments, can develop different intake forms for each unique situation. A form for pregnant women asks different questions from a form for athletes or a form for elderly clients. A form used in a spa asks different questions from a form designed for on-site seated massage. The questions are formulated to reveal possible contraindications. For example, a health intake form in a spa may ask about allergies to shellfish or iodine if the spa uses seaweed-based products or offers seaweed treatments. Anyone allergic to shellfish or iodine is very likely to be allergic to seaweed, and even small amounts of it in lotions or skin care products can cause serious reactions.

You can customize your own forms with your logo, name, address, and phone number. These contact details should be present on every page of every document so that others can contact you easily for additional information, such as in situations where a client's health records are subpoenaed or shared with another health professional.

Overview of a Health Intake Form for Wellness Massage

Let's review the sample wellness health intake form shown in Figure 12-1. It is two pages long and will take clients approximately 10 minutes to complete. The structure of the form and the questions included are up to the individual therapist. This is just one example of many designs, and you're encouraged to look at a variety of health intake forms and then design your own forms to fit your own needs. The school where you train is likely to have a form that is used in classes and in student clinic. The health intake form for a healthcare massage is shown and discussed in Chapter 19.

The first section of the sample wellness health intake form gathers general contact information from the client. It is helpful to know a client's occupation because it often provides clues to a client's muscular tension and postural habits. The second area of the form asks for the client's primary healthcare provider. This information is important if you need a physician's release to provide massage or if a client has an adverse reaction to massage that is not serious enough to warrant a call to emergency services. Sometimes clients don't have primary healthcare providers and wish to leave this section blank. It is okay if the client leaves this section blank, as long as an emergency contact has been listed.

In the third section, clients outline their goals for the session. This information provides a starting point for planning the session with the client. From Chapter 5, you already understand how to use information on medications to adapt the massage to ensure client safety. The questions about pain, tenderness, stiffness, fever, inflammation, and fatigue alerts you that a client's symptoms need further investigation before he or she can receive massage as discussed in Chapter 5. The final section (Current and Previous Conditions) allows clients to quickly provide an overview of their medical history. If the client checks that a condition occurred in the past, it is less worrisome than a current condition. Still, past conditions often signal that greater caution is required. For example, if the client notes hypertension (high blood pressure) in the past, you might want to check the client's blood pressure (Technique 5)

Client Name: _____ Birth Date: _____

Wellness Health Information

Client's Name: _____ Date: _____

Address: _____

Phone: _____ Occupation: _____ E-Mail: _____

Emergency Contact: _____ Phone: _____

Primary Health Care Provider

Name: _____ Phone: _____

Address: _____

Current Health Information

What are your goals for wellness and how can I assist you in achieving these goals?

_____

_____

_____

Please list all the medications, vitamins, and supplements you took today including
over-the-counter medications like cold medications or pain relievers, herbs or homeopathic
remedies:

_____

_____

_____

Please list all the medications you have taken within the last three months including
over-the-counter medications like cold medications or pain relievers:

_____

_____

_____

Have you ever received a massage before? Yes ☐   No ☐

Are you currently experiencing any of the following symptoms? If yes, please mark the
symptom and provide a brief explanation:

☐ Pain _____

☐ Tenderness _____

☐ Stiffness _____

☐ Fever _____

☐ Inflammation _____

☐ Fatigue _____

☐ Other _____

Your Massage Business, 222 Any Street, Suite 300, Any Town, AS, 00990, 222-333-4444, www.ymb.com

Client Name: _____   Birth Date: _____

Current and Previous Conditions

Please check all current and previous conditions and give a brief explanation, if appropriate, in the comments section at the end of the form.

Current   Past

☐ ☐ Headache
☐ ☐ Sleep disorders
☐ ☐ Sinus condition
☐ ☐ Skin condition
☐ ☐ Athlete's foot
☐ ☐ Warts
☐ ☐ Skin sensitivities
☐ ☐ Burns
☐ ☐ Bruises
☐ ☐ Sunburn
☐ ☐ Aversion to scents
☐ ☐ Aversion to oils
☐ ☐ Aversion to cold
☐ ☐ Allergies
☐ ☐ Sensitivities to detergent
☐ ☐ Rheumatoid arthritis
☐ ☐ Osteoarthritis
☐ ☐ Spinal conditions
☐ ☐ Disc conditions
☐ ☐ Lupus
☐ ☐ Tendonitis
☐ ☐ Bursitis
☐ ☐ Fibromyalgia
☐ ☐ Chronic fatigue
☐ ☐ Dizziness
☐ ☐ Ringing in ears
☐ ☐ Head injury
☐ ☐ Mental confusion
☐ ☐ Numbness, tingling
☐ ☐ Neuritis

☐ ☐ Neuralgia
☐ ☐ Sciatica
☐ ☐ Shooting pain
☐ ☐ Depression
☐ ☐ Anxiety
☐ ☐ Panic attacks
☐ ☐ Heart disease
☐ ☐ Blood clot
☐ ☐ Stroke
☐ ☐ Lymphedema
☐ ☐ High blood pressure
☐ ☐ Low blood pressure
☐ ☐ Poor circulation
☐ ☐ Swollen ankles
☐ ☐ Varicose veins
☐ ☐ Respiratory conditions
☐ ☐ Urinary conditions
☐ ☐ Abdominal pain
☐ ☐ Thyroid dysfunction
☐ ☐ Diabetes
☐ ☐ Phlebitis
☐ ☐ Pacemaker
☐ ☐ Contact lenses

Other Conditions: _____
_____
_____

Comments: _____
_____
_____

Client Signature: _____
Date: _____
Therapist Signature: _____
Date: _____

Your Massage Business, 222 Any Street, Suite 300, Any Town, AS, 00990, 222-333-4444, www.ymb.com

Figure 12-1 The primary purpose of the Wellness Health Intake form is to rule out contraindications, indicate when adaptations to treatment might be required, and help you and the client determine appropriate session objectives.

before the massage to ensure that it is within normal parameters. Look up all unfamiliar mediations and conditions to rule out contraindications before starting the massage.

Both the client and the therapist sign and date the form. This demonstrates that the intake process actually took place and that both have reviewed and agreed that the information on the form is up to date and complete. If a different therapist works with the client at a later date, that therapist knows when the original health information was gathered and which therapist to contact in case more information about the client's previous sessions is needed. The health intake form is kept in the client's file and reviewed before every session. If a significant change in the client's health occurs (e.g., if the client is in an accident, sustains an injury, develops a medically diagnosed condition, is prescribed new medications, and has surgery), the client is asked to update the form; otherwise, it is updated annually. The therapist or client can make simple amendments to the form if minor changes in the client's health condition occur (e.g., the client stops smoking or a medication is switched by a physician,). The new entry is dated and the therapist or client initial is beside the date.

Today's Session Form

The form shown in Figure 12-2 is useful in a wellness massage process. The form is completed by the client along with the health intake form. The human figures allow the client to quickly identify areas of pain and particular muscle tension. It also allows clients to mark the regions where they would like to receive massage and the areas they would prefer not to receive massage. A Today's Session form can be used before every massage session to help the therapist and client quickly agree a plan for the massage.

Informed Consent Documents

In Chapter 6, you learned about informed consent, the process by which a fully informed client consents to participate in the massage treatment. To review briefly, informed consent recognizes the legal right of clients to direct what happens to their body. Therapists have an ethical obligation to involve the client in choices related to health and wellness. During the first intake interview, you provide specific types of information, and the client signs a form stating that he or she understands and would like to receive massage. This process protects the client but also helps to establish the boundaries of the therapeutic relationship to protect you. Figure 6-6 provides a sample of an informed consent form. Ensure that the form you develop for your practice covers these areas:

- A definition of massage
- Limitations of massage
- Adverse reactions that can occur with massage
- Your training and experience in massage therapy
- Your business policies and practices including fees
- The expected behavior of the client
- The expected behavior of the therapist

- The rights of the client
- A disclaimer and signature section

Therapists usually hand out forms to clients on a clipboard when they arrive for their first visits to the clinic. Some therapists move clients directly to the treatment room and provide a foot soak and cup of herbal tea to enhance the intake process for a wellness massage. This is optional, and the client might simply fill out paperwork in the reception area. Explain each document to the client and why it is needed before massage is provided. When the client has completed the forms, the interview can begin.

The Health Intake Interview for a Wellness Session

A **health intake interview** is a conversation that occurs between the therapist and the client to gather information that will be used to plan the session. An interview conducted before a wellness session is usually less detailed than an intake interview for a healthcare session. It should be managed efficiently and not cut into the time allocated for the client's massage. In Chapter 7, you learned about the therapeutic relationship. In Chapter 8, you learned about active professional communication practices. Both of these topics directly influence the quality of the health intake interview. If you are uncertain about how to set up and maintain a therapeutic relationship, or if you have not started practicing professional communication skills, reviewing those chapters is recommended. Without first understanding these core skills, it is difficult to conduct an efficient and meaningful health intake interview. The goals of the interview include

- **Put the client at ease and establish rapport:** Rapport is defined as a friendly bond between people based on mutual liking, trust, and a sense that they understand and share each other's concerns. While you don't want to overstep the boundaries of the therapeutic relationship and treat clients like buddies, you should greet them warmly and treat them with respect, friendliness, and compassion. One of the first questions to review on the health intake form is "Have you ever received a massage before?" If the client answers "yes," ask about the experience and what he or she liked about the massage. This can clue you into the client's expectations for the session and help you meet these expectations. If the client answers "no," you should orient the client to how the session will be conducted. New clients may be very apprehensive, and clear descriptions of the draping policy and client's rights often help them relax and develop feelings of trust.

- **Communicate the policies of the clinic to establish the therapeutic relationship:** Review the informed consent form with the client. Don't assume that the client has read it just because it is signed. Briefly describe each section of the form and ensure clients understand the clinic's policies and their rights as a client to stop the session at anytime or to control the massage experience by providing feedback or asking for adaptations to the massage. Discussing the information on the informed consent form helps you establish

Therapist's Name: _____ Date: _____

Wellness Massage - Today's Session

Client's Name: _____ Today's Date: _____

Areas of Focus

Please indicate your current physical experience and the areas where you would like your therapist to focus the massage today by drawing circles on the figure and marking the circles with a letter from the key.

Key
P = Pain
T = Muscle tension
J = Joint stiffness
O = Other (Please describe):
_____
_____
_____

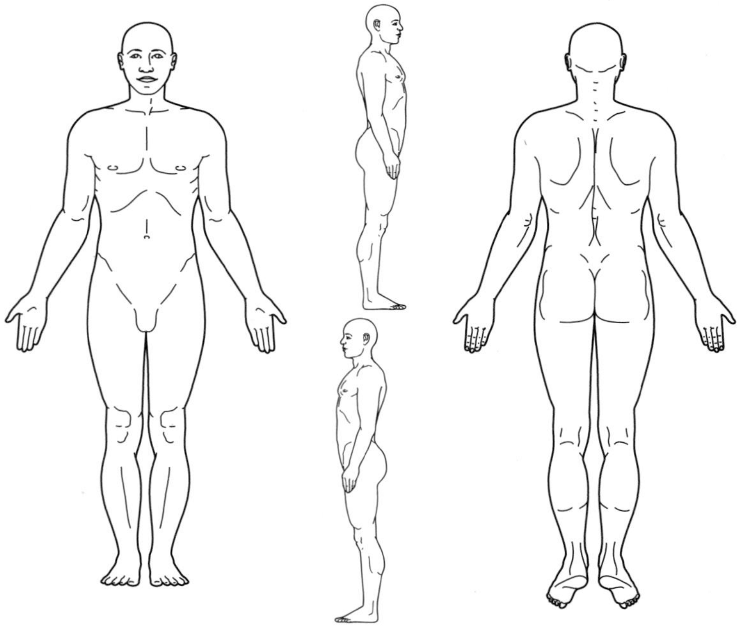

Areas to Massage:

_____Feet
_____Front of the legs
_____Back of the legs
_____Gluteal regions (buttocks)
_____Back
_____Arms
_____Hands
_____Upper chest and shoulders
_____Abdominal region (belly)
_____Neck
_____Face
_____Scalp

Areas NOT to Massage:

_____Feet
_____Front of the legs
_____Back of the legs
_____Gluteal regions (buttocks)
_____Back
_____Arms
_____Hands
_____Upper chest and shoulders
_____Abdominal region (belly)
_____Neck
_____Face
_____Scalp

Client Signature: _____ Therapist Signature: _____

Your Massage Business, 222 Any Street, Suite 300, Any Town, AS, 00990, 222-333-4444, www.ymb.com

Figure 12-2 A Today's Session form can be used before every massage session to help you and the client quickly agree on a plan for the massage.

the therapeutic relationship because it outlines the role of the therapist and the role of the client. It clarifies the scope of practice and limitations of massage, and defines massage as a healthcare profession. This structure often makes clients feel safer about receiving massage and builds their trust that your business is a professional establishment.

- **Clarify information written on the health intake form to rule out contraindications:** Review the health intake form with the client and question the client for more detail about any preexisting conditions or medications that require adaptations in massage. It is appropriate to ask clients to describe the types of side effects they experience from medications and to talk over ways to adapt the massage to better meet their needs. For example, one client experienced increased urination as a side effect of a medication. She needed to take a restroom break at the halfway point in her session. The therapist provided the client with a robe and slippers so she could move between the treatment room and the restroom without having to fully dress and undress again.

- **Physician's release:** In some cases, the therapist may need to contact the client's physician to obtain a physician's release. This takes time that can cut into the massage and frustrate the client. If possible, list conditions that require a physician's release during the booking phone call so the client can bring the release to the massage. Never proceed with a massage if you feel the client has a contraindication or if you feel the client's condition requires a release from a physician. Err on the side of caution. Even if the client is frustrated, you uphold good ethical principles when you make choices that ensure the client's safety. Chapter 5 discusses contraindications, medications, and massage adaptations in depth. It provides a critical thinking model to help new therapists decide whether or not it is safe for a client to receive massage.

- **Determine the client's expectations and goals for the session:** Clients most often seek out wellness massage to relax or reduce minor physical tension, or simply because massage is soothing and pleasurable to receive. Sometimes clients request a massage to relieve intense muscle stiffness or pain from a minor injury. Ask clients to share their expectations of the session with questions like, "How would you like to feel at the end of the session today?" Sometimes clients are very clear about what they want, but sometimes they need the therapist to present some options. For example, you might say, "It sounds like you have no areas that are particularly tense. Would you like me to focus on providing a deeply relaxing and soothing massage? If not, we could go for an invigorating, faster paced massage to get you energized. What do you think would work best for you today?"

- **Identify body regions where the client wants focused massage work:** Often clients hold tension in particular areas and need focused work during the wellness massage. Sometimes other body areas are left out of the session to provide more time for areas that need the most massage.

Ask clients to explain where they would like you to focus, or review the Today's Session form with them to ensure you understand their needs.

- **Identify the body regions the client does not want massaged:** It is important to explain to clients the concept of a full body massage. Some get nervous, "You're going to massage… everything!?" Clarify the areas that are massaged and the areas that are never massaged so clients can relax. Many clients feel nervous about having their gluteal muscles and abdominal muscles massaged. Often they relax when the importance of these muscles in back tension, posture, and free graceful movement is explained. Still, this is the client's choice. Remind clients that they have the right to choose which areas receive massage and which do not.

- **Determine the types of techniques the client likes:** Some clients like deep work while others like a very light touch. Some want the therapist to dig in, even if they experience a bit of discomfort, to work out adhesions and strip muscles. Others want a completely soothing massage and find deep work disruptive to their relaxing session. It is helpful to get an indication of these preferences up front and to share with the client specialized techniques you are trained in. If you are a reflexologist, for example, you might mention that you do skilled foot massage and ask if the client would like to have some extra time on the feet. If you are an expert in energetic bodywork practices, let the client decide if such techniques are used in the session. Many clients don't believe in such practices and expect their massages to take a more traditional form. Using energetic techniques without the client's permission crosses an ethical boundary. A client who has never had a massage will not know what to ask for or what to expect. Spend extra time checking in with the client during the massage to ensure that the techniques feel comfortable.

- **Determine the client's preferences for music and lubricants:** Give some options for music (e.g., classical piano, world rhythms, Japanese flute, even soft rock or contemporary music), or arrange during the booking phone call for the client to bring a CD he or she particularly enjoys. Allow clients to see and smell some lubricant options and explain the differences between them. Some clients don't want any scents, while others enjoy aromas. Usually clients respond more positively to natural aromas like those of herbs or essential oils than to synthetic fragrances and dyes.

By the conclusion of the health intake interview you will likely have a plan forming for how the treatment will begin and progress. Palpation findings during the massage will influence the plan and may require making adaptations. These considerations are discussed later in this chapter.

Post–Wellness Massage Interview

At the end of the massage, when the client is dressed, a second, brief interview is conducted. Ask the client to describe the changes felt in the body as a result of the massage, and document these changes in the client's file (as explained later). Some therapists give their clients self-care suggestions for use at home, such as the application of a warm pack at night before bed, or the use of certain stretches, or self-massage. It's best if the post–wellness massage interview takes place in the treatment room, as you don't want to discuss the client's personal health issues in the hallways or reception area.

Subsequent Wellness Interviews

You will not need to review the information on the informed consent form after the client's first visit and massage, unless you have made significant changes in your business policies and procedures. On subsequent visits, review the client's health intake form and use the Today's Session form (or something like it) to plan the visit. Ask the client verbally if there have been any changes to his or her health or medications taken. Small changes are made to the health intake form with a description, initials, and date. Larger changes require the client to fill out a new health form. Plan the massage by reviewing the Today's Session form or by asking the client to describe the areas he or she would like massaged and the results expected. These interviews are fairly informal and may take as little as 5 minutes. Throughout all interactions with the client, you are gathering data that affects choices about what types of techniques will be used to reach session goals.

Observations

The information you gather through observation of the client and palpation of the client's tissue is called **objective data**. The term *objective* is defined as information that is free of bias caused by personal feelings. Objective data is based on facts and measurements rather than opinions; these are often referred to as *signs*. The use of this term in health care originates in medical phrases such as "vital signs," referring to observable measurements such as heart rate, blood pressure, etc. The massage scope of practice does not involve gathering much data that is truly objective. Often the therapist's personal opinions and beliefs influence visual and palpation findings. The goal is to be as objective as possible when gathering data, but to recognize the limitations of the massage scope of practice.

During all interactions with clients, remain visually alert to gather information that might be useful for session planning. Noticing the ways that clients move, breathing patterns, body language, skin coloration, and gestures can provide a wealth of information that influences the techniques you will use and your approach to the session. At this point in your training, begin to hone your observation skills by viewing clients with these thoughts in mind.

- **Freedom of movement:** Does the client move gracefully and freely? If not, which joints appear to experience limited, uneven, or stiff movement? For example, when the head is turned, is the motion smooth and confidant, or does the client turn slowly and cautiously and twist the upper body with the head? If the client clearly moves the head stiffly, you can bet that he or she will need extra attention paid to the soft tissue around the cervical joints. When the client stands up from the chair in the reception area, is the movement continuous, fluid, and even, or does he or she begin the motion, slow in the middle, catch the body and shift on the feet? Does this rigidity come from the joints of the knees, ankles, or hips, from the lumbar and thoracic vertebrae, or from all of these joints? Much can be learned by watching clients as they get out of their cars in the parking lot, walk to the door of the clinic, sit in the reception area, and move while filling out paperwork and interacting with the receptionist.

- **Symmetry:** Both sides of the body should express a certain degree of regularity and an evenness of proportion. When you look at the client's anterior aspect, do the right and left sides of the client seem balanced? One shoulder or one side of the pelvis may be elevated higher than the other. One eye or ear might seem to sit higher. A tilt in the head might be apparent, or the knees and ankles may seem to roll in or out. When viewed from the lateral aspect, the shoulders might roll forward or the chin jut out. The back may have a pronounced curve in the lumbar spine so that the buttocks stick out (lordosis), or the thoracic spine might exhibit a distinct posterior curve (kyphosis). Notice these irregularities and pay attention to what you feel in the tissue. If something is rolling forward/backward, one group of muscles is likely hypertonic and the opposing group weakened, contributing to the unevenness. See if you can correlate what you see in the client's posture to what you feel in the client's tissue. In Chapter 19, you will learn specific techniques for analyzing posture as needed to assess clients for healthcare massage sessions.

- **Breathing patterns:** In Chapter 10, you learned about bringing breathwork into the massage session. Breathwork is indicated, even in a wellness session, if you note abnormal breathing patterns, as long as breathwork does not cut significantly into massage time. In a normal breathing pattern, the abdominal area is the first to expand during an inhalation. The ribs swell laterally followed by a mild lifting of the upper chest. If the upper chest expands but the movement of the ribs and abdominal area is minimal, this is called upper-chest breathing. If the abdominal area is held tight and the upper chest and ribs compensate by over-expanding, this is called paradoxical breathing. Sometimes breathing rhythms are rapid, shallow, and irregular. Any abnormal breathing pattern indicates the use of diaphragmatic breathing in the session (described in Technique 14)

- **Skin condition:** The skin provides clues about the health of other systems in the body through its color, temperature, and condition. Paleness, which is most easily identified in the lips, nail beds, and mucous membranes, is often caused by reduced blood flow to an area or by lower levels of hemoglobin such as occurs with anemia. Flushed, red skin can signal fever, sympathetic nervous system activation, alcohol consumption, or inflammation. Sometimes the skin takes on a grayish tint and appears dry and drawn. This can indicate dehydration and is often seen with heavy cigarette smokers. When there is not enough oxygen in the circulating blood because of a serious heart condition, or because of chronic breathing problems, the skin takes on a bluish tint called cyanosis. Skin with a yellowish tint (jaundice) can be caused by a number of internal disorders often associated with the liver (e.g., hepatitis). Skin that is bluish or yellowish signals that the client's physician should be called and the session likely postponed until the physician's diagnosis and release are supplied.

- **Level of sympathetic dominance:** Chapter 5 discussed the sympathetic nervous system response to stress and the changes that occur physiologically and psychologically as a result of prolonged stress. Clients often indicate their level of stress (sympathetic dominance) by their behavior. They might speak loudly and rapidly, gesture excitedly, demonstrate more energy and animation than is called for in the situation, or explain a recent event with angry or defensive gestures. Prolonged stress can sometimes cause burnout, causing low energy levels, depression, emotional vulnerability, and decreased physical animation. The client's level of sympathetic dominance can influence the therapist's choices for the massage. For example, deeper work might be replaced by soothing strokes that activate the parasympathetic nervous system to encourage the body to rest and recover. The therapist might bring gentle rocking motions into the massage to encourage entrainment.

- **Body language and gestures:** Much can be learned about clients from their body language and gestures, as discussed in Chapter 8. Pay attention to body language cues, and adapt the interview process and massage to the level of trust and openness displayed by the client. For example, a client who consistently maintains a closed body position during the intake interview may also demonstrate protective mechanisms on the massage table. He or she might keep the arms crossed over the chest when supine, hold the body tense during the massage, and guard during range-of-motion techniques. A therapist can lead clients to greater trust by respecting their need for protection. For example, many clients feel safer beginning the massage in the prone position because their genitals and breasts are underneath them. Cover the client with a thicker blanket or an additional drape to provide more layers of protection. Perhaps you begin the session with a breathing exercise that helps the client connect to the body, and avoid deep work and range of motion (which require greater trust and openness) in the first session. Alternately, a client may demonstrate trust and confidence with body language indicating that you can proceed more rapidly into deep work and use range-of-motion techniques freely.

In a wellness session, all of these observations take place while you interact with the client during the health intake interview.

You might ask the client to demonstrate any movements that feel restricted, but a formal posture and movement analysis are not usually preformed. Instead, these general visual findings inform your overall impression of the client's health and vitality or alert you to a possible contraindication.

Palpation

Palpation is defined as examination by touching. Physicians use palpation to examine patients with their hands or fingertips, feeling for enlarged organs, areas of particular tenderness, abnormal masses, or a regular or irregular pulse. Massage therapists use palpation to assess the client's soft-tissue structures and to feel for changes that occur in the tissue as a result of massage. For example, tissue that is warm or hot to the touch and puffed up with fluid signals inflammation. Cool, clammy skin and tissue that feels flaccid and empty can signal disruptions in nerve innervation or poor circulation. In a wellness session, you palpate and adjust your techniques depending on what you feel in the tissue during the massage. In a healthcare session, palpation might be used in a more systematic way before session planning takes place. In all cases, strong palpation skills are essential or massage therapists. This topic is covered in depth in Topic 12-2.

Concept Brief 12-1
Terms for Assessment and Session Planning

- **Assessment:** A judgment based on an understanding of the situation

- **Session Planning:** The use of information gathered during an assessment to determine goals and techniques

- **Subjective Data (Symptoms):** Information clients tell you about their conditions based on what they feel and their opinions. Gathered through the health intake form and interview

- **Health Intake Form:** A document clients complete before their first session that provides contact details, current health conditions, medications, past health conditions, and health-related goals

- **Health Intake Interview:** A conversation that occurs between you and clients to plan the treatment

- **Objective Data:** Information you gather through observation and palpation

- **Observations:** Data obtained visually based on the client's freedom of movement, physical symmetry, breathing patterns, skin condition, level of sympathetic dominance, body language, and gestures

- **Palpation:** Data obtained through touch based on the client's tissue textures, tone, temperature, and hydration

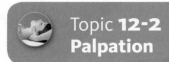

Topic 12-2
Palpation

Palpation is a continuous process in which a massage therapist feels the client's tissue with keen attention to better understand the client's condition, determine treatment goals, compare tissue from one session to the next, choose effective techniques, and adapt techniques if needed during the session. Palpation is both an art and an essential skill. It is used in all levels of massage therapy regardless of whether the therapist works in a spa delivering wellness massage, in a gym with athletes, in a clinic for injury rehabilitation, or in a hospice with elderly clients. This topic explores the sensory receptors that make palpation possible, the objectives of palpation assessments, the types of skills needed for strong palpation, general guidelines for palpating tissue, the layers and anatomical structures that can be palpated, and what might be felt in both healthy and unhealthy tissue.

Understanding Your Palpation Tools

The tools used to palpate the client's tissue include the fingertips, palms, knuckles, forearms, elbows, and even the feet (in massage systems using the feet to apply strokes). These tools provide us with a high degree of palpatory sensitivity because of a number of somatic sensory receptors found in the skin, skeletal muscle, tendons, and joints. These receptors are made up of a single afferent neuron that divides into many fine branches, each ending at a receptor (in a few cases an afferent neuron terminates in a single receptor). Each sensation like light touch, deep pressure, heat, cold, joint position, and pain is associated with a specific receptor type.

- **Light touch:** Conveyed by mechanoreceptors (a class of somatic receptor sensitive to mechanical changes) called Meissner's corpuscles, Merkel's disks, and hair-root plexuses
- **Deep pressure and rough touch:** Conveyed by mechanoreceptors called Pacinian corpuscles, Krause's end bulbs, and Ruffini's end organs
- **Warm and cold temperatures:** Conveyed by thermoreceptors (a type of somatic receptor made up of free nerve endings that detect changes in temperatures)
- **Muscle degree and speed of stretch:** Conveyed by proprioceptors (a class of somatic receptor sensitive to movement) called muscle spindles
- **Muscle contraction and load on tendon:** Conveyed by proprioceptors called Golgi tendon organs
- **Joint movement and position:** Conveyed by proprioceptors called joint receptors, which detect how much of the articular surfaces of joints are touching
- **Pain:** Conveyed by nociceptors (the name means "pain receptor") when tissue damage occurs

Information from somatic receptors passes to the brain stem and thalamus and from there to the somatosensory cortex, an area in the parietal lobe of the brain that processes sensory information.

Palpation skills rely on the responsiveness developed predominantly in the mechanoreceptors that reside in the skin. These are the receptors that are sensitive to touch and pressure, which can be divided in two categories. One category of mechanoreceptor, called rapidly responding receptors, reacts to stimuli with a burst of activity when the stimulus is first felt and again when it is removed. These receptors also respond rapidly to any changes in the stimuli and convey sensations like touch, vibration, movement, and tickle.

The other category of receptor, called slowly adapting receptors, responds to stimuli with continuous unvarying activity throughout the duration of the stimulus. These receptors convey sensations of pressure. Both rapidly responding receptors and slowly adapting receptors can provide precise information about the textures and contours of objects that indent the skin. Many of these highly sensitive receptor types are concentrated in the fingertips. Other receptors convey less specific detail and are involved in relaying information about sensations of vibration, skin stretch, or movement.

While the fingertips and palms are the most sensitive tools for palpation, many therapists also develop finely honed palpation skills with their forearms, elbows, knuckles, and feet. Tools like hot stones used in hot stone massage, or knobs sometimes used with trigger point work, seem to decrease palpation sensitivity initially. Therapists who use these types of tools regularly report that they learn to palpate through the tool and eventually become as responsive to tissue as when not using the tool.

Palpation Objectives

Different types of massage sessions require different levels of palpation, but good massage therapists palpate attentively and continuously throughout all sessions. In a wellness session, the general objective is to palpate in order to adjust techniques appropriately during the massage. You wouldn't want to plow through bound-up tissue as this could cause the client to tighten the muscles in a protective reflex. Similarly, you wouldn't just skim the surface of pliable tissue that needs deeper work. In both cases, a lack of attention to the needs of the tissue could cause the client discomfort or dissatisfaction. A therapist who understands what healthy tissue feels like and can differentiate tissue textures and temperatures can better choose, moment by moment, the techniques that will cause positive changes in the client's tissue and produce results and satisfaction.

In a healthcare massage, where you are likely to work with the client over many sessions, you may conduct a systematic palpation assessment before, during, and after the massage. This includes feeling the quality of the client's movement patterns and using your hands as well as your eyes to assess the symmetry of physical structures. Specific techniques for palpation during a posture assessment and range-of-motion assessment are used to evaluate the tissue and inform session planning (as discussed in Chapter 19). The documentation of presession and postsession palpation findings helps determine the effectiveness of the session and plan techniques for the next session. Palpation findings charted over many sessions demonstrate positive (or negative) changes that occur over time. General palpation objectives include the following:

- Detect irregularity in tissue textures
- Detect irregularity in tissue tone
- Sense differences in tissue temperature
- Notice variations in tissue hydration
- Spot structural asymmetry
- Identify restrictions that are causing reductions in range of motion
- Recognize areas that are painful
- Locate a particular structure, or identify the fiber direction of a muscle, to apply specific techniques correctly
- Distinguish changes in tissue from the beginning of a session to the end of the session or over a series of sessions

Methods to accomplish these objectives will become clear in the following sections.

Palpation Skills

All highly skilled massage therapists palpate continuously, on an almost subconscious level, gathering, interpreting, and responding to data received through their fingers, palms, knuckles, forearms, and elbows. This intense process allows for making moment-by-moment adjustments in the pressure and speed of the stroke to best create positive changes in soft tissue or note changes that occur in the tissue as a result of the session. Palpation skills require the integration of four broader categories of skills: cognitive, kinesthetic, communication, and persistence skills.

Cognitive Skills

Cognitive skills refer to knowledge that informs touch. Without good cognitive skills a therapist might feel every nuance in the tissue but not be able to interpret these feelings to understand the client's condition or make appropriate treatment decisions. Cognitive skills include knowledge of the skeleton and the names and locations of bony landmarks. An in-depth understanding of muscle names, muscle locations, attachment sites, movement patterns, functions, and fiber direction is especially important. It also helps to know about the body's organs, their functions, and their locations.

This includes the position of major arteries, veins, and nerves, which may be superficial in some areas. Build your palpation skills by learning about the structure of the human body. Visualize the structures under the skin, and then find the structures with your hands.

Kinesthetic Skills

Kinesthetic skills refer to the ability to feel nuances in tissue temperature, texture, hydration, tone, and depth. As a student, you may notice that some of your classmates palpate more naturally than others. Some seem to sink into the tissue at just the right depth, while others are either too light or too deep to engage the tissue effectively. Some locate the edges of a muscle effortlessly, while others feel blind to distinguishing features that identify tissue types. Why is this? One reason is variations in anatomy among people.

Studies of both humans and animals find noticeable differences in the size, number, or position of almost all anatomical structures. Students with natural palpation ability likely have higher numbers of sensory receptors per square centimeter of skin leading to greater perceptual ability.[1] Students without this natural ability can still build exceptional skills but may need more effort and practice.

Another factor is attention. Students with strong palpation skills often can put their attention directly into their hands (or forearms, elbows, knuckles, etc.), and focus specifically on what they feel without being distracted. It helps if you use slow movement and sink slowly through layers of tissue. Sometimes novice therapists make the mistake of just poking around with their fingers hoping to suddenly feel something that makes sense. This is irritating to the client and an inefficient method of palpation.

When building your basic kinesthetic skills, it helps to feel the same structure on numerous bodies. Start with a superficial muscle like the deltoid and feel it on both sides of the first body. Move to another body and feel the deltoid again, and then onto a third body, and a forth, and even on a fifth. Each person is likely to express different tissue textures, temperatures, hydration, and tone. By feeling these differences in relationship to one specific muscle, you build your tactile sensitivity.

Communication Skills

Communication skills allow the therapist to name sensations so that perceptions of tissue can be categorized easily. Later in this chapter you learn how to quantify and qualify data as part of documentation. For now, begin to label what you experience in a client's tissue with adjectives like crackly, springy, dry, grainy, pliable, soft, yielding, melting, resistant, and other descriptive words. Don't worry if these terms do not seem "official." The important thing is to refine your personal language of tissue so that you can describe what you feel without hesitation. When you label what you feel, you can better recognize differences in tissue and correlate your palpation findings with visual observations.

One way to build your palpation vocabulary is to use comparative pairs of terms, such as plump versus thin, full versus empty, moist versus dry, smooth versus crunchy, painful versus pain free, concentrated versus diffuse, rigid versus fluid, warm or hot versus cold, taut versus loose, and so on. Go back to the exercise where you palpated many different deltoid muscles. This time describe what you feel in the tissue aloud as you palpate. Ask a second student to palpate and describe aloud what he or she feels. In the early stages, you can learn a lot by listening to how others describe what you have just felt.

Persistence Skills

Therapists with excellent palpation skills likely began as students with poor palpation skills and worked hard until their palpation skills improved. All therapists had to go through a blind period when the body felt like a dense, blank landscape of subtle textures and obscure prominences and depressions. Some students feel frustration while palpating and fail to persist when palpation exercises become challenging. Give yourself permission to feel frustrated, but make a commitment at the same time to keep trying. If you can't feel a particular structure on one client, try to find it on a different client, as variations in their tissue textures might help you identify what you're looking for.

Concept Brief 12-2
Palpation Skills

Cognitive: Your knowledge about the structures of the body that inform your touch

Kinesthetic: Your ability to place your attention in your hands and feel nuances in the client's tissue texture, temperature, tone, and hydration

Communication: Your ability to name and describe what you feel

Persistence: Your ability to keep trying when palpation tasks are challenging

Your knowledge of the body's structure and function, the power to place your attention in your hands and differentiate sensations, and the capacity to describe what you feel in words and to persist when palpation gets challenging enhance your palpation skills. These skills include the ability to:

- Locate a specific structure through touch (e.g., Can you find the teres minor? Can you find the infraspinatus? How do you know you are on the teres minor or on the infraspinatus?)
- Distinguish among different types of tissue through touch (e.g., Can you tell if you are feeling a muscle versus a tendon or ligament? How do you know it's a ligament?)

- Differentiate layers of tissue through touch (e.g., Can you feel the difference between the superficial fascia and the muscle that lies below it? Can you push through the gluteus maximus to identify the piriformis? How do you know you're on the piriformis?)
- Assess the quality or condition of soft-tissue structures through touch (e.g., Can you determine if a muscle is hypertonic, hypotonic, or healthy? Can you tell if a muscle has been under stress for a long period of time or suffered past injury? How do you know?)
- Make comparisons between tissue bilaterally, or session to session, through touch (e.g., Can you feel and describe the difference between the scalenes on the right side to the scalenes on the left side? Can you compare and contrast the feeling of the client's muscle tissue in this session to the same client's muscle tissue in a previous session?)
- Make a distinction between normal and abnormal body rhythms through touch (e.g., Can you determine if the client has a normal or abnormal breathing pattern with your hands? Can you tell if the client's heart rate is elevated?)
- Adapt techniques based on what you feel in the tissue (e.g., Can you move through the tissue lightening and deepening your stroke so that the tissue is engaged but the client feels no discomfort?)
- Describe and document what you feel in the tissue (e.g., Can you feel a muscle and describe what you feel, such as "the muscle feels ropey, crackly, and adhered"? Can you translate your palpation language into proper documentation language [described later in this chapter]?)

The development of these skills takes place over the course of your massage training program and beyond into professional practice.

Palpation Exploration

Structure your palpation practices carefully to develop good skills and make efficient use of time. The more systematic you are now in assessing the client's tissue and gathering data, the easier it will be for you to shift into assessment for healthcare massage in upcoming chapters. A systematic approach to palpation also ensures that you will be more thorough and not overlook important findings. Box 12-2 provides a structure for exploring the layers and rhythms of the body.

Layers and Structures That Are Palpable

When palpating a client's tissue, therapists often work from the superficial layers of tissue into the deeper layers of tissue. This is done for two reasons. First, the sensitivity of light-touch receptors in the hands is diminished for a brief period of time after the hands have been used to apply deeper pressure. You may be more responsive and aware of variations in superficial tissue if you access it first. Second, the client may feel discomfort if you immediately drop into deeper tissue

BOX 12-2 Palpation Exploration

1. Identify one region to palpate and review the anatomical structures present in that region in an anatomy textbook. Make a list of specific structures to identify.

2. Look at the surface area of the region you intend to palpate and visualize the structures of the body laying under the skin in that region. Hold this picture in your mind as you palpate.

3. Ground and center your energy by following your breath and relaxing your body. Place all of your attention in your hands. For now, use the full palmar surface of your hands as you palpate. Later you will use different tools such as your fingertips, knuckles, forearm, and elbow depending on your needs or the particular area where you are working.

4. Explore the superficial tissue first and orient yourself to the landscape of the region by finding specific bony landmarks. These landmarks become your guideposts as you drop deeper into the tissue. Don't force tissue that is resistant by pushing your way into unyielding muscle. Wait for the tissue to relax and only palpate as deep as is comfortable for the client.

5. Palpate "normal" tissue first. If the client complains of tension and pain on the right side, palpate the left, unaffected side first. This gives you a general idea of what "normal" for the client feels like and allows you to more easily distinguish what you experience in the tissue. Even when the client does not report dysfunction, always palpate structures on both sides of the body and draw comparisons.

6. Palpate muscle tissue in at least two different directions. First palpate along the muscle fibers with your hands running the same direction as the fibers. This helps you identify the size and shape of the muscle.

7. Next, palpate across the fibers to identify areas where the tissue becomes stuck, taut, or adhered.

8. Feel the temperature of the tissue and pay attention to regions where coolness or heat is particularly noticeable. Feel the texture of the tissue and describe it out loud. Is it taut, relaxed, smooth, crumbly, crunchy, dry, plump, flaccid, full, alive, empty, or so on?

9. Ask the client to pay attention as you work over the tissue and alert you to areas that feel tender or painful. Notice if you start to identify a recurring texture in tissue with tenderness. One student described the feeling of tender points as "areas where my fingers sink into a hole in the tissue."

and so may brace or guard, decreasing your ability to experience the tissue in its normal state. The layers that can be palpated include just above the body, the skin, the superficial fascia, skeletal muscle layers, and bones. Tendons, ligaments, joint movement quality, lymph nodes, organs in the abdominal cavity, blood vessels, and body rhythms can all be palpated.

Palpation above the Body

When the hands are held just above the body, you can palpate differences in temperature (Fig. 12-3). Some therapists believe they can perceive a delicate resistance that hovers over the client, as if the hands meet a transparent barrier, or that the client's body seems to pull the therapist's hands downward as if the hands and body are magnetized. A region directly over a particular body area can feel like dense air, or empty, thin air. In some Eastern and energetic bodywork traditions, these variations in temperature and sensation are believed to indicate a general overactivity or underactivity in the body area or in the subtle energy fields of the body. Interestingly, some therapists believe that they can associate conditions of hyperactivity, inflammation, trigger points, pathologies, and soft-tissue injury sites with corresponding areas above the body that feel overactive. Cool areas that feel empty or fragile may correspond to conditions of underactivity, including decreased circulation or nerve innervation,

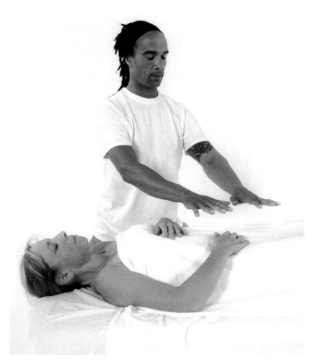

Figure 12-3 When you hold your hands just above the body, you can palpate differences in temperature.

stagnant lymphatic conditions, or flaccid muscle tissue. These types of palpation findings are controversial because they are subjective in nature, and other therapists do not believe that anything besides temperature can be palpated above the body. You are advised to explore this issue with practice clients, teachers, and classmates to draw your own conclusions.

Palpation of the Skin's Surface

When palpating the skin's surface, you might notice if the skin feels dry and crackly (dehydrated) or moist and plump (hydrated) (Fig. 12-4). Bumps, roughness, decreased elasticity, and superficial lines are hints about the client's overall health and vitality. These variations can also signify the client's degree of hydration and provide some indication of what you are likely to find in deeper tissue. Skin color and skin temperature are also noted as the palms make contact with different areas. The client might report that a particular area feels numb or deadened as you pass your hands across the skin's surface. This can be an indication of poor circulation and hypertonic muscles causing decreased nerve activity. Areas where the skin is hot and red suggest inflammation and need further investigation to rule out contraindications. Also notice if bruising or scar tissue is present.

Palpation of the Superficial Fascia

As you probably remember, the superficial fascia connects the skin to the underlying muscle tissue (Fig. 12-5). Palpation of the superficial fascia includes the skin because these two connected structures are lifted away from the fascial sheath

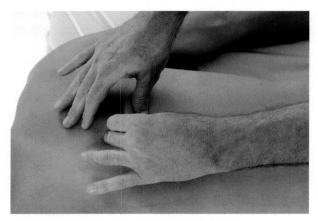

Figure 12-5 Palpation of the superficial fascia will also include the skin as these two connected structures are lifted away from the fascial sheath surrounding the muscle below during techniques like skin rolling.

surrounding the muscle below during techniques like skin rolling. Blood and lymph tissue is palpable in this layer, and you may feel a pulse or small pea-shaped nodules, especially in areas where lymph nodes are concentrated.

The superficial fascia should glide and lift away from the muscular layer easily and evenly. Differences in the amount of lift of the tissue or places where the tissue is "glued down" can be noticed. The fingertips can compress the superficial fascia and glide it over the underlying structures in every direction. If the tissue glides more easily in one direction than another, note this difference. Patterns of tension may start to emerge as you continue to work with the tissue. For example, you might find that the superficial fascia moves easily in a horizontal plane but is restricted when it is moved longitudinally.

Palpation of Skeletal Muscles

Directly under the superficial fascia you encounter the first layer of skeletal muscle. Muscles are layered, and deeper muscles are palpated by dropping through the first layers and in some cases down to the bone (Fig. 12-6). For example, when palpating the skeletal muscle of the upper back, the first muscle you encounter is the trapezius. As you drop through the trapezius you can feel the rhomboids. If you keep going, you may be able to distinguish the erector spinae group. Obviously, pressure must be slow and allow the tissue to melt and relax before dropping to the next layer; otherwise, the client will experience discomfort and tense the muscles to guard the area. One muscle layer should glide easily and freely over the muscle below it. If one muscle sticks to another, note this as an area of adhered tissue.

Muscle areas are easy to differentiate by the way they feel. The belly of the muscle is likely to feel plump and fleshy, and in many cases, the fingers can grasp around the whole muscle belly and lift it (e.g., sternocleidomastoid, triceps). As the muscle transitions into the tendon at the muscle's

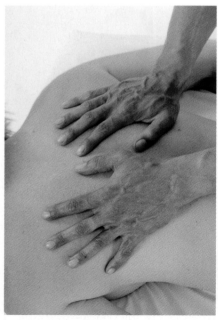

Figure 12-4 When palpating the skin's surface you might notice if the skin feels dry and crackly (dehydrated) or moist and plump (hydrated). Bumps, roughness, decreased elasticity, and superficial lines are hints at the client's overall health and vitality.

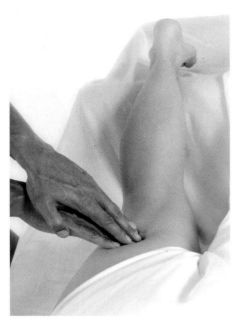

Figure 12-6 Muscles are layered, and so deeper skeletal muscles are palpated by dropping through the first layers, and in some cases down to the bone.

attachment sites, the tissue becomes noticeably smoother and denser. The edges of muscles can be felt, especially where one muscle crosses over another. It is not difficult to feel the edges of muscles in the neck and upper back because changes in fiber direction help differentiate between the trapezius, splenius capitis, splenius cervicis, and levator scapulae.

Notice all the different textures of muscle tissue. Healthy muscle feels plump, springy, full, and pliable, while hypertonic muscle feels dense, hard, uneven, bound, and unyielding. Hypotonic muscle may feel flaccid, limp, and cool. It may feel empty and unresponsive. An area under constant stress or the site of a past soft-tissue injury might feel taut, ropey, stringy, and cord-like. Bands of tissue might form tough, sinewy strands that can literally be plucked like guitar strings. Sometimes metabolic wastes build up in the tissue because of poor circulation, causing the muscle to feel grainy, crunchy, and crumbly. Tender nodules within tight bands of muscle tissue called trigger points may cause pain that refers beyond the palpation site.

Palpation of Tendons and Ligaments

Tendons and ligaments feel denser than muscle tissue because they are made up of higher concentrations of collagen fibers. Muscle fibers run together in a particular direction. This can be felt as a series of small parallel groves; tendons feel smoother. Some tendons are easy to palpate and can help you get a feel for the differences between tendon and muscle. The gastrocnemius attaches to the calcaneus via the calcaneal

tendon (also called the Achilles tendon). The transition from muscle to tendon occurs approximately halfway down the posterior leg. Palpate this region and see if you can feel the changeover from muscle fibers to tendon fibers. Changing the position of the leg by lifting the foot and bending the knee may help you feel these structures, especially when the client plantar flexes and dorsiflexes the foot.

Ligaments have a more uneven fiber configuration than tendons and are always taut, regardless of the position of the joint. A tendon is connected to muscle and so is either taut or relaxed depending on whether it is shortened or lengthened.

Palpation of Bones

Bones feel solid and hard. They have irregular shapes with knobs, grooves, holes, spines, depressions, and angles. Boney prominences help therapists find their way around the body and so are called **bony landmarks**. For example, you can identify the spine of the scapula as the oblique ridge located just below the top of the shoulder on the posterior body. When palpating the spine of the scapula, you know the muscle just above the spine is the supraspinatus, while the muscle just below the spine is the infraspinatus. This bony landmark is key for locating these two muscles of the rotator cuff. Bones also help the therapist determine if the two sides of the body are symmetrical in some assessments. For example, in a posture assessment, you palpate the position of the anterior superior iliac spine (ASIS) for the anterior assessment and the posterior superior iliac spine (PSIS) for the posterior assessment. If the ASIS or PSIS on one side is elevated, this may indicate a tilt in the pelvis.

Palpation of Joints

Joints are most often palpated during range-of-motion techniques where the joint is moved actively or passively. This assessment allows the therapist to feel the quality of the movement. Is it smooth, free, fluid, and full, or is it irregular, restricted, stiff, and shortened? Resisted joint movements assess the muscles around the joint for weakness or uneven firing patterns. Different structures including muscles, tendons, ligaments, and the bones and cartilage that make up the joint itself can become unbalanced or inflamed and cause painful movement, restricted movement, or too much movement (hypermobility). Small fluid-filled sacs called bursae reduce friction between joint structures and can sometimes be felt as balloon-like gelcaps, but usually they are difficult to palpate. You will learn specific techniques for joint palpation during range of motion in Chapter 19.

Palpation of Abdominal Viscera

The liver and large intestine can be palpated in the abdominal cavity by therapists who know the location of organs and approach these structures cautiously. Palpate through the abdominal muscles and intestines to access the psoas muscle, which is an important muscle to massage when clients report low back pain. You will learn how to access and massage this muscle in later chapters (Fig. 12-7).

Palpation of Body Rhythms

Chapter 4 discussed the concept of *entrainment*. To review, entrainment is defined in physics as the process whereby two oscillating systems, which have different rhythms when they function independently, assume the same rhythm. In the body, entrainment can be thought of as the harmonizing and synchronization of different rhythms so that the body finds equilibrium. Biological rhythms such as heart rate, respiratory rate, waking and sleeping cycles, digestive cycles, the urinary excretion of potassium, the menstrual cycle, body temperature changes, and the secretion of some hormones have a natural tempo. When the body is in balance, these tempos become entrained. You will notice that you can feel when the body's rhythms are in harmony. Some of these rhythms are easy to palpate such as the even rise and fall of the abdominal area and chest as the client breathes. The heart rate is detectable at the client's pulse points. Therapists trained in craniosacral therapy learn to palpate the expansion and retraction of the cranial bones and sacrum known as the craniosacral rhythm.

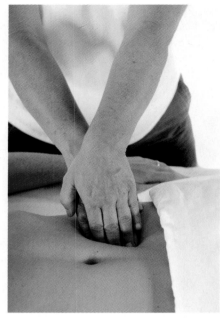

Figure 12-7 Palpating through the abdominal muscles and intestines accesses the psoas muscle, which is an important muscle to massage when clients describe low back pain conditions.

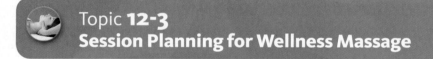

Topic **12-3**
Session Planning for Wellness Massage

Session planning is the process of planning a wellness session and/or using the information gathered during an assessment to set session goals and choose appropriate techniques in collaboration with the client. The purposes of session planning are to ensure client safety, establish realistic client expectations, and guarantee an effective session that meets the client's needs. Although sessions are often considered as either wellness massage or healthcare massage, massage sessions actually occur on a continuum, and the lines between wellness sessions and healthcare sessions are often blurred.

In a strict definition of wellness massage, the client is healthy and seeks massage purely for maintenance or stress management, is on vacation and receiving massage as an enjoyable experience, is specifically seeking relaxation massage, or does not intend to use massage as a regular part of condition management. The client might have a diagnosed condition but still seek out massage purely for relaxation. The condition is considered in session planning only so far as comfort and safety are concerned. Reducing symptoms related to the condition is not part of the session goals. Even if the client receives massage regularly, these sessions are focused on general relaxation and enjoyment and not to cause changes in the condition or symptoms caused by the condition.

Wellness sessions are often standardized, especially when they are delivered in locations like spas or cruise ships. In a **standardized wellness session**, the therapist might be taught a fixed routine that includes enhancers like a foot soak and the application of steamy scented towels at particular points in the session. The same routine is applied to different clients in the same way and adaptations are only made for safety reasons.

Strictly defined, healthcare massage is provided on a regular basis with the intent to cause therapeutic change or as a means to help manage a condition. In-depth assessment and session planning techniques are used to determine treatment goals to improve the client's ability to participate in activities of daily life. If a physician has prescribed the massage, if the therapist is working with a healthcare team to treat the client for a particular pathology, if the treatment takes place in a hospital or hospice setting, if insurance reimbursement is expected, or if the client has a defined medical condition for which he or she is using massage for condition management, the session fits the criteria of a healthcare massage. In this case, the therapist should use a full range of assessment tools before planning the session, as discussed in Chapter 19.

The lines between wellness and healthcare sessions are often blurred because most clients don't know the difference between these two types of massage and they simply want their needs met in an effective manner. Clients visiting a spa on vacation or taking a cruise vacation are more likely to accept and enjoy a standardized wellness session. Clients who wake up with a stiff neck, experience sore muscles from playing basketball over the weekend, have low back pain from cleaning house, or for any other reason feel soreness in their muscles, pain, or high levels of stress are less likely to accept and enjoy a standardized wellness session because they need focused work in particular areas.

One idea to help clients understand their options and to help therapists determine how to manage the session is to describe three categories of sessions. The first two categories (wellness and health care) are defined above. The third category can be called a **customized wellness session** and be placed on the continuum between wellness and healthcare massages. A customized wellness massage can be defined as a massage delivered without an expectation for follow-up sessions but planned to meet the client's healthcare needs within the scope of practice of massage and within the time constraints of one session. The session is not standardized, but enhancing options like a foot soak, aromatherapy, and warm packs can still be used to increase the client's enjoyment. These enhancing options are described in depth in Chapter 15.

This chapter topic explores session planning for a customized wellness massage. The development of standardized wellness sessions is discussed in Chapter 15, while healthcare massage is discussed in depth in Chapter 19 and other chapters related to injury rehabilitation, pathologies, or special populations. In all sessions, the health intake form and health intake interview are used to rule out contraindications and plan necessary adaptations to the session. If you are uncertain how to rule out contraindications, review Chapter 5 before proceeding. Ruling out contraindications is always the first step in planning any type of session.

Planning a Customized Wellness Session

After ruling out contraindications, session planning focuses on using data gathered before, during, and after the session to meet the client's unique wellness goals.

Using Data Gathered before the Session for a Customized Wellness Massage

During the health intake interview, you make general observations about the client's freedom of movement, symmetry, breathing patterns, stress level, and body language. These observations often bring to light a client's massage needs. If you notice a client turning the head cautiously, you know to ask about any neck pain. If the client explains that he or she slept strangely and woke up with a stiff neck, you will focus a good deal of massage time in this area. Perhaps you notice that the client is taking shallow, rapid breaths and you suggest that the session starts with a deep breathing exercise. If the client agrees, you plan to start the session in the supine position so that you can walk the client through the diaphragmatic breathing exercise described in Chapter 10. A client demonstrating high levels of sympathetic dominance is likely to benefit from slow, calming strokes during the opening sections of the massage, while a client with an open body position in good physical health may be ready for strokes that are firm right from the start.

The information the client tells you before the session is very important. You want to understand clients' expectations for sessions, what they hope to feel like at the end of the sessions, and the body areas where they want massage. Clients with a lot of experience receiving massage may have clear expectations and give you specific directions. They might say something like, "I want you to massage my back, the back of my legs, my shoulders, and my neck. I want deep work and I don't like it when I am told to take a breath or when people start moving my arms around." Clearly range-of-motion techniques and breathwork are out! Respect the client's wishes and massage the areas requested. Alternately, the client may have no experience with massage and need guidance. It can be helpful to ask, "What do you know about massage and what do you think massage will be like." This can clue you into clients' expectations, even when they say they have none. The client may say, "I think it will be really soothing, soft and relaxing. I think I'll fall asleep and feel really balanced at the end of the session." You now know that the client will likely respond best to long, soft strokes that allow deep relaxation. You will likely avoid tapotement and deep friction, which might jolt the client out of feeling peaceful.

Clients usually want something specific from the session. Their goals may be realistic or unrealistic. A client who worked all day in the garden and tells you, "I'm sore in every single muscle of my body and I don't want any soreness at the end of the session!" has unrealistic expectations. Explain that you expect that the soreness will be reduced by massage but that there will likely still be some soreness after the session. Ask clients to be as specific as possible about what they want. If they want to relax completely, you are likely to use different techniques than if they want to leave feeling energized.

As noted earlier, it is important to identify the body regions the client wants massaged (or does not want massaged). If a client says I want a full body massage but mentions that the neck and shoulders need lots of work, plan to get to the neck and shoulders early in the massage and make sure to work the area well. Check in with the client before moving on. You could say something like, "Do you feel that your neck and shoulders have received enough work? If they still feel tense, we can continue to spend additional time in this area." The client will say, "Yes, they feel great" and you can move on, or will say, "No, they still feel tense, can you work on them some more?"

New therapists sometimes fall into a routine, get relaxed, and then panic when a client wants the entire session dedicated to one area. Build a variety of skills for each body area and be prepared. Clients sometimes want the entire hour dedicated to certain areas like the feet, face, legs, neck, or back. They sometimes make requests that seem strange to the therapist, but as long as the request is legal, does not require techniques outside the massage scope of practice, and will not put the client at risk, honor the client's request. For example, one client visited a massage clinic twice a week and requested a full body massage performed with only nerve strokes. She enjoyed the sensation of the very light stroking technique and felt that it relaxed her completely. Another client asked for deep, intense work on her feet for the entire hour. This client believed in reflexology and felt that the deep prolonged work on her feet benefited her entire body.

When you feel you understand the client's expectations and know the areas the client wants massaged or does not want massaged, summarize the plan for the session by saying something like, "Okay, I understand. You want me to massage the back of your legs and then spend extra time on your back. I'll turn you over and massage your feet, the front of your legs, and your arms. You want your neck massaged, but you don't want me to touch your face or scalp. Does that sound like a good plan or am I missing something?" Once you and the client agree on a plan, the session can begin.

Using Data Gathered during the Customized Wellness Session for Planning

As the massage progresses, it is likely that the plan you established with the client will evolve or adapt. This might happen because the client's wishes change or because of something you palpate in the tissue. For example, the client may say, "I'm really enjoying this foot massage, would you spend longer on my feet than we originally discussed?" or the therapist might say, "Your shoulders are more tense than I anticipated, could I spend additional time on this area and cut some of the time from your foot massage?"

A client may insist he or she wants deep work, but you may feel that the tissue is resistant and that the client is guarding by tensing the muscles as the stroke begins. You have to find a balance between honoring the client's request and honoring what you feel through palpation. Usually clients are reasonable and responsive if you explain what you are feeling. You might say something like, "Jim, I know you asked for deep work, but as I drop into your tissue it feels like a hard wall and I can see you tense up as if it is painful. I'd like to work more softly for a bit and see if this helps you relax your muscles so that I can work deeper as the session progresses." Hopefully Jim will agree. But he might be insistent and say, "No, I like the deep work, please don't lighten the pressure, in fact, I want you to work deeper." Now you have to decide if you are endangering the client by adhering to his wishes. If you think you might bruise the client, or in any way damage his tissue, you should clarify your boundary and even end the session

if necessary. You might say something like, "Jim, I feel I may bruise you, damage your tissue, or leave you feeling very sore and uncomfortable tomorrow. For these reasons I don't feel I can continue to work on you this deeply. I would like to lighten the pressure so that I am only working as deeply as the tissue allows without you needing to protect yourself by tensing your muscles. If you prefer, we can end the session now and I will only charge you for the first 30 minutes of the massage, because I want to respect your right to have the massage you want, but I also need to respect what I am feeling in your tissue." If, on the other hand, you determine that the client is not in any danger, you can proceed even if he continues to guard by tensing his muscles.

A dilemma might also arise if a client wants prolonged work in one area. In the case of the client earlier who wanted nerve strokes, it is easy to meet the client's needs without concern. But if you are providing deep work on one area of the body for an extended period of time, you may begin to feel that the tissue is "overworked." The tissue may be very red and even hot, and you might become concerned that the client will be sore from the massage later. The best advice is to share your concerns with the client: "Olga, I know we agreed to spend the entire hour on your neck, but your tissue feels as if it has had enough. It's very pliable now but I worry that this much work will cause it to feel stiff and sore tomorrow. What do you think? Would you like me to continue to work on your neck, or perhaps I can massage your feet or arms to finish out the hour?" Unless you feel that you are endangering Olga, it's her call, and if she wants you to continue with her neck, continue.

It is helpful to discuss issue like this with your massage instructor and get his or her recommendations. It can be challenging to balance the right of clients to determine what happens to their body and your duty to "do no harm" as discussed in Chapter 5.

Using Data Gathered after the Customized Wellness Session for Planning

At the end of the session, after the client has dressed, conduct a brief postsession interview. Ask how the client feels as a result of the massage, and note any changes that have occurred such as better breathing or more relaxed body language. Point out your observations to your client. You can say, "When you arrived for your session your arms were clasped across your chest, and you looked pale and tired. Now, your shoulders are relaxed and your color has come back into your cheeks. You look rested and balanced." By alerting clients to these visual changes you help them identify some of the subtler positive effects of massage, and this encourages them to get more massages.

Sometimes when the session ends you find you did not achieve all of the client's goals. The client's can now turn the head without pain but still feels tension in the shoulders, or you massaged the back for an extended period of time and the rhomboids still feel very tense. Acknowledge that progress has been made, and add that more sessions are needed to make lasting change. If the client wants to schedule another appointment, use the information gained from this session to help you plan the next. For example, you might say, "Juan, we made good progress on your back. Let's start with your back during the next session but also include some work on your shoulders and neck to increase your freedom of movement." Clients appreciate therapists who support their goals and think ahead to how those goals might be achieved. Any plans for future sessions should be noted in your documentation of the session, as discussed later in this chapter.

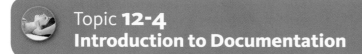

Topic **12-4**
Introduction to Documentation

Documentation (sometimes called charting) is the process of keeping consistent and complete client records and filling out certain forms at the beginning and end of each session. This topic explains the purpose of documentation, gives guidelines for recording sessions, introduces quantifying and qualifying data, introduces SOAP charting, and shows simple methods for documenting a wellness session. While this chapter has dealt mostly with wellness sessions, the information here provides a foundation for all types of documentation including healthcare sessions.

Purposes of Documentation

Professional massage therapists use consistent charting practices to promote client safety, establish the therapeutic relationship, organize assessment data, keep accurate historical records, demonstrate progress, and communicate with a healthcare team, as well as for liability reasons.

Safety

Documentation forms are used not only to rule out contraindications but also to provide a record of the client's reaction to different techniques. If a therapist looks over the client's chart notes and finds an adverse reaction to deep tissue techniques, these techniques would be avoided in the next session. It is impossible to remember all the particulars of a client's condition without documentation. Good chart notes ensure that nothing is left to memory and that you have any important information needed for providing safe, appropriate care to the client.

Establish the Therapeutic Relationship

Chapter 7 described how clients (or therapists) may experience transference or cross professional boundaries. Documentation establishes the boundaries of the therapeutic relationship and keeps the session client focused and treatment goal focused. Because physicians and other healthcare personal routinely document a client's care, documentation also helps to elevate massage and project a professional image.

Organize Assessment Data

Many therapists gather assessment data and write it directly onto the client's chart in a systematic manner. They use the chart to keep the data organized during planning for the session. It also shortens documentation time after the session.

Historical Record

Therapists often see many clients during a busy week or month. Clients tend to assume the therapist will remember everything that happened during their last five sessions. Careful documentation of sessions gives you a historical record of the client's visits, preferences, treatment goals, and outcomes. If the client sees multiple therapists at a clinic, good documentation keeps everyone on the team informed about the client's progress. In some situations, documentation provides evidence of client misconduct and can lead to the expulsion of the client from the clinic. For example, one therapist noted that a client exposed himself and received a warning and reminder about the draping policy. The next session, this client exposed himself with a different therapist and received a warning. Each time the client responded to the therapist's warning and was allowed to continue the session. Documentation showed that the client had a pattern of exposure with new therapists. This information could be used to confront the client and disrupt the unhealthy pattern or to refuse the client future service.

Demonstration of Progress

In as little as one session, clients are likely to see positive results from massage, but sometimes clients with persistent soft-tissue conditions don't recognize the progress they are making. For example, a client with fibromyalgia might feel muscle tenderness and soreness every day. The client may become very frustrated with this constant experience of pain and blame the massage therapist for poor treatment. The therapist reviews the records with the client so that the client can see that he or she is actually making progress. The pain scores have decreased since the initial session, and the client can also see that some functional goals have been achieved.

Before the first session the client could not vacuum the floor without a flare-up, but now the client can vacuum, dust, and clean the bathrooms without the condition getting worse. Sometimes the therapist must be able to demonstrate that massage is effective so that the client's health insurance will continue to reimburse for massage treatment. Through a review of session records you might also be able to discern what treatment techniques your client most often responds to positively.

Communication with a Healthcare Team

If you are working as part of a healthcare team in the treatment of a particular client, good chart notes are essential to the team process of planning future treatment for the client. High-quality documentation is an expectation for every therapist working on a healthcare team.

Liability

Chapter 5 describes the types of insurance claims that have been made against massage therapists. Documentation can prevent a client from getting hurt by alerting you to preexisting conditions that contraindicate some types of techniques. It can also establish a history of high-quality care in the event that a client claims negligence, or bring to light a medication or condition that may be the actual cause of the client's symptoms. Insurance companies usually require therapists to document sessions to be eligible for coverage.

Concept Brief 12-3
Overview of Documentation

- **Purposes:** Client safety, establishment of the therapeutic relationship, historical record, demonstration of progress, communication with a healthcare team, and liability
- **SOAP Chart:** The standard format used by healthcare professionals to document health-related sessions. Broken into different sections to ensure that subjective, objective, assessment, and planning information is captured
- **Wellness Chart:** A simple form used to document wellness sessions when the client is healthy, the massage session is not intended to address a specific condition, sessions are standardized, or sessions are provided purely for relaxation and enjoyment
- **Condensed SOAP Chart:** A form based on the SOAP method but in an abbreviated format. Used for wellness charting or for the documentation of subsequent healthcare sessions
- **Abbreviations:** Used in healthcare documentation because they take up less space on the page and are faster to write

General Guidelines for Documenting Sessions

When documenting any type of session, these basic guidelines are important:
- Write clearly and fill in all areas of the form with information. If an area is not applicable for some reason (unlikely), write NA in the space. This ensures that the document could not easily have been altered in the event it becomes part of a legal proceeding.
- Never use "White-Out" or other correction fluids, correction tape, or erasers to remove documentation mistakes. Cross out the mistake with a single line and initial and date the error.
- Use common medical terms and standard medical or massage abbreviations (described later in this chapter). Describe what you feel in soft tissues using standard terms such as "mild plus hypertonicity" rather than "tissue feels crunchy and bound up."
- State information factually and avoid personal opinions. For example, it would be inappropriate to write, "The tissue is dehydrated because the client is a smoker and doesn't drink enough water" or "The client is not improving because the client fails to participate in self-care activities and continues to eat an unhealthy diet and lie around on the couch."
- Never record personal information about the client that is not relevant to the client's condition. It is enough to note that the client's stress levels are moderate plus because of personal issues without describing the particulars of a divorce, even if the client shares them with you. A client may attribute tense shoulder muscles to the stress caused by conflicts with a supervisor, but on the chart it is adequate to state that shoulder tension is caused by increased work stress. Clients may tell you the stories that they feel are behind many of their symptoms, and it is up to you to distill this down to the simplest terms on the chart. If your records are subpoenaed for a legal proceeding, your clients will appreciate your tact and confidentially.
- Measure every finding and every symptom described by the client with a consistent scale to quantify the data, as described in the next section. Measure findings both before and after treatment. This is the only way that progress can be calculated and documented.

Abbreviations and Symbols

Abbreviations are used in written communication such as SOAP charting and by healthcare providers or the public during verbal communication. For example, people regularly say AIDS and MS rather than acquired immune deficiency syndrome or multiple sclerosis. Abbreviations for words or phrases take up less space on the page and allow the therapist to write more quickly. Most common medical abbreviations can be found in a medical dictionary, but some abbreviations specific to massage may not be included. Therapists may also develop their own abbreviations for common massage terms when standard abbreviations do not already exist. This is fine, so long as a key is provided in case another person must read the chart notes. Symbols are often used on human figures to provide a pictorial representation of what is occurring in the client's body. At the bottom of different types of massage charts a legend is used to provide a key to common symbols used on the human figures. Table 12-1 provides a sample of some common abbreviations and symbols used in massage. You are encouraged to use abbreviations and symbols while you take notes in your classes to build and integrate this important skill.

Quantifying Data

The symptoms a client reports (subjective information) and the signs a therapist observes or palpates (objective information) should always be quantified so that progress or a lack of progress can be recognized and changes made in session planning for customized wellness sessions or healthcare sessions.

The term "quantify" describes *how much* of a sign is present or *how much* of the symptom the client describes. If you observe that one shoulder is elevated higher than the other, you can quantify the elevation by describing it as mild, moderate, or severe in your documentation. By quantifying a sign or symptom in documentation, the therapist can determine if massage is effective and created meaningful changes in the body. For example, you might document that the shoulder elevation is moderate in the first session. At the end of the second session, your documentation states that the shoulder elevation is mild. At the end of the third session, the shoulder elevation might completely disappear. When you look over session chart notes you can verify that the techniques you used are working because the shoulder elevation continued to decrease each session.

TABLE 12-1   Sample Abbreviations Used to Document Massage Sessions

Abdominals	abs	**Massage therapist**	MT
Adhesions	Adh, X	**Medications**	meds
Anterior	ant	**Mild, low**	L
Before	pre	**Moderate**	M
Bilateral	BL	**Myofascial release**	MFR
Change	Δ	**No change**	Δ̸
Constant	const	**Not applicable**	NA
Contraindication	CI	**Numbness or tingling**	≫
Date of injury	DOI	**Pain**	Ⓟ
Decrease, down	↓	**Palpation**	Palp
Deep tissue	DT	**Posterior**	Post
Elevation	Elev, /	**Prescription**	Rx
Energy work	EW	**Reflexology**	reflex
Full body	FB	**Right**	Ⓡ
Gluteal muscles	glutes	**Rotation**	rot, ⬭
Hamstrings	hams	**Severe**	S
Headache	HA	**Short**	⟩⟨
History	Hx	**Spasm**	SP, ≈
Hypertonicity	HT, ≡	**Symptoms**	Sx
Increase	↑	**Tender point**	TeP, •
Inflammation	Infl, ✳	**Treatment**	TX
Left	Ⓛ	**Trigger point**	TP, ⓒ
Long	⟵⟶	**With**	w/
Low back	LB	**Within normal limits**	WNL
Manual lymphatic drainage	MLD	**Without**	w/o
Massage	Ⓜ		

It is important to use consistent terminology when referring to signs or when documenting client symptoms. If a therapist described the shoulder elevation as "kind of high" or "a bit more than regular," it would be difficult to get a clear picture of the elevation. If a therapist documented the client's description of pain as "kind of hurts" or "hurts a lot," it is difficult to demonstrate change. Usually the terms *within normal limits, mild, moderate,* and *severe* are used in healthcare documentation so that all healthcare professionals understand each other. Often these terms are further clarified by a plus (+) sign or minus (−) sign that indicate degrees of mild, moderate, and severe. Normal, mild, moderate, and severe are based on a scale of 0 to 10.

- **Normal (WNL = Within Normal Limits):** Normal represents 0 on a scale or 0 to 10. "Normal" is a subjective term, and everyone's normal is likely to be somewhat different. You can determine the best approximation of normal by comparing the body bilaterally when possible. For example, if one shoulder joint is functional and the other is limited, the functional side is considered normal. The dysfunctional side is compared to the functional side to determine how limited it is (mildly limited, moderately limited, or severely limited). Sometimes the client defines normal for the therapist by describing what the client could do before an injury occurred or a particular tension pattern developed. Symmetry or a lack of symmetry also helps you define normal. The more symmetrical the sides of the body appear, and the more alike their function, the more normal it is. The greater disparity in symmetry, the more abnormal one side is.

- **Mild Minus (L−):** Mild minus represents 1 on the 0 to 10 scale and indicates that the sign (or symptom) is barely detectable and does not limit the client's function in any way. In fact, the client may not be aware of any issue at all. For example, you might notice a pelvic tilt but the client is unaware of the tilt.

- **Mild (L):** Mild represents 2 on the 0 to 10 scale and indicates that the sign is detectable, or that a symptom is experienced, but function is not restricted.

- **Mild Plus (L+):** Mild plus represents 3 on the 0 to 10 scale and indicates that the sign is detectable and noticeable by the client. Function may be minimally influenced.

- **Moderate Minus (M−):** Moderate minus represents 4 on the 0 to 10 scale and indicates the sign is clearly detectable and that function is perceptibly influenced.

- **Moderate (M):** Moderate represents 5 on the 0 to 10 scale and indicates that the sign is clearly detectable and that some modification in activity is required because of a functional limitation caused by the sign/symptom.

- **Moderate Plus (M+):** Moderate plus represents 6 on the 0 to 10 scale and indicates that the sign is obvious and causes a significant modification in some activities because of the amount of physical limitation caused by the sign/symptom.

- **Severe Minus (S−):** Severe minus represents 7 on the 0 to 10 scale and indicates that the sign is obvious and prevents the participation in some activities of daily life because some physical functions are substantially limited.

- **Severe (S):** Severe represents 8 on the 0 to 10 scale and indicates that the sign is pronounced and that participation in many daily activities is substantially impacted by critical functional limitations.

- **Severe Plus (S+):** Severe plus represents 9 on the 0 to 10 scale and indicates that the sign/symptom is pronounced and that participation in most daily activities is substantially impacted by serious functional limitations.

- **Disabled:** Disabled represents 10 on the 0 to 10 scale and indicates that the client is bedridden or unable to participate without assistance in any activities of daily life as a result of the functional limitations.

In wellness massage, therapists are usually working with signs and symptoms in the mild-to-moderate range.

Qualifying Data

The term *qualify* means to attribute a particular quality or characteristic to something. Both subjective and objective information is qualified during documentation in order to capture the nature of a symptom or sign. For example, clients may describe their neck pain (symptom) as achy, shooting, sharp, pinching, burning, numbing, or throbbing. These descriptions help you understand the client's experience right now. As sessions progress, you can continue to check with the client about the neck pain and document how it changes. If it starts out as "deep, intense burning and shooting pain" and progresses to a "slight achy tinge," you can surmise that the techniques used in massage sessions are making a positive difference.

Therapists qualify what they observe and palpate. While moving a client's shoulder passively in flexion, for example, you might describe the quality of the joint this way: "The joint feels moderately restricted when approaching the end of the joint's range of motion." This helps you remember what you experienced during a particular assessment and compare it to what you feel in the current session. While watching a client bend and touch the toes, you might qualify your observation by noting: "Forward flexion of the trunk appears stiff, jerky, and moderately limited." Soft tissue might be described as dehydrated, hypertonic, fibrous, inflamed, adhered, or atrophied.

If you press on an area of the client's body and the client reports that the pressure caused pain, this is considered an objective finding. You would now want to document how much pain was caused (quantify) by how much pressure (quantify) and the characteristics of the pain as described by the client (qualify).

Introduction to SOAP Charting

SOAP stands for subjective, objective, assessment, and plan. This refers to the types of information that you record in each section of a SOAP chart. While there are many types of documentation systems, SOAP charting is a standard format used by physicians, physical therapists, chiropractors, nurses, and other professional healthcare providers, and so is a good system to use.[2] SOAP charting ensures that all relevant information is gathered in an efficient and effective manner. It is the ideal when working as part of a larger healthcare team. Other formats are introduced later in the chapter.

In many wellness massage settings, since SOAP charting may be too formal and time-consuming, abbreviated SOAP formats or other types of charting are used, as described later. Students who take the time to learn the SOAP method develop strong charting skills, which also improve their understanding of assessment techniques. These skills are valuable even if you never plan to provide anything other than wellness massage.

Overview of the SOAP Format

Review the completed sample of a SOAP chart in Figure 12-8. After reading each following section, return to this sample to see the example of what you have read. The sample SOAP chart demonstrates information using charting abbreviations.

At the top of the chart is the therapist's contact details including business address and phone number. The next section asks for basic client information:

- Client's name
- Date (of the massage session)
- Date of Injury: This section is included on a SOAP chart specifically for insurance billing purposes in healthcare massage. If the client was in a car accident, injured on the job, injured in a sporting accident, or hurt in any other situation, the date of the injury is entered on the chart. Even if you do not plan to bill an insurance company for the session, this information is useful as it reminds you that an injury occurred and can help to focus the session. If no injury occurred, enter "NA" for not applicable.
- ID No./DOB: ID refers to the client's insurance identification number. This number is used if an insurance provider is paying for the client's massage treatments. Otherwise, enter the client's date of birth (DOB). This helps positively identify the client. While many clients might have the name Joe Smith, it is unlikely that two Joe Smiths have the same birthday.
- Meds: Meds stands for medication. Enter the client's medications from the health history form and verbally review the list with the client. Ask the client if all medications taken are listed. Writing the list into the SOAP chart is a way to verify that you have reviewed the medications with the client. This information helps protect you in case the client has an adverse reaction to massage because of a medication that he or she did not disclose (highly unlikely, but possible). It also reminds you to pay attention to the client's medication list and update it before each session. If the client has not listed any medications on the health history form, ask if he

or she is taking any medications including over-the-counter medications. If the client says "no," write "no meds per client" in the meds space. Again, this is protection from legal liability in case the client has an adverse reaction to massage because of taking an undisclosed medication.

The main section of the SOAP chart is comprised of the S, O, A, P sections:

- *S* stands for subjective data, including all the information collected on the health intake form and information the client tells you before the session during the health intake interview or during the massage. Subjective data includes the client's goals, symptoms, and activities of daily life that aggravate or relieve symptoms.
- *O* stands for objective data, including all your findings such as visual assessment findings, palpation findings, and test results. You also describe the techniques used during the session and where they were applied. Include the client's response to the treatment.
- *A* stands for assessment data, includes the client's functional goals (ability to perform activities of daily living like cleaning house, picking up children, performing work tasks, etc.), functional limitations (limitations to activities of daily life caused by an injury or pathology), and functional outcomes (meeting functional goals or changes in functional ability).
- *P* stands for plan, including your plan for future massage sessions and the homework or self-care recommendations given to the client.
- The human figures along the side of the SOAP chart are used to make a pictorial representation of objective findings. In future sessions, you can review these figures quickly to note changes that have occurred over time. (At the bottom of the chart is a key to common symbols used on the human figures.)
- The final section of the SOAP chart is the therapist's signature and date. Sign your legal name and include your massage credentials (e.g., LMP, CMT, LMT) after your name.

Following are symbols and abbreviations typically used for notations on the human figures on the chart:

- *TP* = trigger point (a point that refers pain—see Chapter 21). If you discover a trigger point while providing massage, you document it on the human figures using this symbol.
- *TeP* = tender point. If you encounter an area that is particularly tender, you document it on the human figures with this symbol.
- *P* with a circle around it = pain. A circle is placed around the entire area of pain reported by the client or discovered through touch.
- *Infl* = inflammation. If an area is inflamed, this symbol is drawn at its location.
- *HT* = hypertonicity or a region of tension. These lines are drawn to note areas of particular tension. Draw in only pronounced hypertonicities, to avoid filling the entire figure with lines in some cases.

SOAP CHART-M

Therapist's Name: _Any Therapist_

Client's Name: _John Doe_   Today's Date: _Feb 12, 2011_

Date of Injury: _NA_   Client Date of Birth/Insurance ID: _6/9/1970_   Meds: _no meds per client_

S Focus/Health Concerns: Prioritize
↓ Sp Lb, ↓HA ℗, ↓ Sh HF △℗

Symptoms: Location/Intensity/Frequency/Duration/Onset
℗, hd, m– , DD a.m, 2 HR w/wake up
H+, Sh, L+, Const, 1 wk W/ ↑ stress at work
mm Sp, T7-12, m+, intern, 1 wk w/ ↑ workload

Activities of Daily Living: Aggravating/Relieving
A: HA ℗ ↑ w/poor sleep   R: Advil in a.m.
A: Sh HT ↑ w/1 hr drive to wk   R: stretching at desk
A: mm sp ↑ L+ – M+ w/4 hr computer wk   R: warm bath

O Findings: Visual/Palpable/Test Results
Vis: Client up on breathing, looks fatigued, stressed
Pal: see figures

Techniques/Modalities: Locations/Duration
60 min sw ⓜ FB w/focus nk, hd, LB, Sh

Response to Treatment (see △)
Client responds "my HA ℗ is gone!"

A Goals: Long-term/Short-term

Functional Outcomes

P Future Treatment/Frequency
SW ⓜ 1X mo for 2 mo then re eval

Homework/Self-care
↑H₂O
use tennis ball to ↓ sh H+

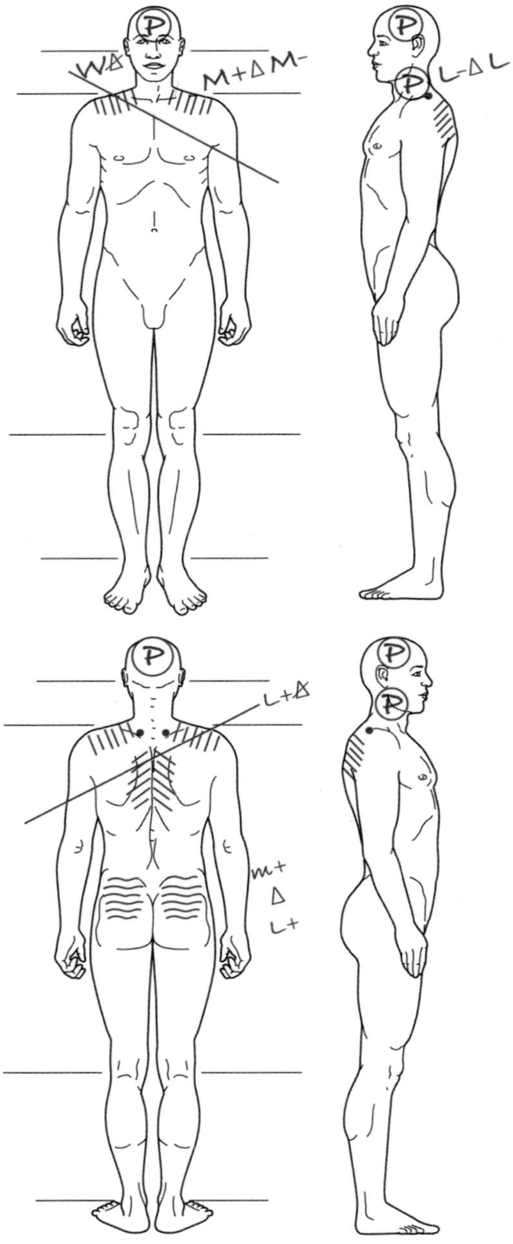

Therapist's Signature _Any Therapist_   Date _2/12/2011_

Legend: ⟳ TP   • Tep   ○ ℗   ✳ Infl   ≡ HT   ≈ SP

✕ Adh   ≫ Numb   ⬭ rot   ╱ elev   ⟩⟨ Short   ⟷ Long

Figure 12-8 Sample SOAP form.

- *SP* = spasm. If a muscle was noted as rigid or spastic or caused splinting to guard an area, this symbol is used to show its location.
- *Adh* = adhesion. Adhesions might be abbreviated with adh or it might be indicated on a figure with an x. Place an x on the figure in any areas where you find pronounced adhesions or stuck tissue.
- *Numb* = numbness or tingling. If the client reports that an area feels numb, tingly, or deadened when you touch it, note that area with this symbol.
- *elev* = elevation. Draw lines to show that one side of the body, like the left shoulder, is elevated above the other.
- *rot* = rotation. This symbol is used to show that a body area like a shoulder or the pelvis is rotated away from normal alignment.
- *Short* = an area shorter than normal. You might use this symbol to note a leg length discrepancy or that muscle spasms are causing an area to draw together and appear shorter than normal.
- *Long* = an area longer than normal. Again this symbol might show a leg length difference or that a muscular group is abnormally lengthened (most likely because the opposing muscles are abnormally shortened).

Some therapists develop their own symbols for noting findings on a chart. This is fine for findings not covered by the standard symbols, as long as the symbol is explained in the legend.

Focus for Today

This section of the form helps you prioritize the client's primary goals for the session and usually relates to the symptoms the client is experiencing. Since you focus the session to meet these goals, you need to understand which is most important to the client. If the client lists headache pain, foot pain, and tenderness in the low back, as which is the client's primary reason for seeking massage today. Sometimes therapists assume they understand a client's goals and work on one area excessively only to learn later that the client would have preferred more time spent in another area.

Because clients have many different reasons for seeking massage, it is best to ask open-ended questions such as these: "How would you like to feel at the conclusion of this session?" "What would you like to focus on today in the session?" "Are there particular areas where you would like me to focus? What are you experiencing in those areas?" "Which area should I work on first?"

In situations when you have a physician's diagnosis and prescription for massage, these external factors will influence the goals for the session. If the physician refers a client to you for healthcare massage related specifically to a rotator cuff injury, for example, it would be inappropriate to massage the client's feet, even if the client reports that the feet are tired and sore. Write the client's goals in simple, precise language in the area provided on the SOAP chart. For example:

- Increase shoulder range of motion
- Decrease low back pain
- Reduce tension in neck muscles
- Increase relaxation
- Decrease stress

The S Section—Subjective Data

As noted earlier, the therapist records subjective data from the client in the S section of a SOAP chart. Most SOAP charts break subjective data into two areas:
- Symptoms
- Activities of Daily Living: Aggravating/Relieving

Symptoms

During the initial health intake interview, get a complete picture of a client's symptoms. Ask clients to identify what they are feeling in their bodies. Many clients want relief from pain, but other conditions such as fatigue, stress, tension, numbness, tingling, joint issues, stiffness, muscle cramping, muscular weakness, losses in range of motion, depression, and anxiety may also be reasons for their visits. Clients might also report symptoms that are out of the massage scope of practice but may be related to stress, such as stomach upset or respiratory issues; while massage can be an effective support strategy, refer the client to a physician for these. Each symptom should then be further clarified in terms of the following characteristics.

LOCATION

Ask clients to point to the exact location of the symptom if possible. If a client just describes leg pain, you won't know if the client means a specific muscle of the thigh, the hip joint, a muscle on the leg, or the knee. With their hands clients can show the entire area of the pain, giving you valuable information about the muscles and other soft-tissue structures involved. Note the location of the symptom in the chart directly after the symptom, using the correct abbreviations.

INTENSITY

Intensity refers to the magnitude of the symptom. Ask the client to rate the symptom according to the scale you explain. Some therapists use a scale of mild, moderate, and severe, adding plus or minus signs when needed. Others use a number scale with 0 representing no symptom and 12 representing the most serious symptom. Be consistent in your use of the scale, asking every client to rate symptoms using the same method. Rate your objective findings using the same scale.

FREQUENCY

Frequency refers to how often the symptom occurs, such as daily upon waking, or flaring up suddenly once or twice a day. It may occur frequently or constantly, or only once a week after a certain activity. List the frequency on the chart directly following the intensity. Terms used for frequency include

- Constant
- Intermittent

- Seldom
- Often
- Daily
- Weekly
- Hourly
- One time a day
- Two times a day
- One time a week

DURATION

Duration refers to how long the symptom lasts. A shooting pain may last 2 seconds and then disappear. A throbbing ache might last for hours or days. A symptom can be felt constantly for months or even years. Note the duration directly after the frequency as shown in the sample SOAP chart.

ONSET

Record the date when the symptom first occurred. Usually an onset is sudden (e.g., because of an injury), or gradual (e.g., because of repetitive mechanical stress or a developing pathology). Be as specific as possible when recording the onset. For example, write "winter of 2000" instead of "a few years ago." Write "the first week of May 2007" rather than "sometime in 2007." If the client can remember, write the exact date. With a sudden onset related to injuries, clients often remember dates, especially if the injury occurred recently. Sometimes clients can't pinpoint a date, or the symptom came on so gradually they can't remember when they first experienced it. Often symptoms are noticeable for some time before becoming painful or troubling enough for clients to seek help.

Briefly record the incident that caused the injury (e.g., fell off ladder). If the injury is due to repetitive mechanical stress, record the action that seems to cause the symptom (e.g., felt with hanging drywall). In healthcare sessions, the incident causing an injury is described in detail. If a client falls from a horse and is diagnosed with a low back sprain-strain, an insurance company or physician may view massage of shoulders, arms, and hands as unnecessary. But if your chart notes reveal that the client fell on the arm and shoulder, massage treatment including these areas will make more sense to the insurance company or physician.

Activities of Daily Living: Aggravating/Relieving

Injuries and pathologies tend to affect a client's ability to perform activities of daily life; these types of limitations are often referred to as functional limitations. Certain situations can aggravate the condition (increase symptoms) or relieve the condition (decrease symptoms).

A computer programmer with a low back injury may be unable to sit to work at a computer for 8 hours a day. After 2 hours of sitting, the injured area becomes uncomfortable (aggravated). After 4 hours the pain has become moderate. After 6 hours the back is so painful the client is unable to drive home. In this case sitting more than 2 hours aggravates the client's low back condition. The client also reports that pain medication and a warm bath later in the day help relieve his symptoms.

In this section of the SOAP chart, record the activities that aggravate or relieve the client's symptoms. Start with activities that are aggravating and record the point (in seconds, minutes, hours, or repetitions) at which symptoms increase. Also note how the client's life is affected. The computer programmer above must work 8 hours to keep the job, but at 6 hours the pain is debilitating. In the sample SOAP chart, these notations are abbreviated, but below they are written out for clarity as examples:

- A: Low back pain increases from mild to mild plus after 2 hours of sitting at the computer. At 4 hours, pain is moderate minus; at 6 hours pain is severe. Client must sit at computer 8 hours for job.
- A: Wrist pain increases from moderate minus to moderate after hammering and sawing for 1 hour. At 3 hours pain is moderate plus and client must stop work. Client works 8 hours of construction daily with approximately 4 hours of hammering and sawing.
- A: Neck tension increases from no tension to mild after 10 minutes of driving. Tension increases to moderate minus after 20 minutes of driving. Client must drive 45 minutes each direction for work.
- A: Leg pain increases from mild to severe in 2 seconds with lifting. Client must lift children as part of normal care.
- A: Back pain increases from mild plus to moderate plus after sitting 2 hours. Client is unable to enjoy movies with her husband for relaxation.

Include any activities the client performs to relieve the symptoms. Clients often take warm baths, use heating packs, take pain medications, stretch, or sleep to relieve their symptoms. Notations about relieving activities can be short and concise:

- R: Warm bath, pain meds
- R: Stretches, nap
- R: Pain meds, massage
- R: Heat pack, yoga class, meditation, massage

The O Section—Objective Findings

As noted earlier, record objective data in the O section of a SOAP chart. This is the data gathered through observation of the client and palpation of the client's tissue before, during, and after the massage. Focus on basic visual data and palpatory data at this stage in your training program. Later on, this section of your SOAP chart may include findings related to posture, pain, and range-of-motion assessment.

Findings: Visual/Palpable/Test Results

Visual data is what you can see, including a client's breathing patterns (e.g., shallow upper-chest breathing), complexion (e.g., pale, flushed), overall vitality (e.g., fatigued, agitated), skin surface (e.g., bruises, wounds, scars, atrophied muscles, skin discoloration), freedom of movement (e.g., client visually stiff and sore, moving with moderate difficulty), and posture assessment.

Palpation data is what you feel. It includes findings about soft-tissue texture (e.g. adhesions, scar tissue, swelling, edema), tone (hypertonic, hypotonic, spasm, guarding, rigid), temperature, which is often related to blood circulation (e.g., cold, warm, hot, or hyperemic, ischemic, inflamed), level of hydration (e.g., dehydrated or dry, hydrated or moist), quality of movement (e.g., weakness, uneven muscle firing patterns, unstable, restricted), and pain elicited by your touch.

Some visual and palpation findings, like skin surface findings, postural asymmetry, hypertonic areas, painful areas, or areas of temperature abnormalities, can be noted on the human figures. Document as much information as possible in this way because you can then rapidly review it before following sessions. Other information must be recorded in written statements in this section.

When documenting objective findings, mark or describe the specific location of the finding and quantify it (e.g., L, M, S). Pain is subjective unless it is caused by your touch. When a client reacts to a massage stroke and tells you that it hurts, explore the quality of the pain, rate its expression, and explain the type of touch that caused the pain. For example: "Sharp, shooting moderate pain with moderate digital pressure to the right middle scalene. Pain referred to the occiput."

Techniques/Modalities: Locations/Duration

This section of the form is for a concise but complete record of the techniques you used during the session, where you applied them, and how long you spent on each area of the body. In a wellness session, for example: "Fifty minutes Swedish massage on the legs, back, arms, and neck. Ten minutes reflexology on the feet." If the session included diaphragmatic breathing, you might write, "Five minutes diaphragmatic breathing exercise, 45 minutes Swedish massage to the back, legs, arms and neck, and ten minutes reflexology on the feet." You can be still more specific when documenting healthcare massage, especially if you used a particular technique to address a specific finding. For example, you might write: "Myofascial release to the back, origin insertion technique to the erector spinae muscles, deep tissue to the adductors, hamstrings, and psoas massage."

Response to Treatment

In a wellness session, the gathering and documenting of objective data is condensed. Time is not usually allotted for a formal assessment, and you simply note and record what you see and feel. If possible, note any changes in findings from the beginning to the end of the session. If you observe no change, note this also. Don't be afraid to document negative reactions to treatment or state that no change occurred. This is valuable information that can help you plan effectively for the next session.

In a healthcare session, on the other hand, the process of gathering objective data is formal and systematic. Often you follow a predetermined system for conducting pre- and postassessments to obtain accurate data and document the client's response to treatment. This process is described in depth in Chapter 19.

When you observe or palpate a finding, rate it using a scale as described previously. For example, you may palpate the hamstring muscles and indicate on the human figures that they are hypertonic with an M− (moderate minus) after the symbol for hypertonicity. You massage the hamstrings with a variety of techniques and gradually the muscle tissue softens and relaxes. At the end of the massage, the hamstrings still feel hypertonic, but much less hypertonic than at the beginning. You use the change symbol next to the first M− and then write L+ to indicate that the hamstrings had mild plus tension at the conclusion of the massage. If the hamstrings don't change at all after the massage, use the symbol denoting no change after the first M−. If you quantify each of your findings and note the changes that occur on the figures or next to your original notations, you don't need to describe them in writing. Yet it is a good idea to describe the client's overall response to the session and any changes the client reports in his or her own words if possible. For example, you might note, "The client reports, 'I feel ten times better. The pain in my back is almost gone and I can turn my head freely. I feel so much more relaxed.'"

The A Section—Assessment Information

Healthcare providers such as physicians, who can diagnose conditions as part of their scope of practice, use the A section of a SOAP chart to draw conclusions from the S and O sections of the chart and diagnose the condition. Because diagnosis is out of the scope of practice for massage therapists, this area of the chart is used to record functional limitations, set goals to overcome functional limitations, and demonstrate progress through the accomplishment of these goals. This is an important process in healthcare massage sessions and is covered in depth in Chapter 19. For now, you can leave this section of the SOAP form blank and focus on providing comprehensive documentation in the S, O, and P sections.

The P Section—Plan

In this section, you document your plan for how you will treat the client in future sessions and record your recommendations for ways the client can improve at home through self-care activities. Record techniques that worked, techniques to try, and techniques to avoid. After choosing techniques to use in the future, determine how frequent and long treatments should ideally be for the client to progress. One client can receive massage once a month for 60 minutes and meet the healthcare goals (e.g., general stress reduction). Another client needs massage more regularly to experience positive change. A massage once a week for 60 minutes would help to reduce chronic muscle tension and poor postural habits. A client who has an injury or pathology that causes intense muscle contracture or functional restrictions may need massage two or even three times a week in 60-minute sessions. If the client cannot remain in a prone or supine position for an entire hour, you may decide to treat the client twice a week in 20-minute sessions. You also need to project how long the client needs treatment at the prescribed frequency and session length. Maybe the client needs two 60-minute sessions a week for 4 weeks and then you will reassess the situation. Each situation is unique and requires you to consider carefully what is needed for the client to improve. Following are examples of entries for this section:

- Swedish massage posterior with myofascial release and deep tissue to the back and hamstrings two times a week for 60 minutes for 3 weeks, and then reevaluate.
- Diaphragmatic breathing and full body Swedish massage one time a month for 60 minutes for 2 months, and then reevaluate.
- Manual lymphatic drainage technique to legs, Swedish massage neck and shoulders two times a week for 30 minutes for 4 weeks, and then reevaluate.

Self-Care Activities

Clients who participate in self-care activities are likely to improve more rapidly. Self-care also teaches the client to be proactive about health and to make choices that facilitate healing and recovery. Recommend self-care activities that will support the client's healthcare goals. Demonstrate for the client how to perform certain activities like stretching and self-massage. For example, if the client is seeking massage for shoulder tension, you might recommend three shoulder stretches to be performed twice during the workday. Common self-care activities include

- Use of a warm pack on chronically tight muscles each night before bed
- Warm baths or baths with Epson salts
- Application of an ice pack
- Lying on a tennis ball to release tight areas on the back
- Stretches
- Simple strengthening exercises
- Modifications in work activity (increased number of breaks, stretches at certain points in the day, etc.)
- Increased water intake
- Self-massage techniques

Upcoming chapters that discuss pathologies and soft-tissue conditions provide recommendations for self-care activities that can be given to clients. For now, give general recommendations like the use of warm packs or baths, increased water intake, and self-massage techniques.

Condensed Formats for Documentation of Wellness Sessions

In the simplest **wellness chart**, the therapist's name appears at the top, followed by the client's name, DOB, and medications (Fig. 12-9). The area under TX (treatment) is used to describe

Wellness Massage Chart

Client's Name: _____ Today's Date: _____

ID#/DOB_____ Meds: _____

TX:_____

_____

_____

Comments: _____

_____

_____

_____

_____

Therapist's Signature: _____

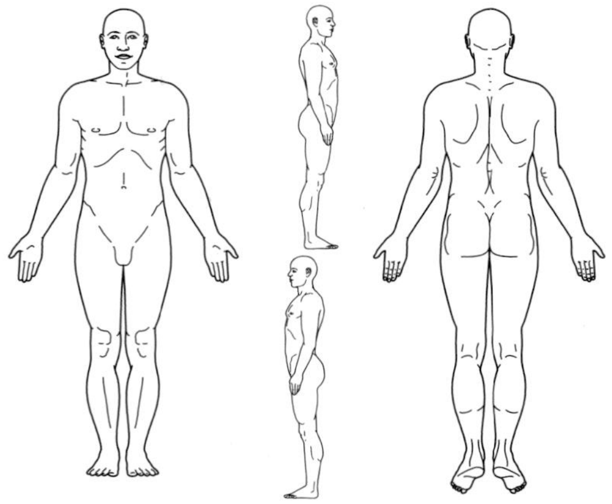

Figure 12-9 Sample wellness form.

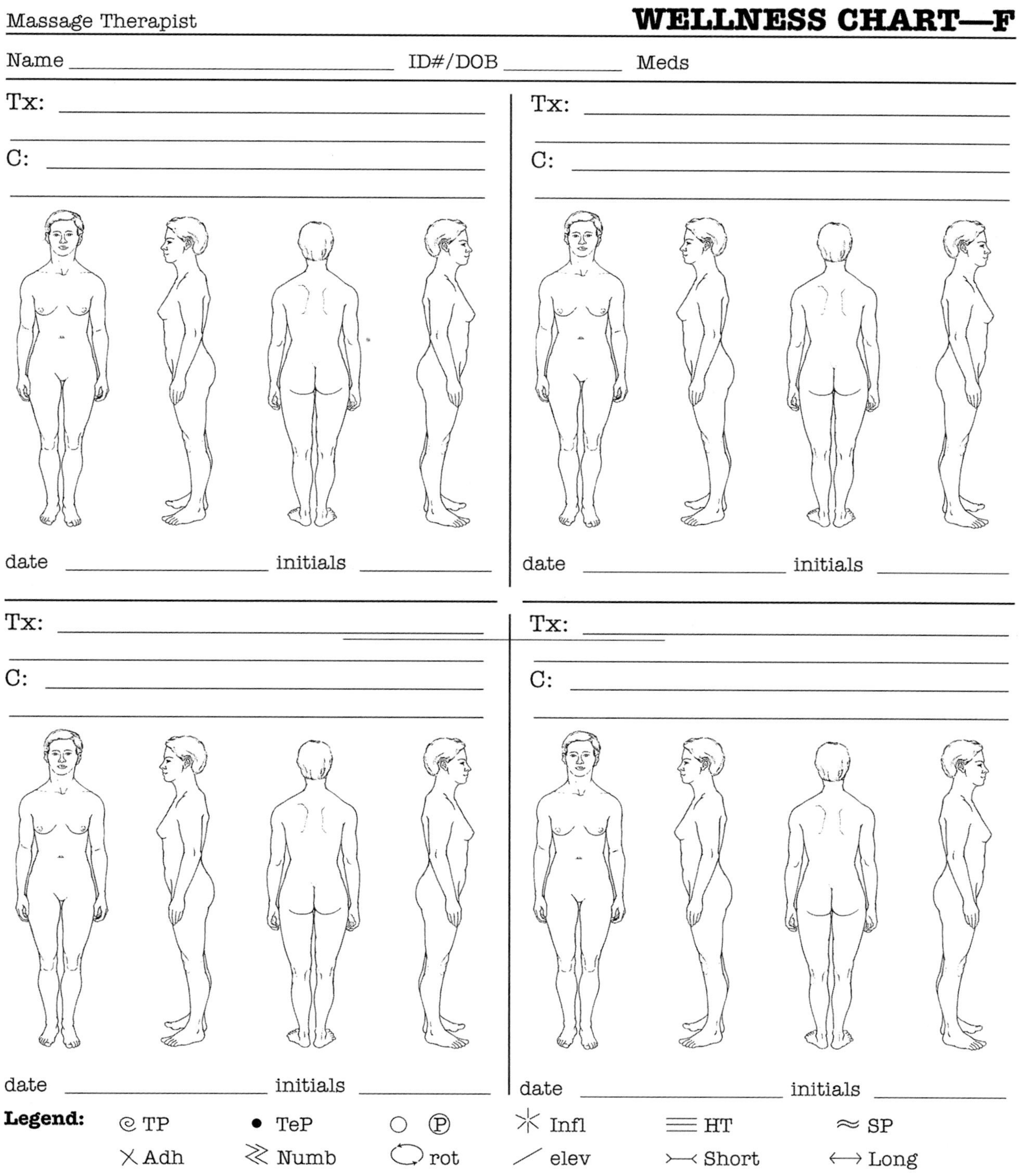

Massage Therapist _____   **WELLNESS CHART—F**

Name _____ ID#/DOB _____ Meds _____

Tx: _____   Tx: _____

C: _____   C: _____

date _____ initials _____   date _____ initials _____

Tx: _____   Tx: _____

C: _____   C: _____

date _____ initials _____   date _____ initials _____

Legend: ℮ TP   • TeP   ○ ℗   ⚹ Infl   ≡ HT   ≈ SP

　　　　　　　✕ Adh   ⋙ Numb   ↺ rot   ⁄ elev   ⊶ Short   ↔ Long

Figure 12-10 Sample condensed SOAP form.

the techniques used and any adaptations made to ensure the client's comfort and safety. The C (comments) section is for recording the client's preferences for lubricants, music, and techniques. Use the figures to chart basic objective findings that may prove useful if the client returns for a second visit or comes regularly for massage. Finally, date and sign at the bottom of the form.

Condensed SOAP forms are useful for documentation of a wellness session (Fig. 12-10) or to document ongoing healthcare sessions as described in Chapter 19. For a wellness session, the client's goals for the session are listed in the S section, while basic objective findings are noted in the O section and on the human figures. Be sure to include the techniques used in the session and the areas where techniques were applied. This record is important if the client returns for another session at a later date. In the A section, you might list one simple functional goal if the client seeks massage for a specific purpose. Perhaps the client wants more flexibility in yoga classes and wants to be able to perform a specific pose. You might leave this section blank and simply write NA for not applicable. In the P section, briefly note any recommendations made for self-care, and then sign and date the form.

As you can see, documenting a wellness session is much easier and quicker than documenting a healthcare session. Sometimes students resist using the full SOAP chart once they are used to a condensed form. To increase your learning and obtain the best possible education, however, you should chart every session collecting as much data as possible on a full

SOAP chart. In this way you will get more feedback from your instructor, and your charting skills will make you a desirable applicant for jobs in a variety of massage settings or encourage keeping excellent documentation in your private practice. You can easily transition to condense wellness forms later on when appropriate.

Concept Brief 12-4
SOAP

- Standard form of documentation used by healthcare providers
- **S** = subjective
- **O** = objective
- **A** = assessment
- **P** = plan

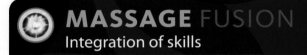

MASSAGE FUSION
Integration of skills

STUDY TIP: Nothing Lost in Translation

When you begin charting, it is helpful to write out everything in longhand on a "scrap" SOAP chart in the proper sections. After the session, rewrite your SOAP chart translating the longhand into abbreviations. This helps ensure that you collect all the relevant information and learn proper abbreviations at the same time. While this is time-consuming at first, it is the surest way to build good skills. Soon you naturally progress to writing in an abbreviated format, and your charting gets faster.

MASSAGE INSPIRATION: Visualization

Therapists with good palpation skills often visualize the structures under their hands. One way to enhance this skill and to better learn the structures of the body is to draw them with washable markers right onto the practice body. For example, view a picture of the abdominal cavity in an anatomy book. Feel for the structures with your hands and use a marker to draw them over your fellow student's abdomen. Feel and draw, and draw and feel. Now, close your eyes and visualize your drawing while you palpate. This helps awaken your tactile sensitivity so that you can feel nuances more readily. This is a great way to learn the location of skeletal muscles and focus your attention on their fiber directions and layers. Start on the back and draw superficial

muscles like the trapezius and latissimus dorsi in red. Draw intermediate muscles like the rhomboids in blue, and deep muscles like the erector spinae group or quadratus lumborum in green. Drawing the muscles in their correct location will require lots of palpation and the guidance of a good kinesiology or functional anatomy book. Have fun!

CHAPTER WRAP-UP

Sometimes when students are introduced to assessment, session planning, and documentation, they first think, "I don't need to learn all that advanced stuff because I'm just going to work in a spa and do relaxation massage." Resistance to the SOAP chart and comprehensive assessment can be so strong you might miss the unique challenges and satisfaction that comes from providing meaningful healthcare massage.

No doubt about it: good assessment, session planning, and documentation are advanced skills, even at this introductory level. These skills don't come as naturally as applying strokes to the body, and they are probably not as fun to learn, but they are absolutely essential for your professional practice.

One of the best ways to start is to embrace the SOAP chart wholeheartedly. Even though it probably seems complicated right now, using the form during health intake interviews will help you focus your questions to obtain the information you need from clients. At first you may end the

⊛ MASSAGE FUSION *(Continued)*
Integration of Skills

massage and then sit down to finish your SOAP chart only to find that you forgot to gather visual data or forgot to ask the client about activities that aggravate or relieve symptoms, or forgot to check whether the client's tissue changed after a massage of a given area. This is normal. As you keep using the SOAP form, you will get more and more efficient at gathering data each time.

Suddenly a curious thing will happen. You will be standing in line at the grocery store check out and notice that you were subconsciously gathering visual objective data about the person in front of you. You will shake someone's hand in greeting and notice the temperature and texture of the tissue without trying to. You will place your hand on a friend's shoulder and feel, without effort, the level of tension and places of adhered tissue, even through your friend's shirt. One day very soon, you will spontaneously start writing all your chart notes and classroom notes using abbreviations, and it will be easy!; All you have to do to experience these wonders is practice and persist. You can do it. You can learn this, and when you do, you will be one step closer to your goal of being an excellent and accomplished professional massage therapist.

Chapter 13

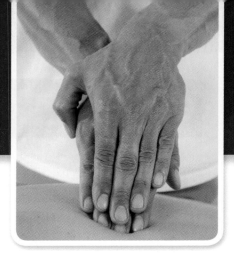

Swedish Massage Techniques

KEY TERMS

effleurage
end feel
friction
joint movements
joint play
petrissage

range of motion
routines
sequencing
synovial joints
tapotement
vibration

LEARNING OBJECTIVES

Having read the chapter and used the related student learning tools, the student will be able to:

1 List two physiological effects from each of the six Swedish massage techniques described.

2 Compare and contrast the effects of a friction stroke applied briskly and lightly with those of a friction stroke applied with slow, moderate pressure.

3 Explain the different effects of applying an effleurage stroke in different directions: away from the heart and toward the heart.

4 Briefly explain the effect of petrissage on Golgi tendon organs.

5 Briefly explain the effect of friction on adhesions.

6 Compare and contrast active, passive, and resisted range-of-motion techniques.

7 Describe the effects of subtle factors such as rhythm, depth, and pacing on the client's massage experience.

hapter 1 introduced you to the history of Swedish massage. Per Henrik Ling of Sweden developed a system of medical gymnastics in the early 19th century that became known as the Swedish Movements. Dr. Johann Mezger gave French terms to these techniques used to loosen and manipulate muscles. In the mid-1800s, the Swedish Movements gained popularity across Europe, and the physician Mathias Roth, who studied with Ling at the Royal Central Institute, published the first book in English on the subject in England. Roth in turn taught the Swedish Movements techniques to the New York physician Charles Taylor, whose brother George in Sweden also studied the Swedish Movements. These two brothers are responsible for bringing the Swedish Movements to America and for promoting their uses and benefits until their deaths in 1899. Over time, some of the Swedish exercises were dropped or evolved as part of physical therapy. Massage therapists emphasized those components of the Swedish Movements that manipulated soft tissue, and gradually the system became known as Swedish massage.[1]

The techniques used in Swedish massage form the foundation of most therapists' massage routine, even those practicing specific different modalities. Swedish massage is sometimes called relaxation massage, but Swedish techniques have many benefits in addition to relaxation. In fact, Swedish massage techniques can be delivered with light, moderate, or deep pressure for a variety of treatment outcomes. Swedish massage still uses the six traditional stroke techniques first named by Mezger. These techniques are effleurage, petrissage, friction, tapotement, vibration, and joint movements (also called Swedish gymnastics or range of motion [ROM]). Each of these techniques is performed with the depth and vigor most appropriate for the individual client. As your skills develop, you may integrate Swedish strokes with other strokes, such as compression strokes introduced as part of sports massage in the 1950s, or with resting/holding strokes often used to open and close massage sessions. These strokes and many other techniques are described in other chapters of this book. For example, myofascial release techniques, which are applied without lubricant, might be used before Swedish techniques, and deep tissue techniques can be used after the body area is warmed with Swedish strokes.

Your goal in this chapter is to learn and practice specific techniques associated with Swedish massage. Novices may want to focus on learning the variations of these techniques and applying them to different body areas. When each specific technique feels natural, the next step is to create smooth transitions between strokes and improve your massage skill subtleties. In upcoming chapters, other techniques are integrated with these Swedish techniques. Before using these techniques with clients, review the contraindications for massage in Chapter 5. Use the techniques learned in Chapter 10 to incorporate good draping, use of breath, and a strong opening and closing in the Swedish massage session.

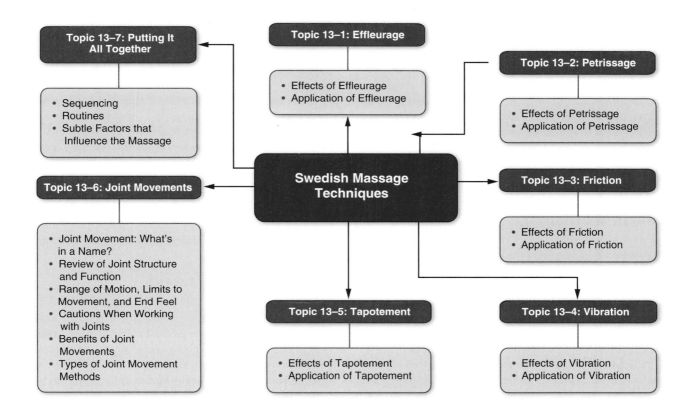

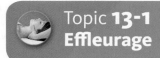

Topic 13-1
Effleurage

Effleurage is a long, gliding stroke delivered with light, medium, or sometimes deep pressure that usually follows the direction of the muscle fibers. The word "effleurage" derives from the French verb meaning "to skim" or "to touch lightly." This stroke is often the first applied to a body area. It is used to spread lubricant, warm the muscles in anticipation of deeper work, and assess the general condition of the client's tissue. Usually effleurage strokes are applied toward the heart (distal to proximal) to assist in venous return and enhance blood and lymph circulation. Interestingly, in some massage approaches like Ayurveda (the traditional medical system of India), gliding strokes are delivered in the opposite direction, outward from the navel, to reenergize the limbs.[2] Proximal-to-distal strokes should be applied lightly to avoid damaging the one-way valves of superficial veins. Effleurage strokes are also used to connect the massage of different body areas and provide a flowing transition between techniques.

The use of effleurage strokes to support venous return and the circulation of blood and lymph is important. You will learn in anatomy and physiology classes that arteries carry oxygenated blood to the body's tissues. Veins carry deoxygenated blood back to the heart to be recirculated after reoxygenation in the lungs. "Venous return" refers to the blood returning to the heart from the veins. When a person is sitting or standing, blood returning to the heart from the lower half of the body must fight gravity. To assist venous return, veins have one-way valves that allow blood to flow only toward the heart. Contractions of nearby skeletal muscles and the pulsing of nearby arteries help push venous blood toward the heart against the force of gravity. During massage, the techniques used to relax muscles also squeeze veins and encourage the movement of blood toward the heart. This decreases the accumulation of metabolic waste and stagnation of the blood and benefits body tissues by helping ensure adequate amounts of oxygen.[3]

Effects of Effleurage

The effects of effleurage on the body vary depending on the stroke's depth, speed, and direction. For example, slow strokes delivered in the same direction as the muscle fibers at a light or moderate depth soothe the body and trigger the parasympathetic nervous system response. Quick strokes delivered in the same direction as the muscle fibers at a light or moderate pressure stimulate the sympathetic nervous system.

Activation of the parasympathetic nervous system response is an important benefit of Swedish massage. The autonomic nervous system coordinates most body functions. It has two divisions: the sympathetic and parasympathetic. Usually but not always, these two divisions have opposing effects that help to regulate homeostasis. The sympathetic division excites an organ, and the parasympathetic division inhibits it. The sympathetic division is associated with the fight-or-flight response, the body's survival alarm system. The parasympathetic division is associated with the rest-and-recover response. When the parasympathetic nervous system response is activated, the body goes into rest-and-recovery mode and conserves energy with a reduction in heart rate and blood pressure, an increase in digestive activity, and other changes allowing the body to refurbish itself. Research has shown that relaxation massage helps reduce anxiety and depression because of the parasympathetic response. Regular massage can help the body deal more effectively with stress, decrease symptoms associated with digestive upset, and reduce pain.[4–6]

Effleurage also affects the skin by rubbing off dead skin cells (desquamation) and creating more pliability in the skin by stimulating sebaceous secretion. It encourages local circulation and lymph flow to improve nutrient and waste exchange in local tissue. As mentioned previously, it supports efficient venous return of blood to the heart. After exercise, effleurage aids tissue recovery and reduces muscle soreness.[7] Effleurage strokes relieve muscle spasms and warm soft-tissue structures to allow more fluidity of movement and length of hypertonic muscle tissue. These strokes also create a pleasurable sensation that facilitates relaxation.

Effleurage is contraindicated for any condition generally contraindicated for massage and over open skin lesions or skin diseases. It should not be applied distal to an area of inflammation, injury, or severe bruising because these conditions may cause fluids to gather in the tissue. Effleurage distal to these conditions might further exacerbate the situation and lead to additional fluid retention. It should not be used repetitively on the limbs of clients with cardiovascular disorders, high blood pressure, or circulatory conditions because it may place weakened or overstressed cardiovascular structures under increased pressure.

Application of Effleurage

The palm of the hand, fingertips, edge of the hand, forearms, knuckles, and thumbs can be used to apply effleurage strokes. The choice often depends on the desired depth and the body area. For example, the forearm obviously would not be used to apply an effleurage stroke to the face; the fingertips are clearly more appropriate. But the forearms may be used for effleurage strokes on the back.

Follow these general principles for the application of effleurage strokes. Undrape the area, and place a moderate amount of lubricant in your hand. Warm the lubricant and apply it to the area in a long stroke that begins at the bottom of the area (distal), travels to the top of the area (proximal), and returns to the bottom of the area (distal) without losing contact with the client. Have your hands open so that the entire surface of the palms and fingers contact the client's tissue, and feel the fullness of the tissue. Notice temperature or texture changes in the tissue. Visualize the direction of muscle fibers running under the skin, and imagine sinking your hands into that muscle. As the tissue begins to warm up, increase the depth of the stroke. Never force your hands into unyielding tissue. Instead, relax and drop into the tissue using the weight of your body rather than the strength of your arm muscles or tense wrists. Pay attention to the rhythm and speed of your stroke. Does the speed of the stroke change the client's breathing pattern? You may notice that as you slow down or speed up, the client's breathing pattern also changes. Now, slow down and explore how slow you can make your stroke. Lighten the pressure of the stroke and explore how soft you can make the stroke. Concentrate the pressure of the stroke and explore how deep you can sink into the tissue. You can apply an effleurage stroke in a number of different ways, as shown in Technique 18.

Concept Brief 13-1
Effleurage

Defined: Gliding stroke.

Primary uses: Apply lubricant, warm tissue, support venous return, activate parasympathetic nervous system response, transition between strokes.

Speed: Slow strokes relax, moderate to fast strokes invigorate.

Direction: Usually toward the heart following muscle fibers.

Depth: Light, moderate, or deep.

Contraindications: Open skin lesions, contagious skin diseases, distal to injury or inflammation, repetitive strokes on limbs of clients with cardiovascular disease, high blood pressure, or circulatory conditions.

Technique 18   Effleurage

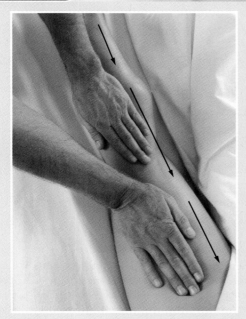

1. General effleurage. On the posterior leg, start the stroke above the heel and run up the entire length of the leg to circle the greater trochanter, and come back down to the heel again.

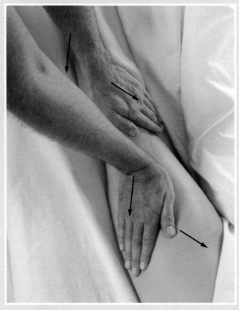

2. In shingling effleurage, use shorter strokes alternated in a continuous motion. (The name comes from the image of shingles overlapping on a roof.)

Continued

Technique 18   **Effleurage** (Continued)

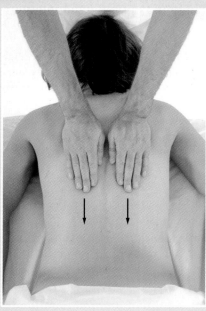

3A. General effleurage on the back. Try the basic effleurage stroke using your hands on the client's back. Begin the stroke at the top of the shoulders and push the tissue toward the sacrum.

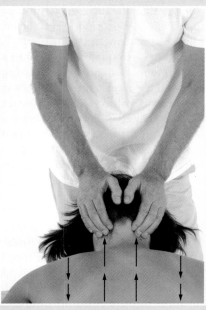

3B. Come around the sides of the sacrum and bring your hands back up along the lateral sides of the body. Bring your hands across the shoulders and halfway down the arms. Finish the stroke at the occipital bone with gentle traction.

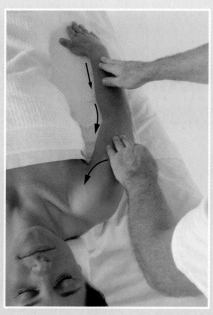

4. Nerve strokes. Very light effleurage strokes relax the nervous system and feel soothing; these are often called "nerve strokes." Gently run your fingertips up and down the lengths of the muscles to practice this technique. This image shows nerve strokes on the arm.

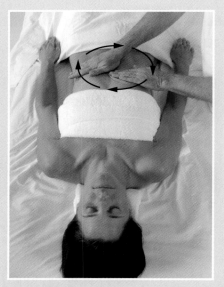

5. Effleurage to the abdominals. Apply a basic effleurage stroke to the abdominal area by circling your hands around the navel in a clockwise direction to facilitate digestion and the elimination of waste products through the urinary system. Use a full-handed stroke with the entire palm and fingers in contact with the tissue.

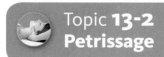

Topic **13-2**
Petrissage

Petrissage is a rhythmic stroke that lifts the muscle off the bone and other muscles, compresses it between the fingers, and rolls the muscle fibers as the muscle falls back into position. The word "petrissage" is from the French verb for "to knead." This technique is often used, after effleurage strokes have warmed the muscle tissue, to stimulate circulation in the muscles, to make soft tissue more pliable, and to break up adhered fibers.

Effects of Petrissage

Petrissage results in many of the same effects as effleurage. Petrissage stimulates sebaceous secretion, thereby conditioning the skin. It stimulates local circulation to warm soft tissue and to improve nutrient and waste exchange. It is particularly suited for decreasing muscle tension. When soft tissue is lifted off the bone and other muscles in a petrissage stroke, the muscle is squeezed and the tendon is stretched. Golgi tendon organs (GTO) are a sensory receptor that monitors changes in muscle tension. The most important function of the GTO is to prevent the strength of a muscle contraction from damaging tendons. When a GTO senses that a strain or tear is at hand (such as when lifting an item that is too heavy), its signal becomes powerful enough to cause an instant reduction in muscle tension. The muscle gives way and damage is avoided. Current research suggests that GTOs are activated during tiny changes in muscle tension, like those caused by petrissage strokes, to send signals through the nervous system that cause a muscle to relax.[8]

Petrissage also plays a role in decreasing adhesions in soft-tissue structures. Adhesions are abnormal deposits of connective tissue that form between surfaces that normally glide over each other. For example, muscles are composed of parallel fibers organized into spirals. Muscle fibers are interwoven and surrounded with connective tissue, referred to together with the term "myofascia" (fascia is a type of connective tissue). Healthy myofascia slides over itself. The myofascia strands, bundles of strands, muscles, and sheets of fascia normally do not stick together. Repetitive stress, incorrect posture, inflammation and injury, dehydration, poor diet, sedentary lifestyle, and other factors can cause dysfunction in connective tissue. The process begins with collagen, which is a component of connective tissue that resembles a cord. Small fibers of collagen form larger strands wound together in a spiral. Each small fiber, the larger strands, and the entire cord can usually slide freely past one another due to lubrication from the ground substance. Ground substance is a viscous fluid with a thixotropic quality. This means that it becomes more fluid when it is stirred and more solid when undisturbed. In unhealthy or injured connective tissue, excessive collagen is deposited randomly instead of in the normal parallel arrangement. Collagen fibers pack together, and additional abnormal cross-links form. Ground substance thickens and fails to adequately lubricate or nourish collagen cords. These collagen deposits are referred to as adhesions. They cause the tissue to become thicker, shorter, and less elastic. Adhesions lead to decreased blood flow, decreased ROM, pain, and decreased function in the area.

When you run myofascial fibers through your fingers during a petrissage stroke, the stroke helps break up adhesive bonds, makes the tissue more pliable, and gives the ground substance a good stirring. Skin rolling is a type of petrissage that lifts the skin and superficial fascia away from the underlying muscle and rolls it through the fingertips. This helps reduce adhesions in the superficial fascia and allows it to glide more easily over the structures below. Petrissage should not be used on atrophied muscles that lack moderate tone because it may damage the tissue. It should not be applied over open skin legions, skin diseases, bruises, acute injuries, inflammation, or varicose veins.

Application of Petrissage

To apply a petrissage stroke, wrap one hand around the tissue, keeping your fingers together as a unit. Lift the muscle away from the bone until you feel it stretch. Roll the muscle through your fingers and out of your hand as your other hand lifts up another section of tissue. Too much lubricant would prevent you from getting a good hold on the muscle, so use very little lubricant for this technique. This rhythmic, kneading action is continued over the entire body area. Petrissage is often referred to as "milking" the tissue of metabolic wastes because of the increase in local circulation.

How much lift and squeeze to use depends on the body area where the stroke is applied. For example, use your fingertips to apply gentle petrissage strokes to the eyebrows and jawline. Use a strong, full-handed stroke to apply petrissage to fleshy areas like the hamstrings. Be careful not to pinch the client or pull on body hair during petrissage. If the client complains that the stroke is pinching, make sure that you lift enough tissue during the stroke. To flush metabolic wastes released from tissue, apply effleurage strokes directly after petrissage.

During the application of petrissage strokes, pay attention to the lift of the tissue and its texture as it runs through your fingers. Is it easy to lift off the bone and underlying muscle, or is it difficult to grasp? When it runs through your fingers is the consistency even and fluid, or are certain areas thick or stuck? Differences in the tissue tell you something about the health of the myofascia and how much massage is needed in a particular area. Check with the client frequently to ensure that the pressure of the stroke is comfortable. Petrissage strokes can be applied in a number of different ways, as shown in Technique 19.

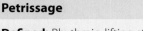

Concept Brief 13-2
Petrissage

Defined: Rhythmic, lifting stroke.

Primary uses: Increase soft-tissue pliability, break up adhesions.

Speed: Regular, moderate rhythm.

Direction: Muscle lifted upward, away from the bone and other muscles.

Depth: Firm but not painful.

Contraindications: Open skin legions, contagious skin diseases, atrophied muscles, bruises, injury or inflammation, varicose veins.

| Technique 19 | Petrissage |

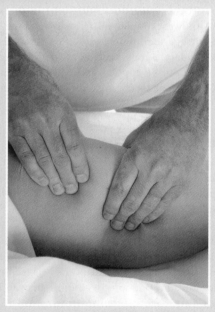

1. Lift the myofascia of the hamstrings with one hand and let it roll through your fingers back into place. While the tissue is rolling out of one hand, lift the myofascia in the next section with your other hand.

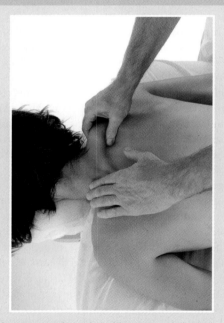

2. Apply petrissage strokes on the back beginning on the low back and working up to the shoulders. You can also petrissage both shoulders at the same time, as shown here.

Continued

Technique 19   Petrissage (Continued)

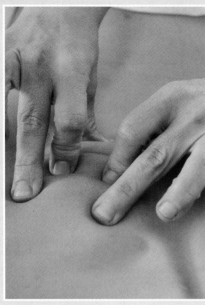

3. Using minimal lubricant, try the skin-rolling technique. Use your thumbs to push the client's tissue away. Your finger pads "walk" ahead of your thumbs to gather up the tissue. Work slowly at first, but as the tissue becomes less adhered you can work faster.

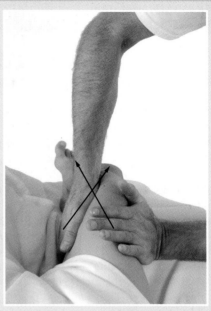

4. "Fulling" petrissage works well on both the anterior and posterior thigh. Grasp the tissue with your entire palms and lift the tissue on both the inside and the outside of the upper leg at the same time. Allow the tissue to roll through your fingers, and repeat the stroke on the next area of tissue.

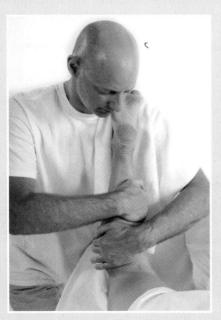

5. Wringing petrissage pulls the tissue together and apart to reduce adhesions and soften the tissue.

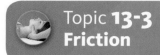

Topic 13-3
Friction

Friction is a heat-producing, chafing stroke applied either with light, brisk strokes (superficial friction) or with depth (circular, linear, or cross-fiber friction). The word "friction" comes from the Latin *frictio* meaning "to rub." In a traditional Swedish progression of strokes, friction is applied after petrissage, using little or no lubricant. It is used to heat the local tissue, break up adhered tissue, and reorganize collagen fibers into parallel patterns allowing for greater ROM. Deep linear friction strokes address connective tissue as the superficial tissue is pushed onto underlying structures and then pulled over the top of these structures, stretching the myofascia.

Cyriax cross-fiber friction is a specific technique developed by James Cyriax in the 1930s to address scar tissue and adhered tissue. As the name suggests, the technique is applied across the fibers of the muscle instead of following the muscle fiber direction. This rapid and deep transverse rubbing creates inflammation in the tissue, which stimulates tissue repair mechanisms. At the same time, connective tissue is reorganized, leading to a breakdown of scar tissue that might otherwise restrict the client's ROM and lead to reinjury. Cross-fiber friction is an advanced technique, often taught as part of orthopedic massage, clinical massage, or treatment massage. It is discussed in greater detail in later chapters.

Effects of Friction

The effects of friction vary depending on the stroke's depth, direction, and speed. Superficial friction is brisk and stimulating. It produces heat in the skin from the resistance between the client's body and the therapist's hands. The heat produced through friction increases circulation and lymph flow to the local tissue. Deep friction is applied parallel to the muscle fibers to separate the fibers so that they can more readily slide over each other and move freely. The myofascia is stretched and broadened, leading to better flexibility and muscular balance. Transverse friction is applied across the muscle fibers to break up an adhesion or scar tissue, although it is usually applied more slowly than the Cyriax cross-fiber friction. Do not use friction strokes over open skin legions, skin diseases, bruises, acute injuries, inflammation, or moderate to severe varicose veins.

Application of Friction

Superficial friction is most often applied with the palms in a quick, light, back-and-forth motion with little or no lubricant. The fingertips, thumbs, knuckles, forearm, elbow, or edge of the hand is used to apply a deep friction stroke. During the application of friction, pay attention to the quality of the client's tissue and how it changes during the treatment. Adhesions feel like stuck tissue that is glued together. Tissue may move freely and then suddenly grab. Sometimes adhesions feel like obvious knots of bound-up tissue that the client may report as an area of mild numbness. Sometimes unhealthy or adhered tissue is not easy to describe or identify clearly. It can feel grainy, crumbly, crackly, or disorganized. It can feel as if it has little elasticity and falls away from the hands. With experience, you will be able to quickly assess a client's tissue. For example, it becomes easy to identify clients who are dehydrated or who are heavy smokers just by the quality of the soft tissue which feels dry and grainy. Friction strokes can be applied in a number of different ways, as shown in Technique 20.

> ## Concept Brief 13-3
> ### Friction
>
> **Defined:** Heat-producing, chafing stroke.
>
> **Primary uses:** Heat tissue, break up adhesions, reorganize collagen fibers.
>
> **Speed:** Slow to very fast.
>
> **Direction:** Parallel to fibers or across fibers (cross-fiber friction).
>
> **Depth:** Moderate to deep.
>
> **Contraindications:** Open skin legions, contagious skin diseases, bruises, injury or inflammation, varicose veins.

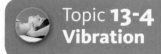

Topic 13-4
Vibration

Vibration is a pulsating, tremor-like or oscillating stroke that stimulates or relaxes the body area or the whole body depending on how it is applied. The term "vibration" comes from the Latin word for "to shake." Vibration is often used

Technique 20 | **Friction**

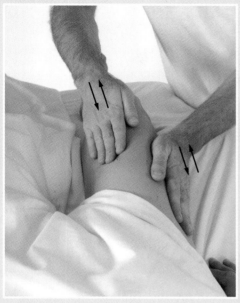

1. Superficial friction strokes are light and brisk to generate heat. Shown here is superficial friction on the upper anterior leg.

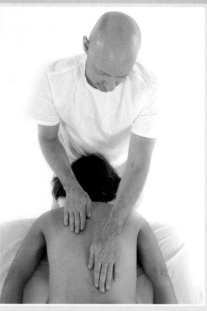

2. Superficial friction strokes can be applied to the back, running with the muscle fibers (as shown) or across the muscles fibers.

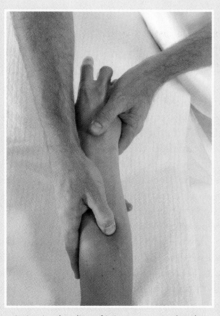

3. This therapist is using deep linear friction to compress, broaden, and lengthen the muscles and tendons of the forearm. Make sure that your fingers or thumbs are straight and supported, because the fingers and thumbs are easily hyperextended during a friction stroke.

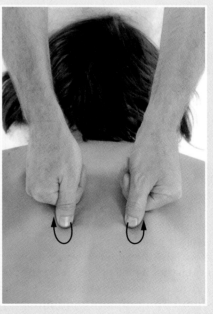

4. This image shows circular friction with the thumbs down either side of the lamina groove. Deep friction strokes can also be applied with the knuckles, reinforced fingers, forearm, elbow, or edge of the hand.

Continued

only in short bursts to a particular area because it can be tiring for the therapist. The shoulders, elbows, and wrists must remain relaxed while the hands vibrate rapidly. Vibration may be fine, coarse, or rocking.

Effects of Vibration

The effects of vibration on the body depend on how the stroke is applied. Initially, vibration is stimulating because it startles

Technique 20   **Friction** (Continued)

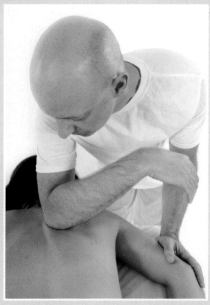

5. A friction stroke is applied with the elbow. Elbow pressure can quickly become too deep for the client. If you use your elbow for a stroke, progress slowly and only to a depth tolerable to the client.

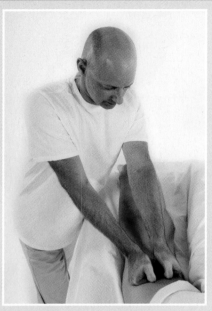

6. Try a linear friction stroke with your knuckles on the hamstrings. Place your knuckles on the posterior upper leg and run them in straight lines up to the gluteal muscles.

the body and briefly activates the sympathetic nervous system. As the stroke progresses, the body relaxes. Sustained vibration to a particular area has a numbing, analgesic effect, reducing pain. Fine vibration is often applied with the fingertips on the abdomen to stimulate peristalsis (the involuntary wave-like contractions that move food through the digestive tract), aiding digestion. Fine vibration can also be used on other delicate areas of the body, such as the face, to relax muscles.

Shaking is a form of coarse vibration in which a muscle group is lifted and shaken to confuse proprioceptors (such as in muscle spindles, as discussed below) so that the muscles relax. Like shaking, jostling is a form of coarse vibration used to prevent muscle guarding of a limb or to encourage general relaxation. Muscle guarding may occur when the client has difficulty relaxing a limb or body area. The client tries to relax but stiffens the area subconsciously. Over time, clients learn how to release a body area to the therapist. If muscle guarding occurs because of an injury, shaking and jostling are contraindicated as this type of "splinting" of an area is appropriate to prevent further injury or pain. Shaking and jostling also encourage synovial fluid production in the joint that aids joint fluidity and health. In this case, the limb is lifted with a slight amount of traction and wriggled back and forth.

Rocking consists of pushing and releasing an area so that it sways back and forth. This soothes the nervous system and relaxes the muscles. The motion may also evoke distant memories of being rocked as a baby and thus be associated with a feeling of being protected and nurtured.

Very rapid vibration can stimulate muscle spindles to cause muscle contractions that tone the muscle, warm the tissue, and increase circulation. Muscle spindles are a type of sensory receptor found in muscle tissue (Fig. 13-1). The two types are primary endings and secondary endings. Regular muscle fibers that produce a contraction are called extrafusal fibers. Muscle spindles that do not produce a contraction are called intrafusal fibers. The muscle spindles are positioned parallel with the other muscle fibers in a fluid-filled capsule embedded within each muscle. Those with primary endings monitor slow and fast changes in muscle length. Those with secondary endings monitor slow changes in muscle length and deep pressure. When a muscle is stretched, the muscle spindle is also stretched and sends a signal causing the muscle to contract. Through this stretch reflex, the muscle spindle helps maintain normal muscle length. Muscle spindles also play an important role in maintaining proper muscle tone and in controlling muscle contractions so that they are smooth and not jerky.[9] According to Thomas Hendrickson in *Massage for Orthopedic Conditions*, emotional upset and anxiety can cause muscle spindles to fire at an accelerated rate, leading to muscle hypertonicity and stiffness.[10] There is some debate as to whether therapists can vibrate their hands fast enough or long enough to cause positive changes in muscle resting length, hypertonicity, and stiffness. Most likely, only professional massage vibrating devices can accomplish this.

Like other Swedish massage strokes, vibration should not be used over open skin legions, skin diseases, bruises, acute injuries, inflammation, or varicose veins.

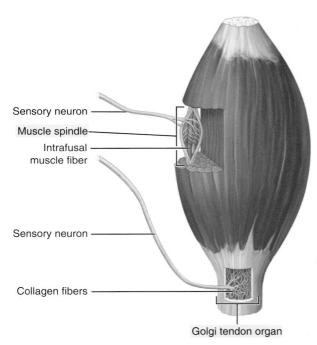

Sensory neuron

Muscle spindle

Intrafusal
muscle fiber

Sensory neuron

Collagen fibers

Golgi tendon organ

Figure 13-1 Muscle spindles are a type of sensory receptor found in muscle tissue. These with primary endings monitor slow and fast changes in muscle length. These with secondary endings monitor slow changes in muscle length and deep pressure. When a muscle is stretched, the muscle spindle is also stretched and sends a signal causing the muscle to contract. Very rapid vibration can stimulate muscle spindles to cause muscle contractions that tone the muscle.

Application of Vibration

Variations in the application methods for vibration are described in Technique 21. Pay careful attention to your body mechanics when performing this stroke. It is easy to

inadvertently tense your shoulders, elbows, and wrists during fine vibration because this technique is difficult until you have gained coordination and practice. Focus on relaxing your shoulders and arms as much as possible. Apply the stroke only for short periods of time to avoid fatigue and allow learning time for your body to adapt.

When using vibration techniques, pay attention to what you see and feel. For example, when the client's body is rocked, it will sway with a particular rhythm. Some clients are easy to push but do not sway back readily. Other clients feel difficult to rock, almost as if they are attached to the massage table. The client's limb may resist being jostled, or it may feel as if the direct vibration stroke is not penetrating the tissue. You might notice that one side of the body rocks in a movement pattern different from the other. All these observations provide information about the client's holding patterns and level of relaxation. Until you gain more experience, you may be unsure how to use this information when developing a session plan. Do not be concerned about this at this point. The important thing is to watch, feel, listen, and think about what you see, touch, and hear. This increased awareness will help you build palpation and assessment skills.

Concept Brief 13-4
Vibration

Defined: Pulsating, tremor-like, oscillating stroke.
Primary uses: Stimulate the nervous system, numb the local area, loosen muscles, stimulate peristalsis.
Speed: Very fast
Direction: Stationary, or parallel to fibers or across fibers.
Contraindications: Open skin legions, contagious skin diseases, injury or inflammation, varicose veins.

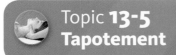
Topic **13-5**
Tapotement

Tapotement is a rapid, rhythmic percussion stroke using the hands in various formations to drum on the client. The name comes from the Old French for "a light blow."

Effects of Tapotement

The effects of tapotement vary depending on the speed, force, and length of the application. Short bursts of forceful tapotement are stimulating to both the local area and the body as a whole, but longer applications tend to relax the body area and body as a whole. Very light tapotement with the fingertips

causes vasoconstriction of superficial capillaries, while moderate drumming applied with the medial sides of the hand causes vasodilation and increased circulation. Brief applications of light percussion help tone atrophied muscles, while long applications of moderate percussion help soothe areas of hypersensitivity. When tapotement is used correctly over the chest or back, mucus is loosened in the chest for easier expulsion.

Tapotement should not be used directly after athletic activity because it stimulates the muscle spindle cells and may cause the muscles to cramp.[11] Tapotement over the kidneys

Technique 21   **Vibration**

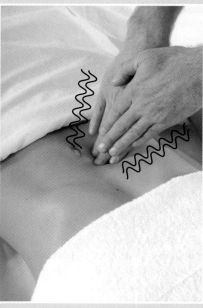

1. To practice fine vibration to simulate peristalsis, overlap your hands with your fingers touching the abdomen. Vibrate your fingers in a clockwise circular direction around the navel.

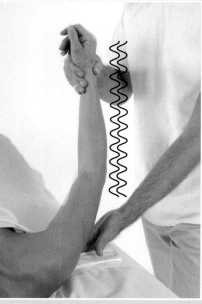

2. To jostle the arm, grasp the client's hand and use your other hand to support the elbow as the arm is lifted. Swing the arm back and forth, keeping a bend in the client's elbow.

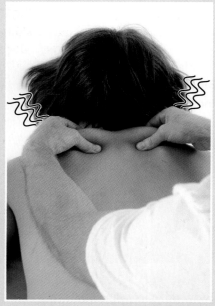

3. Try the shaking technique by picking up the trapezius muscles on either side of the neck. Shake these muscles as shown in the image. Always check to ensure that the technique is comfortable for the client.

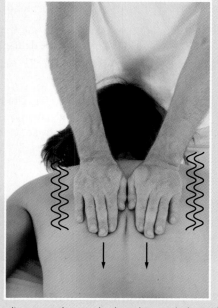

4. With the client prone, place your hands on the upper back on either side of the spine. Compress the tissue and move your hands up and down in an oscillating motion as you move down the back to the sacrum.

Continued

Technique 21   **Vibration** (Continued)

5. To apply the rocking technique, push the client away from you in a rhythmic and soothing series of motions. Move from the upper body to lower body, around the table, and back up to the upper body again.

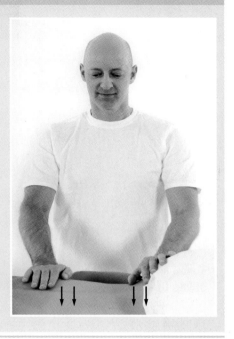

and floating ribs is contraindicated because these structures do not have sufficient protection and may be damaged by the stroke. It should also be avoided on boney areas, especially over the spine, and over bruises and varicose veins. Heavy tapotement strokes should be delivered only over fleshy or heavily muscled areas of the body. Be careful not to bruise or cause discomfort during tapotement. Check with the client regularly to ensure the strokes are comfortable.

Application of Tapotement

You hold your hands in different formations for different types of tapotement. Hacking uses the ulnar side of the hand, while cupping uses the hands shaped like a cup. The hands are held open in slapping, and in pincement the fingertips are used to pick up small bits of superficial tissue. These variations are shown in Technique 22. Tapotement can be applied to dry or oiled skin and even over the drape. It is often called a percussive stroke because it is similar to drumming. Rhythm is very important in the delivery of good tapotement. Irregular strokes that suddenly speed up or slow down can feel irritating to the client's nervous system. The therapist should also move up and down and across the body area fluidly. Avoid overtreating one area, and keep moving the stroke. Keep your wrists and fingers loose during tapotement; with stiff wrists or fingers you may hurt the client or yourself. Tapotement can easily be practiced on a soft surface like a pillow, with music, to improve your rhythm and regularity.

Concept Brief 13-5
Tapotement

Defined	Rhythmic percussion stroke
Primary uses	Promote circulation, increase muscle tone, stimulate the nervous system, loosen mucus for easier expulsion
Speed	Moderate to rapid rhythm
Direction	Stationary, parallel to fibers, or across fibers
Contraindications	Open skin legions, contagious skin diseases, atrophied muscles, bruises, injury or inflammation, varicose veins, over the kidneys, over the spine or boney areas, after athletic activity

Technique 22   Tapotement

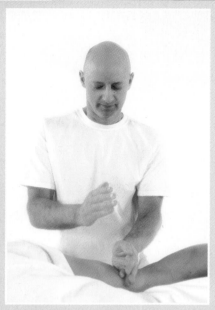

1. In hacking, the ulnar side of your hand is used to strike the client. Keep your fingers and wrists loose, because your fingers will hit each other at the bottom of the stroke.

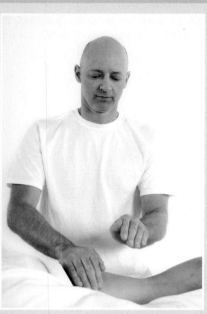

2. With cupping, hold your hands like cups and use in a percussive motion. Check to ensure that the strokes feel comfortable and move up and down and across the body area of the client so that the tapotement is constantly moving.

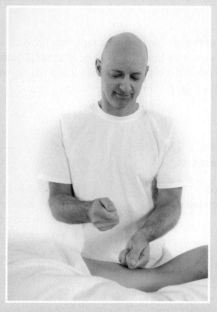

3. To apply a beating tapotement, make your hands into fists. The sides of your fists are used to perform the stroke with a force that is comfortable for the client. Make sure to keep your wrists loose while performing this stroke.

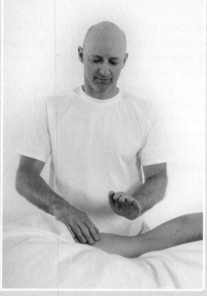

4. With the slapping technique, use your open hands to slap the client briskly and lightly.

Continued

Technique 22   **Tapotement** (Continued)

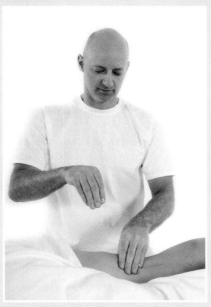

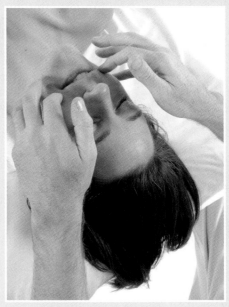

5. To apply the pincement technique, use your fingertips to pick up and then release small bits of superficial tissue in a percussive rhythm.

6. To apply the tapping technique, use your fingertips in a gentle tapotement to any area of the body, especially the face.

Topic **13-6**
Joint Movements

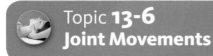

Joint movements involve a complicated process that includes the brain, nerves, muscles, and bones. The simple act of picking up a pencil, for example, requires a complex series of actions and reactions. The brain decides what movement to make and sends a signal through the nervous system to the muscles. The muscles then contract or lengthen to move the joints of the shoulder, elbow, wrist, and fingers so that the arm can reach out and the hand can grasp the pencil. Constant sensory feedback tells the brain where the arm and hand are in relationship to the pencil, and through this feedback the brain adjusts the position of the arm, hand, and fingers until the nerves in the fingers report that the pencil has been successfully grasped and lifted. This all happens in a fraction of a second.

Synonyms of "movement" include "progress," "advancement," "development," "change," and "passage." These concepts also relate to our sense of purpose in the world, as well as to the ability to grasp a pencil and take notes. Consider the saying: "Movement is life, and stagnation is death." In today's world of computers and repetitive work activities, people often hold their bodies in fixed, unchanging positions for long periods of time. The muscles, tendons, and fascia "learn" these new positions, such that the characteristics of being "short," "tense," and "rigid" come to seem normal. This is the stagnation that is the opposite of movement. While a person would literally die only if body organs came to a stop, with diminished muscular movement comes decreased physical expression and diminished psychological expression as well. An important goal for both you and your clients is to achieve both mental and physical fluidity along with free and effortless musculoskeletal movement. Joint movement techniques used as part of Swedish massage are a step in that direction.

Joint Movements: What's in a Name?

Therapeutic movements intended to improve joint flexibility were originally called "gymnastics," and some people still use this term. Joint flexibility techniques are also known as **range-of-motion** (**ROM**) techniques. Some massage therapy texts also use the term "joint mobilization," but that term will not

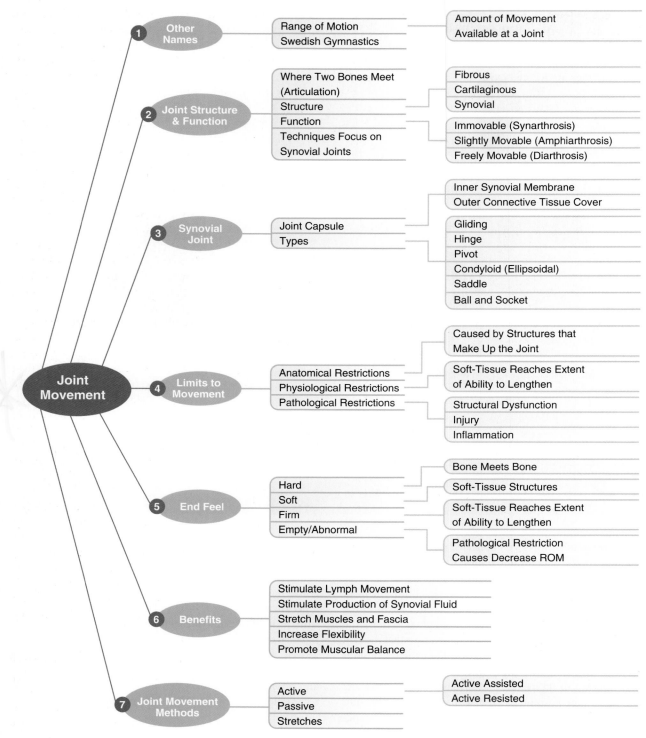

Figure 13-2 Mind map: joint movements.

be used here because some forms of joint mobilization use a high-velocity, low-amplitude thrusting movement. That type of mobilization, used by physical therapists and chiropractors, is outside the scope of practice for massage therapists. To prevent confusion, the terms "joint movements" and "range of motion" are used in this text (Fig. 13-2).

Review of Joint Structure and Function

The following brief review of joint structure and function is intended only as a refresher rather than a detailed discussion as in anatomy and kinesiology classes. Massage therapists are encouraged to learn all they can about joint structure and function and the muscles that move them.

A joint, also called an articulation, is the place where two or more bones meet (articulate). Joints are classified both by the way they are formed (structure) and by the type and degree of movement they allow (function).

Structurally, joints are classified as fibrous, cartilaginous, or synovial. Functionally, joints are classified as immovable (synarthrosis), slightly movable (amphiarthrosis), or freely movable (diarthrosis). For example, the bones of the cranium are held together at joints, called sutures, by dense fibrous connective tissue; sutures are classified as fibrous, immovable (synarthrosis) joints. Slightly movable (amphiarthrosis) joints like the pubic symphysis and the joints between vertebral bodies are called cartilaginous joints because the bones are connected by cartilage. Joint movement techniques focus predominantly on **synovial joints**, which are freely movable (diarthrosis) joints where the bones do not touch each other (Fig. 13-3). The ends of the bones are covered with an elastic, porous connective tissue called hyaline cartilage (or articular cartilage), which creates a smooth gliding surface for synovial articulations. Some synovial joints have additional padding from fat or fibrocartilage between bones (e.g., the medial and lateral meniscus in the knee). Fibrocartilage is different from hyaline cartilage. It is formed by thick bundles of connective tissue that are layered into sheets. It is very strong and very elastic. In areas of high stress, bursae (sacs filled with synovial fluid) help ease movement of the joints and decrease friction.

The bones in synovial joints are surrounded by a tough, connective tissue joint capsule and supported by ligaments and tendons. The joint capsule is composed of an inner layer called the synovial membrane, which secretes synovial fluid and forms a closed sac called a synovial cavity around the ends of the bones. This cavity is filled with viscous synovial fluid. Synovial fluid lubricates the joint, absorbs shock, and reduces friction between moving surfaces. It also contains some white blood cells that remove microbes as well as debris resulting from wear and tear. Hyaline cartilage relies on synovial fluid for nutrients and to remove waste products. Synovial fluid moves in and out of the porous cartilage and circulates around the joint as the joint moves. As long as the joint is moved, the synovial membrane secretes synovial fluid, and the hyaline cartilage remains lubricated and creates new cells. When there is little movement at the joint, the hyaline cartilage dries out and begins to deteriorate.

The outer layer of the joint capsule is formed by tough connective tissue that is continuous with the periosteum of the bones; this tissue allows movement but prevents dislocation of the bones from their normal position in the joint. Ligaments, a type of connective tissue, attach one bone to another. Some ligaments, called intrinsic or accessory ligaments, are interwoven with the joint capsule and thicken it. Other ligaments, called extracapsular or extrinsic ligaments, lie outside the joint capsule, attach directly from one bone to another, and provide additional support to the joint. The ligaments surrounding a joint contain specialized nerve endings that provide sensory information about the position of the joint and its movement. Tendons, which attach muscle to bone, entwine with the joint capsule in certain joints to provide further support. In other situations, the tendons do not entwine with the joint capsule but cross the joint and help to stabilize it.

In general, movement "opens" or "closes" a joint. When a joint is "open," the angle between the bones is reduced, cartilage is the least compressed, and the joint capsule and ligaments are to some degree slackened. Flexing your elbow (such as to touch your nose) "opens" the elbow joint. When a joint is "closed," the angle between the bones is increased, the cartilage is more compressed, and the joint capsule and ligaments are tighter. Bring your hand back to the anatomical position by extending your elbow to experience "closing" this joint.

Gliding joints, such as those between the carpal and tarsal bones in the wrist and ankles, are formed by bones with flattened or slightly curved surfaces that allow the bones to slide over each other, allowing small movements. With such joints, for example, structures in the foot can continually be adjusted slightly to balance the weight of the body.

Hinge joints, such as those between the trochlea of the humerus and the trochlear notch of the ulna at the elbow and in the interphalangeal joints of the fingers, allow movement in one direction (flexion and extension), like the opening and closing of a door.

Pivot joints, such as the joint between the atlas and axis and the joint between the head of the radius and the radial notch of the ulna, allow rotation of a bone. Examples include

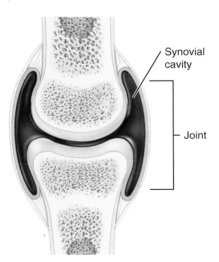

Figure 13-3 Structure of a synovial joint. Joint movement techniques focus predominantly on synovial joints, which are freely movable (diarthrosis) joints where the bones do not touch each other. The ends of the bones are covered with an elastic, porous connective tissue called hyaline cartilage (or articular cartilage), which creates a smooth gliding surface for synovial articulations.

Synovial cavity

Joint

the rotation of the head when you shake your head to say no and the rotation of the forearm that produces supination and pronation.

Condyloid joints (also called ellipsoidal joints), such as the articulation of the metacarpal with the first phalanx of the finger and the articulation of the radius with the scaphoid and lunate (carpal bones in the wrist), are formed when the oval-shaped condyle of one bone fits into the elliptical cavity of another bone. This type of joint allows movement in two directions, including flexion–extension, adduction–abduction, and circumduction where the joint can circulate through flexion and adduction, extension and abduction.

The human body has only one saddle joint: the joint formed by the trapezium of the wrist and the metacarpal of the thumb. The two articulating surfaces of this joint fit together like a rider sitting in a saddle, allowing several types of movement: flexion, extension, adduction, abduction, circumduction, and opposition.

Ball-and-socket joints, such as the articulation between the acetabulum of the hip bone and the head of the femur and between the head of the humerus and the glenoid fossa of the scapula, form when one bone has a ball-like surface that fits into the deep, rounded depression of the other bone. This is the most mobile type of joint, allowing for flexion, extension, abduction, adduction, medial rotation, lateral rotation, and circumduction.

Concept Brief 13-6
Joint Structure and Function

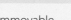

Fibrous (synarthrosis)	Immovable	Example: sutures
Cartilaginous (amphiarthrosis)	Slightly movable	Example: pubic symphysis
Synovial (diarthrosis)	Freely movable	Example: glenohumeral joint

---

Range of Motion, Limits to Movement, and End Feel

ROM refers to the amount of movement that is possible at a joint depending on its structure and condition. If the joint has normal structure and if no pathology exists, then the joint should have full and normal ROM. If the joint has structural anomalies, or if an injury or pathology exists, the joint is likely to exhibit reduced or limited ROM. If the joint's ROM is "normal," the joint can move freely and without pain in all of its actions. If the joint's ROM is restricted for some reason, the joint cannot move freely or without pain in some or all of its actions.

The normal ROM of every joint is restricted by its natural anatomical and physiological characteristics. Anatomical restrictions are restrictions caused by the structures that make up the joint itself. If the bones of a joint are pushed beyond their anatomical stopping point, damage could result. For example, the shoulder joint is formed by the head of the humerus articulating with the glenoid fossa of the scapula. This is a freely movable ball-and-socket joint, but the humerus is prevented from upward displacement by the presence of the acromion and coracoid process of the scapula and the lateral end of the clavicle. These anatomical structures prevent some movement at this joint.

Physiological restrictions typically limit the movement of the joint before anatomical restriction is reached. These usually result when soft-tissue structures like muscles, tendons, and ligaments reach the extent of their ability to lengthen at the end of a joint's ROM. This sensation is referred to as "firm-end feel." It's the place where the therapist feels the structures "push back."

There are three different types of normal **end feel**: hard, soft, and firm. Hard-end feel occurs when bone runs into bone, such as when the elbow is extended and the shape of the joint stops the movement (anatomical restriction). Sometimes the physiological restriction is due to soft tissue getting in the way of movement, such as when the elbow is flexed and the biceps and forearm muscles meet. This is called soft-end feel. Firm-end feel is the most common type of end feel. This is when muscles, tendons, ligaments, and the joint capsule reach the limit of their ability to lengthen without injury.

Pathological restrictions are abnormal restrictions that limit and decrease the joint's ROM because of pain or structural dysfunction. They may result from inflammation and fluid accumulation caused by an injury, adhesions in muscle or fascia, sustained muscular contractions, weakened muscles, degeneration of joint cartilage, tendonitis in a tendon that crosses a joint, or painful inflammation of a bursa. If soft-tissue structures are so tight that they significantly restrict movement before the joint reaches the end of its ROM, or if an injury or pathological condition stops the joint from achieving its full ROM, this is called abnormal-end feel or empty-end feel.

Joint fixation is a term used by chiropractors to describe diminished movement within the joint capsule space. Synovial joints allow a small but precise amount of movement, called **joint play**, which is not under the voluntary control of the client. This "play" in the joint allows for a slight amount of spin, glide, or roll in the joint articulation. Joint play can be palpated during passive joint movements administered by the therapist. For example, if a client flexes the wrist, it will reach a normal stopping point at about 90 degrees. If the therapist flexes the client's wrist passively, it can be moved beyond this 90-degree stopping point. This extra difference is the joint play (also called end play).

You can experience this by adducting and abducting your phalanges. Then flex and extend the phalanges by stabilizing the carpals with your other hand. Now try to rotate one phalange—you'll find you cannot. But you can rotate that phalange somewhat with your other hand; this is the joint's play. Joint play is essential for full, normal ROM and joint health. By lengthening tight muscles and by helping weak muscles to regain their normal firing patterns, massage therapists help restore the muscular balance necessary for normal joint play movements.

Cautions When Working with Joints

Numerous ailments may affect the client's joints and make joint movement techniques either uncomfortable or contraindicated (Table 13-1). Be sure to take a thorough health history and understand the client's physical condition before providing massage. If the client has had surgical replacements or has surgical pins or plates in place to stabilize a joint, the joint is likely more restricted. Joint movements may still be beneficial, but you will need to work more slowly and with greater caution. Never force a joint or use high-velocity thrusting movements or fast bouncing movements that cause the muscles to go into a protective contraction. Joint movement techniques should be relaxing and enjoyable for the client.

Benefits of Joint Movements

Joint movement techniques encourage the movement of lymph, stimulate the production of synovial fluid to lubricate and nourish the joint, increase local circulation, stretch muscles and fascia, and help reeducate the body about its movement potential. These techniques help maintain or increase the client's flexibility, maintain normal joint play, reduce muscle guarding and thereby gain greater kinesthetic awareness, increase relaxation, and improve muscular balance around the joint.[12]

Joint movements are often used as an assessment tool. For example, in active joint movement, the client performs the action, without assistance from the therapist, by contracting muscles and moving the joint through its full available ROM. Active joint movements reveal the client's willingness and ability to move. Always shadow clients to ensure their safety while they carry out the movements. When you shadow clients, you follow their movements to ensure they don't lose their balance or cause more damage to an injury. While the client performs each movement, you analyze it and assess its quality. Is it smooth and effortless? Does it seem shaky and uncertain? Is it stiff and limited? A client with an injury may refuse to move a joint, or may move it only a little and experience more pain. This information helps you determine which soft-tissue structures need attention during the session. Passive and resisted movements also provide information about the client's

TABLE 13-1 Conditions, Contraindications, and Cautions for Joint Movement Techniques

Common Bone or Joint Conditions

- **Avascular osteonecrosis:** Bone tissue is damaged or dies because circulation to that area of bone has been restricted. The head of the femur is particularly vulnerable.
- **Bursitis:** Painful inflammation of a bursa.
- **Dislocations:** A joint injury where the bones that articulate are traumatically separated.
- **Gout:** Deposits of sodium urate cause inflammatory arthritis, particularly in the joints of the feet.
- **Osteoarthritis:** Wear and tear on articular cartilage cause inflammation and degeneration of the joint.
- **Osteoporosis:** The bones are weakened because of endocrine imbalances or poor calcium metabolism.
- **Paget's disease:** Healthy bone is replaced with fibrous connective tissue that fails to calcify, causing pain and weakness.
- **Rheumatoid arthritis:** An autoimmune disease in which the immune system attacks synovial membranes.
- **Septic arthritis:** Inflammation in a joint caused by an infection in the joint capsule.
- **Sprain:** Tears in ligaments from just a few fibers to a complete rupture.

Contraindications

- Any condition contraindicated for massage
- Acute bone injuries (e.g., fracture)
- Recent dislocation
- Acute injuries to muscles associated with the joint (strain)
- Peripheral nerve injuries in associated areas
- Acute sprain
- Rheumatoid arthritis
- Osteoporosis
- Gout
- Avascular osteonecrosis
- Paget's disease
- Surgical reduction of ligaments
- Septic arthritis
- Acute osteoarthritis
- Bursitis
- Evidence of joint swelling, heat, redness, or increased pain with movement

Cautions

- Pins, plates, screws, or rods
- Chronic osteoarthritis
- History of dislocation
- Subacute or chronic *sprain*
- Subacute or chronic *strain*

As you develop your skills and understanding, you can work safely with clients with a broad variety of conditions or situations. While some contraindications are always contraindications (e.g., acute bone injuries), others become cautions with more experience (e.g., osteoporosis and rheumatoid arthritis). The contraindications listed here assume the therapist is a novice.

condition. When used as an assessment tool, ROM is analyzed both before and after the session to assess any changes that have occurred in the tissue as a result of the massage. ROM assessment is discussed in depth in Chapter 19.

Concept Brief 13-7
ROM and End Feel

ROM: Amount of movement available at a joint

Restrictions	Limits to joint movements
Anatomical	Structures that make up the joint restrict movement.
Physiological	Muscles, tendons, ligaments reach extent of ability to lengthen.
Pathological	Abnormal limits caused by structural dysfunction, injury, pathology.
End Feel	**The place where the structures "push back"**
Hard	Bone runs into bone.
Soft	Soft-tissue gets in the way of movement.
Firm	Muscles, tendons, ligaments reach extent of ability to lengthen.
Empty	Structural dysfunction, injury, or pathology prevents full ROM.
Abnormal	Same as empty-end feel

Types of Joint Movement Methods

Joint movement methods are classified as "active" (the client does the movement) and "passive" (the therapist moves the client) joint movements. A variety of techniques fall under these two general headings. Active movements include active-assisted and active-resisted movements. Table 13-2 provides an overview of joints commonly moved during a Swedish massage.

Joint movement methods make the most sense when you understand the structure of the joint, the actions available at the joint, and the actions of the associated muscles. You will build this knowledge throughout your training program. Keep a kinesiology book on hand for reference, and look up each joint and its muscles to become more familiar with these structures. Seeing the direction of muscle fibers and understanding where muscles attach increase one's understanding of joint movement techniques.

Active Joint Movements

In a Swedish massage the client usually wants to relax as much as possible, and therefore passive techniques are most often used (as described later). However, active joint movement combined with massage strokes feels good and gives the massage more substance. Having the client perform a particular movement during a massage stroke can increase the effectiveness of the stroke because the movement lengthens target muscles while the stroke broadens and stretches the muscle fibers. The client benefits from the stimulation of synovial fluid as well as the release of tight muscle tissue. Technique 23 demonstrates some of these techniques.

Active-Assisted Joint Movements

Active-assisted techniques help restore a limited or stiffened joint to a fuller ROM after an injury or a long period of inactivity. First move the joint passively to show the client how the movement should be performed. The client then begins the

TABLE 13-2   Selected Joints That Might Be Moved during a Swedish Massage

Depression of the mandible

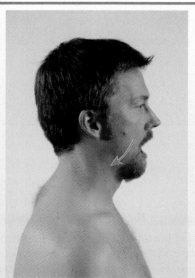

Elevation of the mandible

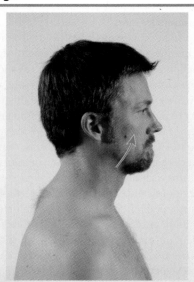

TABLE 13-2   Selected Joints That Might Be Moved during a Swedish Massage *(Continued)*

Neck flexion

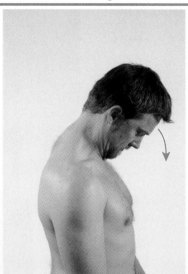

Neck extension

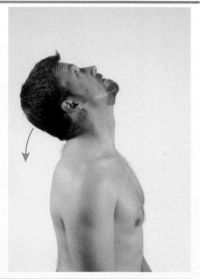

Neck rotation

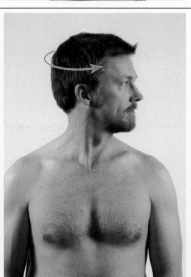

Neck lateral flexion

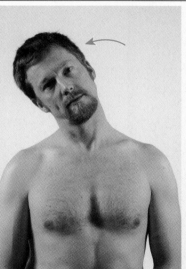

Shoulder flexion

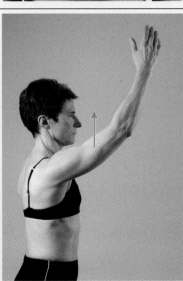

Shoulder extension

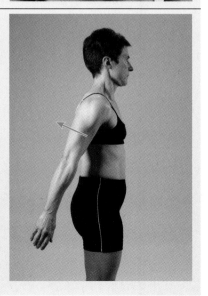

(continued)

TABLE 13-2   **Selected Joints That Might Be Moved during a Swedish Massage** *(Continued)*

Shoulder abduction	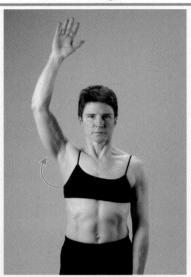	Shoulder adduction	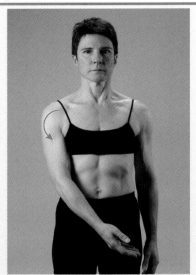
Elbow flexion	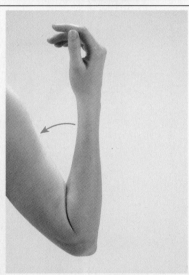	Elbow extension	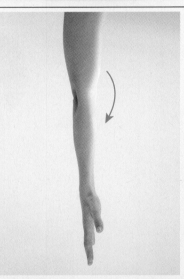
Pronation of the forearm	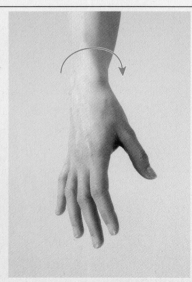	Supination of the forearm	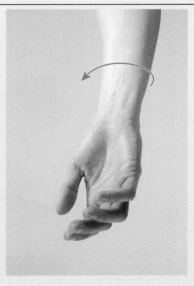

TABLE 13-2   Selected Joints That Might Be Moved during a Swedish Massage *(Continued)*

Wrist flexion 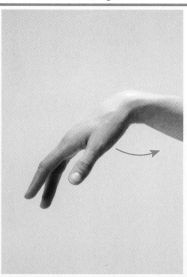		Wrist extension 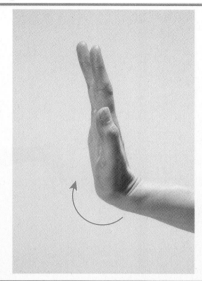
Hip flexion 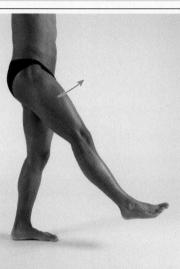		Hip extension 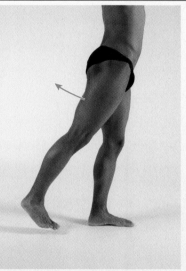
Hip abduction 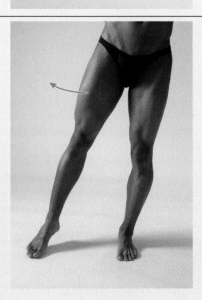		Hip adduction 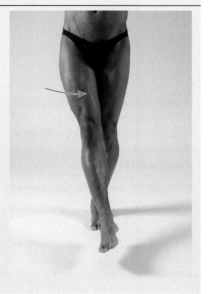

(continued)

TABLE 13-2   Selected Joints That Might Be Moved during a Swedish Massage (Continued)

Knee flexion	Knee extension
Plantarflexion	Dorsiflexion

movement and takes the movement as far as possible, after which you assist the client as needed to complete the movement. This activity is repeated many times to build the client's flexibility and strength. This technique is demonstrated in Technique 24.

Active-Resisted Joint Movements

Active-resisted movements help build the client's strength while taking a joint through its full ROM to lubricate the joint structure with synovial fluid. Sometimes active-resisted techniques help reeducate the muscle so that it can regain its normal firing pattern. This helps promote greater muscular balance at the joint. In an active-resisted technique, the client carries out the movement while you resist the movement. For example, ask the client to abduct the arm. Place one hand directly above the client's wrist and the other hand directly above the client's elbow. As the client performs the movement, you gently resist the movement while allowing it to be completed. Each time the client tries to carry out the movement, add a little more resistance to build up the client's strength. Resisted movements should never be forceful. Clients should not need to exert all of their strength to complete the movement. Think of resistance as just strong enough to make clients work a little harder than normal to complete the movement. This technique is demonstrated in Technique 25.

| **Technique 23** | **Active Joint Movements Paired With Massage** |

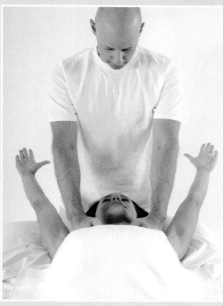

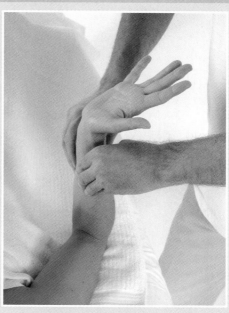

1. Having the client perform a particular movement during a massage stroke can increase the effectiveness of the stroke because the movement lengthens target muscles while the stroke broadens and stretches the muscle fibers. A nice technique for the pectoralis major muscle is the "pec angle" technique. Place your knuckles or palms on the origin of the pectoralis major muscles. Compress the tissue to broaden and stretch the muscles while the client adducts and abducts the arm.

2. This technique broadens and lengthens the flexors and extensors in the forearm. The client actively flexes and extends the wrist while you apply a friction stroke down the flexor and extensor muscles of the forearm.

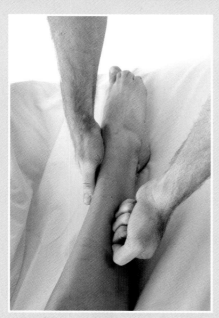

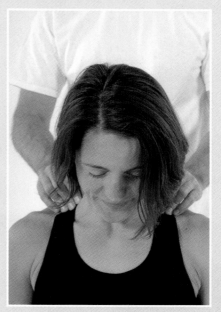

3. Ask the client to point the toes first toward the knee and then toward the area behind the massage table. Apply a friction stroke up either side of the tibia while the client dorsiflexes and plantar flexes the foot.

4. With the client seated in a chair, apply a friction stroke from the occiput down the posterior side of the neck as the client slowly flexes the neck and head.

Continued

| Technique 23 | Active Joint Movements Paired With Massage (Continued) |

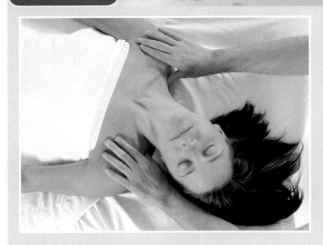 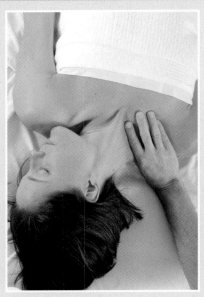

5. Ask the client to laterally flex the neck by touching each ear to the shoulder. Place your hands on either side of the neck and compress the tissue during the movement to broaden and stretch the fibers.

6. Use the same basic hand placement but ask the client to rotate the chin from one side to another. As the head rotates away from your hand, pick up the trapezius and feel it pull out of your hand as rotation lengthens the muscles.

| Technique 24 | Active-Assisted Joint Movements |

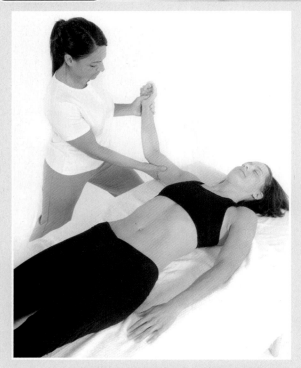 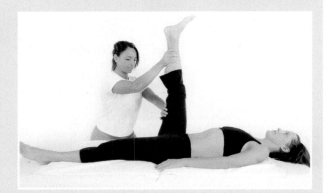

1. Practice active-assisted joint movements by asking the client to abduct the arm (demonstrate the movement first). The client starts to abduct the arm and then you help complete the motion at the end of the joint's ROM.

2. The client begins the motion of hip flexion and you help complete the motion at the end of the joint's ROM.

| **Technique 25** | **Active-Resisted Joint Movements** |

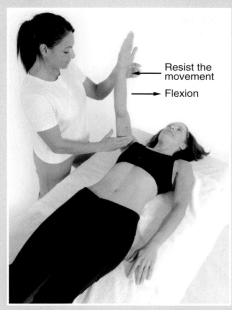

1. Active-resisted joint movements are most often used in ROM assessment and in healthcare massages to build client strength. Later you will learn additional active-resisted techniques. For now, practice resisted shoulder flexion by placing one hand directly above the wrist and the other directly as a guide above the elbow. Ask the client to move the arm into flexion while you resist the movement with the hand above the wrist but allow it to be completed.

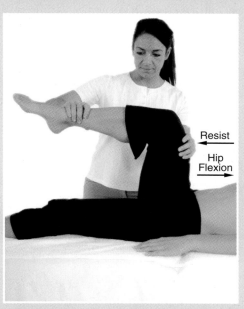

2. Move to the lower legs and practice resisted hip flexion. Place one hand on the client's leg by the ankle to stabilize the leg and hip and the other on the quadriceps directly above the knee. Ask the client to flex the hip.

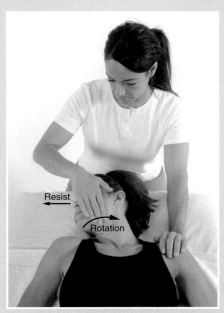

3. Move to the top of the table for resisted neck rotation. Place a hand on the client's chin and gently resist the movement as the client rotates the head to one side and then the other.

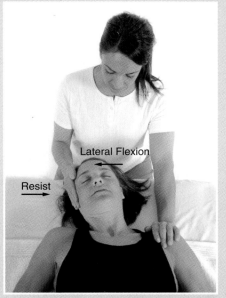

4. For resisted lateral flexion of the neck, place a hand on the side of the client's head and gently resist the movement as the client laterally flexes to one side and the other.

Passive Joint Movements

Passive joint movements are performed while the client is fully relaxed. You move the joint in a number of different directions to stimulate synovial fluid, relax the body, and reduce muscle guarding. Some clients resist passive movements, even when they do not consciously want to resist. It requires a great deal of trust to turn a body part over to someone else. Encourage clients to breathe and release the body area. Usually, over time clients learn how to allow passive joint movements. Passive joint movement is demonstrated in Technique 26.

| Technique 26 | Passive Joint Movement Techniques |

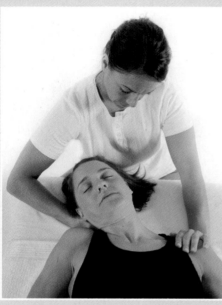

1. Sit at the head of the table and stabilize the shoulder with one hand while the other moves the head and neck into lateral flexion. This movement can be used alone or with a massage stroke.

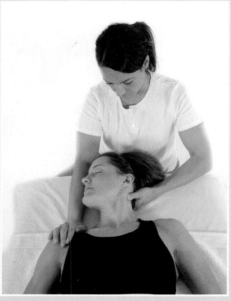

2. Next, stabilize the shoulder with one hand and use the other hand to move the head into rotation. This movement can be used alone or with a massage stroke.

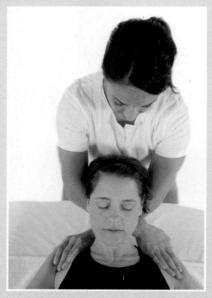

3. To passively stretch the neck into flexion, cross your forearms and place a hand on each shoulder. Lift the head into flexion.

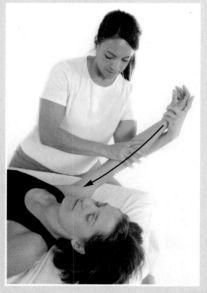

4A. For the "dance of the arms," hold the arm directly below the wrist with one hand and lay the client's arm across your forearm so that the client's arm swings above the head. Stroke down the inside of the client's arm.

Technique 26 | **Passive Joint Movement Techniques** (Continued)

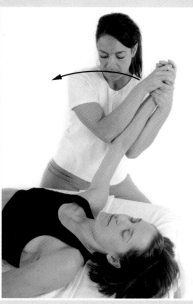

4B. Stroke up the arm and transfer the weight of the arm to your other hand by grasping the arm between your elbows to stabilize it.

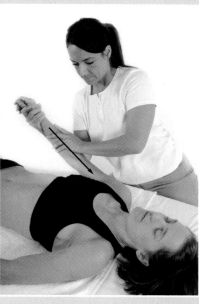

4C. Now lay the client's arm across your forearm and elbow so that it swings down by the client's side, and stroke up the client's arm to the shoulder. Rock the arm back and forth in this dance-like manner until the arm moves freely.

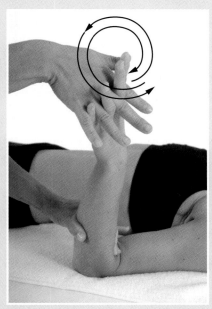

5. Hold the client's arm directly above the wrist with one hand and the client's fingers with your other hand. Move the wrist in clockwise and counterclockwise circles. You might also hold the client's hand in both hands and move the sides back and forth with a scissor-like movement to loosen the gliding joints. Gently pull and twist each finger (not shown).

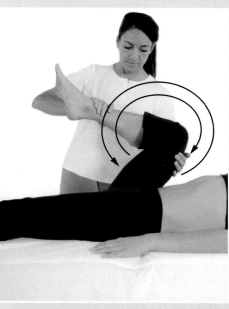

6. To passively move the hip joint with the client supine, hold the client's leg above the ankle with your hand closest to the end of the table, and place your other hand above the knee. Move the client's upper leg first in clockwise circles and then counterclockwise.

Continued

Technique 26	**Passive Joint Movement Techniques** (Continued)

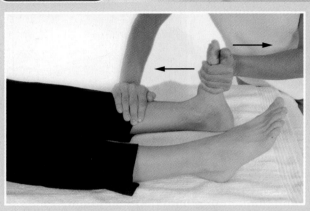

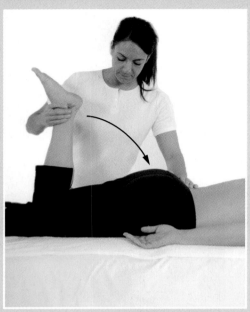

7. With the client supine plantar flex and dorsiflex the foot, and then move the foot in circles first clockwise and then counterclockwise.

8. With the client prone, slowly bring the heel toward the gluteals until you feel resistance and return it to the starting position. Stabilize the thigh with one hand and move the leg in circles with the other.

Passive Stretches

Passive stretches move a joint through its ROM and lengthen muscles, tendons, ligaments, and the joint capsule to increase flexibility. Stretching works well at the end of a massage for a particular body area when the structures are warm and soft. Never bounce the client in the stretch. Bouncing in a stretch can cause microscopic tearing of muscle fibers. This can lead to the formation of scar tissue and additional loss of elasticity. Avoid stretching the client so far as to cause pain because this can lead to tissue damage and a protective contracting of muscle tissue. Stretching the client too fast activates the stretch reflex and may cause more tension in the muscles. To stretch the client, take the joint to firm-end feel and then gently, slowly, and evenly push a little way past firm-end feel. Work slowly and pay attention to the quality of the tissue. Some passive stretches are shown in Technique 27.

The techniques for joint movements illustrated in this chapter are just some of the methods available for each joint. When you learn a technique in one area of the body, be sure to apply it in other areas also. Strive to understand the concept behind the technique so that you can apply it to any area of the body. If it works on the ankle, can it work on the wrist? If it works for the knee, can it work for the elbow? How would this same technique be applied to the hip? Try it and do not be afraid if it takes some time to figure out how to make it feel coordinated. In upcoming chapters, you will see how these solid Swedish skills form a foundation for learning more advanced techniques.

Concept Brief 13-8
Types of Joint Movement Methods

Active	**The client does the movement**
Active Assisted	The client starts the movement and the therapist helps finish.
Active Resisted	The therapist resists the client's movement to build strength.
Passive	**The therapist moves the client**
Passive Stretches	The therapist moves the client's joint slightly past firm end feel.

Technique 27 | **Passive Stretches**

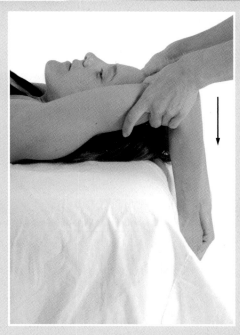

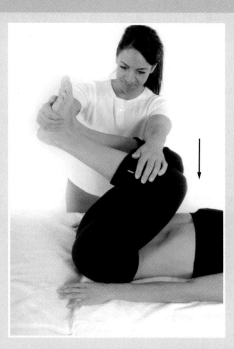

1. For an upper body stretch, ask the client to bring the arms up over the head. Grasp the arms directly above the elbows, and pull them slowly backward keeping the client's arm close to the head. Continue to push the arms down, working slowly, until the client feels a stretch.

2. For a spinal stretch, ask the client to bring the knees up toward the chest. Place your arm across the lower legs directly below the knees, and gently press the knees into the chest to stretch the lower back. From this position, you can also reach up to stabilize the client's shoulder while rolling the knees to the side and down toward the table to stretch the spine (not shown). Repeat the stretch on the other side.

3. In a variation of a spinal stretch, place one leg across the other with the foot flat next to the knee of the flat leg. Press the knee over while lifting the client's shoulder so that a mild twist is experienced in the spine.

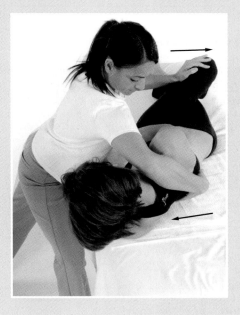

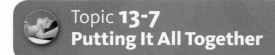

Topic **13-7**
Putting It All Together

When you first begin providing massages to clients, your approach will be somewhat different from how you will later perform massage therapy as a seasoned professional. In the beginning, it is enough to remember a stroke's French name, how it is performed, and why it is used. As you progress, you will learn to think more about the massage session as a whole system rather than the individual components.

Before reading further, review Tables 13-3 and 13-4 to assess your understanding of Swedish skills. Think about the individual strokes, how they tie together, their effects on the body, and how you palpate and adapt the techniques during a massage. The next step is then to understand how to sequence the massage and use the subtleties of massage skills.

TABLE 13-3 **Overview of Swedish Massage Techniques**

Stroke	Defined	General Effects	Contraindication	Variations
Effleurage	A long, gliding stroke usually applied toward the heart.	Desquamation of dead skin cells, increases circulation and lymph flow, triggers parasympathetic nervous system response, supports venous return, relaxation.	Should not be used distal to an area of inflammation or injury; avoid application over open skin legions, skin diseases, or bruises. Avoid prolonged application on the limbs of clients with cardiovascular disorders, high blood pressure, or circulatory conditions.	Superficial, moderate, or deep, shingling technique.
Petrissage	A rhythmic stroke that lifts the muscle off the bone and compresses it between the fingers.	Stimulates sebaceous secretion, increases circulation and lymph flow, activates GTOs to relax muscles, decreases adhesions.	Avoid use with atrophied muscles that lack moderate tone. Do not use over open skin legions, skin diseases, bruises, acute injuries, inflammation, or moderate to severe varicose veins.	Skin rolling, fulling petrissage, wringing petrissage.
Friction	A heat-producing chafing or rubbing stroke.	Superficial friction is stimulating, warming, and increases blood and lymph flow. Deep friction separates muscle fibers and breaks up adhesions and scar tissue.	Do not apply friction over open skin legions, skin diseases, bruises, acute injuries, inflammation, or moderate to severe varicose veins.	Superficial friction, circular friction, linear friction, cross-fiber friction.
Vibration	A pulsating tremor-like or oscillating stroke.	Primarily stimulating, then relaxing; sustained vibration is numbing and analgesic, decreases muscle guarding; fast vibrations can cause muscle contractions and stimulate nerves.	Do not apply vibration over open skin legions, skin diseases, bruises, acute injuries, inflammation, or moderate to severe varicose veins.	Fine vibration, coarse vibration including jostling, shaking, rocking.
Tapotement	A rapid and rhythmic percussion stroke with the hands in various formations to drum on the client.	Short applications are stimulating; longer applications are relaxing. Very light tapotement causes vasoconstriction of capillaries in the local area. Moderate tapotement causes increased circulation. Useful for loosening of mucus.	Do not apply tapotement over the kidneys, over boney areas, especially directly over the spine, or over bruises or varicose veins.	Light, moderate, hacking, cupping, beating, slapping, pincement, tapping.
Joint movements	Movements like flexion, extension, abduction, and adduction performed as part of the massage.	Stimulate the production of synovial fluid to nourish and protect the joint structure. Increase ROM.	General contraindications include acute injuries to bones, joints, muscles, or nerves. Techniques that traction the joint are contraindicated for sprains, rheumatoid arthritis, and hypermobile joints. See specific contraindications in Table 13-1.	Active, passive, and restricted.

TABLE 13-4 Overview of Swedish Massage Considerations

General Benefits

- Desquamation of dead skin cells
- Increased sebaceous secretion to condition skin
- Increased blood and lymph circulation (increased tissue warmth)
- Improved nutrient and waste exchange in local tissue
- Improved venous return
- Decreased muscle spasm, tension, and soreness
- Decreased adhesions in myofascia
- Decreased pain
- Increased ROM and joint health
- Increased relaxation
- Decreased symptoms relating to stress
- Improved muscle tone

Application Choices

The effects of the massage technique on the body vary depending on how the stroke is applied. Pay attention to
- **Technique**: Gliding vs. lifting
- **Depth**: Light vs. deep
- **Speed**: Fast vs. slow
- **Direction**: Toward the heart vs. away from the heart
- **Duration:** Brief application vs. prolonged application

Palpation

Palpation skills increase with more experience. Develop palpation skills by being aware of what you see and feel during the massage session.
- **Visual**: How does the client look (skin color, expression, posture, etc.)?
- **Move**: How does the client move (stiffly, lightly, forcefully, smoothly, etc.)?
- **Touch**: How does the tissue feel (crackly, taut, fluid, hot, cool, clammy, etc.)?
- **Sound:** How does the client sound when he or she communicates (relaxed, sleepy, anxious, fretful, etc.)?

Subtle Factors

- **Intention:** Client centered
- **Contact**: Quality of touch
- **Use of Lubricant**: Use lubricant in moderation. Remove excess lubricant if not absorbed into the skin.
- **Pacing and Leading**: Match the client's pace and then lead the client to more relaxing rhythms.
- **Depth**: Engage the tissue unless a superficial massage is requested.
- **Rhythm:** Use regular patterns or strokes and a regular tempo.
- **Flow and Continuity**: Techniques should flow in an uninterrupted action so the client experiences the constant and steady pressure of your hands.
- **Stroke Length**: Work the length of the muscle or the length of the body area.

Sequencing

Sequencing refers both to the sequence of strokes (the order in which strokes are applied to a given body area) and to the overall sequence of the massage (the order in which body areas are massaged). In Swedish massage, the strokes often follow a defined progression from effleurage to petrissage, to friction, to vibration, to tapotement, with joint movement added as appropriate. Each stroke addresses the tissue in a different way, and the sequence of strokes takes into account the physiological changes that have occurred in soft tissue during the preceding stroke. In a traditional Swedish massage, the therapist might simply deliver each type of stroke to the body area in a predefined order before moving on to the next body area. Alternatively, the order of the strokes might be changed to meet the client's particular needs.

Often a therapist combines different massage systems in a session, which may change the sequencing of the strokes. For example, if myofascial release techniques (discussed in depth in Chapter 20) are being combined with Swedish massage and deep tissue work, myofascial techniques would probably be applied first because they are used on dry skin without lubrication. Deep tissue strokes might be used directly after effleurage, petrissage, and moderate friction, with vibration and tapotement coming after. Another factor determining the sequencing of techniques is the quality of the client's tissue and how quickly it changes. Some clients need a prolonged warm-up, while others are ready for deep work early in the session. Sometimes, areas of taut muscle tissue require work with very specific techniques to reset muscle length and promote better muscular balance. This is why it is important for new massage therapists to continue to develop their palpation skills.

Observe clients and notice how they hold their bodies, their skin coloration and how it changes during the session, and their facial expressions. Listen to clients and notice how their breathing changes during a technique, and listen to sounds they make as the session progresses. Feel the texture of the client's tissue and notice its temperature and pliability. Before long, you will instinctively know which muscles to focus on and which techniques will bring about the greatest positive changes. Your personal rhythm and movements will start to instinctively change so that they harmonize better with the client. Interestingly, although this may feel like instinct, it is in fact a learned skill. Your skill level leads to choices about which body areas to address first, and which body areas to address for a longer time.

When deciding which body areas to address first, be flexible and use your communication skills. There are advantages to starting the massage with the client supine, and other advantages to starting prone. When the massage starts in a supine position, clients can open their eyes and look at you. This is important if the client is new to massage and does not know you. As you can visually check with the client during the first half of the massage, the client gains more confidence and relaxes. Clients also often experience congestion when they are placed face down on the table. On the other hand, if the massage starts in the prone position, the client's sinuses have time to decongest during the second half of the massage when they are in the supine position. This allows the client to leave the session feeling more alert and with less facial puffiness.

TABLE 13-5 **Examples of Different Massage Sequencing**

Example Sequence 1	Example Sequence 2	Example Sequence 3
1. Begin with client prone	1. Begin with client supine	1. Begin with client prone
2. Place warm pack on the lower back	2. Place warm pack on abdominals	2. Place warm packs on hamstrings
3. Open massage with holding strokes	3. Open massage with diaphragmatic breathing exercise	3. Open the massage with holding strokes
4. Massage posterior legs	4. Massage neck and face	4. Myofascial release to back
5. Remove warm pack and place on feet	5. Massage arms	5. Massage back
6. Massage back	6. Massage anterior legs and feet	6. Deep tissue massage back
7. Remove warm pack	7. Remove warm pack from abdominals	7. Remove warm packs from hamstrings and place on back
8. Turn client supine	8. Turn client prone	8. Myofascial release to posterior legs
9. Transition to anterior massage with diaphragmatic breathing exercise	9. Transition to posterior massage with holding strokes	9. Massage posterior legs
10. Massage anterior legs	10. Massage back	10. Remove warm packs
11. Massage feet	11. Massage posterior legs	11. Turn client supine
12. Massage abdominals	12. Close massage with three deep breaths	12. Myofascial release anterior legs
13. Place fresh warm pack on abdominals		13. Massage anterior legs
14. Massage arms and hands		14. Massage abdominals
15. Massage shoulders and neck		15. Psoas release work
16. Massage face		16. Passive hamstring stretches
17. Close massage with holding strokes		17. Passive lower back stretches
		18. Massage neck and upper arms
		19. Close massage with holding strokes

Specific treatment goals may also determine the sequencing of a session. For example, if the client has lower back pain, you might choose to release the hamstrings and adductors of the legs before working the back, and then turn the client supine to finish with psoas work and spinal stretches (discussed in upcoming chapters). In healthcare massages, some regions of the body might not be massaged at all, allowing more time for problem areas.

Most important to sequencing the massage is the information from the client in the intake interview. This process involves designing the session to meet the client's needs. Sometimes it is a little like a negotiation. The client might say, "I want a lot of work on my back and legs." You might say, "Do you only want me to work on these areas, or would you like a full-body massage with extra focus on these areas?" The client might then say, "I want you to work on my back, legs, feet, and neck, with most of the work on my back." You can also suggest areas the client needs to have massaged based on your assessment findings. You and client now have an agreed plan for the session.

The term "full-body massage" often means something different to clients than to therapists. Clients sometimes say they want a full-body massage and then express dismay when their abdominals or gluteals are undraped and massaged. Always be clear about what will happen during the massage by saying things like, "In a full body massage, I massage the legs, feet, arms, back, neck, gluteal muscles (the muscles of the buttocks), abdominal muscles (the muscles of the belly), and the face. Would you prefer I avoid any of these areas?"

While the client's wishes always prevail (unless they are asking for techniques that are contraindicated, illegal, or out of the massage scope of practice), you can educate clients about the benefits of massage for certain areas. For example, clients often feel uncomfortable with the idea of having their gluteals or abdominal muscles massaged. When you take the time to explain the importance of releasing tension in these muscles, the client may feel safe enough to give it a try. The three examples of massage sequences in Table 13-5 demonstrate how diverse sequencing can be. These sequences use some of the techniques described later in this chapter for enhancing a wellness session.

Routines

Routines are a series of strokes that are planned in advance, delivered to body areas in a preset order, and practiced until they flow smoothly together. Some spas and massage clinics develop set routines that are delivered by all of the business's therapists. These standardized wellness sessions often include enhancing extras like the use of warm packs, aromatherapy, and foot soaks to increase the client's sense of luxury and relaxation. Standardized wellness sessions are discussed in Chapter 15. The drawback to such routines is that clients may not get the specific work they want or need for their particular areas of muscular tension. The advantage is that clients know beforehand what the massage will be like and can count on receiving the same massage when they return for another session. When massage is used purely for relaxation, the predictable quality of a set routine can actually add to the client's sense of safety and ability to unwind. The danger for the therapist is that a set routine makes it easy to stop paying close attention to the individual client.

Routines for specific body areas are very useful in relaxation settings. For example, some therapists develop a very effective foot routine that helps them to build a loyal clientele who especially like foot massage. In many spas, the face is massaged while the body is cocooned in a body wrap. A face massage routine that incorporates a variety of strokes is likely to enhance the client's experience. Technique 28

| Technique 28 | Foot Massage |

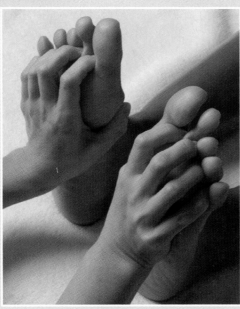

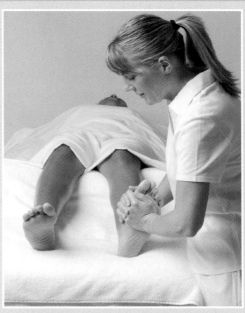

1. In the laced fingers hold, the fingertips of each hand are placed on the plantar surface of the foot, lacing them almost but not actually in between the toes. Hang on the foot as if hanging onto a ledge with just your fingertips.

2. Stand on the lateral side of the foot facing toward the table for the sandwich slide. Slide your interlaced fingers down the medial edge of the client's foot to the heel and then back up to the starting position.

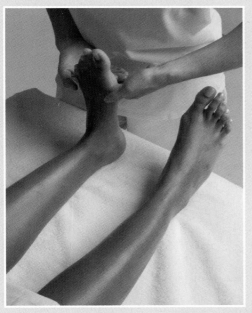

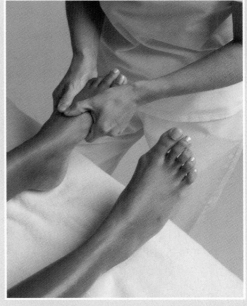

3. Push the foot into dorsiflexion with the edge of your hands placed against the metatarsal heads. Run the edge of your hands down the plantar surface and around the heel, pulling the foot into plantar flexion at the end of the stroke.

4. Starting at the distal part of the foot, use circular motions with your thumbs down the dorsal surface of the foot. Then apply moderate pressure in a circular motion around the ankle with your palms.

Continued

Technique 28   **Foot Massage** (Continued)

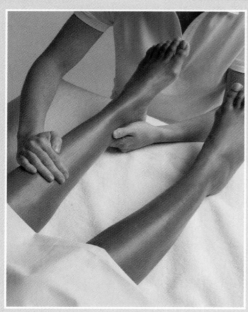

5. Run one hand up the anterior surface of the lower leg and the other down the posterior surface of the lower leg for the Achilles stroke.

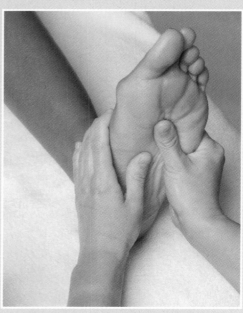

6. Apply circular friction with your thumbs from the heel to the toes.

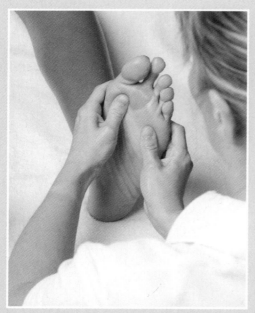

7. Apply thumb friction in a crossing pattern from the bottom of the toes to the heel. When you reach the heel, use circular thumb friction to work back up the foot again.

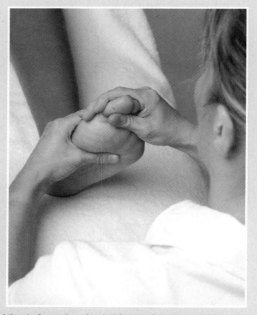

8. Stabilize the foot with one hand while your other rotates all of the toes in a circle. Repeat, this time rotating the toes in the opposite direction. Now twist each toe gently back and forth while gently pulling on it.

Technique 28   **Foot Massage** (Continued)

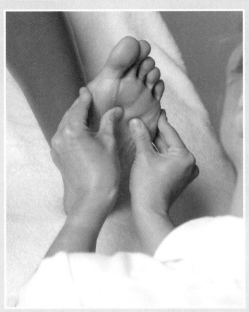

9. With your thumbs on the plantar surface of the foot, circle your fingers down the sides of the foot using firm pressure.

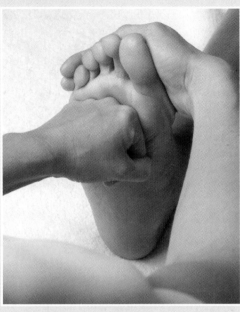

10. Make a fist and place it against the ball of the foot. Your other hand on the dorsal surface stabilizes the foot. Using a rhythmic motion, plantar flex and dorsiflex the foot to loosen it.

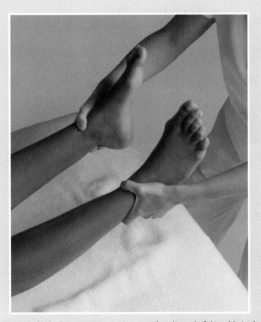

11. To conclude the foot massage session, stand at the end of the table in the center and hold each leg just above the ankle. Lift the legs and bounce them on the massage table three times.

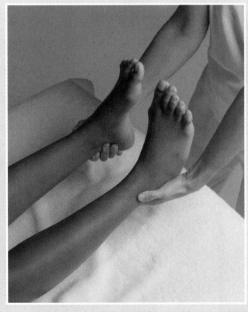

12. Bring your hands around the legs, lean backward, and traction while swinging the legs right and left. This releases the sacroiliac joint and relaxes the lower back.

provides guidance for the application of foot techniques, while Technique 29 demonstrates a basic face massage routine.

The use of routines is not advised for healthcare massage or massage sessions in which the client and therapist have agreed on specific treatment goals. In these cases, you adapt the massage to the client's specific needs and to moment-by-moment changes in the client's soft-tissue structures.

The term "routine" should not be confused with a "treatment protocol" in which a series of techniques are used in a particular order. For example, in trigger point work, the protocol is to warm the area with friction strokes or skin rolling before the trigger point is located and treated. Joint movement and flushing strokes are applied after the trigger point has been treated to help reset the muscle's normal resting length.

Subtle Factors That Influence the Massage

Novice therapists must master individual techniques before trying to combine them in a flowing, integrated professional massage. After mastering these core skills, you can consider how subtle factors like intention, depth, stroke length, and rhythm profoundly influence the client's massage experience.

Therapist's Intention

Chapter 11 describes the importance of centering and grounding before a session. This helps to calm your energy and focus your mind so that you are fully present during the session. Some therapists forget this principle and talk

---

| Technique 29 | Face Massage |

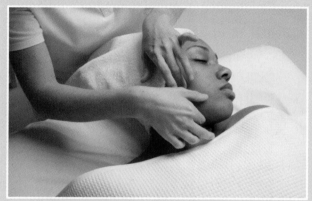

1. Apply a light lotion starting under the chin, coming up around the mouth, around the nose, up the nose to the forehead, and down the sides of the face to the chin. Spread the lotion evenly over the entire face.

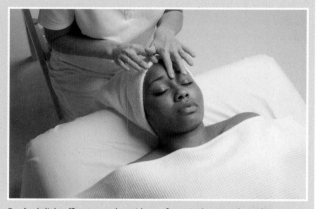

2. Apply light effleurage strokes with your fingertips between the eyebrows.

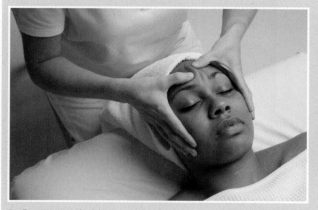

3. Transition into the S-bowing strokes shown here and cover the entire forehead area with this technique.

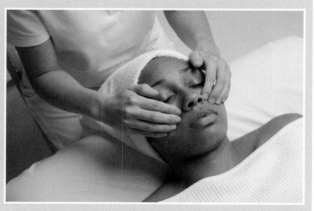

4. Transition to glides down either side of the nose that circle around, and repeat three to six times.

Technique 29   **Face Massage** (Continued)

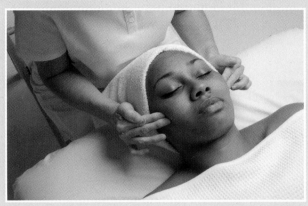

5. Transition into small figure-eights using light fingertip pressure. Glide over the entire face, chin, and forehead with this technique.

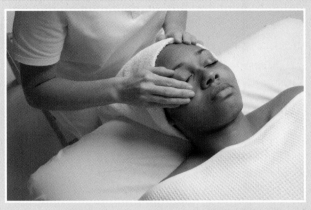

6. Make small circles around the eyes, or alternate your hands to circle one eye and then the other.

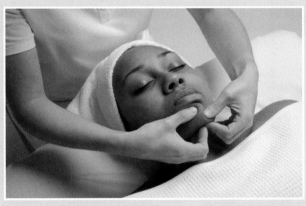

7. Lightly petrissage the jawline and S-bow the chin. Then use a crossed-thumb technique at the chin.

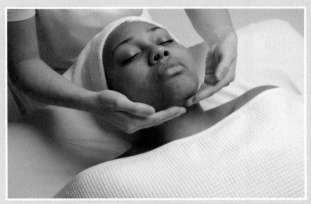

8. With soft hands and relaxed wrists, apply a gentle slapping tapotement to the underside of the jaw. Bring the gentle slapping tapotement up the jawline and cheek area, and then transition back underneath the jaw.

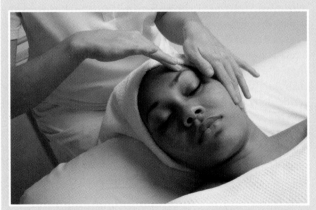

9. Soothe the sides of the face with gentle upward strokes directed toward the top of the client's forehead.

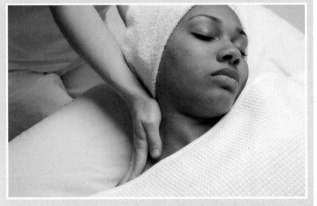

10. Gently massage the outer edge of the ear, and push the ear forward to stretch it. Massage the area directly behind the ear and finish the area by laterally flexing the neck and head to one side during a long stroke down the neck, over the shoulder, and down the arm. Repeat this stroke on the opposite side.

Continued

Technique 29   **Face Massage** (Continued)

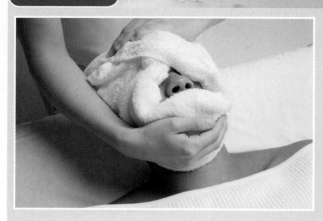

11. Place a steamy rosemary towel over the face for 1 minute to end the face massage routine. Learn about the application of warm steamy towels to enhance relaxation massage in Chapter 15.

loudly, bang into things, fuss with supplies, the drape, or the music, and cause such static in a room that the client cannot completely relax. Before entering the treatment room, take a moment to center and ground your energy. Pay attention to your tone of voice and volume. Talk softly, but not so softly that the client has difficulty understanding your verbal directions. Everything should be ready for the session before the client undresses and moves into position beneath the drape. If music is playing at a pleasant level, if the lubricant is warm and within reach, if extra blankets, bolsters, and draping material are readily available, you are likely to feel more centered and grounded.

When working with a therapeutic intention, maintain appropriate professional boundaries and work in such a way that the client will not experience emotional, physical, mental, or spiritual damage from the session. Therapeutic intention also includes the idea that you are focused only on the session. You are "present," "in the moment," and paying attention to the client's facial expressions, sounds, soft tissue, and communication. When you walk through the door of the treatment room, everything but the client should go away. Set aside all thoughts about paying bills, relationship problems, to-do lists, and plans with friends so that you focus only on the client.

Contact

The quality of your touch is important, and you must think about what your hands are communicating to the client. Warm, soft, dry, open, and confident hands tell the client that you are relaxed and self-assured and know what to do. Cool, damp, uncertain hands tell the client that you are anxious or doubtful about the session. Cultivate confidence in your touch. Do not just touch the client but feel the tissue, open your hands, and sink into the muscle. Once you establish contact, avoid disrupting it. Sometimes novice therapists take their hands off the client repeatedly while transitioning between strokes, or lift their hands off the body to get more

lubricant. Instead try to keep at least one hand in contact with the client at all times. This helps the client to keep track of your presence and the progression of the massage.

Use of Lubricant

In a Swedish massage, most strokes require the use of lubrication to prevent undue friction between your hands and the client's skin. Use the lubricant in moderation. When the client is too slippery, your hands cannot sink into the tissue and manipulate it effectively. After undraping a body area, turn one hand over and place it on the client's skin with the palm side up. Pour a small amount of lubricant into your palm and warm it by rubbing your other hand across it, staying in contact with the client's skin. Turn both hands over and apply long strokes over the entire undraped body area to spread the lubricant. As the lubricant is absorbed into the skin, work the strokes deeper into the tissue. If the skin becomes dry and the strokes start to drag, apply more lubricant (some drag on the tissue is desirable with certain strokes). Again, do not break contact with the client. Keep one hand in contact with the client's skin while warming the lubricant in your hands. If you accidentally apply too much lubricant and it is not absorbed into the skin during effleurage strokes, remove some of the lubricant with a hand towel. It's better to take a moment and remove the lubricant than give a slippery superficial massage of the body area. Most clients do not want to feel oily at the end of the massage. It is a good idea to provide disposable "wet-wipe" towels and a dry hand towel for the client to use at the end of the massage if you use oil for the lubricant. Creams and lotions cause less slip but also feel cooler on the client's skin.

Pacing and Leading

All people have an internal pace or personal "rhythm" that influences how fast they move, how quickly they react, the speed and cadence of their speech, their physical mannerisms, the speed of their thought processes, and even their breathing patterns. At the same time, clients are likely to arrive in a particular state of mind and body (state of being). Perhaps the client encountered bad traffic and is running late. Perhaps the client just came from a yoga class and is feeling balanced. Maybe the client is feeling depressed because of personal issues. Regardless of the cause of the client's mental, emotional, and physical state, try to meet the client halfway and tune in to the client's rhythm and state of being. For example, it may be disconcerting for a mildly depressed client to walk through the clinic doors and encounter the therapist Chirpy Mary Sunshine. Similarly, it may be off-putting for an upbeat client who is enjoying a great day off to encounter the therapist Low Energy Larry.

Therapists can learn to "pace" the massage by matching the first part of the massage to the client. As the massage progresses, the therapist can "lead" the client into more relaxing rhythms. To understand "pacing" and "leading" better, consider one aspect of a counseling and life-coaching technique from neurolinguistic programming (NLP). NLP uses the word "pacing" to describe techniques that build rapport between the counselor and the client. The idea is that people tend to *like* people that they *are like*, so the counselor makes himself or herself *more like* the client. The counselor tunes in to the client's breathing patterns, speech patterns, body language, and personal rhythm. During the session, the counselor uses speech and body language patterns similar to those of the client. When the client is relaxed and when the counselor feels that a rapport has been established, he or she starts to "lead" the client. The counselor breathes with a new pattern and the client follows (so long as good rapport has been established). The counselor slows down (or speeds up) speech and changes his or her body language, and the client follows. All of this is done while the client and counselor are talking about other things. The benefit of this for the client is that these new breathing patterns, body gestures, and/or speech patterns create a "shift" in the client. It is almost as if these new patterns put a person in touch with new internal resources that allow looking at a situation from a new vantage point.[13] NLP is much more complex than this simple description, but this example can help massage therapists think about how they "pace" and "lead" clients.

The goal is to match the client's basic energy levels but not mimic the client or go to extremes of behavior. For a client and therapist both to be bouncing off the walls with hyperactive energy does not do the client any good. Instead, be upbeat but remain grounded until the client can be led to more relaxing patterns. If a client is downhearted, you might still remain positive but subdue your personal energy levels and speak in a quiet voice to respect the client's state of being.

Depth

Massage therapists sometimes call a superficial massage a "fluff and buff." While some clients like gentle massage that only skims the surface of the tissue, most clients want the therapist to sink into the tissue, take hold of the tissue, move the body with confidence, and address tension and any adhered muscle and fascia. This should not mean that you are working so deeply and with so much pressure that the client feels pain. It means that you can feel the quality of the tissue and understand how to engage it properly. Working with appropriate depth is a product of good palpation skills and self-confidence.

To build these skills, pay attention to the way a client's tissue feels and how it changes in different areas of the body. In a Swedish massage, effleurage starts out light and quickly gains depth as the body area softens. Circulation increases in the local area and the tissue begins to "melt," signaling that you can drop deeper into the muscle and fascia. Feel for the "bottom" of the muscle. Think of sinking into a pillow or other soft structure. Drop down and maintain an even pressure as the stroke travels the length of the body area. One way to learn about depth is to practice on clients or fellow students and ask for honest feedback. Ask direct questions like, "Is my pressure deep enough or would you prefer more pressure?" If the client answers "more pressure," sink in and feel what it feels like to sink in. Ask again, "Is this deep enough or should I be deeper?" Keep asking until the client communicates that the pressure is just right. Feel what "just right" feels like and remember that feeling. Remind clients to speak up if something hurts or feels too forceful.

Remember to practice massaging a variety of body types when learning to work with depth. Each body responds to pressure differently, and you must adapt to the tension levels and density of the individual tissue. The more massages you give as a student, the faster you develop these skills. If it happens that you start out working with too much depth and a client complains about the pressure, try to avoid becoming fearful but simply promise yourself to pay more attention to the quality of the tissue. It is okay to work too lightly or too deeply at first. No therapist walks out the training room door and has perfect depth the first time he or she gives a massage. These skills are developed over time, through practice and mindfulness.

Rhythm

Rhythm in massage is a lot like rhythm in dancing. Therapists with good rhythm apply strokes in a regular pattern at a regular pace or tempo. The client relaxes to the rhythm, much as a child relaxes when rocked by a parent. Imagine how petrissage strokes would feel if delivered in an uneven pattern. That sensation may well be distracting and disturbing for the client. Sometimes the rhythm of the massage changes naturally because you change strokes or techniques. Deep work is most often applied very slowly, while tapotement is applied more quickly. You might deliver the first few passes of effleurage at a quicker tempo and then slow down to lead a client into relaxation.

To build good rhythm, think about the regularity of strokes and strive to keep them even in both depth and speed.

Use music to set the pace for the massage, and "dance" the strokes as a training exercise. Check in with your practice clients and get feedback on their perception of the rhythm of the massage. As with all massage skills, rhythm is developed over time and with practice.

Flow and Continuity

Flow and continuity refer to the progression of massage strokes from one technique to another, and from one body area to another. Think of a river streaming over rocks in one unbroken movement. Strokes are like the river water. They should flow in one uninterrupted action so that the client experiences the constant and steady pressure of your hands. A therapist who has not yet developed flow and continuity might pause during strokes, lift the hands off the client, change techniques at the wrong times, and feel disjointed and sporadic.

Changing techniques at the wrong times is a common mistake of novice therapists. For example, it is a bad idea to start with effleurage on the lower leg, shift to tapotement at the lower hamstring, then to petrissage at the upper hamstring, and then back to effleurage on the lower leg. The nervous system cannot process these rapid technique changes and may become hyperalert and irritated. Instead, start effleurage at the lower leg by the ankle, sweep all the way up the leg, and come all the way back down the leg before shifting techniques.

The great ballet choreographer, Balanchine, often choreographed dance sequences in groups of three. He felt that the first time an audience saw a dance sequence, it captured their attention but they did not have time to really see the moves. When the sequence was repeated a second time, Balanchine believed that the audience studied the movement and analyzed the technique. The third time a sequence was danced, the audience could simply enjoy the beauty of the movement. While massage strokes would not be delivered in strict groups of threes, the same philosophy applies. A client needs time to be surprised by a sensation, analyze what is happening, and then settle into enjoyment of the technique.

Stroke Length

A therapist with strong massage skills tends to use long strokes that tie body areas together. He or she will travel the length of a muscle's fibers, or the length of a body area, before changing techniques or lifting the hands away from the client's body. Cutting a stroke short leaves the client feeling oddly frustrated. One area where this happens is on the posterior and anterior leg. Inexperienced therapists often stop short in the stroke because they are taught to be careful of draping and worry that the stroke will become invasive. The stroke should travel all the way up to the gluteals and around the greater trochanter, or all the way up to the anterior superior iliac spine and back again. On the arm, the stroke should travel up to the shoulder or even up to the neck. Understand the muscles and seek to work their entire length whenever possible. Many therapists undrape one or the other side of the client and travel from the foot, up the leg to the back, and then return to the foot again. These strokes build clients' kinesthetic awareness of their body and how different body areas relate to each other.

By learning and integrating the techniques and subtle skills discussed in this chapter, you are preparing for two compatible outcomes. First, you are learning to give an excellent relaxation massage that will help to reduce stress in the client, rejuvenate energy levels, relieve muscular tension, and help the body to find balance. Second, you are building the foundation skills needed to work with the advanced techniques for healthcare massages presented in coming chapters.

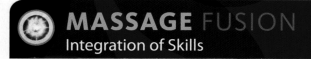

MASSAGE FUSION
Integration of Skills

STUDY TIP: Quiz It!

Visual learner: For this chapter, pretend that you are the instructor writing a quiz on Swedish massage. For each of the seven topics, write one quiz question on a main point. Highlight the answer to your question in the body of the text.

Auditory learner: Make a testing tape for this chapter. As you read through each topic, create a test question from the material and read it into a recorder. After each question, leave 6 seconds of blank space, and then record the answer. When you finish reading the chapter, listen to your tape and try to answer your questions during the 6-second delays.

Kinesthetic learner: For each topic, write a quiz question, but do not write the answers to your questions. When you have finished, take the quiz. Look up the answers to any questions you cannot easily answer.

MASSAGE INSPIRATION: Dance Massage

One of the things that make a great massage is flow. Flow refers to the fluid quality of a therapist's strokes. The speed of the strokes, the amount of body area covered by strokes, the depth of strokes, and the overall rhythm all contribute to flow. A fun way to develop your flow is to practice with dance massage. Pick out 10 favorite songs in any style of music (hip-hop, alternative, jazz, pop, classical, new age, rock, country, etc.)—any style is fine as long as you like

MASSAGE FUSION (*Continued*)
Integration of Skills

the songs (your practice client does not have to like the music—this exercise is for you as the therapist). Then play all 10 songs in a row while giving a massage to a friend, family member, or classmate. The goal is to infuse the massage with the quality of the music. What happens to the massage during a song that is sad and haunting? How does the quality of strokes change? What happens to the massage during a song that is fast or aggressive? Each song communicates something different and affects the massage in a new way. Do not judge whether a song is right for a massage—that's not the point. The point is to feel the music and let it guide your massage as you explore the flow. Therapists often find that listening to music while providing massage improves the flow of the massage and the quality of the strokes. Go with it! Have fun!

MASSAGE INSPIRATION:
Blindfolded Massage

Blindfolded massage helps therapists develop their palpation skills. In this exercise, undrape one body area and then place a blindfold over your eyes. Perform the massage of the body area while blindfolded. The blindfold will keep you from relying on visual clues. It forces you to "see" with your hands. Temperature and texture differences in the client's tissue will become more noticeable. Your hands will mold more fully to the contours of the client's body because the body becomes the guide for the stroke, not your eyes. Blindfolded palpation for the origins and insertions of muscle can also be a useful exercise.

IT'S TRUE! MASSAGE CHANGES BLOOD PRESSURE

A study at the National University of Health Sciences in Lombard, Illinois, found that massage can change a person's blood pressure. The study subjects were 150 adult massage therapy clients with blood pressures lower than 150/95. Each client's blood pressure was measured before and after massage. Researchers had hypothesized that the type of the massage, the length of the session, the body area massaged, and the amount of pressure would all affect the client's blood pressure. And their hypotheses proved true: Swedish massage was found to reduce blood pressure, while sports massage (stimulating) and trigger point therapy (potentially painful) were found to increase blood pressure.[14]

IT'S TRUE! MASSAGE CAN DECREASE THE FREQUENCY OF CHRONIC TENSION HEADACHES

A study at Boulder College of Massage Therapy in Boulder, Colorado, published in the *American Journal of Public Health*, found that muscle-specific massage therapy can reduce the incidence of chronic tension headaches. Massage therapy sessions were designed specifically to address neck and shoulder muscles. Although the intensity of clients' headaches was not affected by the massage, the frequency of headaches decreased for the participants.[15] In a similar study in Finland, 10 sessions of upper body massage were given to 21 female patients. ROM of the cervical vertebrae increased in all directions, and the number of days that patients experienced headache pain "decreased significantly."[16]

CHAPTER WRAP-UP

In this chapter, you learned the names, physiological effects, benefits, cautions, and application methods for Swedish massage techniques. Your palpation skills will develop further as you gain experience working with clients, noticing their movement patterns, feeling their tissue, describing its texture, and engaging tissue during strokes. Gliding strokes produce a different effect on the body from lifting strokes. A stroke applied lightly can relax the client, while deeper strokes require slowing down and paying attention to tissue changes. Fast strokes stimulate the body, and strokes delivered toward the heart aid venous return. Joint movement techniques involve holding and manipulating body areas, requiring a new level of coordination and body mechanics proficiency. As well, you are learning to think carefully about the many subtle factors that affect the client's overall massage experience and to sequence the massage to suit the client's session goals. The quality of your touch, the degree to which you engage tissue, your ability to pace and lead clients, and your overall flow and rhythm are important refinements to your abilities. With these foundation skills, you are ready to learn techniques like myofascial release, deep tissue, and treatment methods.

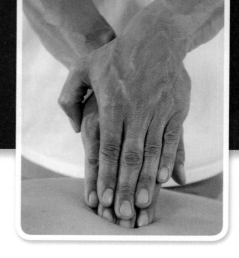

Seated Massage

KEY TERMS

accounts

compression

event massage

massage chair

onsite massage

pin and stretch

seated massage

LEARNING OBJECTIVES

Having read the chapter and used the related student learning tools, the student will be able to:

1 Define the terms *seated massage, onsite massage,* and *event massage*.

2 List three advantages and three disadvantages of seated massage compared to table massage.

3 Describe environments where seated massage can be offered.

4 Explain the general benefits of seated massage for employees in workplaces.

5 Explain the reasons why osteoporosis and previous back injuries or similar conditions require extra caution when clients are in a seated position.

6 Identify the sanitation and safety measures needed for seated massage onsite.

7 Describe adaptations that are necessary for using Swedish massage techniques in seated massage.

8 Compare and contrast the application of rhythmic compression with sustained compression.

Seated massage (also called chair massage) is a massage applied to a fully clothed client sitting in a specialized chair. **Onsite massage** refers to massage taken to clients at their businesses or homes, at events, or situated close to businesses they frequent (often called **event massage** when seated massage is used at an event). Onsite massage is often delivered in a massage chair although it can also be delivered on a massage table. In recent years, the demand for onsite massage has increased because clients are more aware of the benefits of massage and onsite massage is a convenient way to make massage part of a healthy lifestyle. More massage therapists have onsite seated massage accounts as part of their regular massage practice. Topic 14-1 introduces the basics of seated massage, while Topic 14-2 demonstrates how to apply massage techniques to a client positioned in a massage chair while fully clothed. Techniques in this chapter describe how to apply massage to a seated client. You will also learn about ways to use seated massage in your massage career.

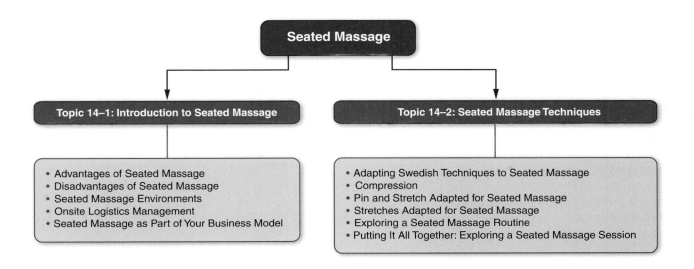

Seated Massage

Topic 14–1: Introduction to Seated Massage

- Advantages of Seated Massage
- Disadvantages of Seated Massage
- Seated Massage Environments
- Onsite Logistics Management
- Seated Massage as Part of Your Business Model

Topic 14–2: Seated Massage Techniques

- Adapting Swedish Techniques to Seated Massage
- Compression
- Pin and Stretch Adapted for Seated Massage
- Stretches Adapted for Seated Massage
- Exploring a Seated Massage Routine
- Putting It All Together: Exploring a Seated Massage Session

Topic **14-1**
Introduction to Seated Massage

This topic introduces the basics of seated massage including the advantages and disadvantages for therapists and clients, the environments where seated massage is practiced, seated massage as part of your career model, and onsite logistics management. Everything you already know about the effects and benefits of massage, cautions and contraindications, body mechanics, and documentation of sessions applies also to seated massage. The differences between seated massage and table massage are pointed out in this chapter, but otherwise you should apply the concepts you already know to this alternative type of massage.

Concept Brief 14-1
Key Terms

Seated massage: Massage applied to a fully clothed client sitting in a special chair (also called chair massage).

Onsite massage: Massage taken to clients at their businesses or homes, at events they attend, or situated close to businesses they frequent.

Event massage: Onsite massage delivered at an event like a music festival, sports event, community fundraiser, or other community activity.

Advantages of Seated Massage

Both seated massage and table massage are beneficial for clients. Because of its portability, seated massage offers a number of advantages over table massage for both clients and therapists in some situations. Clients find seated massage affordable and convenient for their busy schedules. A client can spontaneously stop at a seated "massage bar" in a mall or airport without an appointment and leave relaxed in just 15 to 20 minutes for around $15 (seated massage presently costs around $1 per minute). Compare this to a clinic session for which clients must book an appointment, travel to the business, find parking, remove their clothing, pay $50 to $100 for the session, and travel back home. Although clients typically receive a more deeply relaxing and therapeutic experience from table massage, in some cases this may not be offset by the inconvenience and the cost of the session.

Many companies offer seated massage onsite to employees in the workplace as a nice benefit and as a means to promote employee health (Box 14-1). Seated massage is clinically proven to reduce stress; increase the alertness, speed, and accuracy of workers; and prevent headache pain, burnout, and absenteeism in the workplace.[1–3] Clients sign up and receive 10 to 30 minutes of seated massage on breaks or during lunch. Because seated massage is performed over clothing, a private room is not necessary and techniques require fewer boundary adjustments from clients. Techniques are applied without the use of lubricants, and clients also feel cleaner after a session.

Seated massage is also cost-effective for therapists. Massage chairs are relatively inexpensive, and there is often no fee to set up at a business. This saves the costs of rent and utilities, although there are increased costs for travel and parking. When you bring massage to clients, as opposed to having clients come to an office, you have access to a larger client base. Many therapists also find that a part-time seated massage practice brings new clients into their regular practices because clients are more likely to seek out a full session from a therapist they know.

Disadvantages of Seated Massage

Seated massage has some disadvantages in some situations. You may have difficulty controlling the environment for seated massage at a business or event. The location might be noisy with people talking, children running around, or music blaring. It might be too hot or too cool. You also have less time to conduct a health history interview and establish the parameters of a therapeutic relationship. If you fail to make time for these activities, clients could be injured. Modifications in techniques are required to work over clothing, around jewelry, and without lubricant. Some body areas are not accessible during a seated massage, and therefore certain treatments cannot be given. For example, runners need focus on their quadriceps, hamstrings, and calves. While you can access these muscles to some degree during a seated massage, self-injury from poor body mechanics is more likely. Most therapists end up bending at the waist and squatting to reach these muscles. Range-of-motion techniques, which are effective for runners, are difficult if not impossible to apply to the hips, knees, and ankles when the client is seated. In such instances, both the therapist and the client are better served by table massage.

BOX 14-1 Benefits of Seated Massage in the Workplace

Decreased stress and anxiety

Decreased muscle tension, pain, and headache pain

Increased alertness, speed, and accuracy on tasks

Increased overall health and wellness

Decreased burnout and work absenteeism

Concept Brief 14-2
Key Terms

Advantages	Disadvantages
Portability	Little control of the environment
Convenience	Less time for health history intake process
Affordability	Techniques must be modified
Low overhead	Some techniques won't work
Clean (no lubricant)	Some body areas are not accessible
Access to more clients	Some treatment plans impossible
Helps table practice grow	

Seated Massage Environments

Seated massage can be delivered just about anywhere. One therapist set up her massage chair at a popular beach under a large beach umbrella. Another offers seated massage inside a ski lodge, while a third partners with the owner of a bookstore. In all cases, you should check local regulations and obtain the necessary permits or permissions to set up your chair. Following are some of the environments where seated massage is offered:

1. **Airports:** Seated massage is popular at airports. Carrying heavy bags, sitting in cramped plane seats, and the fatigue of a disrupted sleep schedule cause aches and pains that can be relieved with seated massage.

2. **Community events:** Some therapists set up massage booths or stations at community events like fairs, parades, art festivals, farmers markets, and music festivals. This is a good way to make extra massage income while informing potential clients about your table massage practice.

3. **Conventions:** Conventions bring together large groups of people in a concentrated area, providing a rich opportunity to set up a massage chair and generate income in a short time.

4. **Corporate environments:** Many massage therapists gain corporate accounts to provide seated massage on a weekly or monthly basis to employees. Sometimes the business pays for the massage, and sometimes the employees pay.

5. **Fitness environments:** Seated massage fits in well at gyms, health clubs, fitness centers, and dance studios because people interested in taking care of their bodies are often already aware of the benefits of massage. Seated massage here can also alert people to your table massage practice and broaden your client base.

6. **Health care environments:** Locating your seated massage business at a hospital, hospice, wellness center, or other health care facility can be very rewarding because you bring massage to people who are often highly stressed. You have the opportunity to work on a variety of clients from nurses and doctors to patients and their family members. Each has unique needs that can benefit from the soothing quality of massage.

7. **Malls:** "Massage bars" are increasingly common in malls and large department stores. These high-traffic areas provide access to large numbers of clients who want the convenience of a brief drop-in session.

8. **Natural food stores:** Natural food stores promote healthy living and often offer a space for seated massage, especially in a book or café area. This environment gives you access to a broad range of clients who may also visit your table practice after becoming familiar with your skills.

9. **Sporting events:** At local sporting events such as races and football, basketball, baseball, or soccer games, both spectators and athletes may be interested in receiving massage.

Onsite Logistics Management

When you offer onsite massage, you must create a functional and safe massage environment in a specific location and then ensure the client's comfort and enjoyment. How you organize your space and massage supplies plays a primary role in achieving this end.

Equipment and Supplies

While seated massage could be applied to any person sitting upright in a regular chair or on the floor, professional equipment is important to provide maximum comfort for the client and protect you from injury due to poor body mechanics. Seated massage equipment such as desktop support systems and massage chairs are lightweight, easy to transport, and affordable. Massage equipment companies offer a wide variety of options and accessories including the depth of padding, the color, and the type of vinyl finish in desktop systems and massage chairs. If possible, choose a well-made, highly adjustable system that will last and provide the greatest comfort and safety to clients.

Desktop Support Systems

Desktop (also called tabletop) support systems are less expensive than massage chairs and easy to transport. They are comprised of an adjustable face cradle and chest support pad with a clamp that connects to a desk or tabletop. Clients sit at their desk in a regular chair and lean against the chest pad with their face in the cradle.

Desktop systems are not as functional as massage chairs because it is more difficult to access the client's low back because of the back of the office chair. If the desk or table is against a wall, it can be difficult to comfortably work with the client's arms and hands if you cannot easily position yourself in front or to the side of the client. These systems are effective, however, when massage focuses on the neck and shoulders and when the client is in a wheelchair.

Massage Chairs

A well-designed, high-quality **massage chair** has padding to support the legs, a seat, a chest pad, an armrest, and a face cradle. The chair should be lightweight but strong, and an adjustable seat, chest pad, and face cradle to fit individual clients. The chair is freestanding so that you can easily work from the front, back, or sides of the client.

It takes some practice to learn how to position clients properly in a massage chair. You want the client to feel completely relaxed and supported with the joints flexed but not closed. In Figure 14-1, notice that the client looks cramped and uncomfortable because he is positioned incorrectly.

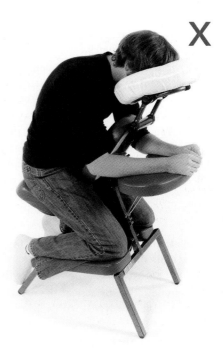

Figure 14-1 Positioning the client in the massage chair. This chair is not positioned correctly, with the chest pad and face cradle adjusted too low so that the client must round his back to fit into the face cradle.

Accessories

Accessories can enhance the seated massage experience for the client or the therapist:

- **Carrying case:** A carrying case protects your massage chair and makes it easier to transport. Most carrying cases have pockets to hold items like face cradle covers or sanitation supplies.
- **Face cradle covers:** Face cradle covers are placed over the face cradle for sanitation reasons and to prevent the client's face from sticking uncomfortably to the vinyl. You can use cloth covers but these must be laundered between clients. Most therapists use disposable face cradle covers, which are easily transported and eliminate the need for laundry.
- **Sternum pad:** Sternum pads are used with large-breasted people, pregnant women, or people with large abdominal regions. They attach to the chest pad to provide additional support and comfort.

Supplies

Some supplies like sanitation products and a first aid kit are essential, while others like a music system are not essential but provide more enjoyment. Box 14-2 has an equipment and supply checklist you can use.

- **Client forms:** Make sure that you always have health intake and informed consent forms on hand, even for seated massage at events. Document sessions on modified SOAP forms or wellness forms created for seated massage (Fig. 14-2). If you regularly work at the same locations, organize your client files so that repeat clients don't need to fill out new paperwork each time. Repeat clients should update their records annually and when health changes occur. Client files can be transported in a small, lockable metal or plastic box. Have clipboards on hand to make filling out forms easier.
- **Money:** Offer your clients as many payment options as possible. Consider offering credit card processing, and carry 1- and 5-dollar bills for making change. Only accept personal checks from clients you work with regularly.
- **Music system:** You may wish to bring a small music system. Some therapists use an iPod or MP3 player with headphones to block out noise from the environment. Remember that clients will have difficulty hearing directions you give them (e.g., "Bring your face out of the face cradle and sit up so that I can stretch your neck"), and that headphones must be sanitized with a disinfectant product between clients.
- **Safety supplies:** Have access to a standard first aid kit in case a client is injured. Have gloves with you to practice universal precautions if necessary.
- **Sanitation supplies:** The surfaces of the massage chair or desktop system should be wiped with a disinfectant product between clients. Disposable sanitation cloths are easy to transport and use onsite, though a spray product and paper towels can also be used. If a hand washing facility is not located nearby, you can sanitize your hands liberally between clients with an alcohol-based gel product.
- **Time:** A clock is needed for monitoring session times and staying on schedule.

- **Enhancers:** You may want to offer soothing amenities like an aromatherapy mist, a microwavable warm pack placed on the shoulders, or bottled water for clients after the massage. Choose enhancers that are cost-effective and easy to transport without stress to your body. Sometimes it is difficult or impossible to provide enhancers at all.

Cautions and Contraindications

Chapter 5 covered sites of caution and contraindications in depth. You already know that contagious diseases (e.g., flu, common cold, or chickenpox), infestations (e.g., lice or scabies), conditions in acute flare-up (e.g., rheumatoid arthritis or hepatitis), and being under the influence of alcohol or illegal drugs are absolute contraindications—for seated massage as well. In other cases, a condition may require a physician's release (severe diabetes, recent surgery, or injury), avoiding that area of the body (e.g., bruise, blister, local sunburn, local inflammation, open wound, or certain skin disorders), or using caution (e.g., a particular medication causes dizziness).

Sites of caution like the kidney region, spinous processes, anterior and posterior triangles of the neck, brachial plexus, and floating ribs are particularly accessible during seated massage. If you are uncertain about how to rule out contraindications, use critical thinking to evaluate adaptations required with medications or areas of caution (Chapter 5).

Back injuries and bone fractures during seated massage have led to insurance liability claims, according to Associated Bodywork & Massage Professionals. In many such claims, therapists had not asked clients for a complete health history and were not aware of preexisting back conditions or osteoporosis (weakened bones). These conditions can contraindicate the use of certain techniques during a seated massage. For example, for a client with osteoporosis, avoid the use of tapotement or strong compression strokes on the back, because these techniques have occasionally caused rib fractures during seated massage. Because the low back is not well supported in a massage chair, techniques that put undue pressure on the spine could cause injury or exacerbate an existing condition.

Concept Brief 14-3
Cautions with Seated Massage

- Contraindications and cautions for table massage are the same for seated massage.
- Areas of caution that are especially exposed during a seated massage include the kidney region, spinous processes, anterior and posterior triangles of the neck, brachial plexus, and floating ribs.
- While rare, bone fractures can be caused by compression techniques and tapotement on clients with osteoporosis.
- Back injuries have occurred due to lack of support for the lumbar region in a seated position when compression techniques were applied forcefully.

Manual Therapist _____ **WELLNESS CHART—SEATED**

Name _____ ID#/DOB _____ Meds _____

Tx: _____   Tx: _____

C: _____   C: _____

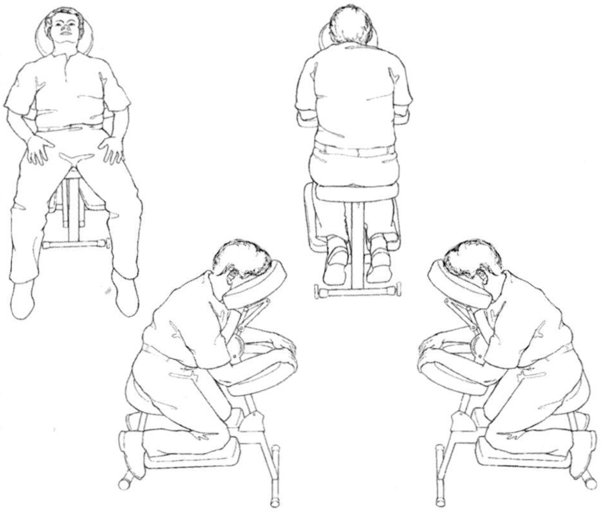

date _____ initials _____   date _____ initials _____

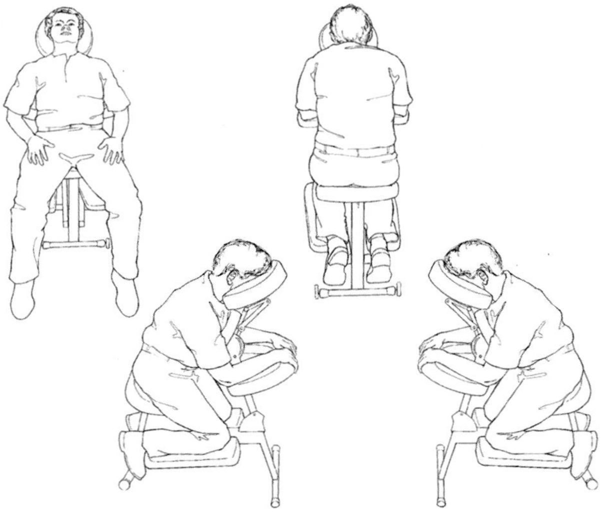

Tx: _____   Tx: _____

C: _____   C: _____

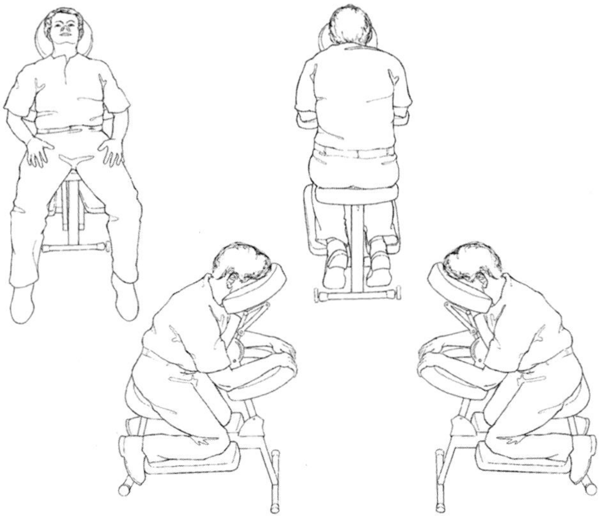

date _____ initials _____   date _____ initials _____

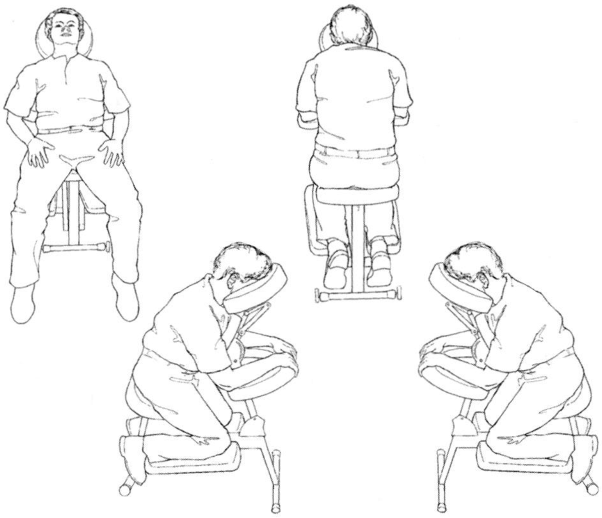

Legend: ℰ TP   • TeP   ○ ℗   ✳ Infl   ≡ HT   ≈ SP
   ⤬ Adh   ≷ Numb   ↻ rot   ╱ elev   ⊱ Short   ↔ Long

Copyright © 2012 Wolters Kluwer Health I Lippincott Williams & Wilkins

Figure 14-2 Wellness form for seated massage.

BOX 14-2 Checklist of Supplies for Onsite Massage

- Massage chair
- Face cradle covers
- Lockable box for client records
- Client forms (health history, informed consent, and treatment records)
- Clipboards
- Change ($1 and $5 bills)
- Credit card processing machine (optional)
- Massage cream (optional)

- Disinfectant wipes or disinfectant spray and paper towels
- Alcohol-based hand sanitizer
- Vinyl gloves
- First aid kit
- Clock
- Snacks for the therapist to prevent low energy and hunger
- Music system (optional)
- Enhancers like microwavable warm packs, aromatherapy mists, bottled water (optional)

Sanitation and Safety

Sanitation and safety were discussed in depth in Chapter 3, but a few points specific to seated massage may be helpful. If possible wash your hands and arms between clients and rinse your mouth with mouthwash in a nearby bathroom. See earlier comments on alcohol-based gel hand sanitizers and disinfecting the massage chair or desktop system before and after sessions.

Only work in locations that are safe, clean, and well lit. Ideally the location has restroom facilities nearby, but this is not always so. Take a cell phone in case you need to call emergency services. Provide water to clients if possible and remain hydrated yourself, especially outdoors in a warm environment. Check that the equipment is safe and in good working order before every massage. All adjustable parts should be tight and secure.

At the end of the session, clients often feel light-headed when they remove their face from the face cradle and stand up. To prevent this, finish the session with a few brief stretches; have clients bring their face out of the cradle and sit up straight for a time before standing.

Organization of the Environment

Organize the environment where you provide seated massage for the greatest possible privacy, safety, and comfort. Divide the area into two spaces. In the first, clients fill in health history forms and pay for sessions. Provide chairs and forms on clipboards. In the separate area clients answer any necessary health-related questions and receive massage. Don't ask clients questions in a way that might be overheard by others. Place completed health forms directly into a locked box after you review them with the client before the massage. Ideally, provide seated massage in a private enclosed area or room. If this is not possible, situate the massage chair so that the client faces away from a public area, or use a screen to increase privacy.

Keep the client's path clear and unobstructed by supply boxes, the chair carrying case, or extension cords. Position clients away from heating and cooling vents whenever possible to avoid discomfort. Check the surrounding environment to ensure that nothing could interrupt the massage or injure the client. For example, during seated massage at a holiday event, a therapist had a giant mock candy cane made of Styrofoam fall onto a client when some children pushed on it. In an outdoor environment, rent a canopy or tent to protect clients from the elements. In all, clients should feel that the space is relaxing, clean, and neatly organized.

Seated Massage as Part of Your Business Model

The business of massage was discussed in depth in Chapter 9, including marketing, promotion, business types, contracts, and other business issues. Seated massage can support your business model in a variety of ways:

- **Main practice:** You may make seated massage your main practice and work full time as an employee for an established business at a location like an airport or a massage bar. Or you might be self-employed and independently set up accounts with local businesses to fill your massage schedule.

- **Diversified practice:** Some therapists practice seated massage as an employee or independent contractor once or twice a week. They offer table massage privately or at a spa or clinic during the rest of the week. A diversified practice helps ensure an income stream and keeps a practice interesting by providing variety.

- **Seated massage to grow a table practice:** You may offer seated massage in a high-traffic area like a mall or gym once or twice a week as a way to meet new potential clients and promote your table practice. This strategy also works well at community events like street fairs or charity events like walk-a-thons, or community sports events like marathons or organized cycle rides.

- **Instant income:** A local event like a big national convention or sports event offers an opportunity to work hard and make additional income. You are likely to be busy throughout the day with new clients and may meet local clients who may come to your table practice.

Fees

Before setting your fees, research the market rate for seated massage in your area by examining what other seated massage businesses are charging per minute of massage. Often clients pay less per minute for longer massages. For example, your fee schedule might look like this:

- 15 minutes: $15
- 20 minutes: $18
- 25 minutes: $22
- 30 minutes: $25

In many situations, you charge each client a fixed fee for the length of massage and collect the fee directly before or after the massage. With business accounts you may collect fees in various ways depending on your contract with the business:

- **Fees from employees:** The business may let you set up your massage chair in its facility but not pay for massage for its employees. Individual employees receiving massage pay you directly.
- **Rent to company—fee from employee:** In rare cases (avoid these if possible), a business charges you a fee to set up in its facility. You then have access to employees, who pay you directly. This type of account is advantageous only with a rich supply of clients ensuring that your day is busy and profitable.
- **A flat fee for a specified time:** The account might pay you a flat fee to provide massage to employees for an agreed amount of time each week or month. This has the benefit of assuring a fixed income and saves you from having to process payments during the workday. A drawback is that many companies require you to invoice monthly and wait up to 30 days for payment.
- **A flat fee per employee:** A company may pay you a specified amount for each employee receiving massage during your scheduled shift.
- **Company–employee split:** A company may pay half the fee for each employee and expect the employee to pay the remaining portion of the fee to you.

Securing Accounts

Many therapists need a number of business **accounts** to sustain their seated massage practice. Begin by identifying prospective businesses where you can offer seated massage. Then get those businesses interested in seated massage, get a commitment from decision makers, promote yourself, and follow through on your obligations.

Identify Prospects

Create a list of businesses or companies that might welcome seated massage in your area. Look for prospects located close to your home. Pay attention to parking and how far you will have to carry your massage chair and supplies. You may choose to focus on a specific type of client (e.g., you want to work with fit people at gyms or office employees). Once you have identified potential accounts, you need to get them interested in seated massage.

Generate Interest

To generate interest in your seated massage business, mail an introductory packet to the owner, manager, or decision maker. The information packet should include a cover letter, a brochure or flyer, a business card, and perhaps one or two articles that explain the benefits of massage in the workplace (see the References for this chapter in Appendix B for examples), as discussed in Chapter 9. Follow up the information packet with a phone call and ask for a meeting.

Obtain the Account

When you meet with the decision maker, be prepared to articulate clearly the following key information:

- **Description:** Describe seated massage and explain how it benefits employees by reducing stress, minimizing repetitive work-related injuries, and promoting general health and wellness. Share one or two examples of research findings related to the benefits of massage in the workplace (see the "It's True" section at the end of this chapter for examples).
- **Schedule:** Provide two or three scheduling options (e.g., once a week, once a month, or bimonthly). It sometimes works well to offer a trial period such as two scheduled days of seated massage at the business and survey the employees to determine their interest (Box 14-3).
- **Logistics:** Explain your space needs and describe the supplies you will bring with you. Emphasize that you are responsible for the supplies, equipment, setup, and cleanup.
- **Cost and payment:** Explain your fees and offer different fee models described above. Describe contract options and how payments can be processed.
- **Credentials:** Outline your credentials and training and provide a copy of your license or certificate if appropriate. Provide a copy of your professional liability insurance.

Usually you present this information informally to one or two people, but in some cases you may be asked to make a formal presentation, as described in Chapter 9. After presenting your information, offer to demonstrate seated massage or give a seated massage to the decision maker. After the demonstration, ask for the account and agree on a start date. Submit your proposed agreement in writing within 5 business days.

Promote Yourself

Once you have secured the account, you have to generate interest from employees and alert them to your schedule. You

BOX 14-3 Survey Questions to Gauge Employee Interest

1. I enjoyed the massage and found it relaxing.
   - Strongly Agree   - Agree   - Neutral   - Disagree   - Strongly Disagree
2. Muscle tension and/or pain and/or any headache pain I felt before the massage is decreased.
   - Strongly Agree   - Agree   - Neutral   - Disagree   - Strongly Disagree
3. I feel alert and ready to accomplish the rest of today's tasks.
   - Strongly Agree   - Agree   - Neutral   - Disagree   - Strongly Disagree
4. I would take part in a massage program at work if it were provided.
   - Strongly Agree   - Agree   - Neutral   - Disagree   - Strongly Disagree
5. I feel I would benefit from a massage program at work if it were provided.
   - Strongly Agree   - Agree   - Neutral   - Disagree   - Strongly Disagree

might place brochures in employee boxes and post a sign-up sheet in the break room. You might give away a free seated massage through a drawing as a way to raise awareness. Other ideas for marketing and promotion are discussed in Chapter 9.

Follow Through

Remember that your attention to professional appearance and personal hygiene, your promptness and sticking to your stated schedule, and the overall quality of service you provide greatly affect how successful you will be with business accounts.

Seated Massage at Local Events

Seated massage can be offered at community events like street fairs, walk-a-thons, music and food festivals, conferences,

conventions and trade shows, and local sporting events. Follow these general steps to organize your efforts:

1. **Schedule:** Identify upcoming events in your area for the year ahead.
2. **Contacts:** Contact event organizers about the process for obtaining a booth or necessary permits to offer your services. Considering partnering with other massage therapists to split the costs and share the workload.
3. **Promote:** Have ample promotional materials available. Consider offering a door prize such as a drawing to win a free session.
4. **Plan carefully:** Consider the logistical elements carefully and plan ahead. Avoid being exposed to extreme elements like direct sunlight or rain. If needed, rent a canopy to provide a safer, more comfortable experience to clients.

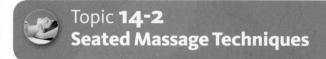

Topic **14-2**
Seated Massage Techniques

With minor modifications, most of the strokes you already know can be adapted for seated massage. A new technique, called compression, is included here, while the pin–and-stretch technique, discussed more in upcoming chapters, is briefly introduced along with some stretches that are easy and effective when applied in a seated position. The end of this section explores how to sequence strokes in a seated massage relaxation routine. Strokes described later can also be adapted for your personal seated massage routine.

Adapting Swedish Techniques to Seated Massage

Chapter 13 described effleurage, pétrissage, friction, vibration, and tapotement. In a seated massage you can use these techniques, but they must be modified because they are applied without lubricant and over clothing. You can use lubricant on areas of skin not covered with clothing, such

| Technique 30 | Adapting Swedish Techniques to Seated Massage |

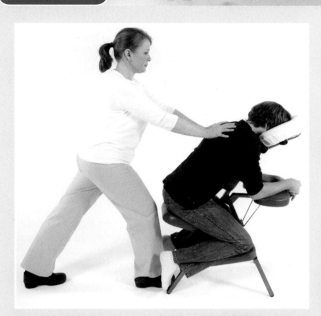

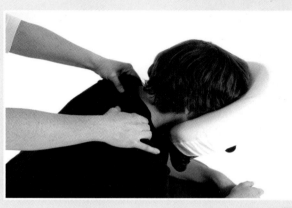

1. Effleurage. In a regular Swedish massage, effleurage is used to warm the tissue and spread lubricant on the skin at the beginning of the massage. In seated massage, it is most often used as a finishing stroke to close a body area. In this image, effleurage is applied up the back and down the client's arms. Effleurage could also be applied up the arms with light strokes to the shoulders or from the ankles up the legs to the hips over clothing. Try applying effleurage to different body areas accessible in the massage chair, and practice transitioning the stroke from a nonclothed body area like the arms over sleeves to the back.

2. Pétrissage. Pétrissage feels good on the shoulders, posterior neck, and upper extremity during a seated massage. It is fatiguing for the therapist's hands and so should be used in moderation during a busy day of sessions. In this image, pétrissage is being applied to the shoulders. Try applying pétrissage to the shoulders, down the back, to the posterior neck, arms, and forearms, and to the thighs and legs over clothing. It can be more difficult to get hold of the tissue and lift it when applied over clothing but it still feels enjoyable to clients.

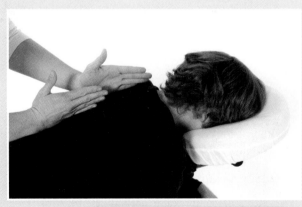

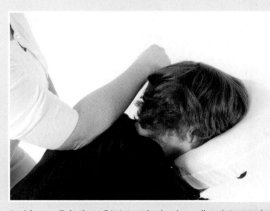

3. Superficial Friction. Superficial friction is useful as a stroke to warm the tissue, even when applied over clothing. In this image, superficial friction is applied to the back. It can also be applied to the shoulders, upper extremities, and lower extremities. Practice applying superficial friction to all body areas that are accessible while the client is seated.

palms

4. Linear Friction. Friction strokes break up adhered tissue and reorganize collagen fibers into parallel patterns allowing for greater range of motion. It is very useful in seated massage. In this image, the elbow is used to apply linear friction to the thoracic region. Try applying linear friction to all of the accessible areas of the body and over clothing. Use your fingers, knuckles, fists, and ulnar edge of your hands.

forearms

Continued

Technique 30   **Adapting Swedish Techniques to Seated Massage** (Continued)

fingertips, fist, knuckles

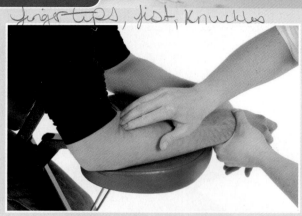

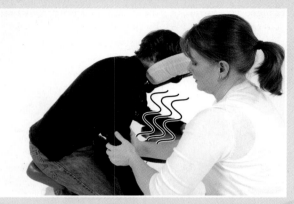

5. Circular Friction. Circular friction moves the tissue in a circular motion to break up adhesions and release tension. This image shows circular friction applied up the forearm muscles with the fingers (Because it is easy to overuse the fingers and thumbs during seated massage, try to use other "tools" whenever possible). Try performing circular friction strokes to all of the accessible areas of the body over clothing using your knuckles, fists, thumbs, and fingers.

6. Vibration. Shaking, rocking, and jostling are forms of coarse vibration that are particularly useful during seated massage. This image shows a jostling vibration on the upper extremity. Try lifting a muscle like the trapezius and shaking it, or rolling the arm back and forth between your hands. Rock the client's body back and forth in the massage chair.

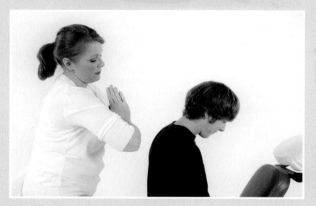

7. Tapotement. Tapotement is easy to apply over clothing and feels invigorating in a seated massage. It should not be used directly after athletic activity because it stimulates the muscle spindle cells and may cause the muscles to cramp. Tapotement over the kidneys and floating ribs is contraindicated because these structures do not have sufficient protection when the stroke is applied with the client in a seated position. It is also avoided on boney areas, especially over the spine. In this image, the therapists have asked the client to sit up out of the face cradle while the hands are held in a prayer position to apply tapotement to the shoulders and down the upper extremity. It's a good idea to have the client sit up out of the face cradle at the end of the session so they don't feel light-headed when they stand up to get out of the massage chair. Try using a variety of hand positions (hacking, cupping, beating, slapping, pincement, and tapping) and applying tapotement at a level comfortable to the client to all accessible body areas except over the kidneys and floating ribs.

---

as the arms, if you and the client choose. Be careful not to get lubricant on the client's clothing or hair, and ensure that your hands and forearms are clean of lubricant before moving back to a clothed body area. Technique 30 describes how to adapt Swedish techniques for seated massage. The contraindications for Swedish techniques are the same whether the client is reclining on a table or seated in a massage chair (see Chapter 13).

Compression

With **compression** strokes, you push the muscle belly directly toward the bone beneath it with a rhythmic pumping action. Compression was identified as a massage technique in the 1950s as sports massage became popular. It is often used in onsite massage like sports massage and seated massage because it does not require lubricant. Sustained compression

strokes are also used, especially in trigger point therapy, to relieve the pain and discomfort of hypersensitive areas in soft tissue.

Effects of Compression

The effects of compression depend on the stroke's depth, speed, and rhythm. Slow, deliberate compression strokes can feel relaxing, while the vigorous compression strokes of sports massage are quite stimulating. Warming muscle tissue and increased blood circulation are primary effects of compression. The stroke temporally prevents blood from flowing through the arterioles and arteries, forcing the blood out of the local tissue. Pressure builds up behind the blockage so that when the blockage is removed, a rush of fresh blood enters the tissue. This improves metabolic waste and nutrient exchange and quickly warms the tissue. Like pétrissage, compression deforms soft-tissue structures, making them more pliable.

In rhythmic compression techniques, the muscle spreads out against the bone beneath it during the stroke, and the muscle spindle cells sense that the muscle is rapidly stretching. They send a signal to contract the muscle to prevent overstretching and potential damage to the muscle. This stimulates the muscle and the nervous system, making compression an appropriate stroke for use directly before a sporting event.[4] Sustained compression, with which the tissue is compressed for a prolonged period of time, is used to reduce trigger points. This type of compression can feel mildly uncomfortable but is an effective method for reducing pain and chronic muscle tension (trigger point techniques are described in Chapter 21).

Application of Compression

The heels of the hands, the fists, the forearms, the thumbs, and the fingertips are used to apply compression strokes. A sustained compression stroke that prolongs the compression is most often applied with the thumbs, forearm, or elbow. Sustained compression and working with trigger points are described in Chapter 21.

During the application of rhythmic compression strokes, pay attention to the client's reaction to the stroke and your body mechanics. First, ensure that the part of your body delivering the stroke is not forcing the tissue. Instead, gauge the amount of give in the tissue and press it only as far as it is willing to go naturally. As the area warms up, more pressure can be used. If the client visibly tenses up each time you compresses the tissue, you are using too much pressure. Experiment with the stroke. How fast can it be? What is the client's reaction to a fast-paced compression? How slow can the compression be? What does it feel like to use the heels of the hand, the fingertips, and the forearm? Technique 31 describes performing compression strokes on a seated client.

> ### Concept Brief 14-4
> **Compression Strokes**
>
> **Rhythmic Compression:** A stroke with which the therapist pushes the muscle belly directly onto the bone beneath it with a rhythmic pumping action.
>
> **Sustained Compression:** A stroke with which the therapist applies direct pressure for a period of time to relieve hypersensitive areas called tender points or to reduce trigger points.
>
> **Effects:** Effects depend on the depth, speed, and rhythm of the stroke. In general, ↑ blood circulation to the local tissue, ↑ muscle warmth, ↑ oxygen and nutrient exchange in the tissue, ↓ muscle tension.

| **Technique 31** | **Compression Strokes in Seated Massage** |

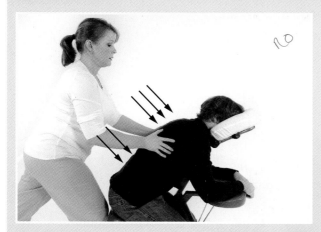

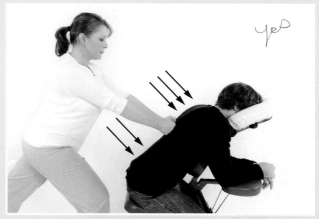

1. Regardless of the part of the body used to apply the stroke (forearm, fist, palms, etc.), the strokes should be applied in a straight line pushing the muscle directly onto the bone beneath it. Strokes should be rhythmic and cover the entire body area at a depth comfortable to the client. This image shows the use of the palms to apply a compression stroke on the back.

2. This image shows the use of fists to apply compression strokes to the back. Try applying compression strokes to all areas of the body that are accessible in a seated position.

Pin and Stretch Adapted for Seated Massage

Pin and stretch refers to a technique in which a muscle is first shortened passively or actively (placed in a shortened position through passive range of motion by the therapist or placed in a shortened position by an active movement by the client), then "pinned" by the therapist's hand at its origin, insertion, or muscle belly, before it is lengthened passively or actively. These types of techniques are used to reset proprioception and lengthen chronically shortened muscle, as described in Chapter 21. Technique 32 demonstrates some basic pin-and-stretch techniques that can be used during a seated massage.

Stretches Adapted for Seated Massage

As described in Chapter 13, passive stretches move a joint through its range of motion to lengthen muscles, tendons, ligaments, and the joint capsule, increasing flexibility. Stretching works well at the end of a seated massage because the muscles are warm and soft and stretching stimulates the client to help transition back to wakefulness. Never bounce the client in the stretch, which can cause microscopic tearing of muscle fibers. This can lead to the formation of scar tissue and additional loss of elasticity. Avoid stretching the client so far as to cause pain, because this can lead to tissue damage and a protective contracting of muscle tissue. Stretching the client too fast activates the stretch reflex and may lead to more tension in the muscles. To stretch the client, take the joint to firm end feel and then gently, slowly, and evenly push a little way past firm end feel. Work slowly and pay attention to the quality of the tissue. Some passive stretches that work well during a seated massage are shown in Technique 33.

Exploring a Seated Massage Routine

Review Table 14-1. The first column lists strokes that work well in seated massage, in alphabetical order. The second column lists the variations of strokes that can be used in seated massage, and the third lists application tools you can use to apply particular strokes. Use this table like a checklist when practicing seated massage, and explore each stroke, each variation, and each application tool thoroughly. Find out what works well, what works with some client body types, and what doesn't work at all for you. Pay attention to your body

---

Technique 32   **Pin and Stretch Adapted for Seated Massage**

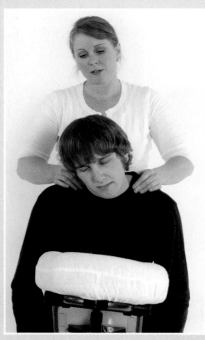

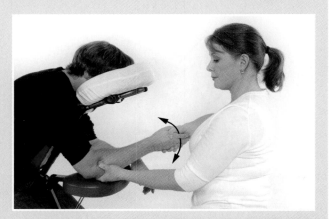

1. In a seated massage, you can work easily with the cervical joints and the joints of the upper extremity. In this image, the client is laterally flexing his neck actively while the therapist compresses the tissue by locking it down on either side of the neck with her hands. Using the same hand position, the therapist can instruct the client to rotate his chin from one shoulder to the other.

2. In this image, the pin–and–stretch technique is used to release the muscles that flex and extend the wrist. The therapist passively flexes and extends the wrist to shorten and lengthen the muscles while pinning the different muscles along their bellies. The therapist then lengthens the muscles by extending the wrist while holding the "pin." This is a particularly useful application for clients with carpal tunnel issues.

Technique 33 | Seated Massage Stretches

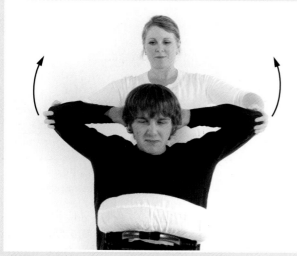

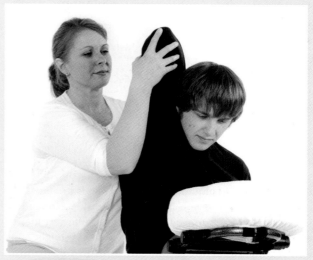

1. Pectoralis Major (lower fibers) and Minor Stretch. The client places his hands on his head with his elbows out to the sides. The therapist grasps the elbows and moves them backward slowly until resistance is felt. Ask the client to exhale as the stretch is performed.

2. Triceps Stretch. The client reaches over his shoulder with his elbow close to his head. The therapist places pressure on the elbow to bring it closer to the client's head while guiding the client's hand down toward his shoulder blade.

3. Neck Stretch. Slowly ask the client to actively move the head and neck into flexion, lateral flexion, and rotation. As the client reaches the end of his range, exert gentle pressure to assist the stretch as shown in this image. Work slowly, gently, and carefully.

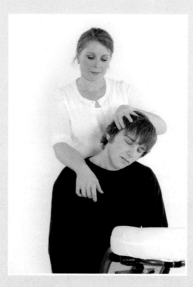

TABLE 14-1   Strokes, Variations, and Tools for a Seated Massage Routine

Stroke	Variations	Tools
Effleurage	Superficial, moderate, deep, shingling technique	Fingertips, palms, and forearm
Friction	Superficial, deep, circular, and linear	Fingertips, thumbs, ulnar edge of hands, forearm, elbow, knuckles, fists
Joint movements and stretches	Active, passive, resisted, assisted	Hands
Pétrissage	Skin rolling, fulling pétrissage, and wringing pétrissage	Fingertips and hands
Pin and stretch	Practice the pin-and-stretch technique shown in Technique 43	Try pinning the muscle with the fingertips, palms, forearm, thumbs, ulnar edge of the hands, knuckles, and fist.
Tapotement	Light, moderate, deep, hacking, cupping, beating, slapping, pincement, and tapping.	Fingertips, palms, ulnar edge of the hands, and fists
Vibration	Fine, coarse including jostling, shaking, and rocking.	Fingertips, palms, and hands

mechanics and use strokes that tire your hands or body only in moderation. When you have completed this exploration process, you are ready to sequence the strokes into a basic outline for a relaxation routine. A general sequence might look like the following, although some strokes should not be used if they are contraindicated for a particular client:

1. Opening: Holding strokes used for three client breaths
2. Compression strokes
3. Pétrissage strokes
4. Friction strokes
5. Pin-and-stretch techniques
6. Rocking the client in the chair
7. Tapotement strokes
8. Effleurage strokes
9. Closing: Stretches

You may notice that effleurage strokes are used toward the end of the sequence and not at the beginning as in Swedish massage. The sequence is different because effleurage strokes don't work as well as compression strokes over clothing to warm the tissue.

Practice the sequence of strokes you choose for your relaxation routine on each body area including the back, neck, shoulders, arms, hands, gluteals, and thighs until it flows naturally and fluidly from one stroke to the next. Having a basic routine worked out gives you a foundation from which to adapt techniques to best fit the needs of a particular client.

Putting It All Together—A Seated Massage Session

Now we can put everything together and walk through a typical seated massage session. The following overview will help you integrate what you know and better plan your own sessions.

1. **Welcome:** Greet the client and briefly explain how the session will proceed. For example, you might say, "If you would like a seated massage, I'll ask you to fill out a health information form. The health form helps me choose massage techniques that are safe for you. After I review the form I'll adjust the massage chair to fit you properly, and you will receive 15 minutes of massage for $15. If you would like a longer session, it is an additional $1 per minute. I'll massage your back, neck, shoulders, arms, and hands during the session, ending with a few stretches of your neck, shoulders, and forearms. After the session I'll process your payment in cash or with a credit card."

2. **Health intake review:** When the client has completed the health form, briefly review it with him or her to ensure all medications and conditions are listed. Make sure you understand the client's unique health picture and have ruled out contraindications before providing massage. Keep the client's health form in a safe, private place where other clients waiting for a session cannot see it.

3. **Orient the client to the chair:** Show the client how to get into and out of the massage chair without touching the chair or face cradle yourself (that would contaminate the chair and require that it be resanitized before the client sits in it). Have the client sit in the chair, and check the position is correct or adjust the chair. If the chair needs adjustment, ask the client to stand up while you adjust the chair, or you may adjust areas of the chair such as the face cradle while the client remains seated.

4. **Massage:** It's a good idea to open the massage by stating the beginning time and the session's ending time to prevent any confusion about length. Otherwise the client may feel anxious that the massage time is being used up with the health intake form or chair adjustment. This also helps the client begin to relax. You might say something like, "Peggy, it is now 12:05 and you have asked for a 15-minute session. I'll finish the massage at 12:20."

5. **Session end:** Use stretches (shown in Technique 33) to end the session. This practice ensures that the client sits up out of the face cradle for a period of time before standing up, decreasing the risk of feeling light-headed and falling or tripping when rising from the massage chair.

6. **Process payment:** When the session ends, allow the client to stand up, and escort the client back to the entry area. State the fee for the session and process the payment. If practical, offer the client a paper cup or bottle of water.

7. **Transition to the next session:** Sanitize your hands and greet your next client. The client can fill out a health form while you wipe the massage chair with a disinfectant and put in place a fresh face cradle cover.

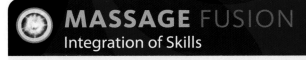

MASSAGE FUSION
Integration of Skills

STUDY TIP: Pay Attention to Your Internal Clock

All people have a personal time of day when they are at their best. Some people jump out of bed refreshed, while others struggle until they've had two shots of espresso. Some people feel sleepy in the afternoon, and others can't sleep until well after midnight. You can optimize your school performance by paying attention to your internal clock. Whenever possible, plan study sessions during periods when you are usually the most alert and awake. If you know you are a "night owl," then don't plan 9 am study sessions. Instead study at night—even late at night. "Early birds" do best when they study in the morning.

MASSAGE INSPIRATION: The Real Thing

If you want a better understanding of massage in the workplace or onsite seated massage, try these activities.

- Observe workplace or onsite seated massage and interview clients at the end of their sessions. What benefits do they feel they received from the sessions?
- Interview one or more professional massage therapists about their onsite seated massage practice. How often do they provide seated massage? How many accounts do they have? What are the benefits—the drawbacks?
- Receive a massage at a seated massage "bar" and reflect on your experiences.

There is nothing like participating fully in the *real thing* to understand it better.

GOOD TO KNOW: David Palmer—Originator of Contemporary Seated Massage

David Palmer is known as the founder and originator of contemporary seated massage. In the 1980s, Palmer invented a specially designed chair that supported people so that they could relax while receiving massage. He believed that massage needed to be "packaged" differently if people were going to embrace it wholeheartedly. If massage was taken to people's workplaces, they would be more likely to give it

a try. About the same time that Palmer was spreading the message about the benefits of onsite massage, businesses began to recognize the benefits of health and wellness programs as a way to decrease workers compensation claims and to lower employee absenteeism. Onsite seated massage was born. More information about David Palmer and his onsite seated massage company, Zubio, is available at www.zubio.com.

IT'S TRUE: Benefits of Massage in the Workplace

Much research supports the benefits of massage in the workplace. In one study, 26 adults were given a seated massage while a control group of 24 adults were asked to relax in a massage chair for 15 minutes, two times per week, for 5 weeks. The massage group demonstrated decreased frontal alpha and beta waves, suggesting enhanced alertness and increased speed and accuracy in math computations following sessions; the control group did not change.[5]

In another study, 15-minute massage sessions were offered to hospital employees. Employees receiving massage reported decreased anxiety, depression, and fatigue and increased vigor following the sessions.[6]

In an Australian study, 15 minutes of back massage was provided to 30 nurses one time a week for 5 weeks. A control group of 30 nurses received no therapy. The psychological stress, cortisol levels, and blood pressure of the nurses were measured weekly. Results showed that massage was a beneficial tool to reduce psychological stress levels in nurses.[7]

CHAPTER WRAP-UP

In this chapter, you learned how to adapt massage techniques you already know for use in seated massage. Seated massage opens up a number of possibilities for you as a therapist and businessperson. You can bring massage to people instead of waiting for people to come to you. You can be mobile and offer massage anywhere you choose as long as it is safe for you and for clients. Work hard to develop a functional basic seated massage routine and use it to entice new clients to try out table massage. Seated massage may be the core skill that ensures your table practice thrives when you become a professional.

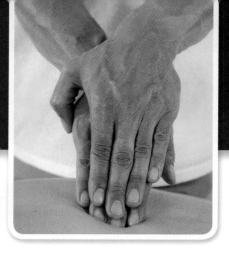

Chapter
15

Spa Therapies and Other Approaches

KEY TERMS

aromatherapy

Basalt

cocoon

dry skin brushing

dry room

essential oil

exfoliation

hot sheet wrap

loofah scrub

reflexology

salt glow

spa therapy

stone massage

sugar glow

wet room

LEARNING OBJECTIVES

Having read the chapter and used the related student learning tools, the student will be able to:

1. Analyze spa treatments and promotional descriptions to make good decisions about scope of practice when delivering spa services.

2. Compare and contrast the removal of spa products in a wet room with the removal of spa product in a dry room.

3. Describe the effects of exfoliation that are similar to the effects of massage.

4. List three contraindications for exfoliation treatments.

5. Differentiate between the procedures for a hot sheet wrap and a cocoon.

6. Explain why remaining with a client at all times during a body wrap is important.

7. List three primary and three accent aromatherapy treatments that might be used in a spa or massage practice.

8. List three contraindications for aromatherapy.

9. Discuss the reflexology belief that there are points on the feet, hands, and ears that stimulate the different regions of the body including glands and organs.

10. State the range of safe stone temperatures for stone massage.

11. Outline the cleaning and sanitation steps therapists take to ensure hot stone massage is sanitary.

This chapter introduces spa therapies and other body-work approaches that are popular with both therapists and clients. Whether you want to work in a spa or offer greater variety to clients in a clinic or private practice, the knowledge and skills in this chapter broaden your understanding of ways to integrate techniques for health and wellness. Topic 15-1 briefly describes the history of spa and scope of practice guidelines before previewing different types of treatments often labeled "spa." You learn to deliver salt and sugar glows, dry skin brushing, loofah scrubs, and body wraps. Topic 15-2 provides an overview of the benefits and effects of essential oils when used with massage or spa therapy. Topic 15-3 explores techniques for a relaxation reflexology routine, while Topic 15-4 demonstrates the many ways that heated stones can be integrated with massage techniques for unique services.

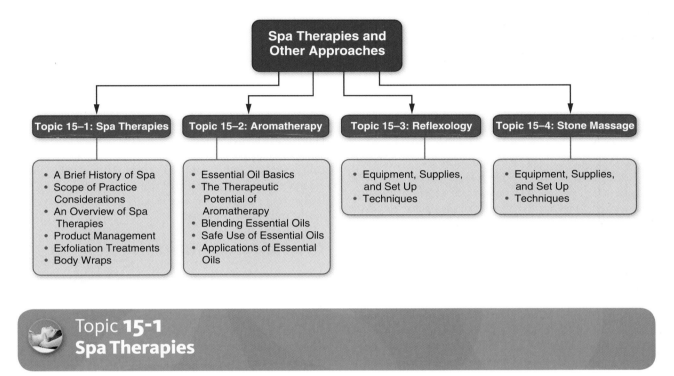

Spa Therapies and Other Approaches

Topic 15–1: Spa Therapies
- A Brief History of Spa
- Scope of Practice Considerations
- An Overview of Spa Therapies
- Product Management
- Exfoliation Treatments
- Body Wraps

Topic 15–2: Aromatherapy
- Essential Oil Basics
- The Therapeutic Potential of Aromatherapy
- Blending Essential Oils
- Safe Use of Essential Oils
- Applications of Essential Oils

Topic 15–3: Reflexology
- Equipment, Supplies, and Set Up
- Techniques

Topic 15–4: Stone Massage
- Equipment, Supplies, and Set Up
- Techniques

Topic **15-1** Spa Therapies

Approaches to **spa therapy** are broad and diverse. While some spa treatments are provided to beautify the skin and are outside the massage scope of practice, many spa treatments have physiological effects in common with massage and enhance a massage practice. A wide range of therapies might be offered in an array of different settings under the title of "spa." This section briefly describes the history of spa therapy, explains guidelines for scope of practice related to spa, introduces common spa treatments, and describes product removal techniques, exfoliation treatments, and body wraps.

A Brief History of Spa

It is hard to pin down the origin of spa therapy. Mineral springs and thermal muds (muds that occur naturally around hot springs that tend to be high in minerals and sulfur) were probably used therapeutically as the earliest civilizations developed. Perhaps the most famous ancient spas were those of the Roman Empire, where public baths were part of Roman culture and served an important social function as well as a means of hygiene. The Romans had a well-developed understanding of hydrotherapy (healing with water), and garrisons were often built around hot springs so that the soldiers could heal their battle wounds using water cures.[1] Water has long been central to spa therapy, and bathing in mineral-rich waters is still a popular way to relax, soothe muscular aches and pains, improve range of motion, and treat many skin disorders.

In the 18th and 19th centuries, Europeans would "take the waters" for common ailments such as rheumatism and respiratory disorders. Often, spas were built in secluded mountain towns near natural mineral springs, providing visitors with spectacular views, fresh clean air, and exercise on nature walks in addition to the benefits of the mineral water. Medical professionals carefully monitored visitors' treatment, and spas as medical retreats became the norm in Europe.

In America, Elizabeth Arden turned her Maine summer home into a beauty and health spa called the Maine Chance in the 1930s. She targeted two groups of woman: middle-aged women trying to recapture youth and "plain" women looking for a means to achieve "beauty in a jar."[2] With cosmetics as her primary product, Arden pioneered the integration of diet, exercise, sports, yoga, facials, massage, beauty training, and pampering into a focused spa program, creating America's version of a retreat spa. Today, Arden's signature Red Door Salons is recognized worldwide.

Unfortunately, spas in the early 1960s developed the stigma of "fat farms" for wealthy woman who wanted to lose weight and detoxify (sometimes from drug and alcohol addictions).[3] The "fat farm" stigma may have slowed the growth of the spa industry for some time, but the concept of an integrated program of fitness, diet, and healthy lifestyle training balanced with pampering treatments and beauty became established. In the 1970s, hair salons seeking to expand their businesses started to offer à la carte spa treatments as well as regular salon services. This transformation of the salon into the day spa took hold, and today 7 of every 10 salons is a day spa.[4]

Scope of Practice Considerations

The rapid growth of the spa industry in the last decade has led to some confusion about scope-of-practice issues between massage therapists and estheticians. In many states, the board of cosmetology has raised concerns that massage therapists are encroaching on the scope of practice of estheticians when they provide such services as seaweed wraps or body polishes. On the other hand, in some states, massage therapists are concerned that estheticians are using massage techniques that manipulate soft tissue while applying products and so are encroaching on the scope of practice for massage therapists. The basis of such concerns is that many of the products used in the spa industry affect circulation, stress levels, and muscle tissue health (general massage scope of practice), as well as the health and appearance of the skin (general esthetics scope of practice). A seaweed wrap could be used for relaxation or as an active treatment to reduce symptoms of fibromyalgia, sore muscles, or low energy (massage scope of practice). A seaweed wrap might also be used to soften, hydrate, and beautify the skin (esthetics scope of practice). Body polishes stimulate circulation and lymph flow, tone muscle tissue, and increase the vital energy of the body as in a classic friction rub (massage scope of practice). They also deep-clean, soften, smooth, and beautify the skin (esthetics scope of practice).

This issue is further complicated because laws and regulations vary widely from state to state. A treatment that is within the scope of practice for massage therapists in some states may be banned for massage therapists in other states. For example, massage therapists cannot cleanse, exfoliate, or mask facial tissue in most states. They can apply creams or lotions (including essential oils) to the face to perform massage. In many states, massage therapists cannot use the word "facial" even when describing a facial massage (they must say face massage). In a few states, however, massage therapists can provide facials but using only certain types of products. Usually (but not always), massage therapists can use an exfoliation product such as salt on the body (except the face) to increase circulation, reduce muscle tension, and relax the body. Products like seaweed and mud can be used to promote changes in soft tissue or for relaxation or revitalization. If you offer spa treatments in your massage practice or deliver them as an employee at a spa, make sure that the promotional descriptions emphasize the benefits of the treatment for the body rather than the skin. If the treatment aims to beautify the skin, it is out of your scope of practice and should be delivered by an esthetician. You should check whether there are any treatments or practices that are not allowed by the laws in your state and that your liability insurance policy covers the treatments you offer.

Overview of Spa Therapies

Massage is the most popular treatment at spas, according to the 2007 International Spa Association Survey.[5] Facials, manicures, and pedicures are also popular. Clients report that they want to focus on health, fitness, antiaging, increased energy, and stress reduction. Many clients visit spas simply to revitalize themselves and give themselves a break from work stresses. Cultural elements that include ayurvedic medicine, Native American wisdom, and Asian influences are used to inspire treatments and create links to the environment and the global community. Going green at spas is a recent trend, with spas offering treatments featuring natural products, organic linens, and recycling. Table 15-1 provides an overview of services commonly offered at spas.

TABLE 15-1 Overview of Common Spa Therapies

The laws, regulations, and scope of practice for professionals working in spas vary widely from state to state. Review the laws in your state before providing any treatments. Also check that a given treatment is covered by your liability insurance. This table provides only an overview and is not comprehensive in terms of treatments or the industry professionals who might deliver them.

Spa Service	Benefits	Likely Industry Professional
Hydrotherapy Specialized showers, steams, baths, saunas, and other applications using water.	The benefits of hydrotherapy treatments depend on the temperature of the treatment, length of the treatment, and the effects of the specialized apparatus that is used in combination with water. See Chapter 16 for details.	Physician, physical therapist, massage therapist, estheticians use specialized baths and showers in the removal of products or to improve the health and condition of the skin.
Full-Body Exfoliation Loofah scrubs, full-body polish, salt glows, sugar glows, dry skin brushing, almond scrub, others. Estheticians can also deliver enzyme peels.	Stimulates circulation, lymph flow, stimulates vital energy of the body, relaxation, revitalization, deep-cleans, removes dead skin cells, softens and refines the skins texture, beautifies the skin	Massage therapist, esthetician Exfoliation has benefits for both skin and body. Massage therapists focus on the benefits for the body, while estheticians focus on the benefits for the skin.

TABLE 15-1   Overview of Common Spa Therapies *(Continued)*

Spa Service	Benefits	Likely Industry Professional
Auto-Tanning Buff and bronze, spray on tans, spray tan booths	Auto-tanning treatments are most often delivered to darken skin color so that the client appears tan.	Massage therapist, esthetician Spray tans and booths can be facilitated by unlicensed or uncertified individuals in most states.
Body Wraps A wide variety including herbal, seaweed, fango, cryogenic, slimming, detoxifying, aromatherapy, others.	The benefits of the treatment depend on the products and techniques that are used during the service.	Massage therapist, esthetician Depending on the desired effects of the application and on the promotional description of the service.
Thalassotherapy Treatments using seawater, seaweed, marine algae, sea air, and diets high in sea products	Thalassotherapy has been used for a wide range of conditions. In general, it revitalizes and detoxifies the body and beautifies the skin.	Massage therapist, esthetician, physical therapist, physician Depending on the desired effects of the application and on the promotional description of the service.
Fangotherapy Treatments using therapeutic mud, clay, and peat	Fangotherapy has been used for a wide range of conditions but especially arthritis and musculoskeletal conditions and to beautify the skin.	Massage therapist, esthetician, physical therapist, physician Depending on the desired effects of the application and on the promotional description of the service.
Spot Treatments Cellulite, back, bust, others	The benefits of the treatment depend on the type of products and techniques that are used during the service.	Esthetician, massage therapist
Foot and Hand Treatments (not pedicures or manicures) Treatments that do not include trimming the nail or cuticle.	Pain relieving, relaxing, revitalizing, stimulates circulation, increases range of motion, can be used to treat soft-tissue pathology like plantar fasciitis.	Massage therapist, certified reflexologist (some states) Estheticians deliver nonpedicure or manicure services to beautify the hands and feet. Massage therapists and reflexologists focus on treatments that relax the body and decrease foot pain. Estheticians focus on the beautification of the skin of the hands and feet.
Pedicures Foot treatments that include trimming the nail and cuticle.	Relaxing, improves the overall health and appearance of the feet, beautifies the feet	Nail technician, cosmetologist estheticians (some states)
Manicures Treatments that include trimming the nail and cuticle.	Relaxing, improves the overall health and appearance of the hands, beautifies the hands	Nail technician, cosmetologist Estheticians (some states)
Massage Swedish, shiatsu, manual lymphatic drainage, craniosacral, lomilomi, Thai, sports, deep tissue, others	The effects of the massage depend on the types of techniques used. In general, massage stimulates circulation and lymphatic flow, relaxes the body, and decreases soft-tissue imbalance.	Massage therapist, physical therapist Sometimes specialized training and certification are required to deliver certain types of massage.
Stone Massage	Warms tissue, stimulates circulation, decreases tension in hypertonic muscles, decreases adhesions, relaxes the body.	Massage therapist
Ayurveda-Inspired Body Treatments Abhyanga, dosha wrap, dosha massage, ubvartana, Indian head massage, shirodhara, pinda abhyanga, pizzichilli, garshan, others	Relax the body, stimulate circulation, revitalize the body, facilitate detoxification of body tissues, bring balance to the body, promote spiritual awareness, create a space for reflection and renewal. See Chapter 17, Topic 17-2, for details	Ayurvedic physician, massage therapist
Ayurveda-Inspired Beauty Treatments Facials, shirodhara, ubvartana, dosha skin wraps, scalp treatments, pedicures and manicures, others	Beautify the intended area using ayurveda principles and products	Ayurvedic physician, esthetician, cosmetologist, nail technician

(Continued)

TABLE 15-1 Overview of Common Spa Therapies (Continued)

Spa Service	Benefits	Likely Industry Professional
Natural and Traditional Forms of Medicine Ayurveda, Chinese traditional medicine, acupuncture, naturopathic medicine, herbal medicine, others	Bring the body into balance, treat a specific condition, or as a preventative to disease	Ayurvedic physician, traditional chinese medicine practitioner, acupuncturist, naturopathic doctor, herbal medicine practitioner
Facials	Deep-clean, smooth, refine, soften, and condition the facial skin and to treat certain skin conditions on the face. Improve the appearance and beautify the skin. Slow the signs of aging.	Esthetician Cosmetologists (some states)
Face and Scalp Massage	Relax the muscles of face and scalp, decrease overall tension, firm and tone the muscles of the face, stimulate the skin and increase local circulation, aid in product penetration, loosen trapped debris in the follicles, facilitate product application to the face or scalp.	Massage therapist, esthetician, cosmetologist
Hair Removal Services Physical depilatories (wax), chemical depilatories (powder, cream, others), electrolysis, electric current tweezers	Remove unwanted hair from the body. Electrolysis is a form of permanent hair removal, while depilatories remove the hair temporarily.	Esthetician, cosmetologist Electrolysis is performed by a licensed electrologist
Nails Includes nail art, gel nails, acrylic nails.	Beautify the hands and the feet, improve nail health, embellish the nails for esthetic purposes.	Nail technician Cosmetologist (some states)
Hair Services Cutting, styling, highlighting, coloring, perming, straightening, conditioning, etc.	Improve the health and/or appearance of the hair. Stimulate the scalp and promote healthy hair growth.	Cosmetologist
Makeup Application	Improve the appearance of the face or camouflage a skin condition or injury such as scaring from burns	Esthetician, cosmetologist
Nutrition Nutrition assessment and/or programming, healthy cooking	Assess the nutritional viability of a client's diet and make recommendations that lead to better nutritional health. Support healing from a specific condition using diet.	Nutritionist Fitness trainer
Fitness Fitness assessment or programming, personal training	Assess the fitness level of the client and to make recommendations that lead to better physical health. Motivate clients to reach their physical goals	Fitness trainer Strength and conditioning specialist
Mind/Spirit Therapies Hypnotherapy, group counseling, counseling, psychotherapy, guided meditation, life coaching, yoga, others	Support the individual in finding inner peace and contentment. Guide personal transformation, create relationships and connections, generate resource states for better living.	Psychotherapists, psychologists, counselors, hypnotherapists, yoga instructors, spiritual instructors, life coaches, others

Product Management

One of the keys to providing spa body treatments is good product management. In upcoming sections, you learn to apply particular products in a series of steps to deliver common spa treatments like body wraps and salt glows. In a **wet room** (a tiled room with drains in the floor that allows services using water to be applied efficiently), a specialized shower is used to remove spa products from the client's body. Showers include handheld showers, standard showers, Swiss showers, and Vichy showers. Always read the manufacturer's instructions for the equipment beforehand. Practice with the shower so that you know how to make the water temperature and pressure comfortable for clients. Wet room equipment used to remove spa products is demonstrated in Technique 34.

Hot, moist towels are often used to remove products in **dry room** environments (facilities that do not include wet room equipment, are not tiled, and do not have a drainage

| Technique 34 | **Wet Room Removal Techniques** |

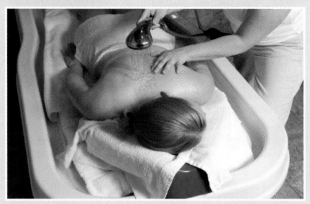

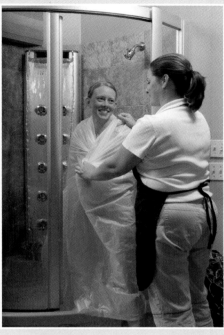

1. Handheld Shower. A handheld shower is used in combination with a wet table for the easy removal of product. Some handheld showers can deliver a pulsating water massage and may also have an attachable body brush for exfoliation. A wet table has a special surface to channel water into a receptacle under the table or a drain in the wet room floor. Hold the shower in one hand and use the other to gently massage products from clients until the client is clean of product.

2. Standard Shower. When you are ready to remove the product from the client's body, ask the client to get off the massage table using the plastic covering used during the wrap as a drape. The client steps into the running shower and passes the plastic back to you so that you can throw it away. Place clean linens on the massage table and tidy the treatment room while the client showers.

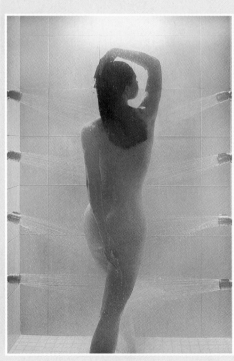

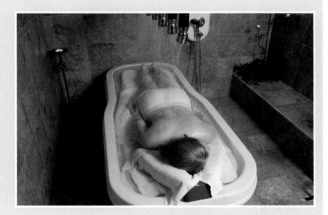

3. Swiss Shower. A Swiss shower surrounds the client with jets of water directed at specific areas of the body. Usually the shower stall has pipes in all four corners with 8 to 16 water heads on each pipe. Adjust the position of the water heads for the client's height. A control panel outside the shower stall allows you to control contrasting warm and cool jets of water. A Swiss shower can be used for product removal, as an active treatment in itself, or to provide the heating phase of treatments like herbal detoxification body wraps.

4. The Vichy Shower. A Vichy shower is a horizontal rod with holes or water heads that rain water down onto the client from above the wet table. Vichy showers are used to rinse spa products off the client, but they can also be used as a treatment in themselves. A control panel allows you to alternate between hot and cool water, which increases the therapeutic benefits of some products and uses the mechanical effects of water to invigorate soft tissue. Vichy showers have an adjustable face guard to keep water from the client's face, although some water invariably gets through. A soft, lightweight washcloth can be used to cover the client's face and protect it from water droplets. Care must be used when moving the client off the wet table because the area around the table may be slippery with water.

system in the floor). To prepare the towels, pull off all tags, fold the towels in half (the long way), and roll them up like a sausage. It is important to remove all tags because they could scratch the client. Place the towels in a hydroculator, hot towel cabinet, or heating unit like the one used for hot stone massage for 20 minutes at 165°F. Wearing thermal gloves, remove a towel from the water, wring it out, and place it in a soda cooler. Close the lid of the cooler and remove the next towel. Keep the lid of the cooler shut as much as possible so that the towels stay hot throughout the treatment.

Towels can be enhanced by adding three to five drops of essential oils to the soda cooler once full of towels. Removing each towel fills the treatment room with a refreshing scent. Most single essential oils such as eucalyptus, rosemary, common sage (*Salvia officinalis*), Spanish sage (*Salvia lavandulifolia*), thyme, and lemon oil smell good, but floral scents like ylang ylang and jasmine are not as pleasant in steam. The

essential oil on the towel is not likely to cause any skin irritation as essential oils are volatile substances and begin to evaporate rapidly when they are placed on the hot towels in the cooler. They will have evaporated before the first towel is used, leaving only some scent behind. Skin irritation is therefore minimized.

Muslin bags filled with fragrant herbs can also be used to scent towels. A muslin bag of herbs is added to the water the towels are heated in. A nice combination is eucalyptus leaf, rosemary, clove buds, and juniper berry. A half a cup of herbs to around 16 quarts of water provides a nice concentration, although more or less herbs can be used according to taste. Towels heated in herbal solutions will be lightly stained. Some therapists color-coordinate their towels for the treatment (e.g., green towels for seaweed treatments, brown towels for mud treatments, and beige towels for herbal infusions) to camouflage any product stains. Dry room removal techniques with hot towels are demonstrated in Technique 35.

Technique 35 — Hot Towel Removal Techniques

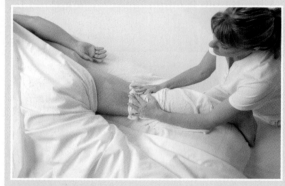

1. Hot Towel Removal—Legs. Remove a towel from the soda cooler and hold it by the edges (because it is hot). Let it cool slightly and place it on the proximal portion of the leg (anterior or posterior). Leave it on the leg and do not touch it again until it cools down (about 30 seconds). Place both hands on the towel and pull it toward the distal portion of the leg and off the foot. Turn the towel over and use the clean side to make another sweep.

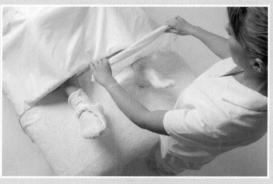

2. Hot Towel Removal—Feet. Place a hot towel around each foot to steam the feet and provide a nice sensation; then remove the product from one foot at a time.

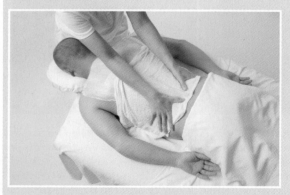

3. Hot Towel Removal—Back. Place the hot towel horizontally on the lower back and allow it to cool slightly without touching it. Place both hands on the towel and pull it toward the client's head. As the towel gets to the neck, pull it off to one side, removing the product from the shoulder without getting it into the client's hair. Turn the towel over and use the clean side to make a second sweep, removing the product from the second shoulder.

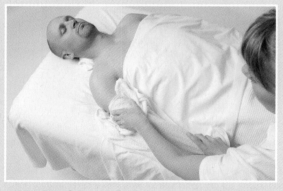

4. Hot Towel Removal—Arms. Place the hot towel vertically on the proximal portion of the arm and pull the towel toward the hand in one sweep. Lift the arm by holding onto the client's hand, and use the clean side of the towel to wipe down the other side of the arm.

Technique 35	**Hot Towel Removal Techniques** (Continued)

5. Hot Towel Removal—Abdominal Area and Upper Chest.
Place the hot towel horizontally on the belly and pull it from the left side to the right side. Turn the towel over and use the clean side to remove product from right to left. Place a hot towel across the upper chest and remove the product by pulling the towel from one side to the other.

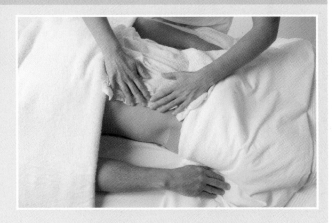

Exfoliation Treatments

Chapter 4 describes how massage desquamates dead skin cells, increases local circulation, and revitalizes the body. **Exfoliation** treatments support these effects when a coarse-textured product or handheld cloth, brush, or mitt is applied to the skin. This brightens the skin by removing the dull top layer of dead cells, causes circulation to increase in the local tissue, improving nutrient exchange and tissue health, and stimulates the nervous system, leaving the body refreshed and rejuvenated. Cautions and contraindications for exfoliation treatments are described in Box 15-1. Common exfoliation treatments include salt or sugar glows, dry brushing, and loofah scrubs.

BOX 15-1 Cautions and Contraindications for Exfoliation Treatments

Cautions: The overuse of manual exfoliation products during a treatment can leave the skin sensitive and inflamed. If such products are used too frequently, the skin will start to thicken and grow leathery. Exfoliation treatments should not be given more than once a week for the best results.
Contraindications: Exfoliation products should not be used on open wounds or broken skin, on clients with chronic skin conditions, on sunburned or inflamed skin, over varicose veins, or within 24 hours of waxing or shaving. Avoid the use of table salt, which has a higher concentration of chloride than sea salt and may burn the client's skin.

Sea Salt and Sugar Glows

In a **salt** or **sugar glow** (also called salt or sugar scrubs), different types of mineral salts (Dead Sea salt, Bearn salt, sea salt, Epson salt, etc.) or sugar (table sugar, brown sugar, raw sugar, etc.) are rubbed across the surface of the skin and then removed with hot, moist towels or a spa shower. Sea salt and sugar glows feel invigorating and desquamate dead skin cells to leave the skin soft and smooth. They can easily be integrated with massage in a dry room to produce a treatment that is popular with clients.

Equipment, Supplies, and Setup

Set up your massage table for a sea salt or sugar glow by placing a large bath towel (about the size of a beach towel) over the bottom massage sheet. The towel catches any excess salt or sugar that falls off the client during the treatment and absorbs dampness from the hot, moist towels used to remove the salt. A top sheet and blanket serve as a drape and keep the client warm. On a nearby worktable place a cheese shaker filled with sea salt or sugar, a bottle of massage oil, a bottle of body lotion or aloe vera gel, a soda cooler holding nine hot, moist hand towels, a bowl of warm water, and two dry hand towels. A popular sea salt or sugar glow procedure is shown in Technique 36.

Dry Skin Brushing

Dry skin brushing is a technique where natural bristle brushes, rough hand mitts, or textured cloths are used to stimulate the sebaceous glands, increase local circulation, remove dead skin cells, and invigorate the nervous system to revitalize the body. Dry brushing can be applied as part of a full-body massage to aid a detoxification program (Technique 37). Each body area is treated in sequence. First undrape and dry brush the area (A). Next, apply a full range of massage strokes with a massage

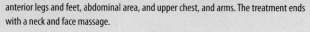

| Technique 36 | A Sea Salt or Sugar Glow Procedure |

It works well to start a glow with the client in a prone position. Follow the steps below for the legs and back, and then turn the client into the supine position and treat the anterior legs and feet, abdominal area, and upper chest, and arms. The treatment ends with a neck and face massage.

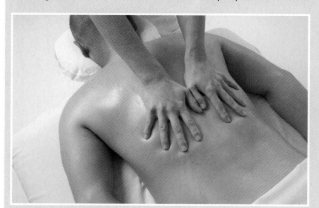

1. Massage. Undrape the body area and apply massage oil with a full range of Swedish strokes. Directly before you apply salt or sugar to the area, add extra massage oil to the skin to prevent skin irritation and client discomfort.

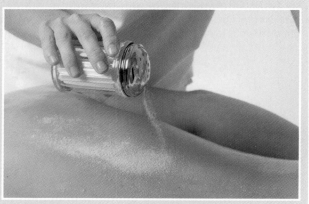

2. Exfoliation. Sprinkle a moderate amount of salt or sugar from the cheese shaker onto the client's body area. Control the application of the product so that the salt or sugar does not get all over the massage table. Work the salt or sugar across the top of the skin with gentle circular strokes to stimulate circulation and remove dead skin cells. Massage therapists often overexfoliate as they tend to work into the muscle rather than keeping the strokes superficial. With coarse crystalline products like salt, this can cause some discomfort to the client. Check regularly with clients to ensure they are happy with the depth of the application and the sensation of the exfoliation.

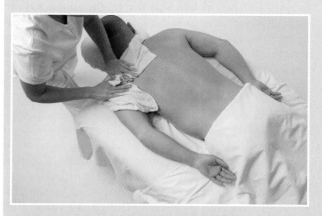

3. Hot Towel Removal. Remove the salt or sugar mix with a hot towel. It should be possible to remove all of the salt or sugar using just one hand towel per body area.

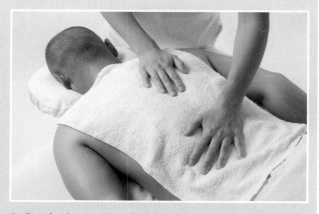

4. Dry. Dry the area with a soft hand towel, redrape the area, and move on to the next body area. You can also choose to finish the body area with the application of body lotion, body cream, or aloe vera gel. This conditions the skin, which may be slightly dry from the salt or sugar, and feels cooling and soothing. When you have completed these four steps for each body area, finish the session by massaging the client's neck and face with massage cream. This rounds out and completes the session so that the client feels the benefits of both the glow and a full-body massage.

lubricant (B1 and B2). Finally, lay hot steamy, herbal infused towels over the area and use the towels to remove any excess massage lubricant to leave the client feeling clean and invigorated (C).

Equipment, Supplies, and Setup

Prepare the table and supplies as you would for a full-body massage. On a nearby worktable, place two natural fiber brushes, rough textured mitts, or fiber cloths. In an enhanced treatment, you might also prepare nine steamy herbal-infused towels and place these in a small soda cooler. Techniques for dry brushing each body area are shown in Technique 37.

Loofah Scrub

The **loofah scrub** (also called a body scrub) is the most invigorating of the exfoliation treatments. It is often paired with uplifting and refreshing essential oils (e.g., eucalyptus scrub and citrus mint scrub) to create inviting smell-scapes that entice clients (a later section describes smell-scapes).

| Technique 37 | Dry Skin Brushing |

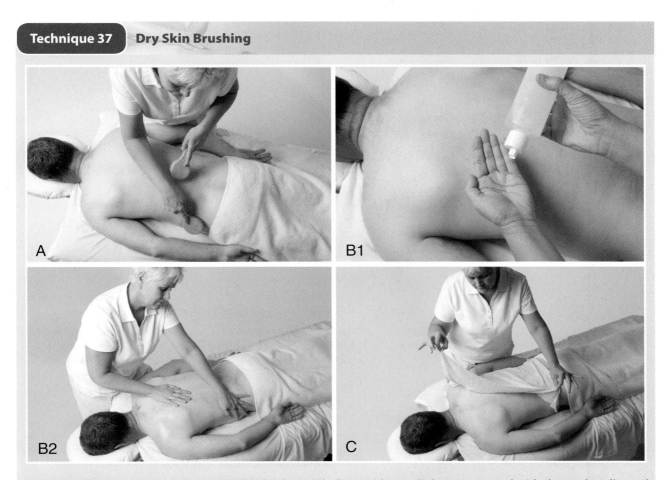

A

B1

B2

C

1. **Dry brushing works best when applied in brisk straight lines with very light pressure and with the strokes directed toward the heart.**

Continued

Technique 37   **Dry Skin Brushing** (Continued)

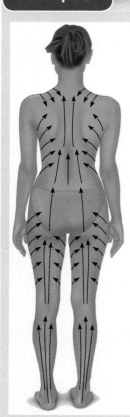

Back:

1. Side to center
2. Sacrum to mid-back
3. Mid-back to shoulders

Posterior leg:

1. Ankle to knee
2. Knee to hip
3. Medial thigh
4. Lateral thigh
5. Ankle to hip

2. Posterior body. Each area of the posterior body is "brushed" in a specific direction to enhance lymphatic flow, cause desquamation of dead skin cells, and increase blood circulation as shown by this diagram. Specifics for brushing each particular area are described here:

1. **Posterior legs:** Brush the posterior leg with overlapping strokes from the ankle to the knee so that the entire area is covered. Brush from the knee to the hip across the top of the thigh with overlapping strokes. To brush the inner thigh, stand at the client's hip facing toward the foot of the table. Place both brushes on the medial aspect of the thigh and pull them toward the outside of the leg in light, rhythmic strokes. To brush the lateral thigh, stand by the knee and run the brushes briskly up the iliotibial band to the hip. To finish dry brushing the posterior leg, brush from the ankle all the way up the leg with long flushing strokes.

2. **The back:** Stand on one side of the client facing across the client's body. Place the brushes on the far side of the client and pull them in light strokes toward the spine, working from both sides of the body. To dry brush the main area of the back, stand at the head of the table and begin the stroke at the sacrum, pulling the brush toward the head of the client.

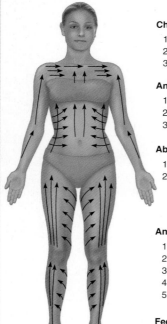

Chest area:

1. Navel to upper chest
2. Armpit to sternum
3. Upper chest

Anterior arms:

1. Fingers to elbow
2. Elbow to shoulder
3. Fingers to shoulder

Abdominal area:

1. Side to center
2. Hip to armpit

Anterior legs:

1. Medial leg
2. Ankle to knee
3. Knee to hip
4. Lateral leg
5. Ankle to hip

Feet:

1. Toes to heel

3. Anterior Body. Just as with the posterior body, brush strokes should be light, brisk, and in the direction indicated by this diagram. Specific areas are bushed as follows:

1. **Anterior legs:** When dry brushing the anterior legs, it is easiest to start with the medial leg, standing at the client's hip and facing toward the foot of the table. Start the strokes by the ankle and work up the leg. Each stroke runs from the medial side of the leg to the midline of the leg. Dry brush the top of the anterior leg by standing at the client's foot and brushing upward toward the knee with light, overlapping strokes. The upper leg is brushed from the knee to the hip in straight, overlapping strokes. The lateral leg is brushed from the ankle to the knee along the peroneal muscles, and from the knee to the hip along the iliotibial band.

2. **Abdominal area:** To brush the abdominal area, stand to one side of the client and brush from the far side of the body toward the centerline. Brush from the hip into the armpit while standing at the head of the table and pulling the brushes upward in a straight line.

3. **Chest:** Stand at the head of the table and brush from below the navel, pulling in a straight line between the breasts with overlapping strokes. To avoid the breast drape, simply lift the brush and "jump" over it. Brush from the armpit up and around the breast, ending at the upper portion of the sternum. Again, jump over the breast drape to keep the flow of the stroke. To finish the chest area, stand to one side of the massage table and brush across the upper chest from one shoulder to the other in a straight line.

4. **Arms:** Brush from the fingers to the elbow and from the elbow to the shoulder. To complete the arms, use long strokes all the way from the fingers to the shoulder.

5. **Feet:** Before brushing the feet, check them carefully for fungal infections. If athlete's foot or any other contagious condition exists, skip the feet to avoid spreading the condition. When brushing the feet, wipe them first with a disposable antibacterial cloth such as a diaper wipe. Brush the feet from the toes down to the heel. Brush firmly to avoid tickling the client, but if the client is too ticklish to tolerate this, skip the feet and move on.

Equipment, Supplies, and Setup

The table is set with a bath towel over the bottom massage sheet to absorb excess water from the application of the body wash product. A top sheet and blanket are used for a drape and warmth. On a nearby worktable, place a bottle of body wash product (any type of foaming bath gel will work), two loofah mitts, a bowl of warm water, two dry hand towels, and a moisturizer. Fill a small soda cooler with nine hot, moist hand towels. The procedure for a loofah scrub is shown in Technique 38.

Body Wraps

A body wrap is a spa treatment in which the client relaxes in warm sheets and blankets while covered in a therapeutic product like seaweed or mud. A large variety of products are used in body wraps depending on the goals of the session. Some products are applied for cosmetic effects by estheticians (e.g., cellulite treatment and skin softening), some by massage therapists for detoxification (e.g., herbal hot wrap), relaxation (e.g., aromatherapy wrap), sore muscles (e.g., Dead Sea mud wrap), and for many other purposes. Table 15-2 outlines some common body wrap types, as well as the benefits and effects of therapeutic products. Box 15-2 provides an overview of general cautions and contraindications for body wraps.

It is especially important to remain with a client at all times during a body wrap to ensure the client's safety. Some clients experience claustrophobia and become anxious or panic stricken when wrapped up tightly. Watch for signs of distress such as rapid breathing or a concerned expression on the client's face. If the client becomes anxious, remove his or her arms from the wrap. If the claustrophobia persists, remove the client from the wrap and modify the treatment.

There are numerous ways to deliver a body wrap, but described here are a basic hot sheet wrap procedure and a basic cocoon procedure. Once you understand how to apply

---

Technique 38   The Loofah Scrub

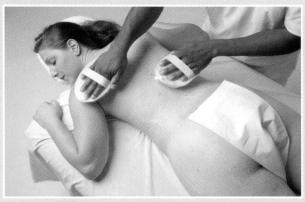

1. Use a gluteal drape so that the entire posterior body can be treated at one time. Apply a foaming body wash with two handheld loofahs to the posterior body using long sweeping strokes beginning at the ankle, progressing up the legs to the gluteals, across the back, and then down the opposite leg.

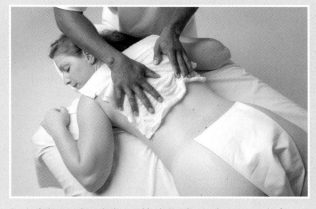

2. Apply hot towels to the legs and back. Use the towels to remove the foaming bodywash product.

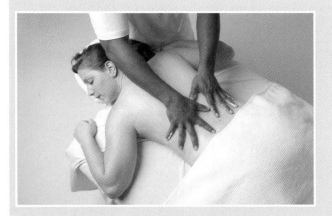

3. Redrape to keep the client warm, and then massage each body area (posterior legs, gluteals, and back) with a moisturizing massage cream. Turn the client and repeat the steps on the anterior body (anterior legs, feet, abdominal area, and arms). End the session with a neck and face massage.

TABLE 15-2   Body Wraps and Products

Type	Product	Product Notes, Effects, and Benefits	Product Preparation
Hot sheet wrap	Herbs	Herbs are chosen based on their therapeutic properties. Herbs to support detoxification include rosemary, juniper, clove, allspice, ginger root, echinacea, goldenrod, lemon peel, nettle, parsley, and sage. Herbs to reduce soreness and stiffness in musculoskeletal structures include eucalyptus, juniper, peppermint, ginger root, clove, bay laurel, pine, thyme, wintergreen and yarrow. Herbs that promote slimming and firming include juniper berry, lemon peel, thyme, fennel seeds, ginger root, dulse, horsetail, parsley, rosemary leaf, and yarrow.	One cup of dried herbs is placed in a muslin bag or tea ball and steeped in the hot water in which the sheets are soaked.
Hot sheet wrap	Milk and honey	Milk and honey is softening and conditioning for the skin and smells warm and homey. It supports relaxation and stress reduction.	Add one or two cups of honey and one or two cups of powdered or full fat milk or buttermilk to the hot water in which the sheets are soaked.
Hot sheet wrap	Juice	Juices like cranberry, pineapple, apple cider, orange, and others brighten and firm the skin, stimulate circulation, smell pleasing, support relaxation and stress reduction. During the holidays, cider, honey, and wine mulling spices make a deliciously aromatic seasonal hot wrap.	Mix one gallon of juice with the hot water in which the sheets are soaked.
Hot sheet wrap or cocoon	Seaweed	Topical seaweed stimulates the thyroid gland and leaves the body feeling energized. It stimulates circulation, decreases muscle stiffness, is useful to reduce the symptoms of fibromyalgia, boosts metabolism, promotes detoxification, and firms the skin. Do not use seaweed on clients with shellfish or iodine allergies because serious reactions might result.	Add two tablespoons to the hot water in which sheets are soaked. For cocoons, mix seaweed powder with warm water or use a gel-based product.
Hot sheet wrap or cocoon	Mud/peat	Therapeutic muds and peats like Dead Sea mud and Moor mud are anti-inflammatory, analgesic, and detoxifying. They are often used for musculoskeletal injury rehabilitation, stiff joints, sore muscles, and general relaxation.	Warm the mud or peat in a hot water bath and mix it to a smooth consistency. Approximately 2 cups of product are needed for a full-body treatment.
Hot sheet wrap or cocoon	Clay	Clay pulls impurities from the skin's surface as it dries and stimulates circulation while conditioning the skin. It is often used to "carry" other therapeutic substances such as essential oils.	Add 1 cup of dry clay to the water in which you soak the sheets for a hot sheet wrap. Mix up about 2 cups of dry clay with warm water for a full-body cocoon.
Cocoon	Emollients	Heavy lipids like shea butter, almond butter, evening primrose, wheat germ, jojoba, hemp seed, and borage oil have natural healing properties that condition the skin and relax the body.	Warm the butter or oil and apply it to the body with a brush in a heavy layer. After the cocoon, use the butter or oil still remaining on the skin as the lubricant for massage.
Cocoon	Essential oils	Each essential oil has specific therapeutic properties for the body when used topically. Oils might be chosen to reduce muscle soreness, promote detoxification, boost immunity, and many other purposes. Usually essential oils are mixed in a carrier like an emollient butter or clay.	Use a total of 12–15 drops of an essential oil blend mixed into an emollient butter, clay, aloe vera gel, or body lotion.
Cocoon	Aloe vera	Aloe vera is usually the main ingredient in sunburn wraps offered at resort spas where often clients have been overexposed to the sun on the first few days of their vacation. It soothes dry skin, ulcerations, chapped skin, eczema, and sunburn.	Usually about 1–2 cups of aloe is mixed with soothing essential oils like lavender, German chamomile, and a drop of cooling peppermint for a sunburn cocoon.
Cocoon	Cryogenic	Cryogenic products are often composed of a clay based with menthol as the active ingredient. Menthol increases local circulation and has a pain-relieving effect. Cryogenic products are most often applied as spot application because they cool the body and the client can become too cold.	Mix the product based on the manufacturer's directions.
Cocoon	Natural elements	Natural foods such as papaya, pumpkin, avocado, honey, yogurt, oatmeal, and cucumber have soothing, revitalizing properties for the skin and are often used in cocoons for skin healing and relaxation.	Often natural products are mashed up and mixed with a clay or gel base before they are applied to the body.

BOX 15-2 Cautions and Contraindications for Body Wrap Treatments

Cautions: Before delivering any type of body wrap, carry out a careful pretreatment health interview with the client to make sure that there are no contraindications for the treatment. Wraps may trigger rapid detoxification of the body, which may result in a headache and nausea. It is normal for clients to experience mild detoxification symptoms. However, if the symptoms are intense or if they occur during the wrap itself, remove the client from the wrap and encourage drinking water and resting at a comfortable temperature. If the client's symptoms persist after being unwrapped or if they get worse rapidly, the client could be in danger and you should consult a physician or call emergency services.

Carefully check for allergies to herbs, essential oils, iodine which is present in seaweed, or other ingredients in the products being used. Never leave the client alone while wrapped. In one case filed with an insurance company, a woman went into anaphylactic shock from an allergic reaction to seaweed. Because she was left alone while wrapped, she could not free herself to seek assistance, and she died on the massage table.

Contraindications: Hot sheet wraps should not be used on children, the elderly, pregnant women, or clients with heart conditions, high blood pressure, peripheral neuropathy, diabetes, poor circulation, or kidney or liver conditions. Hot wraps are contraindicated for those that have recently been in a car accident, suffered a soft-tissue injury, have rheumatoid arthritis, or are contraindicated for massage.

wraps following these two procedures, you can develop multiple body wrap treatments for your private practice or to deliver specific wraps for an employer at a spa or clinic.

Hot Sheet Wraps

In a **hot sheet wrap**, the treatment product (herbs, coffee, milk, honey, seaweed, mud, etc.) is dissolved in hot water. Two muslin sheets (or a sheet and a bath towel) are steeped in the dissolved product and then wrapped around the client. This method is often used for detoxification treatments or where the goal is to stimulate metabolism as part of a weight loss program, to decrease water retention, or to boost immunity. One of the reasons hot sheet wraps are so effective for detoxification is that they elevate body temperature creating an "artificial fever" and stimulating perspiration.

Equipment, Supplies, and Setup

To set up your massage table for a hot sheet wrap, place a wool blanket horizontally across the table so that the long edges fall off either side. A thermal space blanket is placed horizontally on top of the wool blanket. These insulating wrap materials trap body heat and ensure that the wrap is warm enough to cause the client to perspire freely. One bath towel is placed

horizontally at the top of the treatment table, while a second is placed horizontally at the bottom of the treatment table. The towels are wrapped around the client's head and feet to keep body heat inside the wrap. Set the massage table at a lower height so that it is easy for the client to climb onto the table and lie down on top of the hot sheet during the procedure. The table setup for a hot sheet wrap is shown in Figure 15-1.

Dissolve the hot wrap treatment product (herbs, seaweed, milk and honey, etc.) in hot water (165°F) in either an 18-quart heating unit like the one used for hot stone massage or a hydrocollator. Fold two muslin or cotton wrap sheets (or one sheet and one bath towel) into tight squares as shown in Figure 15-2, and place them in the heating product solution for 20 minutes. A clean stone or weight placed on top of the sheets keeps them submerged completely. Never use flannel or jersey sheets for hot sheet wraps because they are difficult to wring out completely and often have hot "pockets" that can burn the client.

Organize a pair of insulated gloves, a small soda cooler, an aroma mist, glass of water with a flexible straw, and light

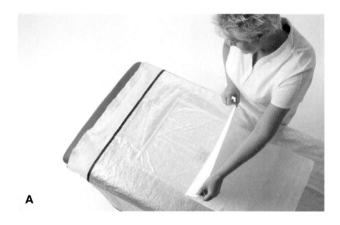

A

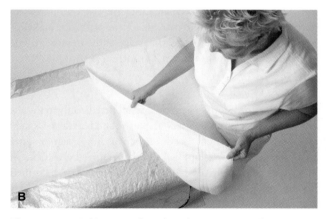

B

Figure 15-1 Table setup for a hot sheet wrap. **A.** The massage table is set from the outermost layer to innermost layer as follows: wool blanket, thermal space blanket (shiny side up), and Fomentek hot-water bottle (optional) covered by a pillow case. The hot sheet will be unfolded on top of the thermal space blanket (and optional Fomentek) immediately before the client gets on the table and is wrapped up. **B.** A bath towel is placed lengthwise over the edges of the blankets on each end of the table. One of these bath towels will be used to wrap up the head and the other to wrap up the feet.

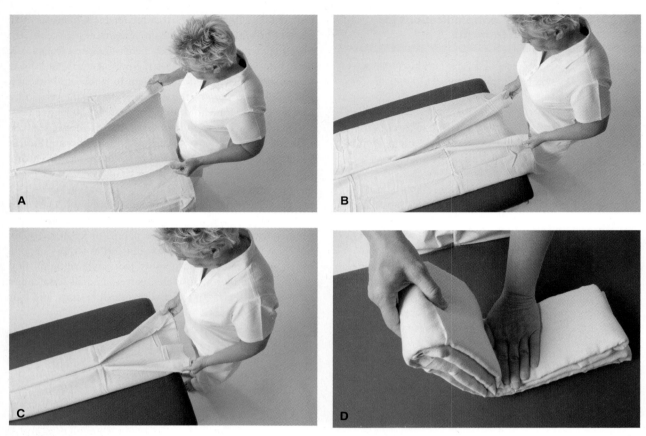

Figure 15-2 A Open the sheet lengthwise across the width of the massage table and fold the long sides into the center. **B, C.** Fold the two new sides into the center until the sheet is long and narrow. **D.** Fold the ends of the long narrow strip into the middle until the sheet is square.

massage cream on a worktable. Offer your client the use of disposable undergarments, or encourage the client to bring an old swimsuit to wear for the session (many products stain fabrics). Ask the client to change into the disposable undergarments or swimsuit, and provide a clean bathrobe and slippers to wear during the preheating stage of the treatment. The procedure for a hot sheet wrap is shown in Technique 39.

Cocoons

In a **cocoon**, the treatment product is applied directly to the client before the client is wrapped in plastic and blankets. Usually an exfoliation treatment like dry skin brushing, a salt or sugar glow, or body scrub is applied directly before the cocoon, as described previously. The different cocoon steps described in Technique 40 can be tried with a variety of products for enjoyable cocoon treatments. You want to explore a number of different procedural steps depending on the facility where the cocoon is offered, the particular product, and the treatment goals for the session. For example, certain types of seaweed are sticky and difficult to remove with hot towels. These products are used only if a shower is available for the removal step. Some therapists use a portable steam canopy instead of wrapping the client in blankets. The warmth of the steam promotes product absorption and keeps the client warm.

Concept Brief 15-1
Common Spa Treatments

- In a **salt or sugar glow**, different types of mineral salts or sugar are rubbed across the surface of the skin with gentle massage strokes.
- **Dry skin brushing** is a technique in which natural bristle brushes, rough hand mitts, or textured cloths are used to stimulate the sebaceous glands, increase local circulation, remove dead skin cells, and invigorate the nervous system to revitalize the body.
- The **loofah scrub** (also called a body scrub) is the most invigorating of the exfoliation treatments.
- In a **hot sheet wrap**, the treatment product (herbs, coffee, milk, honey, seaweed, mud, etc.) is dissolved in hot water. Two muslin sheets (or a sheet and a bath towel) are steeped in the dissolved product and then wrapped around the client.
- In a **cocoon,** the treatment product is applied directly to the client before the client is wrapped in plastic and blankets.

Equipment, Supplies, and Setup

Set up your massage table with a blanket (wool or cotton) placed horizontally so that the long edges fall on either side of the table. If extra warmth is desired, a thermal space blanket can be placed directly on top of the blanket. A plain flat sheet is turned in its normal orientation on the table if the product is removed with hot towels as in the dry room procedure shown in Technique 40. Place a plastic sheet cut to 6 ft over the blanket horizontally. Bath towels are situated at both the top of the table and the bottom of the table horizontally. The table setup for a standard cocoon is shown in Figure 15-3.

On a worktable, place products and equipment for exfoliation (described previously), the treatment product (mud, seaweed, shea butter, etc.) warming in a hot water bath or in a warming unit, two pairs of vinyl gloves, body lotion or massage cream, an aroma mist (described in a later section), a soda cooler with enough hot, moist hand towels to remove both the exfoliation product and the cocoon treatment product, and two dry hand towels. Provide disposable undergarments for the client to wear during the session, and use a heat lamp over the treatment table to ensure the client stays warm. The procedure for a standard cocoon is shown in Technique 40.

Technique 39	**A Hot Sheet Wrap Procedure**

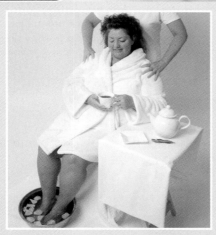

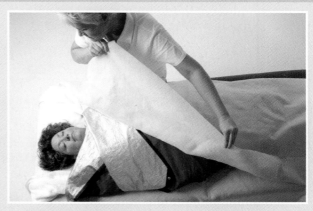

1. Increase Core Body Temperature. There are a number of ways to increase the client's core body temperature before the wrap to ensure the client perspires freely during the wrap phase of the session. Depending on the facility, the client might sit in a sauna or steam cabinet, soak in a warm hydrotherapy or standard soaking tub, or receive a Vichy, Swiss, or standard shower. In a dry room, a warm footbath is often used to preheat the client. Ask the client to sip a cup of warm herbal tea, and place warm packs around the client's shoulders. Use warm instead of hot tea so that the client can drink the tea immediately instead of letting it cool down. The goal is to get the client to perspire before being wrapped, especially if the goal of the treatment is detoxification.

2. The Wrap. While the client is soaking the feet, remove the sheets from the hot water solution. Using heavy insulated gloves, wring the sheets (or sheet and bath towel) out as quickly as possible, and place them in the soda cooler to keep them hot. Remove the client's feet from the footbath and dry them with a towel. Ask the client to stand on one side of the treatment table while you stand on the other side. It is a good idea to describe the procedure so that the client knows what to do at each stage of the treatment. When you are ready, the hot sheet is removed from the cooler and unfolded as quickly as possible on the massage table. It is placed horizontally so that the long edges can be brought up around the client. The client removes the robe (now wearing just disposable undergarments or an old swimsuit) and reclines in the supine position on the massage table while you hold the sheet on one side, looking away to preserve the client's modesty. Clients often find that the sheet feels too hot on their gluteals, so it is a good idea to put a hand towel on the sheet where the gluteals will rest before the client gets on the treatment table. Because men often find the sheet too hot on their genitals (disposable undergarments are very thin), male clients can hold a hand towel in front of their genitals to insulate this area when the sheet is wrapped over them.

Quickly wrap the first hot sheet around the client and pull the second hot sheet (or towel) from the cooler and lay this on top of the first hot sheet. The second sheet is unfolded only as much as needed to completely cover the top of the client. Next, the space blanket and then the wool blanket are quickly tucked around the client. Bring the towel at the top of the table up around the client's head in a "turban drape," and wrap the towel at the bottom of the table around the client's feet. Once the wrap is secure, place a bolster under the client's knees (outside the wool blanket). Throughout the wrapping process, move quickly and efficiently to trap the maximum amount of body heat in the wrap.

Continued

Technique 39 — A Hot Sheet Wrap Procedure (Continued)

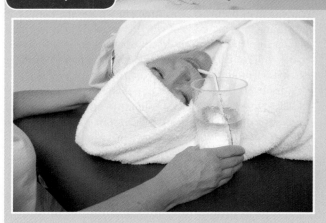

3. Process and Session End. The client usually starts to perspire within 5 minutes of being wrapped up and may continue to perspire freely throughout the treatment. An aroma blend can be misted high over the client's face at various points during the wrap. This cools and calms the client. The face might also be dabbed with a cool cloth. Water is offered through a flexible straw every 3 to 5 minutes during the wrap. The flexible straw allows the client to sip water without lifting the head.

At the end of the wrap (usually 20 to 30 minutes), remove the outer blankets and towels leaving one sheet loosely draped around the client. When the client is ready, help the client sit up and slip back into the robe. Support the client while moving from the massage table to a seat. Once seated, give cool water to sip, and have the client dry off with a hand towel. With most infused or dissolved wrap products, the client will not feel sticky or unclean after the treatment.

A hot sheet wrap might end in a number of different ways depending on your facility or the goals of the session. In the dry room option described above, the client is moved to a chair to sip water and cool down. While the client cools down, put clean massage sheets on the treatment table. Once the client is back on the table, massage with a light cream or gel. A gel-based product works well as it feels velvety and cooling to the client who may still be hot and perspiring slightly. Alternatively, a refreshing body scrub might be applied to remove the impurities released during the wrap and cool the client. If a shower is available, the client might shower while the treatment table is changed over to massage sheets.

Technique 40 — Cocoon Exploration

You have a lot of options when delivering a cocoon procedure. Once you decide on a product, try different application and removal in methods until you find what works best for you. These images show different clients and therapists at different stages in a number of cocoon treatments. You can see that you can mix and match treatment steps with a variety of products for enjoyable cocoons.

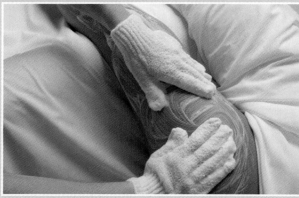

1. Exfoliation. First, choose an exfoliation method from those described early in the chapter, and ask the client to get on the massage table wearing disposable undergarments. The client lies directly on the plastic sheeting. In some cases, it is possible to use standard draping procedures as outlined in Chapter 10. In others cases, the product is messy and would quickly soil the drape, so the client is not draped but a heat lamp is positioned over the treatment table to keep the client warm. Think about how the exfoliation step integrates with the product application step. Usually you exfoliate the posterior of the body and then apply the treatment product before flipping the client and repeating these steps on the anterior body. Some therapists exfoliate the posterior body, flip the client and exfoliate the anterior body, and then ask the client to sit up for the application of the product to the posterior body (shown later). The key is that the client should be supine when they "process" in the wrap. In this image, the therapist is using rough-textured gloves and a body wash for the exfoliation step.

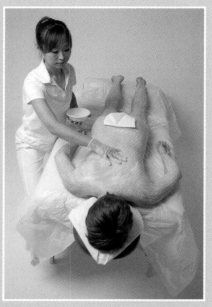

2. Product application option 1. In this image, the therapist is wearing vinyl gloves to apply the product to the client. This is a nice option because the therapist can use a variety of massage strokes with the product acting as a lubricant. This enhances the client's experience. When the client's posterior body is covered in product, the therapist asks the client to flip over. The therapist then removes the first set of vinyl gloves, now soiled with product, exfoliates the anterior body, and then puts on a second set of vinyl gloves and applies the treatment product with massage strokes to the anterior body.

| **Technique 40** | **Cocoon Exploration** (Continued) |

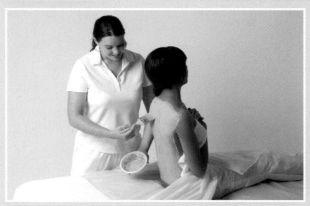

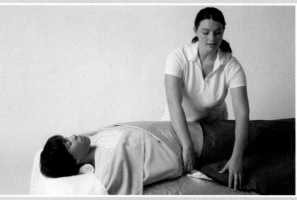

3. Product application option 2. In this image, the therapist has completed an exfoliation treatment on the posterior body, flipped the client over, and exfoliated the anterior body. She then applied product to the lower legs with a paintbrush after asking the client to bend each knee (in order to access the posterior legs with product) and then sit up for the back to be treated with product.

4. Cocoon. Once you have applied product to the client, wrap the client loosely in the plastic (it doesn't have to be snug as in a hot sheet wrap). Next, wrap the blanket around the client and arrange the top bath towel around the head or shoulders and the bottom bath towel around the feet. While the client processes in the wrap (20 to 30 minutes), provide a soothing face massage and foot massage. Water might be offered through a flexible straw, and the client might be misted with an aromatherapy blend. At the end of the cocoon phase, remove the outer blankets from the client but leave the client wrapped in the plastic. You have three different options for product removal and finishing the treatment based on the available equipment and type of product used for the treatment.

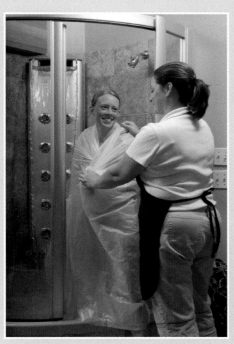

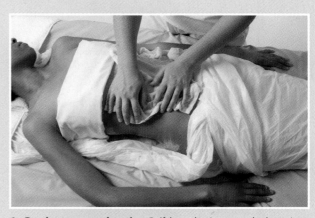

5. Product removal option 1. If a shower or tub is available, leave the client wrapped loosely in the plastic and help him or her to the shower or tub. While stepping into the shower or tub, the client hands the plastic back to you so that you can throw it away. While the client showers or bathes, change the table over to massage sheets. Then provide a full-body massage with a body lotion or rich body cream to finish the session.

6. Product removal option 2. If the product is messy and a shower is not available, the plastic sheeting should be removed completely from underneath the client when cleaned off with hot towels. To remove a plastic sheet, a clean sheet must have been placed under the plastic when the table was made up, as described in the earlier section on setup. Remove the product from the client's arms, upper chest, and abdominal area, and then ask the client to sit up.

Continued

Technique 40   **Cocoon Exploration** (Continued)

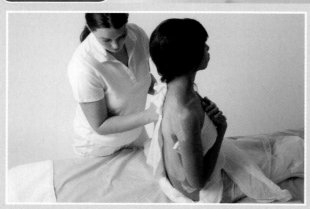

7. Remove the product from the client's back and arms. Roll the plastic sheeting up until it is as close to the gluteals as possible, and ask the client to lie back on the clean massage sheet. Wipe the client's feet clean of product, and ask the client to bend the knees and hold up the feet while you quickly roll up the plastic and place the feet on the clean massage sheet under the plastic.

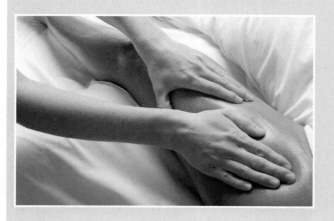

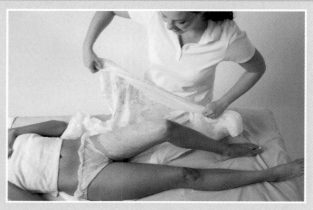

8. Remove the product from both legs with hot towels, and roll the plastic up as high as possible under the gluteals. The client places the clean legs on the massage sheet. Ask the client to lift the hips slightly so that you can remove the plastic completely. Drape the client with a top massage sheet, and finish the treatment with a massage.

9. Product removal option 3. Some products are not messy and are designed to be left on the skin. For example, shea butter is a rich emollient that absorbs slowly into the skin, leaving it soft, conditioned, and hydrated. This product is simply massaged into the body at the conclusion of the wrap phase.

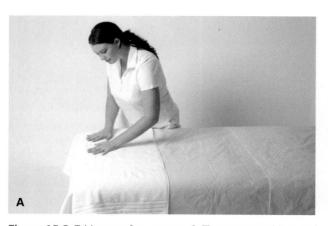

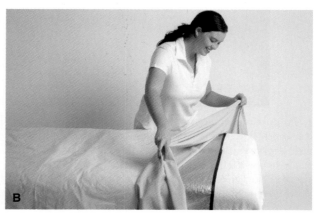

A   **B**

Figure 15-3 Table setup for a cocoon. **A.** The massage table is set from the outermost layer to innermost layer as follows: blanket (wool or cotton), thermal space blanket (optional), and a plain flat sheet in its normal orientation on the massage table (for dry room removal only). On top of this place a plastic sheet turned sideways on the table so that it covers the blanket. **B.** A bath towel is placed across the top and bottom of the plastic sheet at either end of the table to anchor the plastic wrap sheet.

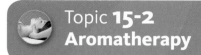

Topic **15-2**
Aromatherapy

Aromatherapy is the use of essential oils (aromatic plant extracts) for health and wellness. Essential oils have pronounced, proven physiological and psychological effects on the body and mind, and thus are equally useful in wellness and healthcare settings. Because aromatherapy is a complex art and science, this section only introduces enough information to start using common essential oils safely to support your work to reduce stress, decrease muscle tension and pain, increase full range of motion in joints, promote deep breathing, and increase the enjoyment of clients during sessions.

Essential Oil Basics

Essential oils are pleasant-smelling substances that come from specific species of aromatic plants (Box 15-3). The oils are extracted from the leaves or needles, twig, bark, flowers, fruits, stems, seeds, roots, or sometimes all parts of the plant through various methods. They are used therapeutically by a wide range of healthcare professionals. Essential oils are highly concentrated. Consider that 1 drop of chamomile essential oil is equal to 30 cups of strong chamomile tea. For this reason, only a small amount of essential oil is needed to provide benefits for the client. In fact, many essential oils have contraindications when used in excess.

Each essential oil is made up of a different mix of chemical components that account for its physiological and

psychological effects. Oils range from having one main component such as sweet birch oil, composed of 98% methyl salicylate, to rose oil, with over 300 main and trace components. This dynamic chemical complexity is what makes essential oils therapeutically valuable and differentiates them from artificial synthetic imitations (Box 15-4).

The consistency of essential oils is more like water than like oil. They don't feel greasy and heavy but are insoluble (do not dissolve) in water and usually float on top of water when added to a bath or combined with water for an aroma mist (described below). They are volatile substances that turn from a liquid to a gas readily at room temperature as they evaporate. Essential oils are attracted to fats (lipophilic) like the adipose layer directly below the skin. They are soluble (dissolve) in fatty substances like the vegetable, nut, and herbal oils used as lubricants in massage.

Compounds from essential oils enter the human body through the skin, where they are absorbed into the capillary network of the circulatory system. The most permeable areas of the body are the armpits, forehead, scalp, hands, feet, and inguinal areas. Essential oils can also enter the body through inhalation. Inhaled essential oil molecules travel down the respiratory tract to the lungs, where they are either absorbed by the mucous membrane lining of the respiratory tract or are transferred to circulating blood in the lungs.

BOX 15-3 The Use of Botanical Names in Aromatherapy

Essential oils are usually listed with a botanical name in literature and on suppliers' lists. This is to prevent confusion because sometimes the common name refers to more than one botanical species or very similar common names are used for different species. For example, the name *sage* can cause problems. Common sage (*Salvia officinalis*) is used differently from clary sage (*Salvia sclarea*) and Spanish sage (*Salvia lavendulaefolia*). Common sage contains up to 42% thujone, a potentially dangerous chemical that is contraindicated for the elderly, pregnant women, clients in a weakened condition, and children. While common sage is not dangerous when applied topically in low concentrations to healthy individuals, it does contain methyl chavicol, which can cause skin irritation. Clary sage contains 75% esters, a type of chemical that supports relaxation and stress reduction and is safe for liberal use. Spanish sage contains camphor and cineol, making it the best of the three oils for respiratory support. Aromatherapists learn these distinctions in order to purchase the best possible essential oils for their needs.

BOX 15-4 Therapeutic-Grade Essential Oils versus Synthetics

Therapeutic-grade essential oils are pure and natural. They have been grown in a defined region from a specific botanical species and cultivated, harvested, and distilled according to internationally defined and accepted methods. Synthetic oils have been produced in a lab to mimic the aroma of natural oils. Usually synthetic oils smell overly sweet and lack the complexity of the aromas of natural plant extracts. This is probably due to the relative chemical simplicity of synthetic oils compared to natural oils. Pure, natural oils are so chemically complex that it is not economically viable to synthesize all of the compounds present. Instead, only the most important aroma compounds are synthesized. Even the best synthetic oils used in perfumery seldom have more than about 30 chemical compounds, compared to 100 to 300 or more present in a natural oil. A seasoned aromatherapist will tell you that clients respond differently to natural oils than to synthetic oils. Often synthetic oils cause headache, nausea, a sore throat, and emotional irritation. Skin sensitivity is seen more readily with synthetic than with natural oils. Use only natural oils when practicing aromatherapy. See the buying guide in Box 1-6 for information that will help you avoid the purchase of synthetic oils.

The Therapeutic Potential of Aromatherapy

Aromatherapy has significant therapeutic potential because each essential oil has a unique combination of chemical compounds that interact with the body's chemistry and thereby affect specific organs, systems, or the body as a whole (physiological effects). For example, the essential oils of German chamomile and *Helichrysum* contain the powerful anti-inflammatory chemical alpha-bisabolol, which makes these oils very useful for decreasing inflammation in the early stages of tissue healing from musculoskeletal injury. Clove bud oil contains a powerful analgesic component called eugenol. When diluted in massage oil, clove bud essential oil is very effective at reducing pain associated with muscular tension. Table 15-3 provides an overview of important physiological effects, the essential oils to which these effects are attributed, and examples of use.

The inhalation of essential oils also triggers an olfactory (smell) response that can lead to powerful mental and emotional behavioral changes (psychological effects).[6] There is

TABLE 15-3   Therapeutic Action/Properties of Selected Essential Oils

Action	Definition	Selected Indications	Selected Essential Oils
Alterative	An agent that corrects disordered body function and supports balance in the body	Stress, recent trauma such as a car accident, as part of a detoxification regime, burnout, anxiety	Lavender, melissa, geranium, fir, juniper berry, petitgrain, lemongrass, valerian
Analgesic	An agent that reduces the sensation of pain	Pain caused by injury, muscle tension, or a pathology	Bay laurel, bay rum, bergamot, birch, cajeput, German chamomile, roman chamomile, clove, coriander, eucalyptus, fir, ginger, jasmine (mild), lavender, lemongrass, sweet marjoram, peppermint, nutmeg, black pepper, rosemary, rosewood (mild), turmeric, wintergreen
Antidepressant	An agent that helps to alleviate depression	Depression, stress, anxiety	Basil, bergamot, geranium, jasmine, lavender, lemongrass, neroli, sweet orange, patchouli, rose, rosewood, clary sage, Spanish sage, sandalwood, vanilla, ylang ylang
Anti-inflammatory	An agent that decreases inflammation	Recent soft-tissue injury, skin irritation or sensitivity, neuritis, tendonitis	Benzoin, birch, camphor (white), German chamomile, frankincense, geranium, *Helichrysum*, jasmine, peppermint, myrrh, bitter orange, sweet orange, patchouli, common sage, Spanish sage, spikenard, tea tree, turmeric, wintergreen, yarrow
Antineuralgic	An agent that relieves or decreases pain from irritated nerves	Neuralgia, neuritis, carpal tunnel syndrome	Bay rum, cajeput, roman chamomile, clove, eucalyptus, *Helichrysum*, Scotch pine
Antirheumatic	An agent that decreases or relieves rheumatism	Rheumatic conditions, stiff, sore muscular conditions	Bay laurel, bay rum, birch, clove, coriander, cypress, eucalyptus, juniper berry, lavender, lemon, lime, nutmeg, Scotch pine, rosemary, thyme, turmeric, yarrow
Antisclerotic	An agent that helps to prevent the hardening of tissue	Scar tissue, adhesions	Lemon, carrot seed
Cicatrisant	An agent that promotes healing through the formation of scar tissue	Soft-tissue injury	Balsam fir, German chamomile, roman chamomile, elemi, eucalyptus, geranium, *Helichrysum*, hyssop, jasmine, juniper berry, lavender, lemon, myrrh, neroli, palmarosa, patchouli, rose, rosemary, clary sage, sandalwood, thyme, yarrow

TABLE 15-3 **Therapeutic Action/Properties of Selected Essential Oils** *(Continued)*

Action	Definition	Selected Indications	Selected Essential Oils
Cytophylactic	An agent that increases the activity of leucocytes in the body thus boosting immunity	Boost general immunity	German chamomile, frankincense, lavender, oregano (caution), rosemary, tea tree
Depurative	An agent that combats impurities in the blood and organs, and aids detoxification	Detoxification treatments, revitalization treatments, dietary support	Angelica, birch, carrot seed, coriander, eucalyptus, grapefruit, juniper berry, lemon, rose, Spanish sage, vetiver
Emollient	An agent that softens the skin	Dry skin, mature skin, dehydrated skin, rough skin	Linden (other oils are not specific emollients but support dry skin—frankincense, myrrh, elemi, rose, lavender)
Expectorant	An agent that promotes the removal of mucus from the respiratory system	These oils can be used for general respiratory support to prevent congestion and aid breathing	Angelica, balsam fir, bay rum, benzoin, cajeput, camphor (white), atlas cedarwood, eucalyptus, fir, frankincense, ginger, hyssop, sweet marjoram, peppermint, myrrh, Scotch pine, Spanish sage, spruce (*tsuga*), tea tree, thyme, yarrow
Hypotensive	An agent that lowers blood pressure	Stress, anxiety	Bay laurel, lavender, lemon, sweet marjoram, neroli, sweet orange, clary sage, Spanish sage, turmeric, valerian, yarrow, ylang ylang
Nervine	An agent that strengthens and tones the nerves and nervous system	Stress, nervous tension, burnout, neuritis, neuralgia	Angelica, basil, *Helichrysum*, hyssop, juniper berry, lavender, lemon, lemongrass, linden, sweet marjoram, peppermint, patchouli, petitgrain, rosemary, clary sage, Spanish sage, spruce (*tsuga*), thyme, ylang ylang
Relaxant	An agent that soothes and relieves tension	Stress, anxiety, insomnia	German chamomile, Roman chamomile, lavender, neroli, nutmeg, sandalwood, vanilla, ylang ylang
Restorative	An agent that revitalizes and strengthens the body	Low immunity, burnout, mental exhaustion, stress	Basil, coriander, lavender, lemon, lime, myrrh, Scotch pine, rosemary, tea tree
Rubefacient	An agent that increases local circulation and is warming. May lead to skin irritation.	Tight muscles, detoxification, muscle pain, and soreness	Birch, camphor (white), eucalyptus, fir, ginger, juniper berry, oregano (caution), black pepper, Scotch pine, rosemary, spruce (*tsuga*), thyme, turmeric, vetiver, wintergreen
Sedative	An agent that sedates or calms the central nervous system, a body system, or the body in general	Relaxation treatments, stress, anxiety, insomnia	Balsam fir, bay laurel, benzoin, atlas cedarwood, German chamomile, Roman chamomile, frankincense, hyssop, jasmine, juniper berry, lavender (balancing), lemongrass, linden, mandarin, sweet marjoram, myrrh, bitter orange, sweet orange, rose, clary sage, sandalwood, spikenard, tuberose, valerian (depresses central nervous system), vanilla, vetiver, yarrow, ylang ylang
Stimulant	An agent that increases the function of a body system or the body in general	Mental and physical burnout, stress, and to revitalize and energize	Angelica, bay rum, bergamot, camphor (white), clove, cardamon, carrot seed, atlas cedarwood (circulatory), coriander, elemi, eucalyptus, fir, geranium, ginger, grapefruit (lymphatic), lavender (balancing), lemon (lymphatic), mandarin (lymphatic), peppermint, nutmeg, neroli (nerve), sweet orange (lymphatic), palmarosa (circulatory), patchouli, black pepper, petitgrain, Scotch pine, rosemary, rosewood (immune), common sage, Spanish sage, spruce (*tsuga*), thyme, turmeric, vetiver (circulation)
Sudorific or diaphoretic	An agent that promotes or increases perspiration	To warm an area, detoxification treatments, sore muscles	Bay laurel, cajeput, German chamomile, Roman chamomile, cypress, ginger, hyssop, juniper berry, sweet marjoram, rosemary, tea tree, thyme, yarrow

credible evidence that agreeable aromas can improve our mood and sense of well-being.[7] This is not surprising because our olfactory receptors are directly connected to the limbic system, the oldest and most emotional part of our brain (Fig. 15-4).

In relaxation massages, therapists commonly use oils that are known sedatives, calmatives, and relaxants. It has been documented that the inhalations of aromas with these properties help people let go of mental, emotional, and therefore physical stress. For example, when the sedative essential oils of lavender, rose, and valerian were dispersed in the air, rats took longer to perform tasks.[8] These oils are known to gently sedate the central nervous system. Oils like lavender, Roman or German chamomile, and sweet marjoram sedate the body and decrease stress because they stimulate the part of the brain known as the raphe nucleus, which causes the release of serotonin. Research shows that ambient lavender increased

sleep and caused better waking moods in elderly patients with psychological disorders who were under long-term treatment for insomnia.[9] During stressful MRI medical testing, a vanilla-like scent was used successfully to help patients relax and to reduce anxiety at Memorial Sloan-Kettering Cancer Center in New York.[10]

Stimulating scents also have their uses in massage and spa therapy. In one study, there was an increase of cerebral blood flow in humans following inhalation of 1,8 cineol, a chemical component present at significant levels in oils like rosemary and eucalyptus.[11] Rosemary, lemon, basil, and peppermint offer a quick energy pickup because they stimulate the locus ceruleus in the brain, causing the release of noradrenalin. People do much better in a task that requires sustained attention if they receive regular puffs of an uplifting aroma.[12] Peppermint, the oil often chosen to promote alert states, enhances the sensory pathway for visual detection, which allowed subjects more control over their allocation of attention. Ambient peppermint aroma increased word learning and recall.[13] You could use this information in your massage practice by applying a stimulating aroma mist to clients at the end of a treatment to help them wake up and return to their normal routine.

The positive emotional effects of agreeable aromas can be used to affect the client's perceptions of you as a therapist, your massage business, or products you sell in your gift shop. In a study to show that scent impacts social relationships, people in photographs were given a higher "trustworthy rating" when the test subjects were exposed to a pleasant fragrance. In a test of shampoos, the product originally ranked last in performance was ranked first in a second test after its fragrance was adjusted.[14] Some key psychological properties of essential oils are provided in Table 15-4.

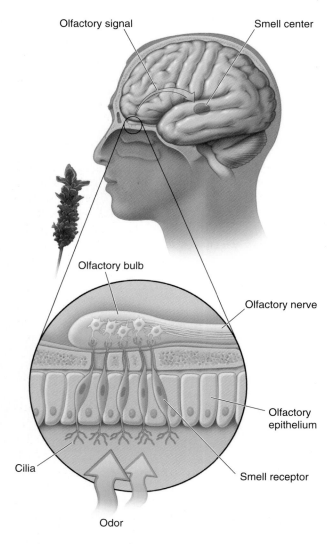

Olfactory signal

Smell center

Olfactory bulb

Olfactory nerve

Olfactory epithelium

Cilia

Smell receptor

Odor

Figure 15-4 The limbic system. Olfactory receptors are directly connected to the limbic system, the oldest and most emotional part of the brain.

Concept Brief 15-2
Aromatherapy Terms

- **Aromatherapy** is the use of essential oils (aromatic plant extracts) for health and wellness.

- **Therapeutic-grade essential oils** are grown from specific botanical species in a clearly defined location, following accepted guidelines for cultivation, harvesting, distillation, and storage.

- **Synthetic oils** are made in a lab and lack the complex chemistry of pure, natural oils. They should not be used in aromatherapy.

- The **actions and properties** of essential oils refer to their effects on the body and mind of the user.

- **Carrier products** are used to dilute essential oils before they are applied to the body.

- The term **concentration** refers to the amount of essential oil in the final volume of massage oil or carrier product.

TABLE 15-4   Selected Psychological Properties of Essential Oils

Anxiety	Roman chamomile, clary sage, geranium, jasmine, lavender, sweet marjoram, myrrh, neroli, nutmeg, patchouli, petigrain, rose, sandalwood, vetiver, ylang ylang.
Calming	Bergamot, German chamomile, clary sage, lavender, myrrh, neroli, petitgrain, vetiver.
Clear thinking	Basil, bay laurel, common sage, eucalyptus, grapefruit, juniper, lemon, lemongrass, palmarosa, peppermint, pine, rosemary, Spanish sage, sweet birch.
Depression	Bergamot, cardamom, clary sage, frankincense, geranium, ginger, grapefruit, jasmine, juniper, neroli, palmarosa, rose, sweet orange, ylang ylang.
Fears and doubts	Bay laurel, cypress, geranium, ginger, lavender, peppermint, rosemary, thyme.
Grief	cypress, neroli, patchouli, rose, spikenard, ylang ylang.
Grounding	Frankincense, ginger, myrrh, nutmeg, patchouli, sandalwood, vetiver.
Indecisiveness	Bay laurel, black pepper, common sage, cypress, ginger, lemon, lemongrass, pine, rosemary, Spanish sage.
Irritability	Atlas cedarwood, bay laurel, bergamot, cardamom, German chamomile, clary sage, frankincense, *Helichrysum*, jasmine, lavender, myrrh, neroli, nutmeg, rose, sandalwood, ylang ylang
Joy	Bay laurel, bergamot, cardamom, clary sage, geranium, grapefruit, juniper, lemon, lime, mandarin, neroli, peppermint, pine, rosemary, sweet orange, ylang ylang.
Mental exhaustion	Basil, bay laurel, cinnamon, cypress, frankincense, geranium, *Helichrysum*, lavender, lemon, peppermint, rosemary, sweet birch, sweet orange.
Renewal	Atlas cedarwood, bay laurel, common sage, eucalyptus, grapefruit, jasmine, juniper, lemon, nutmeg, peppermint, rosemary.

The psychological properties of essential oils noted here are subjective. Each person has a unique response to an oil or blend of oils based on his or her experiences and preferences.

Blending Essential Oils

There are many different ways to approach blending essential oils, but many aromatherapists aim to create essential oil *synergies*. A synergy occurs when the whole is greater than the sum of its parts because the parts are mutually enhancing. Synergistic interactions between chemical compounds of essential oils create a greater spectrum of physiological actions than is possible with a single oil alone. When you combine two, three, or four oils with similar or complimentary therapeutic properties, you create a blend that is more likely to be effective. Because essential oils are chemically complex, however, blending too many at once can muddy the result. Stick to combinations of two to four oils for the best synergies.

For example, to create a synergy for relaxation, fir might be chosen for its alterative action, which helps the body to regain balanced function. Sweet marjoram might be added for its nervine qualities, which help to strengthen and support the overall nervous system. Finally, lavender might be added as a restorative that helps the body cope with burnout and exhaustion. These three oils will have a broader action on stress than fir oil used alone.

You can also use the "action/property" words shown in Table 15-3 to create a synergy. For example, if you want a blend to work as a powerful muscular antispasmodic, you could choose three oils known as antispasmodics, such as Roman chamomile, clary sage, and petitgrain. If you wanted

a blend to work as a powerful diaphoretic (an agent that promotes perspiration) for a detoxification spa treatment, you might choose three or four oils noted as diaphoretics, such as bay laurel, juniper berry, and thyme oil. Sometimes therapists choose oils also for their psychological effects. In this case, two to four oils chosen from categories in Table 15-4 are appropriate. You might choose all the oils for a client because you want them to provide a specific physiological or psychological effect. Alternately, you might offer clients the opportunity to smell a number of different oils and choose what they like best for the session. Before you create a blend of oils, you need to consider carrier products, concentrations, and dosages.

Carrier Products

The term *carrier* (some therapists use the term *vehicle*) refers to the product that is used to "carry" the essential oil to the client. Essential oils are rarely applied "neat" at full strength. Massage therapists most often use expeller-pressed fixed oils as carriers for essential oils delivered in massage. Fixed oils are discussed in detail in Chapter 2. Some fixed oils such as evening primrose, jojoba, wheat germ, and pure vitamin E may be added in small amounts to other fixed oils to enhance the therapeutic properties of these oils or act as natural preservatives (1 tsp of preservative oils to 1 oz of the main fixed oil). Plain, unscented lotion or massage cream, natural gels like aloe vera gel, water (aroma mist, bath, hydrotherapy tub), or steam (sauna or steam room) might also be used as carriers of essential oils.

Carrier products that contain mineral oil, petroleum, lanolin, coconut oil, coco butter, dyes, and synthetic fragrances should be avoided as these components block the absorption of essential oils through the skin, interact unfavorably with the chemicals in essential oils, distort the aroma of essential oils, or cause sensitivity reactions in clients.

Essential Oil Concentrations and Dosages

The term *concentration* refers to the amount of essential oil in the final volume of massage oil or carrier product. Table 15-5 outlines how many drops of essential oil are added to carriers like massage oil, water, or cream for a particular concentration. Figure 15-5 illustrates which concentration to use on a particular type of client or condition. Concentrations of 1% to 4% are standard in the field of aromatherapy and are low enough to insure safety and minimize negative reactions. Concentrations above 4% are used in acute situations or by experienced therapists. Neat (100%) applications are used for spot treatments with specific oils such as tea tree for toe fungus, *Helichrysum* for trigger point therapy, lavender for small burns, or German chamomile for inflammation of soft tissue.

A dosage is the amount of an essential oil that is used in a particular type of application. For example, if you add essential oils to a bath, you wouldn't add 12 drops of essential oil for every ounce of water in the tub because the total amount of essential oil would be very high. Instead you use a set dose of oils: six to nine drops for baths, two to four drops for foot baths, and two drops for hand baths.

Safe Use of Essential Oils

When therapeutic-grade essential oils (oils that are not artificial synthetics) are used at low concentration (1% to 3% or 6 to 18 drops to every fluid ounce of carrier product) and applied topically, negative reactions are minimal. Potential undesirable effects may occur if the oils are used inappropriately or without understanding their properties. Before using any essential oil, identify any possible contraindications for its use by checking safety data and comparing it to the information on the client's health intake form.

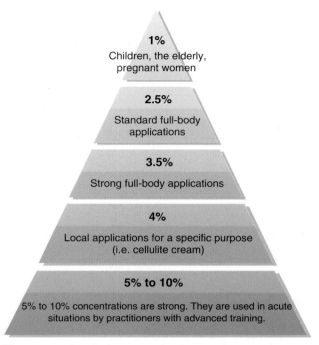

Figure 15-5 Standard concentrations in aromatherapy.

It is out of the massage therapy scope of practice to recommend the internal use of essential oils because they are potentially toxic when taken internally in doses larger than those used therapeutically by doctors. For this reason, oils must be kept out of the reach of children and not used internally. Some oils contain chemical components that may cause liver or kidney irritation when used for prolonged periods of time (even when they are applied topically). The general rule of thumb is that an oil should not be used continuously longer than 2 weeks to prevent sensitization of the kidneys, liver, or skin.

It is believed that most essential oil compounds may pass through the placenta to the developing fetus during pregnancy. It is also possible that certain essential oils may disrupt the delicate hormonal balance of the body and cause unwanted effects during pregnancy. With the exception of mandarin and lavender (1% concentration), the use of essential oils should be avoided with pregnant clients by those without formal training in aromatherapy.

The most likely undesirable effect you might see when using essential oils is skin irritation or phototoxicity. Skin

TABLE 15-5 Concentration of Essential Oil (EO) in Carrier Product

Carrier	EO 1%	EO 2%	EO 2.5%	EO 3%	EO 4%
½ oz	3 drops	6 drops	7.5 drops	9 drops	12 drops
1 oz	6 drops	12 drops	15 drops	18 drops	24 drops
2 oz	12 drops	24 drops	30 drops	36 drops	48 drops or ½ tsp
4 oz	24 drops	48 drops	60 drops	72 drops	96 drops
8 oz	48 drops	96 drops	120 drops	144 drops	192 drops

irritation is rare if you stick to standard concentrations of 1% to 3% of therapeutic-grade oils (irritation is more likely with synthetic oils). When large amounts of certain oils are used topically, or when oils are used with heat (e.g., stone massage, hot pack, and hot sheet wrap), irritation is more likely to occur.

The term *phototoxicity* refers to an increased sensitivity to sunlight. Oils containing compounds called coumarins and furocoumarins increase the skin's tendency to burn. Clients should avoid sun tanning and tanning booths for 24 hours after the application of these oils. Box 15-5 lists oils that should be avoided or used with particular caution.

BOX 15-5 Essential Oils to Avoid or Use with Caution

Essential Oils to Completely Avoid

Bitter almond, boldo leaf, buchu, yellow camphor, brown camphor, sassafras, calamus, horseradish, mugwort, mustard, pennyroyal, rue, savin, savory, tansy, thuja, wormseed, wormwood

Essential Oils to Avoid with Pregnancy

Aniseed, basil, birch, wintergreen, cedarwood, clary sage, cypress, geranium, sweet fennel, jasmine, juniper berry, sweet marjoram, myrrh, peppermint, rosemary, common sage, thyme, hyssop

Essential Oils That Are Skin Irritants

Ajowan, cinnamon bark, cinnamon leaf, sweet fennel, cassia, clove leaf, clove bud, costus, oregano, basil, fir needle, lemongrass, lemon verbena, melissa, peppermint, thyme

Essential Oils to Avoid with Clients Who Have High Blood Pressure

Pine, hyssop, rosemary, common sage, thyme

Essential Oils to Avoid with Clients Who Are Taking Homeopathic Remedies

Rosemary, eucalyptus, peppermint

Essential Oils to Avoid with Clients Who Have Epilepsy or a History of Seizure

Sweet fennel, bitter fennel, common sage, hyssop, basil

Essential Oils to Avoid with a History of Estrogen-Dependent Cancer

Aniseed, basil, birch, wintergreen, cedarwood, clary sage, cypress, geranium, sweet fennel, jasmine, juniper berry, sweet marjoram, myrrh, peppermint, rosemary, common sage, thyme, hyssop

Essential Oils That Are Phototoxic

Bergamot, lime, bitter orange, lemon, grapefruit, sweet orange, mandarin, ginger, angelica root

---

When essential oils are exposed to light, heat, and oxygen, their chemical compositions are altered (oxidation) and their therapeutic properties may change. To slow the rate of oxidation, oils should be kept in dark bottles with as little air at the top of the bottle as possible. They should be stored in a box in the refrigerator and replaced if they have not been used within 2 years. Citrus oils oxidize more rapidly than other oils and should be replaced within 6 months to a year.

Applications of Essential Oils

Aromatherapy can be viewed as the primary treatment or used as an accent to increase the pleasure derived from the session. Even the simplest aromatherapy application can benefit a client immensely by decreasing stress and boosting the effects of massage. The methods of application described below focus on some of the common ways that essential oils are used in a massage practice or spa. Table 15-6 lists 21 versatile oils and 21 blends made from those oils for easy adoption at a massage clinic or spa. Box 15-6 provides a basic buying guide to help you avoid the purchase of synthetic oils and ensure your aromatherapy blends are therapeutic grade.

Primary Aromatherapy Applications

A primary aromatherapy application is a treatment in which aromatherapy is the focus of the session. In this case, the massage, bath, steam, sauna, or wrap is used as the medium by which aromatherapy is applied for therapeutic benefit.

Aromatherapy Massage

In a classic aromatherapy massage, you meet with the client during a "formal" aromatherapy consultation in which the client fills out a health history form and together you discuss the client's expectations for aromatherapy and healthcare goals. A custom blend of essential oils is created specifically for the client to address his or her physiological and/or psychological needs and applied in a full-body Swedish massage. Some therapists let the client pick all of the oils for the blend, believing that clients are drawn only to oils that will support them in their particular healing process. Other therapists take the opposite approach and choose oils that the client mildly dislikes. The assumption in this case is that the client is "out of balance" with what is needed for wellness and that wellness will happen slowly as the client develops an affinity to the oil or blend. Usually, choosing oils for the blend is a joint process between the client and the therapist. You suggest oils that have physiological or psychological effects that would support the client's healthcare needs, and the client shares likes and dislikes, until you are both satisfied with the oils chosen. You then check for contraindications before creating the final blend of oils.

Some spas choose not to offer custom blending but create a series of premade blends from which the client chooses.

TABLE 15-6   Twenty-one Versatile Oils and 21 Easy-to-Use Blends

21 Versatile Oils	These blends are formulated at a 2% concentration for use in 1 oz of carrier product (12 total drops to 1 oz of carrier). They are composed of the 21 starter oils at the left.
Bay laurel (*Laurus nobilis*)	Muscle ease: bay laurel (3), rosemary (1), lemon (6), juniper berry (2)
Bergamot (*Citrus x bergamia*)	Breathe easy: eucalyptus (3), lemon (7), thyme (2)
Clary sage (*Salvia sclarea*)	Mother to be: lavender (5), mandarin (7)
Cypress (*Cupressus sempervirens*)	Clarity: thyme (1), grapefruit (9), cypress (2)
Eucalyptus (*Eucalyptus radiata*)	Rain: cypress (5), thyme (5), geranium (2)
Frankincense (*Boswellia carteri*)	Equilibrium: clary sage (3), neroli (2), bergamot (7)
Geranium (*Pelargonium graveolens*)	Girl power: clary sage (2), lavender (6), geranium (1), frankincense (3)
German chamomile (*Matricaria recutita*)	Body boost: lemon (4), thyme (1), bergamot (4), lavender (3)
Ginger CO$_2$ extraction (*Zingiber officinale*)	Purity: juniper berry (3), grapefruit (8), thyme (1)
Grapefruit (*Citrus x paradisi*)	Revitalize: bergamot (6), rosemary (2), lavender (4)
Jasmine (*Jasminum officinale L. form grandiflorum*)	Ocean: rosemary (3), frankincense (7), ylang ylang (2)
Juniper berry (*Juniperus communis*)	Zen: ylang ylang (2), ginger CO$_2$ (2), mandarin (8)
Lavender (*Lavandula angustifolia*)	Renew: German chamomile (1), rosemary (2), clary sage (4), lavender (5)
Lemon (*Citrus x limon*)	Shimmer: bay laurel (3), ylang ylang (1), bergamot (5), frankincense (3)
Mandarin (*Citrus reticulata*)	Meditation: frankincense (4), jasmine (1), ginger CO$_2$ (2)
Neroli (*Citrus x aurantium*)	Energy: peppermint (1), thyme (4), bay laurel (4)
Peppermint (*Mentha x piperita*)	Summer: neroli (2), lavender (4), bergamot (6)
Rose (*Rosa x damascena*)	Refresh: peppermint (1), eucalyptus (2), lemon (8), geranium (1)
Rosemary (*Rosmarinus officinalis*)	Moon mist: jasmine (2), grapefruit (10)
Thyme linalol type (*Thymus vulgaris*)	Relax factor: rose (1), clary sage (2), mandarin (6), frankincense (3)
Ylang ylang (*Cananga odorata*)	Circulate: ginger CO$_2$ (2), grapefruit (9), juniper berry (1)

BOX 15-6 Buying Guide to Avoid the Purchase of Synthetic Oils

To ensure that you are buying pure and natural essential oils rather than synthetics, pay attention to these signs of poor quality:

- The oils are being sold at very low prices or all the oils are being sold at the same price.
- The supplier does not know or supply the botanical name and location where the oil was grown and produced.
- The oils are sold in clear bottles (the oils should be sold in cobalt or brown bottles to protect them from exposure to light).
- Oils like rose, jasmine, sandalwood, melissa, *Helichrysum*, and neroli are being sold in large sizes (1/2 to 1 oz). These oils are so costly to produce that 1 oz of rose essential oil may cost up to $400. Usually these oils are sold in 1, 2, or 3 mL sizes (1 mL equals 20 drops).
- The supplier sells honeysuckle, cherry, pear, lilac, or banana "essential oil." Because these plants do not produce an essential oil, these aromas are produced only as synthetics. They are not be carried by authentic aromatherapy suppliers.

This gives the client more massage time for the same amount of money. It also enhances retail opportunities as clients often become attached to a blend and will purchase the body wash, body lotion, and room mist that match the aroma of their massage oil.

To create a blend for massage, add 12 to 18 total drops of essential oils (2% to 3% concentration) chosen for their physiological and/or psychological properties to 1 oz of massage oil or cream. Use a 1% concentration (six drops per ounce of carrier) when massaging the elderly, children, or pregnant women. Four percent blends (24 drops in 1 oz) can be used for spot treatments such as trigger point therapy or for specific conditions. At the conclusion of the massage, send the client home with the remainder of the oil so that it might be used for self-care in the bath or as a support blend (described below).

Aromatherapy Baths

A hydrotherapy tub is a specialized soaking unit that has multiple air and water jets, as described in Chapter 16. Essential oils (six to nine drops) can be added to the hydrotherapy tub or to a standard soaking tub for therapeutic baths. Sometimes the oils are added simply for the pleasure of their aromas, or they can be used to treat sore muscles, stress, insomnia, low immunity, depression, irritability, or a variety of other conditions. The drawback to using essential oils in a bath is that the oils will "pool" on the top of the water. When the client gets into the bath, the oils stick to the area that enters the water first or pool around exposed area and may cause skin irritation. For this reason, it is best to dilute the oils in carrier oil and massage the blend into the client's skin. After the massage, allow the client to soak in a warm tub enjoying the fragrance of the oils and allowing for greater skin absorption. Sometimes essential oils are added to an emulsifier, which disperses them in the body of the water to prevent pooling.

Aromatherapy Wrap

Aromatherapy body wraps can take many forms. The oils for the wrap might be chosen to provide a physiological effect (e.g., detoxification, decreasing muscle soreness) or for their effects on the mind, emotions, and spirit. Aromatherapy wraps provide time for contemplation, where the body and mind can be still, rest, and reflect while surrounded by inspiring and uplifting aromas.

Essential oils might be mixed into a number of different carrier products including seaweed, clay, heavy emollients like shea butter, and aloe vera gel. In the simplest aromatherapy wrap, the client is cocooned in blankets at the end of an aromatherapy massage to relax while the essential oil blend continues to be absorbed through the skin. In the aromatherapy wrap shown in Figure 15-6, essential oils are mixed into melted shea butter, painted on the body with a brush, and left to be absorbed while the client is wrapped in warm blankets. At the end of the wrap, the excess shea butter/essential oil mix is massaged into the skin. Aloe vera gel mixed with German chamomile, lavender, and one drop of peppermint essential oil is applied to the skin with a brush or atomizer for an effective sunburn wrap. Essential oils might also be added to body milk (very light and watery lotion) and misted on the body with an atomizer before the body is wrapped. Use a maximum of 18 drops of essential oil total in a body wrap session.

Aromatherapy Sauna or Steam

Essential oils that support the respiratory system are effective when used in the steam room or sauna. In one study, 96 patients suffering from chronic bronchitis showed significant clearing of the airways as well as reduced infection levels when inhaling vapors of camphor and menthol, and particularly oils of eucalyptus and peppermint. The oils improved the function of the lungs and bronchi by reducing mucus congestion and decreasing chest infections, colds, and influenza; when inhaling essential oils in steam, smaller doses are more effective than large amounts of oils.[15] Pine, rosemary, eucalyptus, and thyme oil work well in both a sauna or steam room. Floral oils like ylang ylang, jasmine, rose, and neroli should not be used in a sauna or steam room because they tend to cause headaches when used in close, hot environments.[16] Some steam rooms or cabinets have a special holder in which essential oils are placed, or the oils can be placed directly onto the floor at the edges of the steam cabinet or room (three to six drops). In the sauna, add the oils to the water that is ladled on the heat source (three to six drops). Oils added to the heat source in a sauna must always be mixed in water because essential oils are potentially combustible and could "pop" or flame up if added plain.

Accent Aromatherapy Applications

Accent applications use aromatherapy enhancements to add therapeutic value to a treatment and to increase the pleasure the client derives from the session. A variety of accents might be used during a client's visit to a spa or massage clinic.

- **Diffuse oils:** Diffuse essential oils in your business or treatment room to fill the space with clean, fresh aromas that enhance the client's perception of the business or service. A commercial nebulizing diffuser available from aromatherapy suppliers is the best choice if the aim is to eliminate microbes and promote a clean, healthy living or working space. Nebulizing diffusers have a glass chamber that should be cleaned with alcohol once a day to keep the apparatus functioning well. Follow the manufacturer's directions. Earthenware burners, electronic fan diffusers, or items like lamp rings can be used to scent a room and are available at natural food stores.

- **Hand inhalations:** At the beginning of the treatment, place one drop of an essential oil or blend of oils between your hands and rub them together to generate heat. Now hold your hands over the client's nose while the client takes a deep breath (Fig. 15-7). Use sedative oils like lavender, neroli, or hyssop at the beginning of the massage and stimulating oils like peppermint, rosemary, or eucalyptus at the end of the massage.

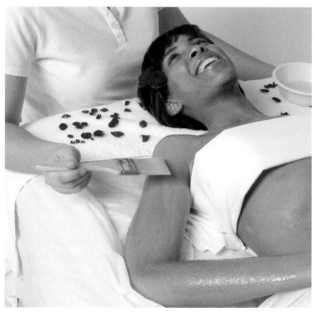

Figure 15-6 This image shows the application of melted shea butter and essential oils before a body wrap.

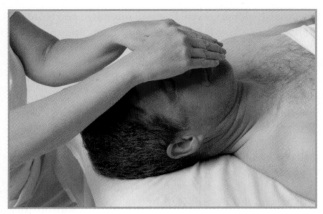

Figure 15-7 At the beginning and/or end of the treatment, place a drop of essential oils between your hands. Rub your hands together and then hold them in an arc over the client's nose while he or she takes a deep breath.

- **Tissue inhalation:** Place one drop of an essential oil on a tissue and tuck the tissue into the bottom of the face cradle to enhance the client's experience while in the prone position. One small drop of eucalyptus is a good choice for clients who easily get congested during massage.
- **Steamy aromatic towels:** Scent hot, moist towels with essential oils and use these towels to remove products or as an accent during massage or spa services, as described earlier.
- **Aroma mists:** To create an aroma mist, add 12 drops of an essential oil blend to 1 oz of filtered water in a bottle with a fine-spray top. Aroma mists have a number of different uses in a massage clinic or spa setting. They might be used as air purifiers and fresheners, linen fresheners, mood enhancers, skin toners, or body coolers. At the beginning of the treatment, spray a fine mist in a high arc over the treatment table to fill the room with a relaxing aroma. At the end of the

session repeat the mist with a stimulating blend to wake the client up and signal the end of the massage or spa treatment. Aroma mists make nice take-home gifts for clients as they can use them to refresh the car or to mist at any time as an olfactory link to the relaxation they experienced in their massages.

- **Support blends:** A support blend is a synergy of essential oils mixed into a lotion or oil base that is given to the client to use as a form of self-care. Essential oils might be chosen to give the client an energy boost, to calm a client who is feeling anxious, as a link to a positive affirmation or new life choice (e.g., quit smoking, take a break, eat healthy), or as a pleasant reminder of the visit to the spa or massage clinic. The blend can be used at any time by the client in a variety of ways and provides a simple way to bring aromatherapy into the client's life. Clients can rub it on their hands and then hold their hands over their nose for a simple inhalation. They can spread the blend over the anterior neck, down the sternum, under breast tissue, and behind the neck where lymph nodes are close to the surface, for a gentle immunity boost. They can rub the blend all over the body and take a bath or wear the blend throughout the day as a personal perfume.
- **Smell-scapes:** A smell-scape is an "aroma landscape" that is planned for a massage or spa treatment. Different aromas are used to engage the client's olfactory interest throughout the session. For example, a citrus salt glow includes citrus essential oils. If you use the same aromatherapy blend throughout the session, the client will register the aroma consciously for the first 10 minutes or so and then forget about it. If you want citrus aromas to be an integral part of the treatment, you keep all of the aromas in the same category (e.g., citrus oils) but change the aromas regularly. You might begin with a hand inhalation using lemon oil and then apply massage with a mandarin and lime blend. An aroma mist of grapefruit rounds out the smell-scape.

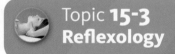

Topic **15-3**
Reflexology

Reflexology is a therapy based on the belief that there are points on the feet, hands, and ears that stimulate the function of different parts of the body including the glands and organs. It is most often used as a preventive therapy to soothe the nervous system, reduce stress, improve circulation, and create the optimum internal environment for balanced energy, rest, and recovery so that the body can draw on its natural ability to heal and revitalize itself. (The Massage Fusion section at the end of the chapter describes reflexology certification.)

Modern reflexology owes its development to the American doctor William Fitzgerald, who developed a comprehensive

method for working the feet in the early 20th century. Dr. Fitzgerald discovered that when he applied pressure to the feet, other areas of the body were affected. He called his work zone therapy and mapped out 10 zones in the body that could be accessed by manipulating the feet or hands (Fig. 15-8). Fitzgerald taught that when a zone on the feet or hands is manipulated, any gland or organ falling in the path of that zone is positively affected.

Eunice Ingham, an American physical therapist, became interested in Fitzgerald's methods. She worked on a variety of patients over a number of years and kept detailed notes

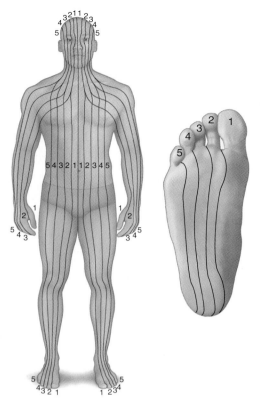

Figure 15-8 The 10 zones of the feet.

on her findings. She charted each body area on the foot and through trial and error created an intricate map that shows the placement of reflex points for each gland and organ in the body. She is credited by many as being the first person to create an "anatomical" model of foot reflexes in which the feet are a mirror image of the body (Fig. 15-9).

In general, when a client reports to the therapist that one area of the foot or hand is tender, the therapist gives that area focused attention. While the pressure applied to the area is firm, it should not feel unbearable. Areas of tenderness relate to what reflexologists consider "congestion" in the corresponding glands and organs of the body. Remember that the foot is a complex structure, prone to adhesions, hypertonicities, and inflammations, just like the rest of the body. Congestion in an area does not necessarily indicate pathology, and you should be careful not to alarm the client by relating tenderness specifically to a particular organ or gland.

While the hands, ears, and feet can all be manipulated to improve health and well-being as part of reflexology, the feet receive the most attention. The feet are considered very important because of their rich supply of superficial nerve endings (7,000 in each foot) in an intricate structure that consists of 26 bones, 33 joints, 19 muscles, and 107 ligaments. In modern societies, people often choose shoes for fashion and not for comfort, leading to foot pain and hip, knee, and low

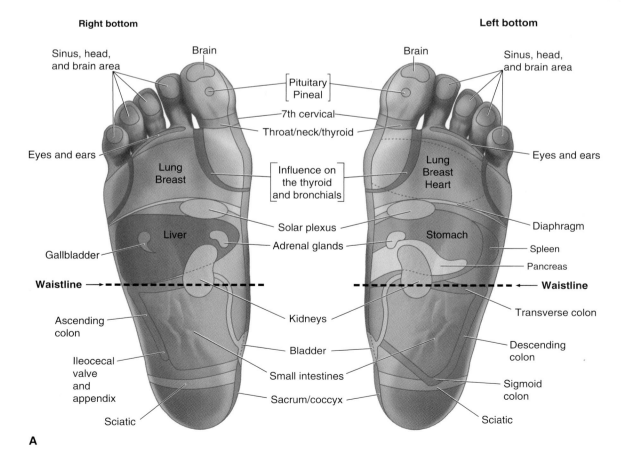

Figure 15-9 Reflexes on the feet. **A.** Reflexes on the bottom of the feet.

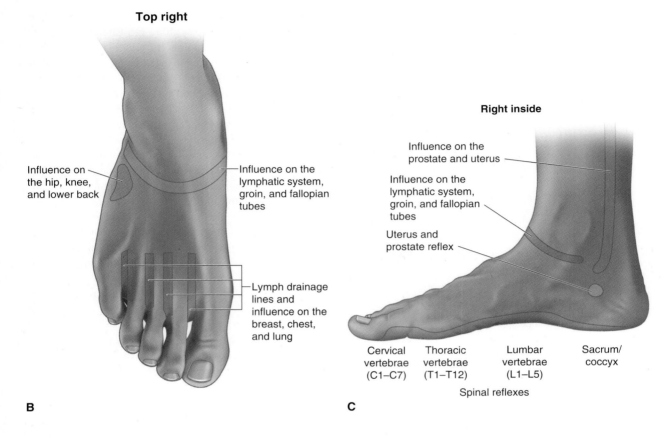

Top right

Influence on the hip, knee, and lower back

Influence on the lymphatic system, groin, and fallopian tubes

Lymph drainage lines and influence on the breast, chest, and lung

B

Right inside

Influence on the prostate and uterus

Influence on the lymphatic system, groin, and fallopian tubes

Uterus and prostate reflex

Cervical vertebrae (C1–C7)

Thoracic vertebrae (T1–T12)

Lumbar vertebrae (L1–L5)

Sacrum/ coccyx

Spinal reflexes

C

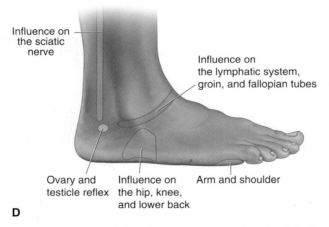

Right outside

Influence on the sciatic nerve

Influence on the lymphatic system, groin, and fallopian tubes

Ovary and testicle reflex

Influence on the hip, knee, and lower back

Arm and shoulder

D

Figure 15-9 *(Continued)* **B.** Reflexes on the top of the feet. **C.** Reflexes on the medial side of the feet. **D.** Reflexes on the lateral side of the feet.

BOX 15-7 Cautions and Contraindications for Reflexology

Cautions: Use caution when working with older adults, who are on multiple medications, and clients who have compromised circulatory systems. Reflexology techniques should be used only on such individuals with light pressure to avoid overstimulation and accelerated elimination symptoms such as nausea, diarrhea, or headache. While negative responses are rare, clients may experience a variety of reactions to reflexology techniques. During the session, clients may have muscle cramping in their legs and feet, their feet and hands may perspire, and they may feel mildly nauseous or headachy. Some clients respond to reflexology by falling into a deep sleep during the session. Others experience involuntary jerks of the arms and legs as the nervous system "unwinds." In all cases, monitor the client's comfort level and make necessary adjustments to the degree of pressure you use in the treatment.

Contraindications: If a client has pitted edema, broken bones, advanced or poorly treated diabetes, neuropathy, deep vein thrombosis, infections, ingrown toenails, painful corns, gout, warts, or athlete's foot in the area of the lower leg and foot, foot massage and reflexology are contraindicated.

back conditions. In addition, circulation tends to stagnate in the feet because they are furthest from the heart. Inorganic waste materials such as uric acid and calcium may turn to crystalline deposits that can build up in the bottom of the feet. Reflexologists focus on working every surface of the foot to decrease muscle tension and pain, increase circulation, loosen the foot so that it is more flexible and mobile, and stimulate the flow of vital energy through the body.

Clients find that reflexology is deeply relaxing and enjoyable to receive, reduces foot pain, and leaves the body revitalized. Cautions and contraindications for reflexology are described in Box 15-7.

Equipment, Supplies, and Setup

The massage table is set with massage sheets and a blanket, similar to regular massage. A bath towel is situated horizontally at the bottom of the treatment table where the client's feet will rest. Provide a pillow for the client's head. On a nearby worktable, place antiseptic wipes like diaper wipes, foot cream, hand sanitizer, and a dry hand towel. Methods for applying reflexology are shown in Technique 41, and a reflexology relaxation routine is demonstrated in Technique 42.

Technique 41 | **Reflexology Techniques**

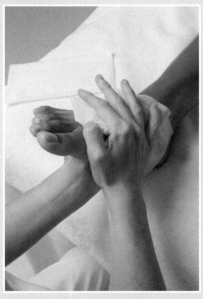

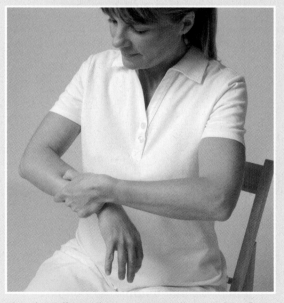

1. Cleansing the Feet. Cleansing is required before a reflexology session for hygienic reasons. In the simplest cleansing method, wipe off the client's feet before the massage with disposable cleansing wipes such as a diaper wipe. Another simple method is to wet your hands in a bowl of warm water and apply a foaming cleanser to the feet while the client relaxes on the treatment table. The cleanser is removed with hot towels. A 10-minute footbath accompanied by a seated shoulder and neck massage is often paired with a reflexology session to warm the tissues of the feet, relax the body, and enhance the treatment.

2. Thumb Walking. The most common technique used in reflexology is thumb walking. To thumb-walk a zone or reflex point, use the edge of your thumb in an inchworm motion to take small "bites" out of the area you are working. The pressure is steady and firm. To practice the technique, walk your thumb up your forearm.
Finger walking: Finger walking is similar to thumb walking except that the edge of your index finger is used and the pressure is usually gentler. To practice the technique, walk your finger up your forearm.

Continued

Technique 41   Reflexology Techniques (Continued)

3. Hook and Back Up. The hook and backup technique is used to stimulate a specific point. Apply direct pressure to the point with your thumb and then pull your thumb back slightly to hook the point (think of taking the slack out of the tissue). Now, slide your thumb into its original position and again place direct pressure on the point with your thumb. You might also rotate your thumb on the point or hold the point with direct pressure to stimulate it.

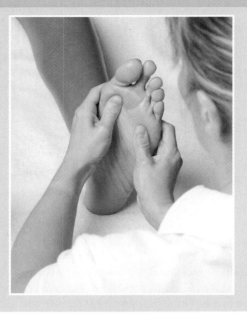

Technique 42   Reflexology Relaxation Routine

Technique 42 demonstrates one approach to a reflexology relaxation routine, but sessions can and should be customized for the individual client. Start with the following steps 1 to 7, and then focus on specific points in a systematic manner, designing the reflexology routine to suit the client. For example, if a detoxification routine is indicated, steps 1 to 7 are applied to the feet, and then you thumb-walk or use direct pressure on the kidney, spleen, stomach, and colon points on the plantar surface of the left foot; the kidney, liver, gallbladder, and colon points on the plantar surface of the right foot; and on the lymphatic points on the dorsal surface of the foot (Fig. 15-9). If a respiratory support routine is indicated, you follow steps 1 to 7 and then thumb- or finger-walk the reflex points associated with the sinuses and lungs.

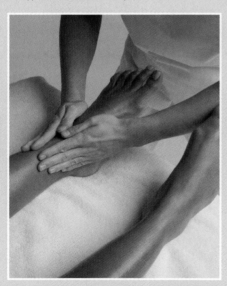

1. Massage the Feet. Use 10 to 20 minutes of foot massage to warm the feet, increase circulation, and relax the client. A foot massage routine is demonstrated in Chapter 13, Technique 28. When you complete the foot massage, remove all excess lubricant from the feet with a hot, moist towel or diaper wipe. Cleanse your hands with an alcohol-based hand sanitizer. The client's feet and your hands must be dry or your thumbs and fingers would slip over the reflex points instead of grabbing them.

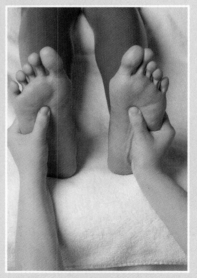

2. Solar Plexus Hold. Sit down while holding one foot in each hand. Position your thumbs so that they rest on the point directly below the ball of the foot known as the solar plexus point on each foot. This point is associated with deep breathing and opening the chest region. Ask the client to take three deep breaths and hold this point with firm pressure.

Technique 42   **Reflexology Relaxation Routine** (Continued)

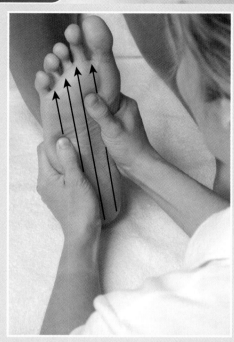

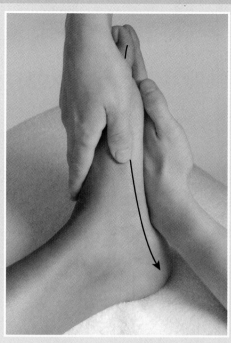

3. Clear the Zones. To clear the zones, thumb-walk each zone from the heel to the top of the toe in that zone. It may take two or three passes over a zone before you start to feel the tissue soften. If you find an area of particular tension, thumb-walk it repeatedly to increase circulation and soften the tissue. The goal of clearing the zones is to ensure that the entire plantar surface of the foot is soft, warm, and stimulated.

4. Spinal Walk. Using Figure 15-9, identify the spinal reflexes. They are on the inside of both feet at the medial edge of zone 1. Thumb-walk from the heel to the base of the big toe. Turn the hand over and support the plantar surface of the foot. Thumb-walk from the base of the big toe to the heel. Repeat the stimulation of the spinal reflexes until the tissue softens.

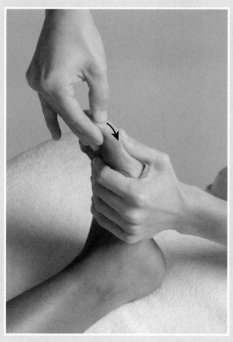

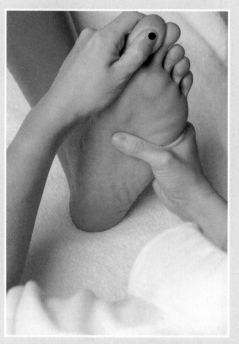

5. Thumb-Walk the Toes. Support the foot with one hand and thumb-walk the toes with the other hand in a technique sometimes referred to as "biting." Bite the big toe first (in five passes, with 15 bites a pass) and work down to the little toe (three passes, with 10 bites a pass). To finish the toes, roll the knuckle of a finger over each of the brain reflexes at the top of each toe.

6. Pituitary Press. Hook and back up on the pituitary reflex point or hold the point with direct pressure up to 2 minutes.

Continued

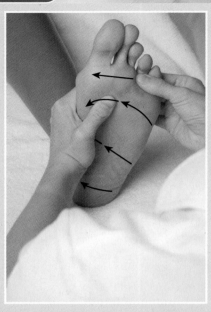

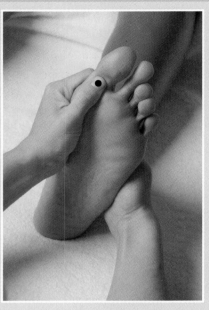

7. Thumb-Walk the Horizontal Lines. The horizontal lines on the plantar surface of the foot include the shoulder line, diaphragm line, waist line, and pelvic line. Thumb-walk each line horizontally from zone 5 to zone 1 and then again from zone 1 to zone 5. In a longer reflexology session, the areas between the lines can also be thumb-walked in a cross pattern so that the entire plantar surface of the foot is stimulated along the horizontal lines.

8. Thyroid Press. Thumb-walk the area associated with the thyroid point, and then hook and back up on the area at the base of the big toe. You can also hold this point with direct pressure up to 2 minutes.

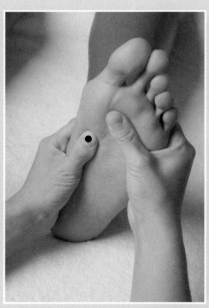

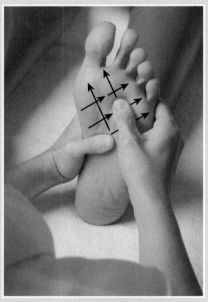

9. Adrenal Gland. Apply direct pressure up to 2 minutes to the adrenal gland reflex, which is located below the solar plexus, above the kidney, and toward the medial side of the foot.

10. Thumb-Walk the Lungs. Beginning at the diaphragm line in zone 5, thumb-walk diagonally across the lung reflexes to the base of the big toe. Next, thumb-walk from the diaphragm line in zone 1 to the base of the little toe. Thumb-walk from the diaphragm line in zone 4, diagonally across the lung reflexes, to the base of the second toe. Thumb-walk from the diaphragm line in zone 2 diagonally, across the lung reflexes, to the base of the fourth toe. Support the foot and hold it upright and open with the hand that is not thumb walking. When you finish walking the lung reflexes, take hold of the solar plexus point on both feet and take three deep breaths together with the client. Cover the foot you just worked on, and repeat the routine on the other foot. At the end of the reflexology session, take hold of the solar plexus point and "balance the energy" between both feet with focused intent before ending the session.

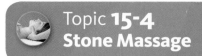

Topic **15-4**
Stone Massage

In **stone massage**, both hot and cold stones might be combined with selected massage techniques to produce unique sessions that meet the needs of a variety of clients. Stones are regularly incorporated with massage for relaxation, injury rehabilitation, and energy balance; to apply deep tissue techniques; to apply reflexology techniques; and integrated with many other types of massage. For example, in a relaxation stone massage, the stones are heated and applied with long, flowing Swedish strokes. Large, flat stones are placed on points of tension to increase circulation to the local tissue and relax muscular tension. These "placement" stones also help to draw the client's attention to an area to support body awareness and deeper muscle release.

For a massage meant to invigorate and energize the body, a hot stone might be held in one hand and a cold stone in the other, or the area is heated first with hot stones and then massaged briskly with cold stones. This "contrast therapy" feels refreshing and stimulating without being too cold or uncomfortable. Hot stones are also used to apply deep tissue and trigger point methods. The stones protect the therapist's hands while bringing heat directly to a particular area of muscle tension or band of taut tissue.

Because reflexology causes repetitive stress to therapist's thumbs, stones can be used instead of the thumbs to activate the reflex points on the feet and hands while also stimulating the point with heat.

Many practitioners have an instinctive and deeply held belief that stones have their own peculiar "energetic stamp" that can be used to balance the body's natural healing mechanisms. Hot or cold stones are often used in a number of energetic bodywork practices such as polarity therapy, chakra balancing, guided meditation, and other techniques.

As you can see, specialized approaches to stone massage may evolve when therapists experiment with stone techniques. In one example, a therapist wanted to use hot stone massage to bring balance and calm to emotionally disturbed children. She developed her own unique approach to stone massage that incorporated a number of different ideas including polarity therapy with stones, aromatherapy, placement stones, vibration with the stones, and gentle clicking of the stones. Her routine calmed and captivated her young clientele, and she developed a series of practical techniques she taught parents to use at home. This is just one of the innovative ways that therapists are using stones for relaxation and healing. Cautions and contraindications for stone massage are described in Box 15-8.

Equipment, Supplies, and Setup

The delivery of stone massage requires an investment in additional equipment and the careful organization of the treatment room to ensure a flowing delivery of techniques

---

> **BOX 15-8 Cautions and Contraindications for Stone Massage**
>
> **Cautions:** Hot stone massage increases circulation and lymph flow in the same way as a standard massage, but because of the heat involved, clients tend to react more strongly to stone massage. This can produce a positive result, such as deep muscular release, or a negative result, such as accelerated detoxification with symptoms like nausea and headache.
>
> Do not work with stones heated to temperatures above 140°F at any point during the treatment because either you or the client could be burned. Your hands will quickly grow accustomed to the heat, and soon hot temperatures will feel only warm. For this reason, the temperature of the stones must be constantly monitored using a thermometer.
>
> Placement stones are placed on top of the client's drape and not directly on the client's skin. A large bath towel provides enough protection so that the stones do not burn the client but at the same time allows the warmth of the stones to penetrate through the drape to the client.
>
> **Contraindications:** Any condition contraindicated for regular massage is also contraindicated for stone massage. Acute illness, fever, circulatory conditions, sunburned skin, broken or inflamed skin, recent soft-tissue injury, advanced or poorly treated diabetes in which tissue is unhealthy and circulation is decreased, edema, thrombus, deep vein thrombosis, gout, heart disease or a serious heart condition, high blood pressure, neuropathy, high-risk pregnancy, renal diseases, rheumatoid arthritis, varicose veins (site contraindication), and intolerance to heat are all contraindications.

(Fig. 15-10). Stone sets for massage vary in the number and size of stones included. An ideal stone set contains about 55 basalt stones of various shapes and sizes. The stones in a massage set can be categorized as "placement stones" and "working stones." Placement stones are larger and rougher than working stones. They are placed on the body, over a drape, to heat an area and to relax the client with their weight:

- **One sacral stone:** The sacral stone is the largest stone in the set. It is placed on the sacrum in the posterior layout or on the belly in the anterior layout.
- **Four large oblong stones:** The four large oblong stones are slightly smaller than the sacral stone and are used in the posterior layout to heat up the erector muscles on either side of the spine. In the anterior layout, they are placed up

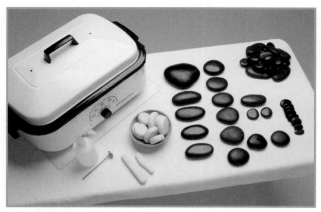

Figure 15-10 Stone massage equipment. The equipment shown here includes a heating unit, 55 basalt stones, marble stones, a latte thermometer, and a spray bottle with alcohol for quick clean up or for cooling the stones.

the centerline of the body and at the origins of the pectoral muscles.

- **Six to eight back stones**: The back stones are placed on the upper areas of the back above the large oblong stones during the posterior layout, and are used as additional placement stones on areas deemed important by the individual therapist.

- **Two palm stones**: The palm stones are placed in the client's hands after they have been smoothed with massage oil (or else they feel dry).

- **Two foot stones**: The stones for the feet are about the same size as a back stone with a flat side that fits easily into the arch of the foot. They are held in place on the foot by being wrapped and tied on with terry strips or with hand towels.

- **Eight toe stones**: Eight small stones are placed between the client's toes. It is a good idea to have a large set for big feet and a small set for small feet. The toe stones must be cooled before they are placed between the toes because this tender, bony area is sensitive to heat. **Working stones**: These stones are usually smoother than placement stones and fit comfortably in the hands of the therapist. It is useful to have a variety of sizes that can be used for different techniques. It is also helpful to have at least two stones with a sharper point that can be used for trigger point or reflexology techniques.

Basalt stones are the main type of stones used in hot stone massage because they hold heat well. Basalt is formed from the solidification of molten magma such as from a volcano. It is tumbled to smoothness in riverbeds or on ocean shores over thousands of years. Some stone suppliers machine tumble stones to smoothness; these are fine as long as the stones are not "glazed" with a sealant to make them look shiny. The glaze prevents the stones from absorbing heat properly.

Marble is often used for cold techniques in stone massage. In its natural state, marble feels cool to the touch because it absorbs heat rapidly. Marble is cut into disks for use in stone massage. While marble stones are visually pleasing and have a unique texture, they are not strictly necessary for cold stone

therapy. Cooled basalt stones work just as well, are easier to obtain, and are less expensive.

A very practical type of heating unit for stone massage is an 18-quart heating unit as shown in Figure 15-10 (18 quarts is the right size for full-body stone massage). A smaller roaster oven or Crock-Pot can be used if you plan to use only a few stones in the treatment. Fancy, decorative heating units are also available from spa and massage suppliers. The heating unit is placed on top of a bath towel to absorb any water splashes as the stones are removed. A white plastic dish mat (cut to size) is then placed in the bottom of the heating unit, and the stones are arranged on top of it. The white dish mat helps the stones to stand out against the otherwise dark interior of the heating unit. This makes them easier to see in the low light of the treatment room and prevents the stones from making a scratching noise on the bottom of the heating unit as they are removed.

The most efficient way to arrange the stones is to place them in the order that they will be pulled out of the heating unit. The sacral stone is placed in the upper right-hand corner of the unit, with the four large oblong stones in front of it. In the next row are the back stones, palm stones, foot stones, and toe stones. The toe stones are placed in a small mesh bag so that they do not get lost under other stones during the treatment session. On the left-hand side of the roaster are the working stones in a pile. Some therapists split their working stones into four or five mesh bags holding prearranged sizes and shapes of stones. This makes it easy to quickly pull the right stones from the heating unit.

Before use, stones are warmed in water heated to 120°F to 140°F. The best water temperature for most clients and therapists is 130°F to 135°F At 120°F, the stones are warm and comfortable, but they cool so quickly that it is difficult to maintain any flow in the massage. At 140°F, the stones would be too hot for many clients and too hot for many therapists to hold in their hands. Never use stones heated above 140°F because you could burn the client.

A bowl of ice water containing four to six working stones (or marble discs) is placed on the worktable. These stones are used for the "vascular flush" or to provide a contrast to hot stones.

A pitcher of cold water is placed close to the heating unit in case the stones get too hot and need to be cooled quickly. Alternately, you could mist the stones with alcohol from a spray bottle to quickly cool them if they are too hot for immediate use. A thermometer is used at all times to monitor the temperature of the water in the heating unit. A digital thermometer is easiest to use because you can fix the part with the digital readout to the outside of the heating unit and read it from a distance while the attached probe is in the water. A set of thermal gloves and a strong slotted spoon are placed to the side of the roaster. The gloves are used to pull the placement stones from the roaster during the posterior and anterior layouts. The slotted spoon lets the water drain out and makes it easier to remove the stones from the hot water in the heating unit.

A bottle of expeller-pressed massage oil is placed on a rolling cart along with six to eight dry hand towels. Sunflower or hazelnut works well, though many different types of cold pressed or expeller-pressed oils can be used. Stone massage does not work well with a massage gel or cream product. These products leave a sticky residue on the stones and turn the water in the roaster cloudy.

The massage table is laid with sheets and a large bath towel over the top sheet. The bath towel is necessary as an insulating layer to prevent burning from placement stones.

Concept Brief 15-3
Stone Temperatures

- 120°F to 125°F: Stones are lukewarm.
- 125°F to 130°F: Stones are warm.
- 130°F to 135°F: Stones are hot but not uncomfortable.
- 135°F to 140°F: Stones are very hot—they can be used only if they are moved rapidly until they cool.
- 140°F and above: Stones are too hot for use and will burn the client.

Cleaning and Sanitizing Stone Massage Equipment

After a session, remove the stones from the heating unit and spray them on both sides with alcohol. Dump out the water in the roaster and wipe the interior of the roaster with alcohol. At the end of the day, wash the stones with hot soapy water, rinse, and allow them to dry completely. The roaster should be rinsed out and sprayed with alcohol. If the stones become sticky or gummy, they can be soaked overnight in a covered container filled with rubbing alcohol. The stones can also be cleaned in a dishwasher; make sure that the stones are secured because they may damage the unit if they become dislodged and fall. Alternatively, they can be soaked overnight in baking soda, water, and lemon juice and then rinsed in the morning.

Box 15-9 outlines some common mistakes that novice therapists make when first practicing stone massage. Technique 43 describes how to use placement stones effectively, and Technique 44 explains basic stone massage techniques. An outline of a relaxation stone routine is provided in Box 15-10.

Technique 43	Placement Stone Layouts

1. Posterior Layout. In the posterior layout, stones are removed from the heating unit and placed on the body in a particular order. The following order works well, but you can use any order you want.

1. Place the sacral stone over the coccyx of the client rather than directly over the sacrum, because it provides a slight traction on the back that feels good.

2. Place the four large oblong stones on either side of the spine directly above the sacral stone. Place the back stones the rest of the way up the spine.

3. The foot stones are wrapped in towels and tied around the arch of each foot. To do this, fold a towel in half across its length and slip the stone into the pocket created in the folded towel. The towel is then tied around the client's foot with the stone placed directly over the arch.

4. The two palm stones are oiled and slipped into the client's hands by lifting the drape and placing a stone in each palm. If the stone is too hot, the client may not be able to hold it, so a washcloth can be placed across the client's hand for protection.

5. Once the stones have been placed on the client, take a moment to ground and center by pressing on the sacral stone to increase the client's perception of weight and warmth. As you press down, take three deep breaths with the client. This creates a nice transition between the placement of the stones and the massage. Some therapists tap four to six times ceremonially on the sacral stone to open the session.

Note: Stones are never placed on bare skin. They are always placed on top of insulating materials like a thick bath towel. This image is shown without a drape to help you visualize proper placement

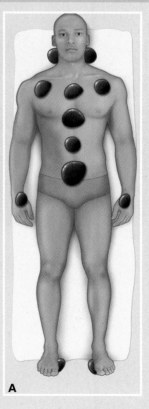

A

Continued

Technique 43 **Placement Stone Layouts** (Continued)

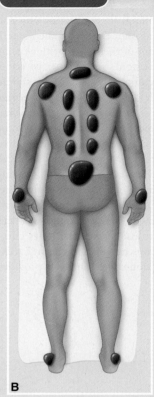

B

2. Anterior Placement. On the anterior body, this placement order and positioning work well:

1. The sacral stone is placed over the navel to act as a belly stone.

2. Two large placement stones are positioned up the centerline of the body.

3. The two remaining large placement stones are placed above the origin of the pectoralis minor muscle on either side of the body.

4. The feet are wrapped with fresh foot stones, and toe stones are placed between the toes. It is important to cool the toe stones sufficiently because they can feel uncomfortably hot in the bony, unprotected area between the toes.

5. Two fresh palm stones are oiled and placed in the client's hands. Some clients like to bring their hands around the edges of the blanket and rest their hands over the belly stone (sacral stone) instead.

6. A warm stone on the forehead or over the eyes feels very nice. However, when stones are left positioned on the face for an extended period, clients tend to tense their neck muscles to keep the stones from sliding off as their body moves during the massage. If you choose to place stones on the face in the anterior layout, leave them only a short time and make sure that they have cooled significantly before you apply them to delicate facial tissue.

7. Before beginning the anterior massage, press down on the two stones placed at the pectoralis minor muscles while taking three deep breaths with the client. This helps to create a smooth transition into the second half of the massage. Some therapists gently tap ceremonially four to six times on both of the pectoralis minor stones at the same time to begin the anterior routine.

Note: Stones are never placed on bare skin. They are always placed on top of insulating materials like a thick bath towel. This image is shown without a drape to help you visualize proper placement

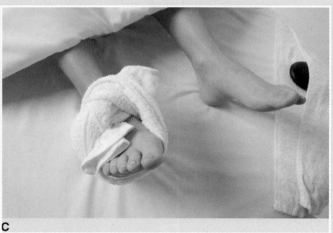

C

3. Detail of Wrapping the Feet with Stones. The foot stones are wrapped in a towel and tied around the arch of each foot. Fold the towel in half across its length and slip the stone into the pocket that is created by the folded towel. The towel is then tied around the client's foot in either the prone or supine position with the stone placed directly over the arch.

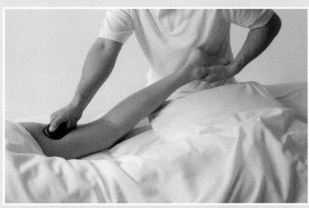

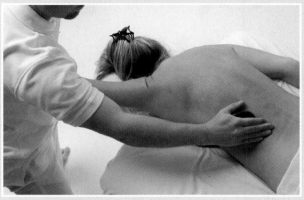

1. Introduction of the Stones to the Client's Body. Apply oil to the client's skin with Swedish massage strokes, and then pick up a stone in each hand. Move the stones briskly over the skin to begin the massage. Do not place the stones directly on the skin and hold them still while asking, "Is this too hot?" If you did that, they would feel too hot and the client would be tense for the rest of the massage. The important thing is to keep the stones moving briskly over the skin and keep flipping them (as described below) until they begin to cool. The client will adapt to the temperature of the stones after three or four passes, and you will be able to slow the strokes and drop deeper into the tissue.

2. Stone Flipping. You will notice that the side of the stone next to the client cools more quickly than the side of the stone touching your hand. To keep the stone temperature even for the client, flip the stone over at the end of a long stroke. When the stones are very hot, you need to flip the stone repeatedly to protect your own hands (the stone is static heat for the therapist while it is moving for the client). To flip a stone, pick up one end with your thumb and turn the stone over while it is in motion. With practice, flipping the stones becomes easy and natural.

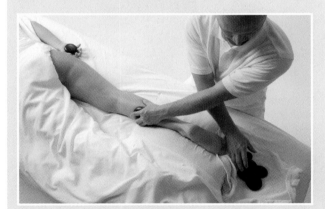

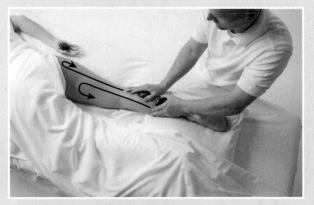

3. Stone Transitions. The smooth transition from a stone that has cooled to another that is hot is an important technique to master for flowing stone massage. Keep one stone moving as you take the other off the body and drop it in a predetermined place. Pick up a fresh, hot stone from the same area and place this new stone on the body. Keep the new stone moving while you repeat the transition with the other hand.

4. Long Strokes with the Stone Flat. Long strokes (effleurage with stones) are used when a stone is first introduced to a body area and when transitioning between different types of strokes. The stones are placed flat against the body and passed up the length of the body area and down again without losing contact. If an area is particularly bony, lighten the stroke over the area. Stones will glide over bony areas as long as there is enough oil on the skin. Pay attention to avoid knocking the stone accidentally into a bony prominence. It helps to palpate the tissue around the edges of the stone by keeping your fingertips on the skin surface. This helps you judge the appropriate depth for the stroke.

Continued

Technique 44   **Stone Massage Techniques** (Continued)

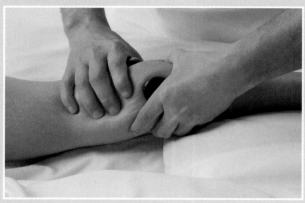

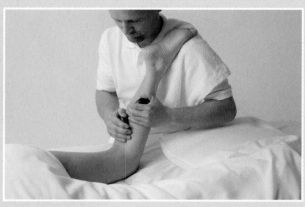

5. Stone Petrissage. Holding a small stone in each hand, use your fingers to lift the tissue as you would in a normal petrissage stroke.

6. Wringing with Stones. Holding a medium-size stone in each hand, use it in a cross motion, lifting the tissue at the top of the stroke where your hands meet.

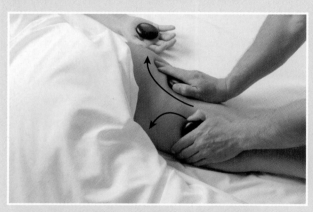

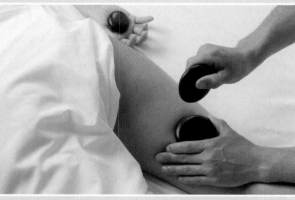

7. Rotation of a Stone with Compression. Holding a medium-size working stone flat against the body area, rotate it in a half circle toward the outside of the body while applying pressure to the stone. The stroke can be performed with one hand or in alternating two-handed strokes. It is particularly useful on fleshy areas such as the hamstrings.

8. Stone Vibration. Place a large stone against the body area and use a smaller stone to tap it. This creates a pleasant sound and a gentle vibration. Some therapists open their massage routine by tapping on the sacral stone before they massage the legs. Another nice idea is to gently tap both edges of a warm stone placed under the neck and pulled back to traction the occiput. This creates a vibration throughout the head and face that feels relaxing for some clients.

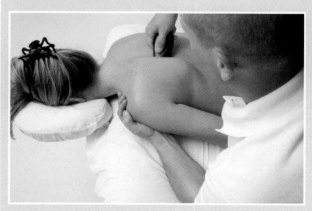

9. Deep Tissue with the Edge of a Stone. The edge of a stone is placed on the area to be worked. As the client exhales, the stone is pressed into the area. This technique is particularly useful around the scapulae.

Technique 44   **Stone Massage Techniques** (Continued)

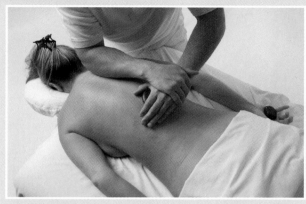

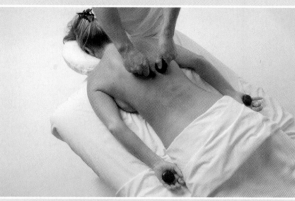

10. Deep Tissue with the Flat of the Stone. Place the stone flat on the client's tissue and use it to warm the tissue ahead of a deep tissue stroke with your elbow. A nice variation for the posterior leg is to hold a medium-size stone in each hand while standing at the posterior knee. Push your forearms forward on either side of the posterior knee, and then bring them back again. As the stones come back, they are placed onto the skin and separated. One stone goes toward the foot, while the other goes toward the hip. They are then brought back together again and the stroke is repeated.

11. Friction with Stones. Stones can be held in the hands and used in place of the thumbs or fingers for friction strokes. A number of friction strokes can be performed using the lamina groove as a guide. Press two stones into the lamina groove on either side of the spine, and run the stones slowly down the back with moderate pressure toward the sacrum. You can also stand on one side of the client and place the edge of a stone in the groove on the opposite side of the spine. Press downward and then flare the stone outward. This is a small movement that nevertheless feels intense to the client. Work slowly and carefully while building your palpation skills with stones. Running stones quickly or roughly over the spinous processes feels uncomfortable for the client and may cause an injury.

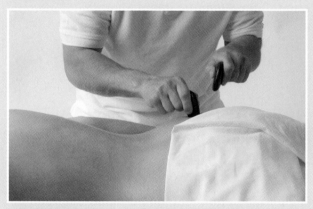

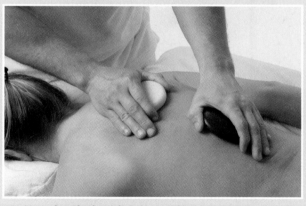

12. Stone Tapotement. Hold a stone in each hand and use them to apply gentle tapotement strokes on various areas of the body.

13. Vascular Flush with Stones. Hold a hot medium-size stone in one hand and a cold medium-size stone in the other hand. With the hot stone leading, run both stones over the body area in long brisk strokes. This feels stimulating and invigorating and is a nice way to finish a body area before redraping and moving on.

Continued

| **Technique 44** | **Stone Massage Techniques** (Continued) |

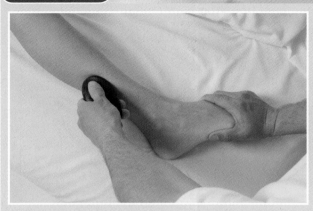

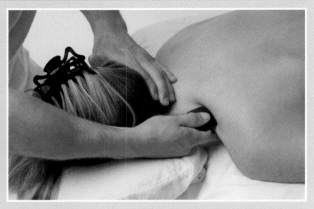

14. Stone Massage on the Anterior Leg. The bony anterior lower leg can be a tricky place for stone massage. Keep the stones on either side of the tibia where they access the many attachment sites for the extensors of the ankle and toes. In a nice technique for the peroneus and tibialis anterior muscles, the lower leg is held in medial rotation and a hot stone is worked up the lateral side of the leg. A stone can also be held on one side of the tibia while the foot is passively dorsiflexed

15. Stone Massage on the Neck in the Prone Position. The upper fibers of the splenius capitis, the trapezius, and the suboccipitals can be accessed when you sit at the head of the table and bring the stones up the lamina groove and out toward the mastoid processes or down into the trapezius muscles as shown here. To reach the suboccipitals, use a deeper, more specific pressure.

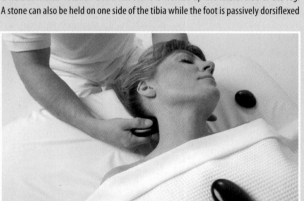

16. Stone Massage on the Neck in the Supine Position. Stone massage on the anterior regions of the neck works best when the head is rotated to one side or the other. This opens up the neck so that the stone can flow without becoming stuck in flesh. On the anterior neck, the stone should be kept in a flat position for the client's safety.

BOX 15-9 Common Mistakes Therapists Make with Stone Massage

The delivery of stone massage requires much attention to details. Therapists often make the following common mistakes when they are learning stone massage. Pay attention to these issues to ensure your own safety and to provide flowing and enjoyable sessions for clients:

Shoes: Always wear shoes when giving a stone massage. The client might sneeze and send placement stones flying onto your feet, or you might accidently drop a stone on your own foot.

Body mechanics: Some therapists "death-grip" a stone during a stroke, position their wrists at extreme angles, or watch the stone as it moves over the body and begin to hunch over clients. While stones can feel slippery, it is best to trap the stone against the client's body with your palm and reach your fingers around the stone so that they contact and palpate the client's tissue. Some techniques do require the therapist to grip the stone. In this case, take care to grip without straining your hands. Watch the position of your wrists when using stones so that they remain as straight as possible during a technique. Any technique that causes strain to your body should be reevaluated and either changed to avoid unnecessary stress or eliminated from your routine.

Roaster speed versus body speed: In stone massage, you work at two different speeds: "roaster speed" and "body speed." A therapist with good roaster speed is fast and focused when removing stones from the heating unit. The minute the therapist's hands leave the client, the therapist moves into high gear, removes the next set of stones from the roaster, and returns to the client. Then the therapist shifts to a slower body speed. The pace becomes slow and relaxing again. The therapist is able to instantly become

BOX 15-9 Common Mistakes Therapists Make with Stone Massage *(Continued)*

grounded and centered as the hands make contact with the client's body and start to massage.

Remove enough stones: Therapists new to stone massage sometimes do not remove enough stones from the heating unit for the body area they are working on. They pull two or three stones, walk to the client, undrape the area, massage, and soon the stones are cold. They must now walk back to the heating unit and swap the cold stones for hot stones. Instead, they should remove a minimum of 8 to 10 stones for each body area. Stones start to cool the moment that they are used on the client's body, but when they are to one side of the client wrapped up in a towel, they remain relatively hot. If you pull enough stones at one time, you

don't have to walk away from the client as often and your massage will be smoother.

Draping: Before placing any stones on clients, check the client's drape. In both the supine and prone positions, pull the drape up toward the top of the client's body so that there is excess over the shoulders. Many clients' shoulders slope downward. This is especially true of woman with larger breasts. Placement stones tend to roll or slide off these clients with the slightest movement. If you have excess drape at the top of the table, you can bring it up and around the stone to create a pocket to hold the stone in place. The drape is then anchored with another stone.

BOX 15-10 Sample Outline of a Stone Massage Relaxation Routine

1. Place the stones in the posterior layout.
2. Massage the posterior legs.
3. Remove the back stones.
4. Massage the back.
5. Remove all the stones from the client's body.
6. Have all the stones reheating in the roaster.
7. Turn the client into the supine position.
8. Place the stones in the anterior layout.
9. Massage the anterior legs and feet (remove the toe stones).

10. Remove all the stones from the midline of the body except the belly stone.
11. Massage the arms.
12. Massage the abdominals (optional).
13. Massage the neck and face.
14. Remove all the stones from the client and end the session.

MASSAGE FUSION
Integration of Skills

STUDY TIP: Botanical Name Flash Cards

Serious students of aromatherapy learn the botanical names of the plants from which essential oils are extracted. A great way to learn these names is to create flash cards. For example, write the common name "lavender" on one side of the card, and on the other side, write the botanical name *Lavendula angustifolia*. Usually the botanical names of plants are Latin and are pronounced just as spelled.

GOOD TO KNOW: Reflexology Certification

To become a certified reflexologist requires specialized training. In some states, a specific license is required to practice as a reflexologist, but in other states, reflexologists must be credentialed as massage therapists before they can practice.

Massage therapists who are not reflexologists can use "reflexology techniques" during sessions but should not claim to be reflexologists. The American Reflexology Certification Board (ARCB) is an independent testing agency. It requires students to take a hands-on reflexology course of no <110 hours and to complete 90 postgraduate treatment sessions that are properly documented using ARCB forms. To obtain the certification, students then sit for a 300-question written exam and a practical skill test. Find out more about the ARCB at www.arcb.net.

MASSAGE INSPIRATION: Spa Party

A fun way to practice your spa skills is to host a "spa party." Get a group of massage friends together and develop a menu of simple spa services such as a salt glow, seaweed gel cocoon (seaweed gel is easier to remove with hot towels than seaweed powder mixed with water), reflexology foot treatment, and hot stone massage. Organize aromatherapy

(Continued)

accent treatments and appetizers. With a plan in place, invite family and friends to come and find out what you are learning in school by being a guest at your spa party. Many therapists offer spa parties on their menu of services when they graduate and become professionals.

IT'S TRUE! SEAWEED IS THERAPEUTICALLY ACTIVE

Seaweed has been well researched in Europe and especially in France for its therapeutic effects when applied topically. The studies of seaweed show that it contains large amounts of polysaccharides, which have a range of biological activities, including antithrombotic, anticoagulant, anticancer, and antiviral effects.[17] Seaweeds have high concentrations of vitamins A, B_1, B_2, B_3 B_5, B_{12}, C, D, E, and K. They also contain polyphenols and carotenoids, which play a role in protecting the body from oxidative stress.[18] Brown seaweeds, the type most commonly used in spa treatments, stimulate metabolism, raise body temperature, increase local circulation, and facilitate detoxification because of the effect of iodine on the thyroid.[19] Remember to avoid seaweed on clients with shellfish, iodine, or seafood allergies.

CHAPTER WRAP-UP

Massage students tend to "take sides" when it comes to spa therapies, aromatherapy, and reflexology. Some "love it" and immerse themselves in aromas, products, and all aspects of wellness approaches that are pampering and luxurious. Some "hate it" and view such approaches as fluffy, beauty focused, and ineffective for helping clients make long-term positive changes in the health of their muscle tissue. In fact, spa and wellness approaches are complex. They involve all the things that therapists love and hate, but more than that, they are therapies with immense therapeutic potential. As you continue to learn about different spa products, especially natural products like therapeutic mud and seaweed, you find that spa treatments can and do increase circulation; decrease muscle tension, soreness, and pain; and leave the body feeling revitalized. If you work with aromatherapy, you will be amazed at the responses clients have to essential oils. If you have practiced any of the treatments described in this chapter, you have probably already realized that spa, aromatherapy, reflexology, and stone massage require attention to detail. You have to organize and manage not just your massage oil but also various treatment products and other equipment to deliver meaningful sessions. Commit to learning these standard spa treatments and unique approaches to wellness, just like you have committed to learning massage techniques. Whether you practice in a spa or in a home office, your clients will appreciate and benefit from your knowledge of these complex and dynamic approaches to wellness.

Chapter

16

Hydrotherapy

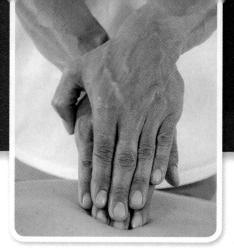

KEY TERMS

buoyancy

compress

friction treatments

homeostasis

hydrostatic pressure

hydrotherapy

mechanical effect

pack

paraffin

plaster

reflexive effect

therapeutic bath

therapeutic shower

LEARNING OBJECTIVES

Having read the chapter and used the related student learning tools, the student will be able to:

1 Define the term *hydrotherapy*.

2 List the characteristics of water that make it useful as a therapeutic application.

3 Compare and contrast the hydrostatic effects of hydrotherapy applications with the mechanical effects of hydrotherapy applications.

4 Classify the uses of hydrotherapy as they relate to both wellness and health care environments.

5 Define the term *homeostasis*.

6 Distinguish between the effects of hydrotherapy applications applied close to body temperature and the effects of hydrotherapy applications applied at greater temperature differences.

7 Distinguish between effects that occur with longer applications of heat and cold and effects that occur with shorter applications of heat and cold.

8 List the key effects of hot, cold, neutral, and contrasting temperatures.

9   Identify safety guidelines and sanitary methods of hydrotherapy used in a massage setting.

10   Discuss three contraindications to cold and hot temperatures.

11   Explain two methods of applying hydrotherapy applications in either a wellness or health care setting.

Hydrotherapy is the external use of water for health and wellness. This chapter explores hydrotherapy and its integration with massage in both wellness and health care settings. The effects of hydrotherapy applications are the same even when the focus of sessions in these settings is different. In a wellness setting like a spa or massage practice focused on reducing stress and promoting enjoyment of sessions, hydrotherapy is most often used to relax the body with hydrotherapy baths, showers, and steams and saunas.

In spas, hydrotherapy is also used as part of the beautification process by estheticians. A particular product might be applied to the legs to improve the appearance of cellulite. Specialized water applications like a Swiss shower or Scotch hose might then be used to activate the product or stimulate the skin and circulation as part of the session.

In health care settings, hydrotherapy is applied to support changes needed in the body for the management of a particular pathology or condition, and to rehabilitate musculoskeletal tissue after injury. In a health care setting, a sauna or steam room might be used as part of the client's treatment plan. If a client has a sports injury, ice packs are likely to be applied to the area to reduce inflammation. As the client's injury heals, heat applications might be used to soften scar tissue and improve range of motion as the client returns to full function.

Topic 16-1 identifies the therapeutic characteristics of water that make it useful and beneficial for clients. The physiological, psychological, and reflexive effects of hydrotherapy are explained in Topic 16-2, before hydrotherapy applications are demonstrated in Topic 16-3. Whether you choose to provide wellness massage and relaxation or work in a health care setting providing condition management or injury rehabilitation, you are likely to use hydrotherapy regularly to promote healthy changes in soft tissues. A solid understanding of hydrotherapy principles and application methods is essential to your work as a professional massage therapist.

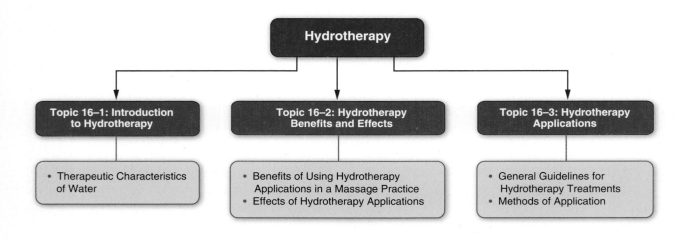

Topic **16-1**
Introduction to Hydrotherapy

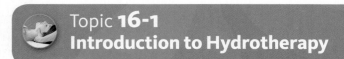

The term *hydrotherapy* originates in two Greek words, *hydro,* meaning water, and *therapeia,* meaning therapy. It is an external application of water as a liquid, solid, or vapor for therapeutic purposes.

The use of water in healing dates back before recorded history, and many cultures around the globe have traditions that include hydrotherapy. North American Indian tribes, for example, used a special hut or a covered sweat lodge built partly into the ground. Large stones were heated in a fire and taken inside the hut where they were sprinkled with water to warm the air, causing the body to perspire as a means of purification. There is evidence that every major U.S. hot spring was used at some point by an Indian tribe.[1] Native Americans considered hot springs to be sacred, neutral ground. Warriors could rest by hot springs to heal battle wounds without worry of attack from another tribe.

Early civilizations often had a version of the spa bath, which combined some form of social interaction with cleanliness. The *hamam* (bath) became popular in Islamic countries around 600 AD after Muhammad recommended sweat baths for spiritual cleanliness. Later, hamams became central to the community both as a place of spiritual retreat and for socializing with friends. Bathers would stop first at the *camekan*, a small court of changing cubicles surrounding a fountain, before entering the *hararat* (hot marble baths). Bathers would receive a vigorous massage or kese (exfoliation with a rough cloth) on a raised marble platform above the wood or coal furnaces used to heat the *hararat*.[2]

As mentioned briefly in Chapter 15, the baths of the Roman Empire are probably the most famous in history. The central role of public baths in Roman culture led to a well-developed understanding of hydrotherapy, and garrisons were often built around hot springs so that the soldiers could heal their battle wounds. By 43 AD, the Roman public viewed the baths as a way to relax and maintain health, and by the early 5th century AD Rome alone had 900 baths.

The medical benefits of hydrotherapy were advanced in Europe by two natural healers who developed their methods in the early 1800s. Many of these methods are still used today as part of hydrotherapy. The first was the Austrian Vincent Priessnitz (1699–1852), who promoted "the cold water cure." This "cure" consisted of drinking large amounts of cold water, bathing in cold water, a simple diet, and physical activity in the open air. Priessnitz used the cold water cure to care for a personal injury that doctors of the time thought untreatable. In 1826, Priessnitz opened a water cure establishment at Grafenberg in the mountains of Silesia, where his ideas were adopted by many prominent physicians.[3]

The second natural healer was Father Sebastian Kneipp (1824–1897), a Bavarian priest who was said to have cured himself of pulmonary tuberculosis by bathing in the icy Danube and "shocking" his body into health. In one of his many books, *My Water-Cure* (1894), Kneipp writes, "Being a priest, the salvation of immortal souls is the first object for which I wish to live and die. During the last 30 or 40 years, however, the care for mortal bodies has absorbed a considerable portion of my time and strength." Instead of administering last rites to the gravely ill, he used water and herbs to cure them. Kneipp's healing system, which combined physical exercise, simple food, hydrotherapy, and herbs, forms the basis of modern naturopathy. He is well known for the "wet-nightshirt" treatment that involved wearing a shirt that had been dipped into water with salt or hay flower. He also introduced classic methods of friction like salt glows and body wraps, which are widely used today in spas.[4]

Today, hydrotherapy applications are used successfully to treat a broad range of conditions and are particularly useful for musculoskeletal problems. Modern research proves what people throughout the ages have always known: water has healing characteristics that change the way we feel mentally, emotionally, and spiritually.

> ### Concept Brief 16-1
> **Hydrotherapy History**
>
> **Cultures around the world have traditions that include hydrotherapy.**
> - **Native Americans**—Sweat lodge for purification
> - **Islamic countries**—Hamam for spiritual and physical cleansing
> - **Romans**—Highly developed understanding of hydrotherapy—900 baths in Rome
> - **Vincent Priessnitz (Austrian)**—the "Cold Water Cure"
> - Father Sebastian Kneipp (Bavarian)—Frictions, wet sheet wraps, use of herbs

Therapeutic Characteristics of Water

Water is a unique substance that covers more than 70% of the earth's surface and provides natural beauty in oceans, rivers, rain, waterfalls, and snow. The human body is 55% to 60% water, and tissues like lean muscle (75%), blood (95%), and bone (22%) contain significant amounts of water. Water also has a number of characteristics that make it useful as a therapeutic application. Water is versatile and changes forms, dissolves other *therapeutic* substances, exerts hydrostatic pressure, causes buoyancy, and absorbs and transfers hot and cold temperatures.

Water Is Versatile and Changes Forms

Water is a liquid that can easily be changed into ice or vapor. It is therapeutically useful in all its forms. As a liquid, water is applied in baths and showers or used to heat special packs, called hydrocollator packs, that bring moist heat directly to a specific body area. Ice packs and ice massage cool heated tissue and reduce inflammation, while saunas and steam rooms use water in a vaporized form to promote perspiration and detoxification.

Water Dissolves Other Therapeutic Substances

Water is known as the "universal solvent" because it dissolves so many other substances. Many of the known elements found on earth are dissolved in seas and lakes. For example, people all over the world have noticed that they feel revitalized from a day at the beach and swimming in the ocean, where seaweeds and minerals dissolve in the water making it a rich, therapeutic soup. Many different substances can be dissolved from a solid to a liquid form for absorption through the skin. Substances like clay, minerals, powdered seaweed, ground oatmeal, and a variety of herbs are routinely dissolved in water and applied to the body in baths and body wraps as part of hydrotherapy.

Water Exerts Hydrostatic Pressure

Hydrostatic pressure is a term that refers to the amount of pressure exerted by a liquid when the liquid is at rest. In other words, water has weight. If you have swum underwater, you have probably noticed that the deeper you go, the more pressure you feel in your ears from the accumulated weight of the water above you. If you stand neck deep in water, there is greater hydrostatic pressure on the lower part of your body (deeper) than on your upper body. Hydrostatic pressure pushes blood and fluid from the lower body into the thorax. This characteristic of water has been used effectively to treat edema in the extremities caused by many different conditions. Pregnant women who exercise in water find that hydrostatic pressure reduces lower leg edema, decreases the occurrence of varicose veins, improves general blood circulation, and stabilizes blood pressure.[5]

Water Causes Buoyancy

Buoyancy refers to floating in water. When immersed in water, your body displaces water and there is an upward thrust of water that lifts you. This is why you feel weightless when you swim. The water you displaced supports the weight of your body. Exercising in water reduces the stress on joints, tendons, and bone that would occur with the impact of the body moving on a hard surface. People who have arthritis, are elderly, or have recently undergone surgery for a musculoskeletal condition benefit from movement in a buoyant environment.

Water Absorbs Hot and Cold Temperatures

Water can be heated or cooled to specific temperatures for therapeutic application to the body. Topic 16-2 later in this chapter describes the effects of hot and cold temperatures on the structures and functions of the body. As you likely already know, hot applications increase local blood circulation, warm soft-tissue structures, relax tense muscles, and soften muscle tissue. Cold applications decrease local blood flow to an area and increase muscle tone.

Water Transfers Hot and Cold Temperatures

Water effectively transfers hot and cold temperatures to the body in two different ways. When heated or cooled water makes contact with your body, it transfers its warmth or coolness to your body through *conduction* (the transfer of hot or cold temperatures through direct contact). Water is more effective at transferring hot or cold temperatures than is air, which is why moist heat feels hotter than dry heat.

Convection is the process by which hot or cold temperatures are transferred via air or gas. For example, it feels colder when the wind is blowing (wind chill) than when the air is still. Saunas are an example of the transfer of temperatures via air; water poured over hot rocks turns quickly into a vapor, which evaporates into the air and warms it. These general characteristics of water are the foundation for the mechanisms by which hydrotherapy is effective.

Concept Brief 16-2
Therapeutic Characteristics of Water

- Water is versatile and changes forms (water, ice, and vapor).
- Water dissolves other therapeutic substances (minerals and plant materials).
- Water exerts hydrostatic pressure (weight of water).
- Water causes buoyancy (lift of displaced water).
- Water absorbs hot and cold temperatures.
- Water transfers hot and cold temperatures (conduction = direct contact, convection = via air).

Topic 16-2
Hydrotherapy Benefits and Effects

Hydrotherapy applications support many of the benefits and effects of massage and can improve the results clients experience from the massage session. The benefits of hydrotherapy include the pleasure and comfort clients receive through hydrotherapy applications. The effects of hydrotherapy usually depend on the temperature of the application and the delivery method (bath, pack, shower, etc.). This section considers the benefits of hydrotherapy applications in massage practice and their physiological, psychological, reflexive, and mechanical effects. Specific hydrotherapy for the treatment of different stages of inflammation during the healing process from musculoskeletal injury is discussed in Chapter 22.

Benefits of Using Hydrotherapy in a Massage Practice

The use of hydrotherapy applications in both wellness and health care settings increases clients' enjoyment of sessions, offers soothing comfort, ensures that clients stay warm, and provides a useful means of empowering clients to manage many conditions through self-care practices.

A recent study suggests that feelings of warmth are associated with a sense of relaxation and well-being. Researchers have found that sensations of warmth alter neural circuits controlling cognitive function and mood, influencing serotonin levels. So whether you are lying on a warm beach in the Caribbean, sitting in a sauna or hot bath, or even working up a sweat through exercise, your brain chemistry changes and your mood is enhanced.[6]

Many clients begin to feel cold as a session progresses. A warm hydrocollator pack on the feet or low back can warm the client and increase the client's enjoyment of the session. A hydrotherapy tub immersion (bath) with soothing additives like essential oils or herbs after a massage boosts the benefits of the massage and prolongs the pleasure the client experienced during the session. At the same time, dead skin cells desquamated during the massage and impurities released from the skin are removed, leaving the client feeling clean and revitalized.

In both wellness and health care settings, therapists often suggest that clients use hydrotherapy applications at home for self-care. Use of hot packs on tight shoulder muscles at the end of a workday can help the client maintain the lengthening effects achieved through a massage session. Regular Epson salt baths help reduce stress, decrease muscle soreness, and improve sleep. Cold packs are applied during the early stages of inflammation to reduce swelling and heat in the tissue and speed the healing process. The simple act of taking a warm bath at night can serve as part of a stress-reduction regimen. These general benefits complement the significant physiological and psychological effects of hydrotherapy applications.

Effects of Hydrotherapy Applications

Understanding hydrotherapy's effects on the body begins with the concept of homeostasis. **Homeostasis** is the relative constancy of the body's internal environment. The body's internal environment includes the extracellular fluid that bathes cells. From this fluid cells receive oxygen and nutrients, and into this fluid cells excrete wastes from their metabolic activities. The health of each cell and an organism's survival depends on the ability of the organism to sustain a relatively constant internal environment. If the internal environment is disturbed to the extent that it can't adjust, such as by prolonged exposure to cold and hypothermia, death of cells and potential death of the organism result.

Humans are able to maintain internal environmental stability because intricate regulatory mechanisms continually monitor and correct the body's internal environment by adjusting physiological functions.[7] The body's core temperature is relatively constant, even in the face of widely varying external environmental temperatures, because of this ability. For example, the body produces heat when the core becomes too cool, and increases heat loss when the core starts to overheat. Hydrotherapy applications are designed to change the internal environment of the body by applying temperatures above, close to, or below that of the body's normal temperature (97°F). The physiological effects of hydrotherapy occur as a result of the body's attempt to return to a constant internal state. For example, a common physiological effect of the application of heat is vasodilatation of blood vessels and increased blood flow to the local area, which moves warm blood out toward the periphery, cooling the core of the body. A common physiological effect of cold is decreased local edema and decreased pain. The edema is reduced through vasoconstriction of blood vessels, which drives warm blood back to the core ensuring the core maintains the proper temperature. As a result, pain is reduced by a decrease in nerve conduction velocity. Three key factors influence the degree to which the body is affected by hydrotherapy applications:

- **The greater the temperature difference between the body and the hydrotherapy application, the greater the physiological effect on the body.** If a client is placed in a bath at 97°F (close to normal body temperature), neither the therapist nor the client will notice much of a physiological difference (although a mild tonic effect occurs with neutral applications). If the same client is placed in a bath at 110°F, the physiological changes in the body will be readily apparent to both. The pulse rate increases, the skin flushes, body temperature rises, metabolism picks up, the blood becomes more alkaline, and white blood cells increase in number. The client may feel nervous or even agitated by the application and will probably want to get out of the hot water.

- **The length of the hydrotherapy application influences the physiological effect on the body.** A client placed in very cold water (32°F to 55°F) will have two very different reactions based on the length of the treatment. If the application is brief (<1 minute), blood vessels will constrict to prevent heat loss. A short time later, blood vessels will dilate as the body attempts to warm itself and prevent tissue loss at the periphery. Muscle tone is increased, and there is an initial spike in blood pressure and respiratory rate. The client is likely to report feeling refreshed and invigorated. If the application is longer than 1 minute, the client's blood vessels constrict as the body attempts to move blood to the core to keep the core temperature consistent. After about 20 to 30 minutes of continuous cold, vasodilation occurs, which increases circulation (Box 16-1), although not above the baseline when the cold was first applied. The physiological processes of the body are depressed, and if the client is not removed from the cold water, death could result.

- **The larger the body area treated, the greater the physiological effect on the body.** Hydrotherapy applications can be used over the entire body or locally. If the body is immersed in a bath, as in the examples above, the effect is more profound than if a cold pack is applied to one local area, say the hamstring. If the cold application is a full-body immersion, the hunting reaction described in Box 16-1 is potentially deadly because heat from the body's core is used to delay tissue loss at the periphery. If the cold is applied just to the hamstrings, the hunting reaction acts as a pump

BOX 16-1 The Hunting Reaction

The hunting reaction involves alternating cycles of vaso-constriction and vasodilatation. When an ice pack is applied to an area, the body undergoes a series of distinct physiological responses. In the first phase, the blood vessels constrict and blood flow to the area is reduced. This decreases local edema and causes the skin to appear pale. In the second phase, the body attempts to warm the area through vasodilatation that increases circulation. If the cold persists, vasoconstriction resumes and the cycle repeats itself with irregular sequences in an apparent "hunting" for an equilibrium of skin temperature. The benefits of the hunting reaction are that vasodilation phases flush the area with fresh blood, bringing nutrients and oxygen to the tissue. Vasoconstriction phases squeeze the blood out of the tissue, removing many metabolic wastes, before another vasodilation phase again flushes the area with fresh blood.

to flush out metabolic wastes in tissues and bring fresh oxygen and nutrient-rich blood to the area.

The effects of hydrotherapy applications can be understood in terms of six primary categories, which overlap and interrelate

- Physiological effects
- Psychological effects
- Reflexive effects
- Mechanical effects
- Effects from dissolved substances
- Effects from specific temperatures

A combination of different types of effects usually occurs simultaneously during a hydrotherapy application. For example, different temperatures cause physiological effects, and dissolved substances, like herbs, can influence the psychological impact of an application.

Physiological Effects

As mentioned earlier, many of the effects of hydrotherapy occur because the body responds to temperatures above or below normal body temperature in an effort to maintain homeostasis. Hydrotherapy applications have a strong effect on blood circulation, causing vasodilation of blood vessels in some instances and vasoconstriction of blood vessels in others. Certain applications can shift blood from one area of the body to another or cause cycles of vasoconstriction and vasodilation that flush the local tissue of metabolic wastes by bringing fresh nutrient- and oxygen-rich blood into an area, pushing blood back out, and repeating the process. In this way, metabolic wastes are removed from the area, leaving the tissue healthier. Certain types of applications cause an increase in blood pressure and heart rate, while others cause it to decrease.

The skin is also directly impacted by hydrotherapy applications because sensory receptors are responding to all the textures and nuances of feeling created by the application and

sending rapid signals to the brain. Overheating the body, as in a sauna treatment or hot immersion bath, stimulates the sweat glands, which helps the skin excrete metabolic wastes from the body. Metabolic wastes that have accumulated in the adipose layers under the skin can be metabolized and released during this process, helping the body to naturally detoxify.

Concept Brief 16-3
Physiological Effects of Hydrotherapy

- Homeostasis is the relative constancy of the body's internal environment.
- Hydrotherapy seeks to change the internal environment of the body.
- Physiological effects occur as a result of the body's attempt to maintain homeostasis.
- When the body is hot, it attempts to cool itself.
- When the body is cold, it attempts to warm itself.

Psychological Effects

While the psychological effects of water and hydrotherapy applications are not always as clearly defined as physiological effects, you have only to contemplate your feelings as you visualize a warm tub full of water, the delights of a swimming hole on a hot summer day, or the feel of warm sea mist on your face to understand water's psychological impact. Most people love water. In fact, maps of the world's population show that most of humanity lives near water. People gather along coastlines, along the course of rivers, and on islands. Popular vacation spots are often located on bodies of water.[8] Water holds an important place in myth and legend and is often viewed as a transformative power. Artemis in Greek mythology ruled the tides as the goddess of the moon. She also personified the unconscious depths of the human mind, which are associated with water. Rituals of purification often involve water, as it is a substance that washes away dirt from the body and in some religions cleanses the soul. Many cultures believe that life sprang from water and that special waters impart youth and renewed beauty. Water can represent an important passage through difficulties to renewal of the spirit. All of these conscious and subconscious factors can be at play during hydrotherapy sessions and benefit clients through the pleasure they receive through interaction with water.

Reflexive Effects

Hydrotherapy applications can produce **reflexive effects** (sometimes called a consensual response) that occur because of a nervous system reaction to the treatment. Reflexive effects happen in an area removed from the point of local application, usually between the skin and the viscera, although heat applied to one limb will increase circulation in the other limb. The reflex relationship between the skin and the internal organs is due to a segmental connection. Both receive sensory innervation from the same segment of the spinal cord. For example, heat applied to the abdomen causes the activity of the intestines to decrease. A hot or cold application to the sternum affects the function of the esophagus. A cold application to the head stimulates mental activity, while the application of a cold pack to the sacrum or feet causes dilation of the uterine blood vessels.[9]

Mechanical Effects

When water is pressurized in a spray, shower, hydrotherapy jet, or whirlpool, the force of the water on the skin's surface and on the muscle tissue below manipulates the tissue for a **mechanical effect**. The body may respond to the sensation of water striking the tissue defensively at first, causing muscle tone to increase. Gradually the body relaxes into the sensation of the pressurized water and muscular tension is reduced, circulation is improved, and overall body function and vital energy are increased.

The hydrostatic pressure of water (described in Topic 16-1) can be considered to exert a mechanical effect on body tissue. Recall that water exerts more pressure on body areas that are deeper in the water. This effect can be used to squeeze fluid from the lower extremities to the thorax; for example, exercising in water reduces edema in the lower legs. In some types of hydrotherapy applications, fluids are pulled from the upper body to the lower body. A classic example is the use of a hot foot bath to decrease congestion in the sinuses due to a cold. The hot water pulls fluid down toward the feet and out of the head. In folk medicine, migraines are treated with a warm foot bath and an ice pack on the back of the neck. The dilation of blood vessels in one body area reduces the fluid congestion in another area.

Another type of mechanical effect of hydrotherapy applications occurs with classic friction rubs like salt glows, wet skin brushing (like the dry skin brushing described in Chapter 15 except the skin is dampened with water or vinegar), or cold mitt friction. The mechanical action of the rough-textured product, brush, or mitts against the skin causes local circulation to increase as the friction generates heat in the tissue.

Effects from Dissolved Substances

In Topic 16-1 you learned that water is called the universal solvent because it dissolves many other substances such as minerals and plants, creating a therapeutic "soup." For example, the Dead Sea is an ancient landlocked sea whose water has been slowly evaporating over the centuries, producing a highly concentrated natural salt solution. After bathing in the Dead Sea, people often report a feeling of increased energy and well-being as well as soft skin. The main mineral elements in Dead Sea water are chlorine, magnesium, sodium, calcium, potassium, and bromine.[10] Research on the usefulness of bathing in the Dead Sea confirms that it benefits a variety of skin conditions because it improves the barrier function of the skin.[11] It is also used to reduce inflammation from musculoskeletal

injuries including back injuries,[12] improves the function of joints effected by both rheumatoid and osteoarthritis,[13,14] and decreases the severity of symptoms associated with fibromyalgia.[15] Additives dissolved in water may have physiological or psychological effects that enhance and support the benefits of the hydrotherapy application. For example:

- **Herbs:** When herbs are soaked in water, many of their chemical components are transferred to the water along with their therapeutic properties. Red clover, lavender flowers, chamomile flowers, powdered oatmeal, comfrey, elderflower, and calendula petals soothe skin irritation and are used to improve many skin conditions. Juniper berries, ginger root, clove bud, allspice, rosemary, and sage warm the body and support perspiration for detoxification treatments. A wide range of herbs and herbal products are used in combination with hydrotherapy applications. Visit spa and massage supplier Web sites to research your options.

- **Milk:** Milk, powdered milk, buttermilk, and cream can be dissolved in water to soften and condition the skin.

- **Minerals:** Minerals in salts like those from the Dead Sea, regular sea salt, or Bearn salt from the mineral springs of the Pyreness Mountains of Southern France dissolve in water, allowing the minerals to be absorbed by the skin to improve both the texture of the skin and overall body function. Epson salts are inorganic mineral salts that help the body detoxify and increase general circulation. They are well known for use with sprains, strains, and sore, fatigued muscles. They also relax the body and are useful for insomnia.

- **Seaweed:** Seaweed contains many bioactive compounds that can be absorbed through the skin and used by the body to support overall body function. Seaweeds have high concentrations of vitamins A, B_1, B_2, B_5, B_{12}, C, D, E, and K. They also contain polyphenols and carotenoids, which play a role in protecting the body from oxidative stress. Brown seaweeds such as *Laminaria*, *Sargassum*, *Fucus*, and *Ascophylum* species stimulate metabolism, raise body temperature, and affect cell membrane transport, facilitating detoxification. All seaweeds contain some amount of iodine, which influences thyroid activity. For this reason, do not use seaweed with clients who have iodine, shellfish, or seaweed allergies or who take thyroid medications.

- **Essential oils:** Essential oils do not dissolve in water, as noted in Chapter 15, but they are commonly added to baths, saunas, and steam rooms to increase the therapeutic benefits of these applications. Review the aromatherapy section of Chapter 15 for specific information on essential oils to use in such treatments.

Effects from Specific Temperatures

Different reflexive and physiological effects depend on the temperature of the water applied to the body. Table 16-1 provides an overview of common water temperatures used in hydrotherapy, while Table 16-2 summarizes the effects of hot and cold temperatures. Hot, cold, neutral, and contrasting temperatures are used in hydrotherapy applications.

TABLE 16-1   Degrees of Hot and Cold in Hydrotherapy

Degrees of Hot and Cold			
Neutral to Very Cold		**Warm to Very Hot**	
Neutral	90°F–98°F	Warm	98°F–100°F
Cool	70°F–90°F	Hot	100°F–104°F
Cold	56°F–70°F	Very hot	104°F–110°F
Very cold	32°F–56°F	Too hot (don't use)	110°F and above[a]

[a]Some products like paraffin (122°F to 126°F), Parafango (120°F to 126°F), and therapeutic mud and peat (115°F) are applied at temperatures above 110°F. These products transfer the heat slowly to the body area and so do not burn the client.

Effects of Heat

The physiological responses of the body to heat result from the body's attempt to prevent a rise in body temperature. Brief applications stimulate the body, while applications of longer duration sedate the body. The use of external applications of heat for therapeutic purposes is sometimes referred to as thermotherapy.

When heat is applied to a client with a full-immersion bath, steam bath, sauna, hot pack, or partial bath such as a foot bath, the peripheral blood vessels dilate and the client begins to perspire. The blood flow to the area where hydrotherapy is applied increases significantly and flushes the tissue. The heart rate, pulse rate, respiratory rate, and overall rate of metabolism rise, which increases the consumption of oxygen in the tissues. The rise in core body temperature creates an artificial fever which in turn stimulates the

TABLE 16-2   Effects of Heat and Cold

Effects of Heat and Cold	
Hot	**Cold**
• Perspiration	• Decreased local blood flow
• Increased local blood flow	• Decreased tissue metabolism
• Tissue will flush	• Decreased edema
• Increased heart rate	• Increased numbing
• Increased pulse rate	• Decreased pain
• Increased metabolism	• Initial increase in respiratory rate
• Increased O$_2$ consumption in body tissues	• Initial increase in heart rate
• Increased white blood cell count	• Initial increase in blood pressure
• Stimulates immune system	• Respiratory rate, heart rate, and blood pressure gradually drop
• Relaxes muscles	• Increased muscle tone
• Decreased muscle spasm	• Short applications stimulate
• Increased range of motion	• Long applications sedate
• Decreased pain	
• Short applications stimulate	
• Long applications sedate	

immune system and causes the body's white blood cell count to increase, inhibiting the growth of some bacteria and viruses. The higher blood flow to the area relaxes muscles, reduces muscular spasm, increases the extensibility of collagen, "melts" the superficial fascia, increases the range of motion in joints, reduces pain, and is generally relaxing.

Effects of Cold

The physiological responses of the body in reaction to cold result from the body's attempt to prevent a decrease in body temperature. Like heat, brief applications stimulate the body, while applications of longer duration sedate the body. The use of external applications of cold for therapeutic purposes is sometimes referred to as cryotherapy.

Cold penetrates more deeply into the tissues than heat because vasoconstriction causes a decrease in local circulation and tissue metabolism. There is also a decrease in leukocytic migration through the capillary walls, which aids in the reduction of edema and pain. Initially, there is an increase in respiratory rate, heart rate, blood pressure, and muscle tone. These gradually drop if the application of cold is prolonged. The reduction of nerve conduction velocity leads to a numbing effect that significantly reduces pain. If the cold persists, vasodilatation and circulation are briefly stimulated.

Clients often have difficulty with cold applications and pass through distinct stages that might feel uncomfortable. The first stage is a sensation of cold, which progresses to a feeling of itchiness or tingling. As the cold continues, the tissue feels as if it is aching and burning. Eventually numbness replaces the uncomfortable feelings and the client relaxes in the later stages of the treatment.

Effects of Neutral Temperatures

Neutral applications are administered at or close to normal body temperature and produce a tonic and balancing effect in most clients. These types of applications are used to soothe the nervous system and can be an effective treatment for insomnia, nervous irritability, anxiety, or depression. Neutral applications are sometimes used at the beginning or end of a hot or cold application to help the body ease into or out of more extreme temperatures. The use of external applications for therapeutic purposes at temperatures close to the body's normal temperature is sometimes called neutrotherapy.

Effects of Contrasting Temperatures

Contrasting applications involve applying a heat application and then a cold application to the same body area in an alternating sequence. This creates a *vascular flush* in which the tissues are "pumped" free of metabolic waste buildup due to the alternating vasoconstriction and vasodilatation of the peripheral blood vessels. Often the treatment uses a pattern of 3 minutes of heat to 1 minute of cold in three cycles. The treatment always ends with a cold application to prevent congestion in the local tissue. Sometimes a longer rotation is used with a ratio of 10 to 15 minutes for the hot application followed by 10 to 15 minutes of a cold application. Again, the treatment ends with a cold application. When using packs to apply heat and cold, it works well to place a cold pack on the area of injury and a hot pack proximal to the injury site close to the cold pack. This relaxes the client and makes it easier to tolerate the cold pack. Contrasting applications are used with immersion baths, partial baths, showers, and packs.

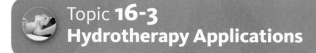

Topic **16-3**
Hydrotherapy Applications

This section discusses how to clean and sanitize hydrotherapy equipment, how to recognize contraindications and adapt sessions to ensure client safety, and how to apply common hydrotherapy treatments.

General Guidelines for Hydrotherapy Treatments

Before you can offer hydrotherapy treatments, you should understand general guidelines for ensuring your client's health and safety. Areas that require particular attention include the sanitation of hydrotherapy equipment and protocols that reduce the transmission of germs and disease, safety issues, and cautions and contraindications to hydrotherapy services.

Cleanliness and Sanitation Guidelines

In Chapter 3, you learned how to prevent the transmission of disease by properly cleaning and sanitizing the treatment room and paying attention to your own hygiene and hand washing habits. Hydrotherapy equipment often requires rigorous cleaning and sanitation between treatments. Showers, tubs, steam rooms, wet tables, and soaking basins must be cleaned, sanitized, and dried between clients. Soaking basins without jets are simply washed with hot, soapy water, dried, sprayed with alcohol, and left to air-dry. If the soaking basin has jets, it must be flushed with an approved disinfectant. Modern hydrotherapy tubs usually come with a self-cleaning function that makes sanitizing the tub jets easier. You put a concentrated disinfectant (formulated by the manufacture of the tub) into a special holder and then push a button. At the end of the cleaning cycle you simply dry the tub. Small, one-person steam cabinets should be completely wiped out with an antiseptic between clients. For larger steam rooms or steam showers, the floor and seats should be sanitized between clients, but the walls can be left until the end of the day. The floor and walls around hydrotherapy equipment must also be cleaned with an approved disinfectant and dried after each use. Pay particular attention to handrails and door handles (e.g., the handle of the steam cabinet). Bath mats, bath towels, robes, washable slippers, and hand towels are changed between clients.

Clients should shower before entering hydrotherapy treatment pools to decrease the spread of waterborne infections. The client's hair should be secured or covered with a cap before using hydrotherapy equipment including tubs, steam rooms, wet tables, or showers. In the event of body fluid "spills" (e.g., the client suddenly gets sick and vomits on a wet table), follow the procedures for universal precautions outlined in Chapter 3.

Safety Guidelines

Specific safety issues must be considered before you offer hydrotherapy treatments:

- **Equipment:** Check hydrotherapy equipment regularly to ensure it is working properly. Maintain the equipment according to the manufacturer's recommendations. Don't allow bare electrical cords in wet rooms or any areas where they might be exposed to water. Identify hot equipment with a sign so that clients don't inadvertently touch it. For example, the outside of a hydrocollator can get very hot, and the heating units for saunas should be surrounded with a grate.

- **Health history intake:** Hydrotherapy applications cause profound physiological changes in clients' bodies. Do not provide any hydrotherapy applications until you have conducted a thorough health history intake process, identified cautions, and ruled out contraindications.

- **Preparation:** Install handrails around showers, wet tables, and hydrotherapy tubs to ensure clients have something solid to hold on to when they get into, out of, or onto and off hydrotherapy equipment. Invest in robes and disposable or washable slippers so that clients can move about in warmth and comfort. Don't allow clients to walk around the facility barefoot. Foot funguses can be spread in this manner, and the client is more likely to slip on a tile floor and sustain an injury.

- **Water spills:** Water is often sloshed about during a hydrotherapy treatment. For example, the area around a wet table usually gets wet and slippery. Before allowing clients to exit hydrotherapy equipment, take a moment and dry the floor with a hand towel.

- **Oils and lotions:** Clients who have had a massage or who arrive at the clinic or spa covered in body lotion, cream, or body oil should shower before using hydrotherapy tubs, saunas, pools, or steam rooms. The oil or heavy cream can block perspiration and make it more difficult for the body to detoxify. Clients are more likely to slip when getting into and out of hydrotherapy equipment when covered in lubricants. Lotions and oils might interact with a treatment product (such as mud, seaweed, and essential oils) and decrease the effectiveness of the session, or the client might leave a sticky residue on seats and equipment making cleanup more difficult.

- **Prevent chills:** Clients who are wet and exit either cold or hot treatments may suddenly become chilled. As clients exit hydrotherapy tubs, wet tables, steam rooms, and saunas, wrap them in towels or a robe and get them entirely dried off as soon as possible. Pay attention to the temperature of treatment rooms and the facility so that clients stay warm.

- **Cold clients never respond well to cold treatments:** If a client is cold, don't put him or her into a cold treatment (e.g., cold plunge) or apply a cold application. Warm the client before applying cold.

- **Dizziness and low blood sugar:** Clients sometimes feel a slight dizziness at the conclusion of the session, or low blood sugar may cause shakiness. Make sure clients stay hydrated during sessions by offering them water at regular intervals. Have packaged food items like fitness bars on hand in cases of shakiness. Educate clients not to eat a heavy meal before a hydrotherapy session.

- **Temperatures:** Use a thermometer to check the water temperature in hydrotherapy tubs and permanently mounted temperature gauges to monitor the temperature in saunas and steam rooms. Never rely on how hot or cold an application "feels" to you. Use a thermometer to ensure you are working at the correct temperatures.

- **Timers:** In some situations, the client should receive a particular type of treatment only for a fixed amount of time. Use timers with alarms to monitor the client's session time. If you rely on a clock you may forget to check the start time and leave a client in an application for too long, endangering his or her health.

Cautions and Contraindications

When used properly, hydrotherapy is safe for most clients. Like massage, hydrotherapy treatments can be contraindicated completely, be contraindicated without a physician's release, contraindicated at a particular location on the client's body, or require adaptive measures and increased therapist vigilance. For example, in many full-body hydrotherapy treatments such as immersion in a hot bath, you can decrease the cardiovascular load on the client by using warm and cool applications rather than hot and cold ones. The closer the temperature of the application to the client's body temperature, the less intense their response will be.

In general, hydrotherapy is contraindicated for individuals who have serious heart, circulatory, nervous system, or systemic conditions. Open wounds and skin rashes are also contraindications for using extremes of hot or cold. The length of time that the client is exposed to the treatment depends on the client's overall state of health and vitality. Children, those in a weakened condition, the elderly, and those with mental challenges, may be contraindicated for full-body treatments like saunas, steam rooms, and immersion baths. Children have thinner skin and become overheated or chilled more easily than adults. Elderly clients have less subcutaneous adipose tissue and may be burned by topical hot applications or chilled more easily as a result. Blood vessels may not function efficiently, such that repeated cycles of vasodilation and vasoconstriction may place a heavy burden on the circulatory system.

If the client seems healthy enough to benefit from such treatments, or if treatments are conducted under the supervision or direction of a physician, start slowly. Begin with 10-minute sessions and progress up to 15-minute sessions. Healthy individuals can remain in saunas, steam rooms, and baths 20 to 30 minutes. Very cold applications longer than 20 minutes are not recommended for any client because of the risk for tissue damage, frostbite, or even hypothermia. A client who is already cold will not benefit from a cold treatment.

If a client feels light-headed, nauseous, headachy, or dizzy, stop the treatment and monitor him or her while relaxing in a quiet environment at a normal temperature with a glass of water. If the client's symptoms increase or persist, consult a physician. If symptoms increase rapidly, contact emergency services because the client might be in danger. Specific cautions and contraindications for hydrotherapy applications are outlined in Table 16-3.

Methods of Application

Common methods of application include hot, warm, or cold packs, local applications like ice massage and mustard plasters, therapeutic showers and immersion baths, hot-air baths, friction treatments, and specialized body wraps. In a wellness setting, hydrotherapy is most often used to relax the client, revitalize the body, or remove a treatment product like mud or seaweed. In medical spas, certain types of wellness centers, many European spas, massage clinics, and private massage practices, hydrotherapy applications might be used for relaxation but also for condition management or injury rehabilitation.

Hydrotherapy Packs and Compresses

A **pack** is any local hydrotherapy treatment (hot, warm, cool, or cold) that uses a gel pack, hydrocollator pack, fomentation pack (moist heat), or commercially made chemical pack. Some packs are electric, some are heated in the microwave, some are chilled in a freezer, and some require specialized equipment. Probably the most effective hot pack is the hydrocollator pack shown in Technique 45. This type of pack has a canvas casing filled with either silicon granules or clay

TABLE 16-3   Cautions and Contraindications for Hydrotherapy

Acute inflammation	Warm and hot applications can increase swelling in injured tissue and thus are contraindicated. Cold applications are indicated.
Allergies	Check for allergies to any substances you dissolve into the water for the session. Allergies to iodine and shellfish indicate an allergy to seaweed or products containing seaweed. Clients might also be allergic to herbs or essential oils, though this is rare.
Artificial devices	Hot or cold applications should not be applied over pacemakers, defibrillators, medication pumps, implants, or artificial devices. Hot and cold applications may be indicated for use with hip and knee replacements.
Asthma	Avoid the use of cold applications on clients who have asthma. Ensure that clients with asthma do not get chilled or walk from a hot environment like a sauna to a very cool or cold environment like an air-conditioned hallway. Movement from very warm to cool environments can trigger asthma attacks.
Athletes	Athletes tend to have very low body fat and may be easily burned by topical hot applications or chilled by cold applications. Use caution and monitor athletes carefully during sessions.
Autoimmune conditions	Autoimmune conditions can flare up causing contraindications for hydrotherapy applications, or a hydrotherapy application might trigger a flare-up. Ask for a physician's release before providing hydrotherapy.
Cancer	Some types of cancer and cancer treatments cause the client to experience a condition that would not indicate hydrotherapy. In other cases, hydrotherapy may prove beneficial. Discuss the particular treatment with the client's physician and obtain a physician's release before providing hydrotherapy treatments.
Children	Children have thinner skin and become overheated or chilled more easily than adults. Avoid the use of extreme temperatures with children, shorten applications, and monitor children closely. Don't apply hydrotherapy applications to infants or very young children except under the guidance of a physician.
Decreased ability to sense hot and cold	Some pathologies and conditions including arteriosclerosis, nerve injuries, diabetes, spinal cord injuries, neuropathy, and multiple sclerosis decrease the client's ability to determine if something is too hot or too cold. In many situations, the extremities are site contraindicated or you can choose warm and cool as opposed to hot and cold temperatures.
Diabetes	Diabetes can lead to cardiovascular diseases and affect the blood vessels in the legs and feet depending on how the condition has been managed and its severity. Consult with the client's physician to determine if hydrotherapy applications are contraindicated, are site contraindicated, or require adaptations. Obtain a physician's release before providing hydrotherapy.
Elderly clients	Elderly clients are more likely to have less adipose tissue and so are prone to burns or chills from hydrotherapy applications. The heart and circulatory system may not be strong enough to cope with the cardiovascular load caused by full-body applications. If the client seems healthy enough to benefit from hydrotherapy, consult with the physician and obtain a physician's release.
Heart disease	Clients with heart disease such as coronary artery disease or congestive heart failure are likely to be contraindicated for hot, full-body treatments like sauna and steam room use or baths. Medications may alter the way the heart functions, contraindicating cold applications. Consult with the client's physician and obtain a physician's release.
History of stroke	Clients with a history of stroke are contraindicated for full-body hydrotherapy such as saunas, baths, and steam rooms. Local, moderate applications such as a warm pack are likely to be safe. Consult with the client's physician and obtain a physician's release.
HIV/AIDS	The suitability of hydrotherapy applications for clients with HIV/AIDS depends on the condition of the individual. Consult with the client's physician and obtain a physician's release.
Hypersensitivity to hot or cold	Usually treatments can be modified to temperatures that are warm and cool if the client has a hypersensitivity to hot or cold. Hydrotherapy treatments should not be unpleasant, and you can adjust temperatures to suit the client's preferences.
Hypertension	At the beginning of both hot and cold full-body hydrotherapy applications there is an initial spike in blood pressure that may be dangerous for some clients. Additionally, clients are likely to be on medications that affect the way in which they respond to hydrotherapy. Modify temperatures to warm and cool, consult with the client's physician, and obtain a physician's release before providing hydrotherapy.

(Continued)

TABLE 16-3   Cautions and Contraindications for Hydrotherapy (Continued)

Hypotension	Hot or cold full-body hydrotherapy applications may cause fainting in clients with hypotension. Modify temperatures to warm and cool, consult with the client's physician, and obtain a physician's release before providing hydrotherapy.
Lymphedema	Hot applications are contraindicated. Neutral and cold applications may be indicated depending on the condition of the individual client. For example, exercise in pools close to normal body temperature can be helpful. Consult with the client's physician and obtain a physician's release before providing hydrotherapy.
Medications	Clients on various prescription medications may respond adversely to hydrotherapy applications. Consult with the client's physician and obtain a physician's release before providing full-body hot or cold hydrotherapy (local applications are usually not contraindicated).
Mental conditions	Hot or cold full-body hydrotherapy applications should be provided to clients with mental conditions only under the direction of a physician.
Multiple sclerosis	Hot applications can increase symptoms in people living with multiple sclerosis and are therefore contraindicated. Neutral and cool applications are indicated.
Obesity	Because of the load on the cardiovascular system, and because of the way in which adipose tissue holds heat and cold, extreme hot or cold applications are contraindicated. Warm and cool applications are more appropriate. If the client's condition is weakened, consult with a physician and obtain a physician's release before providing hydrotherapy.
Osteoarthritis	In some cases, cold applications have caused an increase in symptoms in clients with osteoarthritis. Use cool applications or use short applications of cold, and monitor the client's responses carefully. Warm to hot applications are generally indicated.
Phlebitis	Hydrotherapy is contraindicated except under the direction and supervision of a physician.
Poor kidney function	Cold applications are contraindicated.
Pregnancy	Hot full-body applications including baths, showers, saunas, and steams are contraindicated. Hot local applications to the abdominal region are contraindicated. Cool or warm applications are usually not contraindicated, but it is best to consult with the client's physician and obtain a physician's release.
Raynaud syndrome	Cold applications are contraindicated.
Rheumatoid arthritis	Hot and cold full-body applications are contraindicated. Warm local applications are contraindicated. Neutral and cool local applications are safe.
Seizure disorders	Full-body hot or cold applications are contraindicated.
Skin conditions	Burns including sunburn, open wounds, rashes, and skin infections are contraindications for both full-body and local hydrotherapy applications. Because some skin conditions benefit from hydrotherapy, you should consult with the client's physician and obtain a physician's release if the condition is pronounced or covers a large body area.
Thyroid disorders	Regular hot or cold full-body applications are contraindicated for clients with thyroid disorders. Local applications are generally safe.
Varicose veins	Varicose veins are site contraindications for hot and cold packs. If the client has severe varicose veins, full-body applications like hot or cold baths may be contraindicated. Consult with a physician if you are unsure about the correct way to proceed with the client.

particles that can hold moist heat for up to 30 minutes. These packs are submerged in water kept at 165°F in a specialized heating unit called a hydrocollator. Hot and warm packs are most often used to relax tense muscles, keep the client warm and comfortable, or soften tissue before massage.

Gel-filled commercial packs or homemade ice packs can be used effectively as cold packs. In fact, large bags of frozen peas make an effective cold pack because the small size of the peas feels lighter on an injury site than ice in a plastic zip-lock bag or large ice cubes. Gel-filled packs are also useful because they don't freeze in a solid block and can be shaped to fit a body area. Cold packs are an effective treatment for acute inflammation or after a massage treatment using friction techniques. Methods for using and applying packs are demonstrated in Technique 45.

Compresses are wet cloths soaked in warm, hot, cool, or cold water (sometimes with additives dissolved in the water), and wrung out before they are applied to the skin. They are used to provide comfort or enhance the enjoyment of a session. A cool compress might be placed over a client's forehead while wrapped in a detoxification wrap. Alternatively, a warm compress might be applied to the back of the neck while a

Technique 45 | Application of Hydrotherapy Packs

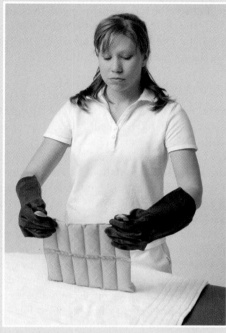

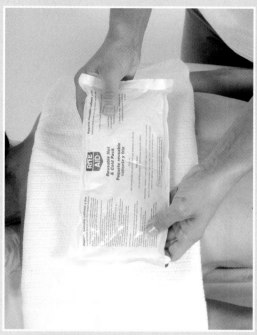

1. Hot pack. Remove the pack from the hydrocollator using tongs or thermal gloves and wrap it in a minimum of four to six layers of thick towels. Place the bundle on the area to be treated for up to 20 minutes. Monitor the pack constantly by lifting it every 5 minutes to check the skin for extreme redness so that it does not burn the client. Clients should never lie on top of hydrocollator packs.

2. Cold pack. Apply cold packs on top of a thin layer of insulation (rather than the thick layer used with a hot pack) for up to 20 minutes.

cold pack is placed on a shoulder injury. The compress helps the client deal more easily with the cold of the cold pack.

Local Applications

You might use a variety of local hydrotherapy applications for condition management or injury treatments. Ice massage, mustard plasters, castor-oil packs, and paraffin dips are popular. Ice massage is massage provided with ice. A paper cup is filled with water and frozen. The edges of the cup are then peeled away while the base of the cup is left intact. Hold on to the base of the cup while applying the ice to the affected area in a circular motion. Ice massage of an area can last up to 20 minutes and is used to reduce inflammation during the acute inflammatory stage, or to cool tissue after using intensive heat-producing techniques like friction.

The term **plaster** refers to herbal pastes (herbs mixed with either water or oil) that are spread on a particular body area or onto a piece of cloth that is then applied to a particular body region. Mustard plasters are warming and useful for the treatment of osteoarthritis, poor circulation, back stiffness, joint stiffness, and general muscular aches and pains. To make a mustard plaster, mix 1 tsp of mustard seed powder

and 4 tsp of wheat flour with warm water until you have a paste of medium consistency. Spread the paste onto a muslin or cotton cloth, and place it over the region being treated. Because a mustard plaster gets hot and can even blister the skin, monitor it constantly. Cover the plaster with a warm pack to increase the therapeutic benefits of the application. Mustard plasters can irritate sensitive skin.

Castor-oil packs and castor-oil applications have been used in both European folk medicine and ayurvedic medicine (the traditional medical system of India) for centuries to increase blood and lymph circulation, relax tight muscles, reduce pain, ease joint stiffness, and break down scar tissue. Castor oil is extracted from castor beans and is high in the fatty acid ricinoleic acid. It is believed to support natural detoxification in the body. Apply castor oil to the affected area in a thick layer, and cover it with plastic wrap. Place a hand towel and an electric heating pack over the top of the plastic. The castor-oil "pack" can be left in place for 30 to 45 minutes.

Paraffin is a waxy substance obtained from the distillates of wood, coal, petroleum, or shale oil. It is used to coat the skin and trap heat and moisture at the skin's surface. This increases circulation and softens the local tissue, which improves joint mobility and decreases pain. A paraffin dip is

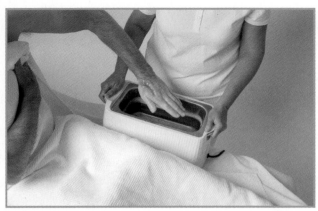

Figure 16-1 Paraffin dip. In this image the client sits up on the massage table for his hands to be dipped in paraffin. He will then relax in the supine position and the paraffin will remain while his legs and neck are massaged. It will be removed directly before the massage of his hands and arms.

an effective treatment for chronic arthritis, tight muscles, and painful joints. It also leaves the skin soft, and it feels warm and sumptuous. To apply paraffin to the hands or feet, first wash the area to be dipped or mist the area with alcohol so that it is properly sanitized. Dip the hand or foot into the paraffin, and allow the paraffin to harden slightly before dipping the area again. Dipping up to five times should be sufficient.

Wrap the paraffin-covered hand or foot in cellophane wrap or a plastic bag before placing it into a heated mitt or a warm towel. To remove the paraffin, simply peel off the cellophane wrap together with the wax all in one piece. The hands can be dipped while the client is on the table in the prone or semi-reclined position. The feet can be dipped while the client is on the table in the supine position (Fig. 16-1).

Therapeutic Baths

Therapeutic baths (sometimes called balneotherapy) encompass a range of different hydrotherapy methods including footbaths, whirlpool baths, steam baths, saunas, full-immersion baths, partial baths, and sitz baths (Table 16-4). Hydrotherapy tubs with multiple air and water jets are designed for professional use and full-immersion baths. Additives are often used with baths to increase their therapeutic benefits.

Footbaths ease foot fatigue or pain, cleanse the feet, warm the body, and relax the client in preparation for a massage. Sometimes they are used therapeutically to draw fluids down toward the feet, as in a footbath delivered to reduce sinus congestion. Massage therapists often use footbaths as a complimentary treat for the client while the client fills out paperwork before the session. Some clinics encourage clients to arrive early and relax with a footbath in a quiet room where soothing music, a cup of warm herbal tea, and dim lights help

TABLE 16-4 Therapeutic Baths

Bath Type	Location	Temperature	Time	Indications
Partial	Feet	Warm to hot (98°F–110°F)	10–20 min	Cold feet, menstrual cramps, arthritis, gout, migraine headache, insomnia, sinus congestion, relaxation, to warm a chilled client, to warm a client in preparation for a detoxification treatment
		Cool to cold (98°F–55°F)	1–15 min	To revitalize and stimulate the body, to cool the body, to reduce inflammation from an injury to the feet or lower legs
		Contrasting hot (110°F–115°F) with cold (50°F)	2 min hot and 1 min cold—three rounds, and end with cold	Poor circulation, repair stage in the inflammatory process for a lower leg injury such as an ankle sprain, to revitalize and stimulate the body
	Hand	Warm to hot (98°F–110°F)	10–20 min	Cold hands, arthritis, hand fatigue, hand or arm injury in the maturation stage of inflammation
		Cool to cold (98°F–55°F)	1–15 min	Inflammation from acute injury, hand fatigue
		Contrasting hot (110°F–115°F) with cold (50°F)	2 min hot and 1 min cold—three rounds, and end with cold	Hand or wrist injury in the repair stage of the inflammatory process, hand fatigue, arthritis

TABLE 16-4   Therapeutic Baths *(Continued)*

Bath Type	Location	Temperature	Time	Indications
Paraffin dip	Feet or hands	Hot (122°F –126°F)	15–20 min	Hand, wrist, foot, or ankle soreness or stiffness, poor circulation, to warm tissue and aid scar tissue reduction in the repair or maturation stage of the inflammatory process for injury, hand or foot fatigue, cold hands or feet
Full-body immersions	Whole body	Warm to hot (98°F–110°F)	5–20 min	To relax muscle tissue, soften fascia, increase circulation, for relaxation (warm) and to decrease pain
		Cool to cold (98°F–55°F)	1–2 min	To stimulate and revitalize the body, to cool the body after a hot treatment
		Neutral (94°F–98°F)	10–20 min	To reduce anxiety, insomnia, depression and to provide gentle revitalization
Epson salt bath	Whole body	Warm (98°F–104°F)	15–20 min	Sore and stiff muscles or joints, general fatigue, insomnia, anxiety, general detoxification
Oatmeal bath	Whole body	Warm (98°F –104°F)	15–20 min	Skin irritation, skin conditions, rashes, itchy skin, to soften the skin
Baking soda bath	Whole body	Warm (98°F–104°F)	15–20 min	Skin irritation, skin conditions, rashes, itchy skin, to soften the skin
Sea salt bath	Whole body	Warm (98°F–104°F)	15–20 min	General revitalization and detoxification, as part of the rehabilitation process for a soft-tissue or bone injury
Mustard bath	Whole body	Warm (98°F–104°F)	15–20 min	Sore and stiff muscles or joints, back pain, general detoxification
Herbal bath	Whole body	Warm (98°F–104°F)	15–20 min	Effects depend on the herbs are used in the bath; skin soothing, muscle soothing, revitalizing, and sedative herbs might be chosen
Aromatherapy bath	Whole body	Warm (98°F–104°F)	15–20 min	Effects depend on the oils used in the bath; skin soothing, muscle soothing, revitalizing, and sedative oils might be chosen
Thalasotherapy bath (seaweed)	Whole body	Warm (98°F–104°F)	15–20 min	To promote weight loss and detoxification, for general fatigue or mental burnout, to stimulate circulation and firm skin, and to revitalize the body
Fangotherapy bath	Whole body	Warm (98°F–104°F)	15–20 min	Sore and stiff muscles, joint pain, back pain, to soften and condition skin
Steam bath	Whole body	104°F with 100% humidity	5–20 min	To warm the body, for detoxification, to increase circulation, for sore or stiff muscles, for joint stiffness or pain, for general relaxation, to unblock congested skin, for certain skin conditions
Sauna	Whole body	145°F–200°F with 6%–8% humidity	5–20 min	To warm the body, for detoxification, to increase circulation, for sore or stiff muscles, for joint stiffness or pain, for general relaxation, for certain skin conditions

release tension. A therapist might start every massage with a 5-minute footbath while the client's neck and shoulders are massaged in a seated position.

Whirlpool baths contain turbines that mix air with water. The agitated water is directed at specific body areas so that soft tissues are manipulated by the force of the water hitting the body.

Steam baths, steam showers, steam cabinets, and saunas are considered hot-air baths because the client is "bathing" in water vapor. Steam baths use steam to facilitate perspiration and help the body to detoxify. Steam baths are often applied before another treatment to warm and relax the muscles, or before the application of a particular product. They are also used to clear the sinuses and respiratory congestion, or to clear clogged and congested skin.

Saunas combine hot air (160°F to 210°F) with low humidity to stimulate metabolism, increase core body temperature, and facilitate detoxification. They are useful as a support treatment for a number of different conditions. For example, people living with chronic fatigue syndrome often experience debilitating feelings of fatigue, musculoskeletal pain, and low-grade fever. One study found that regular use of a sauna improved these symptoms significantly.[16] The humidity in a sauna must not be allowed to drop below 10% or else the hot air will start to dry out the mucous membranes of the respiratory system. Like a steam bath, a sauna can be used to preheat the body in preparation for another treatment.

Partial baths involve the submersion of body areas like the feet, legs, arms, or hands into baths of water heated to specific temperatures. A sitz bath is a type of partial bath in which the

---

| Technique 46 | **Application of Therapeutic Baths** |

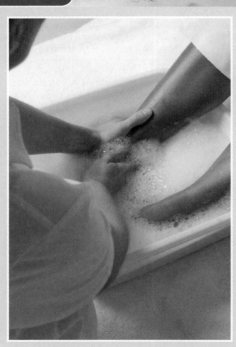

1A. Footbath. Prepare the foot soak by placing warm (not hot) water in a soaking basin. One or two additives like ½ cup of Epson salt (for foot pain), ½ cup of sea salt (energizing), bubble bath (cleansing), herbal infusions (detoxifying), 3 drops of essential oil (properties based on the oil), or powered milk (relaxing) add to the experience. Place the basin in front of a comfortable chair on top of a bath towel. A cup of warm herbal tea on a side table is a nice touch. The client relaxes with the feet in the soak while you massage the shoulders, neck, and scalp. It works well to have the client change into a robe before the soak; otherwise, having to roll up pant legs can be inconvenient and defeat the purpose of the soak, which is to relax the client. At the conclusion of the soak, ask the client to lift the feet from the basin. Remove the basin, and have the client place the wet feet on the preset bath towel. Dry the client's feet by bringing the bath towel up and around the feet. Then move the client to the massage table.

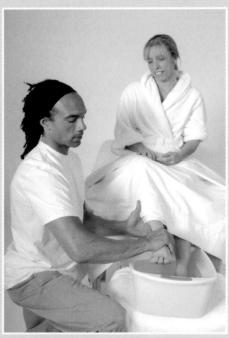

1B. Some therapists deliver the soak with the client seated on the massage table. This way the client can simply lean back and the session can start. Notice that the client wears a robe and that the drape is placed over the client's lap. The client then removes the robe under the drape and hands it to you.

Technique 46 **Application of Therapeutic Baths** (Continued)

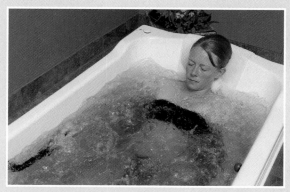

2. Full-immersion bath. Ask the client to change into a swimming suit or disposable undergarments for the bath. As you fill the tub, monitor the temperature with a thermometer so that the bath is hot, warm, neutral, cool, or cold depending on the treatment goals. Help the client into the tub. If the application is hot, it is useful to have the client get into the tub when it is half full of warm water, and then fill the tub the rest of the way with hot water to the desired temperature. Place a towel behind the client's neck for support, and set the timer.

Professional hydrotherapy tubs have an underwater massage hose that uses air pressure aimed at specific body areas to improve circulation and lymph flow. Begin the underwater massage by pointing the hose at the plantar surface of the foot, and work your way up and over the top of the foot in small circles. Continue up the medial leg and then return to the foot and repeat the process, this time working up the lateral leg. Then direct the airflow from the hose from the distal area of the body toward the proximal area of the body. Work up the lateral leg, and ask the client to shift slightly to the side so that the gluteals and back are treated. Treat both sides of the lower body before moving to the upper body. Ask the client to sit low enough in the water for the shoulders and neck to be treated; the hose will splash if it is not kept under the surface of the water.

3. Steam cabinet. Place a towel on the seat and floor of the steam cabinet, and ask the client to change into a swimsuit or disposable undergarments for the session and to take a shower to remove oils or lotions from the skin. When the client sits in the cabinet, close the door. Place a towel around the client's neck to keep steam from escaping out the top of the cabinet. Set the timer for the session based on the client's health and treatment goals. At the end of the session, offer the client water, and wrap the client quickly in a robe or towel to prevent chilling.

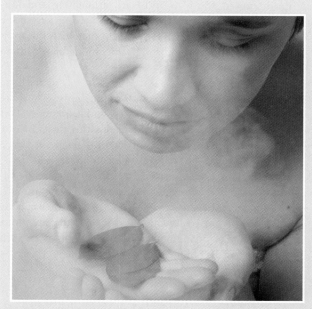

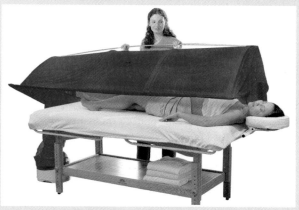

4. Steam room. Ask the client to change into a swimsuit or disposable undergarments for the session and to take a warm shower to remove any lotions or oils. The client relaxes in the steam room for a session length based on the client's health and treatment goals. At the end of the session, offer the client water and wrap them quickly in a robe or towel to prevent chilling.

5. Steam canopy. A steam canopy fits over the top of a wet table or massage table and can be used in place of a blanket or thermal space blanket for body wraps (see Chapter 15 for details of body wraps). Cover the massage table with a plastic table protector and a large bath towel. With the client relaxing on the towel, lower the canopy into place. Wrap a towel around the client's neck to prevent steam from escaping out the top of the canopy, and set the timer for the session based on the client's health and treatment goals. At the end of the session, cover the client in a robe or towel to prevent chilling, and offer a glass of water.

Continued

Technique 46 Application of Therapeutic Baths (Continued)

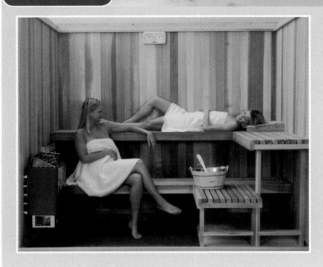

6. Sauna. Ask the client to change into a swimsuit or disposable undergarments for the session and to take a warm shower to remove any lotions or oils. Place a bath towel on the sauna seat, and have the client sit or recline on the towel. Set the timer for the session based on the client's health and treatment goals. At the end of the session, the client can take a cool, warm, or graduated shower to cool down. Wrap the client in a robe or towel to prevent chilling, and offer a glass of water.

patient sits in water that comes up to the navel but no higher. Naturopathic doctors use it to treat reproductive or urinary disorders.

Methods for applying footbaths, full-immersion baths, steam baths, and saunas are demonstrated in Technique 46.

Therapeutic Showers

Chapter 15 introduces the use of **therapeutic showers** for product removal. Technique 34 in that chapter demonstrates the use of a Swiss shower, Vichy shower, handheld shower, and standard shower. Therapeutic showers use hot, warm, cool, or cold temperatures to facilitate desired physiological and reflex effects. Often they are used to warm the body in preparation for another treatment or to cool the body at the end of a treatment. Swiss and Vichy showers have control panels with which you can manage the temperature of the water. In a standard home shower in which the client controls the water temperature, the temperature will not be exact or provide the same benefits.

Hot showers (100°F to 104°F) are stimulating and pain relieving. They might also be used to raise the core body temperature of the client in preparation for another service like an herbal detoxification wrap. A hot shower begins at 100°F. As the client acclimates to the temperature, it is gradually increased. A healthy client may tolerate very hot temperatures up to 110°F, but the temperature should not exceed 110°F. The hottest temperature that is safe and tolerable for the individual client is held for 2 minutes and then decreased rapidly to a neutral temperature to end the shower.

A graduated shower is used to cool the body after a prolonged heating treatment like a steam bath or sauna. The water temperature begins at 102°F and is increased quickly to the tolerance of the client. The elevated temperature is held for 2 minutes and then lowered at intervals. Each interval is held for 1 to 3 minutes. The final ending temperature is in the range of 80°F to 85°F. This temperature is held for 4 minutes to finish the shower.

Cold showers (56°F to 70°F) are stimulating and toning for muscles and skin. They are often used to refresh the body after the application of a treatment that heats the body. They are short and used only on healthy individuals with no contraindications.

Hot and cold contrast showers stimulate metabolism, increase circulation, and revitalize the body. They are effective for fatigue, mental burnout, and low energy. Hot and cold temperatures are reversed for three sets of one interval each; the timing per interval ranges from 1 to 3 minutes. The treatment ends on the cold-water setting.

A Scotch hose directs a strong stream of water at the client to increase circulation, stimulate function, tone muscles, decrease pain, and decrease congestion in a particular body area. It is an effective treatment to use on areas that are prone to stagnation (e.g., poor circulation). Application of a Scotch hose is shown in Technique 47.

Friction Treatments

Chapter 15 introduced **friction treatments**. Salt glows, dry skin brushing, and loofah scrubs all trace their origins back to the traditional methods of Sabastian Kneipp. Kneipp's classic

Technique 47   **Scotch Hose Application**

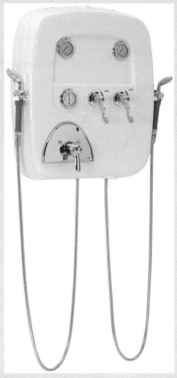

1. This is the type of Scotch hose used in a spa.

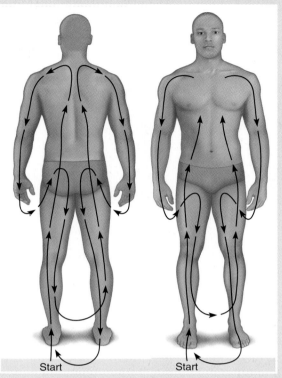

Start   Start

2. Ask the client to change into a swimsuit and then stand at the end of the wet room holding onto the handles attached to the wall. Direct the pressurized stream of water over the client's body in the sequence as shown in this diagram. Start with a warm water temperature, and graduate to hot for 1 minute. Then shift between contrasting hot and cold temperatures. The pressure of the hose can also be controlled based on the client's level of comfort with the pressure. Avoiding the breasts and face, use long smooth movements from the feet to the shoulders.

frictions were carefully chosen for each patient. Frictions could be delivered soft and dry with the palms flat, covered in powder, buffed across the skin to warm and invigorate, or wet and brisk, with water, vinegar, or rubbing alcohol mixed with salt. Cold mitt friction is still widely used to prevent colds, boost immunity, increase circulation, increase endurance, and invigorate the body. Review Techniques 36, 37, and 38 in Chapter 15 for the application of salt glows, dry skin brushing, and loofah scrubs. Technique 48 in this chapter demonstrates cold mitt friction.

Body Wraps

Like frictions, body wraps originated in Kneipp hydrotherapy. One of his most famous body wraps was the cold, wet sheet wrap. Kneipp believed that this treatment strengthened the patient's body so that it could overcome a disease or resist diseases. Kneipp's patients lay on a cold wet sheet or were covered with a cold wet sheet, and then wrapped in blankets for up to an hour.[4] The patient would experience a vascular flush effect in which body temperature was elevated so that the patient perspired. Kneipp used cold, wet sheet wraps successfully for menstrual cramps, digestive complaints, fever, weakness, lower back pain, and general revitalization. Review Techniques 39 and 40 in Chapter 15.

Technique 48 Cold Mitt Friction

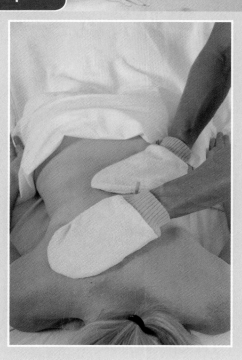

The client reclines on a massage table under a drape beginning in either the prone or supine position. Place the terry mitts on your hands and dip them into ice water. Rub the client vigorously over the selected body area with a back-and-forth motion. Then rub the area dry with hand towels, and drape the area just treated. Move onto the next body area. Depending on the client's health and the treatment goals, you may treat one body area or many areas in a session. If the client is shivering and cold, end the treatment.

Concept Brief 16-4
Hydrotherapy Applications

Pack: A hot, warm, cool, or cold application using a commercial product placed on the body

Compress: A cloth that is dipped in hot, warm, neutral, cool, or cold water, wrung out, and placed on the body.

Ice massage: Massage of a body region or area with ice.

Plaster: The application of an herbal paste to a body region.

Paraffin dip: The submersion of the hands or feet into a waxy substance called paraffin to trap heat at the surface of the skin and warm the tissue and joints.

Therapeutic baths (balneotherapy): Whirlpool, steam, sauna, full-immersion and partial baths in which the entire body or a body region is soaked in water (often with dissolved substances) at specific temperatures.

Therapeutic showers: Swiss showers, Vichy showers, handheld showers, regular showers, and Scotch hose treatments are applied to the body at specific temperatures to manipulate soft tissues through the striking of water on the body and the heating or cooling of the body to create effects based on the body's maintenance of homeostasis.

Friction: Salt glows, dry or wet skin brushing, cold mitt friction, and loofah scrubs stimulate the skin, blood circulation, and lymph flow when applied to one body area or the entire body.

Body wraps: Sheets are soaked in dissolved substances like herbs at specific temperatures and wrapped around the body to achieve specific therapeutic effects.

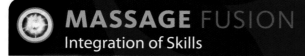

MASSAGE FUSION
Integration of Skills

STUDY TIP: Fact Sheets

When you start to provide treatments with fixed protocols, like many of the treatments that make up hydrotherapy, it is helpful to develop one-page fact sheets that outline pertinent information about the treatment. For example, write these headings equally spaced down one side of a blank page: Indications, Cautions, Contraindications, Temperature Range, Time Frame, and Procedural Steps. Now title the page with the name of the treatment, such as Full-Immersion Hot Bath, and write the key information under each heading. Keep these fact sheets in a binder. They are useful when preparing for an exam and may prove even more valuable when you finish school and deliver the treatment at a clinic or spa.

MASSAGE INSPIRATION: Self-Care with Hydrotherapy

Many of the hydrotherapy treatments you provide clients at a spa or massage clinic you can try at home. For example, get in the shower and gradually increase the water temperature until it is as hot as you can tolerate it safely for 2 minutes; then rapidly turn the shower to cold for 1 minute. Repeat this cycle three times and end with 1 minute of cold. Get out of the shower and dry off briskly. How do you feel? You can learn a lot by playing with different temperatures at home and keeping track of your physiological and psychological reactions in a journal. Remember to check your own health history for contraindications and check with your physician before experimenting if you think any of the treatments might cause you to experience adverse reactions.

IT'S TRUE! HYDROTHERAPY IMPROVES PHYSICAL PERFORMANCE FOR PEOPLE WITH OSTEOARTHRITIS

Researchers studied 152 older persons with chronic symptomatic hip or knee osteoarthritis to determine if hydrotherapy or tai chi classes were more helpful in managing their symptoms. Pain, physical function, general health, psychological well-being, and physical performance were assessed at 12 and 24 weeks in both the hydrotherapy group and tai chi group. While both groups had improved scores, the hydrotherapy group showed significantly greater improvement at 12 weeks. Furthermore, the hydrotherapy group continued to demonstrate improvements at 24 weeks, while the tai chi group remained relatively the same. Researchers noted that this difference probably occurred because the hydrotherapy group had regular session attendance, while 40% of the tai chi group missed multiple classes.[17]

CHAPTER WRAP-UP

One predominant theme has run throughout this chapter: most people like water. They like to swim in it, they like to soak in it, they like to stand in it, they like to have it sprayed on them, and they like the moist, comforting warmth of a hot pack on their shoulders, lower back, feet, and just about everywhere else. Water generally conveys a sense of wellness and health. It simply makes most people feel better. Think about this as you enter your massage career. Whether you work in a clinic, a fancy spa, a chiropractor's office, or a private practice, and whether you practice wellness massage or health care massage, many clients like water—and this gives you a powerful way to boost the benefits your clients receive from your massage sessions. Offer to apply a warm or hot pack to a client's low back, even if they don't have low back pain. Offer a foot soak to a client as they fill out health intake forms, even if they don't have sinus pressure or tired feet. Offer to place a cool compress on a client's forehead on warm days. Offer free paraffin dips to a client, even if they don't have arthritis. Most people like water, and water is good for people, and now you know how to use water therapeutically.

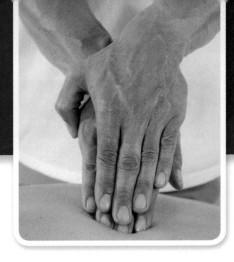

Eastern Approaches

KEY TERMS

abhyanga

acupoints

Asian bodywork therapy

ayurveda

channels

Chinese four pillars of examination

dosha

essential substances

five elements

Indian head massage

kapha

meridian system

pitta

prana

qi

shiatsu

taila

Thai massage

tuina

vata

yin and yang

zang-fu system

LEARNING OBJECTIVES

Having read the chapter and used the related student learning tools, the student will be able to:

1   Define terms related to Chinese medicine concepts, including yin and yang, essential substances, five elements, the zang-fu system, and the meridian system.

2   Discuss the functions and relationship of yin and yang in nature and the human body.

3   Compare and contrast the five elements in the traditional Chinese medicine model and in the ayurveda medicine model.

4   Describe the pathway of one of the twelve primary channels.

5   Identify two assessment methods unique to the traditional Chinese medicine model.

6   Explain the application of three different techniques used in Asian bodywork therapies.

7   Define key terms associated with core concepts of ayurveda, including doshas, prana, marma points, and abhyanga.

8   List two characteristics of each dosha.

9   Compare the application of massage techniques for a kapha as opposed to a vata.

10 Explain the application of three different techniques used in ayurvedic bodywork.

Eastern approaches to massage and bodywork are based on traditional medical systems that view the body differently than in Western medicine (Box 17-1). While many Eastern techniques share similar treatment methods with Western-based approaches, they are applied with different intent. This chapter first presents core concepts in traditional Chinese medicine (TCM) that underlie Asian bodywork therapies. Selected techniques from three Asian bodywork systems are described. Ayurvedic bodywork is covered in Topic 17-2, which teaches an abhyanga (Indian massage) and Indian head massage routine. This broad overview of Eastern approaches provides a basis for students to begin exploring areas of interest within Asian and Indian bodywork systems. Understanding Eastern approaches broadens your perspective on massage and may inspire specialization in your practice.

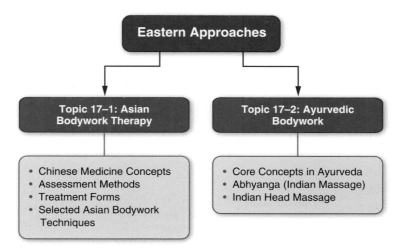

BOX 17-1 West Versus East

The Western view of the body is radically different from the Eastern view. To apply Eastern approaches properly, it is important to understand the differences in these two views.

- **The Western view of the body:** The Western view of the body is based on the Western medicine model and can be described by the words "reductionist" and "mechanistic." Reductionism is the tendency to explain a complex set of facts, phenomena, or structures by another, simpler set. This tendency comes from the Greeks, who separated medicine from magic and explored the anatomy of the body through dissection. As they developed their ideas, they split the human away from the environment, the brain and thinking away from the body and feeling, and even the body's organs and systems away from other organs and systems. They broke down the human body into its simplest parts to better understand each individual part. In the process, many would argue that an understanding of the whole and how it fits into the greater whole of the universe was lost along the way.

- Western medicine also tends to be mechanistic in its approach (where the body is viewed as a machine that can be "fixed" just as a car is fixed at an auto shop) and body systems are studied independently. Early Western medicine wanted to explain illness, build a body of scientific knowledge, and develop precise, repeatable methods for eliminating disease or malfunctions of body structures.[2] With the invention of the microscope and evidence that pathogenic microbes caused disease, Western medicine became very focused on destroying disease-causing agents, alleviating the body's symptoms with prescription medications, or repairing structural dysfunction or damage through surgery. When symptoms are gone, the body is perceived as "healthy," even if drugs are used continuously to mask symptoms or improve physiological function.

- **The Eastern view of the body:** In Eastern medical models like traditional Chinese medicine (TCM) and ayurveda, the view of the body could be described with the words "unified," "holistic," and "balanced." Each human has an intimate relationship with his or her environment on every level. Changes in the natural world including the cycles of the seasons and variations in geographical regions influence the body physically, mentally, emotionally, and spiritually. The body is viewed as a miniature version of the universe, and the same energies that make up the universe make up the human body.

- The Eastern medical models are also holistic in their approach to health care. They emphasize the need to look

(Continued)

BOX 17-1 West Versus East (Continued)

at the whole person, including an analysis of the physical, nutritional, environmental, emotional, social, mental, spiritual, and lifestyle values of the patient. Everything has energetic value in the Eastern worldview. Food can increase strength and energy flow or cause blockages. Activity levels can increase energy flow, block it, or deplete it. The quality of relationships can promote the balanced flow of energy or disrupt it. When energy flow is blocked or disrupted, disease can take root.

- Balance is another concept prevalent in the Eastern medical models. For example, in TCM, the integrity of the body

and its relationship to its environment is based on an understanding of Yin and Yang. Yin represents water, quiet, substance, and night, while Yang represents fire, noise, function, and day. These two parts of a unified whole are polar opposites and must be carefully balanced to maintain health. In ayurvedic medicine, balance is achieved when people make an effort to live mindfully and make choices that promote harmony for their particular body–mind–spirit constitution.

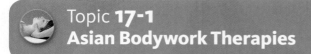

Topic 17-1
Asian Bodywork Therapies

Asian bodywork therapy (ABT) is a general term used to describe a number of different forms of bodywork that have developed over the centuries in Asian countries and more recently in the West. The treatment principles, goals, and methods used in Asian bodywork therapies are based on concepts from TCM. One needs to understand the basics of TCM in order to apply techniques of Asian bodywork systems appropriately and to gain a broader prospective on the use of touch for health and wellness. This section explores key concepts of TCM and sample techniques from tuina (Chinese massage), shiatsu from Japan, and Thai massage.

Chinese Medicine Concepts

TCM is an accepted medical system used throughout modern East Asia and practiced alongside Western medicine in China's hospitals and clinics. It is recognized in the United States as a form of complementary and alternative medicine (CAM). Rooted in the ancient philosophy of Taoism, TCM originated in the Yellow River (Huang Ho) region of China some 5,000 years ago and spread via ancient trade routes across China, the Korean peninsula, Japan, and Thailand, as described in Chapter 1.

According to the 2007 National Health Interview Survey, which asks questions about the use of various CAM therapies, an estimated 3.1 million U.S. adults had used acupuncture (a common treatment method of TCM) in 2007. While the exact number of people who use TCM in the United States is unknown, a survey conducted in 1997 estimated that approximately 10,000 practitioners served more than 1 million patients each year.[1] According to the National Center for Complementary and Alternative Medicine (NCCAM),

scientific evidence for TCM's effectiveness is limited. The use of acupuncture is supported by a significant body of evidence and is considered safe, as are some Chinese herbal remedies. Other Chinese herbal remedies have demonstrated little effectiveness, and still others may not be safe.[1]

Chinese medicine is a complex system based on broad principles that affect how symptoms are perceived and treatment is prescribed by Chinese medicine doctors. These concepts underlay the theory and practice of Asian bodywork therapies; they include yin and yang, the essential substances, the five elements, the zang-fu system, the meridian system, and acupoints. Specific assessment methods and treatment forms impact the practice of Asian bodywork therapies.[2]

Yin and Yang

The ancient Chinese sought to understand the principles governing the natural world. They observed that interdependent opposing forces caused motion and change in nature (e.g., night is followed by day, water extinguishes fire, and the heat of summer is replaced by the cold of winter). They named these opposing forces **yin and yang** and developed specific ideas about their characteristics and interaction (Fig. 17-1).[3]

All Phenomena Can Be Classified as Yin or Yang

All phenomena can be classified as either yin or yang based on observable properties related to "fire" and "water." This classification system occurred because the ancient Chinese viewed fire and water as exact opposites in nature. Yang is defined by the properties of fire, and any object or phenomena that have characteristics similar to fire—warmth, brightness, excitability, lightness, activity, or a tendency to rise—are described as yang. Yin is defined by the properties of water, and any object

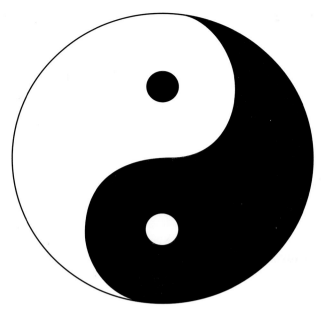

Figure 17-1 The symbol for yin and yang. Yang is defined by the properties of fire, and any object or phenomena that have characteristics similar to fire—warmth, brightness, excitability, lightness, activity, or a tendency to rise—are described as yang. Yin is defined by the properties of water, and any object or phenomena that have characteristics similar to water—cold, dim, heavy, moist, or a tendency to sink—are described as yin.

TABLE 17-1   Yin and Yang Correspondences

Yin	Yang
Anterior	Posterior
Chronic	Acute
Cold	Hot
Community	Competition
Concave	Convex
Contraction	Expansion
Dark	Light
Deep	Shallow
Earth	Heaven
Feminine	Masculine
Inferior	Superior
Inhibited	Excited
Interior	Exterior
Lethargic	Energetic
Matter	Energy
Medial	Lateral
Moist	Dry
Moon	Sun
Numb	Inflamed
Passive	Active
Slow	Fast
Static	Transforming
Substantial	Nonsubstantial
Water	Fire

or phenomena that have characteristics similar to water—cold, dim, heavy, moist, or a tendency to sink—are described as yin. Some of the traditional correspondences of yin and yang are presented in Table 17-1.[4]

Yin and yang represent both opposing objects (e.g., yin represents the earth below, and yang the heavens above) and the opposing aspects of the same object (even as the earth is characterized as predominantly yin, it has yang properties). Although everything has some yin and some yang in its makeup, the predominance of one set of properties over the other determines the object or phenomena's classification.

Yin and Yang Are Interdependent

Yin cannot exist without yang and yang cannot exist without yin. They are interdependent. Through their evolving relationship of opposition, they create unity and underlie all of the necessary changes that occur in the natural environment all around us and within our bodies. The properties associated with yin and yang are absolutes and do not change, but the yin and yang properties of any object or phenomena are relative (changing based on the circumstances) and variable (able to change and prone to change). In any object or phenomena, the aspects of yin and yang are in a continuous state of motion. This is described in Chinese medicine as a mutually consuming and supporting relationship. The consumption of yin results in the supporting of yang. The consumption of

yang results in the supporting of yin. For a fire to exist, both yin and yang must be present. The yin logs nourish the yang flames. This consuming and supporting interaction requires a dynamic balance. Under normal conditions, yin and yang both support and restrain each other (when the logs run out so does the fire), but under abnormal conditions, the harmonious interplay between yin and yang is disrupted and one aspect becomes excessive, while another becomes insufficient.

When we contemplate nature or any phenomenon, we can see that yin and yang are not static and constantly transform into each other. When the consuming/supporting relationship between the two aspects reaches a certain point, yin transforms into yang or yang transforms into yin. For example, after hard exercise (activity = yang), an athlete stops and relaxes (rest = yin). The cycles of the seasons where temperatures change from the intense heat of the summer to the cooler temperatures of the fall, to the extreme cold of the winter, to the warming of spring demonstrate the transformation of yin into yang and yang into yin in the natural world.

In addition, yin can be subdivided into yin and yang, as can yang, and this process of subdivision can go on infinitely. For example, day and night are opposites: day is yang and night is yin. Both day and night can be subdivided into yin and yang parts. The morning of the day is viewed as the yang part of the day, while the afternoon is viewed as the yin part of the day. The period of time right before midnight is the yin part of the night, while the period of time right before the dawn is the yang part of the night.

Yin and Yang and the Human Body

The interdependence of yin and yang is expressed in the human body by the idea that substance corresponds to yin and function corresponds to yang. The solid structures of the body, like organs and blood, are predominantly yin in nature, while the transport of fluids or transformation of substances into energy is yang in nature. Each body structure can be classified as yin or yang and further subdivided. In a healthy body, yin and yang uphold and restrain each other (there is a balance between consuming and supporting) to maintain a dynamic equilibrium, but if there is a predominance or deficiency of one or the other aspect, this equilibrium is lost and disease or dysfunction can result. Imbalances might be caused by pathogenic factors the body encounters in nature that influence the balance of yin and yang or by dysfunction in the body that results in changes to the body's strength and resistance, allowing disease to take root.

Concept Brief 17-1
Principles of Yin and Yang

Opposition: Yin and yang are opposite forces or aspects that together create unity.

Interdependence: Yin cannot exist without yang and yang cannot exist without yin.

Consuming/supporting relationship: The consumption of yin results in the support of yang. The consumption of yang results in the support of yin.

Intertransformation: Under certain circumstances or at a particular point in the consuming/supporting relationship, yin can transform into yang or yang can transform into yin.

Infinite divisibility: Objects and phenomena can be infinitely divided into yin and yang aspects. Yin can be infinitely divided into yin and yang, and yang can be infinitely divided into yin and yang.

The Essential Substances

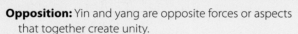

The Chinese believe that the body contains five **essential substances** known as qi, jing, shen, blood, and body fluid.

Qi

Qi (pronounced "chee") is also written as *chi* and as *ki* in Japanese. Qi is the energy that underlies everything in the universe. In the human body, qi is vital life force energy. As condensed and consolidated energy, it forms matter to give the body its shape and substance. As dispersed energy, it provides the momentum behind all physiological and psychological processes. In the body, qi has five primary functions:

- **Transformation:** Qi is constantly passing from one state to another. The food we eat (a form of energy) is converted by body functions (a form of energy) into the cells that make up structures (muscle, organ, blood—a form of energy), and into physical movement (a form of energy) or mental activity (a form of energy).

- **Movement:** Qi empowers voluntary physical movements such as walking as well as involuntary movements such as respiration, the constant beat of the heart, and digestion. The transportation of the human body through life processes such as birth, growth and development, decline and death are functions of qi.

- **Stabilization:** The structural integrity of the body is a function of qi. Qi holds the shape of the body, the blood in vessels, and the organs in their places.

- **Protection:** In the Chinese view, the body is composed of electrically conductive substances (bioelectricity) that generate an external energy field around the body (often referred to as an electromagnetic field). Qi protects the body through the defensive functions of the immune system and through the energetic barrier created by the electromagnetic field and the physical barrier of skin against factors like wind, cold, heat, damp, and pathogenic organisms.

- **Warmth:** The regulation of body temperature and metabolism are functions of qi.

If we view the body as an energetic system, as Eastern cultures do, it makes sense that outside forms of energy such as the changing of the seasons, the nutritional value of food, the quality of the air, pathogens, or environmental factors like cold and damp could alter the flow of qi in and around the body to influence health and wellness. Disharmony of qi arises because of

- **Deficient qi:** There is not enough qi to form body substances or carry out body functions.

- **Collapsed or sinking qi:** There is not enough qi to contain body substances or maintain the structures of the body in their proper orientation.

- **Stagnant or excess qi:** There is an obstruction in the flow of qi through the body, and it becomes slow or stuck in one area where it accumulates and stagnates.

- **Rebellious qi:** Qi flows in the wrong direction or in the wrong way.

In Asian bodywork therapies, the goal of treatment is to promote the harmonious flow of qi through and around the body to positively influence health and wellness.

Concept Brief 17-2
Qi

- Pronounced "chee" (also written as chi and ki)
- The energy that underlies everything in the universe
- Human body = life force energy
- Functions: transformation, movement, stabilization, protection, warmth

Jing

The Chinese word "jing" translates to "essence" and refers to an essential substance of the body that is believed to reside in the kidneys and governs a person's physical condition and development processes including gestation, birth, growth, maturation, decline, and death. High-quality jing provides vitality, longevity, and fertility. Lifestyle choices or periods of overexertion can deplete jing, leading to premature aging, age-related diseases, infertility, and other diseases and conditions. Jing can be strengthened and maintained through conscientious living and the participation in activities, like bodywork, that cultivate qi.

Shen

The Chinese word "shen" translates to "spirit" or "psyche" and refers to an essential substance of the body that is believed to reside in the heart. Associated with the personality and the ability of the mind to form ideas, shen influences social relationships, will, intellect, and emotions. If shen is not in harmony, this leads to muddled thinking, loss of will, and forgetfulness.

Blood

The Chinese concept of blood is different from the Western concept of blood. Blood is viewed as an extension of qi that originates in the heart and bone marrow. Blood transports the nourishment of food qi and provides a moistening and lubricating function for the internal tissues and organs. Blood is moved by qi, and qi is nourished by blood.

Body Fluids

Body fluids like saliva, perspiration, mucus, tears, and synovial fluid are considered an essential substance of the body. They lubricate tissues, muscles, tendons, organs, the skin, and hair. Light, clear fluids are called *jin*, while thicker, yellowish fluids like cerebrospinal fluid are called *ye*.

The Five Elements

The ancient Chinese developed the theory of the **five elements** as an analogy to better understand the systems of the natural world, including the system we know as the human body.[3] The five elements are wood, fire, earth, metal, and water. Each of these elements corresponds to colors, climatic factors, growth and development, motions or patterns of movement, seasons, flavors, body organs, sense organs, tissue types, and emotions (Table 17-2). These elements and their correspondences share the same kind of energy (qi). The five elements also manifest as particular physical, mental, emotional, and spiritual characteristics in people. Understanding the five elements and their correspondences provides practitioners of Asian bodywork therapies clues that can influence bodywork treatment goals and techniques.

TABLE 17-2   Five Elements Correspondences

Element	Color	Climate	Development	Season	Flavor	Organ	Sense Organ	Tissue	Motion	Emotion
Wood	Green	Wind	Germination	Spring	Sour	Liver (Zang) Gallbladder (Fu)	Eyes	Tendon	Spreading out freely	Anger
Fire	Red	Heat	Growth	Summer	Bitter	Heart (Zang) Small intestine (Fu)	Tongue	Vessel	Flaring upward	Joy
Earth	Yellow	Damp	Transformation	Late summer	Sweet	Spleen (Zang) Stomach (Fu)	Mouth	Muscle	Promotion of growth and nourishment	Pensiveness or over-thinking
Metal	White	Dry	Reaping	Autumn	Pungent	Lung (Zang) Large intestine (Fu)	Nose	Skin and hair	Purification and solidity	Grief
Water	Black	Cold	Storing	Winter	Salty	Kidney (Zang) Urinary bladder (Fu)	Ears	Bone	Flowing downward	Fear

Wood

In nature, wood is a yang element and corresponds to spring, a time of germination when seeds sprout and the landscape starts to green and spread outward freely. Fruits are still unripe and sour, and the climate is windy and changeable as temperatures start to warm up after the cold of winter. In the human body, wood is analogous to tall, lean, and muscular body types; high physical activity; and creative, productive, and authoritative personality types. If the wood element is balanced, a person demonstrates benevolence, patience, and compassion. If the wood element is unbalanced, a person may be prone to irritation, anger, and belligerence or alternatively, timidity, rigidity, or indecisive behaviors.

Fire

In nature, fire is a yang element and corresponds to the heat of summer and flaring growth. Fire is experienced in the bitter tastes of coffee and dark chocolate and in the warm hues of reds, deep oranges, and dark yellows. In the human body, fire is analogous to delicate, pointed features, ruddy complexions, curly hair, thinning hair or baldness, and quick, coordinated movements. Personality characteristics associated with fire include a tendency toward high emotion, animated and articulate communication, a sociable and outgoing nature, and multitasking. If the fire element is balanced, a person demonstrates love, passion, joy, insightfulness, and confidence. If the fire element is unbalanced, a person may be prone to guardedness, vulnerability, a need to control situations excessively, or apathy.

Earth

In nature, earth corresponds to late summer and the transformation from one season to the next. Earth is characterized by dampness and moist conditions, the sweetness of candy, and the hues of yellow colors. In the human body, earth is analogous to a tendency toward weight gain, to solidity of the hips and legs, to a large head, wide jawline, and yellow-hued complexions. Personality characteristics associated with earth include stability, groundedness, practicality, loyalty, and supportiveness. If the earth element is balanced, a person demonstrates integrity and adaptability. If the earth element is unbalanced, a person may demonstrate selfishness, needy behavior, stubbornness, or a tendency toward overthinking and excessive worrying.

Metal

In nature, metal is a yin element and corresponds to autumn, the dryness of the cooling air, and the letting go of outdoor enjoyments for indoor activities. Metal is characterized by the pungent, spicy flavors of Indian or Mexican food, grief, twilight, and crying. In the human body, metal is analogous to triangular shapes seen in those with broad shoulders, or angled, sculptured features, an abundance of hair, deliberate movement, and pale complexions. Metal manifests in personality characteristics like rational thinking, methodical planning, and reserve. If the metal element is balanced, a person demonstrates clear thought processes, good organization, inspiration, and receptiveness. If the metal aspect is unbalanced, a person may demonstrate a tendency toward vanity or self-deprecation, zealousness, or despondency.

Water

In nature, water is a yin element and corresponds to the cold of winter, the color black, night, and the salty taste of foods like potato chips. In the human body, water is analogous to long bone structures, long torsos, soft features, and smooth movements. The personality characteristics of water include the ability to go with the flow and adapt to surrounding circumstances. If the water element is balanced, a person demonstrates wisdom, concentration, fearlessness, and flexibility. If the water element is unbalanced, a person may demonstrate a tendency toward emotional numbness, intense conservatism, recklessness, or inertia.

Interaction and Relationships of the Five Elements

The five elements interact to maintain the healthy function of a system (Fig. 17-2). No element acts in isolation. A change in one element causes a change in all the other elements so that the condition of one part reflects the condition of the other parts of the system. In the human body, harmonious relationships between the five elements are important for health and wellness. If one element overly promotes another or exerts undue control over another, an imbalance results. Disease is the result of a destructive relationship among the five elements.

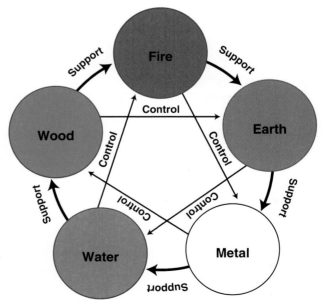

Figure 17-2 Interaction of the five elements. A change in one element causes a change in all the other elements so that the condition of one part reflects the condition of the other parts of the system.

PROMOTING RELATIONSHIPS

The sheng cycle might also be referred to as the promoting cycle, creation cycle, generation cycle, or mother–son relationship. In this cycle, one element supports the next in a specific direction and order. The "mother" element promotes the "son" element. Wood promotes fire, which creates ash that becomes earth. In this way, fire promotes earth. Earth gives birth to metal (deep in the earth metals are formed), which then finds its way to the surface in trace amounts in water. Water nourishes trees and the cycle continues.

CONTROLLING RELATIONSHIPS

The ko cycle might also be referred to as the acting cycle or the control cycle. In this cycle, one element controls another to prevent unrestrained growth. Metal controls wood (think of an ax). Fire is extinguished with water, while the earth is controlled by wood, which loosens the dirt of earth with its roots and creates ground cover that prevents erosion. Fire melts metal, and earth can be used to obstruct water.

Both cycles are in motion simultaneously and produce a relatively stable situation. Promotion is needed for birth and development, and control is needed for equilibrium and harmony. If any one element becomes too strong, it might overpromote another element or overcontrol another element, throwing the system out of balance. If one element is too weak, it may fail to properly promote or control another element, also throwing the system out of balance.[4]

The Zang-Fu System

Zang means organ in Chinese. In Chinese medicine, the organs of the body are understood differently from in Western medicine. Organs are not viewed as separate structures with purely physiological functions, but rather as energy networks that include the channels that interconnect different areas of the body, as described a little later. Organs in the Chinese model may have psychological and spiritual functions in addition to their physiological functions. Other structures including the skin, muscle, tendon, bone, and the sense organs are also considered by Chinese medicine to function as organs.[5]

There are two classes of organs in Chinese medicine. Zang organs are yin and solid organs, including the heart, liver, spleen, lung, and kidney. They function to maintain a full and vital supply of qi in the body. If they fail, qi becomes stagnant and disease can result. Fu organs are yang and hollow organs, including the gallbladder, stomach, small and large intestine, urinary bladder, and triple burner. The triple burner (also called triple heater or triple warmer) is a term found in the oldest texts of TCM. The upper burner corresponds to the thoracic cavity and is associated with respiration. The middle burner corresponds to the upper part of the abdominal cavity and is associated with digestion. The lower burner corresponds to the lower abdominal cavity and is associated with elimination. While the triple burner is not associated with an actual organ (you could not find it if you dissected a body), it is believed to play an important role as a mechanism of metabolism. The function of the fu organs is to digest food, absorb nutrition, and eliminate wastes. If they do not clear themselves regularly and remain full of unusable materials, disease can result.

The **zang-fu system** (Table 17-3) is a concept of the organs as an interdependent network in which organs oppose or restrain each other as well as promote and unify each other. Each zang organ is paired with a fu organ. These pairs are believed to operate in accordance with the theory of yin and yang. The zang organs also depend on each other and are believed to function in accordance with the five elements theory. For example, the heart governs blood while the lung governs qi. Good blood flow produces abundant lung qi, which in turn assures that the blood will circulate normally. When there is balance and harmony between the function of the zang-fu organs, health and wellness result.

The Meridian System

The **meridian system** is an energy network composed of channels, collaterals, and their associated zang-fu organs, sense organs, and tissues. The channels are pathways or routes where qi flows, and the collaterals are interconnecting branches that link the channels to the internal zang-fu organs and the external tissues of the skin, tendons, and muscles in a network. The primary function of the system is to transmit energy (qi) to different areas of the body and to regulate the function of the zang-fu organs and body tissues.

Channels

In the traditional texts of Chinese medicine, the meridian system is viewed as a conduit for both the flow of qi and blood.[6] This often causes confusion because **channels** don't have an actual physical structure (e.g., they are not like blood vessels or nerve pathways—you could not find them in a dissection of the body). Instead, qi is compared to beams of light and the pathway created by the light is the channel. Turn on a flashlight and view the distance it travels. The path it creates (the channel) would not exist without the light (qi).

The channels can be compared to power lines. They carry energy to their associated organs and tissues. If the energy flow to a particular organ is deficient, the organ becomes underactive and can't maintain normal function. Similarly, if the energy flow to a particular organ is excessive, the organ becomes overactive and may "burn out" or become completely depleted. In both cases, the overall condition of the body is thrown out of balance and disease can take root. Channels are located in specific places, and qi flows through channels in a specific pattern and direction. Most often, channels run parallel to major blood vessels and nerves, and so channels, blood vessels, and nerves affect each other's function. For example, if qi is blocked in an area, there is usually decreased circulation of blood in the region affecting local organs and tissue including muscles. Channels in a healthy body regulate the function and relationship of zang-fu organs. If qi is blocked or disrupted, the

TABLE 17-3   The Zang-Fu Organ System

Zang Organs	Fu Organs	Tissues	Sense Organs	Storage of	Emotion
Heart	Small intestine	Vessel	Tongue	Consciousness	Joy
Function: Governs the blood and vessels, controls mental activities.	Function: Receives and contains water and food. Converts food to useful substances.				
Liver	Gallbladder	Tendon	Eye	Soul	Anger
Function: Stores blood and controls volume of blood in circulation. Regulates flow of qi, which helps to regulate emotional activities. Stores the soul. Controls the condition of tendons. Closely linked to the eyes and eye conditions.	Function: Stores bile (a refined liquid formed by surplus liver qi). Helps to promote the smooth flow of qi and blood.				
Spleen	Stomach	Muscle	Mouth	Intention	Pensiveness
Function: Digestion, assimilation, and distribution of nutrients and water. Keeps blood in blood vessels. Stores intention. Controls the limbs and flesh.	Function: Digestion and storage of food and water.				
Lung	Large Intestine	Skin	Nose	Vitality	Grief
Function: Control of qi. Respiration. Controls the downward flow of fluid and stores vitality.	Function: Governs body fluid.				
Kidney	Urinary bladder	Bone	Ear	Determination	Fear
Function: Growth and development of the body and controls reproduction. Stores vital essence (the material which forms the basis of life). Produces marrow, regulates water in the body, helps to coordinate respiration, and stores determination.	Function: Determine usable (or clear) fluid from unusable (turbid) fluid. Eliminate unusable fluid.				

channels can transmit imbalances and so the entire system is impacted, allowing disease to occur.

THE TWELVE PRIMARY CHANNELS

The twelve primary channels of the meridian system are the main trunks that carry qi to different areas of the body. They are shown with their acupoints in Figure 17-3. The channels are named after their associated organ and paired in the same way as zang-fu organs are paired. The liver channel is paired with the gallbladder channel and the stomach with the spleen, and so on. The twelve paired channels occur symmetrically on both sides of the body. Each channel starts or ends in the hands or feet, and each channel connects to an associated organ or sense organ somewhere along the channel's pathway. Each meridian thus controls qi associated with the organ for which it is named. Those channels associated with zang organs are yin channels and carry the interior energy of the body. Those channels associated with fu organs are yang channels and carry the exterior energy of the body. Each channel pair is dominated by the energies of one of the five elements.

Six of the twelve channels flow qi through the lower half of the body passing through the legs and feet; they are known as the "foot channels." The yin channels of the foot include the kidney, liver, and spleen channels. The yang channels of the foot include the bladder, gallbladder, and stomach channels. The other six channels flow qi through the upper half of the body passing through the arms and hands; they are known as "hand channels" (Table 17-4). The yin channels of the hand include the heart, pericardium, and lung channel. The yang channels of the hand include the small intestine, triple burner, and large intestine channels. Each of the 12 channels flows in a fixed direction where it meets another channel and transfers qi. The orderly flow of qi creates a cycle lasting 24 hours (Fig. 17-4).

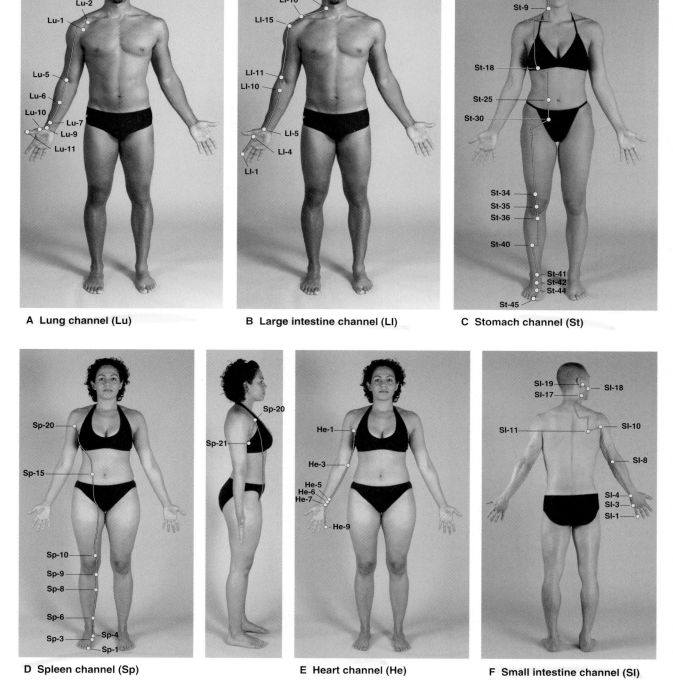

A Lung channel (Lu)

B Large intestine channel (LI)

C Stomach channel (St)

D Spleen channel (Sp)

E Heart channel (He)

F Small intestine channel (SI)

Figure 17-3 The 12 primary channels of the meridian system are the main trunks that carry qi to different areas of the body. They are shown with their acupoints in this image.

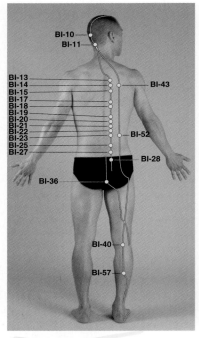

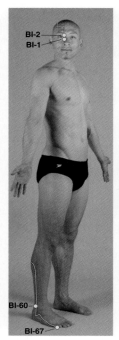

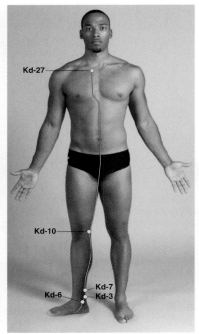

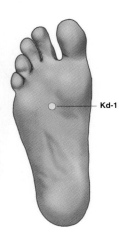

G Bladder channel (Bl)

H Kidney channel (Kd)

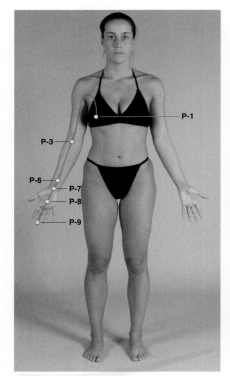

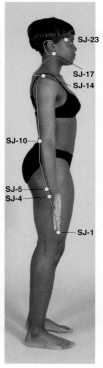

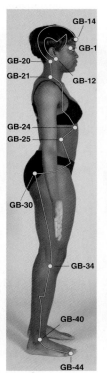

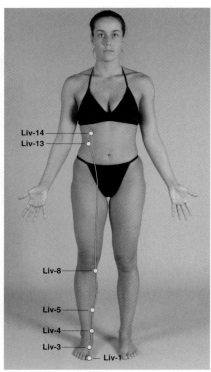

I Heart Protector channel (P)

J Triple Heater channel (SJ)

K Gallbladder channel (GB)

L Liver channel (Liv)

Figure 17-3 *(Continued)*

TABLE 17-4   Overview of 12 Principal Channels

Location	Yin Channel (Medial Side)	Yang Channel (Lateral Side)	Direction of Qi Flow
Upper extremity (hand channels)	Lung channel	Large intestine channel	The yin channels of the hand start in the chest and flow qi to the hand where they connect with the yang channels of the hand. The yang channels of the hand start from the hand and flow to the head where they connect with the yang channels of the foot.
	Pericardium channel	Triple burner channel	
	Heart channel	Small intestine channel	
Lower extremity (foot channels)	Spleen channel	Stomach channel	The yang channels of the foot start from the head and flow qi to the foot where they meet the yin channels of the foot. The yin channels of the foot start from the foot and flow qi to the abdomen where they meet the yin channels of the hand.
	Liver channel	Gallbladder channel	
	Kidney channel	Urinary bladder channel	

An understanding of the twelve primary channels is important for applying techniques in Asian bodywork therapies because the musculoskeletal system is closely related to the channels. An Asian bodywork practitioner who understands the pathways of channels can make connections to seemingly unrelated systems and identify important areas for bodywork. For example, the bladder channel connects to the small toe, lateral aspect of the foot, the ankle, the posterior aspect of the leg, the gluteal and sacroiliac region, the occiput, central frontal region, and the inner canthus of the eye.

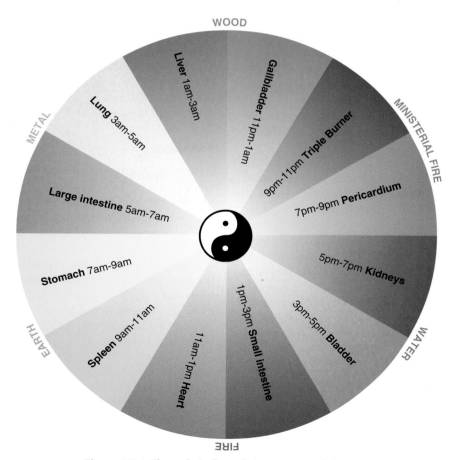

Figure 17-4 The orderly flow of qi creates a cycle lasting 24 hours.

A client with symptoms such as itchy eyes, headache pain, low back pain, or muscle spasms in the gastrocnemius is likely to benefit from bodywork along this channel.

Acupoints

Acupoints (also known as *qi xue* meaning "energy cavities" in Chinese, qi-points in Tuina massage, or *tsubo* meaning "body points" in Japanese) are places along channels where qi can be accessed and manipulated to improve qi flow. Asian bodywork therapies manipulate disordered qi at acupoints to bring qi back into balance, to promote normal flow of qi, to cause a particular therapeutic effect, and to encourage general health and wellness. TCM notes 365 acupoints on the body, but modern research has identified up to 2,000 points. On average, about 150 points are commonly used by acupuncturists.[4]

Acupoints might be thought of as gateways to the body's energy system. They interface with the environment to draw energy into the point or expel energy out of the point. They might be wide open, somewhat open, or barely open depending on their function and condition. They can be palpated as indentations or sunken hollows, small raised nodules, or taut areas in skin, fascia, and muscle. Many people liken them to trigger points and note that the location of trigger points often corresponds to the location of many acupoints.

The location of acupoints along a given channel is traditionally calculated through a measurement unit called a cun (pronounced chun) from anatomical landmarks. A cun is the length of the client's thumb at its widest point. Three cun is equal to the breadth of four fingers. The general location of acupoints is shown in relationship to the twelve primary channels in Figure 17-3. While the Chinese rely on precise measurements from anatomical landmarks when locating acupoints, the Japanese use palpation skills and the sensation of *de qi* (contacting qi).[7]

Acupoints are usually manipulated in combinations based on the therapeutic properties of individual points or because specific combinations create a synergistic effect. Points are coordinated through various methods to create equilibrium. For example, superior and inferior points might be combined, as might proximal and distal, anterior and posterior, right and left, and yin and yang points. Many different methods might be employed to stimulate acupoints to harmonize qi, including acupuncture (the use of needles), acupressure (the use of finger pressure), moxibustion (the burning of a particular herb over selected acupoints), the application of seeds, pellets, and magnets, and the use of a skin-scraping technique called gua sha.

Assessment Methods

TCM practices assessment methods from the standpoint that the interior condition of the body can be detected from examination of the exterior of the body.[8] TCM doctors and many Asian bodywork practitioners use a systematic approach to assessment consisting of four key methods called the **Chinese four pillars of examination,** which involve observation, listening, asking, and touching. Doctors and practitioners use different levels of assessment based on their training and scope of practice.

Observation

Doctors and practitioners use observation skills to determine the person's general condition. A person's posture, movement patterns, expression, complexion, skin color, and tongue condition provide information on qi imbalances. For example, an obese person might suffer from a yang deficiency, while a very thin person might suffer from a yin deficiency. A tendency to be very active and not be able to sit still points to excess yang, while a tendency to be very sluggish or fatigued points to excess yin. In another example, the practitioner might observe a person's expression and see a sparkle in the eyes, quick responses to questions, and clear speech. This type of expression indicates a "vigorous spirit" showing that qi is not damaged and that the organs are in good condition. If the spirit is vigorous, then a disease is likely mild. If a person has dull eyes, slow responses, and a weak voice, however, this indicates a lack of vitality and the disease may be more serious.

Tongue diagnosis is highly regarded in TCM because the tongue is viewed as a mirror of the heart and a reflection of the condition of the spleen and stomach. It also connects through various channels directly and indirectly with the zang-fu organs. Tongue diagnosis is a complex art form, but in one simple example a healthy tongue is light red, not overly dry or moist, and covered by a thin white coating of evenly spread granules. Compare this to a tongue that is pale, which indicates a deficiency of yang qi, or an overly red tongue, which might indicate an excess of qi.[9]

Listening

Doctors and practitioners of Asian bodywork therapies listen carefully to the quality of a person's speech, breathing sounds, and digestive sounds. A person who speaks energetically in high-pitched tones may suffer from a condition of excess heat, while a person who speaks in a weak, low-pitched voice may suffer from a qi deficiency. Breath sounds can indicate a variety of conditions. For example, feeling smothered in the chest and deep sighing can indicate the stagnation of qi because of a sluggish liver, while faint breathing or shortness of breath indicates qi deficiency. Digestive sounds like hiccupping and belching also indicate an abnormal flow of qi, excesses, or deficiencies.[4]

Asking

Asking the person about major complaints, the duration of symptoms, past medical history, family history, lifestyle, and diet provides clues that can help doctors or practitioners develop treatment plans in the same way that interviews help massage therapists plan sessions. TCM doctors use a series of questions developed over many centuries of practice, called "The Ten Questions." The Ten Questions gather detailed information about the development of symptoms, illness, or disease.[3] Topics are

1. The severity and frequency of fever and chills
2. Perspiration, and if it occurs: when it occurs, and how much it occurs
3. Pain, and if it occurs: in the head, trunk, or limbs
4. Sensations that are felt in the chest and abdomen
5. The frequency and color of stools and urination
6. The quality and amount of appetite
7. The quality and amount of thirst
8. The previous history of illness or disease
9. The onset and development of the present symptoms, condition, or disease
10. Questions specific to the special needs of women and children

Touching

The TCM doctor palpates the temperature of areas of the body such as the hands and feet, feels for rigidity or suppleness in the chest and abdomen, determines if abnormal lumps or masses are present in the abdominal area, and notes any areas of edema. Pulse diagnosis is an important method for understanding the circulation of qi and blood through the channels and vessels and the condition of the internal organs in TCM. The pulse is palpated on the wrist in an area called the *cun kou*, which is divided into three regions (Fig. 17-5). On the right hand the radial pulse corresponds to the lung, spleen, stomach, and kidney, while on the left hand the radial pulse allows the condition of the heart, liver, and kidney to be assessed. TCM doctors feel the rhythm, frequency, strength, smoothness, depth, and amplitude of the pulse to determine imbalances.[3]

Asian bodywork practitioners like shiatsu practitioners may focus on palpation to identify areas of kyo and jitsu. Kyo and jitsu refer to the quantity and quality of ki

(qi) levels in meridians (channels). Kyo defines a situation where ki is deficient and weak, while jitsu defines a situation where ki is excessive and overly strong. A kyo–jitsu imbalance can be detected visually through observation of the body and through palpation. Kyo can be observed or palpated as concave depressions of body areas or structures and hollow impressions in tissue and as soft, spongy, or flaccid tissue, which feels cool, cold, numb, or deadened. When pressure is applied to kyo areas, the client experiences sensations of dull pain that tend to feel good because energy is being given to the area. Jitsu can be observed or palpated as bulging areas or protrusions and as tissue that is firm, tight, or hypertonic. Tissue is warm, hot, and hyperactive and feels overly reactive, sensitive, and tender. When pressure is applied to jitsu areas, the client may experience sharp, intense pain.[7]

Concept Brief 17-3
Chinese Four Pillars of Examination

Observation: the person is observed to determine his or her general condition. Tongue diagnosis is one of the methods used during observation.

Listening: doctors and practitioners of Asian bodywork therapies listen carefully to the quality of a person's speech, breathing sounds, and digestive sounds.

Asking: doctors and Asian bodywork practitioners ask the person questions about symptoms and lifestyle.

Touching: the use of palpation helps the doctor or Asian bodywork practitioner determine areas for treatment.

Treatment Forms

The overall goal of TCM is to support the body so that it can remain balanced and adaptable regardless of changing environmental conditions. If an imbalance occurs, TCM seeks to

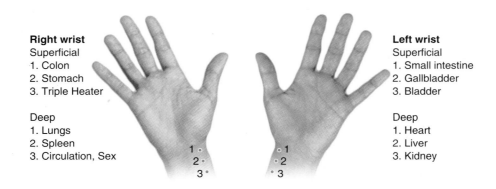

Right wrist
Superficial
1. Colon
2. Stomach
3. Triple Heater

Deep
1. Lungs
2. Spleen
3. Circulation, Sex

Left wrist
Superficial
1. Small intestine
2. Gallbladder
3. Bladder

Deep
1. Heart
2. Liver
3. Kidney

Figure 17-5 Cun kou and pulse diagnosis. The pulse is palpated on the wrist in an area called the *cun kou,* which is divided into three regions.

correct it before disease can take root. Alternately, if the body is already fighting a disease, the goal is to correct the imbalance so the body can heal itself. The goal of treatment is to maintain or restore the balance between parts of the body and between the body and its environment for optimal health and wellness.

Originally, bodywork was one form of treatment used by TCM doctors along with a number of other treatment forms. Currently, many treatment forms are practiced independently with the goal to promote balance and harmony in the body.

- **Acupuncture:** Small needles are inserted into specific points on the patient's body to increase or balance the flow of qi.
- **Asian bodywork therapies:** Bodywork methods like shiatsu (Japanese massage) and tuina (Chinese massage), among many others, are used to support the balanced flow of qi through the channels.
- **Chinese food therapy:** Dietary recommendations are made according to TCM principles and the client's condition using information related to the five flavors. When the five flavors are in balance, the body maintains optimal health and wellness.
- **Chinese herbal medicine:** Over 500 herbs are prescribed individually or in combinations (herbs in combination contain between 3 and 25 different plants) to create harmony and balance in the body and for their medicinal properties. For example, the use of mushrooms like reishi and shiitake is used to boost immunity.
- **Cupping:** Cupping is a bodywork therapy in which glass cups are heated and placed on the skin. With cooling, the cup suctions the skin, pulling tissue up into the cup. Sometimes the cups are combined with massage oil and slid across the back in a form of massage.
- **Gua sha:** The name *gua sha* means to "scrape away fever." A sharp edge such as a ceramic Chinese spoon, animal horn, piece of jade, or metal cap with a rounded edge might be applied in long pressured strokes over lubricated skin. A piece of ginger root soaked in rice wine might be applied in strokes down the spine to alleviate fatigue from heavy physical labor.
- **Moxibustion:** Moxa is the term used to describe dried Chinese mugwort (*Artemisia vulgaris*) herb. It is burned on acupoints to warm the body and increase the flow of qi and blood. Sometimes the moxa is rolled into a tube and then lit and held at acupuncture points or placed on the end of an inserted needle.
- **Qigong:** Qigong is a form of meditation and exercise that uses slow movements and breathing techniques to promote the harmonious flow of qi in the body and improve overall health and function.

With this broad overview of concepts and methods used in TCM, you can apply this understanding to the application of selected Asian bodywork techniques.

Selected Asian Bodywork Techniques

The American Organization for Bodywork Therapies of Asia (AOBTA) is a professional membership organization that promotes ABT and serves Asian bodywork practitioners and schools. Forms of ABT recognized by AOBTA include acupressure, Amma, AMMA Therapy, Chi Nei Tsang, Jin Shin Do, Nuad Bo' Ran (traditional Thai massage), tuina, and five distinct approaches to shiatsu (Zen, integrative eclectic, Japanese, macrobiotic/barefoot, and five element).

AOBTA recognizes bodywork forms that originate from Chinese medicine theory and defines ABT as

> The treatment of the human body/mind/spirit, including the electromagnetic or energetic field, which surrounds, infuses and brings that body to life, by using pressure and/or manipulation. Asian bodywork is based upon Chinese medical principles for assessing and evaluating the body's energetic system. It uses traditional Asian techniques and treatment strategies to primarily affect and balance the energetic system for the purpose of treating the human body, emotions, mind, energy field, and spirit for the promotion, maintenance, and restoration of health.[10]

The scope of practice for Asian bodywork practitioners as defined by AOBTA is broader than that of a massage therapist. Asian bodywork practitioners use the Chinese four pillars of examination, as described earlier. Treatment includes touching, pressing, or holding the body along meridians or on acupoints with the hands. Stretching, the external application of medicinal plants or foods, hot and cold therapies, and dietary or exercise suggestions may be included. Cupping, gua sha, moxibustion, and other methods or modalities are allowed when applied by properly trained practitioners. To find out more about AOBTA, visit www.aobta.org.

The goal of this section is to explore three Asian bodywork therapies (tuina, shiatsu, and Thai massage), and explain the application of some useful Asian bodywork techniques. Each of these bodywork systems is complex and requires in-depth study and training for mastery. Proper assessment and the discovery of imbalances in yin and yang, the five elements, and qi flow are essential to effective treatment choices in Asian bodywork. There is not room here to explain the methods and analogies each of these systems use to accomplish a thorough assessment. Therefore, the aim here is to give you a taste of these systems to stimulate a desire to learn more through dedicated textbooks or training. Many of the techniques presented here are isolated from the framework of a comprehensive session and thus have lost the integrity of the particular Asian bodywork form. Still, all of these techniques integrate nicely with Western techniques and can be added to your repertoire to increase the variety of ways you meet massage treatment goals.

Tuina

Tuina, also spelled *tui na*, is a bodywork form practiced as part of TCM for over 4,000 years and based on principles of Chinese medicine as outlined in the previous section. *Tui* means "push," and *na* means "grasp" in Chinese, conveying the vigorous and firm quality of this massage system where squeezing, compression, kneading, and joint movements are used to positively manipulate qi. Tuina is focused on releasing tension in muscles, ensuring smooth movement at joints, and promoting the balanced flow of qi through the channels.

Tuina is applied with the client fully dressed and without the use of a massage lubricant. Most practitioners request that clients wear loose, comfortable cotton clothing, because synthetic fibers in newer materials are believed to disrupt the flow of qi. The client sits upright in a chair or reclines on a massage table for the session. As with many Asian bodywork therapies, the focus of the session is on reinstating the balanced flow of qi through the twelve primary channels (meridians) by manipulating acupoints (in tuina the points are referred to as qi-points). In tuina, two additional channels, the ren and du channels, are also manipulated to balance qi. These are unpaired channels that encircle the head and trunk along the midline (Fig. 17-6). Tuina practitioners massage the pathways of particular channels to clear all blockages of qi. While qi-points usually feel a little tender, points that feel particularly tender are likely to indicate an underlying energetic problem and require increased focus. Sample methods from tuina are demonstrated in Technique 49.

Shiatsu

Shiatsu is a bodywork form from Japan based on principles of TCM as outlined earlier. The name *shiatsu* is composed of the Japanese words *shi* meaning "finger" and *atsu* meaning "pressure," translating literally to finger pressure. Finger pressure is the primary technique used in shiatsu, but the palms, hands, elbows, knees, and even the feet might also be used to deliver pressure to body areas. Stretches are used to loosen joints. Like other Asian bodywork therapies, shiatsu aims to promote the uninterrupted flow of ki (ki is Japanese for qi) through the channels (often called meridians) by manipulation of tsubos (Japanese for pressure points or acupoints) to improve health and wellness.

Working from the hara is a concept unique to shiatsu, referring to the use of the practitioner's own ki to stabilize the ki of the client. The term *hara* means abdominal region or belly. The practitioner's hara is the source of his or her ki and brings strength and purpose to the session. All of the therapist's movements and power originate from the hara and protect the therapist's body from overexertion. Hara also describes a person's ability to achieve goals and actualize ideas. Someone who works hard to accomplish a particular

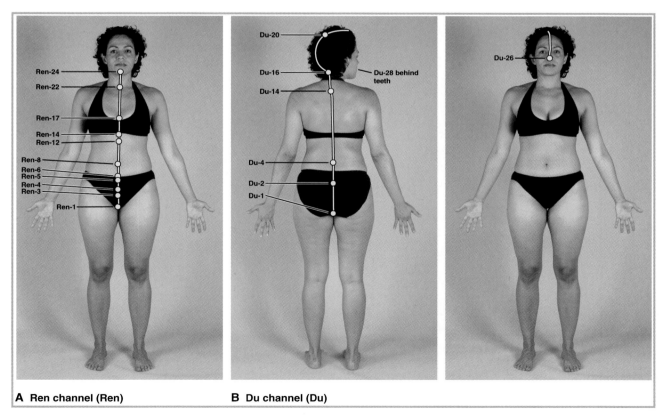

A Ren channel (Ren)   **B Du channel (Du)**

Figure 17-6 In tuina, two additional channels, the ren and du channels, are also manipulated to balance qi. These are unpaired channels that encircle the head and trunk along the midline.

Technique 49   **Sample Methods from Tuina**

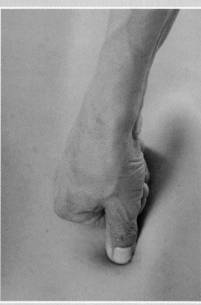

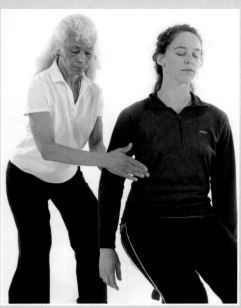

1. Work with One Thumb. This technique can be applied to any area of the body and along channels to improve the flow of qi. It is applied by making a loose fist that supports a flexed or extended thumb. Place the surface of the thumb (the lateral surface, tip, or medial surface of the thumb might all be used) on the body area, and alternately flex and extend the thumb so that the thumb surface "rocks" over the body area being treated. Repeat the application until the areas is completely treated and the tissue starts to soften.

2. Cuo Technique. The Cuo technique is also referred to as "foulage" and is most often applied to the extremities or upper torso region. The practitioner's hands are placed on either side of the area and rubbed back and forth rapidly so that the area twists with the movement. This technique is believed to regulate the flow of blood and qi, lubricate joints, and relax muscles.

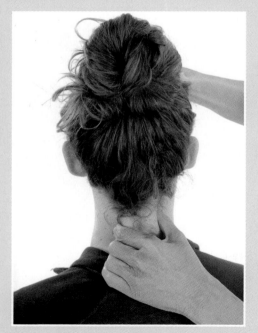

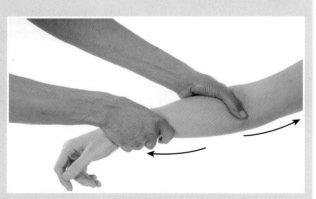

3. Grasping Technique. Use one or two hands to slowly lift tissue in a particular region. Lift the tissue until all the slack in the tissue is removed. Continue to lift the tissue as you slowly pull and twist it back and forth. Repeat this application to the same region until the tissue starts to soften. It is believed to improve consciousness, expel excess wind and cold, promote blood circulation, and relieve pain.

4. Bashen Technique (Pull-Extend). In this technique, the ends of a joint are pulled in opposite directions with even force at a slow pace for a prolonged period. On the extremity, pull the arm out from the shoulder, then grasp the hand and pull on the hand while pushing the forearm back toward the elbow. Finally, pull each finger while holding directly above the wrist and pushing the tissue above the wrist toward the elbow.

task is said to have good hara. People with good hara are not intimidated by setbacks and persist even when circumstances are difficult. Aligning energy in the hara helps to harmonize the body, mind, emotions, and spirit of the practitioner to deliver the best possible treatment for the client.

Shiatsu is applied to a fully dressed client without a massage lubricant. Clients are encouraged to wear loose-fitting cotton clothing to promote the flow of ki and so that the practitioner can more easily sense the flow of ki through the clothing. During the session, the client reclines on a mat placed on the floor, and the practitioner uses a kneeling or squatting stance to apply techniques (Fig. 17-7). Some sample methods from shiatsu are demonstrated in Technique 50.

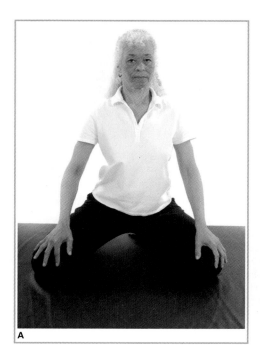

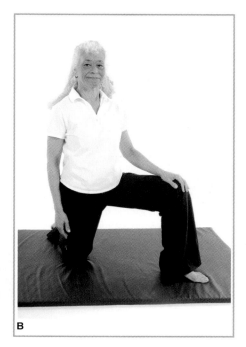

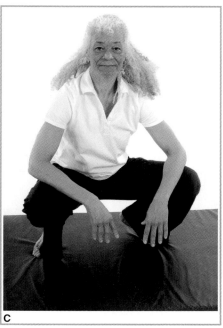

Figure 17-7 During a shiatsu session the client reclines on a mat placed on the floor, and the practitioner uses a kneeling or squatting stance to apply techniques. **A.** Wide kneeling. **B.** Half kneeling. **C.** Squatting.

Technique 50 | **Sample Methods from Shiatsu**

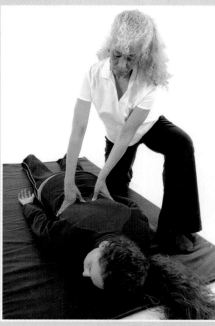

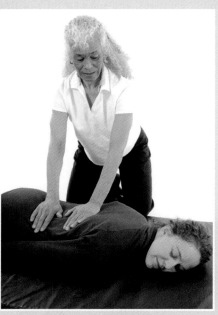

1. Thumbs Down Bladder Channel. Starting just below the base of the neck on either side of spine (about 1½ thumb widths lateral to the vertebral column), adjacent to the spinous processes, press your thumbs into the client's tissue. Retract the stroke and glide just a little way down to the point where you are adjacent to the next set of spinous processes, and repeat the stroke. Continue working down the sides of the spine to the sacrum. Make sure you adjust your position as you work so that your back is in a straight line, your hara is open and expanded, and your shoulders are positioned directly over the stroke so that you use your body weight and not strength to apply the technique.

2. Baby Walking. Kneel next to the client facing across the client's back. Place your hands on the client's back and allow your weight to drop through your palms. Now move your hands over the client's back as if you were a baby crawling on all fours. You can walk all over the back and posterior legs, but avoid placing direct downward pressure on areas of caution (described in Chapter 5).

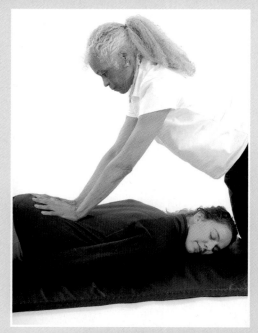

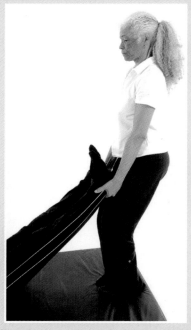

3. Retreating Cat. Position your body at the top of the mat, by the client's shoulder and facing toward the client's feet. Glide your hands down either side of the client's spine until your hands reach the client's gluteal muscles. Press down on the gluteal muscles to stretch the back. Now "walk" backward with your hands from the client's gluteal muscles to the shoulders. Repeat this process three or four times.

4. Heel Pulling. Position your body so that you are standing at the end of the mat by the client's feet. Lift the feet up to your waist by grasping the feet under the heels and lifting them slowly and steadily upward. Hold the feet in this position so that the client experiences a stretch in the low back.

Thai Massage

Thai massage is part of the broader practice of traditional Thai medicine, which has four branches: herbal medicine, nutritional medicine, spiritual practice, and massage (massage is called *nuad bo'rarn* in the Thai language). Thai medicine is heavily influenced by ayurveda (see Topic 17-2), the traditional medical system of India. Jivaka Kumar Bhaccha (also called Shivago Komparaj) was believed to be a contemporary of the historical Buddha and the primary physician in the community that gathered around the Buddha 2,500 years ago in India. He migrated to Thailand with other Buddhist monks, bringing ayurvedic influences with him. Thai massage is also influenced by TCM theories spread via ancient trade routes and with the migration of people between China and Thailand.

An important concept in Thai massage is that of "wind" derived from both the ayurvedic model of vata and the Chinese model of feng. Wind is viewed as a component of the universe and of the human body that regulates the body's activities. When wind is in balance, the body

- Digests and assimilates foods properly
- Eliminates wastes effectively
- Breathes deeply and effectively
- Thinks clearly and processes sensory information appropriately
- Has the desire to lead an active and fulfilling life
- Is vital and healthy for procreation
- Lives a long life

When wind is out of balance, disease is likely to take root or develop from mild symptoms into a serious condition.

Thai medicine adopted the idea that the body is a manifestation of universal energy and that energy (Thai uses the term "prana" from ayurveda) travels on pathways called sen, which are closely related to the meridian system of Chinese medicine. There are 10 primary sen pathways that connect the abdominal region, where wind (vata) is held in the lower abdominal cavity, to the rest of the body.

Thai massage is applied to a fully clothed client without massage lubricant. During the session, the client reclines on a mat while the practitioner applies techniques slowly with mindfulness. Sample methods from Thai massage are demonstrated in Technique 51.

Technique 51	**Sample Methods from Thai Massage**

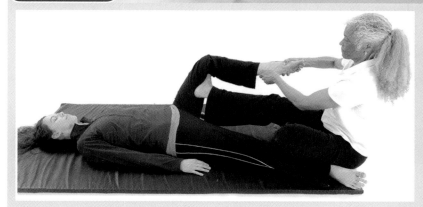

Posterior thigh press/stretch. Position your body on the mat with the client's foot in both hands and your foot (toes pointing laterally) against the client's thigh just below the popliteal fossa. Hold the client's leg at a 90-degree angle and press your foot into the client's thigh while pulling at the ankle and stretching the client's toes downward. Move your foot one position lower on the client's thigh (the foot moves toward the mat) and repeat the stretch, and then again move one position lower on the client's thigh to repeat the stretch.

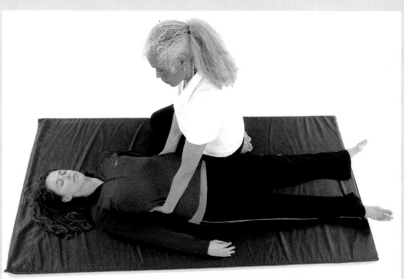

Torso lift. Position your body on one side of the client by the ASIS. Place your hands on both sides of the client just below the ribs and lift with both hands, bringing the client's low back off the floor. Hold this position for a breath, and then repeat the lift two or three times.

Continued

Technique 51	**Sample Methods from Thai Massage** (Continued)

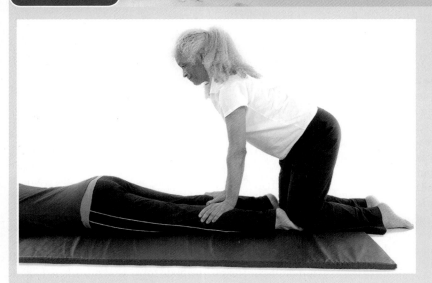

Walking palm press. With the client in the prone position on the mat, place your knees on the bottoms of the client's feet. Press your palms on the Achilles tendon and retract the stroke. Palm press all the way up the posterior of the leg to the gluteal muscles.

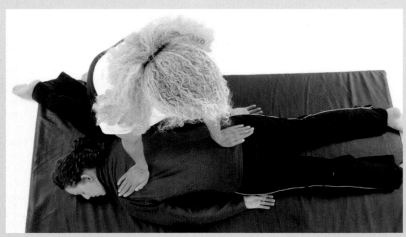

Diagonal back stretch. Place one hand on the client's scapula and the other on the PSIS on the opposite side of the back. Press down with both hands so that the back is elongated. Repeat the stretch on the other side of the client.

Topic **17-2**
Ayurvedic Bodywork

Ayurveda is both a traditional medical system and a philosophy that offers keys for creating harmony and balance in life. Ayurveda developed in Southern India and Sri Lanka, with early texts written before the 5th century bc. In Sanskrit, "ayur" means life and "veda" means knowledge.[11] Like TCM, traditional ayurveda includes many elements of practice that require years of careful and dedicated study. The ayurvedic physician is trained in eight branches of traditional therapies that are integrated into a holistic practice to treat the person's body, mind, and spirit. These branches include surgery, medicine, gynecology, pediatrics, toxicology, ear, nose, and throat, rejuvenation, and virilification therapy (treatments that improve fertility). In each of these branches, detoxification, diet, yoga, herbal medications, external treatments like massage, and meditation play a role in the healing or strengthening process. Ayurvedic bodywork methods are part of the broader practice of ayurvedic medicine but can be used by massage therapists as stand-alone treatments to relax, rejuvenate, and balance the body for better health and wellness. An overview of ayurvedic bodywork treatments is provided in Table 17-5. This section explores core concepts in ayurveda, abhyanga (Indian massage), and Indian head massage.

Core Concepts in Ayurveda

Like TCM, ayurvedic medicine is a complex system based on a holistic and traditional worldview. The concepts that underlay ayurvedic medicine influence how ayurvedic bodywork is applied to clients and includes an understanding of the five elements, the three doshas, prana, and a basic knowledge of marma points. There is not room here to describe some of the

subtler concepts used in advanced ayurvedic bodywork, such as an understanding of koshas (subtle energy bodies), dhatus (body tissues), srotas (channels), nadis (like meridians), and the chakra system. While the techniques and routines in this chapter are immediately applicable in sessions and can be integrated with skills you already possess, this chapter should be viewed as your first exploratory steps into a bodywork system you could spend many years to master.

The Five Elements

The foundation of traditional ayurveda is based on the belief that everything in the universe is composed of five elements (called panchamahabhutas). These elements or eternal substances (similar to the concept of the five elements in TCM)

TABLE 17-5 Traditional and Ayurveda-Inspired Body Treatments

Name	Brief Description	Main Indications
Shirodhara	A thin, thread-like drizzle of refined sesame oil is poured across the forehead to bring calmness of mind, body, and spirit.	Aggravated vata, insomnia, and anxiety
Udvartana	An invigorating massage delivered with the application of a herbal paste.	Increased circulation, cleanses, exfoliates, and tones the skin, stimulates weight loss, supports detoxification, good for kaphas
Garshan	One or two therapists briskly massage the client wearing raw silk gloves.	Increased circulation, toxin removal, weight loss, used to increase energy, good for kaphas
Swedana	This is an herbal steam bath usually given after a massage.	Detoxification, balancing for vata and kapha types
Vishesh	A firm massage using deep strokes and squeezing movements.	Detoxification, muscle soreness, particularly indicated for kapha types
Pizzichilli	Large amounts of warm oil are poured over the body while two or more therapists perform massage.	To decrease muscle pain and to bring flexibility to joints, indicated for vatas but contraindicated for pitta types
Pinda	The client is massaged by one or two therapists who hold muslin bags full of rice, milk, and herbs. This leaves the client very relaxed and the skin smooth.	Indicated for dry, rough skin; very relaxing and has a particular and unmistakable fragrance; cooling for pittas
Kati basti	A massage using heat and specific medicated oils to address lower back pain.	Lower back pain, rigidity of the lower spine
Abhyanga	A massage performed by one, two, or more therapists working in synchronicity. The strokes are varied depending on the dominant dosha of the client.	To bring balance to the doshas, to increase circulation, and aid detoxification
Bindi	Bindi means "point or origin." Spas combine different elements to make their own unique bindi treatment. These elements might include a hydrosoak, botanical mask, exfoliation, and herbal wrap.	To bring balance to the doshas, to increase circulation and detoxification, and to smooth the skin
Dosha wrap	Like the bindi treatment, spas mix and match elements for this wrap. It usually includes a custom blend of oils for the client's dosha, an exfoliation, massage, and wrap in warm towels or sheets.	To bring balance to the doshas, to increase circulation and detoxification, and to smooth the skin

TABLE 17-6 **The Five Elements (Panchamahabhutas)**

The Five Elements (Panchamahabhutas)					
Element	**Body Part**	**Senses**	**Quality**	**Taste**	**Action**
Space (also called ether)	Relates to spaces in the body, e.g., mouth, nostrils, abdomen, respiratory tract, cells	The ears—sound	Smooth, soft, subtle, porous, nonslimy	No taste	Creates softness, lightness, and porosity
Air	Relates to movement, e.g., muscle, pulse, respiration, peristalsis, movement in cells	The skin—touch	Rough, light, dry, cold, soluble	Astringent and slightly bitter	Creates lightness, dryness, and emaciation
Fire	Relates to metabolism, digestive processes, and intelligence	The eyes—Sight	Rough, bright, heating	Pungent	Creates an increase in temperature, burning sensations, improved eyesight, improved digestion
Water	Relates to plasma, blood, saliva, digestive liquids, mucous membranes, and cytoplasm	The Tongue—Taste	Cold, fluid, moist, heavy, slimy, emollient, purgative	Sweet with astringent, sour, saline	Creates moisture, glossiness, increases fluid content
Earth	Relates to bones, teeth, nails, muscles, tendons, skin, hair, cartilage	The nose—smell	Heavy, dull, thick, firm, immobile, compact, strong, rough, emollient, purgative	Sweet	Creates firmness, strength, hardness

help explain the nature of the universe. They are space (sometimes referred to as ether), air, fire, water, and earth. Each of these elements has specific qualities that intermix in the body and, when combined with the soul, form a unique individual. The five elements relate to different parts of the body, to the senses that help us interpret the world, and to particular actions that produce change (Table 17-6).[12] Specific combinations of the five elements make up the three doshas (tridoshas).

The Three Doshas (Tridoshas)

The **doshas**, known individually as vata, pitta, and kapha, are viewed as vital body energies and as the energies that underlie all things in the world. In nature, the doshas govern the qualities of different times of the day or night and different seasons or climates (Fig. 17-8). In the body, each dosha governs specific physiological functions.

Vata is the strongest of the three doshas and combines the elements of space and air. The word *vata* means "to move" or "to enthuse." Vata is the dosha most likely to become unbalanced because of this tendency toward movement. It governs both the physical and mental movements of the body including thought processes, the circulation of blood, the conduction of impulses in the nervous system, the elimination of wastes, and muscular movements like walking, lifting, and speaking. The vata season is autumn and early winter and any day that is cold, dry, and windy. Each dosha has its own qualities. Vata qualities are described as dry, light, cold, subtle, unstable, rough, clear, and transparent.

In Sanskrit, **pitta** means "to heat" or "to burn." It is considered the dosha of transformation and is composed of the elements of fire and water. Its functions include digestion, heat production, appetite, intellectual tasks, vision, the softness and suppleness of the body, and the imparting of color to the body. The pitta season is middle and late summer, or any day that is hot or humid. Pitta qualities are described as hot, sharp, bright, liquid, slightly oily, sour, and pungent.

Kapha is the most stable of the doshas, and this stability functions as both physiological and psychological strength in the human body through anabolic or building processes, mucus membranes, phlegm, fat, and the lymphatic system. The kapha season is late winter and spring, or any day that is cold, wet, dull, and still. Kapha is the dosha that is the least likely to go out of balance. Kapha qualities are described as heavy, cold, soft, viscous, sweet, stable, and slimy.

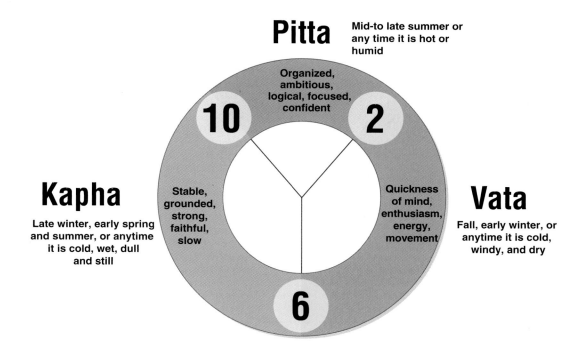

Pitta Mid-to late summer or any time it is hot or humid

Organized, ambitious, logical, focused, confident

10

2

Kapha

Late winter, early spring and summer, or anytime it is cold, wet, dull and still

Stable, grounded, strong, faithful, slow

Quickness of mind, enthusiasm, energy, movement

Vata

Fall, early winter, or anytime it is cold, windy, and dry

6

Attention and attunement to the natural world and its rhythms is one way to keep the doshas in balance. In Ayurveda, time, the seasons and the phases of life are governed by the doshas. Through mindfulness to the dosha clock and dosha season, greater harmony, balance, and health are achieved.[1]

Wake up: It is best to wake up during vata time (by 6:00 AM) to start the day with vata qualities (quick and energetic). Sleeping into kapha time (past 6:00 AM) gives the day kapha qualities (slow and heavy).

Exercise: Exercise is best during the early phases of kapha time (6 to 10 AM and 6 to 10 PM) because the body will be at its strongest and have the most stamina. Exercise during the middle of the day tends to aggravate pitta and can lead to feelings of irritability.

Work: Focus, organization, planning, and clear communication are at their best during pitta time from 10:00 AM to 2:00 PM. In the evening pitta cycle from 10:00 PM to 2:00 AM, pitta qualities enhance the dream state.

Main meal: Pitta governs metabolism and the absorption of nutrients from food. For this reason, it is important to eat the main meal during the middle of the day during pitta time, around 12:00 noon. Digestive processes slow during kapha time, so avoid eating anything heavy after 6:00 PM.

Sleep: To fall asleep quickly and to have a sound sleep throughout the night, ayurveda recommends bed before 10:00 PM (before kapha time ends).This allows a complete night's rest before the next kapha cycle begins.

Figure 17-8 A dosha mindful day. In nature, the doshas govern the qualities of different times of the day or night, and different seasons or climates.

Dosha Profiles

The way that the doshas combine in a person governs body type, mental and emotional characteristics, personality, and the types of diseases most likely to develop. While every person has elements of all three doshas, one is usually dominant. This unique dosha combination is referred to as a person's doshic prakriti (constitution).[13]

In the simplest terms, a person is healthy when the three doshas are in a state of balance. An unbalanced dosha state (vikrti) allows disease to take root. When people practice ayurveda, they are mindful of the activities and life choices that aggravate and pacify their particular prakriti. This allows a person to make choices that promote balance and harmony, and thereby decrease stress and disease.

While a person may have a dominant dosha, this does not mean that the doshas are static. Like yin and yang and the five elements in TCM, the doshas are in a constant state of transition. A certain situation may aggravate one dosha but pacify another dosha. For example, a person might have physical, mental, and emotional traits that indicate that he or she is decidedly a kapha (prakriti) but the current condition and symptoms demonstrate that he or she has a pitta imbalance (vikrti). Dominate dosha profiles are described in Boxes 17-2 to 17-4.

BOX 17-2   Vata Profile

Body	Mind/Emotions	Factors that Pacify	Factors that Aggravate	Diseases Associated with Aggravated Vata
Thin or angular	Restless, sensitive, and flexible mind	Quiet time	Rainy, cold, or windy weather	Arthritis
Short or tall	Short-term memory precise, but long-term memory weak	Chanting or calming music	The seasons of fall and early winter	Rheumatoid arthritis
Skin and hair tend to be dry and rough		Massage with warm sesame oil	Vata-decreasing foods (foods that are cold, dry, light, bitter, and astringent including raw vegetables, dried fruits, red meat, stimulants such as coffee or soda, dried beans)	Musculoskeletal disorders
Teeth large	When balanced: Creative, enthusiastic, artistic, open-minded	Warm, natural colors		Paralysis
Mouth small and thin		Sweet, gentle, and calming scents		Cardiovascular disorders
Eyes dull and dark		Vata-decreasing foods (food that is rich, oily, and moderately spicy including dairy products, grains, natural sweeteners like honey, cooked vegetables, sweet, sour, and heavy fruits, chicken, seafood, and turkey, herbs and spices)		Digestive disorders
Highly active	When unbalanced: Emotionally insecure, anxious, fearful, unstable		Physical overexertion	Constipation
Difficulty gaining weight			Irregular eating and snacking between meals	Diarrhea
Sleep little or sleep easily disrupted		Regular sleep	Lack of sleep	Foot diseases and disorders
		Structured routine	Mental overstimulation	Mental instability
		Grounded and creative exercise like gardening and dance	Emotional upset	

BOX 17-3   Pitta Profile

Body	Mind/Emotions	Factors That Pacify	Factors That Aggravate	Diseases Associated with Aggravated Pitta
Medium build	Aggressive	Soft music	Hot or humid weather	Burning sensations in the body
Gain or lose weight easily	Sharp mind and clear memory	The sound of water	Mid to late summer	Impaired vision
Hair may gray or fall out prematurely	Articulate in communication	Cool colors with blue, green, or cream hues	Hot rooms or being overdressed in a warm environments	Skin disorders and itching skin
Hot, sweaty body	Ambitious, organized, focused	Pitta-decreasing foods (basmati rice, oats, wheat, unprocessed sugars like maple syrup, vegetables that are not spicy, grapes, raisins, apples, nuts in moderation, chicken, turkey)	Irregular meals	Ulcers
Experience intense hunger pains	Emotionally intense and prone to irritability or jealous behavior		Increased water intake	Pitta-increasing foods (foods that are salty, sour, light, pungent, or too oily, and acidic foods including cheese, yogurt, hot peppers, tomatoes, garlic, onion, citrus fruits, tofu, peanuts, fish, red meat)
Light blue or gray eyes that tend to redden when strained			Excessive mental activity	
Fair skin with prominent freckles, birthmarks, or moles	Perfectionist, decisive, impatient		Long periods indoors	
Pointed nose and chin	When balanced: Confident, bold, brilliant	Increased water intake	Alcohol consumption	Jaundice
Sleep soundly		Walks by water or in cool forests	Uncommitted relationships	Excessive perspiration and foul body odor
Like strong foods that are sweet, bitter, or intensely flavored	When unbalanced: Irritable, aggressive, impatient, critical	Stable relationships		

BOX 17-4 Kapha Profile

Body	Mind/Emotions	Factors That Pacify	Factors That Aggravate	Diseases Associated with Aggravated Kapha
Tall and solidly built or short and stocky with a large frame	Mind absorbs information slowly	Regular exercise	Wet, cold, dull, or still weather	Weight gain or obesity
Tendency to gain weight	Strong long-term memory	Regular mental stimulation	The seasons of late winter and early spring	Skin irritations
Hair is thick, soft, dark, and oily	Speak slowly and consider their position on a topic carefully	Change of routine	Kapha-increasing foods (foods that are heavy,	Anorexia
Round faces with large expressive eyes	Loyal, patient, compassionate with a loving and emotionally secure nature	Kapha-decreasing foods (foods that are light, dry, warm, spicy, bitter, and astringent including most grains, vegetables, light fruits like apples, pears, and berries, beans, and spices)	oily, cold, sweet, salty, or sour including dairy products, sweets, sweet fruits like avocados, bananas, coconut, and citrus fruits, nuts, red meat, dark meat, oily fish, salt, cold carbonated drinks)	Disorders caused by excess mucus
Full mouth with small, white teeth				Goiter
Pale skin that is often oily	Stable and grounded with steady personality			Indigestion
Steady appetite and slow metabolism	Difficulty managing change or making changes			Allergy and asthma (in traditional ayurveda these two disorders as well as chronic eczema are believed to be inherited from life in the womb)
Like bitter, pungent, and sharp tastes	When balanced: Content, supportive of others, loving, and affectionate	Bright colors	Lack of exercise	
Sleep soundly and for long periods	When unbalanced: Sleep too much, overindulge in food, lazy, and may exhibit greedy, possessive behaviors	Upbeat music Relationships that encourage appropriate autonomy	Overeating Too much sleep and taking naps Overdependence on loved ones Not allowing change	Diabetes (starts as kapha and exacerbates pitta and vata in later stages) Sinus problems

Prana

Prana is spiritual, physical, and mental energy. This vital energy is the fundamental life force of the body and the source of all knowledge. From the Sanskrit for "breath," prana flows through a network of subtle energy channels that can be likened to the Chinese concept of meridians, called nadis. The breath is the main medium that Prana uses to enter the body. It enters the body on the inhalation and leaves the body on the exhalation of breath. When the body is healthy, prana flows continuously, creating vigor, life, spirit, passion, and self-determination. Too little prana in the body is often experienced as a feeling of being stuck, a lack of motivation, or fatigue. This type of depressed state can lead to illness. Stress can affect the amount of prana and the way it flows through the body, leading to a condition where disease can take root.

Ayurvedic therapies are a form of communication with Prana. For example, the attitude of the therapist is as important as the way that strokes are applied. Sincerity, a sense of wonder, honor for the client and for the self, and respect for the beauty of ayurveda are believed to lead to positive outcomes in the session. As the therapist applies pressure or begins a stroke, he or she exhales through the mouth (not the nose, as is done in meditation) and becomes the prana quality he or she wants to give the client. A client who has aggravated pitta may need "cooling." An image of a quiet pool of water might be generated in the therapist's mind. The therapist imagines the water as self while exhaling and beginning a stroke. The image of the water will affect the quality of the stroke and this, in turn, affects the therapist's communication with Prana. It sounds mysterious, but the important point is that the therapist has clear positive intent for each stroke or technique.

Marma Points

Marma points are energy centers in the body that are traditionally used with Indian massage and ayurvedic healing.[14] The name *marma* means secret, hidden, and vital, providing clues to the nature of these points. Marma points connect the physical body with subtle energy bodies and often relate to specific organs or body areas. Marma point therapy is believed to enliven pure consciousness in the body, harmonize the flow of prana, and stimulate a spontaneous healing response. They are massaged in order to restore the body to normal function, balance the body's energies, and either energize or relax the body as necessary for improved health.

Marma points are located on the body by taking finger measurements from identifiable starting points. An individual's marma points are specific to his or her body. For this reason, the client's fingers are traditionally used to do the measuring.[15] The general locations of marma points are shown in Figure 17-9, while techniques for working with marma points are described in Technique 52.

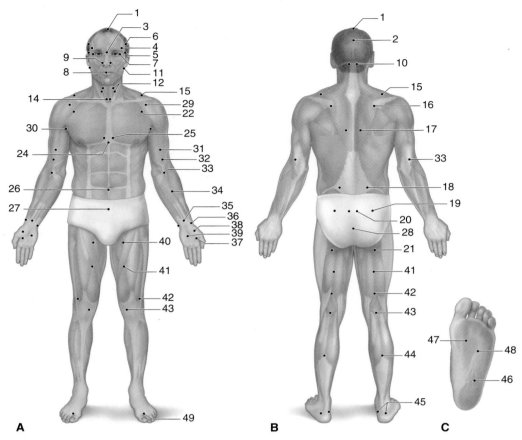

Figure 17-9 Marma points are located on the body by taking finger measurements from identifiable starting points. An individual's marma points are specific to his or her body.

Technique 52 — **Stimulation of a Marma Point**

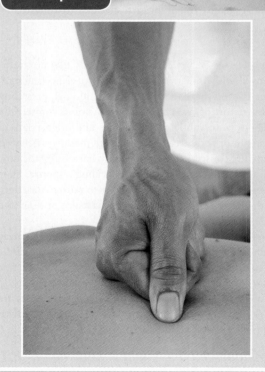

Marma points are primarily massaged with the thumb (sometimes with the fingertips, knuckles, fist, palm of the hand, or heel of the foot) after a drop of warm oil or a specific taila has been applied to the point. Most often, the point is massaged in clockwise circles to strengthen and tone the tissue, but sometimes counterclockwise motions are used. Direct pressure for 1 to 3 minutes can be used to stimulate a point. Often the therapist begins at the center of the point and makes ever-larger circles until the entire point has been massaged for 3 to 5 minutes. The pressure should be firm but not hard. If the client experiences any discomfort, the pressure on the point is too deep.

Concept Brief 17-4
Core Concepts in Ayurveda

The five elements: The foundation of traditional ayurveda is based on the belief that everything in the universe is composed of five elements (called panchamahabhutas). These elements are space, air, fire, water, and earth.

The three doshas: The doshas, known individually as vata, pitta, and kapha, are viewed as vital body energies and as the energies that underlie all things in the world.

Prana: Prana is spiritual, physical, and mental energy. This vital energy is the fundamental life force of the body and the source of all knowledge.

Marma points: Marma points are energy centers in the body that are traditionally used with Indian massage and ayurvedic healing.

Abhyanga (Indian Massage)

In India, massage is part of daily life, and it is common to see mothers, with a blanket spread across the ground, massaging their children in the open marketplace or to see women chatting and massaging each other's shoulders. Self-oiling and self-massage are also common practices. **Abhyanga** is the Sanskrit word for oil massage, which might be delivered by one, two, or more therapists working together in a coordinated manner on a client. The strokes and massage oils vary depending on the dosha of the client and the dosha characteristics of the day or season.

India is a large country, and the techniques used in massage vary in different regions. There are, however, five general strokes used in traditional massage. These strokes are sweeps, tapping, kneading, rubbing, and squeezing.[15] These Indian massage methods are described in Technique 53. They should be delivered at particular speeds and depths in order to bring the client's dosha into balance.

The Vata Massage

Vata qualities are described as dry, light, cold, subtle, unstable, rough, clear, and transparent. The massage for a vata or client with a vata imbalance should be oily (balances dry), firm (balances light), warm (balances cold), smooth (balances rough), and precise (balances subtle). Strokes are long and flowing with firm pressure and an even rhythm. Irregular movements, abrupt transitions, fussy and inefficient draping, tapotement, and pressure that is either too deep or too light aggravate vata. The appropriate massage oils for vata include

sesame, olive, almond, and ghee (clarified butter). Extra oil might even be applied to the body and allowed to soak in after the massage of a particular body area has concluded. Warm packs, like flaxseed packs heated in a microwave, might be used to provide extra warmth during the massage. Applying warm oil to the abdominal area and covering it with a heated towel and then a warm pack is particularly comforting for vatas. Grounding elements like the placement of warm stones on the feet or on areas of muscular tension (heavy balances light, warm balances cold) pacify vata.

The Pitta Massage

Pitta qualities are described as hot, sharp, bright, liquid, slightly oily, sour, and pungent. The pitta massage must be moderate in temperature or cooling (balances hot), smooth (balances sharp), dark (balances bright), precise (balances liquid), and varied. A pitta client may become critical and aggravated if he or she feels the therapist is not grounded and focused on the massage. The massage rhythm must be slow and calming because too many fast movements are irksome. Light or cooling oils are used in moderation. The appropriate massage oils for pitta include coconut, sunflower, safflower, and ghee (clarified butter). Warm packs and heavy blankets are only used if the day or treatment room is particularly cold.

The Kapha Massage

Kapha qualities are described as heavy, cold, soft, viscous, sweet, stable, and slimy. The massage for a kapha is the most stimulating and the least oily of the dosha massages. This massage must be vigorous (like a sports massage), fast paced, warming, firm, and nonoily. In a traditional ayurveda setting, massage for kaphas might be done with powders, alcohol, or silk gloves (a massage with silk gloves is called gershan) to avoid adding more oil to the kapha constitution. Lightweight oils or warming oils are used when a dry massage is not desired. Appropriate massage oil for kaphas includes safflower, apricot kernel, sunflower, sesame, and mustard oil used in moderation. Like vatas, kaphas need warmth and can be heated with hot water bottles and warm packs.

Taila

Abhyanga often uses medicated herbal oils called tail or **taila** (*tila* means sesame oil). To make taila, a base oil such as sesame or coconut oil is cooked with herbs to infuse the oil with the properties of the plant. The herbs used in taila tend to be tonic or nervine, and the oil is often (but not always) named after the main herb in its recipe. Sometimes a full-body massage is performed with taila, and sometimes specific marma points are massaged with a particular taila to treat a symptom or condition. In one example, the respiratory system might be supported by massaging the

Text continued on page 525

Technique 53   Traditional Indian Massage Strokes

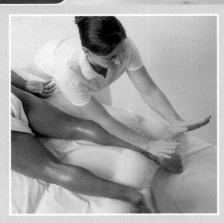

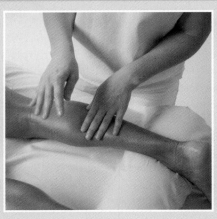

1. Sweeps. Sweeps (similar to effleurage) are applied from the navel out toward the distal areas of the body in brisk, straight strokes. On the legs, the sweep starts at the greater trochanter and ends at the feet. On the upper body, the sweep starts at the navel, sweeps up to the shoulder ("jump" the breast drape on female clients), and then sweeps down to the hands. Sweeps are used to "open" and "close" a body area and are repeated up to 25 times on one area. Sweeps warm the tissue, revitalize the limbs, and feel invigorating.

2. Tapping. Tapping (similar to light tapotement) is used to awaken the body, alert the nerve endings, and increase circulation. It is done with open palms and relaxed fingers.

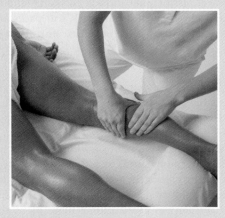

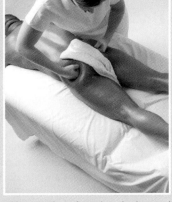

3. Kneading. Kneading (similar to petrissage) is performed at a depth that is tolerable to the client. The area is kneaded thoroughly and completely before the therapist moves on to another technique or body area.

4. Rubbing. Rubbing (similar to friction) can be done on dry skin (except for vatas) or performed with oil. It can be deep (applied with the knuckles or thumbs) or light and superficial (applied with the fingertips). It can be performed quickly or slowly. Although some specific techniques rub in a counterclockwise direction, most often the rubbing is in clockwise circles. Often marma points are stimulated during the rubbing application (see Technique 52 on the stimulation of marma points).

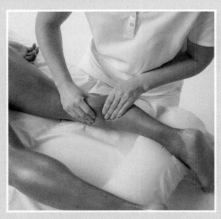

5. Squeezing. Using both hands, the therapist lifts an area of muscle with a squeezing and crossing torque-like motion. In bony areas such as the fingers and toes, a combination of squeezing and twisting is used to mobilize the area. To finish the fingers and toes, a drop of oil is placed on the finger so that it fills the gap between the nail and the flesh.

two amsaphalaka marma points (one on each of the upper medial boarders of the scapula #16) with strong clockwise circles using mahanarayan taila (mahanarayan taila is a combination of 14 herbs and sesame oil that is used for muscle or joint pain and to support the respiratory system). A variety of taila and taila for the different doshas can be purchased from specialist ayurveda stores, which are easy to find online using the search phrase "ayurveda massage supplies."

Essential Oils for Dosha Blends

Essential oils can also be used to make dosha-pacifying blends or to anoint a specific marma point. Heating oils are indicated for pacifying vata and kapha. These are commonly spicy oils such as ginger (*Zingiber officinale*), nutmeg (*Myristica fragrans*), pepper (*Piper nigrum*), thyme (*Thymus vulgaris*—linalol type), and cinnamon (*Cinnamomum verum*). Sweet oils, such as the floral oils of rose (*Rosa x damascena*), ylang ylang (*Cananga odorata*), jasmine (*Jasminum officinale* form *grandiflorum*), and neroli (*Citrus x aurantium* "amara"), or cooling oils, such as German chamomile (*Matricaria recutita*), and yarrow (*Achillea millefolium*), pacify pitta but aggravate kapha. Root oils, which are energetically grounding, are good for vatas. These oils include ginger (*Zingiber officinale*) and angelica (*Angelica archangelica*). Many oils are neutral and balancing for all of the doshas. This group includes lavender (*Lavandula angustifolia*), clary sage (*Salvia sclarea*), and frankincense (*Boswellia carteri*). Some of the oils indicated by ayurvedic therapists are quite strong (e.g., cinnamon and basil) and should only be used in a diluted form (6 to 12 drops to 1 fl oz of carrier oil is recommended).

If the season or conditions of the day are decidedly of one dosha, any individual, regardless of his or her dominant dosha or dosha imbalance, might be given a massage with an oil blend that pacifies the qualities of the day. For example, if the day is cold, dry, and windy, a vata-pacifying blend and warm packs might be used on all clients. This is because even a person with dominate pitta will be cold on such a day and need vata qualities pacified to feel in balance.

An Abhyanga Routine

As mentioned previously, one, two, or more therapists can perform abhyanga. In the ayurveda-inspired routine described in Technique 54, two therapists work together in synchrony with a specific series of strokes. One therapist could just as easily deliver this routine simply by applying each of the strokes to each body area.

You and the other therapist who deliver this routine must decide who will be the leader and who will be the follower. The leader sets the pace of the massage strokes and never leaves the client's body; the leader always maintains contact with the client in some way. The follower gets everything that is needed for the treatment (e.g., extra oil, hot herbal towels, and an eye pillow) and follows the leader's pace.

Indian Head Massage

Indian head massage is an art form that is deeply relaxing and rejuvenating. In a typical session, the head, neck, and shoulders are massaged; marma points are stimulated; and the scalp and hair are oiled and invigorated.

The thin, sheet-like muscles of the scalp move the scalp, ears, and eyebrows. The thin, small muscles of the face create the movements that lead to facial expression. Everyday these muscles get a workout, and tension in facial and scalp muscles can play a significant role in tension headache pain or pathologies such as temporomandibular joint syndrome. Indian head massage is indicated for neck tension, tension headache, face tension, relaxation, stress reduction, and revitalization. The ultimate goal is to soothe and comfort the mind and to bring the body into harmony through the senses. Techniques for Indian head massage are demonstrated in Technique 55.

Technique 54 **Synchronized Abhyanga Routine**

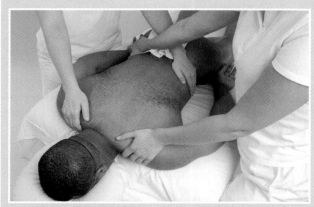

1. Ground and Center. Begin the session with a footbath and Indian head massage as described in Technique 55. Match the speed and depth of your strokes and use warm packs, special taila, essential oils, or other features to the dosha of the individual client. This description assumes that you are acting as the leader during the session. Bolster the client in the prone position and adjust the drape (use a gluteal drape) to allow access to the back and the posterior legs at the same time. Move to one side of the table while the follower moves to the other side. Match your breathing to the client's breathing and cross your hands and place one hand on a hip and one hand on a shoulder. The follower joins in.

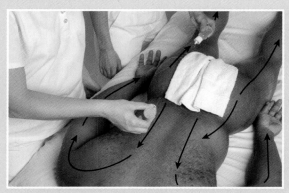

2. Application of Oil to the Posterior Body. Apply oil from the lower back, up the back, down the arm to the hand, back up the arm, and down the back to the hip on one side. At the same time, the follower applies oil from the hip, down the leg to the foot, and back up the leg to the hip on the same side. Repeat this process on the other side.

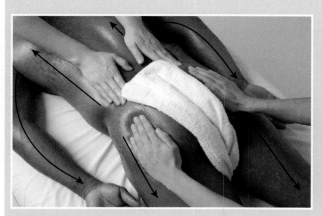

3. Spreading the Oil in Tandem. Work the oil across the upper body while the follower works oil across the legs until it is even. You spread the oil from the lower back, up the back, and down to the hands. At the same time, and with the same rhythm, the follower spreads the oil from the hips to the feet. Your hands should be on the lower back (at the beginning of the stroke) at the same time that the follower's hands are at the hips (the beginning of the stroke).

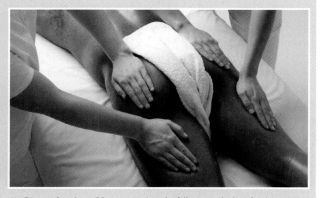

4. Posterior Leg Massage. Join the follower at the hips for the posterior leg massage. Watch each other carefully so that massage strokes are occurring in the same area at the same time. Each stroke begins at the greater trochanter and moves toward the feet. (The energy is "pushed" out from the core of the body, the navel, toward the extremities, in this case the feet). Begin the sequence with 20 to 25 straight sweeps, and hold the foot at the end of the last stroke. Progress from straight sweeps to the tapping technique, followed by kneading, rubbing, and finally squeezing. Marma points can be incorporated into the routine at the discretion of the leader or treatment designer. End the posterior leg sequence in the same way it began, with 20 to 25 straight sweeps, and hold at the foot on the last stroke.

Technique 54 **Synchronized Abhyanga Routine** (Continued)

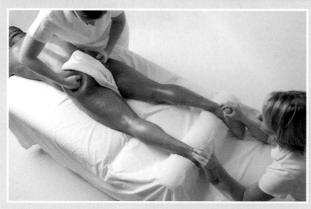

5. Gluteal Massage. After completing the massage of the posterior legs, the follower holds both feet to ground the client's energy while you massage the gluteals. Eventually, the follower joins in on one side of the gluteal massage to make a smooth transition into the back.

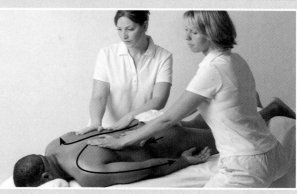

6. Back Massage. Stand on either side of the table at the hips facing toward the head of the client. Apply the five traditional strokes simultaneously starting at the lower back, running up the back to the shoulder and down the arm to the hand. Begin with 20 to 25 straight sweeps, and hold at the hand on the last stroke. Progress from the straight sweeps to the tapping technique, followed by kneading, rubbing, and finally squeezing. Marma points can be incorporated into the routine at the discretion of the leader or treatment designer. End with another 20 straight sweeps, and hold at the hand on the last stroke to end the back sequence.

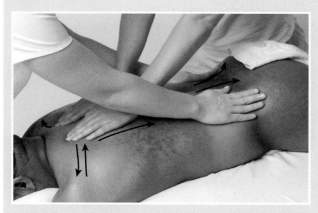

7. Creative Back Massage Strokes. As part of the back routine, you can develop a number of creative tandem strokes. One method is for each therapist to do a deep tissue stroke starting at the top of the spine and running down to the sacrum on either side of the spine. Another enjoyable stroke is to do effleurage strokes in a rhythmic and crossing sequence as shown in this image.

9. Spreading the Oil in Tandem. You spread the oil in an even layer on the upper chest, neck, and down the arms. At the same time, the follower spreads the oil in an even layer on the lower legs

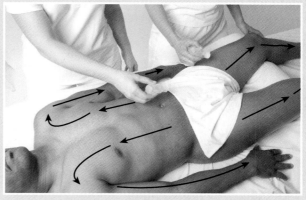

8. Application of Oil to the Anterior Body. Turn the client into the supine position, bolster him or her for comfort, and use a breast drape for females and an anterior pelvic drape. The follower moves to the client's feet. You turn the client's head to one side and apply oil down the neck and across the shoulder. At the same time, the follower applies oil to the foot (same side) and up the leg. Repeat this procedure on the opposite side.

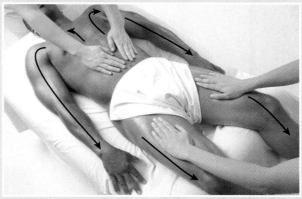

Continued

Technique 54 **Synchronized Abhyanga Routine** (Continued)

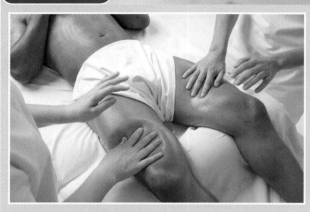

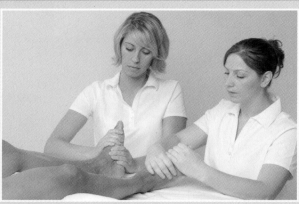

10. Anterior Leg Massage. You move to stand at one hip facing toward the feet, and the follower stands at the other hip facing the feet. Again the energy is pushed out from the navel toward the feet with the five strokes performed simultaneously (sweeps, tapping, kneading, rubbing, and squeezing). End with 20 to 25 straight sweeps and a hold at the feet.

11. Foot Massage. You take one foot and the follower takes the other foot and together you massage them with the same series of strokes (see Topic 16-5 for ideas). Another option is to move to the top of the table and place your hands on the client's shoulders while the follower massages the client's feet. At the end of the foot massage, the follower grasps both feet and holds them with thumbs on the Talahridaya (heart or center of the foot) marma (#48). Interestingly this is called the solar plexus point in reflexology. It is believed to pacify vata and ground and center the body.

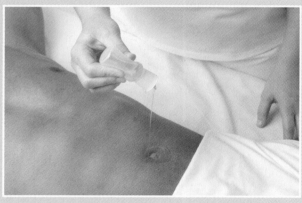

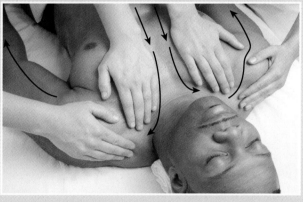

12. Abdominal Massage. Move to the abdominal area and fill the navel with oil. Work the oil around the abdominal area while the follower continues to press the feet and stabilize the client's energy.

13. Upper Body Massage. The follower moves with you to the upper body when the abdominal massage is complete. Stand on either side of the client and apply oil from the chest and down each arm simultaneously. Spread the oil in an even layer working from the abdominal area, up to the upper chest, and down the arms to the hands with straight sweeping strokes (20 to 25 times). If the client is female, "jump" the breast drape when it gets in the way of your stroke.

14. Massage the Arms. Each of the traditional strokes (sweeps, tapping, kneading, rubbing, and squeezing) is carried out on each arm simultaneously starting at the glenohumeral joint and working down to the hand. End with straight sweeps (20 to 25 times) and hold at the hand on the last stroke.

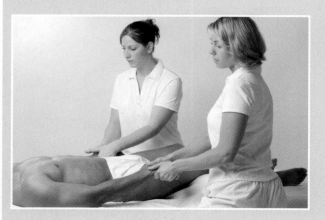

Technique 54   **Synchronized Abhyanga Routine** (Continued)

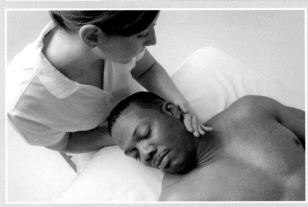

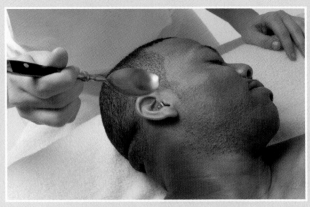

15. Neck and Face Massage. Move to the head of the table and massage the client's neck and face, while the follower moves to the bottom of the table to ground the client's energy through the Talahridaya marma on the bottoms of the feet.

16. Karna Purana. A nice way to end the treatment is to pour oil from a spoon into the ears. Oiling the ears is called karna purana. It is practiced to relive itching or dryness in the ears, to settle the vata dosha through the sense of hearing, and to relax the mind and body. A towel is placed under the client's head, and the head is then rotated to one side so that the ear can be filled with a spoonful of warm sesame oil. The area around the ear is gently massaged and the client is encouraged to open and close his or her mouth two or three times. In most states, it is out of the scope of practice for massage therapists to massage inside the ears of a client, so only the outer area of the ear is massaged. The head is rotated to the other side and the procedure is repeated on the other ear. The oil in the first ear will run out onto the towel under the client's head. Repeat the process on the other ear. The client can then dry the ears with a tissue.

Technique 55   **Indian Head Massage**

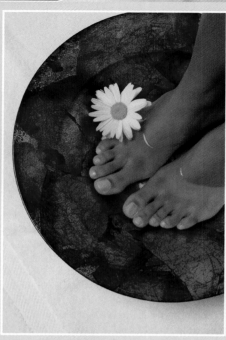

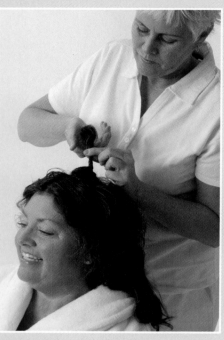

1. Foot Soak. A foot soak signifies the spiritual element of welcoming and purifying the client. Herbs or essential oils can be used to enhance the foot soak. The client relaxes in the foot soak while you massage the head, neck, and shoulders. The follower periodically fills the foot soak container with more warm water and washes, exfoliates, and massages the client's feet while they soak.

2. Oiling the Simanta and Krikatika Marmas. The simanta (summit) marma falls along the lines of the sutures of the skull and thus covers a large area. The first point to oil in this area is found by measuring eight finger widths up the head using the point between the brows as a starting point. A generous amount of sesame oil is poured on this spot, and then the hairs are lifted and twisted to stimulate the point. The second point to oil is found at the point where the client's hair forms a whorl. After the point is oiled, the hairs over this point are lifted and twisted to stimulate the marma. Between these two points is Adhipati (Overlord #1), which is located at the top point of the skull. This marma has a ruling action over the simanta marma and controls the seventh chakra, pineal gland, and nervous system. Oil and stimulate this point with hair twisting. To oil the krikatika (joint of the neck #10) marmas, the client is asked to bring the head forward so that the chin sits on their chest. The points are directly beneath the occipital protuberance on each side of the neck. Oil and stimulate these points with hair twisting.

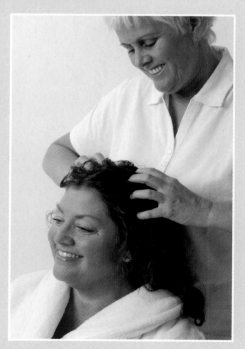

3. Zigzag Fingers. Using zigzag finger movements, work the oil evenly through the hair and into the scalp. Go back to each of the points that were oiled, and use gentle circular finger friction in clockwise circles to release the energy and tension in these areas.

Technique 55 | **Indian Head Massage** (Continued)

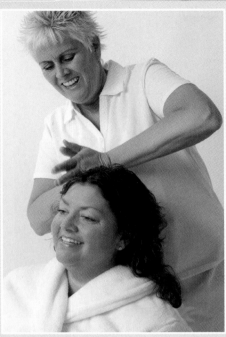

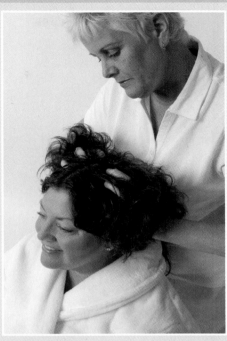

4. Pounding. Place both hands together in a prayer position. While keeping the wrists loose and flexible, use the edge of the joined hands in a tapotement-like action over the entire head.

5. Circular Finger Friction—Scalp. Reaching up under the client's hair, massage the entire scalp with gentle circular finger friction.

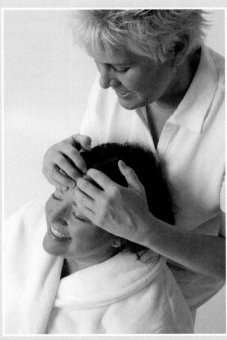

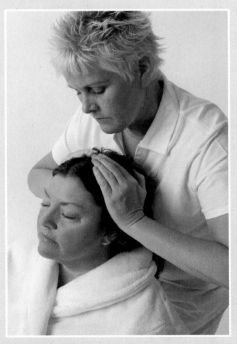

6. Circular Finger Friction—Face. The forehead, above and behind the ears, and the base of the skull are also massaged with circular finger friction. The point between the brows, down the sides of the nose, under the eyes, under the cheekbones, and then down around the edges of the mouth and across the lower part of the cheek are massaged with circular fingers.

7. Skull Squeeze Position 1. Interlace the fingers over the top of the skull and press the hands together gently. Repeat this four to six times working over the anterior and posterior sections of the skull.

Continued

Technique 55   **Indian Head Massage** (Continued)

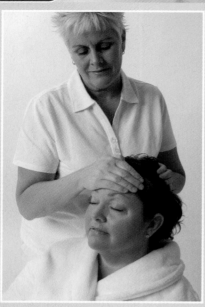

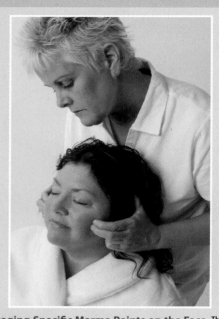

8. Skull Squeeze Position 2. Place one hand on the forehead and the other at the back of the head, and repeat the skull squeeze.

9. Massaging Specific Marma Points on the Face. There are two marma points called Phana (A Serpent's Hood #9) on the side of each nostril. These points can be massaged with strong circular strokes to decrease headache pain, sinus pressure, and congestion. Usually the whole side of the nasal bone is treated. The Apanga marma (Looking Away #7) points are located on the outer corner of the eye and are massaged to relieve headaches due to eye strain. These points also help to clear the upper sinuses. Shankha (Conch #6) is the name of the point located on each temple. These points aid sleep and are associated with directing energy to the brain. The points named Utkshepa (What is Cast Upward #5) reside above the ears and are gently massaged to calm vata and the mind. Just above the center of each eyebrow is a point called Avarta (Calamity #4), which is massaged to decrease vata and improve energy and adaptability. The Sthapani marma (What Gives Support #3) resides between the eyebrows and is often called the "third eye." This point is associated with the sixth chakra, prana, the mind, senses, and the pituitary gland.

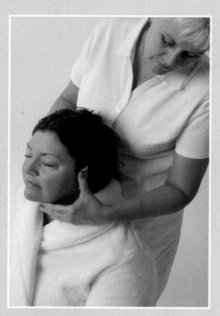

10. Ear Massage. Rub oil into the external regions of the ear, pulling the ear backward as the oil is applied. Pull the lobe in a downward and backward direction, and then pull the lobe across the opening of the ear to stretch it. After the head massage, massage the shoulders and upper arms of the client, pulling the robe off the shoulders (but leaving it to cover the rest of the body). When the massage of the head and shoulders is complete, the client's feet are removed from the foot soak and dried by the follower before the client is moved to a treatment table for another ayurvedic treatment such as abhyanga.

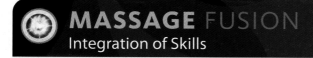

MASSAGE FUSION
Integration of Skills

STUDY TIP: Make It Personal

To learn anything, you must feel interested in it, have a basic understanding of concepts, and spend time processing the subject matter. With Eastern concepts this process can be particularly important. To apply Eastern concepts, you have to make the analogies about energy, the makeup of the universe, and the flow of qi or prana personal. As you contemplate this material, pay careful attention to yourself. Can you feel a place in your body where energy is blocked? Can you identify events in nature that represent the relationship between yin and yang? Can you palpate a tender area on your arm, leg, or back and associate it with an acupoint or marma point? The more you can engage these concepts at a personal level, the easier they will be to understand and apply.

MASSAGE INSPIRATION: Get Some New Culture!

It's fun to learn about other cultures, and the more you know about Eastern cultures the easier it is to apply Eastern concepts in your bodywork practice. Plan some activities that expose you to the Eastern worldview. You might see a subtitled film from India or China. You might attend a yoga or meditation class or practice martial arts. Maybe you visit the local art museum to view a collection of Eastern artifacts. These activities will help you create connections between pieces of information in your classes. As you make connections, write them down in a massage journal so that they continue to inspire your massage practice, even after you graduate.

CHAPTER WRAP-UP

If you were raised in a Western culture, Eastern concepts of medicine and bodywork can seem very strange at first, and you might want to simply reject them because they don't match your worldview. This is a normal reaction but may cut you off from ideas and techniques that could inspire and inform your developing practice. You have probably noticed already that many of these "new" Eastern techniques are surprisingly like the "old" Western techniques you already know. It's interesting to contemplate that people in many different areas of the world were developing similar ways to use touch therapeutically. Isn't it amazing that comparable methods developed despite the very different cultural viewpoints of people about bodywork? As you continue to progress through your studies, think about your perspective and how it is changing. In the early days of your studies, you probably couldn't apply the idea of qi or prana to your massage. Today, these are concepts that you understand and can explore as you deliver massage. Each concept you learn changes you in some way: changes your thinking, changes your hand placement, changes the questions you ask clients to plan session goals, and changes how you understand the world and bodywork.

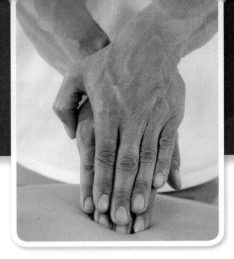

Energetic Approaches

KEY TERMS

biomagnetic field

energy

energy medicine

human energy field

infrared radiation

polarity

polarity therapy

reiki

therapeutic touch

vibration signature

LEARNING OBJECTIVES

Having read the chapter and used the related student learning tools, the student will be able to:

1. Define the term "energy" as it relates to energetic bodywork practices.

2. Describe the concept of a biomagnetic field and its relevance to energetic bodywork practices.

3. Outline the levels of practice in the energetic bodywork system called reiki.

4. Discuss what happens in a typical reiki session.

5. Explain the general principles behind the practice of polarity therapy.

6. Match body areas to negative, positive, or neutral charges.

7. Relate the goals of a typical therapeutic touch session.

8. Outline the steps therapists follow in a typical therapeutic touch session.

In general, energetic bodywork systems seek to harmonize the flow of energy throughout and around the body allowing the body to find emotional, spiritual, and physical balance. This balanced state encourages the body's healing mechanisms to correct disordered body systems or functions. The body is able to focus its resources on healing itself. In some cases, energetic systems attempt to "jump start" a healing response from the body and trigger the body to attack a pathogen or correct a dysfunction.

Many energetic bodywork systems evolved from traditional medical systems such as traditional Chinese medicine and ayurvedic medicine. These systems focus on the balanced flow of life force energy (qi in Chinese, ki in Japanese, prana in ayurveda) through and around the body and how life choices and the external environment can influence energy flow to either promote or inhibit health and wellness, as described in Chapter 17.

You will notice that these systems are very different from the systems described in previous chapters of this textbook. The focus is not soft-tissue structures like muscle and tendon, and most techniques could not be classified as massage strokes. This is not to say that energetic bodywork systems don't use touch, but rather to point out that the effects of touch are focused on facilitating energy flow so that the body (including muscles, tendons, and bones) has the resources it needs to heal itself.

Energetic bodywork systems should not be integrated within a massage session without the informed consent of the client (review Chapter 6, for a discussion of informed consent). This means you would not practice energy techniques on massage clients without their express written consent that they are seeking energetic methods of treatment. In many cases, complaints have been filed with state massage therapy boards or with professional organizations because therapists used energy work in massage sessions. Clients in these cases were not seeking energy work, wanted more traditional soft-tissue manipulation, or held personal beliefs in conflict with the beliefs of a particular energetic system.

Energetic bodywork systems are among the most controversial of bodywork practices because the existence of energy fields in and around the body has been difficult to verify or measure. Therapeutic effects from these systems are equally difficult to convincingly demonstrate because observed benefits are often attributed to a placebo effect. Still, energetic bodywork systems are popular with many massage therapists and clients, and new research is supporting the theory of an energetic system of the body and the ability of human touch to influence it for better health. This chapter will first introduce ideas that support the practice of energetic bodywork and then present the basics of three systems of energetic bodywork: reiki in Topic 18-2, polarity therapy in Topic 18-3, and therapeutic touch in Topic 18-4.

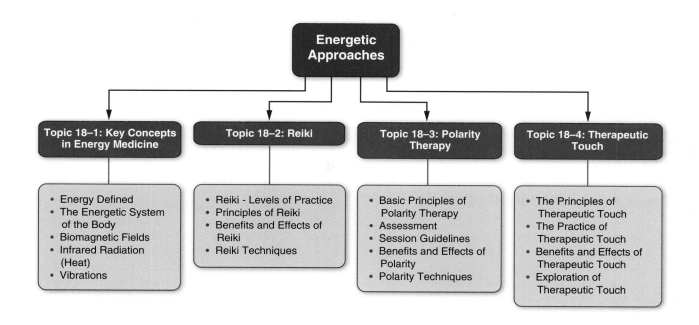

Topic **18-1**
Key Concepts in Energy Medicine

Energy medicine is one of five domains of CAM therapy identified by the National Center for Complementary and Alternative Medicine (NCCAM). Energy medicine can take many different forms, and the philosophies behind particular approaches can vary widely. Well-known energy medicine systems commonly practiced by massage therapists include polarity therapy, reiki, therapeutic touch, Healing Touch, Zero Balancing, Attunement Therapy, Bach Flower Remedies, Body Talk, Pranic Healing, Quantum Energetics, SHEN Therapy, Barbara Brennan Healing Science, and Zen Body Therapy. Other energy medicine systems (some used by physicians and physical therapists) employ mechanical vibrations (including sound), electrotherapy (the use of electricity for healing), visible light, magnetism (use of magnets and the fields they create), and monochromatic radiation such as the use of laser beams. The key concepts in energy medicine help us understand why some practices might demonstrate efficacy in the promotion of health and wellness.

Energy Defined

Energy is typically defined as the exertion of power or a capacity to do work, taking the forms of kinetic energy, potential energy, chemical energy, electrical energy, and others. In physics, energy is described by the amount of work that can be performed by a *force,* and the types of energy (thermal, gravitational, sound, light, and electromagnetic) are named after the related force. These definitions help us to understand a broad concept of energy and may apply to the way the term is used in certain energetic bodywork systems. Energetic bodywork systems often use the term *energy* to refer to types of energy fields that originate within the body or from sources outside the body and their use for healing, health, and wellness.

The Energetic System of the Body

Many energy medicine systems base their practices on a belief in an energetic system of the body. Michel Gauquelin, author of *Cosmic Clocks* writes, "The scientist knows that in the history of ideas, magic always precedes science, that the intuition of phenomena anticipates objective knowledge." An intuitive belief in an energetic system of the body dates back thousands of years and shows up in many medical traditions. As described in Chapter 17, traditional Chinese medicine describes the flow of qi (life force energy) through the body via channels called meridians. Chinese medicine doctors influence the flow of qi through various methods that include touch therapies to promote health. In ayurvedic medicine from India, vital life-force energy is known as prana, from the Sanskrit word for "breath." Prana flows through a network of energy channels called nadis. When the body is healthy, prana flows continuously creating vigor, life, spirit, passion, and self-determination. Many Native American cultures believe in a manifestation of divine spirit in living beings, which is very similar to the concept of life force in Asian traditions. In Lakota this spirit is known as ni, while in Navajo it is called nilch'i. A balance of the energy of divine spirit in the body gives a healthy person a sense of purpose and wholeness that manifests in ethical behavior, strong connections to family and community, and a harmonious relationship with nature. These are just three examples of similar concepts of an energetic system of the body present in healing methods from around the world.

When we think about the body's anatomy and physiology, it's easy to view the body as an energetic system. At the chemical level, charged ions that occur in the body, such as sodium, potassium, chloride, calcium, and magnesium, create biological electricity. There is an electrical potential difference between the interior and exterior of a cell. An electrical charge is created as cell membranes temporarily depolarize and then repolarize because of the different concentrations of ions inside and outside of the cell. This is the process that allows nerves to conduct signals from one place to another and to signal muscles to contract. Each beat of the heart begins with a pulse of electricity through the heart muscle. Electrical depolarization occurs in slow waves across the skin in response to injury. These injury potentials are believed to trigger tissue repair.

The current predominant belief held by many energetic bodywork therapists is that energy is produced by body structures, including cells, tissues, organs, and organ systems, transferred from place to place in the body, and projected as a field around the body. In many ways, this energy system could be thought of as a communication system of the body. The body uses energy to communicate well being, balance, and health, or to communicate injury, imbalance, dysfunction, and disease. When energy becomes blocked in one area of the body, perhaps in an area of weakness, it disrupts the harmonious flow of energy and communication in the rest of the body's energy system. Unless the flow of energy is returned to normal, the area of weakness is likely to get weaker, or a more serious pathology could take root. Energy medicine systems believe that a therapist using his or her hands or other tools can improve the flow of energy through the body so that the body enters an optimal healing state.

At various points in this book, we have discussed the Western medicine view of the body and talked about the idea that Western medicine is mechanistic and divides the body into parts that can be "fixed" like a car in an auto shop. Western medicine is also focused on eliminating disease or symptoms with drugs. This pragmatic approach to the body has yielded amazing advances in our understanding, but it also discounts or ignores less measurable phenomena, such as an energetic system of the body. Western medicine recognizes some aspects of an energetic system of the body and uses them for diagnosis. For example, an electroencephalogram is a test that measures and records the electrical activity of the brain. Certain conditions, like seizures, are recognized by changes in the normal patterns of the brain's electrical activity. An electrocardiogram (EKG) measures and records the electrical activity of the heart. The speed and rhythm of the heart and the strength and timing of electrical signals demonstrate the overall health and function of the heart. Abnormalities in EKG measurements are used to diagnose many heart conditions.

While the measurable electrical patterns of both the brain and heart hint at a larger energetic system, Western medicine has yet to fully explore the possibility that an energetic system exists and that its balanced function is essential for health and wellness. However, energy medicine has recently become the subject of investigations at some academic medical centers, and new research is supporting the "intuition of phenomena" embraced by ancient medical traditions.[1]

Biomagnetic Fields

A magnetic field is a force field in the region around a magnet or an electric current. It is characterized by a detectable magnetic force and magnetic poles. A magnetic force is exerted between the magnetic poles, producing magnetization. Magnetic poles are the places in the magnetic field where the force is most intense. As noted above, the body produces its own electrical activity. Wherever there is biological electrical activity, a **biomagnetic field** results (Fig. 18-1).

The heart produces the strongest electrical and magnetic activity of any tissue in the body. The pulsating magnetic field produced by the heart spreads out in front of and behind the body indefinitely into space. The further out from the body, the weaker the field and soon it gets lost in the "noise" created by other environmental fields. Other organs, such as the brain, nerves, and muscles, also create biomagnetic fields that spread out into surrounding tissues and past the perimeter of the skin into the space around the body. Researchers have confirmed that every physiological process in the body produces electrical charges and therefore resulting alterations and fluctuations in the biomagnetic fields. Because biomagnetic fields extend out from the body, the fields of people standing close to each other interact even if the people are not physically touching.[2]

Pulsed electromagnetic fields (fields generated through electrical medical devices) are often used for healing musculoskeletal and skin conditions.[3,4] In a series of studies

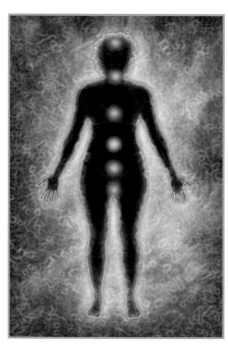

Figure 18-1 Representation of a biomagnetic field. A magnetic field is a force field found in the region around a magnet or an electric current. The body produces electrical activity. Wherever there is electrical activity, a biomagnetic field results.

conducted at the Colorado School of Medicine in Denver, a SQUID detector (superconducting quantum interference devices that measure small magnetic fields) was used to measure the biomagnetic fields emanating from a practitioner's hands when she used an energetic bodywork system called therapeutic touch (described later in this chapter). As the practitioner fell into the meditative state used during healing work, the SQUID detected a strong increase in the biomagnetic field coming from the practitioner's hands, which pulsed in such a way that the field swept through a range of frequencies during the session. In further studies, people who were untrained in therapeutic touch were unable to produce the same strength of biomagnetic pulses.[5] While the study was not designed to prove that healing was taking place, biomedical researchers note that biomagnetic fields in the same frequency range as those emitted by the practitioner are used to stimulate healing in soft-tissue and bone injury.[6]

Infrared Radiation (Heat)

Infrared (from the Latin *infra*, meaning "below" red, referring to the visible light spectrum of colors that are just within the red end of the spectrum) or heat radiation is defined as electromagnetic radiation of a wavelength longer than that of visible light but shorter than that of radio waves. As described in Chapter 16, heat is used for healing. In addition, infrared radiation has been used successfully to stimulate wound healing and stimulate bone remodeling when applied with a low-level laser.[7,8] Some energetic bodywork practitioners use the heat from their hands as a form of general infrared healing to help the body achieve an optimal internal state. For example, qigong masters are able to project measurable amounts of infrared radiation from their palms in a practice called "facilitating qi" shown to increase cell growth and protein synthesis as well as cell respiration.[9] Heat can also be absorbed from the environment in a practice called "inhibiting qi," which slows metabolism.

Vibrations

Everything in nature vibrates. In a human body, every atom, molecule, cell, tissue, and organ vibrates as it conducts its functions. The sum of these individual vibrations creates a unique whole-body **vibration signature**. Essential oils, herbs, crystals, flower essences, sound, light, homeopathic remedies, and other people vibrate and produce a specific vibration signature. Everything that vibrates emits a frequency (sound or light) or a range of frequencies that reflect a particular vibratory character. We can think of these vibrations and the frequencies they produce as an intricate song. Therapists who practice energy medicine speculate that good nutrition, regular exercise, the avoidance of toxic substances, satisfying relationships, and stress reduction activities allow the body to "sing a song" of health. Alternately, poor nutrition, a sedentary lifestyle, the accumulation of toxins from processed foods or habits like smoking, or an injury cause the body's vibrations to become unbalanced and produce discordant

"notes" that allow disease or dysfunction to result. Research demonstrates that the vibrations and energy fields produced by the hands of a therapist are in the range of frequency that influences regulatory processes in the body of another person.[10] Furthermore, substances like essential oils or homeopathic remedies and applications like light or sound therapy produce an electromagnetic vibration signature that may stimulate the defense and repair mechanisms of the body to speed healing or fight off a disease.[11]

Concept Brief 18-1
Blood Pressure

Energy: types of energy fields that originate within the body or from sources outside the body.

Energetic system of the body: Energy is produced by body structures and body functions and projected as a biomagnetic field around the body.

Biomagnetic field: The electromagnetic field produced as a result of the body's electrical activity that is projected into the space around the body.

Infrared radiation: Heat radiation used for healing, in this case the heat produced by the practitioner's hands.

Vibrations: Everything in nature vibrates at a particular frequency. The vibrations from a therapist's hands are believed to be in a range that promotes healing and balanced function.

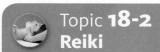

Topic 18-2
Reiki

Reiki is composed of two Japanese words. *Rei* is roughly translated to mean "higher intelligence" and *ki* is the word for "life-force energy." Reiki is an energetic approach to health and healing in which a reiki practitioner places his or her hands on or above a recipient or heals from a distance. This therapy was developed in Japan in the early 20th century by Mikao Usui, a schoolteacher who later opened a reiki training center where the reiki healing tradition was passed down to others. One of Usui students was Dr. Chujiro Hayashi, who studied with Usui in 1825 and made numerous adaptations to the reiki system. Hayashi trained Hawayo Takata, who later opened a clinic in Hawaii and brought reiki to the west. Most practitioners in the West trace their lineage to Takata.

Reiki — Levels of Practice

Takata developed three levels of training that reiki practitioners undertake in order to practice reiki or teach it to others.

1. Level 1 or first-degree reiki training teaches hand placement for hands-on healing, light touch, or placements for hands held just above the body. During the first-degree training, students receive four initiations (also called attunements or empowerments) that are believed to remove energetic blockages, open the student to the unified reiki source energy, and allow the student to act as a conduit for that energy in healing sessions.

2. Level 2 or second-degree reiki training teaches healing over a distance with no direct contact with the recipient. Symbols, passed down from Mikao Usui, are empowered in a special initiation and used as part of the healing session. The symbols are believed to connect reiki practitioners with primordial consciousness that creates a connection to the unified reiki source energy.

3. Level 3 or third-degree reiki training teaches master reiki practitioner skills so that practitioners are able to initiate and train more students.

Reiki practitioners view each level as a chance to deepen their connection to their concept of a unified reiki source energy and bring their lives into greater balance. While progression through the levels can be achieved quickly, the practice of reiki and a practitioner's relationship to reiki are viewed as ever evolving.

Principles of Reiki

Reiki practitioners seek presence, or the ability to live in the moment and be highly aware and sensitive to what is happening around them. Mikao Usui passed down five principles or affirmations that help practitioners remain personally balanced and present and promote an evolving relationship to unified reiki source energy. The five principles of reiki are believed to help practitioners cultivate and facilitate the flow of energy to others.

1. **Just for today, I will not be angry.** This principle reminds the practitioner that anger at others or at self creates blocks that prevent the free flow of energy through the body and the ability to act as a conduit of reiki source energy for others. This principle asks the practitioner to be aware of held anger and actively seek to release it and find peace of mind.

2. **Just for today, I will not worry.** This principle reminds the practitioner that worry leads to energy deficiency and fatigue, which in turn leads to illness or disease. Practitioners are reminded not to worry about future events or about the results of the session for the recipient. If the practitioner is worried for the recipient or the session outcome, it becomes impossible to allow uninterrupted vibrations from reiki source energy to flow. Instead, a sense of faith is cultivated and trust is placed in the unified reiki source energy.

3. **Just for today, I will be grateful.** This principle reminds the practitioner to pay attention to the manifestation of abundance all around and to be attentive to the ways in which the universe nurtures, supports, and provides for fulfillment. Practitioners with a sense of thankfulness and gratefulness experience fewer blockages in their own energy and are better able to allow the flow of reiki source energy to others.

4. **Just for today, I will do my work honestly.** This principle reminds the practitioner to live a life of honor and to support self and family respectfully, without harming or cheating others. Honor is believed to be held in the gut where energy can be cultivated or depleted. By living honestly, the practitioner is able to generate and allow the uninterrupted flow of reiki source energy.

5. **Just for today, I will be kind to every living thing.** Kindness builds on kindness and positive energy builds on positive energy. By practicing this principle, the practitioner allows the flow of reiki source energy to spread out, without limitation, to all people.

The five reiki principles are viewed as the foundation of practice that lead to the cultivation of greater energy and effectiveness. They ensure that practitioners remain balanced in life and are able to use the abilities they receive during initiations to channel the flow of reiki source energy in positive ways.

Benefits and Effects of Reiki

Practitioners of reiki regularly report that recipients experience a feeling of increased well being, deeper relaxation, and improved sleep after sessions. Like most therapies that employ touch, reiki likely reduces stress and supports improved health for any condition exacerbated by stress. While a study conducted in Sweden did not focus on reiki specifically, researchers found that the use of gentle touch led to significantly lower levels of anxiety in patients placed in intensive care units.[12] One study conducted in Wales indicates that adults with chronic pain had mild reduction in pain perception after reiki sessions,[13] and another noted that oncology nurses at Children's Hospital in Boston believed that reiki helped patients feel more peaceful and experience less pain when they practiced it on patients regularly.[14]

However, it should be pointed out that overall, research data on reiki are limited and the findings are inconclusive. In a systematic review of research to evaluate the evidence for the effectiveness of reiki, researchers identified 205 potentially relevant studies with nine randomized clinical trials that met the researchers' inclusion data. Two of the randomized clinical trials suggested beneficial effects of reiki for depression as compared with a sham (placebo) control, while one noted that there were no differences between the sham and reiki for depression. For functional recovery from stroke, there were no differences between the control and the test group reported for reiki. There were no differences for the control and the test group in a study to determine if reiki was effective for reducing anxiety in pregnant women undergoing amniocentesis, or for diabetic neuropathy and pain. A further study failed to show significant effects of reiki for anxiety and depression in women undergoing breast biopsy compared with conventional care.[15] More clinical testing is needed to determine the evidence-based effects and benefits of reiki.

Reiki Techniques

In the reiki tradition, a practitioner must be empowered with "attunements" provided by a reiki master in order to channel reiki source energy for healing. For this reason, specific techniques are not taught here, but a general session is described.

In a typical reiki session, a client lies down on a massage table in a relaxed position dressed in loose, comfortable clothing. The practitioner places his or her hands on the client in various positions (between 12 and 20 different hand positions might be used), or holds the hands above the client over particular body areas for 3 to 5 minutes before moving to the next hand position. Some practitioners use a fixed set of hand positions while others use their intuition to guide them to where hand positions are needed. If the client has a particular injury or an area of dysfunction, the hands might be held directly on or over the area for up to 20 minutes. In some cases, second-degree practitioners use symbols believed to enhance the strength of a session or allow reiki to be used at a distance.

Concept Brief 18-2
Reiki

- Reiki is an energetic approach to health and healing in which a reiki practitioner places hands on or above a recipient or heals from a distance.

- There are three different levels of training practitioners undertake in order to work with clients, heal from a distance, or "attune" other therapists to universal reiki energy.

- Five principles of reiki are believed to help practitioners cultivate and facilitate the flow of energy to others.

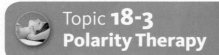

Topic 18-3
Polarity Therapy

Polarity therapy is an energy-based system that aims to address the body, mind, and spirit of the client through energetic bodywork, diet, exercise, and improved self-awareness. Dr. Randolph Stone, a naturopathic physician, osteopath, and chiropractor who emigrated from Austria to America in the early 1800s, developed polarity therapy because he was disillusioned by the "mechanistic" approach (viewing the body as a machine that can be fixed in the same way that a car is fixed) to the body practiced in Western medicine. Stone traveled widely exploring traditional medical systems and their views of body energetics. The Indian system of ayurveda (Chapter 17) formed the basis for Stone's ideas about the **human energy field** (see the earlier section on biomagnetic fields). He was also influenced by reflexology, described in Chapter 15.

Stone believed that diet, movement, sound, touch, attitudes, relationships, life experiences, trauma, injury, and environmental influences affect the human energy field. The balanced flow of energy in and around the body is the foundation of good health. Disease results when energy is blocked, fixed because of stress or injury in a particular region, or unbalanced. Polarity therapy aims to find blockages of unbalanced energy, release or rebalance it to promote normal flow patterns, and maintain the human energy field in an open, adaptive position.

Basic Principles of Polarity Therapy

The term **polarity** is use in both electricity and magnetism. It is helpful to understand polarity in terms of electrical wiring to better understand how Stone believed energy flowed in the human body. Imagine two points or objects, which are connected by a wire that carries an electric current. One of the points or objects (poles) has more electrons than the other. The pole with more electrons is said to have negative polarity; the other pole is assigned positive polarity. Electrons flow from the negative pole toward the positive pole in what we understand as an electric current. The movement of an electric charge produces a magnetic field. So, in polarity therapy, the belief is that both life energy and biomagnetic energy are flowing at the same time. The movement of electric charge is life energy, and the biomagnetic field it creates is known in polarity therapy as the human energy field.

It is also helpful to think about a magnet. A magnet has two poles of opposite polarity held together through a neutral balanced middle point. Two magnets are attracted by their opposite poles, and each repels the same pole of the other magnet.

In the human body, polarity is functioning at a cellular level (e.g., every cell is positive, negative, or neutral) and more broadly in terms of the way that energy is believed to move through the body. Polarity therapy is based on the idea that the flow of energy in the body can be rebalanced by using the attraction and repulsion of the positive and negative forces in the body through a neutral middle point.

Flow of Energy

In polarity therapy, energy is believed to flow throughout the entire body and around the body at every level from positive to negative regions (Fig. 18-2).

- The head is positive.
- The sacrum is negative.
- The feet are negative.
- The joints are neutral.
- The right side is positive.

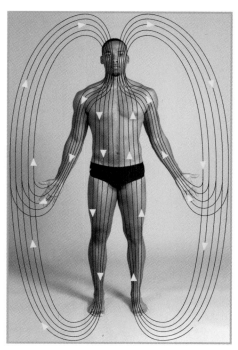

Figure 18-2 In polarity therapy, energy is believed to flow throughout the entire body and around the body at every level from positive to negative regions.

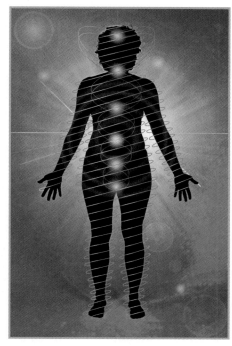

Figure 18-3 Chakras and the flow of energy in polarity therapy. The five elements are also associated with five key chakras, or energy vortexes, that are located down the centerline of the body.

- The left side is negative.
- The little finger and the middle finger are positive.
- The ring finger and the index finger are negative.
- The thumb is neutral.
- The little toe and the middle toe are positive.
- The second and the fourth toes are negative.
- The big toe is neutral.

Life energy flows vertically, horizontally, and in spirals from the top of the body in a downward direction and from the center of the body in an outward direction. Five vertical columns of energy flow on each side of the body. The energy lines on the right side of the body flow down the anterior of the body and up the posterior of the body. The energy lines on the left side of the body flow up the anterior of the body and down the posterior of the body.

Five Elements and Chakras

Dr. Stone associated each of the energy lines with one of the five elements from ayurveda. The elements are space (ether), air, fire, water, and earth. Stone borrowed aspects of ayurveda but didn't incorporate the entire ayurvedic system into his concepts related to polarity therapy. For this reason, there are differences between Stones ideas and what you might read in a dedicated ayurvedic textbook.

The five elements are also associated with five key chakras, or energy vortexes, which are located down the centerline of the body (Fig. 18-3). Chakras are believed to have neutral

energy and spin in a clockwise direction that disperses energy both upward and downward forming the vertical energy lines of the body. A dual spiral of energy moving from the head downwards is called the caduceus current and connects the chakras, which are associated with specific organs, physiological functions, and vibrational qualities.

- The first chakra is associated with earth, elimination, the bladder, and the rectum and has the lowest level of vibration.
- The second chakra is associated with water, genitals, the endocrine system, and emotions.
- The third chakra is associated with fire, digestion, the stomach, and the bowels.
- The fourth chakra is associated with air, circulation, the heart, and the lungs.
- The fifth chakra is associated with space (ether), hearing, the voice, and the throat and has the highest vibration of the five chakras in Stone's system.

Reflexes of the Hands and the Feet

Dr. Stone believed that energy could be balanced using the hand and foot reflexes (described in Chapter 15). He defined a reflex as a point along an energy current which, when stimulated, affects the energy of other places along the same current (Fig. 18-4). This concept of a reflex is in accordance with William Fitzgerald's idea of zone therapy. The focus of the therapist's hand contacts is to stimulate the energy along the zones and then to balance the energy

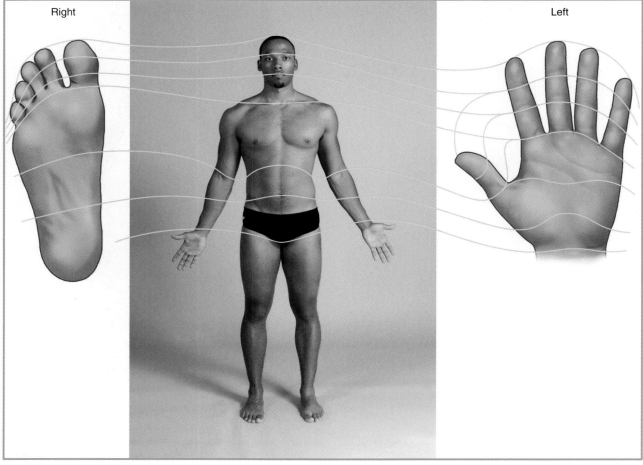

Right

Left

Figure 18-4 Reflexes of the hands and feet in polarity therapy. Dr. Stone defined a reflex as a point along an energy current which, when stimulated, affects the energy of other places along the same current.

directly over the region of the body where a blockage is suspected. Technique 58, later in this chapter, demonstrates the use of foot and hand reflexes to balance the energy in this manner.

Diet, Exercise, and Attitudes

Polarity therapy is a holistic system that advocates a healthy diet, regular exercise, and attention to attitudes and thinking patterns.

- **Diet:** Dr. Stone often used the ayurvedic understanding of foods based on dosha imbalances (what he called *the three principles*) to treat energy blockages and poor health. For example, if vata, or the air principle, is out of balance the polarity therapist would suggest foods to pacify vata. If pitta, or the fire principle, is out of balance the therapist would suggest foods to pacify pitta.

- **Exercise:** Dr. Stone outlined the regular practice of specific exercises in his book, *Easy Stretching Postures for Vitality and Beauty*. In this system, rhythmic movement is used in specific positions to stimulate the body's energy fields.

- **Attitudes:** Dr. Stone believed that thoughts are very fast vibrations of energy that initiate actions that produce the results of those thoughts. Dr. Stone proposed that a positive state of mind is essential for good health and negative thinking is the initial cause of disease. Affirmations are used throughout the day to send positive vibrations throughout the body and to attract positive forces to the body.

Concept Brief 18-3
Polarity Therapy Concepts

- The biomagnetic field that surrounds the body is called the human energy field.

- Energy flows from positive to negative regions in the body and can become unbalanced, blocked, or fixed because of poor diet, injury, or other disturbances.

- Dr. Stone, the founder of polarity therapy, borrowed concepts from ayurveda and reflexology.

Assessment

Polarity therapists use different approaches to assess clients and determine where energy is blocked or fixed. Some therapists use one method for assessment while others use a combination of methods.

- **Interview:** The therapist interviews the client to find out about present conditions, symptoms, physical sensations, emotional balance, stress levels, and thought patterns. The information gained during the interview is used to choose appropriate hand contacts to affect the energy that flows through an affected region.

- **Intuition:** An experienced therapist might palpate the energy flow of the client by holding his or her hands a few inches off the body and noticing areas of warmth or coolness and areas that pull or push the hands toward the body or away from the body. The therapist might also palpate the client's tissue to determine where pain or tenderness is experienced. The therapist uses this information about energy flow to choose hand contacts he or she believes will benefit the client.

- **Reflexes:** The therapist palpates the reflexes of the hands and the feet to determine areas of blocked or fixed energy. Tender areas of the hands and feet indicate areas that need attention. If the reflex point on the foot is sorer than the same point on the hand, the blockage or the fixation is considered a chronic condition. If the reflex point on the hand is more tender than the same point on the foot, the condition is believed to be more acute.

- **Five elements:** The five elements combine into three doshas (vata, pitta, and kapha). While Dr. Stone referred to the three doshas as the three principles, he used a method similar to ayurveda to determine dosha (principle) imbalances. Once a dosha imbalance is identified, an appropriate series of hand contacts can be chosen to bring the body into balance.

- **Left/right symmetry:** Polarity therapists usually find that an area that is tender or painful on the left side is also tender and painful on the right side. Both sides need to be treated in order for the energy to be balanced.

- **Anterior/posterior symmetry:** An area that is sore or painful on the posterior of the body is often also sore and painful on the anterior of the body. The particular region should be treated both anteriorly and posteriorly to balance the body's energy.

- **Joints:** Joints are neutral points where life energy intersects. As a result, energy often becomes congested around the joints of the body leading to painful points that need to be addressed during sessions.

Session Guidelines

During the delivery of sessions, polarity therapists follow some basic guidelines to ensure treatments are comfortable for the client and as effective as possible.

- **Focus of treatment:** The focus of treatments is on life energy and not on a specific disease, condition, or injury.

The therapist uses hand contacts to free blocked or fixed energy knowing that the body can heal itself more easily if energy is flowing freely. Therapists do not equate areas of blocked energy to a specific pathology or medical condition. People in weakened conditions or pain may be more susceptible to suggestion and develop additional complications as a result of a therapist's comment. It is, of course, out of the scope of practice of a massage therapist or polarity therapist to diagnose client conditions.

- **Therapist attitudes:** Your attitude should be positive, relaxed, and loving. Focus on trusting the process and allowing the session to progress naturally. If you dislike a person or feel negative energy toward a person, you should not practice polarity therapy on that person. Similarly, if you are going through a time of personal turmoil or experiencing mental or emotional anxiety or upset, put off the session until you feel calm, centered, and positive.

- **Therapist energy:** If your energy is depleted because you are overly tired, sick, or distracted, put off the session until you feel rested, well, and focused.

- **Atmosphere of the treatment room:** The treatment room should be warm, clean, quiet, and comfortable. A massage table is often set up with a cloth surface that the client can recline on and a blanket for warmth.

- **Clothing:** Both therapists and clients should wear loose, comfortable clothing made from natural fibers and remove shoes, jewelry, and metal objects such as belt buckles or change from pockets. Metal is believed to interfere with the flow of life energy.

- **Use of breath:** Both clients and therapists are encouraged to take long, slow, deep breaths throughout the session.

- **Cautions/contraindication:** Do not place your hands directly on an injured or an inflamed area. In this case, hold your hands about 2 to 3 inches above the area instead of using a direct contact.

Benefits and Effects of Polarity Therapy

Polarity therapists note that clients have a variety of reactions to polarity. Some experience profound relaxation, while others have physical "unwinding" where the arms and legs jerk as the nervous system decompresses. Still others experience emotional releases and strong body sensations or imagery. Like most energetic approaches to bodywork, polarity therapy is indicated for any condition exacerbated by stress and is a reliable means to promote relaxation. Polarity therapists report that sessions are useful for pain reduction and to speed recovery from injury or illness, but the research to support these claims is limited and mostly anecdotal.

Polarity Techniques

You already know that when the positive and negative poles of two magnets are put together, they attract each other. The therapist places his or her hands in such a way to use this attraction of positive to negative to balance the flow of energy in the client's body. Two contacts are made at the same time either with the hands, the fingers, or a combination of hands and fingers. The hands can actually make contact with the client's body or be held slightly above body areas. A positive contact is made with the right hand or the middle finger, which is stimulating, while a negative contact is made with the left hand or the index finger, which is sedating. Your right hand (positive) is placed on the left side of the client's body (negative) and your left hand (negative) is placed on the right side of the client's body (positive). If you are working along the centerline of the body, your left hand (negative) is placed toward the top of the body (positive) and your right hand (positive) is placed toward the bottom of the body (negative). If an area is painful, it is common for a polarity therapist to place the left hand on the area of pain and the right hand opposite to the pain on the posterior, anterior, or side of the body. Technique 56 demonstrates the exploration of common polarity hand contacts in a complete routine that is useful for stress reduction and overall body balance. Technique 57 explores the high movement of life energy that flows through the coccyx, navel, and base of the occiput for simple but effective polarity contacts. Using foot and hand reflexes to balance energy or to treat an area of blocked or fixed energy is shown in Technique 58.

Concept Brief 18-4
Polarity Therapy

- Polarity therapy is an energy-based system that aims to address the body, mind, and spirit of the client through energetic bodywork, diet, exercise, and improved self-awareness.

- The movement of an electric charge produces a magnetic field. So, in polarity therapy, the belief is that both life energy and biomagnetic energy are flowing at the same time. The movement of electric charge is life energy, and the biomagnetic field it creates is known in polarity therapy as the human energy field.

- Polarity therapists use different approaches to assess clients and determine where energy is blocked or fixed. An interview, the experienced therapist's intuition, principles from ayurveda, the reflexes on the hands and feet, or an understanding of body symmetry might be used.

Technique 56 — Exploration of Polarity for Body Balance

The series of hand contacts outlined here are designed to be provided in a particular order (follow the picture sequence) to bring general polarity balance to the body and promote stress reduction and relaxation. The posterior of the body is treated first with the client in the prone position, and then the client is asked to turn into the supine position. Bolster the client as you would for a massage. As you begin the session, take a moment to focus your intention and attitude so that your thoughts are positive. Regularly check in with yourself to ensure your focus and attitude remains positive throughout the session. Keep your own spine in a relaxed position and avoid bending at the waist. The hand contacts you make with the client are very light. In fact, it works well to hold your hands just slightly off the client's body area. There is no set length of time to hold a position. Maintain each hand contact as long as you feel an exchange of energy or until your intuition tells you to move.

As you release one position and move into the next, exhale and re-center your own energy. Take long, slow, deep breaths throughout the session and regularly remind your client to do the same. Pay attention to what you feel in your hands, the images that arise during the session, and your client's responses. Ask your client to give you good feedback about his or her experiences at the end of the session.

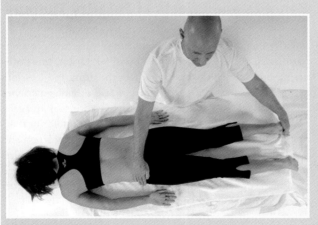

Posterior positions 1 and 2

From posterior position 1 on the right side of the table with your right hand on the client's left hip and your left hand on the client's right foot, walk around the table and repeat this holding position from the opposite side. You are now on the left side of the table with your left hand on the client's right hip and your right hand on the client's left foot.

Technique 56   **Exploration of Polarity for Body Balance** (Continued)

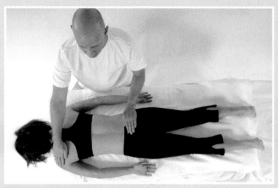

Posterior positions 3 and 4

From posterior position 3 on the right side of the table with your right hand on the client's left shoulder and your left hand on the client's sacrum, walk around the table and repeat this holding position from the opposite side. You are now on the left side of the table with your left hand on the client's right shoulder and your right hand on the client's sacrum.

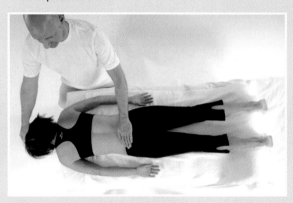

Posterior position 5

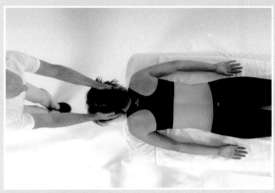

Posterior position 6

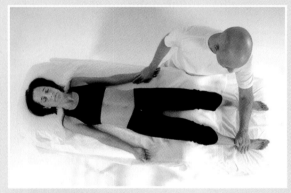

Anterior positions 1 and 2

From anterior position 1 on the right side of the table with your right hand on the client's left hand and your left hand on the client's right ankle, walk around the table and repeat this holding position from the opposite side. You are now on the left side of the table with your left hand on the client's right hand and your right hand on the client's left ankle.

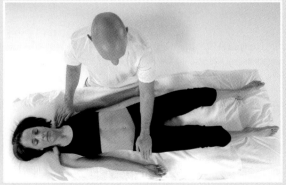

Anterior positions 3 and 4

From anterior position 3 on the right side of the table with your right hand on the client's left shoulder and your left hand on the client's right hip, walk around the table and repeat this holding position from the opposite side. You are now on the left side of the table with your left hand on the client's right shoulder and your right hand on the client's left hip.

Continued

| Technique 56 | **Exploration of Polarity for Body Balance** (Continued) |

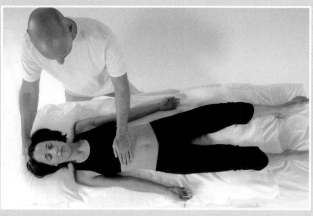

Anterior position 5

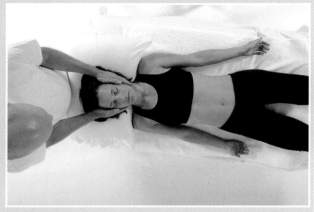

Anterior position 6

| Technique 57 | **Polarity for the Coccyx, Navel, and Base of the Occiput** |

The coccyx, navel, and base of the occiput are believed to be areas of high life-energy movement and are very receptive to polarity treatment.

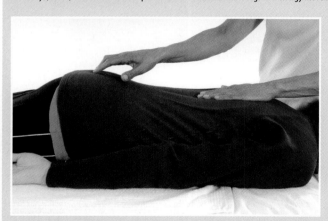

1. The Coccyx. The coccyx is located at the end of the spine and has the highest degree of negative charge of any area of the spine. The middle finger of your right hand can be placed directly over the coccyx, with your left hand placed on any area of pain above the right hand along the centerline of the body. This is a simple and effective way to ease pain from low-back conditions, labor related to childbirth, or general tension due to stress.

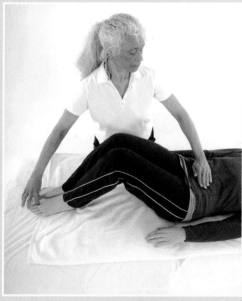

2. The Navel. The navel is a central area of life energy and can be used to connect and polarize both the superior regions and inferior regions of the body. For example, with the client positioned supine, with the knees together and bent and the big toes touching, hold the big toes of both feet with your right hand and place your left hand over the navel. This position is believed to send strong energy to the center of the body to aid in lower abdominal and pelvic disturbances. Alternatively, you can send a strong flow of energy from the center of the body to the head by placing your right hand on the navel center and your left hand under the posterior of the neck.

| **Technique 57** | **Polarity for the Coccyx, Navel, and Base of the Occiput** (Continued) |

3. The Base of the Occiput. The base of the occiput is located at the top of the spine and has a strong positive charge. Use this point to polarize sore spots inferiorly. For example, place your left hand on the base of the occiput with the client in the prone position. Your right hand holds any sore areas on the feet, legs, joints, or back.

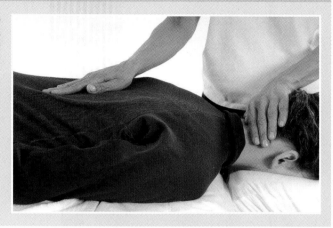

| **Technique 58** | **Polarity Balance of Energy Using Foot and Hand Reflexes** |

While foot reflexology is usually performed with the client in the supine position, during a polarity session if the blockage is on the posterior of the body, the client is positioned prone for the treatment. Review the reflexology figures in Chapter 15. These figures provide information on the location of specific foot and hand reflexes.

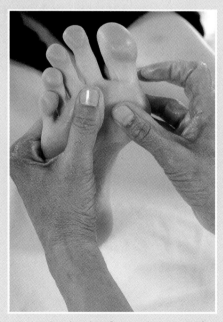

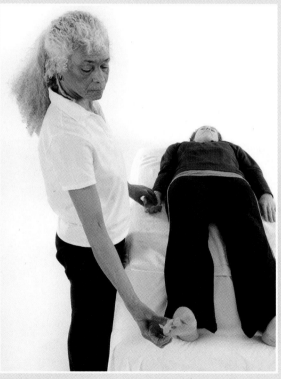

1. Assessment. Stimulate the reflexes on the hands and feet to determine areas of tenderness or pain. These areas relate to blocked or fixed energy flow. When you have identified the areas that need to be balanced, follow the same series of steps for each reflex point and its associated body region.

2. Hand Contacts of the Foot and Hand. Contact a tender point on a foot (the right foot and hand corresponds to the right side of the body, and the left foot and hand to the left side of the body) with your thumb. With your other thumb, contact the same spot on the client's hand. Hold these points until your intuition tells you that the energy is balanced.

Continued

Technique 58   **Polarity Balance of Energy Using Foot and Hand Reflexes** (Continued)

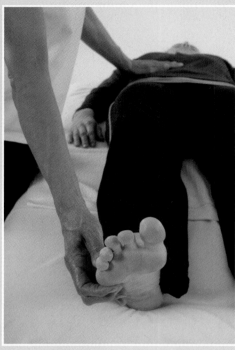

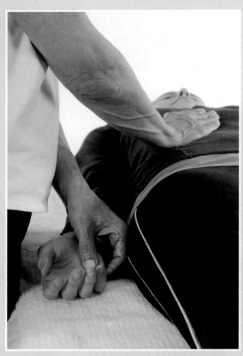

3. Hand Contacts With the Affected Region and Foot. Remove the thumb from the hand and use your fingers to make contact with the region of the imbalance. For example, if you have identified that the liver reflex of the right foot and hand is tender and you have been holding the liver reflex on the right foot and hand, remove your thumb from the liver reflex of the hand and place your fingers directly over the liver on the anterior of the body. At the same time, continue to hold the point on the foot and gently stimulate that point with your thumb.

4. Hand Contacts With the Affected Region and Hand. Now contact the hand reflex with your thumb and place your fingers over the affected region of the body. Stimulate the hand reflex with your thumb while you hold the position. When you finish, move on to the next reflex that demonstrates tenderness.

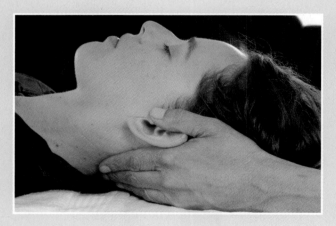

5. Finish the Session. When you have balanced all of the tender points you identified on the hands and the feet, finish the session by cradling the head. The thumbs rest by the client's ears and the fingers rest down the sides of the neck. Hold this position until the client feels energetically relaxed.

Topic **18-4**
Therapeutic Touch

Therapeutic touch is an energetic healing method that aims to balance and increase the body's energy as a way to support health and wellness. The body is viewed as an energetic system that has a natural thrust toward health and healing that can be rebalanced or redirected when necessary to combat injury and disease. Therapeutic touch recognizes a body, mind, and spirit connection and understands the ability to think, feel, sense the world intuitively, and take action as an energetic character with a particular rhythm and pattern in each person. When this rhythm and pattern are disrupted or out of sync, the body is more susceptible to disease and injury or less likely to heal itself effectively. Therapeutic touch seeks to reestablish and integrate the aspects of the body's natural energy character to promote health and wellness.[16]

Developed by Dolores Krieger, a professor at New York University School of Nursing, and Dora Kunz, a natural healer, in the 1870s, therapeutic touch is based on the age-old practice of "laying on of hands" but without a religious or cultural connotation. Originally taught to Krieger's graduate school nursing students, Krieger's research and professional writing helped to spread the popularity of the technique among nurses throughout the United States. While therapeutic touch is predominantly practiced by nurses at hospitals and health centers today, it is slowly finding its way into the massage and bodywork profession because there is a growing body of clinical research that demonstrates its effectiveness.

The Principles of Therapeutic Touch

Therapeutic touch is based on a belief in a human energy field and on universal energy available to all people. This system also promotes the idea of order as an underlying characteristic of the universe and of human beings that allow the body, mind, and spirit to act as a coherent whole. Healthy function relies on the ability of the body to maintain order or return to order if order is disrupted. Dora Kunz believed that each person has a human energy field that interacts with the human energy field of other people and with the larger universal energy field of our natural world. In the therapeutic touch system, the human energy field is separated into several components:

- **The physical field** is associated with the physical body and has a particular rhythm signature. When the body is healthy, there is a normal exchange of energy between all the systems of the body. When the body is injured, diseased, or healing from an event like surgery, the body's physical energy field is disordered and may need assistance to return to its natural rhythm.

- **The emotional field** is associated with feelings and interacts closely with the physical field. When we feel happy we experience increased energy, while sadness can cause an inward draw of energy and fatigue. The emotional field is believed to move outward and so can affect the energy of other people because it becomes part of the shared universal field that connects all people.

- **The mental field** is associated with what we think and affects both the emotional and the physical fields. Negative thought patterns sap energy from the emotional and the physical fields, leading to fatigue that leaves the body open to injury or disease. Positive thought patterns ensure that the emotional and physical fields have plenty of free-flowing energy to draw upon.

- **The intuitional field** of each person is part of a universal intuitional field shared by all people that provides a sense of connection to our environment and other beings. It provides us with insight and instantaneous recognition of truth, and inspires our ability to innovate and create. When the physical, emotional, and mental fields are interacting harmoniously, we can tap more easily into intuitional energy.

When all of these components of the human energy field are interacting according to the natural rhythm of a person, then health and wellness are expressed and the body has stored resources that help it fight off disease, avoid injury, and interact with others to evolve and grow. If a person is unhealthy, injured, or is fighting a disease, the components of the human energy field can get out of sync and the body lacks the energy resources it needs to heal effectively. Therapeutic touch practitioners believe that they can help increase the energy in a person's system to support health and healing.

Concept Brief **18-5**
Principles of Therapeutic Touch

- There is a human energy field surrounding each person.
- There is universal energy available to all people.
- The human energy field of one person can influence the human energy field of another person.
- Good health relies on the ability of the human body to maintain order or return to order if order is disrupted.
- Therapeutic touch seeks to increase the energy in a person's system to support healing processes.

The Practice of Therapeutic Touch

Therapeutic touch practitioners follow a specific series of steps when providing sessions to clients.

- **Centering:** The goal of centering is to quiet the mind and emotions, set an intent to benefit the client, and focus on the session by setting aside the concerns of the external world. Practitioners are mindful of maintaining their energetic boundaries. They remain aware of the client's emotions, pain, anxiety, or other physical and emotional sensations, but avoid attaching to the outcome of the session or overidentifying with the client and losing their calmness.

- **Assessment:** During an assessment, the therapeutic touch practitioner moves his or her hands above the body to sense the flow of energy. Usually, the fully clothed client is seated in a chair. The assessment proceeds in a downward direction from the head toward the feet, first on the anterior region of the body and then on the posterior region. Practitioners report that healthy energy feels soft, warm, rhythmic, and flowing. Blocked areas feel cooler, "sticky," or slow. When the practitioner encounters an area where the energy is low or deficient, a sucking or a pulling sensation might be experienced.

- **Balancing the energy field:** Balancing the energy field is sometimes referred to as "unruffling." To balance the energy field, a therapeutic touch practitioner moves his or her hands in long, slow, rhythmic, downward sweeping motions about 3 inches off the client's body, projecting the state of calm achieved during centering. If the energy is balanced correctly, the client enters a deeply relaxed state in which breathing slows and the hands and the feet feel warm. If the client feels light-headed or anxious, the energy has not been balanced correctly. A practitioner using an incorrect rhythm or speed of "strokes" sometimes causes this.

- **Directing the energy:** Directing the energy is sometimes referred to as "modulation." Injury, disease, trauma, or other forms of compromised health deplete the client's energy so that he or she does not have the necessary resources to heal effectively. In the final step of a therapeutic touch session, the practitioner directs universal energy to the client to boost his or her energy systems so that energy can reorganize itself and find its natural rhythm and flow. When directing energy, the practitioner places the hands about 3 inches off the body over regions where energy feels depleted. He or she might visualize a light or a specific color flowing from universal energy, through self to the client and then flooding the client's body before exiting through the client's feet. As the energy field of the client is treated, it begins to feel even and expanded.

- **Balancing the energy field:** To close the session, a therapeutic touch practitioner balances the energy field a second time to integrate all aspects of the session. He or she holds the intent that the client is healthy and that the energy and body are organized and whole.

- **Integration of the session:** Therapeutic touch sessions usually last 10 to 15 minutes but can also be expanded or shortened based on the practitioner's intuition. Once the practitioner has finished balancing the energy field the second time, the client is encouraged to sit quietly so that the body, mind, and spirit can process and integrate the session.

Benefits and Effects of Therapeutic Touch

Therapeutic touch practitioners notice that sessions increase client relaxation and are beneficial for any condition exacerbated by stress. The benefits of therapeutic touch for reducing anxiety in a hospital or clinical setting before stressful testing are well documented.[17] Therapeutic touch also demonstrates the ability to reduce the experience of both acute and chronic pain. For example, in a study of 60 patients with headache pain, participants were divided into two groups. The test group received a therapeutic touch session. The control group received a sham treatment. 90% of the group receiving therapeutic touch sessions reported a decrease in headache pain with an average pain reduction score of 70% reduction. In the control group, 80% reported a reduction of pain but with a pain reduction score of only 37%.[18] In another study, therapeutic touch prolonged the intervals between the administration of analgesics to people in pain, and reduced the anxiety and pain experienced by burn patients.[19] While a review of the research suggests that therapeutic touch demonstrates higher levels of effectiveness than Reiki, more research is needed to clarify the significance of findings for anxiety and pain reduction.[20]

Exploration of Therapeutic Touch

There is no official certification process to become a therapeutic touch practitioner in the United States. However, therapeutic touch is not massage and should not be practiced as part of a massage session; Chapter 6, discusses why energetic systems should not be mixed with nonenergetic systems without the client's informed consent. Most often, therapeutic touch is practiced as an extension of another healthcare profession, such as nursing, or in therapeutic touch sessions delivered by massage therapists trained in therapeutic touch. You can explore some of the techniques of therapeutic touch in Technique 59 and use them in a general way to better understand concepts of energetic bodywork and your own sensations and intuition as you work with energy. If therapeutic touch is a modality that interests you, contact The Nurse-Healers Professional Associates International (the official organization of therapeutic touch) to find out about training opportunities. Contact details are listed in the Massage Fusion section of this chapter.

Concept Brief 18-6
Therapeutic Touch

- Therapeutic touch is an energetic healing method that aims to balance and increase the body's energy as a way to support health and wellness.

- Therapeutic touch is based on a belief in a human energy field and on universal energy that is available to all people.

- Therapeutic touch practitioners follow a specific series of steps when providing sessions to clients. The steps are centering, assessment, balancing the energy field, directing the energy, re-balancing the energy field, and time for the client to integrate the session.

| Technique 59 | Exploration of Therapeutic Touch |

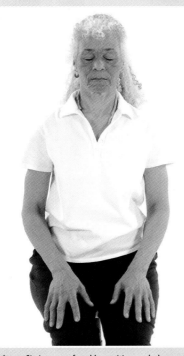

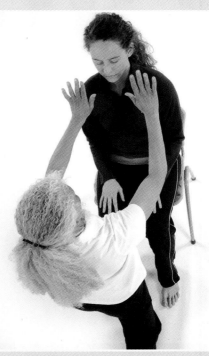

1. Centering. Sit in a comfortable position and close your eyes. Turn your attention inward and disregard any distractions from the outside world. Focus on long, slow deep breaths and pay as much attention to the space between your breaths as to the inward and outward flow of air. Let your attention move to the area of your heart and ask yourself to provide an image of peacefulness. You may instantly have an image appear or you may need to generate a peaceful image. Maybe it's a still mountain lake, a tree with wide green branches, a hummingbird hovering in the blue sky, or any other image that comes into your mind that represents peace, calm, and stillness. Think of this peaceful feeling as being yourself, and affirm "I am this peace." When you feel you are connected to your peace, inner quiet, and calm you are ready to explore what you feel during "assessment."

2. Assessment. Hold your hands about 3 inches from the fully clothed client who sits in a comfortable chair. Start on the anterior side of the client, and move your hands in a slow, steady downward motion toward the feet. Notice any sensations you experience in your hands or any intuitions you have about the client's energy field. Healthy flow of energy is often experienced as soft, warm, and flowing. Blocked energy may present itself as coolness in a particular region or energy that feels "sticky" or slow moving. An area of depleted energy may pull your hands toward it. Once you complete the anterior assessment, repeat the downward movement of your hands on the posterior side of the body.

Continued

Technique 59   **Exploration of Therapeutic Touch**

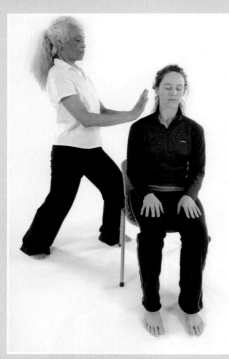

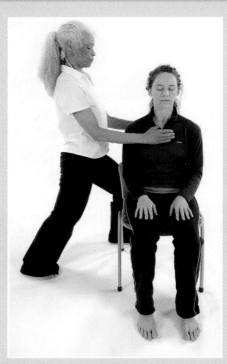

3. Balancing the Energy Field. Pay attention to the sensations you experience as you explore balancing the client's energy field. Use long, slow, rhythmic, downward sweeping motions of your hands about 3 inches off the client's body. The client should enter a relaxed state where breathing slows down and deepens and the hands and feet feel warm. If the client experiences feelings of light-headedness, discomfort, or anxiety, the speed and the rhythm of your "strokes" may be "off." Re-center your energy, project feelings of calm and peacefulness to the client, and slow your strokes while keeping them rhythmic and moving in a downward direction.

4. Directing Energy. During the assessment exploration, you may have found areas where the energy felt depleted. Hold your hands over these areas and imagine energy flowing from a great universal source through you to the client. You might imagine the energy as a white light or as a color that floods the entire system of the client and moves out through the feet. Therapeutic touch practitioners believe that the color white, cobalt blue, and purplish-blue are the most healing colors. When your intuition tells you that the client's energy field is expanded and smooth, return to step 3 and re-balance the client's energy field. Encourage the client to relax for an additional 10 minutes to ensure the body has time to process and integrate the session.

 MASSAGE FUSION
Integration of Skills

STUDY TIP: Conduct an Interview

A great way to explore energetic bodywork practices is to interview practitioners or therapists about the type of energetic system they use. Here are some interview questions to get you started:

1. Can you describe for me the energetic bodywork system you practice?
2. Why did you choose this system of energetic bodywork over other systems?
3. Why do you feel this system is effective? What are the general mechanisms that create effects in the body?
4. In your experience, how have clients been affected by sessions and what types of conditions or diseases have you worked with?
5. What is the most challenging aspect of offering this type of bodywork?
6. What is the most rewarding aspect of offering this type of bodywork?

MASSAGE FUSION (Continued)
Integration of Skills

MASSAGE INSPIRATION: Explore Your Biomagnetic Field

It's easy to experience your biomagnetic field and even to "feel" the fields of other people. Try this. Rub your hands together vigorously and then hold them a few inches apart. Move them closer together and then further apart and notice the sensations you experience. Have a classmate rub his or her hands together and place one hand between your two hands. Move your hands closer to his or her hand and then further apart and notice the sensations you experience. Many people report feeling warmth, coolness, tingling, vibrations, or the feeling of being drawn closer or pushed away.

GOOD TO KNOW: Energetic Approaches Resources

International Association of Reiki Professionals (IARP): www.iarp.org.
World Reiki Association: www.worldreikiassociation.org.
American Polarity Therapy Association: www.polaritytherapy.org.
Nurse Healers Professional Associates International (the official Therapeutic Touch association): www.therapeutictouch.org.

CHAPTER WRAP-UP

As we discussed at the beginning of the chapter, energetic bodywork systems are among the most controversial of bodywork practices because the existence of energy fields in and around the body has been difficult to verify or measure. Therapeutic effects from these systems are equally difficult to convincingly demonstrate, because benefits are often attributed to a placebo effect. In your classes, you will likely get the chance to "play" with energy and explore its effects. You have the opportunity to determine what you think and feel about energy work. Maybe you love it and get a burst of energy when you give it or receive it. Maybe it leaves you perplexed because you think you feel something happening, but you're not completely sure what it is or if it is related to the session. Perhaps you think it's all a bunch of hogwash and you just want to get back to practicing treatment massage techniques. Whatever your feelings, write them down to capture them. As you progress through your schooling and when you are out in the real world practicing massage, it is likely that you will encounter situations where something shifts for the client and you have no explanation for it. It is also possible that energy work is the only type of treatment the client can tolerate in certain situations. For example, in one instance a client had been in a car accident and went the next day for a massage. Her body was so flared up and tender that actually touching the client was impossible. Instead, the therapist obtained the client's informed consent to apply energy work and used polarity holds for the session to help the client relax and rebalance. The client reported that the polarity session not only helped her relax her muscles but also helped her feel emotionally balanced and less traumatized. Remember what Michel Gauquelin, wrote in *Cosmic Clocks*. He said, "The scientist knows that in the history of ideas, magic always precedes science, that the intuition of phenomena anticipates objective knowledge." So ask yourself: "What does my intuition tell me about energy work?"

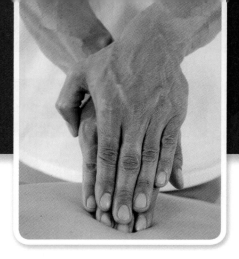

Chapter

19

Assessment, Treatment Planning, and Documentation for Healthcare Massage

KEY TERMS

client self-care

functional goals

functional limitations

functional outcomes reporting

gait

hyperkyphosis

hyperlordosis

pain assessment

postural dysfunction

posture

posture assessment

range-of-motion assessment

scoliosis

soft-tissue rehabilitation

LEARNING OBJECTIVES

Having read the chapter and used the related student learning tools, the student will be able to:

1 Compare and contrast intake forms and intake interview questions for a wellness massage with those for a healthcare massage.

2 Compose three functional goals for oneself or classmates acting as clients.

3 Describe a postsession intake interview specific to healthcare massage.

4 List two reasons to conduct a pain assessment.

5 Discuss the relevance of questions in a pain questionnaire.

6 Distinguish between ideal posture and postural dysfunctions.

7 Outline the views and boney landmarks used during a posture assessment.

8 Explain the purpose of active range-of-motion, passive range-of-motion, and resisted range-of-motion assessments.

9 Outline the stages of health on a continuum.

10 Describe the phases of soft-tissue rehabilitation.

11 Construct a treatment plan using evaluation data.

Throughout many chapters, this textbook has differentiated between wellness massage and healthcare massage. Wellness massage is discussed in detail in Chapters 10 and 12. Healthcare massage (also referred to as treatment massage, rehabilitative massage, therapeutic massage, or similar terms) is massage that addresses chronic soft-tissue holding patterns that lead to dysfunction, soft-tissue injury, or chronic pain. Methods used in healthcare massage include advanced assessment procedures and a variety of techniques such as hydrotherapy, myofascial release, deep tissue, and some remedial exercises (e.g., resisted range of motion).

Often, this type of massage is provided in a healthcare setting such as a hospital, chiropractor's office, sports medicine clinic, or physical therapy office, and it may be supervised by a physician, chiropractor, physical therapist, or athletic trainer. Sports massage for athletes is considered healthcare massage because the massage therapist supports the training and recovery process by including goals such as increased flexibility, increased strength, and the prevention of injury. Healthcare massage also includes massage for clients with an illness other than soft-tissue conditions or who have experienced some physical, mental, or emotional trauma for which they are receiving medical treatment. Massage is often provided in this case for condition management to decrease some symptoms and improve quality of life. Examples include massage in a hospital for cancer patients, massage for patients in a psychiatric ward, and massage for terminally ill patients in a hospice setting. In these cases, a physician or mental health professional develops an overall treatment plan for the patient that includes massage. The massage therapist is supervised to ensure that the techniques used are appropriate for the patient's overall treatment goals. This chapter introduces assessment procedures, treatment planning processes, and documentation practices that are specific to healthcare massage and builds on the techniques and critical thinking skills described in Chapter 12.

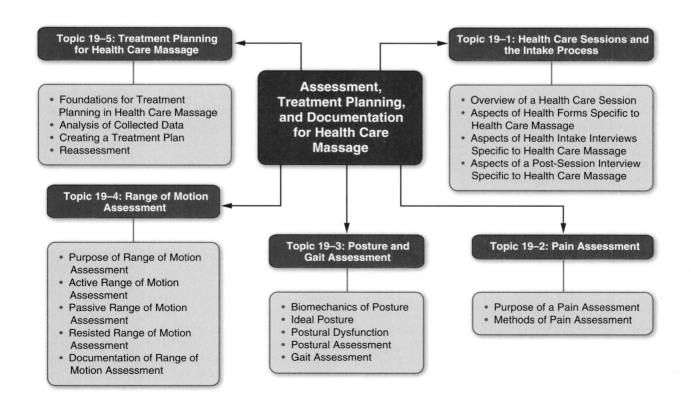

Topic 19–5: Treatment Planning for Health Care Massage
- Foundations for Treatment Planning in Health Care Massage
- Analysis of Collected Data
- Creating a Treatment Plan
- Reassessment

Assessment, Treatment Planning, and Documentation for Health Care Massage

Topic 19–1: Health Care Sessions and the Intake Process
- Overview of a Health Care Session
- Aspects of Health Forms Specific to Health Care Massage
- Aspects of Health Intake Interviews Specific to Health Care Massage
- Aspects of a Post-Session Interview Specific to Health Care Massage

Topic 19–4: Range of Motion Assessment
- Purpose of Range of Motion Assessment
- Active Range of Motion Assessment
- Passive Range of Motion Assessment
- Resisted Range of Motion Assessment
- Documentation of Range of Motion Assessment

Topic 19–3: Posture and Gait Assessment
- Biomechanics of Posture
- Ideal Posture
- Postural Dysfunction
- Postural Assessment
- Gait Assessment

Topic 19–2: Pain Assessment
- Purpose of a Pain Assessment
- Methods of Pain Assessment

Topic 19-1
Healthcare Sessions and the Intake Process

This topic considers the sequence of events that often occur in a healthcare massage, in advance of later chapter sections presenting specific assessment techniques. It also covers documentation related to intake interviews, functional goal setting, and client self-care.

Overview of a Healthcare Session

The sequence of events in a healthcare massage is often the same as in a wellness massage, as discussed in Chapter 10. Described here are additional events that do not occur in a wellness massage but are specific to healthcare massage. Every situation is unique, however, and every session does not follow this exact sequence. For example, a client in a hospital receiving massage for condition management might not benefit from a posture and gait assessment. These issues are discussed later in this chapter.

BOX 19-1 Sequence of Events in a Healthcare Massage

- Client greeting and completion of intake forms including pain questionnaire
- Tour of the facility
- The intake interview
  - Review policy and procedures
  - Rule out contraindications through a review of health forms
  - Score a pain questionnaire
  - Discuss client symptoms
  - Discuss functional limitations and goals
  - Discuss client expectations
- Physical assessment
  - Posture and gait assessment
  - Range-of-motion assessment
  - Palpation assessment
- Formulation of the treatment plan
- Implementation of the treatment plan during massage
- Postmassage physical assessment
  - Posture and gait assessment
  - Range-of-motion assessment
- Recommendation of client self-care activities
- Collect the fee (if applicable)
- Schedule the next appointment
- Say goodbye
- Complete chart notes

Box 19-1 outlines the events in a general healthcare massage typically related to a soft-tissue injury. The greeting, the tour of the facility, and the aspects of the interview related to policy and procedures, ruling out contraindications, and client expectations are often the same as in a wellness session. Clients still fill in paperwork, but the health history form is likely to be more comprehensive, and other intake forms such as a pain questionnaire might also be used, as described in upcoming sections. Healthcare sessions focus primarily on functional limitations, setting functional goals, and massage treatments that will help the client return to full function. Physical analysis such as a posture and gait assessment and range-of-motion assessment are conducted before finalizing the treatment planning process and transitioning into the massage. After the massage, the therapist conducts a postmassage physical analysis that may include a posture, gait, and range-of-motion assessment. The pre- and postassessments can be compared to explore the effectiveness of the massage treatment. The therapist may also want to suggest client self-care activities, such as the application of a hot pack or specific stretches to use between sessions.

Aspects of Health Forms Specific to Healthcare Massage

The health intake form for healthcare massage (Fig. 19-1) is generally longer than a form for wellness massage. With a wellness massage, the client may come once a month for relaxation or come to a clinic once while on vacation in the area and never return again. With healthcare sessions, however, the therapist is likely to work with a client regularly in an effort to achieve treatment goals over many sessions. You are also more likely to interact and share information with others on the client's healthcare team. The form shown here is one example that works well. You can adapt forms or create your own to best address the types of healthcare massage you offer.

The first section of this sample healthcare form is like that of a wellness form and gathers general contact information. The second section gathers information about the client's healthcare team. The client might list contact information for a physician, physical therapist, chiropractor, psychologist, acupuncturist, traditional Chinese medicine doctor, or other healthcare providers who manage the client's condition or symptoms. Recall the release of information form discussed in Chapter 6. Clients must give their permission for their health information to be shared with other healthcare providers on their teams.

On the second page of a typical form, the client prioritizes current health concerns and notes the severity of symptoms (mild, moderate, or severe) and whether they come and go (intermittent) or occur continually (constant). The client

(Text continued on page 561)

Client Name: _____ Birth Date: _____

Health Information

Client's Name: _____ Date: _____

Address: _____

Phone: _____ Occupation: _____ E-Mail: _____

Emergency Contact: _____ Phone: _____

Health Care Providers

Name:_____Occupation: _____

Address: _____

Phone: _____Fax:_____

Name:_____Occupation: _____

Address: _____

Phone: _____Fax:_____

Name:_____Occupation: _____

Address: _____

Phone: _____Fax:_____

Name:_____Occupation: _____

Address: _____

Phone: _____Fax:_____

Release of Information

Client name, _____
give my permission for (therapist's or business name) _____
to share or exchange pertinent information with my other health care providers listed above. This
agreement begins on _____(date) and ends on (date when the agreement needs to be
renewed) _____. I understand that this permission can be revoked at any time either
verbally or in writing.

_____Date:_____

Client or Guardian Signature:

Your Massage Business, 222 Any Street, Suite 300, Any Town, AS, 00990, 222-333-4444, www.ymb.com

Figure 19-1 The health intake form for healthcare massage is generally longer than a form for wellness massage, as this sample shows.

Client Name: _____ Birth Date: _____

Current Health Information

Please prioritize your current heath concerns and
check all boxes that apply.

1._____

☐ Mild ☐ Moderate ☐ Severe

☐ Intermittent ☐ Constant

Activities that aggravate this symptom:

_____

_____

_____

Activities you use to relieve this symptom:

_____

_____

_____

Currently this condition is:

☐ Getting worse ☐ Getting better ☐ No change

Treatment received: _____

_____

3._____

☐ Mild ☐ Moderate ☐ Severe

☐ Intermittent ☐ Constant

Activities that aggravate this symptom:

_____

_____

_____

Activities you use to relieve this symptom:

_____

_____

_____

Currently this condition is:

☐ Getting worse ☐ Getting better ☐ No change

Treatment received: _____

_____

2._____

☐ Mild ☐ Moderate ☐ Severe

☐ Intermittent ☐ Constant

Activities that aggravate this symptom:

_____

_____

_____

Activities you use to relieve this symptom:

_____

_____

_____

Currently this condition is:

☐ Getting worse ☐ Getting better ☐ No change

Treatment received: _____

_____

4._____

☐ Mild ☐ Moderate ☐ Severe

☐ Intermittent ☐ Constant

Activities that aggravate this symptom:

_____

_____

_____

Activities you use to relieve this symptom:

_____

_____

_____

Currently this condition is:

☐ Getting worse ☐ Getting better ☐ No change

Treatment received: _____

_____

Your Massage Business, 222 Any Street, Suite 300, Any Town, AS, 00990, 222-333-4444, www.ymb.com

Figure 19-1 *(Continued)*

Client Name: _____ Birth Date: _____

Functional Limitations

Please list the daily activities that are limited by this condition, or those activities you once performed but cannot perform now because of this condition (i.e., pick up grandchildren, jog, work on a computer, clean the house, garden, etc.)

1._____

2._____

3._____

4._____

5._____

6._____

7._____

8._____

9._____

10._____

List the self-care routines you use to feel better (i.e., heat pack, hot bath, pain medications, etc.)

1._____

2._____

3._____

4._____

Medications

Please list your medications including over-the-counter medications, vitamins, herbs or other supplements. Please provide the dosage that you take each day, the reasons why you take the medication and any side effects you experience:

_____

_____

_____

_____

_____

_____

_____

_____

_____

_____

_____

_____

Please list any surgeries, injuries or major illnesses including the dates and treatment received:

Surgeries:_____

_____

_____

Injuries: _____

_____

_____

Major Illnesses: _____

_____

_____

Your Massage Business, 222 Any Street, Suite 300, Any Town, AS, 00990, 222-333-4444, www.ymb.com

Figure 19-1 *(Continued)*

Client Name: _____ Birth Date: _____

Current and Past Conditions

Please check all current and previous conditions and give a brief explanation, if appropriate, in the comments section at the end of the form.

Current **Past**

Current	Past	Condition
☐	☐	Headache
☐	☐	Sleep disorders
☐	☐	Sinus condition
☐	☐	Skin condition
☐	☐	Athlete's foot
☐	☐	Warts
☐	☐	Skin sensitivities
☐	☐	Burns
☐	☐	Bruises
☐	☐	Sunburn
☐	☐	Aversion to scents
☐	☐	Aversion to oils
☐	☐	Aversion to cold
☐	☐	Allergies
☐	☐	Sensitivites to detergent
☐	☐	Rheumatoid arthritis
☐	☐	Osteoarthritis
☐	☐	Spinal conditions
☐	☐	Disc conditions
☐	☐	Lupus
☐	☐	Tendonitis
☐	☐	Bursitis
☐	☐	Fibromyalgia
☐	☐	Chronic fatigue
☐	☐	Dizziness
☐	☐	Ringing in ears
☐	☐	Head injury
☐	☐	Mental confusion
☐	☐	Numbness, tingling
☐	☐	Neuritis

Current	Past	Condition
☐	☐	Neuralgia
☐	☐	Sciatica
☐	☐	Shooting pain
☐	☐	Depression
☐	☐	Anxiety
☐	☐	Panic attacks
☐	☐	Heart disease
☐	☐	Blood clot
☐	☐	Stroke
☐	☐	Lymphedema
☐	☐	High blood pressure
☐	☐	Low blood pressure
☐	☐	Poor circulation
☐	☐	Swollen ankles
☐	☐	Varicose veins
☐	☐	Respiratory conditions
☐	☐	Urinary conditions
☐	☐	Abdominal pain
☐	☐	Thyroid dysfunction
☐	☐	Diabetes
☐	☐	Phlebitis
☐	☐	Pacemaker
☐	☐	Contact lenses

Other Conditions: _____

_____

_____

_____

Comments:_____

_____

_____

Therapist Name: _____

Date:_____

Therapist Signature: _____

Your Massage Business, 222 Any Street, Suite 300, Any Town, AS, 00990, 222-333-4444, www.ymb.com

Figure 19-1 *(Continued)*

describes the activities that aggravate the symptom and make it worse, and any activities that help relieve symptoms. If clients wish to list numerous health concerns, supply them with additional pages.

Functional limitations are daily activities that are limited by a condition or a symptom. A client lists these limitations on page three of the sample form shown here and describes self-care routines used to decrease symptoms. Clients often lose the ability to do small tasks that have great meaning to them, because of an injury or the onset of a condition. For example, Sarah, a 62-year-old grandmother, could pick up her grandchildren and carry them around without limitation before she was in a car accident. In the accident, she sustained a whiplash injury and now can't lift her grandchildren, even once during a day, without her neck pain increasing from mild to moderate. After any lifting, her neck pain persists sometimes for 2 or 3 days and is relieved only by warm packs and pain medication. Sarah's primary goal is to be able to lift her grandchildren without increased neck pain. Knowing this functional limitation and the importance of Sarah's grandchildren in her life will help you focus on treatment goals that address Sarah's neck pain.

Page three of this form is also used to gather information about medications, past surgeries, injuries, and major illnesses. Like page 2 of the wellness form, page 4 of the healthcare form provides a broad overview of a client's medical picture and is signed and dated by the therapist.

Overview of a Health Check-In Form

A health check-in form (Fig. 19-2) is used by some therapists before every healthcare massage session to get an up-to-date picture of a client's symptoms, the severity of symptoms, and any limitations the client is experiencing in activities of daily life. This form may also reveal improvements or setbacks from the previous session. You can use a health check-in in a written format as shown in Figure 19-2, or a form that allows clients to quickly chart their symptoms on human figures (Fig. 19-3).

Human figure illustrations can be used by clients to show pictorial representations of their symptoms or by therapists to document visual and palpation findings. This form is different from that used in a wellness session. The client draws circles around areas where they experience a symptom, indicates the type of symptom with a letter, and notes the severity of the symptom experience with a second letter. Pain in an area is noted with a P, while joint or muscle tension is noted with a T, and numbness or tingling is noted with an N. If the symptoms are mild, an L is used (to denote low pain, tension or numbness); moderate symptoms are indicated with an M, and an S indicates severe symptoms. Other ways of indicating symptoms and severity can also be used. The client is asked to describe any current functional limitations.

One benefit of this type of documentation is that it is quick and easy to use and simple to read. If clients are asked to document their symptoms on human figures before every session, the therapist can tell at a glance if the client is making progress. The number and the size of circles should decrease, and the symptom ratings (L, M, S) should be lower. Fewer functional limitations should be listed. This type of documentation also shows if the client is getting worse or developing new symptoms. Over time, these forms provide invaluable information for treatment planning.

Aspects of Health Intake Interviews Specific to Healthcare Massage

The initial healthcare session interview can be fairly complex and involve much physical assessment (e.g., posture, gait, range of motion, palpation). As with the wellness session described in detail in Chapter 10, you are likely to begin with a review of policies and procedures, a discussion of the client's general medical information to rule out contraindications to massage, and a review of the informed consent form. If the client's condition causes pain, it is useful to ask the client also to fill in a pain questionnaire (discussed in Topic 19-2).

In all cases, gather and record detailed information about the client's symptoms, location, severity, occurrence, onset, and exacerbating or relieving activities. This process is described in depth in Chapter 12. In a healthcare session, you are more likely working with a client who has suffered an injury (e.g., car accident, sports injury, or repetitive stress injury) or has a diagnosed condition (e.g., fibromyalgia, rheumatoid arthritis, cancer, anxiety disorders, etc.). You may have a prescription from the client's physician to provide massage or a referral from another healthcare professional. These members of the client's healthcare team may specify some of the treatment goals for massage. For example, a client may be sent to a massage therapist specifically to decrease muscle tension in the hamstrings, erector spinae muscles, and psoas muscles. This will be stated on the client's prescription from the treating physician. In any case, you should discuss and record the client's functional limitations and work with the client to list functional goals. If the client's needs seem broader than the prescription, you may need to discuss the case with the physician with the client's consent.

Functional Outcomes Reporting

Functional outcomes reporting is a form of SOAP or chart notes that focus on the client's ability to function in activities of daily life. As the therapist, you document the client's functional limitations and work with the client to develop meaningful functional goals. Treatment focuses on helping clients reach their functional goals so that they can perform necessary activities without increased symptoms and participate in activities of value to them.

Functional Limitations

Functional limitations are defined as any restriction or impairment of basic functions. Basic functions include

Therapist Name: _____ Date: _____

Health Check-In

Client's Name: _____ Today's Date: _____

Date of Injury: _____ Client Date of Birth/Insurance ID: _____

Current Symptoms & Limitations

Please prioritize your current symptoms and describe the limitations you are experiencing today:

1._____ ☐ Mild ☐ Moderate ☐ Severe

Limitations: _____

_____

_____

_____ ☐ Mild ☐ Moderate ☐ Severe

Limitations: _____

_____

_____

_____ ☐ Mild ☐ Moderate ☐ Severe

Limitations: _____

_____

_____

_____ ☐ Mild ☐ Moderate ☐ Severe

Limitations: _____

_____

_____

Comments

_____

_____

_____

Therapist Signature: _____ Date: _____

Your Massage Business, 222 Any Street, Suite 300, Any Town, AS, 00990, 222-333-4444, www.ymb.com

Figure 19-2 Health check-in form in written format. A health check-in form is used by some therapists before every health-care massage session to get an up-to-date picture of a client's symptoms, the severity of symptoms, and any limitations the client is experiencing in activities of daily life.

Therapist Name: _____ Date: _____

Health Check-In

Client's Name: _____ Today's Date: _____

Date of Injury: _____ Client Date of Birth/Insurance ID: _____

Current Symptoms & Limitations

Please prioritize your current symptoms by drawing a circle around the location and adding letters to the figure to indicate the type of symptom and its severity.

Key
P = Pain
T = Muscle/joint stiffness/tension
N = Numbness or tingling

L = Symptom Mild
M = Symptom Moderate
S = Symptom Severe

List and describe
current limitations:

_____
_____
_____
_____
_____
_____
_____
_____
_____
_____
_____
_____
_____
_____

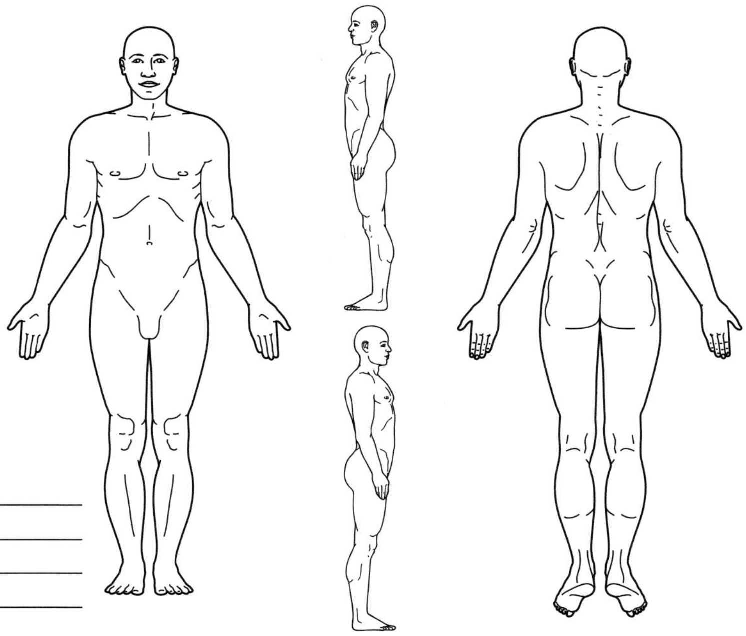

Comments

_____
_____
_____

Therapist Signature: _____ Date: _____

Your Massage Business, 222 Any Street, Suite 300, Any Town, AS, 00990, 222-333-4444, www.ymb.com

Figure 19-3 Health check-in form in human figures format. In this version of a health check-in form, the client can quickly chart their symptoms on human figure illustrations.

seeing, hearing, speaking, walking, standing, sitting, carrying, lifting, walking up and down stairs, moving the arms, legs, trunk, or head, or grasping and holding objects. Functional limitations impact a client's ability to participate in activities of daily living. Primary activities of daily living include getting around inside the home, getting in and out of bed, bathing, dressing, eating, getting a full night's sleep, and going to the toilet. People must also be able to keep their homes clean, get around outside the home, use the telephone, pay bills, shop for food, prepare food, care for children, drive cars, and perform employment tasks. People participate in additional activities that hold meaning and value in their lives. They may take walks with friends, garden, ride bikes, dance, take yoga classes, go to movies, paint, and any number of other activities in which they bond with friends and family members and participate in the larger community.

An injury or pathology that causes functional limitations that restrict people's ability to participate in activities of daily life can impact them on many levels. Physically, they can't do what they once were able to do. This can make them feel weakened emotionally, which can influence their mental patterns. If they can't get out and connect with people normally, they may feel spiritually inhibited, lonely, and isolated. Limitations can range from minimal but annoying to completely debilitating, and it can sometimes be hard for others to truly understand and empathize with another's feelings about a physical restriction. For example, after a fall while cycling, Steve finds he can't run more than 5 mi without knee pain. At 6 mi the pain increases to a moderate-minus pain and at 8 mi to a moderate-plus pain. At 10 mi he has to stop running. To most people this individual seems highly functional, but Steve is a marathon runner, and these limitations seriously impact his ability to participate normally and fully in his life.

When the therapist focuses on comprehending a client's functional limitations and how these limitations impact the client's activities of daily life, the therapist is better able to provide guidance in the goal-setting process.

Functional Goals

Functional goals are written before session goals to define the particular activities the client would most like to accomplish in daily life without a significant increase in symptoms. Review the information the client provides in the S section of the SOAP chart, particularly the section where the client describes activities that aggravate the condition. Aggravating activities often relate to work or life duties such as driving to work, sitting at a computer, or caring for children. Often, clients must participate in these activities to maintain some normalcy in life. You should also question clients about activities that have recreational or social value for them and add to their life's meaning. Ask the client to prioritize two or three activities that are particularly important. Set goals involving these activities.

The acronym SMART is used as a reminder to write useful goals that lead to reliable outcomes. In functional goal setting, keep these factors in mind when writing goals:

- **Specific:** The goal should relate directly to an activity of daily life and be as specific as possible. For example, "housework" is broad, but "vacuuming the floor twice a week" is more specific. "Child care" is broad, but "lifting a child in and out of a car seat" is specific.
- **Measurable:** Goals must be quantified and qualified in order to demonstrate progress. To quantify the goal, describe how much of the activity should be performable. For example, "lift 5 lb onto a conveyer belt for 1 hour three times during the day," or "run 3 miles," or "lift 30 lb toddler in and out of a car seat twice a day," etc. To qualify the goal, describe what the client should feel like at the completion of the activity. For example, "with no increase in pain," or "with only mild increase in pain," or "with no noticeable increase in muscle tension," or "with mild stiffness and soreness."
- **Attainable:** Guide the client toward setting goals that are realistic in relationship to the client's current condition. If the client experiences increased pain from moderate-plus to severe when driving 2 mi daily to work, it is unrealistic for the client to expect that he or she will have no pain with driving to work in a short time frame. A more attainable goal would be "to drive 2 miles daily to work with a smaller increase in pain from mild to moderate in 2 weeks; in 3 weeks drive 2 mi daily to work with moderate-minus pain."
- **Relevant:** The goal should feel relevant and meaningful to clients so that they feel motivated to participate in their own health care through self-care activities and make a commitment to massage treatment.
- **Time-bound:** Help clients set both long- and short-term goals. Long-term goals are commonly reached within 30 to 60 days, while short-term goals are written for a 7- to 14-day period. The goal should be as specific as possible. For example, "run 3 miles with moderate-minus knee pain in 12 days" rather than "run 3 miles with moderate-minus knee pain in about 3 to 4 weeks."

When the client has set one to three functional goals with your help, write the goals down in the A section of the SOAP chart. Write both a short-term goal and a long-term goal for the same functional limitation. When the client reaches a particular goal, it is documented as a functional outcome of treatment. Figure 19-4 shows a SOAP chart with functional goals and the functional outcome the client has already achieved.

Aspects of a Post-Session Interview Specific to Healthcare Massage

In a healthcare massage, you perform the same assessments after the session that you performed before the massage session. For example, if you conducted a posture and

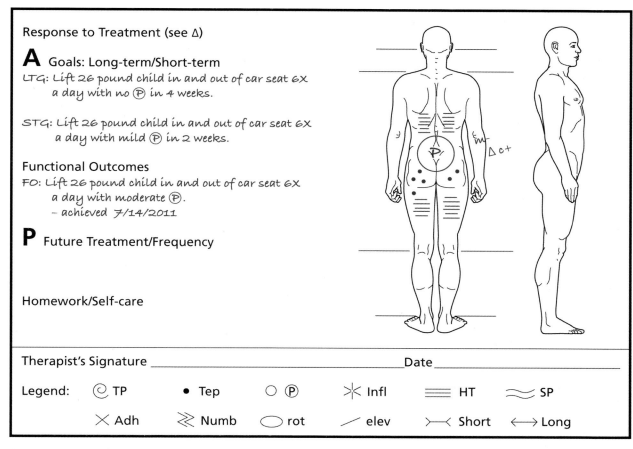

Response to Treatment (see Δ)

A Goals: Long-term/Short-term

LTG: Lift 26 pound child in and out of car seat 6X a day with no ℗ in 4 weeks.

STG: Lift 26 pound child in and out of car seat 6X a day with mild ℗ in 2 weeks.

Functional Outcomes

FO: Lift 26 pound child in and out of car seat 6X a day with moderate ℗.
– achieved 7/14/2011

P Future Treatment/Frequency

Homework/Self-care

Therapist's Signature _____ Date _____

Legend: ℃ TP   • Tep   ○ ℗   ✳ Infl   ≡ HT   ≈ SP

× Adh   ≫ Numb   ◯ rot   ╱ elev   ⟩─⟨ Short   ⟷ Long

Figure 19-4 SOAP chart section with functional goals and functional outcomes. When the client has determined one to three functional goals with your help, write the goals down in the A section of the SOAP chart. Write both a short-term goal and a long-term goal for the same functional limitation. When the client reaches a particular goal, it is documented as a functional outcome of treatment.

range-of-motion assessment before the session, you conduct a second posture and range-of-motion assessment after the session. This way you can document and compare the results of the two identical assessments to determine if your treatment improved the client's condition. At the end of testing, summarize for the client your findings during assessments, your reasons for your treatment choices, and the results you observed. Ask clients to describe their experience and document their statements. For example, you might write, "The client reports that her headache pain decreased from moderate to mild-plus." The client can also give you valuable feedback about the locations where massage felt particularly needed and the techniques that felt especially effective. Review the client's functional goals and discuss which aspects of the massage treatment felt like they were helping the client achieve goals. When you have discussed all aspects of the session results that are relevant, help the client take power in the healing process by providing some ideas for useful self-care activities he or she can use at home to increase the results from sessions.

Concept Brief 19-1
Functional Outcomes Reporting

Functional limitations: Daily activities that are limited by a condition or a symptom.

Functional goals: Particular activities the client would most like to participate in without a significant increase in symptoms.

Functional outcomes: Functional goals achieved by the client and related to benefits from regular healthcare massage.

Client Self-Care

Chapter 12 introduced self-care activities for clients. Recall that **client self-care** activities are actions the client performs that aid in recovering from an injury or managing a condition or disease. You want to suggest self-care activities that are simple enough for the client to remember and easy enough to fit into a busy life. These activities may include:

- **Hydrotherapy:** Depending on the injury and its stage in the inflammatory process, you might suggest the use of ice packs; warm or hot packs; cool, warm, or hot baths; or Epson salt baths. For example, if the client has hypertonic muscles in the back and neck that contribute to headache pain, the application of a hot pack to the area in the evening, accompanied by gentle neck stretches, can be very helpful for loosening the area and improving muscle tissue health.

- **Stretches:** Static postural positions held during repetitive activities such as sitting hunched at a computer during work hours can exacerbate a client's condition. Suggest one or two easy stretches the client can do to release muscle tension in specific areas throughout the day. For example, "Eduardo, three times during the work day, sit up straight in your chair and stretch your neck to each side by bringing your ear directly to your shoulder."

- **Self-massage:** Encourage clients to purchase massage bars or self-massaging tools to use daily to release muscle tension in target areas.

- **Rest/breaks:** Clients who work at jobs that involve manual labor can be encouraged to take regular breaks or to take naps to decrease fatigue and relax the body.

- **Referrals:** Depending on the client's condition, you might refer the client to another health professional such as a fitness trainer or physical therapist to help the client build strength in weakened muscles.

Record suggested self-care activities in the homework section listed under the P in many SOAP chart formats. At subsequent health interviews, follow up with self-care and document the activities clients are using to improve their health.

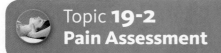

Topic 19-2
Pain Assessment

Clients seeking healthcare massage are often in pain. Pain can be caused by a soft-tissue injury or as a symptom of a variety of conditions such a fibromyalgia or arthritis, among many others. Pain is an unpleasant feeling that signals actual or potential injury to the body and that has both physical and emotional components. Physically, pain results from sensory nerve stimulation. Emotional factors influence how pain is perceived both consciously and unconsciously, making pain a highly personal, individual experience. The experience of pain can range from a mild, localized sensation of discomfort to general, diffuse discomfort, to agony. This section describes pain assessment methods and provides some practical tools for measuring the client's perception of pain. The anatomy of pain is discussed in greater detail in Chapter 23.

Purpose of a Pain Assessment

Pain assessment involves a number of methods that can be used to describe a client's experience of pain at a given point in time. Pain assessment has a number of benefits and uses:

- **Inform treatment planning:** Understanding the location, quantity, and quality of a client's experience of pain is essential for choosing appropriate techniques and methods for a session.

- **Prove injury:** In situations where a client must prove injury or loss of function due to a condition or disease to an insurance provider, court, or employer, pain assessment provides documentation that is useful for the case.

- **Demonstrate progress:** Regularly conducted pain assessments can demonstrate to a referring physician and an insurance company that massage treatment is reasonable

and necessary, ensuring that the client can continue treatment until fully healed.

- **Encourage clients:** Because healing processes can be lengthy, clients often feel discouraged as they cope with the changes to their lives brought about by injury or disease. Sharing improvements demonstrated through regularly conducted pain assessments helps clients recognize their improvement.

Methods of Pain Assessment

Questionnaires, analog measures, or combinations of these two methods are easy to use in a massage practice. Ask clients to complete your pain assessment form on their first visits. Direct clients to complete the entire form and to describe their current experiences of pain (what they feel right now). Review the form and question clients about their answers if needed when determining treatment plans. Re-administer forms every six to eight sessions, and keep the results in the client's file. A number of different methods of pain assessment are used in health professions, including:

- **Analog measures:** Analog measures have extremes (no pain vs. extreme pain) on the ends of a continuum line. Clients place a mark on the line to indicate their experience of pain in a visual scale. Analog measures also use verbal scales (mild, moderate, severe) and numerical scales (0 to 10), although visual scales are believed to be more reliable. Figure 19-5 illustrates different types of analog measures. Analog measures are often used on pain questionnaires.

- **Area-specific pain and disability indexes:** Two indexes are widely used in healthcare professions to capture the experience

Figure 19-5 Analog measures.
A. Visual. **B.** Verbal. **C.** Numerical.

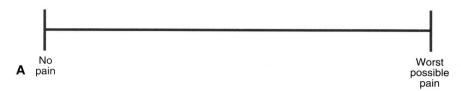

Mark the place on the line that best demonstrates your experience of pain.

A No pain — Worst possible pain

Circle the word that best describes your experience of pain.

No pain	Just noticeable	Weak
Moderate	Uncomfortable	Strong
Excruciating	Severe	Intolerable

B

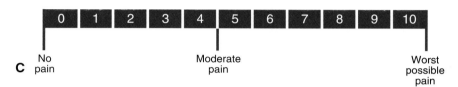

Choose the number that best demonstrates your experience of pain.

| 0 | 1 | 2 | 3 | 4 | 5 | 6 | 7 | 8 | 9 | 10 |

C No pain — Moderate pain — Worst possible pain

of pain related to the low back or the neck: the Oswestry Low Back Pain and Disability Index and the Vernon-Mior Neck Pain and Disability Index. Both indexes are scored by assigning a value to each answer (0 to 5) in the 10 different sections of the index. The scores are added together and multiplied by 2 to determine an overall disability rating. Pain and disability indexes are also readily available for other areas of the body, such as the shoulder or knee. Conduct an online search using the search phrase "pain assessment tools" to find indexes that works best for your practice or a particular client.

- **Functional Rating Index:** The Functional Rating Index, which is not specific to any body area, is widely used in healthcare professions. It captures pain data related to function for any injury or condition. It is often the easiest to adopt and use in a massage practice.

Concept Brief 19-2
Pain Assessment

- Pain assessment involves a number of methods that can be used to capture a client's experience of pain at a given point in time.
- Questionnaires, analog measures, or combinations of the two are easy to use to capture pain data in massage practice.
- Conduct pain assessments every 6 to 8 weeks during client re-evaluations to record changes in the client's pain history that hopefully demonstrate that massage treatment is effective and necessary.

Topic **19-3**
Posture and Gait Assessment

The term **posture** refers to the arrangement of the body's parts in space, in other words, the body's position. Gait is the client's walking pattern. Posture and gait assessment are regularly used in healthcare massage to gather information that guides treatment choices. This section explores the basic biomechanics of posture and gait, postural dysfunctions, and assessment procedures for findings that can be used in the treatment planning process.

Biomechanics of Posture

The human skeleton comprises long bones and a multi-jointed spine. Joints are strapped together by ligaments, and the whole structure is held erect against the forces of gravity with coordinated muscle activity. Reflex mechanisms that are "hard-wired" into the neural system of the brainstem and spinal cord control the muscles maintaining posture. For example, consider that the skeleton is a tall structure poised on a rather small base. Its center of gravity is quite high, located just above the pelvis. For the body to remain stable, the center of gravity must be maintained within this base or the structure will topple. Even in situations of unstable equilibrium, people are able to maintain their balance because of postural reflexes and the unique characteristics of postural muscles.

Postural muscles (also called tonic muscles) are composed of slow-twitch, red fibers that can sustain a semicontracted state for long periods of time and have high levels of endurance because their fibers fire not in unison but rather in segments. As one section contracts, another relaxes, so that the muscles share the workload of holding the body upright against gravity. If joints in the body become misaligned for any reason, these muscles become hypertonic and the body produces additional connective tissue to help the muscles brace and compensate for these misalignments. Over time, the tissue becomes unhealthy and trigger points form, which can lead to chronic pain conditions.

Massage supports good posture by helping to balance muscles so that the body can more easily achieve alignment and relaxed, coordinated movement.

Ideal Posture

When the skeleton is aligned properly, bones assume their normal and correct position at joints, which are held in place by strong, healthy ligaments. The muscular system is balanced (some muscles are not too tight while others are not too weak), and the body can disperse the forces of gravity efficiently and stand or move with little effort.

Ideally, gravity acts in an equalized line on the physiological curves of the spine, but very few people actually have perfect posture. As well, posture is not static and fixed. It is dynamic and adaptive, allowing the body to move and function in a variety of circumstances and conditions.

Although people are not perfectly symmetrical, the body should demonstrate horizontal and vertical consistency. The greater the degree of lack of symmetry in the left and right sides of the body, the greater is the potential for injury or dysfunction.

A person with good posture looks symmetrical and moves gracefully (Fig. 19-6). The nose, chin, sternum, spine, and navel align vertically down the center of the body. Bilaterally from the anterior view, the eyes, ears, shoulders (acromion process), pelvic girdle anterior superior iliac spine (ASIS), fingertips, knees (patella), and outer anklebones (lateral malleoli) align on the same horizontal level.

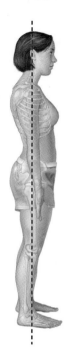

Figure 19-6 Ideal posture. When the skeleton is aligned properly, bones assume their normal and correct position at joints, which are held in place by strong, healthy ligaments. The muscular system is balanced (some muscles are not too tight while others are not too weak) and the body is able to disperse the forces of gravity efficiently and stand or move with little effort.

Bilaterally from the posterior view, the ears, shoulders, superior angle of the scapulae, pelvic girdle posterior superior iliac spine (PSIS), fingertips, and lateral malleoli align on the same horizontal levels. When viewed from the side (lateral aspect), an imaginary vertical line runs through the center of the ear, through the center of the glenohumeral joint, through the bodies of the lumbar vertebrae, through the center of the greater trochanter of the femur, through the center of the tibiofemoral joint, and through the talocrural joint.

When the alignment of body parts such as the joints are altered, the stresses on the body change, and this can lead to a variety of biomechanical problems. Soft tissues and bones must respond to these changes or be damaged.

Postural Dysfunction

Postural dysfunction can be simply defined as any position of the body that exerts undue strain on body structures including joints, ligaments, fascia, muscle, nerves, blood vessels, and bones. Dysfunctional body positions cause adaptations that lead to unhealthy tissues and a variety of other complications. Postural muscles must brace misaligned joints to maintain the body's erect posture. This causes some muscles to become chronically shortened, hypertonic, and prone to the development of trigger points. Other muscles become chronically overstretched and weakened, leading to microtrauma that causes an inflammatory response and pain. Fascia and connective tissue become dense and adhere, while nerve fibers and blood vessels are compressed under taught soft tissue. Postural dysfunctions can be classified as either functional or structural.

Functional postural dysfunctions refer to changes in soft-tissue structures like muscles, fascia, and connective tissue like ligaments and tendons. This type of dysfunction responds well to massage treatment because the therapist can lengthen shortened muscles and use techniques that help strengthen weakened muscles to support the body so it can find better balance. Stress to associated blood vessels and nerves is reduced, and tissue health improves.

Structural postural dysfunctions are pathological processes or genetic abnormalities that cause changes in the shapes of bones, placing soft tissue like ligaments and muscles under greater stress. While massage therapists cannot correct the shape of bones, they can help the soft tissues of the body achieve greater health and balance as these structures attempt to brace against misalignments.

Factors that Influence Posture

The previous section defined postural dysfunction as any position of the body that exerts an undue strain on body structures. Many factors can influence posture and lead to postural dysfunction. The following factors often contribute to how a person holds the body and moves through space.

- **Heredity:** Genetic factors such as the shape and physiology of tissues can influence posture. In addition, some conditions of the spine that lead to postural dysfunction are linked to a person's genetic makeup.
- **Disease:** Any disease that affects muscle tone, joints, the bones, or neurological function or that causes pain is likely to impact posture. For example, muscular dystrophy is a group of genetic diseases that cause a progressive atrophy of skeletal muscles leading to a loss of muscular strength, disability, and deformity. Rheumatoid arthritis is an autoimmune disease affecting the synovial membranes of joints. The inflamed tissue releases enzymes that erode cartilage and cause the joint to become deformed over time.
- **Habits:** People develop movement patterns early in childhood that can persist into adulthood and lead to postural dysfunctions. For example, think of slouching teenagers. Some habits develop from work life such as the head-forward and rounded-shoulders position caused by hunching over a computer screen.
- **Environment:** A person's environment can influence posture especially if it causes repetitive actions that place undue stress on muscles and joints. Sitting for long periods of time in a poorly constructed or improperly adjusted office chair can lead to postural positions that cause low back problems.
- **Injury:** When one area of the body is injured, other areas compensate, and often these compensational patterns become habitual. Any injury that affects the position of a joint, movement, or structures including bones, muscles, ligaments, and tendons or that causes pain is likely to influence a person's posture and movement.

- **Lifestyle:** Past chapters have discussed the effects of a sedentary lifestyle on muscles and fascia. We know that good nutrition, regular exercise, and activities to reduce stress support the overall function of the body. Any lifestyle choice that impacts overall health or that leads to weakened muscles is likely to influence posture.
- **Compensation patterns:** The body is highly adaptive. It makes whatever changes it needs to stay as functional as possible. A person who suffers a knee injury is likely to place more weight on the uninjured leg. Even when the injury is completely healed, this person may continue walking with a slight limp out of habit. This compensation pattern places undue strain on the uninjured leg, pelvis, and spine. These types of patterns influence posture.
- **Mental and emotional state:** A person's thoughts, attitudes, and emotional state can impact posture. Think about the position the body acquires when a person experiences grief. Often, the chest sinks and the shoulders become rounded while the forehead tilts toward the ground. Even when the person overcomes the grief and moves into a happier mind and emotional state, the postural habit may remain and impact the balance of the body.

Common Postural Conditions

When viewing the client from the side, you will notice three visible spinal curves (Fig. 19-7): in the lumbar region, in the thoracic region, and in the cervical region. A fourth curve, created by the sacrum and the coccyx and called the coccygeal curve, is not visible.

Before birth and when an infant is born, the spine is in flexion, so the thoracic curves (and the accompanying coccygeal curve) are considered *primary* curves. When infants begin to hold up their heads, the cervical curve begins to develop. When they start to sit up and walk, the lumbar curve develops. These curves are considered *secondary* curves.

If the spine has too little curve, it is likely to be more rigid and inflexible. If the spine has too much curve, it is likely to be unstable. The position of the pelvis plays an important role in determining the degree to which the spine curves. If the pelvis is rotated anteriorly, this rotation increases the lumbar curve and the thoracic and the cervical curves also increase to brace against the forces of gravity. If the pelvis is rotated posteriorly, the lumbar curve is decreased and the thoracic and the cervical curves also decrease, giving the spine a flattened appearance. Hyperlordosis, hyperkyphosis, scoliosis, and head-forward position are common postural conditions encountered by massage therapists.

Hyperlordosis

Hyperlordosis (also called lordosis) is an abnormal increase in the lumbar curve of the spine (Fig. 19-8). Hypertonic iliopsoas muscles and rectus femoris muscles due to prolonged postural positions such as slouching or standing on hard surfaces for work often cause this condition. Contributing factors include wearing high-heeled shoes, abdominal muscles weakened through disuse or because of abdominal surgery, obesity, and pregnancy. Hyperlordosis may contribute to the development of other postural conditions, such as hyperkyphosis and head-forward position. Muscles that are hypertonic include the erector spinae, quadratus lumborum, iliopsoas, rectus femoris, tensor fascia latte, and the adductors. Muscles that are overstretched and weakened include the gluteus maximus muscles, the abdominal muscles, and the hamstrings.

Hyperkyphosis

Hyperkyphosis (also called kyphosis) is an abnormal increase in the thoracic curve of the spine (Fig. 19-9) that causes a humpbacked appearance. Prolonged postural positions such as hunching, sleeping in a tightly curled fetal position, or sitting hunched at a computer, or pathologies including osteoporosis and ankylosing spondylitis (a condition that causes fusion of the spine in a hyperkyphotic position) cause this condition. Other postural conditions such as sway or flatback (evidenced by tight hamstrings and abdominal muscles), shoulder protraction (shoulders rolled anteriorly), and head-forward positions accompany or contribute to the development of hyperkyphosis. When hyperkyphosis is accompanied by a head-forward position, which is common, the muscles that are hypertonic include the sternocleidomastoids, upper trapezius, suboccipitals, levator scapulae, scalenes, pectoralis major and minor, subclavius, serratus anterior, and anterior intercostals. Muscles that are overstretched and weakened include the rhomboids, middle trapezius, erector spinae in the thoracic region, longus capitis, and longus cervicis.

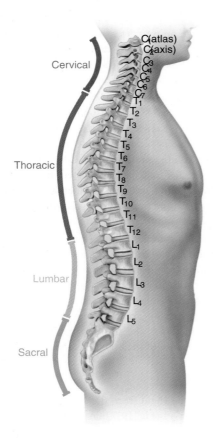

Figure 19-7 Normal spinal curves. When viewing the client from the side, you will notice three visible spinal curves. There is a curve in the lumbar region, in the thoracic region, and in the cervical region. A fourth curve, created by the sacrum and the coccyx and called the coccygeal curve, is not visible.

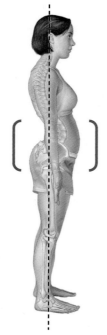

Figure 19-8 Hyperlordosis (also called lordosis) is an abnormal increase in the lumbar curve of the spine.

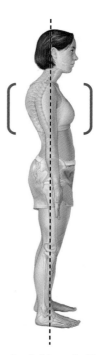

Figure 19-9 Hyperkyphosis (also called kyphosis) is an abnormal increase in the thoracic curve of the spine that causes a humpbacked appearance.

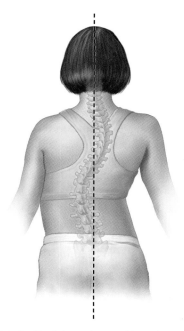

Figure 19-10 **Scoliosis** is an abnormal lateral curve of the spine.

Scoliosis

Scoliosis is an abnormal lateral curve of the spine (Fig. 19-10). It may be either functional or structural. Functional scoliosis is caused by imbalances in the feet or legs (e.g., one leg is shorter than the other), imbalances in the right and left psoas muscles, or imbalances caused by right- or left-handedness that lead to a lateral pelvic tilt or a pelvic rotation that places stresses on the spinal column causing it to distort laterally. Functional scoliosis can be resolved or improved if the factors causing the imbalances are eliminated.

Structural scoliosis is caused by spinal deformities, usually genetic or congenital, that cause vertebrae to rotate and the ribcage to shift. Factors leading to structural scoliosis include abnormal muscle spindle reactions, imbalances in the labyrinth of the inner ear, abnormally sized structures (e.g., the right halves of the vertebral bodies, ribs, and humerus are larger than the left, while the left femur, fibula, clavicle and skull bones are larger), malnutrition, growth and sex hormones, and muscle imbalances. While massage therapists cannot change structural deformities, they can aid in decreasing pain and improving muscle health in people living with structural scoliosis.

In both types of scoliosis, the muscles on the concave side of the curve will be hypertonic, and muscles on the convex side of the curve will be overstretched and weakened.

Abnormal Head and Neck Positions

Abnormal head and neck positions are postural dysfunctions that lead to disordered flow of blood, lymph, and spinal fluid in the cervical region (Fig. 19-11). Structural deformities, hypertonic muscles, or weakened muscles can lead to painful neck conditions, trigger cervical disk disorders, or cause an increased risk of arthritis. Common abnormal head and neck positions include:

- **Head-forward position:** Head-forward position (also called forward head) is an abnormal posture in which the head is positioned forward of its correct alignment. Over time, this position of the head places strain on the cervical spine that may lead to disk problems. Prolonged postural positions such as slumping or hunching over a computer screen as well as conditions including injury, structural deformities, osteoporosis, hyperkyphosis, and arthritis can cause it.
- **Military neck:** Military neck refers to a postural dysfunction in which the cervical curve is abnormally decreased or absent, causing the posterior of the neck to appear elongated. The name originates from the position soldiers maintain while at attention. The sternocleidomastoid, longus capitis, and longus colli muscles tend to be hypertonic in this condition.

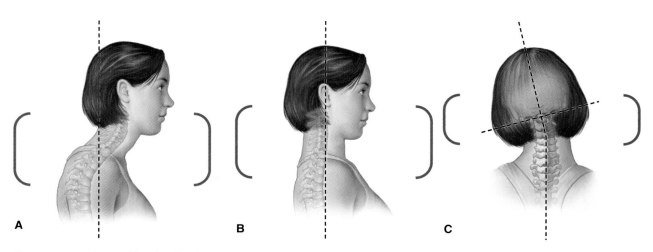

A B C

Figure 19-11 Abnormal head and neck positions are postural dysfunctions that lead to disordered flow of blood, lymph, and spinal fluid in the cervical region. **A. Head forward position. B. Military neck position. C. Lateral head tilt position.**

- **Lateral head tilt:** Lateral head tilt refers to a condition in which the head is maintained to one side or the other with a slight lateral flexion. This head position is often caused by a compensation for a weakness in one eye or the other. The sternocleidomastoid, scalenes, upper trapezius, and levator scapula muscles on one side are likely to be hypertonic.

Concept Brief 19-3
Common Postural Conditions

Hyperlordosis (lordosis): An abnormal increase in the lumbar curve of the spine.

Hyperkyphosis (kyphosis): An abnormal increase in the thoracic curve of the spine.

Scoliosis: An abnormal lateral curve of the spine.

Head-forward position: An abnormal posture in which the head is positioned forward of its correct alignment.

Military neck: An abnormal posture in which the cervical curve is decreased or absent.

Lateral head tilt: An abnormal posture in which the head is maintained to one side or the other with slight lateral flexion.

Posture Assessment

While the basic definition of posture is important, a broader understanding of the term *posture* is helpful. Posture is generally described not just as the position of the body but also as an *attitude, a stance, a cultivated position,* or *a pose that conveys attitude.* A person's posture tells the story of his or her life. It reveals relationships among thoughts, feelings, lifestyle, work habits, beliefs, and values. When we look thoughtfully at a person's posture, we have an insight into his or her world and can use this insight to support meaningful session planning.

Assessment Procedure

During a **posture assessment,** you evaluate the symmetry of boney landmarks, document your findings, and then analyze these findings to determine which soft-tissue structures need your focus during the session. You may add your findings from the posture assessment to findings from other methods of assessment, such as range-of-motion testing and palpation.

Equipment and Client Dress

A posture grid, plumb line, and footprint board are helpful assessment equipment to have if you intend to focus on healthcare massage (Fig. 19-12).

- **Posture grid:** A posture grid is a large, lined chart posted on a wall in the treatment room. The bottom of the grid should touch the floor, and its height should be taller than

the average adult client. The client stands in front of the grid during the posture assessment, and the lines of the grid help you identify muscular holding patterns that affect posture (e.g., one shoulder higher than the other). Sometimes, photos are taken in front of the grid to document progress over a series of sessions.

- **Plumb line:** A plumb line is a string with a weight fastened to one end. The string is attached to the ceiling and hangs in a perfect vertical line all the way to the floor; it should come all the way to but not actually touch the floor. Like the posture grid, the plumb line provides a reference point for assessment of a client's posture.

- **Footprint board:** A footprint board shows where the client should stand in relationship to the plumb line. Two lines intersect between the footprints marked on the board. One line is drawn from front to back and used during anterior and posterior assessment. The other is drawn from left to right and used for lateral assessment.

If you do not have these tools, you can still assess the client's posture against a bare wall and with palpation. Ideally, the client should wear a swimsuit or underwear during the assessment so that clothing does not distort your observations.

Evaluation and Documentation of Posture

During the posture assessment, you evaluate four views of the client (anterior, posterior, and both lateral views) and use boney landmarks as reference guides to determine the degree

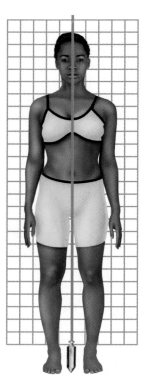
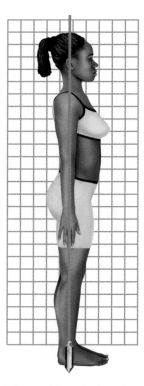

Figure 19-12 A posture grid, plumb line, and footprint board are helpful assessment equipment to have in your massage practice if you intend to focus on healthcare massage.

of symmetry in the body. Some therapists also observe clients from a position standing on a chair and looking down on them from a superior view. Develop a system for how you systematically complete the assessment. For example, you may choose to start with an anterior view and look at the body from the feet up. Alternately, you might start with the posterior view and look at the body from the head down. It is helpful to palpate bony landmarks as well as observe the body. This provides the best possible information on which to base your treatment plan and facilitates your correlation of tight or weak muscles with postural dysfunctions. Document each of your findings as you progress through the assessment, using lines to depict elevations and arrows in the direction of rotations (Fig. 19-13). Any observation that cannot be depicted with symbols on human figures is described in writing in the O section of a SOAP chart (review Chapter 12 for details).

ANTERIOR VIEW

Position the client so that the plumb line falls in front of the client directly between the feet. Instruct the client to place the weight evenly on both feet, look straight ahead, and let the arms hang relaxed at the sides. Starting with the feet, carefully observe the client using specific boney landmarks to determine the degree of symmetry on the left and the right sides of the body.

- **Feet:** How does the client naturally position the feet? Are one or both feet turned inward (pes varus), indicative of an internal rotation of the femur, or are one or both feet turned outward (pes valgus), indicative of an external rotation of the femur? Is the medial longitudinal arch of one or both feet decreased due to pronation (pes planus), or is the medial longitudinal arch of one or both feet increased due to supination (pes cavus)? Observe and palpate the levels of the medial and lateral malleoli to help you determine if the feet are pronating or supinating.

- **Knees:** How are the client's knees positioned? Rotation of the lower limbs occurs at the hip sockets. For example, medial rotation of the lower limb is often caused by hypertonicities in the adductor muscles of the inner thigh, while lateral rotation is often (not always) caused by hypertonicities in gluteal muscles and the deep lateral rotators of the thigh. Does the client demonstrate a knock-kneed (valgus) or bowlegged (vagus) pattern? Are the superior surfaces of both patellae aligned horizontally? Are there "bulges" on the medial sides of the knees? This can indicate that soft-tissue structures are bracing the knees against gravity due to misalignment of the bones of the legs.

- **Anterior thighs:** While examining the knees, also compare the size, shape, and orientation of the quadriceps muscles. Are the muscles well toned? Do any of the muscles appear to be pulling in particular directions? Are there pronounced differences between the right and left thigh? Does an imaginary straight line run from the center of the hip joint anteriorly to the center of the patellae?

- **Anterior superior iliac spine:** Palpate the levels of the ASIS and both iliac crests. Feel for an anterior pelvic tilt

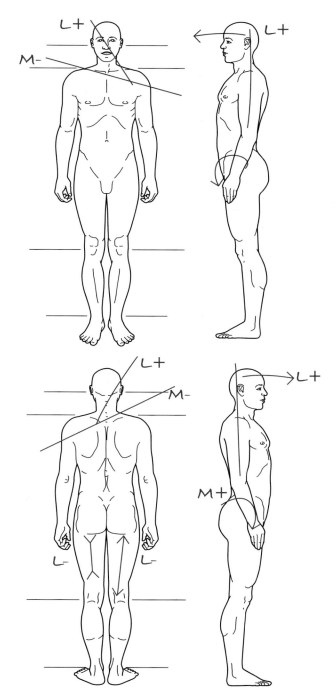

Figure 19-13 Document each of your findings as you progress through a posture assessment, using lines to depict elevations and arrows in the direction of rotations as shown here.

where the ASIS tips forward, or a posterior pelvic tilt where the ASIS is tipped back. The pelvis can also rotate forward and backward in a horizontal plane. Palpate to feel if one ASIS is positioned forward of the other. If the pelvis is rotated laterally, one hip may seem to be hiked up while the other is depressed.

- **Fingertips:** Stand back and evaluate the tips of the fingertips and their relationships to each other. Does one set of fingertips fall higher up on the thigh than the other? Is one hand rotated medially while the other is neutral? How do the arms hang? Are they straight or flexed at the elbow? What is the distance of the arms and hands from the sides of the body? Is it the same on both sides?

- **Sternum:** Check the position of the sternum and determine if it is lifted or depressed. What is the general shape of the chest? Do the left and right sides match, and is the client's breathing pattern relaxed and even?

- **Clavicles:** Are the clavicles horizontal? How similar or dissimilar are their positions in relationship to each other? Compare the height of the left and right shoulder. If one or both shoulders are elevated, the scalenes, upper trapezius, and lower trapezius muscles are likely shortened.

- **Head:** Use the ears (external auditory meatus), mandible, and two sides of the neck to determine if the head is tilted to one side or rotated to one side. Are the ears on the same horizontal plane? Is the mandible tilted to one side or the other? Are the two sides of the neck the same length? Notice the muscles of the neck. Hollows above the clavicles indicate that the scalene muscles are shortened. One sternocleidomastoid muscle may be more pronounced than the other.

POSTERIOR VIEW

Position the client so that the plumb line falls behind the body and directly between the feet. Observe, palpate, and document your findings using these landmarks:

- **Feet and legs:** Observe the position of the medial and lateral malleoli and the longitudinal arches of both feet from the posterior view, and compare your findings to what you discovered during the anterior assessment. Notice the Achilles tendons. Is one thicker than the other? Are they vertical or do one or both pull in a particular direction? Are the calves of equal size and shape on both sides? Palpate the levels of the fibular heads. Are they even? Are the hamstrings of equal size and shape on both legs? If you noticed varus or valgus tendencies from the anterior view, how do those findings relate to what you see from this view?

- **Posterior superior iliac spines:** Palpate the positions of the PSIS, the levels of both greater trochanters and both iliac crests, and correlate your findings with what you observed and palpated in the anterior view. Are the gluteal folds at the base of the buttocks horizontally aligned? If not, this can help you identify a pelvic tilt or a leg length difference.

- **Spine and trunk:** Use the plumb line or visualize a line running down the spine and notice the size and shape of the left and right sides of the body. Is the musculature on one side more developed than the other? Check for possible scoliosis.

- **Scapulae:** Observe and palpate the position of the scapulae by first assessing the inferior angles and their relationship to one another and to the spinous processes. Are the scapulae retracted, protracted, depressed, elevated, or rotated upward or downward? For example, do the scapulae lie against the body or do the inferior angles "wing" outward? This can indicate shortened rhomboids, trapezius, teres minor, infraspinatus, and lat muscles. Look at the muscles surrounding the scapulae and palpate these muscles to determine hypertonicities and weaknesses.

- **Acromioclavicular joints:** Observe and palpate the position of the acromioclavicular joints and notice their degree of horizontal symmetry.

- **Head:** Observe the relationship and position of the external auditory meatus and the level of the base of the occiput. Compare your findings when viewing the head and neck in the anterior position with this position.

LATERAL VIEWS

Position the client so that the plumb line falls in front of the client. You want the plumb line to fall slightly anterior to the lateral malleolus. Ideally, the plumb line aligns just anterior to the lateral malleolus, just anterior to the head of the fibula, directly through the head of the greater trochanter, and in a line with the acromion and the external auditory meatus (review earlier Fig. 19-6). Look first at the right side and then at the left side to determine if any of these landmarks fall anterior or posterior to the plumb line. Palpate structures such as the greater trochanter to better determine its position.

- **Knees:** You may notice that the knees are locked, flexed, or hyperextended.

- **Pelvis:** The pelvis might be tipped anteriorly or posteriorly. A rotated pelvis shows up in a lateral view because you will see one ASIS visible anterior to the other.

- **Spine:** Assess the spinal curves and determine if any of the curves seems increased or decreased. Notice the sacral, lumbar, thoracic, and cervical curves and palpate to determine if any vertebrae are projecting outward or drawn downward.

- **Trunk:** Notice the position of the trunk and check for rotations. For example, if one shoulder is visible anterior to the other, this indicates a rotation.

- **Shoulders:** The shoulders might be protracted, retracted, or situated in a neutral position.

- **Head:** The head might be tilted or pushed forward or backward.

Concept Brief 19-4
Body Areas to Examine in a Posture Assessment

Anterior View	Posterior View	Lateral View
Feet	Feet	Knees
Knees	Legs	Pelvis
Thigh	PSISs	Spine
ASI	PSIS	Trunk
Fingertips	Spine	Shoulders
Sternum	Trunk	Head
Clavicle	Scapulae	
Head (ears, mandible)	Acromioclavicular joints	
	Head (ears)	

Interpretation of Findings

To finalize your assessment, do one final scan of the body and notice the overall muscular balance. Think about the balance between opposing muscle groups. If the hamstrings are hypertonic, for example, you may find the quads have less than optimal tone. Perhaps the muscles around the scapulae are bound and the chest muscles are weak. Obtain one last view (often call the superior view) of the client by standing on a chair and looking down on him or her. This view helps you verify any rotations of the head, shoulder, pelvis, feet, or knees. Your goal is to identify muscles that are hypertonic and to lengthen shortened tissue, reduce trigger points in areas that are chronically bound, often from bracing the body against gravity, and then apply techniques that strengthen weakened muscles so that the body can find greater balance and freedom of movement. Table 19-1 provides a basic overview of muscles to investigate for hypertonicities based on general postural dysfunctions.

Gait Assessment

Gait is a person's walking patterns. Gait assessment is the observation of a client's walking patterns to gather information for treatment planning. Gait assessment can be a simple process used to confirm findings from a posture assessment and to identify areas of tension or stiffness that might be addressed in a massage session. Some health professionals, such as athletic trainers or physical therapists, might use a more detailed and complex process while training athletes for peak performance or during a rehabilitation process. The better your understanding of muscles, joints, and movement patterns, the easier it is to recognize muscle weaknesses based on how people holds themselves while walking.

Biomechanics of Gait

Ideally a person's gait is smooth, coordinated, rhythmic, and graceful with the body held erect, head up and eyes looking forward, and the thumb facing forward as the arms swing in opposition to the legs. The toes should point forward and not turn medially or laterally when the foot is placed on the ground. A person's step length is the distance between the point of first contact with one foot to the point of first contact with the other foot. Stride length refers to the point of first contact with one foot to the next point of contact with the same foot. In the two phases of the gait cycle, the foot is in contact with the ground and bearing weight (stance) or is swinging through and not bearing weight (swing) (Fig. 19-14).

TABLE 19-1   Postural Conditions and Shortened Muscles

Postural Condition	Muscles That May be Chronically Shortened
Pes varus (feet turn inward) with a valgus alignment of the knees (knock-knees)	Adductors, gluteus medius, gluteus minimus, tensor fascia latae
Pes valgus (feet turn outward) with a vagus alignment of the knees (bowlegged)	Gluteus maximus, iliopsoas, piriformis, deep lateral rotators
Pes planus (decreased medial longitudinal arch due to pronation)	Peroneal muscles
Pes cavus (increased medial longitudinal arch due to supination)	Tibialis anterior, tibialis posterior
Anterior pelvic tilt	Iliopsoas, rectus femoris, erector spinae, quadratus lumborum
Posterior pelvic tilt	Rectus abdominus, gluteus maximus, lateral rotators, hamstrings
Lateral pelvic tilt	Gluteus medius, quadratus lumborum, abductors on the side with the elevation, adductors on the side that is depressed
Hyperlordosis	Iliacus, psoas major, rectus femoris, quadratus lumborum
Hyperkyphosis	Muscles that extend the neck, pectoralis minor, anterior deltoid
Scoliosis	Erector spinae and paraspinal muscles on the concave sides of the spinal curves
Shoulder elevation	Scalenes, upper trapezius, lower trapezius
Shoulder rotation (medial)	Anterior deltoid, trapezius, pectoralis major and minor, teres major, serratus anterior
Shoulders retracted (scapulae pulled back)	Rhomboids, trapezius, teres minor, infraspinatus, latissimus dorsi
Head forward	Scalenes, splenius capitis, upper trapezius, semispinalis capitis
Military neck	Sternocleidomastoid, longus capitis, longus colli
Head tilted laterally	Sternocleidomastoid, scalenes, upper trapezius, levator scapula

Gait Cycle

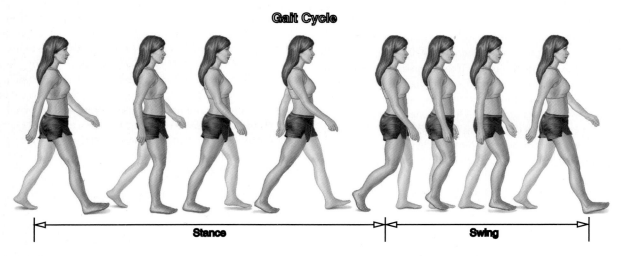

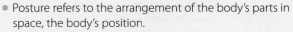

Figure 19-14 In the two phases of the gait cycle, the foot is in contact with the ground and bearing weight (stance) or is swinging through and not bearing weight (swing).

1. **Stance phase:** The stance phase begins with the heel strike of one foot, which leads to a load response as the foot flattens out, bearing the weight of the body. The foot is in a natural pronation and the trunk is aligned over the weight-bearing leg. The hip and knee extend as the pelvis falls slightly over the swinging leg. As the hip, knee, and ankle flex, the heel comes off the ground and the body's weight is shifted to the other leg. The stance phase of the gait cycle is complete when the toes come off the ground.

2. **Swing phase:** The swing phase begins when the toes leave the ground. The hip, knee, and ankle flex as the weight of the body is repositioned over the leg in the stance phase. The hip flexes and medially rotates as the knee moves into extension and the ankle dorsiflexes and supinates as the leg prepares to re-enter the stance phase with initial heel contact.

Assessment Procedure

Ideally, the client should be dressed in undergarments or a swimsuit and barefoot for the assessment. You need an area big enough for the client to walk freely while you observe gait anteriorly, posteriorly, and from both lateral views. Instruct the client to walk at a normal pace, and notice the motion and position of the feet, legs, pelvis, spine, trunk, shoulders, and head. Notice if the feet and/or knees rotate medially or laterally, if the client slaps his or her feet down on the heel strike (which can indicate weakness in the muscles that dorsiflex the foot), and if the pelvis dips latterly or anteriorly and posteriorly during the gait cycle. Record your findings in the O section of a SOAP chart in written notation, and use your observations to determine muscular imbalances. For example, weakness in hip adductors can allow the leg to rotate during the initial part of the swing phase, while a person with loss of coordination is likely to keep the feet farther apart while walking to increase stabilization. You can also analyze clients' shoes for wear patterns that indicate how their weight is distributed when walking or standing.

Concept Brief 19-5
Overview of Posture and Gait Assessment

- Posture refers to the arrangement of the body's parts in space, the body's position.
- The biomechanics of posture are complex. Even in situations of unstable equilibrium, people are able to maintain their balance because of postural reflexes and the unique characteristics of postural muscles.
- While people are not perfectly symmetrical, the body should demonstrate horizontal and vertical consistency.
- Postural dysfunction is any position of the body that exerts undue strain on body structures. Common postural dysfunctions include hyperlordosis, hyperkyphosis, scoliosis, and head-forward position.
- During a postural assessment, evaluate four views of the client (anterior, posterior, and both lateral views) and use boney landmarks as a reference guide to determine the degree of symmetry in the body.
- Gait assessment is the observation of a client's walking patterns in order to gather information for treatment planning.
- In the two phases of the gait cycle, the foot is in contact with the ground and bearing weight (stance) or is swinging through and not bearing weight (swing).

Topic **19-4**
Range-of-Motion Assessment

Chapter 13 introduced the topics of range of motion, limits to movement, and end feel. By this point in your massage training, you are likely well versed in these concepts. If you need a refresher, review that section of Chapter 13. This topic builds on that information and adds to an understanding of active, passive, and resisted joint movements used as an assessment tool.

Purpose of Range-of-Motion Assessment

Recall that the term *range of motion* refers to the amount of movement that is possible at a joint based on its structure. The normal range of motion of every joint is restricted by its natural anatomical and physiological characteristics. Anatomical restrictions are restrictions caused by the structures that make up the joint itself, such as bones and joint capsules. Physiological restrictions usually result when soft-tissue structures like muscles, tendons, and ligaments reach the extent of their ability to lengthen at the end of a joint's range of motion. This sensation is referred to as "firm end feel." It's the place where you will feel the structures "push back." Physiological restrictions typically limit the movement of the joint before an anatomical restriction is reached.

Pathological restrictions are abnormal restrictions that limit and decrease the joint's range of motion because of pain or structural dysfunction. Inflammation and fluid accumulation from an injury such as a sprain or strain, adhesions in muscle or fascia, sustained muscular contractions, weakened muscles, degeneration of joint cartilage, tendonitis in a tendon that crosses a joint, and inflammation of a bursa may all cause pathological restrictions. The purpose of **range-of-motion assessment** is to evaluate the client's ability to move and to identify any pathological restrictions present in a particular joint. Usually, only one or two joints are tested during an assessment. These joints usually relate to an area of injury or an observed postural dysfunction or are assessed because the client mentions pain and dysfunction in a particular joint during the health intake interview.

Active Range-of-Motion Assessment

During assessment of active range of motion, the client performs the movements available at a particular joint while the therapist evaluates the client's broad functional capacity, including willingness to move, general muscle strength and tone, coordination, and available range of motion. Active range of motion is the most general range-of-motion assessment method because during active movement both contractile tissue (muscle and tendon) and inert tissues (e.g., bursa, fascia, nerves, etc.) are affected. If the client experiences pain when performing a movement, any of these tissues could be damaged and causing the problem.

Active range of motion is performed before passive or resisted range of motion because if the client is not willing or able to move due to pain, other testing might be unnecessary or even contraindicated. If a particular movement markedly increases pain, assessment with passive or resisted range of motion might further stress tissues. The steps for performing an assessment using active range of motion are described in Technique 60.

Passive Range-of-Motion Assessment

In passive range-of-motion assessment, the therapist moves the client's joint through its normal motions and appraises the condition of the movement and pain levels. Inert tissues are evaluated throughout the movement; you should hone your sensitivity to movement patterns and movement quality so that you can identify fascial restrictions and crepitus. Crepitus is a grating, crackling, or rasping sound or sensation experienced under the skin of certain areas and in joints. In soft tissue, crepitus is caused by gas, most often air that has infiltrated an area. In joints, crepitus can indicate cartilage wear in the joint space.

Contractile tissues are assessed at the end of the joint's range of motion as muscle and tendons reach their ability to elongate. You move the joint to the end of the client's active range and then apply a slight overpressure to evaluate end feel. Overpressure can be described as the sensation of applying a gradual or gentle stretch to the tissue. If soft-tissue structures are so tight that they significantly restrict movement before the joint has reached the end of its range of motion, or if an injury or pathological condition stops the joint from achieving its full range of motion, this is called an abnormal or empty end feel. The steps for performing an assessment using passive range of motion are described in Technique 61.

Resisted Range-of-Motion Assessment

In resisted range-of-motion assessment (also called manual resistive tests), the client performs the selected joint motion while the therapist applies light resistance in the

Technique 60   Assessment with Active Range of Motion

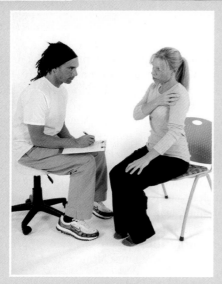

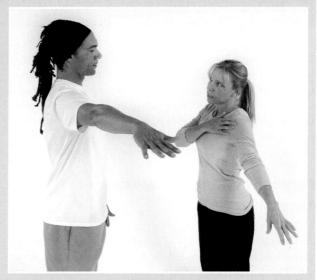

1. Determine the Joint and the Movements to Evaluate. During the health history interview, the client is likely to report which area of the body is causing pain and loss of function. If the client indicates that certain movements cause severe pain, there is no need to put the client through the distress of testing these motions. If, however, the pain is mild to moderate, assess the movements to document baseline information. Test both sides of the body even when only one side is affected. This way you can better determine what the client's "normal" looks like. Active range of motion can be performed in a number of different body positions (seated, standing, prone, supine, side lying) as long as a position doesn't limit a client's ability to move a joint in its full range.

2. Assess the Movement. As the client performs the movement, observe the motion carefully. Note when the movement causes pain, how much pain it causes, and where the pain is located. Capture the quality of the movement and note if it is smooth and coordinated, stiff, weak, clumsy, rigid, or difficult. Is the client compensating or guarding during the movement? Ask the client to describe what he or she experiences and feels while moving. Identify the structures involved in the movement and use this information to formulate some ideas about what might be causing pain and dysfunction. The more you understand biomechanics, kinesiology, and anatomy and physiology, the better you will be at determining which structures are implicated in a movement dysfunction. Make sure to carefully document all of your findings. It is helpful to show the client the movement you would like performed by demonstrating the movement properly yourself. Sometimes, you can give the client verbal directions such as, "Lift your arm out to the side like this and take it as far as you can without undo pain."

---

opposite direction of the muscle's concentric action so that the client contracts the muscle isometrically. The muscle contraction does not need to be maximized for the therapist to be able to evaluate the tissue. Resisted range of motion is used to determine the functional capacity of muscles and tendons during muscle contraction. Because the contraction is isometric, no movement occurs, and the therapist can rule out inert tissues as the problem if pain results. The strength of muscles and the strength loss due to motor nerve compression are often revealed by resisted range-of-motion assessment. The steps for performing an assessment using resisted range of motion are described in Technique 62.

Concept Brief 19-6
Range-of-Motion Assessment

Active ROM: Client performs the movement—This assesses the client's willingness and ability to move contractile and inert tissues.

Passive ROM: Therapist moves the client's joint—This assesses inert tissues throughout the movement and contractile tissues at end feel with overpressure.

Resisted ROM: The therapist resists the client's active movement—This assesses the functional capacity of muscles and tendons.

Technique 61   Assessment with Passive Range of Motion

Passive range-of-motion assessment evaluates inert tissue during movement and contractile tissue at the end of the joint's range of motion as these tissues approach the end of their ability to elongate. As with active range-of-motion assessment, test the unaffected side first to determine the client's "normal" movement pattern. Hold the body area gently but firmly and move it in clean patterns of movement. Ask the client to relax completely and allow you to move the joint without guarding the area. Pay attention to what you feel as you move the area, including sensations of fascial binding, muscle tension causing restriction, or crepitus. As you approach the end of the joint's range, assess end feel and determine if there are pathological issues related to the joint as you apply a slight overpressure. Ask the client to describe what he or she feels as you move the joint. If the client feels pain, note when in the movement the pain occurs or how much the pain increases with movement. If the pain is severe, there is no need to continue the testing for that particular movement. Identify the structures involved in the movement to determine which structures might be involved in dysfunction. Carefully document all of your findings in the client's SOAP chart.

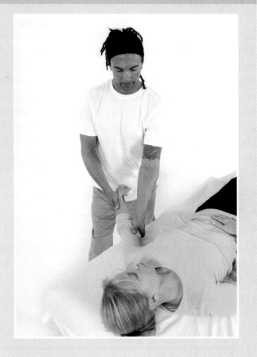

Technique 62   Assessment with Resisted Range of Motion

Because resisted range-of-motion assessment evaluates contractile tissue, it works well to have the client's body positioned in such a way that you can assess the target muscle when it is in the middle of its contraction (i.e., half-way through its range of motion). If applicable, test the unaffected side first to establish the client's "normal" muscle contraction. Place the client's body area in the proper position (half-way through its range of motion for the target muscle) and ask the client to hold this position while you resist the movement. The contraction is held only long enough to determine if there is pain or weakness with the movement. Avoid "strength contests" with clients. The muscle does not need to make a maximum force for the evaluation to be accurate. As you resist the client's movement, notice any weakness or unevenness in strength. If the client reports that the test causes pain, the injury is likely in the muscle or tendon. Weakness indicates neurological issues, motor nerve lesions, or systemic diseases. Weakness without pain may indicate a muscle-tendon rupture. If weakness is pronounced, refer the client to a medical specialist for further evaluation.

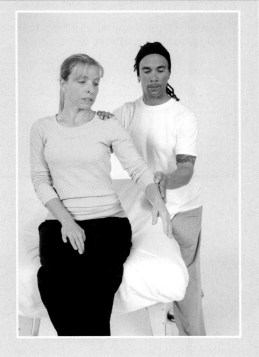

Documentation of Range-of-Motion Assessment

Range-of-motion testing is performed and documented both before and after the session to identify the level of dysfunction and verify progress brought about by massage intervention (Fig. 19-15). Periodic re-testing demonstrates continued progress for the client, other members of a healthcare team, or an insurance provider. It helps you recognize when a treatment plan is effective or needs to be re-evaluated for potential changes. The range-of-motion chart shown in Figure 19-15 provides structure for the testing. In the section labeled Pretest, note the following:

- The position of the client
- The type of test
- The joint you are assessing
- The actions at the particular joint that you evaluated
- Whether the range of motion was increased (hypermobile), decreased (hypomobile), or within normal limits
- The level of pain with movement
- The quality of the movement, such as rough, smooth, segmented, stiff, crepitus, etc.

BOX 19-2 Weakness Scale

Weakness is graded on a scale of 0 to 5 during resisted range-of-motion assessment.

- **0:** No contraction. No neurological activity in the muscle.
- **1:** Slight contraction. Slight neurological activity in the muscle.
- **2:** Low-strength contraction. Severe dysfunction in muscle contraction.
- **3:** Fair contraction. Range of motion achieved actively but no range of motion possible against resistance.
- **4:** Good contraction. Strength deficit evident.
- **5:** Normal contraction.

Any details that you feel are important can be described in narrative form in the O section of the SOAP chart. Weakness is often rated on a scale of 0 to 5 (Box 19-2) and can be included in the O section of the SOAP chart. After the massage session, repeat the test to determine how range of motion changed due to your treatment.

PRE-TEST 3 Initials ___KL___ Date ___07/27/2011___
Position of patient: prone, sidelying, sitting, (standing,) supine, other:_____

Type of test: (active,) active assisted, passive, resistive, other:_____

Joint: (C-spine,) T-spine, L-spine, hip, knee, ankle, shoulder, elbow, wrist, other:_____

Action	Quantity ↓ or ↑		Rate Pain		Rate Quality	
	®	Ⓛ	®	Ⓛ	®	Ⓛ
flex	WNL		L		smooth	
ext	WNL		L		smooth	
Lat flex	M+	L+	M-	M-	L+	L+
Ro+	M+	L+	M-	L-	M-	L+

PRE-TEST 3 Initials ___KL___ Date ___07/27/2011___
Position of patient: prone, sidelying, sitting, (standing,) supine, other:_____

Type of test: (active,) active assisted, passive, resistive, other:_____

Joint: (C-spine,) T-spine, L-spine, hip, knee, ankle, shoulder, elbow, wrist, other:_____

Action	Quantity ↓ or ↑		Rate Pain		Rate Quality	
	®	Ⓛ	®	Ⓛ	®	Ⓛ
flex	⟋		⟋		⟋	
ext	⟋		⟋		⟋	
Lat flex	M-	L-	M	M	L-	L-
Ro+	M-	L-	L+	L	L+	L-

Figure 19-15 Range-of-motion testing is performed and documented both before and after the session to identify the level of dysfunction and verify progress brought about by massage intervention.

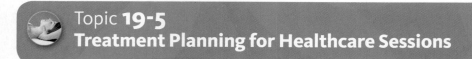

Topic **19-5**
Treatment Planning for Healthcare Sessions

Treatment planning for healthcare sessions is more complex than for wellness sessions. The client is likely to have a diagnosed condition or injury that affects your treatment choices. This section provides a foundation for treatment planning

by exploring the continuum of health, the rehabilitation process, methods for assessing the data you have gathered, ideas for how to create a treatment plan, and the reassessment process.

Foundation for Treatment Planning in Healthcare Sessions

Shared massage knowledge and research have documented the positive effects of massage for many conditions and client populations. In a healthcare massage session, you should match the treatment goals to the client's current level of health, functional goals, and particular condition. To do this, it is helpful to understand the continuum of health and the basic rehabilitation process for soft-tissue injuries.

Continuum of Health and Massage

Massage can be indicated for comfort care, condition management, therapeutic change, or health maintenance, depending on the client's health level. Before you read about how massage is indicated for particular client groups or specific conditions in Chapters 23 and 24, it is helpful to consider the continuum of health and identify the role massage can play for clients in each stage along the continuum. This understanding improves your critical thinking foundation when choosing appropriate treatment goals and techniques for the session.

Health can be viewed as a continuum where each person exists somewhere between two extremes (Fig. 19-16). Notice that the fields on Figure 19-16 flow into and out of each other. They are not fixed or static, because health is usually in constant flux. On one end of the spectrum are terminal illness and the dying process. On the other end are good health and optimal health. A client with a serious injury is likely to get better and move up the health continuum as his or her condition improves. On the other hand, a client with optimal health might one day sit down on the sofa, eat potato chips all day, and take up smoking. It won't be long before this client moves down on the health continuum. Health and wellness are constantly shifting, sometimes based on daily choices and activities, sometimes based on unexpected events (e.g., a car accident or sports injury). When contemplating

the continuum, keep in mind that although we often see the expression of poor or good health on a physical level, mental attitudes, emotional disturbances, coping resources, interpersonal relationships, stress levels, and spiritual influences also likely affect a client's state of health or disease. Remember also that as therapists we assess a client's health to help us make treatment choices, but we never judge a client's health. We accept clients as they are and never make any comments that might make them feel they are being judged. Massage therapists must also avoid stepping outside their scope of practice by not making nutritional or fitness recommendations to clients.

General massage treatment goals can be placed on the health continuum to match the client's needs in each area. This helps therapists think about treatment outcomes that are realistic for the client and achievable in a session. When reviewing the continuum and the general massage treatment goals, we must also acknowledge the limitations of this model. No model can capture the complexity of health and disease that therapists often see during the course of their professional practice. Avoid becoming locked into one mode of thinking about health, but remain flexible and adapt to each client's unique health history and personal health goals. View this model as one way to examine health issues, but not as the only way. Use it to think about health critically and to maintain a curiosity about health-related issues.

Terminal Illness, The Dying Process, and Comfort Massage

People on this end of the health continuum are most likely to continue to deteriorate, but good care can ease the end-of-life process. People who are dying may express concerns about being abandoned or losing control of their body functions, and worry about loved ones who will be left behind, be concerned about their appearance as they lose hair or develop dark circles under their eyes, or express regret about a long-ago wrong they may have done to another. In many

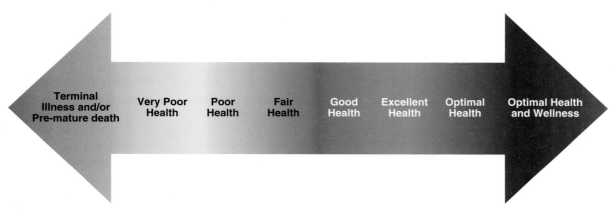

Figure 19-16 Health can be viewed as a continuum where each person exists somewhere between two extremes. General massage treatment goals can be placed on the health continuum to match the needs of clients in each area. This helps therapists think about treatment outcomes that are realistic for the client and achievable in a session.

cases, people who are terminally ill or dying are coping with physical pain and emotional distress. As their condition worsens, they may experience prolonged periods of sleepiness as their overall energy declines. Breathing changes may occur suddenly, with periods of rapid breathing and periods when breathing stops and then starts again. Appetite is likely to be depressed, and hallucinations may occur (seeing people or reliving scenes from the past).

In situations of serious illness, severe injury, terminal illness, or the dying process, massage provides comfort and reassurance. The massage might consist only of laying the hands on areas of the client's body to soothe anxieties before a medical procedure. Sometimes, it can be a foot massage that feels pleasurable and provides a break in the hospital routine. Sometimes, it is just holding the client's hand and sitting with the client, listening if needed, or remaining silent. In most cases, touch with loving care can promote calm, provide a respite from intense emotion or pain, and raise the spirits of the client, even if only temporally.

Pathology with High Life Impact and Condition Management

In this position on the continuum, a pathological or chronic condition significantly impacts the client's life. This might occur because of the nature of the pathology or because the condition is in an acute stage of inflammation or has flared up. For example, the difficulty with voluntary muscular control and unusually weak muscles of people living with cerebral palsy affects the activities they can undertake at all times. This is the nature of the condition. A person with rheumatoid arthritis, on the other hand, may experience minimal impact on the activities of daily life while the disease is in a subacute or chronic stage. During a flare-up or in the acute stage, the disease can cause pain and inflammation that completely incapacitate the person for a period of time.

Massage treatment goals in this range of the health continuum are based on the client's overall state, particular pathology, and current symptoms. Massage might be given for comfort, as described in the previous section, or may be used for condition management. When used for condition management, massage is not expected to cure the disease or alleviate the condition; rather, it is applied to reduce some symptoms or improve the body's ability to cope. For a client with cerebral palsy, for example, massage might be used to stretch and strengthen muscles. A client with rheumatoid arthritis in the subacute or chronic stage benefits from the release of tight muscles around affected joints, leading to greater range of motion.

Pathology with Moderate-to-Minimal Life Impact and Therapeutic Change

Many people live with pathologies and chronic conditions that exert moderate-to-minimal impact on their activities of daily life. A client with chronic tension headaches might be in excellent physical health until a headache hits. The headache may debilitate the client for an afternoon, but the next day the client is fine. A client living with fibromyalgia might experience constant, low-level soreness in muscles. This client may avoid some activities as a result or find that cleaning the house causes a flare-up and a day in bed with intense muscle tenderness.

Massage in this stage of the continuum is used for condition management or for therapeutic change. A person living with fibromyalgia might seek massage for condition management to decrease pain and fatigue or for a brief respite because massage temporarily reduces muscle soreness. Similarly, a client with osteoarthritis may have better range of motion with a monthly massage. In certain situations, the use of regular massage might decrease the occurrences of flare-ups. For example, people who experience regular migraine headaches have found that their number of headaches in a month decreased when they received regular relaxation massage.[1]

A client with tension headaches might seek massage for therapeutic changes. In this instance, massage is a tool to promote change in the client's physical, mental, emotional, or spiritual health. If massage sessions focus on the neck and shoulder muscles and on reducing trigger points in these areas, the tension headaches might completely disappear. A computer programmer who is diagnosed with carpal tunnel syndrome might seek massage as part of a rehabilitation program. Similarly, a client seeking greater physical ease and improved posture might incorporate massage into an overall wellness plan. A runner with tight hamstring muscles might visit a massage therapist to focus on releasing leg muscles as part of injury prevention or to improve recovery time from intense training sessions. Massage goals for therapeutic change focus on creating meaningful muscular and postural alterations for clients and helping clients improve their health.

Dysfunctional Health and Therapeutic Change

In this range of the continuum, a person is not sick and may not have a diagnosed condition but is not healthy. Fatigue, digestive disturbances, headaches, sleep disturbances, moderate-to-serious muscular tension, aches and pains, colds and flu are experienced regularly. Stress levels tend to be high, emotional coping skills may be low, and mental attitudes can tend toward the negative. Often, a person in this range of the continuum teeters on the edge of developing conditions like high blood pressure, irritable bowel syndrome, or a repetitive stress injury. Alternatively, a person in this stage of the continuum could make small lifestyle changes that could dramatically improve his or her health.

Massage in this stage can often create meaningful therapeutic change through stress reduction. Massage can also play a role in helping clients have moments of greater ease in their bodies, which can provide the mental, emotional, and physical space to make lasting changes in their dedication to their own health and wellness.

Functional Health and Therapeutic Change

This stage of the continuum is characterized by fair energy levels, few sleep disturbances, occasional but mild digestive disturbances, and muscular tension that may be persistent but do not prevent normal daily activities. Physical fitness is average but not exceptional. Colds and the flu may be experienced periodically. Stress levels are moderate, mental attitudes are generally good, and emotional coping resources are variable.

Again, massage for stress reduction may be the intervention a client needs to create positive life changes that lead to better health. Massage can boost immunity levels and improve breathing patterns and posture. These changes alone could reduce a client's muscle tension and improve sleep and energy levels.

Good Health and Therapeutic Change or Maintenance

In this range of the continuum, the client has good energy levels, good physical fitness, a healthy diet, good posture with minimal muscle pain and tension, and a positive, upbeat attitude; he or she may practice stress management activities. Sleep and digestive disturbances are insignificant or nonexistent.

In this case, massage might be used to move the client to even better health or to maintain the health level already achieved. Perhaps the client has a monthly massage as part of a stress management plan. Perhaps the client views massage as a treat once a week to boost energy levels and keep muscles fluid. Massage might be applied for maintenance and still result in positive therapeutic change.

Optimal Health and Maintenance

In this range of the continuum, the client has exceptional physical fitness and high energy levels. Ease and grace characterize this client's posture and movement patterns. The client eats a healthy diet, sticks to a consistent sleep schedule, and manages stress efficiently. The client's attitude is upbeat and positive, and he or she feels balanced emotionally and spiritually. Maintenance massage is used to preserve physical ease and as part of a healthy lifestyle.

As you continue the process of assessing clients, ruling out contraindications, and picking treatment techniques to balance muscular tension, promote better posture, or address the condition of an injury, consider the continuum of health and massage for comfort care, condition management, therapeutic change, or maintenance as a useful starting point for defining treatment goals. Massage can play a positive role in the health care of most people as long as the treatment goals of the session are realistic and match the needs of the client.

> ### Concept Brief 19-7
> ### Massage and General Treatment Goals
>
> **Comfort care:** Gentle massage or laying-on of hands to ease pain, bring comfort, and provide reassurance for serious illness, terminal illness, or the dying process.
>
> **Condition management:** Massage is not expected to cure the pathology but is used to reduce some symptoms or improve the body's ability to cope.
>
> **Therapeutic change:** Massage is used as a tool to promote change in the physical, mental, emotional, or spiritual health of the client.
>
> **Maintenance:** Massage is used to help the client maintain their present state of well being as part of a healthy lifestyle.

Soft-Tissue Rehabilitation Process

In Chapter 22, you will learn about the stages of inflammation in the soft-tissue healing process and will explore common types of soft-tissue injuries, treatment goals, and suggested techniques. During the treatment planning process, this information is valuable for ensuring that massage sessions are effective. The **soft-tissue rehabilitation** process is briefly outlined here to help you better understand treatment planning for healthcare massage.

- **Phase 1: Acute stage of the healing process.** In the early stage of the rehabilitation process, the tissue is likely red, hot, and swollen, and some bruising may be present. Muscle spasms likely splint the area, and pain radiates from the injury site into the surrounding area. The client may be unwilling to move the affected joint during active range of motion or may move it very carefully. During this stage, treatment goals focus on reducing swelling, pain, muscle spasms, and sympathetic nervous system firing and on retaining any available pain-free range of motion. Clients are cautioned to rest the area and practice self-care to prevent re-injury.

- **Phase 2: Repair stage of the healing process.** In the second stage of the rehabilitation process, the redness, swelling, and heat have mostly disappeared and any bruising has turned from dark colors like red, purple, and black to lighter shades of yellow, green, and brown. Muscle spasms have decreased or disappeared, and pain is localized to the injury site. Range of motion and mechanical function in the affected joint are still decreased. During this stage, treatment goals focus on increasing circulation to improve tissue health, decreasing trigger points and adhesions in affected tissues, promoting proper scar tissue formation, increasing range of motion, and encouraging clients to continue self-care regimes.

- **Phase 3: Maturation stage of the healing process:** In the third stage of the rehabilitation process, pain, swelling, bruising, and muscle spasms have disappeared but the client has not yet regained full range of motion or mechanical strength. If the tissue is stressed because the client resumes activities too quickly, pain, stiffness, and mild swelling may reappear and the healing process might stall. During this stage, the treatment goals focus on reducing trigger points and adhesions, increasing range of motion, re-balancing muscles (lengthening shorten muscles and strengthening weakened muscles), reducing scar tissue, increasing strength, and treating compensating structures.

Rehabilitation for soft-tissue injuries focuses on correctly identifying the healing stage of the tissue, choosing methods appropriate to that stage, and encouraging client self-care that protects against re-injury.

Analysis of Collected Data

To plan a healthcare massage session, you analyze the data you have collected, prioritize needs and goals, and then make decisions about what techniques to use and the order to apply them during the massage. You also adapt the session to make the massage safer for the client if you have identified cautions or contraindications. Following are a recap of the types of data you have collected and some suggestions for forming treatment goals and choosing techniques.

- **Healthcare referral**: Clients coming for healthcare massages are often referred by a physician, physical therapist, or chiropractor. The healthcare professional is likely to indicate the type of treatment the client is expected to receive. The healthcare professional may request specific techniques or specific locations to focus the massage treatment. Use this information to guide your decisions about treatment goals and techniques. For example, if the healthcare provider asks you to reduce adhesions and trigger points in the trapezius muscle, this doesn't mean that you can't massage related structures, but reducing adhesions and trigger points is the primary focus. If your chart notes indicate that you massaged the hamstrings and low back for most of the session, the healthcare provider is unlikely to refer to you again because you failed to address the primary purpose of the client's visit.

- **Health intake form**: As discussed in Chapter 12 and earlier in this chapter, health intake forms provide a broad picture of a client's health history and current status. They also provide facts about the cause of an injury (e.g., a fall from a horse), the progression of a condition (e.g., fibromyalgia for 3 years with an increase in muscular pain 6 months ago), the current care the client is receiving, and whether it is working or not working. Use these forms to help you formulate questions for more in-depth inquiry, to rule out contraindications, and to anticipate adaptations for the session based on functional limitations (e.g., the client cannot be positioned on the back) or medications.

- **Pain assessment**: The use of a pain questionnaire or other method of pain assessment provides information about the location, quantity, and quality of the pain the client is experiencing, right now, before the session begins. In some cases, this information might signal a contraindication (e.g., the client is experiencing severe neck pain but has not been assessed by a healthcare provider), or be used to adapt positioning during the session (e.g., the client's pain increases from mild to moderate when lying prone in a face cradle), or to modify techniques (e.g., the client's fibromyalgia pain is moderate and only gentle techniques are tolerable at this time). In other cases, the information becomes an indicator that treatment is working (e.g., pain has regularly decreased over the last three sessions) or not working (e.g., pain has remained the same or increased over the last three sessions).

- **Health intake interview**: Chapter 12 discussed the types of questions you might ask during a health intake interview. While many of these questions also apply in an interview for a healthcare session, this type of interview focuses more specifically on gathering data about functional limitations and helping the client set functional goals. These functional goals will direct your treatment plan. For example, a client who has suffered multiple soft-tissue injuries from a car accident may have various locations that need massage attention. While you are likely to give some attention to each of these areas, the client's primary functional goal is to be able to lift the right arm to shoulder height in order to wash his or her hair. Knowledge of this goal alerts you to the need to focus a good deal of time on massage of the shoulders, upper chest, upper back, and neck.

- **General observations**: As is discussed in depth in Chapter 12, be alert to the client's body language, skin tone, breathing patterns, vocal patterns, quality of movement, facial expressions, and overall expression of fatigue or energy. In many cases, these general observations help you make choices about the depth and vigor of the techniques you choose. A client whose voice, skin tone, energy levels, and facial expressions indicate fatigue and high emotion is probably not in a physical or emotional condition to tolerate trigger point work even if this is indicated in your overall treatment plan. On this particular date, the client is more likely to benefit from soothing massage focused on reducing overall pain, fatigue, and muscular tension.

- **Posture analysis**: The goal of posture analysis is to help you identify muscles that are hypertonic and shortened or hypotonic and weakened. Use this information to guide your thinking about which muscles may need trigger point work, warm hydrotherapy applications, massage to address adhesions, or muscles that need strengthening.

- **Gait analysis**: Like posture analysis, gait analysis helps you identify muscle imbalances and muscles that are hypertonic or weakened. Use your findings to supplement those of the posture analysis and aim to lengthen and soften hypertonic, shortened muscles while strengthening weakened muscles.

- **Range-of-motion assessment**: The purpose of range-of-motion testing is to evaluate the client's ability to move and to identify any pathological restrictions present in the joint. It helps you determine if contractile or inert tissues are the cause of the restriction and focus your treatment on specific structures.

• **Palpation assessment**: In Chapter 12, you learned about palpation assessment. A systematic approach to palpation helps detect irregularities in tissue texture, tone, temperature, and hydration. Through touch, you can identify tissue restrictions that are causing reductions in range of motion and recognize when areas are painful in response to external pressure.

You may not use all these assessment methods for every client. Pick the assessment methods depending on the client's overall condition, whether they have a diagnosed disease or injury, and what you know and don't know about their physical signs, symptoms, and limitations. Box 19-3 provides some questions to ask as you analyze your assessment data and formulate a treatment plan.

Creating a Treatment Plan

To create the client's treatment plan, consider all the data you have gathered, trust your intuition, consult with the client to ensure his or her participation in the choices made about treatment, and formulate a plan to decide which locations and structures you will address and which techniques you will use to meet treatment goals. Before beginning this process, ask yourself three key questions:

• Do I have the skills and knowledge necessary to work with this client safely and effectively?

• Should this client be referred to another healthcare professional for analysis and treatment before receiving massage?

• Should this client be referred to another healthcare professional to receive analysis and treatment in addition to massage? If yes, to which professional?

If you feel ready and able to work with the client, it can be helpful to follow a structured process for writing up a treatment plan:

1. Review the client's functional goals and prioritize the body locations and specific structures to be addressed in order to improve the client's functioning to meet functional goals.

2. List specific session/treatment goals and techniques for each location or structure that needs massage intervention. For example, treatment goals may include decreasing muscular tension in the trapezius, rhomboids, and erector spinae group. Treatment techniques may therefore include

---

BOX 19-3 Questions to Guide the Formulation of a Treatment Plan

1. What are the primary facts of this case? What do you already know about the client's condition that might guide your choices, such as what happened, what's the time frame, and at what point are you entering the client's care process?

2. If there is a referral from another healthcare professional, does it give you specific directions on locations to work or techniques to use?

3. Based on the continuum of health, does the client need comfort massage, condition management, therapeutic massage to promote change, or maintenance massage?

4. If the client has a soft-tissue injury, what stage of inflammation do the signs and symptoms indicate (see Chapter 22, the section on the inflammatory response, for details)?

5. Does the health intake form indicate a need for caution or adaptations in the session? If yes, what cautions or adaptations are needed? If the client has not been referred to you by another healthcare professional, do you have any reason to believe that massage could endanger the client of that the client should be referred to another health professional before you provide massage treatment?

6. If the client is taking medications, have you identified and researched whether any of these medications require adaptations to the massage treatment? If so, what adaptations are needed?

7. Is the client in pain? If so, where is the pain located, how severe is the pain, and what is the quality of the pain? How will the client's current experience of pain influence the massage treatment? What adaptations will you make?

8. What are the client's functional goals? Which locations of the body or specific structures need attention for the client to be able to conduct the activities of daily life that are important to him or her?

9. What do your general observations tell you about the client's overall condition, emotional state, and energy levels? What level of depth and vigor of techniques can the client tolerate based on your observations?

10. During posture and gait assessment, which muscles seemed particularly tight and short? Which seemed weakened? Did a particular structure or group of structures seem particularly imbalanced? If so, what structures seemed to need the most attention?

11. Did the range-of-motion assessment indicate any pathological restrictions in a particular joint? If so, to the best of your knowledge are the restrictions caused by inert tissue, contractile tissue, or both? Which structures require massage intervention to improve range of motion and decrease pain?

12. In your palpation assessment, which structures demonstrated texture, temperature, tone, or hydration irregularities? Which areas of the body or which structures felt particularly restricted?

using a hydroculator pack to the upper and lower back while massaging the hamstring muscles to warm the tissue, myofascial massage followed by Swedish massage to the selected structures, followed by deep tissue massage and trigger point work in the trapezius.

3. Plan the sequence of locations where you plan to work. In the example above, the therapist is planning to work the posterior legs first while heating up the muscles on the client's back with a hydroculator pack.

4. Think carefully about the sequence of locations you plan to work, the treatment goals you hope to achieve, and the techniques you want to use. Then, ask yourself what effects will each technique achieve? Is there a better way to achieve the desired effect? Could any of the techniques cause adverse reactions? What adverse reactions might the client experience?

5. List any cautions or adaptations you need to make to ensure the client's safety.

6. Talk over your plan with the client and make adjustments based on his or her concerns, feedback, or additional data providing during the conversation.

7. Implement your plan and track your results.

Treatment plans are not static. They are always changing based on the results you document at the end of the session and over a series of sessions. Strive to regularly review your session data and make refinements to your plan as sessions progress. Consult clients to determine if they have ideas about their sessions and which techniques they find particularly effective.

Reassessment

The initial health history intake process can be quite lengthy. While you won't conduct such a thorough assessment before and after each massage session, some specific testing can help fine tune the treatment planning for each session. Periodically conduct an in-depth reassessment using the same procedures you used in the client's initial visit. This allows you to identify changes that have occurred over the course of numerous sessions. Often, reassessment is scheduled every six to eight sessions. After reassessment, evaluate your findings and determine whether your treatment plan is working effectively. Adjust the plan as needed to better meet treatment goals, and proceed with the new plan until the next reassessment.

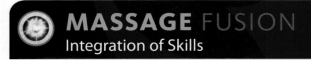

MASSAGE FUSION
Integration of Skills

STUDY TIP: Book It

When you practice posture, gait, and range-of-motion assessments on classmates and clients in your student clinic, keep an anatomy or a kinesiology book close by. Take the time to look up regions of the body and identify which muscles are shortened, which are weakened, and which are producing movement at particular joints. While this process may take some time during your initial efforts, as you continue to hone your skills you will get faster at making the connections among tension patterns, movement patterns, and particular structures.

MASSAGE INSPIRATION: A Trip to the Mall

There is no better way to view a range of postures and gait patterns than to visit your local mall and watch people. Take multiple SOAP charts and practice charting the posture and gait patterns you see all around you. Go with a classmate and discuss what you see, and share ideas about which muscles you would massage if the person came to you for a session. See if you can spot common postural dysfunctions like hyperlordosis, hyperkyphosis, and scoliosis.

IT'S TRUE!

There is good evidence that massage is an effective way to reduce pain in a variety of settings. For example, in a randomized, controlled trial, test subjects with muscle pain from various sources were placed into three groups. One group was the no-treatment control, while another received light-touch massage, and the third received deep-tissue massage. Deep massage decreased pain 48% over light touch at 27%. Overall, the researchers determined that massage is effective at reducing muscle pain symptoms from 25% to 50% depending on the type of pain.[2]

CHAPTER WRAP-UP

This chapter is a turning point. You have successfully navigated through chapters that teach you foundation knowledge, skills, and abilities, which you have applied to wellness massage. Now these foundation skills become your stepping stone to working with clients with medical conditions and injuries. This chapter provides you with the tools you need to make good treatment planning decisions through in-depth assessment. Upcoming chapters consider advanced massage techniques like myofascial release and deep tissue massage, neuromuscular therapy, massage for injury, chronic pain conditions, and pathologies, and massage for special populations. At this point, you are drawing on information from a variety of classes and sources and applying it to new situations and client types. It's an exciting time because all of the pieces of the massage puzzle are coming together as you get closer to graduation and your career as a professional massage therapist!

Chapter 20

Myofascial and Deep Tissue Approaches

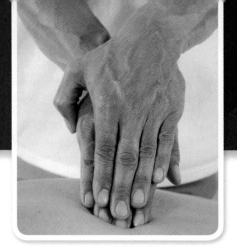

KEY TERMS

collagen

connective tissue

deep tissue massage

fascia

ground substance

myofascia

piezoelectricity

tensegrity

therapeutic edge

thixotropy

viscoelasticity

LEARNING OBJECTIVES

Having read the chapter and used the related student learning tools, the student will be able to:

1 Describe the structure of muscle and its relationship with fascia.

2 Explain the concept of thixotropy and explain how this phenomenon relates to ground substance.

3 Summarize the process whereby structures that should be functionally separate become "glued together."

4 Using the concept of tensegrity, predict the possible ramifications of a tight Achilles tendon for other areas of the body.

5 Contrast the location of the superficial fascia with the deeper fascial layers.

6 List three causes of myofascial dysfunction.

7 Describe three effects of myofascial techniques.

8 Give an example of one assessment technique that can be used to identify myofascial restrictions.

9 Summarize basic guidelines for the application of myofascial techniques.

10 Recall the primary goal of deep tissue work and explain the way in which deep tissue massage helps to achieve this goal.

11 Give an example of an assessment technique that might be used to identify muscle imbalance.

12 Summarize basic guidelines for the application of deep tissue massage.

The term **myofascia** comes from *myo* (from the Greek *mys*) meaning muscle and the Latin word *fascia* meaning a bandage. This chapter investigates the inseparable nature of muscle and fascia and explores ways to manipulate myofascia for greater freedom of movement, increased muscular balance, reduced pain, and better overall health. Topic 20-1 briefly describes the structure and the function of connective tissue, especially fascia, and explains its properties and their implications for massage. Topic 20-2 identifies the effects of myofascial massage, provides guidelines for the delivery of myofascial work, and demonstrates some specific techniques. In Topic 20-3, you learn that the primary goal of deep tissue work is to elongate chronically shortened tissue to promote greater muscular balance. Some specific approaches to deep tissue manipulation are demonstrated. Myofascial techniques and deep tissue work are regularly integrated with Swedish massage. While many of these techniques are used in a relaxation massage, this chapter focuses more on the delivery of healthcare massage for the needs of the individual client.

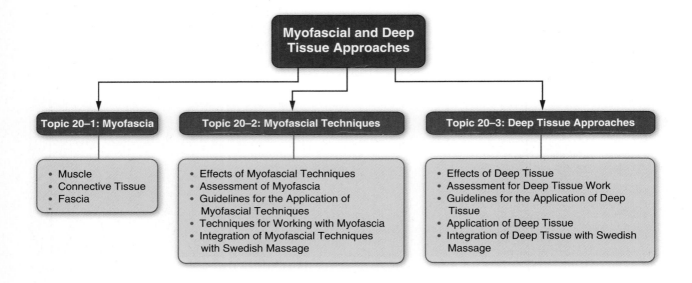

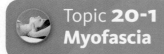

Topic **20-1**
Myofascia

Muscle and **fascia** are intimately associated. Understanding fascia broadens our perspective on the way in which balanced or unbalanced movement occurs and how patterns of tension emerge and influence both the local region and the distal regions of the body. It is impossible to contract muscle tissue without involving connective tissue. It is impossible to massage a muscle without massaging fascia. This section of the chapter explores connective tissue, especially fascia, in terms of its relationship to muscle and all the cells in the body. Understanding the interconnectedness of muscle and fascia is essential for the effective application of myofascial techniques and deep tissue massage.

Muscle

You already know a great deal about muscle structure and function from anatomy, physiology, and kinesiology classes.

Important here is the basic structure of skeletal muscles. In skeletal muscles, thousands of long, cylinder-shaped fibers called myofibers (muscle fibers) lie parallel to one another. Myofibers are made up of very fine fibers called myofibrils that run lengthwise and consist of even smaller structures called myofilaments. Each myofiber is encased in fascia called the endomysium. Groups of myofibers are bundled together into fascicles by sheets of fascia called the perimysium. Individual muscles are formed by groups of fascicles wrapped in fascia called the epimysium. The muscle's layers of fascia merge at both ends of the muscle and thicken into tough tendons that attach the muscle to the connective tissue covering of the bone (the periosteum). At every layer of muscle, fascia wraps fibers, groups of fibers, and the entire muscle organ, and then weaves the muscle into tendon and to the connective tissue covering bone (Fig. 20-1).

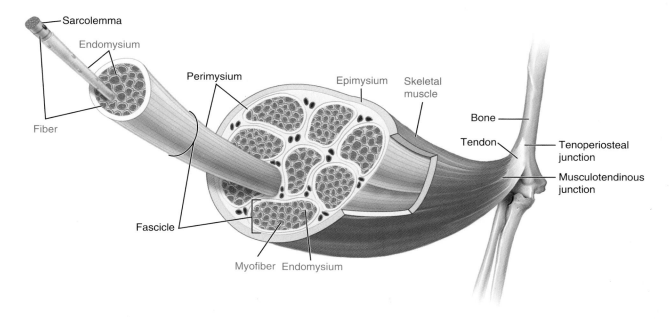

Figure 20-1 Structure of skeletal muscle.

Concept Brief 20-1
Structure of Muscle

1. Myofilaments → myofibrils = myofibers (fascial wrap = endomysium)
2. Bundles of myofibers = fascicles (fascial wrap = perimysium)
3. Groups of fascicles = muscle (fascial wrap = epimysium)
4. Fascia merge at either end of muscle to tendons to attach muscle to bone

Connective Tissue

Connective tissue is widely distributed throughout the body and in various forms creates the body's supportive network. Types of connective tissue include fascia, bone, cartilage, ligaments, tendons, joint capsules, the periosteum of bones, blood, and adipose tissue. This section focuses on fascia, the type of connective tissue that plays many important functions in the body and directly impacts the body's ability to move freely through space.

Components of Connective Tissue

Connective tissue varies in density, thickness, strength, elasticity, and rigidity depending on where it occurs in the body and its form. It has a consistency ranging from a watery sol state, to a semifluid sol state, to a viscous gel state, to the solid crystalline structure of bone. These differences mainly depend on the varying ratios of cells, ground substance, and fibers that are the primary components of connective tissue. The ground substance and fibers, which are outside the cells, are often referred to as the matrix.

Connective Tissue Cells

Fibroblasts (fibro = fiber + blast = maker) are the most abundant cells in connective tissue and produce the connective tissue matrix of ground substance and fibers. Fibroblasts are especially abundant in dense connective tissue such as ligaments, tendons, fascia, and joint capsules. Fibroblasts are key in tissue repair and are highly active during growth or healing processes. Their activity increases when soft tissues are placed under mechanical stress, and they are directly responsible for creating scar tissue and adhesions.

Mast cells are another component of connective tissue and often found along blood vessels where they produce heparin and histamine. Heparin is an anticoagulant that prevents blood from clotting, while histamine acts as a vasodilator and increases capillary permeability during an inflammatory response when tissue is injured or placed under stress. When you massage myofascia, mast cells initially respond to the pressure of strokes as if the tissue is being damaged, increasing circulation in the local region.

Macrophages, plasma cells, and leucocytes occur in connective tissue and provide immune defense, while adipocytes (fat cells) store fat and provide padding around kidneys, joints, and the body as part of the superficial layer of fascia.

Ground Substance

Ground substance is a fluid produced by fibroblasts that looks like egg white and surrounds all the cells in the body to support cellular metabolism. It provides nutritional support to cells while binding them together and providing a medium though which substances can be exchanged between blood and cells. It also serves as a lubricant and spacer between collagen fibers to keep them from sticking together. The composition of ground substance can fluctuate from location to location, from a fluid state to a thick, gel-like consistency. This phenomenon is called thixotropy. Massage can influence the consistency of ground substance.

Connective Tissue Fibers

The three different types of fibers found in the connective tissue matrix are collagen, elastin, and reticular fibers. **Collagen** is a protein that forms the tough rope-like strands that make up the fibrous content of skin, fascia, tendons, ligaments, cartilage, bone, blood vessels, and organs. Collagen strands are arranged in a variety of ways depending on where they occur in the body. Sometimes, they are crisscrossed to form a sheet-like structure, or piled on top of each other in layers. They might occur as parallel formations or knit into a sweater-like web. The proportion of collagen fibers and the state (between sol and gel) of ground substance differ depending on how the connective tissue is used. In healthy connective tissue, ground substance lubricates the collagen strands so that they can slide over each other without sticking and catching.

Elastic fibers are yellow and made of the protein elastin. These long, thin, crosslinked fibers can be stretched to one-and-one-half times their resting length and provide the elasticity of skin, blood vessels, and lung tissue, where elastic fibers are found in high concentrations. Reticular fibers are formed from smaller, more delicate collagen strands that cross over each other to create intricate and extensive networks that support skeletal and smooth muscle cells and nerves and that provide the framework for soft organs like the spleen and the lymph nodes. They are often found in basement membranes, lymphoid tissue, and adipose tissue.

Properties of Connective Tissue

As mentioned, connective tissue occurs in many forms based on the ratios of ground substance, cells, and fibers in its makeup. The thixotropic, viscoelastic, piezoelectric, and adhesive properties of connective tissue allow it to be altered, either positively or negatively, by lifestyle choices, chronic stress, injury, and massage techniques that manipulate soft tissue.

Thixotropy

Thixotropy is a phenomenon in which gels become more fluid when they are stirred up and more solid when they are undisturbed. The ground substance in connective tissue, especially fascia, has the unique ability to move between a more fluid sol state and a viscous gel state. Regular exercise, physical labor, stretching, proper hydration, and good nutrition promote a fluid sol state in fascia. The heat created in the tissue by movement warms and "stirs" the ground substance. On the other hand, a sedentary lifestyle, poor hydration, poor nutrition, little physical movement, and tissue trauma related to injury cause

the ground substance to cool, thicken, and enter a stiffened gel state. A stiffened gel state might lead to a decrease in range of motion, patterns of tension in tissue that lead to postural imbalances, a greater risk for injury, pain, and overall lethargy. The application of massage techniques that lift, twist, compress, vibrate, and stretch the tissue mechanically stir the ground substance and raise energy levels in the tissue. This leads to greater range of motion, an environment where cellular metabolism is enhanced, a decreased fascial tension that may lead to better posture, the possibility of greater release and length in muscles, and less risk for injury, pain, and lethargy (Box 20-1).

Viscoelasticity

The term **viscoelasticity** comes from words parts meaning viscous (thick, sticky, gummy) and elastic (stretchy, expandable, flexible). If a substance is viscous, it will become deformed when an outside force manipulates it and will remain deformed. Imagine pressing your fist into a piece of clay. The clay will flatten and remain flattened. If a substance is elastic, it will deform when manipulated by an outside force but then snap back into its original shape when the outside force is removed (think of stretching and releasing a rubber band). The viscoelasticity of connective tissue makes it plastic, whereas muscle is elastic. When connective tissue is deformed by an outside force like massage techniques or by stretching, the tissue will remain in the deformed state after the outside force has been removed for a certain period of time and then slowly return to its original shape. For example,

BOX 20-1 Conceptual Models of Connective Tissue

1. Marmalade provides a good conceptual model for connective tissue. The thick gelatinous base of marmalade is like ground substance, while the pieces of orange peel represent protein fibers. If you place marmalade in the refrigerator, it becomes thicker because it is cold. When marmalade is warmed, it becomes more fluid. This mirrors the thixotropic properties of connective tissue.

2. Fascia can be compared to a full body sweater. Pulling one area affects the entire sweater network. This is why pain in one area may be caused by a structural dysfunction in a region that seems unrelated.

3. Fascia as a grapefruit: Cut a grapefruit in half. Notice that the white pith that forms the inner skin of the grapefruit and connects the skin to the fruit also breaks the grapefruit into sections and interweaves the fruit with delicate supporting branches. In fact, each tiny bulb of fruit is encased in a thin membrane. The grapefruit provides a good conceptual model for understanding how superficial and deep fascia entwine to provide support to muscles, organs, blood and lymph vessels, nerves, and all body cells.

if the techniques you use elongate chronically contracted tissue, the tissue will remain elongated for some period of time after the massage. Regular massage and adaptations in movement patterns can lead to positive long-term changes in the shape and length of fascia. Some types of connective tissue have more elastin fibers in their makeup (the connective tissue that forms the lungs, for example, or the more elastic ligaments that occur between the vertebrae) and so are less plastic and more elastic.

Piezoelectricity

Piezoelectricity means "pressure electricity." It refers to the ability of living tissue to generate electrical potentials in response to mechanical deformation. Mechanical deformation that might cause piezoelectricity includes activities like walking, running, dancing, or any weight-bearing movement, or the manipulation of soft tissue or bone as might occur during a massage or a chiropractic session. Research has demonstrated that keratin, elastin, collagen, hyaluronic acid (found in connective tissue), and the actine and myosin in skeletal muscles exhibit piezoelectric properties.[1] It is believed that these electrical potentials stir ground substance and improve the health of connective tissue. One common example is the use of electrical machines that simulate piezoelectricity and increase osteogenesis to speed the healing of fractures.[2] During massage, soft tissue is electrically stimulated in a positive way by techniques, and this leads to improved tissue health.[3]

Adhesiveness

Collagen is formed by fibroblasts as a long chain of amino acids. Because of the tension created by atomic attraction and repulsion in proteins, these amino acid chains twist to the left creating a long corkscrew shape. These single chains float about as fragile incomplete collagen spirals until they come into contact with other spirals and then start to coil around each other (this time to the right) in groups of three, creating a three-stranded helix. Hydrogen molecules are attracted to the oxygen radicals that stick out from the sides of the individual protein strands and attach to the oxygen radicals, forming hydrogen bonds that hold the helix together and give collagen its great strength. Now fully formed within the fibroblast, the new collagen molecule is secreted into the ground substance as a separate unit to take on whatever form is needed in the local area. As people age, or because of injury, postural habits, habitual movement patterns, lack of movement, or soft-tissue stress, collage fibers start to pack more tightly together, increasing hydrogen bonding. This thickens and binds the tissue causing a decrease of range of motion, postural imbalances, structural tension, and increased possibility for injury. In fact, two structures that are designed to be functionally separate but which reside side by side may become "glued" to one another so that they don't slide over each other freely (e.g., two muscles). Bodywork, physical therapy, and movement re-education all help to break or prevent unnecessary hydrogen bonding to promote greater freedom in the myofascia network.

Concept Brief 20-2
Connective Tissue

Types:
Fascia, bone, cartilage, ligaments, tendons, joint capsules, periosteum, blood, adipose tissue

Components:
  Cells: Fibroblasts, macrophages, plasma cells, mast cells, adipocytes, leucocytes

  Ground Substance: Produced by fibroblasts with egg white consistency.

  Fibers: Produced by fibroblasts—three types
  Collagen = protein that forms rope-like strands = very tough

  Elastic = stretchy protein

  Reticular = delicate form of collagen

Properties:
  Thixotropy: Phenomenon where gels become more fluid or more solid

  Viscoelasticity: Viscous + elastic = plastic quality of connective tissue

  Piezoelectricity: Ability of tissue to generate electrical potentials in response to mechanical deformation including massage.

  Adhesiveness: Packing of collagen fibers and increased hydrogen bonding that occurs in response to tissue stress

Fascia

Fascia has more ground substance than other forms of connective tissue, which causes it to move between a sol and gel state easily when manipulated by massage techniques. The superficial layer of fascia is often compared to a knit sweater that wraps the entire body to explain how fascia links all body regions together. Tension in one area of the body sweater influences freedom of movement and function in all other areas. For example, massage therapists often report that clients complain of pain in a particular region. The massage therapist massages all of the structures in that region over numerous massage sessions, but the client doesn't improve significantly. Why not? More often than not, the pain is being caused by structural tension in a region removed from the area where the pain is experienced. The fascial network disperses the stress caused by the mechanical dysfunction throughout its web. In order to decrease the pain, the therapist must address the root cause of the pain. This means that the therapist must identify the tension pattern, wherever it is occurring, and correct that imbalance to decrease the client's pain.

Functions of Fascia

Fascia performs many important functions in the body including structural integrity, protection and shock absorption, immune defense, and cellular exchange processes.

Structural Integrity

Fascia maintains the structural integrity of the body in many ways. It separates individual structures without losing the cohesion between them. We see this in the way that fascia wraps individual muscle fibers, fascicles, and individual muscles and then weaves them to tendons to attach muscles to bone. When you think of fascia, imagine a continuous network of connective tissue that links all of the different organs and regions of the body into wholeness. It provides the underlying supportive structure of blood vessels, lymph vessels, and nerves, defines the shape of organs, and tethers them in their proper places within the organism. Many authors comment that if all of the body's organs, the blood vessels, the nerves, the muscles, and even the skeleton were removed, the remaining fascia would provide a comprehensive outline of the human form.

Tensegrity

Tensegrity, a term coined by architect and designer Buckminster Fuller, has been adopted by massage therapists and bodyworkers. Fuller's architecture was based on a geometrical model in which structures maintain their integrity because of a balance of continuous tensile forces throughout the building.[4] Tensile forces refer to stretching forces (tension) pulling at both ends of a structure. Fuller was famous for the geodesic dome, in which a network of intersecting triangles distributes the stresses of gravity across the entire structure, making the whole dome stronger as a complete unit than the individual components are on their own (Fig. 20-2).

Compare this tensegrity model to a brick wall. The brick wall is formed when bricks are stacked one on top of another and cemented together, transmitting the weight of the structure to the earth. The forces are compressive as opposed to tensile. Not long ago the body was viewed like that brick wall, and it's easy to understand how this misconception occurred because the head is stacked on the vertebrae, the vertebrae are stacked on each other, the femurs are stacked on the tibial bones, and the tibial bones are stacked on the calcaneus and talus bones. In this model of the body, stress to one structure is localized. For example, a light pole could fall on a part of our brick wall and only damage one small section of the wall. Similarly, a shoulder injury was viewed as an injury that affected just the shoulder region.

If we view the body as a tensegrity structure, however, we better understand the relationship of all body parts to each other and recognize that a shoulder injury is not localized to the shoulder region but affects every other body structure on some level. In the tensegrity model, muscles, tendons, and fascia provide the continuous tensile forces that maintain the upright structure of the skeleton against the forces of gravity and allow changes in tension to create movement. The head and neck form an inverted triangle connected to the triangle created by the shoulders and trunk and to the triangle created by the pelvis (Fig. 20-3). The configuration of these triangles disperses gravity and absorbs and distributes compressive forces.

Ida Rolf was the first to help us understand that when myofascial tension is balanced, the body is best able to

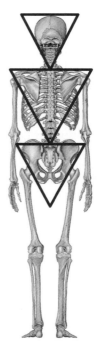

Figure 20-3 As in a geodesic dome, the sum of the triangles created by the angles of the human body as a whole are stronger than the individual pieces. The configuration of these triangles disperses gravity and absorbs and distributes compressive forces.

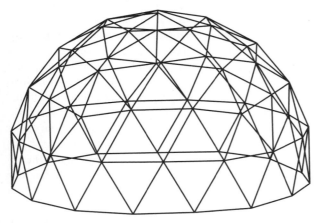

Figure 20-2 A geodesic dome is composed of a network of intersecting triangles that distribute the stresses of gravity across the entire structure, making the whole dome stronger as a complete unit than the individual components are on their own. The geodesic dome can be compared to the human body because both are tensegrity structures in which balanced tensile forces create stability.

disperse and effectively use the forces of gravity. If one set of muscles exerts tension in one direction, the opposing muscles must exert tension in the opposite direction or the structure may begin to bow and demonstrate postural misalignment. The two sets of tensile forces must be equal or balanced for optimal function. Uneven tension places the entire structure under pressure and weakens it. The goal of massage is to ensure balanced tension so that the support beams (skeleton) and cables (muscles and connective tissue) can maintain their structural integrity.

Concept Brief 20-3
Tensegrity

- Balance of continuous tensile forces = stretching (tension) at both ends
- Muscles + connective tissue = continuous tensile forces on skeleton
- Opposing muscles = sets of tensile forces: opposing tensile forces must be equal for balance and optimal function
- One set tensile forces excessively strong + other set weak = structure misalignment and stress
- Aligned inverted body triangles disperses gravity, absorbs shock, distributes compressive forces
- All body parts are related to each other and affected by each other (injury is not localized)

Protection and Shock Absorption

The adaptability and variation of connective tissue in different regions allows it to play a fundamental role in protecting the body from dangerous forces. For example, in the periphery, the fascia tends to be thicker and denser. When a body area is under repeated stress, thickened fascia starts to replace muscle to cope with the heavy load. The viscoelastic properties of fascia and other connective tissue allow it to act as a shock absorption system throughout the body. This shock absorption goes beyond the function of cartilage like the meniscus in the knees or the fibrocartilage disks between the vertebrae. The fascial support system dampens and disperses the forces to which the body is subject, buffering organs and diffusing compressive energy along multiple channels to minimize its impact.[5]

Immune Defense

Earlier we discussed the components of connective tissue and explained that macrophages, plasma cells, and leucocytes occur in connective tissue. These immune system cells fight pathogenic organisms and infections in the ground substance of connective tissue. Deane Juhan points out in *Job's Body* that compartments of fascia throughout the body assist in preventing the spread of infections, diseases, and tumors because each compartment attempts to contain destructive agents and wall them off from other compartments.[6] Some researchers note that certain internal conditions may negatively affect the quality of ground substance, and this may cause the cells its supports to become dysfunctional, pathological, or malignant.[7] In addition, the immune function of the ground substance is altered, leaving the body vulnerable to disease and infection. Massage improves the quality of ground substance and thereby supports immune function.

Cellular Exchange

The ground substance of connective tissue is in contact with most cells in the body and makes up a good part of the intercellular fluids where many metabolic exchanges take place. Nutrients are passed from capillaries to cells and wastes are passed from cells to capillaries for removal across these fluid spaces. Good nutrition and proper hydration are important to maintain the health of ground substance to facilitate cellular exchanges. This is one reason massage therapists often suggest that clients increase water intake when healing from a soft-tissue injury.

Location of Fascia

We already know that connective tissue occurs throughout the body. Fascia is often described as occurring in layers or at specific depths in the body, but in reality fascia occurs at every layer because the body is a three-dimensional structure. For ease of discussion, this text describes a superficial layer of fascia and the deep layers of fascia. A brief look at fascial planes, bands, and chains helps us understand how myofascial tension in one body region affects the local area and also the function of distant but related regions.

Superficial Fascia

As the name suggests, superficial fascia occurs just below the skin and anchors the skin to underlying structures. It covers the body in different thicknesses depending on the location. On the back of the hand and top of the foot it is thin, while on the abdominal wall it is thick. The superficial fascia is composed of areolar connective tissue (remember that areolar refers to tissue that is loosely and irregularly arranged) and adipose tissue with arteries, veins, lymph vessels, and nerves running through it.

Deep Fascia

Deep fascia surrounds organs and muscles, carries nerves and blood and lymph vessels, and wraps these structures so that they can glide over each other without sticking to each other. As already discussed, the interweaving fascia wraps each muscle and penetrates into the interior of the muscle before forming the tendons that join muscle to the periosteum of bones. In the limbs, muscles that share similar functions and nerve supply are located in compartments that are defined by thick sheets of fascia. These fascial wraps limit the outward expression of contracting muscle bellies and so help act as a pump that pushes blood in veins back toward the heart. At the wrist and ankle, the fascia forms thick retinaculums to lock down tendons. Broad, flat tendon sheets like the thoracolumbar aponeurosis and the iliotibial tract interweave the superficial fascia to deep fascia.

Myofascial Planes, Bands, and Chains

Various authorities illustrate the organization of myofascia by describing the planes, bands, and chain-like patterns it forms. Examining this organization of myofascia gives therapists insight into the way that fascia helps support the body and disperses tension and compressive forces. We can see how an imbalance in one plane, band, or chain can affect many structures including veins, arteries, lymph vessels, local organs, and joints.

Horizontal Myofascial Planes

Fascial sheets converge at joints where tendons, ligaments, joint capsules, and the periosteum of bones lead to interlacing and thickening of the fascia. Each joint line creates a horizontal pattern of fascia that runs both superficially and deeply (Fig. 20-4). Imagine tension and adhesions in any of these horizontal planes to understand how an entire joint or region might experience pain, restricted circulation, fluid accumulation, and decreased range of motion.

FASCIAL BANDS

In the *Endless Web*, authors Dr. Louis Schultz and Dr. Rosemary Feitis identify superficial fascial bands that they liken to the thickening of the retinacula of the ankle or

the wrist.[8] Some of these bands correlate with the horizontal myofascial planes described previously, but while the horizontal planes run deep, these bands reside in the superficial layer of fascia (Fig. 20-5). The authors note that fascial bands restrict fat deposits and so show up as contours or rolls of adipose tissue. Now imagine any of these bands being tightened. It's not hard to understand the effect on breathing that might occur if the chest band is stiffened, or that headache pain might result if the band around the eyes is rigid. We know from earlier discussions about the bodymind connection that the suppression of emotion causes body armoring. Imagine that each of these bands is a piece of body armor, and it becomes easy to understand how massage can cause emotional release to occur as the band is loosened.

Myofascial Chains

In *Anatomy Trains*, Thomas Myers shows how myofascia creates long chains, both superficial and deep, from the foot to the top of the head on both the anterior and posterior body (Fig. 20-6). For example, the superficial front lines run on both sides of the midline from the dorsal surface of the toe phalanges to the tibialis anterior muscles, to the subpatellar tendons, up the rectus abdominis muscle, to the sternalis and sternochondral fascia, to the sternocleidomastoid muscles (SCMs), ending at the scalp fascia. Mechanical tension is communicated along these lines, demonstrating how dysfunction in one region can influence function in a seemingly unconnected region. In Figure 20-6, it is easy to see that the anterior front lines and posterior back lines have a synergistic relationship. What happens if excess tension in the front lines pulls the fascia down and forward? It makes sense that this will bunch up the fascia of the back lines, leading to neck and shoulder problems, a collapsed chest causing breathing problems, and low back issues. Imagine tension in the back fascial lines. It makes sense that a tight Achilles tendon might lead to multiple problems such as plantar fasciitis, a

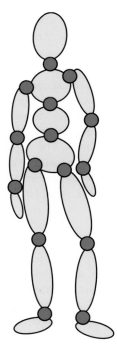

Figure 20-4 Fascial sheets converge at joints where tendons, ligaments, joint capsules, and the periosteum of bones lead to interlacing and thickening of the fascia. Each joint line creates a horizontal pattern of fascia.

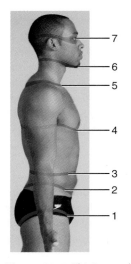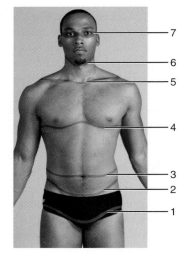

Figure 20-5 This image shows the body bands or body retinacula described by Louis Schultz and Rosemary Feitis in *The Endless Web*.

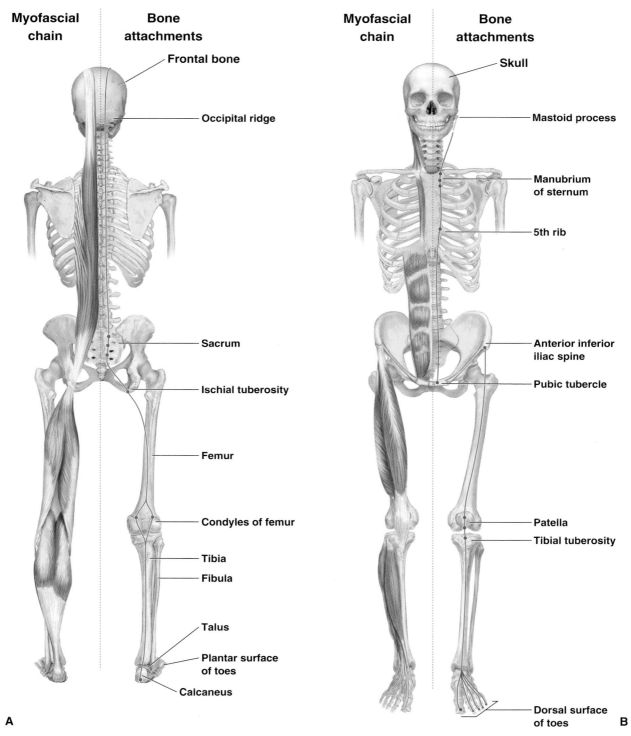

Myofascial chain	Bone attachments		Myofascial chain	Bone attachments

Figure 20-6 The superficial back line **(A)** and superficial front line **(B)** described by Thomas Myers in *Anatomy Trains*. Myers also describes lateral lines, spiral lines, arm lines, functional lines, and the deep front line. Working with this concept of myofascia can illuminate treatment options and help the therapist identify the causes of myofascial pain or tension.

hamstring tear, low back pain, and even a tension headache.[9] Understanding the connected nature of myofascia means that we never look at an injury as localized. Instead, we view the injury as something that happens to the entire body, and we address compensating regions with as much vigor and focus as the injury site.

Myofascial Dysfunction

While we have briefly discussed myofascial dysfunction and why it occurs at various places, it is helpful to review some common causes. Note that any and all of the issues described here, as well as other issues not described here, might contribute to myofascial dysfunction. Usually, more than one issue is present at any given time, complicating the issue. For example, a client might have both a repetitive stress injury and a poor diet that will influence myofascial balance and the healing process.

- **Postural habits**: Postural habits like a head-forward position, slumped shoulders, or hyperextended knees creates tension that can lead fascia in certain areas to thicken while some muscles assume static positions to brace the body. When the myofascia around joints becomes unbalanced, the joint structure may function from a position of misalignment, leading to pain or injury.

- **Diet**: Poor nutrition and dehydration can affect the quality of the ground substance of connective tissue, causing it to thicken, cool, and settle into a gel state. Hydrogen bonds attach tissues together, leading to a decreased range of motion and an increased susceptibility to injury. Poor quality ground substance can lower a body's resistance to pathogens and leave it open to disease.

- **Repetitive mechanical stress**: Repetitive stress such as might occur on a job can create stress and trauma in tissue that leads to adhesions and thickening of fascia. Nerves, blood vessels, and lymph vessels might be compressed by the tightened tissue, impacting circulation and further complicating the condition.

- **Injury**: When skin, muscle, tendon, ligament, or fascia is injured, the healing process involves tissue remodeling with collagen fibers. These fibers are distributed in the crisscross arrangement of adhesions and scar tissue. While gaps in tissue are filled and areas of mechanical stress are reinforced, this process shortens and binds the tissue, creating imbalances and tension. Additionally, nerves, blood and lymph vessels, and organs in the region can be impaired, leading to chronic pain conditions, loss of function, restricted movement, and the possibility of re-injury (tissue injury and repair is discussed in depth in Chapter 22).

- **Chronic stress**: Chemicals released as part of the flight-or-fight response, especially cortisol, cause changes to connective tissue and weaken connective tissue structures. Cortisol inhibits the activity of fibroblasts and reduces their number in connective tissue. Wounds, fractures, muscle strains, tendon sprains, and joint injuries are less likely to heal correctly in a body exposed to chronic stress.

- **Lifestyle**: A sedentary lifestyle and habits like smoking can change the body's internal chemistry and influence the quality of ground substance. This might cause tension patterns to develop, the thickening of ground substance leading to a gel state in connective tissue as well as susceptibility to illness and disease.

Concept Brief 20-4
Fascia

Greater amount of ground substance = ↑ thixotropy

Functions: Structural integrity, protection, shock absorption, immune defense, cellular exchange

Location:

Superficial = just below the skin

Deep = at all layers of the body providing framework for organs and tissues

Horizontal planes of fascia = places where fascial sheets converge at joints

Fascial bands = superficial fascia in horizontal strips that restrict fat deposits

Myofascial chains = connect foot to top of head—anterior and posterior—superficial and deep.

Dysfunction caused by postural habits, diet, repetitive mechanical stress, injury, chronic stress, sedentary lifestyle

---

Topic 20-2
Myofascial Techniques

This section explores massage techniques, often called myofascial release, which work directly with fascia to promote pain-free movement and postural balance. The effects of myofascial techniques on the body are described along with general assessment techniques for identification of myofascial restrictions, guidelines for the application of myofascial techniques, specific techniques for reducing myofascial restrictions, and integrating myofascial work with Swedish massage.

Effects of Myofascial Techniques

While the focus here is specifically on certain myofascial techniques, note that Swedish massage and many other massage and bodywork methods also affect fascia. Myofascial techniques are applied in specific ways to take advantage of the thixotropic, viscoelastic, and piezoelectric properties of connective tissue to reduce myofascial restrictions and promote pain-free and balanced motion. The myofascial techniques included here promote these general effects:

- **Melt ground substance**: The warmth of the therapist's hands melts thickened ground substance, making it easier to "stir" it with techniques that lift, compresses, twist, and raise energy in the tissue. When the ground substance becomes more sol, stagnant fluids are more easily exchanged with fresh fluids, improving ground substance health and the health of associated cells.

- **Increase piezoelectricity**: The electrical potentials created by the piezoelectric properties of connective tissue and muscle tissue are stimulated, leading to increased soft-tissue health.

- **Reduce fascial restrictions**: Myofascial techniques break the hydrogen bonds between fibers that have become closely packed together. Separate structures that were once adhered can again slide over one another smoothly. Elongating shortened myofascia takes advantage of the viscoelastic properties of fascia to create long-term changes in the tissue, allowing associated muscles to achieve their maximum length and range of motion. As muscular tension is balanced, the body regains optimal form and function.

- **Decreased adhesions**: Myofascial techniques help to break the hydrogen bonds that hold adhesions together. Collagen fibers distributed in crisscross arrangements are returned to their healthy parallel alignments along the lines of mechanical stress, allowing greater range of motion and improved muscular balance.

- **Reduce stress**: Myofascial release is pleasurable to receive and may feel very relaxing, triggering the parasympathetic nervous system response. Chronic stress is reduced, helping body chemistry normalize and thereby reducing the effects of cortisol and other stress-related chemicals on body tissue.

Assessment of Myofascia

Before you can assess your client's fascia, play with it to get a feel for it. This is easy with the superficial fascia. Start by picking up the skin on your own hand and then lifting it in multiple places as you work up your forearm. The skin pulls up easily in some places and is more difficult to lift in others. If it weren't attached by fascia to deeper structures, you could pull it off. When you lift the skin, you are also lifting the superficial fascia.

Fascial restrictions can occur anywhere in the body and show up in postural asymmetry. Use the skills you learned in Chapter 19 to identify areas where postural imbalances are causing some myofascia to bunch and pack down. Focus your work on these restricted areas. Three techniques are particularly useful for identifying fascial restrictions: fascial gliding, slow skin rolling, and passive range of motion (Technique 63).

Guidelines for the Application of Myofascial Techniques

Different authorities on myofascial techniques offer varying perspectives on working with myofascia effectively, but certain common principles emerge for the application of myofascial techniques:

- **Comfort and safety**: Myofascial techniques should not feel painful, although the client may feel a burning sensation (described below). If pain is experienced, make sure you are applying the techniques correctly and that the client doesn't have a strain, sprain, or other condition that contraindicates massage. If massage is contraindicated, myofascial techniques are contraindicated. Any skin condition that would be exacerbated by pulling on the skin contraindicates myofascial release in the local region.

- **Use of lubricant**: Use very little or no lubricant during the application of myofascial techniques. Using lubricant makes it difficult to "grab" the fascia and stretch it. Instead of engaging fascia, your hands slip over the surface of the skin. If the client's skin is very dry or fragile, or if he or she complains that the burning of myofascial work feels too uncomfortable, use a small amount of lubricant to make the strokes more comfortable and to prevent tissue tearing.

- **Depth**: Lighter work engages the superficial layer of fascia while deeper pressure accesses deeper fascial layers. Work at a level that is comfortable for the client while maintaining clear intent and visualization of the structures you seek to affect.

- **Take out the slack**: When you apply a technique, you will drop into the tissue, depending on the level of fascia you seek to address, and then take the slack out of the tissue. Removing all of the slack in the tissue and then holding this stretch engages the tissue.

- **Work in all directions**: Once you have engaged the fascia, stretch it one direction, such as longitudinally, and then on the next pass stretch it horizontally. Now stretch it at oblique angles. Work in all directions to ensure that the tissue is free of restrictions.

- **Feel the burn**: The client may report feeling a burning sensation as you hold a fascial stretch. As long as this burning sensation is not too uncomfortable, this is a good sign that hydrogen bonds are breaking and the tissue is unwinding. Increased hyperemia is perceptible in the tissue after myofascial techniques are applied.

- **Avoid tissue compression**: When you engage the myofascia, you are taking the slack out the tissue in order to stretch it. Even when working with deep fascia, the motion of your hands is not to compress the tissue into the structures beneath it or to the bone. While you may drop your fingers, palms, or even forearm into the tissue to engage the myofascia at a particular depth, once you have reached the appropriate depth your intent is to move your hands apart or pull the tissue in a particular direction—not to drop deeper in order to compress muscle.

Technique 63	**Identification of Fascial Restrictions**

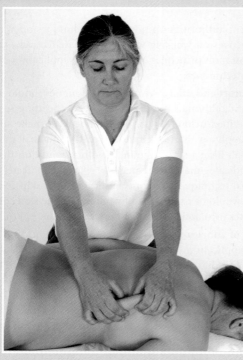

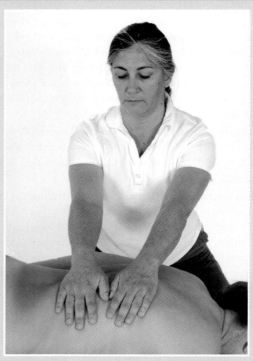

1. First, slowly roll the skin in all directions, noting places where the fascia thickens or sticks to underlying structures. This image shows the therapist getting a lot of "lift" in the tissue. Only lift the tissue as far as it will go without causing the client discomfort.

2. Next, place your hands on the area to be assessed and move the superficial fascia and skin over the underlying structures in all directions. Identify areas where the skin and superficial fascia sticks or becomes resistant. In this image, the therapist is pulling the tissue back toward her body to assess restrictions. If it is appropriate for the particular body region, drop into a deeper layer of tissue and repeat the fascial glide assessment.

3. Finally, apply what you learned about joints, end feel, and passive range of motion in Chapter 13. When fascial restrictions limit a joint, the joint "pushes back" before normal anatomical or physiological barriers are reached. In this image, the therapist is taking the slack out of the fascia with her right hand while she moves the shoulder joint passively to feel for restrictions. Move joints passively to assess possible fascial restrictions around particular joints.

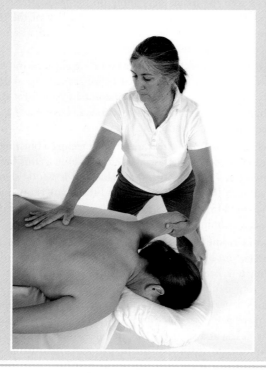

- **Work slowly:** The viscoelastic property of fascia suggests some specific methods for working with tissue during a massage session. If the tissue is dense or feels thick, cold, and viscous, slow down and warm the tissue fully before dropping into deeper structures. If you drop too deep too fast, the tissue will resist or sustain microtears and the client is likely to brace against your strokes. If you apply techniques that stretch the tissue, apply the stretches slowly because tissue generates greater tension when the rate of the stretch is faster and injury is therefore more likely. Release in myofascia doesn't happen automatically and you may find that you need to hold a particular stretch 2 to 5 minutes. Maintain the stretching motion of a technique until you feel the tissue "melt" and give way. When you release the tissue and move out of a technique, go slowly so as not to cause shock to the tissue.

- **Let the tissue guide you:** The tissue may start to release in a given direction and you will feel a sensation that is often described as tissue unwinding. Allow the tissue to guide you. If it wants to move in a particular direction, allow it to release in that direction. Let go of your preconceived ideas about where the stretch needs to occur and follow the path of the unwinding tissues. It can feel pretty exciting when the tissue starts to lead you, but don't feel disappointed if tissue unwinding doesn't happen every session or with every body.

- **Use passive and active movement to reset proprioception:** When you have finished working on a particular body area, use passive range of motion to re-educate the myofascia about its potential for movement. At the end of the session when the client is fully dressed, have him or her take the different joints through full available range of motion actively. For example, have the client move his or her neck through forward flexion, extension, lateral flexion, and rotation. If you don't reorient the client to full movement patterns, the proprioceptors may not reset and may limit the client's amount of movement. The new freedom achieved during the session may be lost.

Techniques for Working with Myofascia

Following are some key techniques for working with myofascia, but these are not all of the recognized myofascial techniques a massage therapist might use. Additional techniques are covered in upcoming chapters, but others are omitted because they are best reserved for continuing education classes once you have mastered your core massage curriculum and practiced professionally for a certain period of time. The broad categories of techniques demonstrated here include myofascial skin rolling, gross myofascial stretches, and focused myofascial stretches. Passive range of motion is used at the conclusion of work on each body area, while active range of motion is used at the very end of the session to re-educate proprioception.

Myofascial Skin Rolling

The first technique to use in myofascial work, skin rolling, you already know. The difference here is that you do not use lubricant and you will be watching for fascial restrictions and working very slowly. Roll the skin along the fiber direction of the muscle tissue and cover the entire body area (e.g., skin roll the entire back region, or the entire posterior leg). Next, skin roll horizontally across the fibers of the muscle tissue. Now skin roll at oblique angles to the muscle fibers. Roll the skin in the entire area fully so that the tissue is warm and pliable before moving on to the next myofascial technique. Notice that the skin has developed red tracks where you passed over the tissue. This hyperemia is a positive sign that the ground tissue is warmed and moving toward a sol state. Skin rolling is shown in Technique 19 (Pétrissage) in Chapter 13.

Gross Myofascial Stretches

Techniques broadly categorized as gross myofascial stretching include arm and leg pulling and crossed-hand stretches. As the name suggests, these techniques address broad fascial restrictions and help the therapist identify particular areas that need more focused work. Arm pulling is demonstrated in Technique 64 and leg pulling in Technique 65, and crossed-hand stretches are shown in Technique 66. Arm and leg pulling with a client in a side-lying position is not shown here but is another effective way to apply this technique. Contraindications for arm pulling include acute or subacute sprains, strains, or injury in the regions of the shoulder, elbow, or wrist. Leg pulling is contraindicated if the client has acute or subacute sprains, strains, or injury in the region of the hip, knee, ankle, or back. Any local condition such as a skin condition or edema that might be exacerbated by these techniques is also contraindicated, as is any condition that would contraindicate massage. Work slowly and within the comfort level of the client at all times.

Focused Myofascial Stretches

A number of different techniques can be categorized as focused myofascial stretches. While gross stretches reduce fascial restrictions in broad sheets, focused stretches hone in on particular areas, address the denser fascia around joints, work with deeper fascia in a particular area, or release the tissue of a particular muscle. Focused myofascial stretches include fascial spreading (Technique 67), fascial torquing (Technique 68), fascial cutting (Technique 69), and fascial bowing (Technique 70).

Passive and Active Range of Motion

Passive range of motion is used at the end of work on a particular body area. Passive joint movement is described in Chapter 13, and shown in Technique 26 in that chapter. At the end of the session when the client has finished dressing, have the client actively move joints through their full range of motion. This takes as little as 5 minutes and can dramatically improve the long-term effects experienced from the session.

Technique 64	Myofascial Arm Pulling

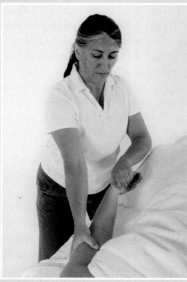

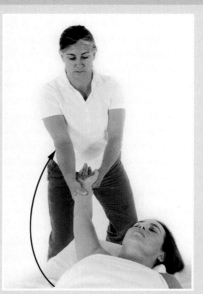

1. With the client supine, grasp the client's hand with both of your hands and stand at the client's thigh with the client's arm adducted (don't pull the arm up so that it is in slight flexion—keep all movements in clean lines) and the wrist in a neutral position. Place your weight on your back foot and lean back so that there is just enough traction for resistance to be felt with the client's elbow fully extended. Hold this position until the tissue releases (2 to 5 minutes). Avoid bouncing or jiggling the arm. Keep the traction steady and consistent. Now, while maintaining the traction with one hand, stabilize the arm above the elbow with the other and fully supinate the forearm until you meet resistance (shown), and hold the stretch against resistance until the tissue gives. You can also supinate and hold, release to neutral, and slowly supinate and hold multiple times until the tissue becomes malleable. Now repeat this process with pronation, making sure the arm is continually in traction. With the arm in constant traction and the elbow fully extended, begin to spread the palm of the client's hand, holding various positions until the tissue melts.

2. Slowly abduct the arm maintaining constant traction and spreading the palm while the arm stays in a clean line of movement. When an area of tension is experienced, stop and hold the position, increasing the traction slightly until a release is felt. When the arm reaches a 90-degree angle, bring the arm down slightly toward the floor to open up the chest. Move slowly, and when resistance is felt, stop and hold the position until the tissue gives. Do not move the arm in such a way that the client arches the back or experiences discomfort. The movement does not need to be big to be effective. Allow the arm to flex and rotate as you bring the arm up over the client's head. Traction the arm in a straight line by placing your weight on your back foot and leaning back while spreading the palm.

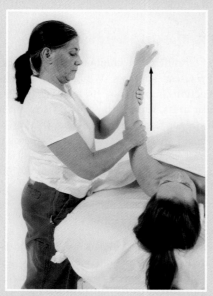

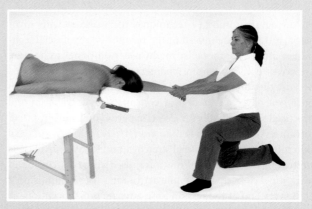

3. Change your hand position so that one hand grasps the client's arm above the elbow and one hand grasps the client's arm below the elbow. Flex the arm and lift the shoulder joint off the treatment table while maintaining steady traction (as shown). Hold this position until the tissue releases. Move the arm across the client's chest while continuing to traction upward. Use the fingertips to encourage the scapula to travel around the ribcage into protraction. Allow the elbow to flex as you hold the arm in horizontal adduction until the tissue releases.

4. When the client is in a prone position, repeat the arm pulling and palm spreading procedure. As the arm reaches 90 degrees of abduction, allow the arm to rotate as you traction it in front of the client's head. Wait for the release of the tissue.

Technique 65   Myofascial Leg Pulling

1. With the client in the supine position, grasp under the heel with one hand and on top of the foot with the other. The client's leg will be fully adducted with the knee and foot pointing up. The leg can be slightly lifted off the massage table. Lean back and traction the leg steadily until the tissue releases slightly (as shown). Don't bounce the leg up and down or jiggle it. The pressure should be steady and only as much as to meet the resistance in the tissue. Avoid pulling so hard that a client slides on the table or braces his or her muscles. Continue to traction the client's leg while using the foot and ankle to place the leg in lateral rotation (the knee should track in the same direction as the foot) until you feel resistance. Hold the position until the tissue softens. Continue to traction the client's leg while using the foot and ankle to place the leg in medial rotation until you feel resistance. Make sure that the knee tracks with the foot. You want the entire leg to rotate, not just the lower leg.

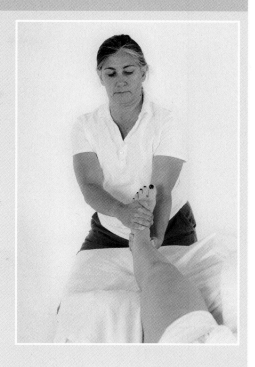

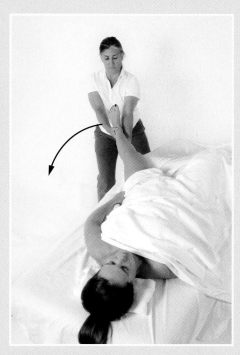

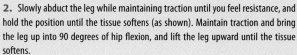

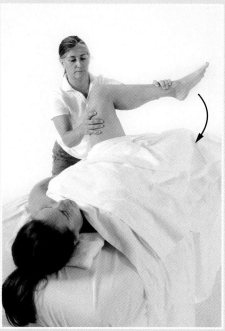

2. Slowly abduct the leg while maintaining traction until you feel resistance, and hold the position until the tissue softens (as shown). Maintain traction and bring the leg up into 90 degrees of hip flexion, and lift the leg upward until the tissue softens.

3. Allow the knee to flex, and press the leg slowly into internal rotation holding any place resistance is felt (as shown). Work very slowly and only within the comfort level of the client. While stabilizing the leg above the knee, move the leg into external rotation and hold until the tissue softens. Place the leg in a neutral position on the massage table and dorsiflex the foot until resistance is felt. Hold the stretch until the tissue releases. Now plantar flex the foot, and hold.

Technique 66   Crossed-Hand Stretch

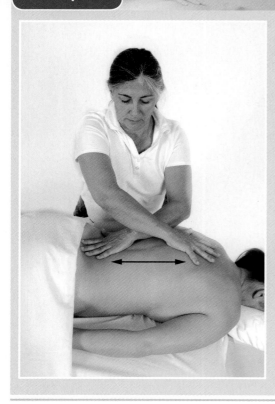

1. Cross your forearms and place your hands with your fingers pointing in opposite directions on the area in focus. Use the heels of your palms, your palms, and your fingers to engage the tissue and take the slack out of the fascia. One forearm and one hand might also be used. Hold the stretch until the tissue softens. The crossed-hand stretch can be applied superficially or deeply as determined by the therapist. This image shows a crossed-hand stretch on the back, but this technique can be used on any region of the body.

Technique 67   Fascial Spreading

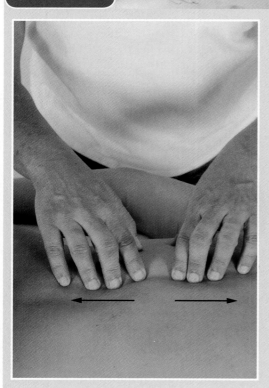

1. This technique can be applied in a few different ways. In this image, the fingers are placed side by side and separated to stretch a very specific area of fascia. You might also lock down one area of fascia with one hand while using the other to push the tissue away, taking slack out of the fascia and creating a stretch. The fascia could also be pulled toward you. For example, you might stand at the head of the massage table and pull the fascia of the gluteals and low back toward you. Fascia might also be pushed away from you; for example, the fascia between the shoulders and midback might be pushed toward the sacrum.

Technique 68 | Fascial Torquing

1. Lift the tissue until the slack is removed from the tissue, and deform the tissue slowly by torquing it back and forth and holding the tissue in a torqued position until the tissue softens. Release the tissue and then re-engage the tissue, and repeat the stroke until the tissue feels malleable. This stroke can feel intense and should be applied slowly with attention to the client's comfort level.

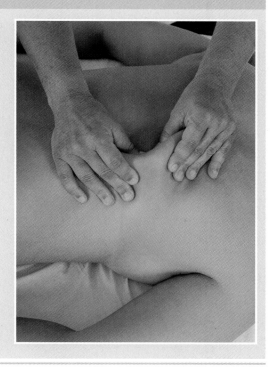

Technique 69 | Fascial Cutting

1. Use reinforced fingers, a knuckle, or the edge of one hand to outline muscles or bones at progressively deeper levels. In this image, the therapist is cutting up the lamina groove. The fingers, knuckle, or edge of the hands can be pushed away from you or pulled toward you depending on the body area being treated.

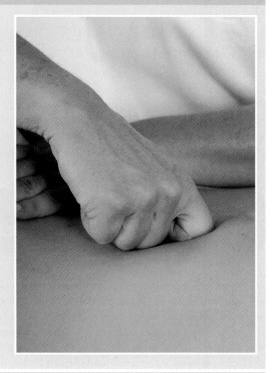

Technique 70   **Fascial Bowing**

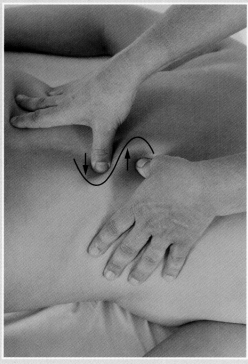

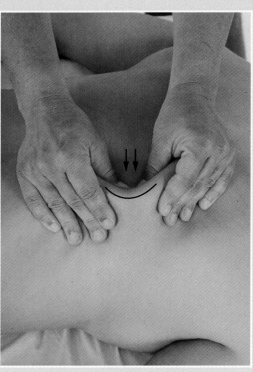

1. S-bowing is a technique in which the thumbs, fingers, or hands face each other and cross to create an S shape. Hold the deformed tissue in the S shape until you feel the tissue soften.

2. C-bowing is a technique in which the hands are used to deform the tissue in the shape of a C. It can be used both superficially and deeply on many regions of the body.

Integration of Myofascial Techniques with Swedish Massage

Often, therapists integrate myofascial techniques with Swedish massage or other massage systems like deep tissue massage, neuromuscular massage, and trigger point therapy. Myofascial techniques call for the absence of lubricant and are therefore applied first. Next Swedish techniques are used, and finally the area is passively stretched. For example, on the posterior legs you might apply skin rolling working in all directions. Then, you might use leg pulling and crossed-hand stretches before moving into more focused fascial techniques. Lubricant is applied to the skin before Swedish techniques are delivered, and then you finish the area with passive stretches. The order in which body areas are addressed depends on your preferences, the client's preferences, and the session goals.

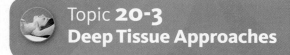

Topic 20-3
Deep Tissue Approaches

As the name suggests, **deep tissue massage** (also called deep pressure massage) is directed at the deeper myofascial structures of the body. Deep tissue massage is not really an independent system or even a separate technique. It is better described as a way to approach soft-tissue structures. At any time, and during any type of massage, a therapist should be able to slow down and work more deeply when localized tension is encountered. This section discusses the effects of deep tissue massage, assessment that informs deep tissue work, guidelines for the application of deep tissue massage, application of deep tissue massage, and how to integrate deep tissue work into a Swedish massage.

Effects of Deep Tissue Massage

In Chapter 13, you learned about friction. Because deep tissue massage uses deep friction strokes, the effects of deep friction apply to deep tissue massage. Earlier we discussed the effects of myofascial techniques and explained that they help to stir ground substance and improve its quality, increase piezoelectricity to improve the health of connective tissue, and reduce fascial restrictions and adhesions so that functionally separate structures don't stick together. These important effects also apply with deep tissue work, but with deep tissue massage the primary focus is to improve muscular balance by reducing the stress on the body caused by chronically shortened tissue. Your approach to the tissue focuses on identifying and lengthening chronically shortened tissue to help the body achieve greater muscular balance.

Goal: Muscular Balance

We know that myofascia can become chronically shortened for many reasons, such as poor posture, repetitive work stress, a sedentary lifestyle, poor diet and dehydration, or injury. Chronically shortened tissue disrupts the symmetry of balanced muscular tensions working on the skeleton and places the entire myofascial network under increased stress, as discussed earlier. From your study of kinesiology and anatomy, you understand how paired groups of muscles alternately contract or lengthen to move the bones to which they are attached. The interaction of opposing muscles is complex because the muscles must work in a coordinated manner to produce smooth movement in both directions. The agonist concentrically contracts to shorten the muscle, with the antagonist eccentrically contracts to control the movement at the joint while lengthening. You can imagine what happens if one of the closely related muscles becomes excessively strong or weak. The balance between the muscles is upset and suddenly new stresses are placed on the related joints and, through the fascia network, on all body structures. When a therapist uses deep tissue techniques effectively, the uneven pulls on the skeleton are corrected and the body experiences greater ease of movement and less structural stress through muscular balance.

Assessment for Deep Tissue Work

An important component of client assessment for deep tissue work is the health intake interview. Ask clients to describe previous injuries, surgeries, and medical conditions. Much can be learned about the ways in which the body compensated for these conditions by exploring with clients how they felt and moved before the condition and how they feel and move as a result of the condition. Oftentimes, these differences are illuminated by functional limitations to activities of daily life.

Posture and gait assessments are probably the most important tools for planning a session using deep tissue methods. In general, you are looking for postural asymmetry that indicates regions where myofascia is chronically shortened or chronically weakened. Note these areas on a SOAP chart and focus the massage to address restrictions in the shortened tissue.

Another method for assessing which structures require focus using deep tissue methods is range-of-motion testing. This assessment method helps you determine the client's current level of function using active, passive, and resisted range of motion to determine healthy or dysfunctional end feel, muscle length, and muscle strength. Functional limitations, posture and gait assessment, and muscle testing are discussed in Chapter 19.

Palpation before, during, and after the massage provides invaluable information about myofascial restrictions, patterns of tension, and the overall health of the myofascia. Use an anatomy or a kinesiology book to review the region where you are working, and visualize the muscle layers and fiber directions as you work. As you feel fiber direction changes and move from one muscle to the next, identify in your mind's eye the individual muscles and play along their borders, outlining their borders if possible with your strokes. As you reach the ends of muscles, feel for differences between muscle and tendon. Tendons feel smooth and dense. Ligaments feel taut, even when muscle is at rest.

Guidelines for the Application of Deep Tissue Massage

Follow these guidelines to reach your primary goal with deep tissue massage, which is to seek muscular balance. These guidelines remind therapists to remain attentive at all times to the current status of the tissue, how it is changing, and the comfort level and safety of the client.

- **If pain, no gain:** It is a common misconception that deep tissue massage is painful to receive and that the pain must be endured so that the tissue can be forcefully elongated. Instead of thinking "no pain, no gain," think "if pain, no gain." When people experience pain, they contract their muscles to protect themselves. Elongation of tissue cannot be achieved if the client is bracing against the stroke.

- **Safety:** In Chapter 5, you learned about sites of caution and contraindications. Never apply deep pressure over sites of caution. Instead, lighten your pressure and then re-engage the tissue at a deep level when you have cleared the site of caution. The client's overall condition and medications being taken may contraindicate deep tissue methods. Review the client's health history carefully and use good critical thinking skills to determine whether the client can benefit from deep tissue massage. Review Chapter 5 if you are unsure how to use critical thinking to rule out contraindications.

- **Integrate techniques:** Before dropping into the deeper layers of the myofascia with deep tissue methods, warm the tissue so that it is mobile and pliable with lighter myofascial techniques and Swedish massage. A session should never be composed entirely of deep tissue methods, which could overwhelm the client's system. Clients who are "overworked" may feel nausea during or directly after the session, may feel headachy during or directly after the session, and are likely to be sore and exhausted the next day. By integrating a number of different techniques, you ensure that the client's system can respond positively to the deep tissue methods you use.

- **Be present and communicate often:** During the application of deep tissue methods, you must remain present and responsive. Visualize the tissue under your hands to stay attuned to it and recognize when it is "inviting you deeper" or when it is "asking for more time." Regular communication with the client is important. In a general Swedish massage delivered for stress reduction, you usually communicate with the client a few times during the session to gauge the client's reaction, but too much communication could mar the client's relaxation. When using deep tissue massage, both you and the client should be focused on the changes occurring in the tissue and communicate about these changes regularly.

- **Use of lubricant:** Deep tissue work requires you to slow down and drop into deeper myofascial layers. If there is too much lubricant on the skin, you will slip over the surface of the skin and have difficulty working at the right depth. If, after the application of Swedish massage, the skin is too oily for deep work, use a dry towel to absorb the excess lubricant before attempting to drop into the tissue.

- **Slow down and wait for the tissue to release:** Deep tissue is applied slowly with keen attention to the tissue and the way in which it is changing. Drop into the tissue and intend for the tissue to soften and release, and for your forearm, elbow, knuckles, reinforced fingers, or supported thumbs to progress through the fibers of the myofascia as the prow of a boat moves through water. If you are working at the correct depth and remaining responsive to the tissue, it will slowly start to "open" and you will feel your elbow, knuckles, fingers, or thumb melt into the tissue and advance.

- **Never force resistant tissue:** Some therapists develop the habit of plowing through resistant tissue. If the tissue resists, make sure that it is warmed up sufficiently and then drop down to the point of resistance and wait for it to let go. If you truly listen to the tissue and are patient, it is likely to release and allow real progress to be achieved during the session.

- **Find the therapeutic edge:** For every client, there is a particular pace and depth of deep tissue manipulation that allows for the greatest possibility of therapeutic change in the tissue. The **therapeutic edge** can be defined as the place where the client feels the "good hurt." The client experiences some pain, but the pain feels right, appropriate, and good because along with the pain is the feeling of tissues releasing and tension patterns diminishing. Work that is too light can feel disappointing and leave the client's tissue "irritated" because it was not engaged with enough depth. Work that is too deep causes a defensive resistance in the tissue and leaves the tissue feeling violated or invaded. If you have solid palpation skills, you are more likely to be able to find the optimal pace and depth for each individual client and work on the client's therapeutic edge.

- **Work in layers:** Avoid changing the depth of your work sporadically and jumping between layers of tissue during the application of deep tissue methods. The nervous system can become overstimulated by such rapid changes, leaving the client restless or slightly irritated by the work. Instead, work in even patterns at progressively deeper layers as the client's tissue releases.

- **Work at oblique angles:** In some situations you might drop straight down into the tissue, but most often you apply pressure at an angle no >45 degrees. The use of oblique angles ensures that blood vessels, lymph vessels, and nerves won't be pinched against a bone. This also allows you to use your body weight effectively without undue stress on your joints.

- **Work origins and insertions as well as muscle bellies:** Novice therapists sometimes apply deep tissue manipulation to muscle bellies but avoid the use of deep tissue around the origin and insertion points of muscles. Many of these areas require you to remain responsive to tissue changes and adjust your pressure accordingly, but as long as the client expresses no discomfort, work in these areas is valuable. For example, deep pressure on long tendons can stimulate Golgi tendon organs to support myofascial release.

- **Place muscles in lengthened positions when possible:** It can be helpful to place a muscle in a lengthened position before the application of deep tissue massage to facilitate the elongation of tissue. For example, you might use one hand to plantar flex the ankle while applying a deep tissue stroke up the muscles of the anterior leg. Similarly, you might rest the arm above the head supported by a pillow in a slightly flexed position while applying a deep tissue stroke to the triceps.

- **Work the entire length of muscles:** When you apply a deep tissue stroke, start at one end of a muscle, group of muscles, or body area and work the entire length of the muscle, group of muscles, or body area. It can be disconcerting for the nervous system if you stop and start strokes that don't follow the structural lines of the body.

- **Use the breath:** Chapter 10 describes the basics of breathwork for massage. Remember that a client can support the release of adhered tissue with breathing. As a muscle is lengthened, as you move from the origin of a muscle to its insertion during a stroke, or as you move from distal body areas to proximal body areas, encourage the client to take a full breath and then exhale as the stroke is performed. If an area is particularly painful or tense, the client can use breath to decrease the sensation of pain. The use of the diaphragmatic breathing exercise described in Chapter 10 and demonstrated in Technique 14 in that chapter can help ease the strain on overworked scalenes and shoulder muscles and prepare the client to use his or her breath effectively during the session.

- **Use of passive and active movement:** Earlier, passive movement was described as the last technique applied to a body area, with active movement used at the very end of the session. These techniques help alert proprioceptors that new movement patterns are available and are important to reach and maintain treatment goals.

- **Watch for signs of emotional release:** Chapter 7, discussed body armor and emotional release. Because deep tissue work effectively breaks down body armor, emotions may surface during the course of the massage. If you are uncertain how to recognize signs of emotional release and manage an emotional release process, review Chapter 7.

Application of Deep Tissue Massage

Good body mechanics factor prominently in the ability to deliver deep work and remain responsive to tissue. Review Chapter 11, to refresh your good practices, especially if you feel stress in any joints or muscles while you work. Remember to use your body weight to achieve deeper pressure, and don't rely on strength from the muscles of your back or arms. Deep work is not hard work as long as you pay attention to your body and make adjustments to facilitate ease and efficiency. The strategies described here include lengthening strokes, muscle stripping, a modified pin and stretch technique, friction, and muscle separation. Because the psoas and iliacus muscles are a bit tricky to work with, the later Technique 75 demonstrates some techniques for massaging these deep muscles.

Lengthening Strokes

Lengthening strokes compress the tissue parallel to muscle fibers in a gliding motion that works from the origin of a group of muscles up the length of the muscles or body region in order to return a contracted muscle to its fundamental resting length along broad planes of structural tension. This stroke is applied with the forearms, knuckles, heel of the palms, or reinforced fingers and is the most common type of stroke used to apply deep tissue. The lengthening stroke is shown in Technique 71.

Muscle Stripping

Muscle stripping is similar to a lengthening stroke because it involves gliding compression. The primary difference is that muscle stripping is often used on one specific muscle from the muscle's origin to its insertion. For example, a lengthening stroke might be applied to one side of the back from the gluteal muscles up the erector spinae group and quadratus lumborum, across the rhomboids, splenius capitis and cervicis, over the upper fibers of the trapezius, and then down across the deltoid. Muscle stripping can be applied from the origin of the quadratus lumborum to its insertion with precision. A second muscle-stripping stroke can then be applied from the sacrum up the erector spinae group, while a third stroke might progress across the multifidi and rotatores muscles using the lamina groove as a guide. Don't be confused if this looks a lot like friction. It is friction, but its friction performed in a very specific way. Muscle stripping is shown in Technique 72.

Modified Pin and Stretch

A later chapter describes a true pin and stretch technique to help reset proprioceptors. A modified pin and stretch is useful as a deep tissue application strategy. One hand anchors a region, while the other moves either toward the anchoring

| Technique 71 | Deep Tissue Lengthening Strokes |

1. This image shows a lengthening stroke being applied to the back with the therapist's forearm. The stroke begins on the gluteals superior to the greater trochanter and progresses up the quadratus lumborum and erector spinae group. The therapist uses the entire forearm to apply this broad pressure. As she reaches the rhomboids, she will move onto the edge of her elbow to pass between the transverse processes on one side and the scapula on the other to finish the stroke around the shoulder. Lengthening strokes can also be applied with reinforced fingers or knuckles.

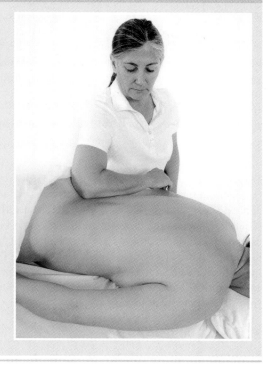

Technique 72   Muscle Stripping

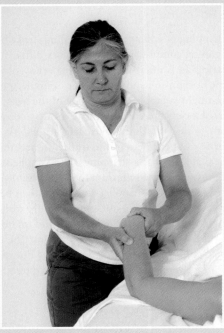

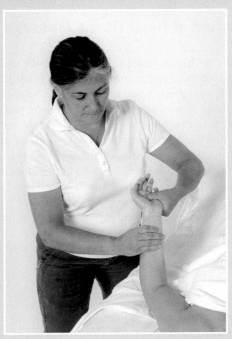

1. Notice that the flexors on the forearm are held in a lengthened position while the therapist strips with her thumb from the tendinous insertions of these muscles up to the common flexor tendon from the medial epicondyle of the humerus. Usually muscle stripping is used on one specific muscle, but in this case it is easy to strip multiple muscles at one time.

2. The same technique can be used on the extensor muscles by flexing the wrist and turning the forearm over.

hand or away from it. For example, while a lengthening stroke is applied up one side of the back with the forearm, the hand that isn't working locks down the myofascia at the sacrum, taking the slack out of the myofascia so that the lengthening stroke is more effective. Alternatively, to lengthen the tibialis anterior, you might place and hold the foot in plantar flexion while stripping from the knee toward the plantar flexed foot, thereby encouraging the length achieved by the passive motion you apply. The modified pin and stretch is shown in Technique 73.

Friction

Friction strokes are described in Chapter 13. All deep friction (circular, linear, and crossfiber or transverse friction) can be applied as part of deep tissue massage. In this case, these techniques are applied more slowly and deeply than in Swedish massage. Friction techniques are useful for both tendinous insertions of muscles and on muscle bellies, where they break up adhered tissue and promote healthy collagen production and alignment. Review Technique 20 in Chapter 13 to refresh your understanding of friction.

Muscle Separation

Muscle separation is a technique in which strokes are applied specifically to separate individual muscles that have become adhered due to increased hydrogen bonding and adhesions, as described earlier in this chapter. To separate adhered muscles, you might grab one muscle and roll it away from another, or you might outline its borders with progressively deeper strokes to break the bonds where muscles overlap or run in parallel. The use of active or passive range of motion while performing grasping and stripping techniques is also effective. The separation of muscles is shown in Technique 74.

Working with the Psoas and the Iliacus Muscles

The psoas and iliacus muscles (referred to collectively as the iliopsoas) play important roles in hip flexion and in stabilizing the low back. The psoas originates from the bodies and transverse processes of the lumbar vertebrae, while the iliacus originates from the iliac fossa and sacral ala. Both insert on the lesser trochanter. Many low back problems related to spinal rotation and lordosis are associated with the level of tension in the psoas and with the balance between the two psoas muscles (if one psoas is weak and the other is hypertonic, the tight psoas places rotational and side-flexion forces on the spine). Tension in the iliacus may disrupt the balance of the sacrum.[10] It is important to include massage of these muscles in treatment plans for low back issues. Methods for accessing and massaging these muscles are shown in Technique 75. Be sure to

Technique 73 **Modified Pin and Stretch**

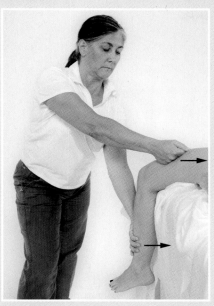

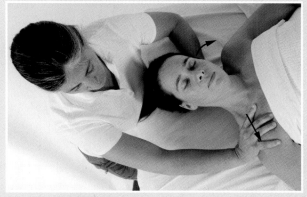

1. In this image, the therapist is anchoring the quadriceps muscles with one hand while applying a lengthening stroke with the other. By dropping the leg off the table, the therapist is also able to lengthen the quadriceps with one leg while applying this stroke.

2. The client's head is positioned to the left to lengthen the right lateral flexors. The therapist anchors the upper fibers of the trapezius and levator scapula with the hand that is bringing the neck into passive lateral flection. The other hand applies a lengthening stroke to further stretch the neck muscles.

Technique 74 **Muscle Separation**

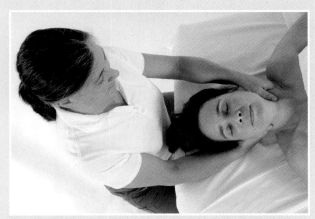

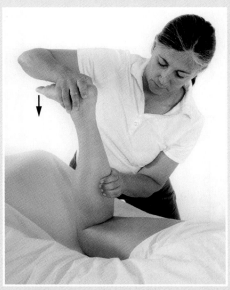

1. The SCM can easily stick to the other muscles beneath it. In this image, the therapist is picking up the SCM to separate the muscle. Hold this position until you feel the muscle soften.

2. The therapist in this image is using her fingers to separate the fibers of the gastrocnemius while holding the foot in dorsiflexion during the stroke. This places the gastrocnemius in a lengthened position. The therapist could also pick up the gastrocnemius to separate it with the client's leg in a bolstered position. You may notice that the therapist's body mechanics have become altered during the application of the technique. Be careful with your own body mechanics while applying these strokes, and avoid bending at the waist and tilting your head to watch the stroke.

Technique 75 **Massage of the Iliopsoas Muscles**

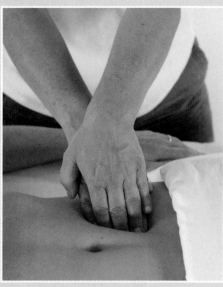

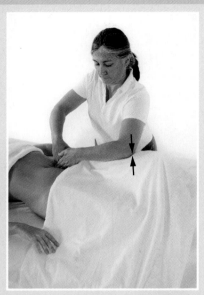

1. With the client supine and not bolstered and the abdominal area undraped, draw an imaginary line from the navel to the anterior superior iliac spine (ASIS). Find the point on the imaginary line that is halfway between the navel and ASIS. Place the fingertips of one hand on this point, and use the fingertips of the other to reinforce them. Ask the client to inhale, and when the client exhales gently drop your fingers into the tissue working at a slight angle with your fingers pointing toward the spine. Work very slowly and carefully. It will likely take three to four breaths to drop your fingers all the way to the psoas. The psoas lies just lateral to the abdominal aorta, so if you feel a strong pulse move your fingers laterally to get off the aorta.

2. When you are deep in the tissue, drop your forearm down and ask the client to flex the hip slightly (the movement should be small) into the resistance you are placing with your arm on the thigh. If you are in the right spot, you will instantly feel the muscles contact under your fingers. Now work your fingers in short longitudinal strokes along the fiber direction of the muscle. Then, work your fingers in short strokes transversely across the fibers of the muscle. This technique can also be used with the client in the side-lying position.

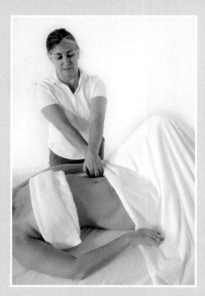

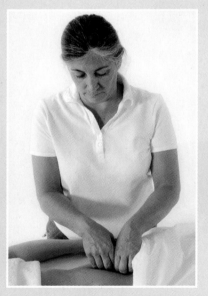

3. With your fingers still in place, ask the client to slowly flex the hip and drag the foot along the table as the knee comes up toward the chest. Compress the muscle fibers with your fingers, and then ask the client to lower the leg flat to the massage table. Repeat this action two to three times. Ask the client to slowly wave the foot (lateral and medial rotation) back and forth while you compress and strum with your fingers the fibers of the psoas. Exit the tissue very slowly.

4. With the client supine and not bolstered, place your fingertips side by side on the iliac crest. With a curling motion, bring your fingertips around the medial edge of the iliac fossa to rest on the iliacus. Ask the client to flex the hip (the movement can be small) and you will instantly feel the iliacus contract. Gently massage the muscle across its fibers by sliding your fingertips in small strokes inside the rim of the iliac fossa. Now, make small longitudinal strokes with your fingers as the tissue softens. Ask the client to slowly flex the hip and drag the foot along the table as the knee comes up toward the chest. Compress the fibers of the iliacus during both the contraction and the release as the client's leg relaxes back to the table. Again, this technique can also be used with the client in the side-lying position.

| Technique 75 | **Massage of the Iliopsoas Muscles** (Continued) |

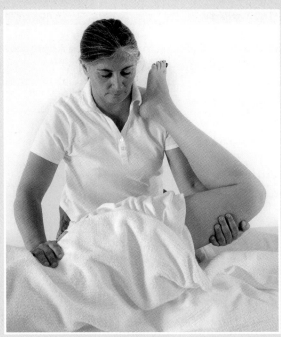

5. There are a number of ways to stretch the iliopsoas after it has received massage, but it works well to roll the client into a side-lying position and grasp the thigh with one hand while stabilizing the pelvis with your torso and other hand. Pull the thigh back so that the leg comes into extension. Alternatively, the client can be placed in a prone position. The therapist grasps under the thigh just above the knee. With the foot moving straight up toward the ceiling, lift the thigh taking the hip into extension until you feel resistance.

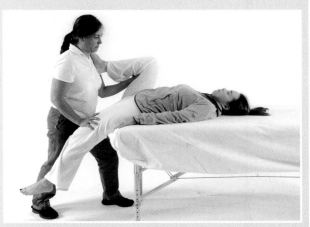

6. At the end of the session, you can stretch the iliopsoas with the client dressed (if clothing allows). The client is positioned at the end of the massage table. The therapist gently presses on the thigh above the knee to take the hip into extension until resistance is felt.

review the sites of caution for the abdominal and thigh regions in Chapter 5 before trying these techniques. Do not perform iliopsoas massage on pregnant women. Women who are menstruating may find this work too uncomfortable to tolerate.

Integration with Swedish Massage

Deep tissue massage is integrated easily with both myofascial techniques and Swedish massage. All three types of massage are often used in one session, even a session promoted as a relaxation massage. After you undrape a body area, apply myofascial techniques without lubricant. Next, place lubricant on the skin and warm the tissue with effleurage, pétrissage, and lighter friction strokes. When the tissue is warm and pliable, work on deeper layers using deep tissue methods, and then finish the body area with vibration, tapotement, and joint movement.

Many therapists use full-body strokes to connect body regions and address myofascia in broad planes. For example, after massaging the posterior legs and back, you might finish the posterior body with a lengthening stroke that begins at the ankle, passes over the gastrocnemius and soleus muscles, over the hamstrings, over the gluteal muscles and then up the erector spinae group, and around the shoulder to end with a sweep down the deltoid and arm. This type of stroke connects the entire span of the body and helps clients sense their full length. Remember to end the session with 5 minutes of active range of motion so that clients learn and integrate their new level of movement capability.

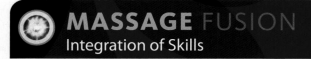

MASSAGE FUSION
Integration of Skills

STUDY TIP: List Assist

ACTIVE LEARNERS: hear it! see it! say it! write it! do it!

Students often pick up one or two new techniques and use them regularly but forget about other techniques and may never incorporate a full range of strokes into the massage. It's also important to follow the guidelines for the application of new techniques because it ensures that you develop good habits and apply the techniques correctly. To check that you are using all the new techniques you have learned and applying them correctly, copy the information in Tables 20-1 and 20-2 onto two separate poster boards. Tack these posters above your massage table when you practice your techniques on classmates. Refer to the information before, during, and after the massage of a body area to check that you have used a full range of techniques and applied them correctly. The action of making up the poster board, saying the information out loud regularly, and then practicing with the information fresh in your mind will help you memorize it and integrate it into your practice. Use this study tip for any new techniques you learn.

GOOD TO KNOW: Resources to Learn More

A number of excellent resources for myofascial and deep tissue work can help you to explore these techniques in more depth. Check out these books:

- Travell and Simons. *Myofascial Pain and Dysfunction—The Trigger Point Manual*. Baltimore, MD: Lippincott Williams and Wilkins, 1999.

TABLE 20-1   Checklist for Myofascial Application

Techniques to Try	Guidelines
Myofascial skin rolling	Ensure client comfort
Arm pulling	Safety—no if skin condition
Leg pulling	No lubricant or little lubricant
Crossed-hand stretch	Take out the slack
Fascial spreading	Work in all directions
Fascial torquing	Burning feeling okay—hyperemia okay
Fascial cutting	Avoid tissue compression
Fascial bowing	Work slowly—wait for release Follow the tissue release Use passive and active movement

TABLE 20-2   Checklist for Deep Tissue Approaches

Techniques to Try	Guidelines
Lengthening strokes	If pain, no gain
Muscle stripping	Lighten up over sites of caution
Modified pin and stretch	Warm the tissue—don't overwork client
Friction	Stay present and responsive
Muscle separation	Communicate often Seek muscular balance Minimal lubricant Slow down—wait for release Never force resistant tissue Find the therapeutic edge Work in layers Work at oblique angles Work origins, insertions, and bellies Place muscles in lengthened positions Use breath Use passive and active movement Watch for emotional release

- Barns. *Myofascial Release—The Search for Excellence*. Available at www.myofascialrelease.com/store/books.asp. Accessed June 2008.
- Schultz and Feitis. *The Endless Web—Fascial Anatomy and Physical Reality*. Berkeley, CA: North Atlantic Books, 1996.
- Myers. *Anatomy Trains—Myofascial Meridians for Manual and Movement Therapists*. Churchill Livingstone. New York. 2002.
- Juhan. *Job's Body—A Handbook for Bodywork*. New York: Station Hill, Barrytown, Ltd., 1989.
- Riggs. *Deep Tissue Massage: A Visual Guide to Techniques*. Berkeley, CA: North Atlantic Books, 2002.

MASSAGE INSPIRATION: Fascia as Plastic Wrap

Take a piece of plastic wrap and have a classmate wrap your arm in it. Tighten the wrap over one joint (shoulder or elbow), and then move your arm. What happens to your movement pattern? Fascia is like one large piece of plastic wrap. The lubricating nature of ground substance allows fascia fibers to slide over each other, but when ground substance cools the fascia starts to stick to itself, just as plastic wrap sticks to itself. Eventually freedom of movement is inhibited, which leads to more cooling of ground

MASSAGE FUSION *(Continued)*
Integration of Skills

substance and more sticking of fascia. It can be fun and informative to use long sheets of plastic wrap over a body area and then practice your myofascial release techniques. You can see the plastic stretching, just as fascia stretches.

IT'S TRUE: fascia as contractile tissue? what? no way! maybe!

This chapter discusses the current understanding of fascia and notes that fascia is plastic and not contractile. It connects and separates structures, distributing gravitational forces and forces related to posture and movement throughout the body. It adjusts to mechanical tension generated by muscle activity or external forces it doesn't actively contract. New research could change some of these views in the future if they are verified. A German study concluded that there is some evidence to suggest that fascia may be able to actively contract in a smooth-muscle-like manner and thereby influence musculoskeletal dynamics. The research team discovered contractile cells in fascia and cited an in vitro study that demonstrated autonomous contraction of the lumbar fascia of a human. Further, temporary contractions were stimulated via drugs in rat fascia in another in vitro study.[11] If future research confirms these findings, this could improve our understanding of musculoskeletal pathologies and the role of myofascial techniques in their treatment. For massage therapists, physical therapists, and chiropractors, the idea that fascia could contract is revolutionary. In fact, it's mind blowing!

CHAPTER WRAP-UP

If you studied this chapter carefully, you have a stronger grasp of the properties of connective tissue and really understand the interconnectedness of muscle and fascia. As you begin to apply myofascial and deep tissue techniques and integrate them with Swedish massage, you will notice that your sessions are more effective and you will see differences in posture and movement in as little as one treatment. Understanding myofascia is often an "Ah!" moment for students when what you feel under your hands starts to make sense on a new level. As one student, who was also a dancer, put it, "Knowing about fascia changes everything I know about movement and the limitations of my body. It changes everything I know about how to prepare for a performance and everything I know about how to massage other dancers." A professional massage therapist once commented, "Connective tissue was my transformative moment! Before that I did massage but I didn't really get it. When I learned about fascia in school it didn't make an impact, but after graduation I took a continuing education class in myofascial release and, wow, it happened. I felt my exchange partner's myofascia suddenly let go and it was like sinking into butter. It was the most amazing feeling. I always mark that massage as the point where I truly became a massage therapist."

For some students, the feeling of myofascia melting may take some time, but it is a goal worth working toward. Pay attention to what you feel, and visualize the structures under your hands as you work. Attune to the client's breath and rhythm. Apply the guidelines you have learned and be patient. When it does happen you may very well say, "This is the moment I am truly a massage therapist."

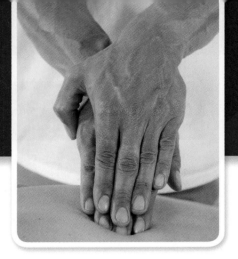

Chapter 21

Proprioceptive and Neuromuscular Approaches

KEY TERMS

Golgi tendon organs

muscle spindles

neuromuscular therapy

proprioceptors

proprioception

reciprocal inhibition

sarcomeres

stretch reflex

tendon reflex

trigger points

LEARNING OBJECTIVES

Having read the chapter and used the related student learning tools, the student will be able to:

1   Describe the proprioceptors and mechanisms related to the stretch reflex, tendon reflex, and reciprocal inhibition.

2   Explain considerations for the application of selected proprioceptive techniques.

3   Define the term *neuromuscular therapy,* and outline the origins of this form of therapy.

4   Define the term *trigger point,* and list three characteristics of trigger points.

5   Compare and contrast an active trigger point with a latent trigger point.

6   Explain the mechanisms related to the formation of trigger points, and identify four factors that can contribute.

7   Construct a plan to locate four trigger points on a practice body.

8   Predict three symptoms a client with trigger points might exhibit.

9   Explain two techniques that are used to deactivate trigger points.

It is safe to say that every person, at some point in his or her life, has suffered from muscles that feel tight and cause stiffness and soreness that lead to a decrease in freedom of movement. This chapter looks at a number of techniques that address short, tight, sore muscle tissue, and the interplay of neurological responses that cause problems or can be manipulated to reduce problems. The term **proprioception** comes from the Latin *proprius*, meaning "one's own," and the word perception.[1] It refers to the position of the body in space and the relationship of body parts to one another and to the environment around them. Proprioceptors include the Golgi tendon organs and muscle spindle cells. In Topic 21-1, you will learn how to stimulate these sensory neurons to cause positive changes to muscle tone and length. Topic 21-2 explores the relationship between the nervous system and the muscular system and how muscle health is affected through the deactivation of trigger points. The techniques in this chapter will expand the range of tools you can use to address muscle tension, postural dysfunctions, pain, soft-tissue injury, and chronic musculoskeletal dysfunction.

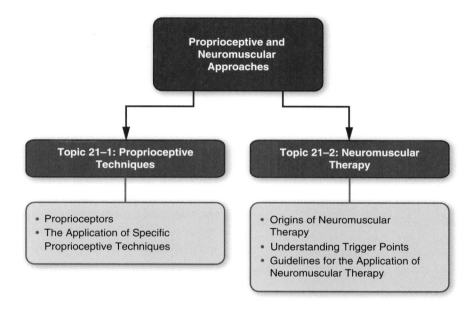

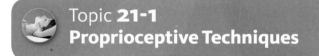

Topic **21-1**
Proprioceptive Techniques

Several bodywork systems (e.g., proprioceptive neuromuscular facilitation, muscle energy technique, and others) have been developed based on the idea that **proprioceptors** like Golgi tendon organs and muscle spindles can be manipulated to reset muscle tone and resting length to improve muscular balance and function. In some cases, techniques strengthen weakened muscle and help to facilitate normal muscle contraction and better range of motion. This section introduces key techniques that focus on proprioceptors as a means to improve muscle health.

Proprioceptors

Chapter 4 described how proprioceptors in muscles, tendons, and joints can be manipulated with certain techniques to alter muscle tension patterns and re-educate muscles about proper resting lengths. Bodywork techniques like those described here take advantage of somatic reflexes that help ensure smooth coordinated movement and protect muscles and tendons from damage. To understand the effects of these techniques, let's first review the stretch reflex, tendon reflex, and reciprocal inhibition.

Muscle Spindles and the Stretch Reflex

The **stretch reflex** is mediated by proprioceptors called **muscle spindles** that are located in the muscle belly and that monitor muscle length. Muscle spindles send information in the nervous system that helps control muscle movement by detecting the amount of stretch placed on a muscle. They protect the muscle from being overstretched and play a role in setting muscle tone.

When a muscle is stretched very rapidly, or overstretched, the muscle spindles are activated by gamma motor neuron activity and directly stimulate alpha motor neurons, causing the muscle to reflexively contract, thereby protecting the muscle from tearing. Sedentary habits, work conditions, stress, injury, and many other factors can cause muscles to lose their "memory" of their proper resting length in relationship to other muscles. Often, gamma motor neuron activity becomes hyperactive, and muscle spindles needlessly increase muscle tension, causing hypertonicity and shorter resting lengths. Some proprioceptive techniques employ voluntary isometric contractions that shorten the muscle belly, thereby "unloading" muscle spindles and reducing the rate at which gamma motor neurons fire to reduce muscle tone and reset muscle length.[2]

Golgi Tendon Organs and the Tendon Reflex

The **tendon reflex** is mediated by proprioceptors called **Golgi tendon organs** that monitor muscle tension and tendon strain. Golgi tendon organs are located in tendons near where the tendon joins with muscles. If a muscle contracts too strongly, such as when lifting a heavy load, the muscle and the tendon could be damaged. When Golgi tendon organs sense that a muscle contraction is straining a tendon, they are activated and cause the inhibition of the muscle's motor units, stopping the contraction and causing the muscle to relax. Many proprioceptive techniques stretch tendons in such a way that Golgi tendon organs reflexively relax the muscle.

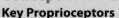
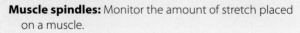

Concept Brief 21-1
Key Proprioceptors

Muscle spindles: Monitor the amount of stretch placed on a muscle.

Golgi tendon organs: Monitor muscle tension and tendon strain.

Reciprocal Inhibition

Reciprocal inhibition refers to a reflex mechanism in the body that ensures coordinated movement between groups of opposing muscles. For one muscle to contract during movement, the contraction of the opposing muscle must be inhibited, because people cannot move if both opposing muscles contract at the same time. When the agonist contracts to perform the movement, the antagonist muscle is stimulated to relax slightly to allow the contraction of the agonist. Some proprioceptive techniques employ this reflex mechanism for therapeutic purposes to decrease muscle spasms and hypertonicities in a target muscle.[3]

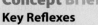

Concept Brief 21-2
Key Reflexes

- **Stretch reflex (muscle spindles):** Protects the muscle from being overstretched and damaged.
- **Tendon reflex (Golgi tendon organs):** Protects against tendon damage.
- **Reciprocal inhibition:** Ensures coordinated movement through inhibition of the antagonist muscle's contraction.

The Application of Specific Proprioceptive Techniques

Massage therapists find that the application of proprioceptive techniques enhances the benefits and effects clients experience from massage. While these techniques are most often used in healthcare sessions to achieve specific treatment goals, many can also be used successfully in wellness sessions because they are comfortable and enjoyable to receive. As you begin to integrate a variety of techniques in your sessions, keep some basic principles of sequencing in mind:

- **Broad to detailed to broad:** Often, therapists sequence techniques so that they open sessions and body areas with broad, general strokes like effleurage to warm the tissue and introduce the client to their hands and quality of touch. Broad techniques are followed by more detailed work, such as the trigger point application included later in this chapter. Finally, the therapist returns to the application of broad techniques to help the body integrate the work and to tie the body area or a group of body areas together.

- **Superficial to deep to superficial:** Usually, therapists sequence techniques so that they work the superficial tissues first and gradually move into deeper work as the body relaxes and accepts the therapist's hands and the pressure of strokes. At the end of a body area, the therapist is likely to return to superficial work to flush the tissue (e.g., effleurage strokes applied toward the heart).

- **Get the client moving:** Often, passive movement, passive stretching, and active movement are incorporated into the protocol for a particular technique. The use of passive movement, stretching, and active movement can be employed during every massage, especially when proprioceptive techniques are used to reset muscle resting lengths. At the end of the treatment of a particular body area, take a moment to passively move any joints through their full available range of motion. As long as it is appropriate and not contraindicated, gently stretch muscles at the joint's end range. Then, when the client is fully dressed, ask him or her to actively move any joints where you performed treatment. This helps the body integrate new information about forgotten movement patterns and helps to re-educate muscles about new length and ease of motion.

Golgi Tendon Organ Release

Golgi tendon organ release is a technique developed with physical therapy methods. It is useful as a means to reduce muscle spasms and hypertonicity, especially in muscles with long tendons such as the Achilles' tendon and hamstring tendon at the ischial tuberosity. Review Technique 76 for a demonstration of its application.

Contract Relax, Hold Relax, and Postisometric Relaxation

Three similar techniques were developed in the 1940s related to proprioceptive neuromuscular facilitation and muscle energy technique systems. In these techniques, the target muscle is first contracted and is then passively lengthened to increase muscle length and range of motion. In the contract-relax technique, you identify a target muscle and slowly and gently move the body into a position that places the muscle in a lengthened position at the point where the tissue "pushes back" or exhibits resistance (usually due to muscle tension). Instruct the client to "hold this position while I try to move you." The client contracts the target muscle while you resist the movement. In this technique it is okay for the muscle to contract concentrically

(contract while shortening), but the movement you allow to occur at the joint should be minimal. The client continues to contract the muscle, and you continue to hold the position for 5 to 10 seconds. Instruct the client "to relax fully," and as the client relaxes, take the target muscle into a passive stretch until you feel the tissue again "push back." Repeat the process three or more times. Each time the process is repeated, the tension barrier (the point where the tissue pushes back) should be extended, demonstrating that muscle tone is reducing and muscle length is increasing. Note that the client should fully contract the muscle but not so strongly that it is impossible for you to resist the movement. This method is shown in Technique 77.

The hold-relax technique is performed in exactly the same way as contract-relax but with a small variation. In this case the muscle is contracted isometrically (without any movement occurring at the joint), so the client is directed to use a mild contraction so that the therapist has no difficulty resisting the movement. This ensures that the therapist can hold the client in position without movement occurring at the joint. Hold-relax is demonstrated in Technique 78.

In the 1980s, Karel Lewit developed a technique called postisometric relaxation. It is very similar to contract-relax and hold-relax. The difference is that Lewit advocates the use of gentler client contractions, specific breathing patterns, and eye movements to facilitate the phases of the technique. Review Technique 79 for a demonstration of this technique.

Technique 76   Golgi Tendon Organ Release

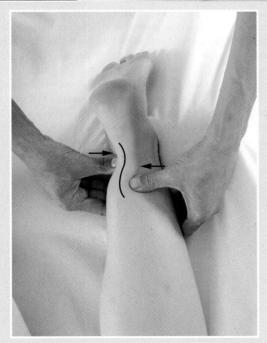

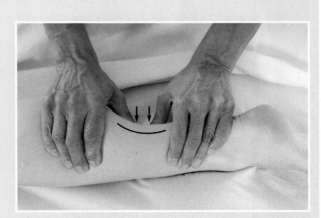

1. Use your thumbs or fingers to apply an S-bow (review Chapter 20 for details) on the tendon where it joins with the muscle.

2. You can also apply a C-bow. Hold the S-bow or C-bow for 30 seconds or longer with moderate-to-deep pressure. Repeat the application up to three times.

Technique 77 · Contract-Relax

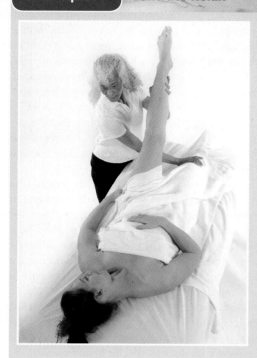

In this image, the target muscles are the hamstrings. The therapist has placed the hip in flexion at the point where the client's tight hamstring muscles create a tension barrier. The client is instructed to contract the hamstrings while the therapist resists the movement. The therapist instructs the client to relax completely and then passively stretches the hamstrings until the next tension barrier is reached.

Technique 78 · Hold-Relax

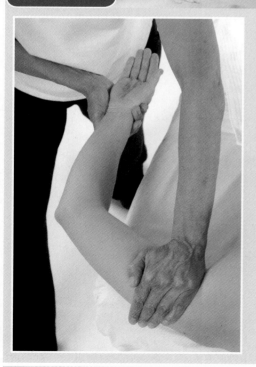

In this technique, the target muscle(s) is first contracted and is then passively lengthened to increase muscle length and range of motion. In the hold-relax technique, you identify a target muscle or muscles, in this case the lateral rotators of the shoulder, and slowly and gently move the body into a position that places the muscle in a lengthened position at the point where the tissue "pushes back" or exhibits resistance (usually due to muscle tension). Instruct the client to "hold this position while I try to move you." The client contracts the target muscle while you resist the movement. The muscle is contracted isometrically (without any movement occurring at the joint), so the client is directed to use a mild contraction so that the therapist has no difficulty resisting the movement. The client continues to contract the muscle and you continue to hold the position for 5 to 10 seconds. Instruct the client to relax fully, and as the client relaxes, take the target muscle into a passive stretch until you feel the tissue again "push back." Repeat the process three or more times. Each time the process is repeated, the tension barrier (the point where the tissue pushes back) should be extended, demonstrating that muscle tone is reducing and muscle length is increasing.

Technique 79   Postisometric Relaxation

The therapist has passively moved the hip in flexion to the point where the client's tight hamstring muscles create a tension barrier. The client is instructed to contract the hamstrings gently against the therapist's resistance while inhaling slowly for 10 seconds. The therapist instructs the client to relax completely while exhaling and moving the eyes in the direction of the stretch, while the therapist passively stretches the hamstrings until the next tension barrier is reached.

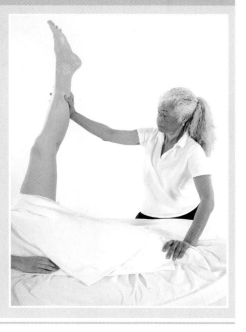

Reciprocal Inhibition

Reciprocal inhibition is a reflex mechanism of the body that inhibits the contraction of antagonist muscles while agonist muscles are contracting, to ensure coordinated movement (one group contracts while the opposing group relaxes). In the technique named reciprocal inhibition, this reflex is used to reduce spasm or tension in the target muscle. The target muscle(s) is identified and the antagonist(s) of the target muscle(s) is contracted isometrically for 10 seconds against resistance from the therapist. The client is instructed to stop the contraction and relax fully while the therapist passively moves the target muscle into a deeper stretch and then into its action. Review Technique 80 for a demonstration of this method.

Contract-Relax-Antagonist Contract

Contract-relax-antagonist contract is a cycle that uses elements of postisometric relaxation (contract-relax) and reciprocal inhibition to lengthen muscles that are chronically shortened while decreasing adhesions and hypertonicities. This method is demonstrated in Technique 81.

Origin and Insertion Technique

Origin and insertion technique is applied to activate the Golgi tendon organs in muscles with shorter tendons. It reduces muscle spasm, hypertonicity, and adhesions. Apply the technique by making small with-fiber strokes using the fingers or thumbs

Technique 80   Reciprocal Inhibition

In this case, the target muscle is the gastrocnemius (a muscle that plantar flexes the foot). The client is isometrically contracting the dorsiflexors against the therapist's resistance. Hold this position for 10 seconds and then ask the client to relax while you stretch the target muscle (gastrocnemius). You can repeat this process up to three times.

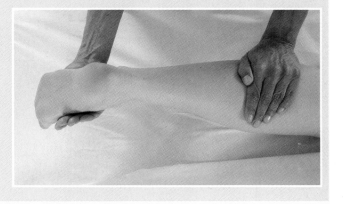

Technique 81 — Contract-Relax-Antagonist Contract

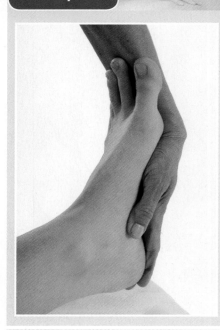

In this image, the therapist is focusing on the gastrocnemius with the client in the supine position. The therapist places one hand on the heel and forearm on the ball of the foot. The client actively contracts the dorsiflexors and the therapist assists the motion. The therapist then instructs the client to not allow movement. The client contracts the plantar flexors to resist the movement of the therapist pushing the foot further into dorsiflexion. The contraction is held for 5 seconds and then the client is instructed to relax. The cycle is repeated three to five times.

at the muscle's origin. The pressure is moderate to deep and applied slowly. Then, repeat the technique using cross-fiber strokes. Cover the entire surface of the area where the muscle originates with the technique. Next, move to the muscle's insertion and apply both with-fiber and cross-fiber strokes to the entire area of the insertion. This method is shown in Technique 82.

Muscle Approximation

Muscle approximation is a physical therapy technique that decreases muscle spasm and hypertonicity by unloading muscle spindles. With slow, deliberate pressure and movement, grasp both ends of a muscle and push the muscle together. Muscle approximation is shown in Technique 83.

Technique 82 — Origin and Insertion Technique

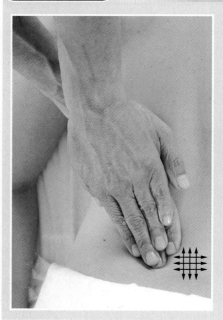

Origin and insertion technique is applied to activate the Golgi tendon organs on muscles with shorter tendons. It reduces muscle spasm, hypertonicity, and adhesions. Apply the technique by making small with-fiber strokes using the fingers or thumbs at the muscle's origin. The pressure is moderate to deep and applied slowly. Then, repeat the technique using cross-fiber strokes. Cover the entire surface of the area where the muscle originates with the technique. Next, move to the muscle's insertion and apply both with-fiber and cross-fiber strokes to the entire area of the insertion.

Technique 83 | **Muscle Approximation**

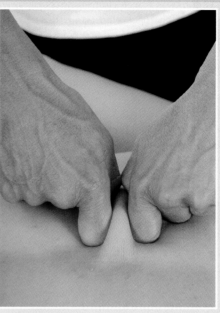

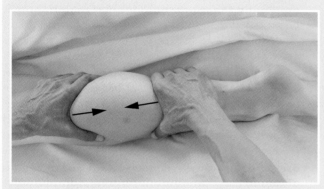

1. Muscle approximation is a physical therapy technique that decreases muscle spasm and hypertonicity by unloading muscle spindles. With slow, deliberate pressure and movement, grasp both ends of a muscle and push the muscle together. In this image, the therapist applies the technique to the gastrocnemius muscle.

2. In this image, the therapist applies muscle approximation to a segment of the erector spinae group by using the knuckles of each hand to push the origin and insertions toward one another.

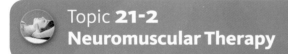

Topic **21-2**
Neuromuscular Therapy

Neuromuscular therapy (NMT) is a form of bodywork that aims to locate, treat, and prevent chronic pain associated with myofascial **trigger points**. Many healthcare professionals, including massage therapists, athletic coaches, physical therapists, chiropractors, osteopaths, nurses, dentists, and occupational therapists, use techniques derived from NMT. This section briefly discusses the origins of NMT, explains the basics of the development of trigger points, provides guidelines for the application of NMT, and previews some key NMT techniques. NMT is an advanced massage system, and the goal here is only to introduce practical methods you can add to your massage technique toolbox. Continuing education classes are recommended if you find this technique useful.

Origins of Neuromuscular Therapy

Ideas that lead to similar systems of treating soft-tissue pain associated with trigger points emerged in the mid-1930s and early 1940s. In Europe, Stanley Lief and Boris Chaitow developed a system called neuromuscular techniques.[4] In America, Raymond Nimmo and James Vannerson published a newsletter titled *Receptor Tonus Techniques* in which they described methods for addressing "noxious nodules" in muscle.[5] A number of different osteopaths, naturopaths, medical doctors, researchers, physical therapists, and massage therapists contributed to the development of similar protocols and methods known by the names neuromuscular techniques, NMT, and trigger point therapy, among others in Europe and America. Names most familiar to massage therapists include Leon Chaitow, John Sharkey, Paul St. John, and Judith DeLaney.

Dr. Janet Travell and Dr. David Simons deserve special mention for their landmark book *Myofascial Pain and Dysfunction: The Trigger Point Manual Volume 1—The Upper Half of the Body,* and *Volume 2—The Lower Half of the Body.*

Janet Travell (1901 to 1997) was an American physician who spent her life exploring the mechanisms of myofascial pain and dysfunction. She was appointed White House Physician during the Kennedy and Johnson administrations and published over 40 articles about her research in medical journals, beginning in 1942.

David Simons was Travell's long-time colleague who began his career as an aerospace physician. Intrigued by Travell's work, he retired from the Air Force and began an informal apprenticeship under her guidance. As a research scientist, he was rigorous in the objective documentation of myofascial pain and was the driving force behind the completion of their trigger point books.

Travell and Simon's trigger point manual introduced substantial research related to myofascial pain syndromes. Based on this research, they describe their theories about how trigger points develop, how they impact particular muscles and the body as a whole, and methods to release trigger points to promote better health and function. This work provided in-depth, rigorously referenced data to inform massage and bodywork practices and provided relevance, background, and structure to NMT.

Understanding Trigger Points

Travell and Simons define a trigger point as a "hyperirritable spot in skeletal muscle that is associated with a hypersensitive palpable nodule in a taut band" (Fig. 21-1). Trigger points exhibit a number of characteristics that help us differentiate them from other soft-tissue injuries or dysfunctions:

- **Trigger points feel like nodules:** As a massage therapist, you can feel trigger points in soft tissue as small rounded structures that can be described as nodules, knots, bound tissue, lumps, or pea-like masses that range in size from a pinhead to a lump the size of a knuckle.

- **Trigger point nodules are hypersensitive:** Trigger points are susceptible to any additional stress in the region where they are located and are easily upset by touch. Clients may wince or pull away when you apply a stroke in a region where there are trigger points.

- **Trigger points cause hyperirritability in local tissue:** The hypersensitivity of trigger points causes the tissue in the region of a trigger point to become hyperirritable. For example, the area may overreact to a brief increase in physical activity that might occur with a day of yard work or housework. Muscles in the region may spasm, circulation is decreased, and pain is increased.

- **Trigger points are found in taut bands of muscle tissue:** Trigger points are found in taut bands of muscle. Taut bands are groups of tense muscle fibers surrounding trigger points. Small muscles tend to create taut bands that feel like wiry strings, while larger muscles produce areas that feel like ropes or cables.

- **Trigger points cause symptoms locally and in regions distant to the point:** Pain and tenderness are likely specifically at the nodule and also possibly referred to other areas of the body. This means that pain felt from a trigger point might radiate out into broader regions of the body. Travell and Simons mapped predictable referral patterns for common trigger point locations. For example, trigger points in the triceps muscle can cause pain up into the shoulder and trapezius and down to the wrist (Fig. 21-2).

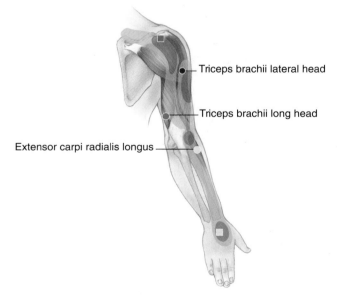

Figure 21-2 Pain felt from a trigger point might radiate out into broader regions of the body. Travell and Simons mapped predictable referral patterns for common trigger point locations. For example, trigger points in the triceps muscle can cause pain up into the shoulder and trapezius and down to the wrist.

Triceps brachii lateral head

Triceps brachii long head

Extensor carpi radialis longus

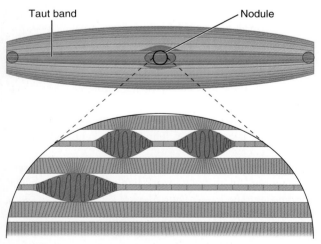

Taut band

Nodule

Figure 21-1 Travell and Simons define a trigger point as a "hyperirritable spot in skeletal muscle that is associated with a hypersensitive palpable nodule in a taut band."

Concept Brief 21-3
Trigger Point Defined

A trigger point is a hyperirritable spot in skeletal muscle that is associated with a hypersensitive palpable nodule in a taut band.

Types of Trigger Points

Trigger points are classified based on their qualities as active, associated, attachment, central, key, latent, primary, and satellite. Myofascial trigger points refer to trigger points that occur in muscle or fascia, but trigger points might also occur in cutaneous, ligamentous, periosteal, or other nonmuscular tissue.[6]

- **Active:** An active trigger point causes pain even when the client is at rest and not receiving stimulation through palpation. Clients recognize active trigger points as the source of pain.

- **Associated:** An associated trigger point is a trigger point in one muscle that occurs in tandem with a trigger point in another muscle. Both trigger points often originate from the same mechanical or neurological cause. Sometimes, one trigger point leads to the formation of the associated point.

- **Attachment:** As the name suggests, this type of trigger point forms at places where muscle attaches to bone. They might occur at the musculotendinous junction or at periosteal insertions.

- **Central:** Central trigger points form near the center of the muscles fibers and are associated with dysfunctional motor endplate activity (described in more detail later).

- **Key:** This type of trigger point activates one or more satellite trigger points. It is often identified as a key trigger point only after it has been deactivated, because its deactivation causes the deactivation of satellite points.

- **Latent:** A latent trigger point causes pain when it is palpated but is not recognized by the client as a primary cause of their pain or limited range of motion.

- **Primary:** This is a central trigger point activated by acute trauma or by chronic overuse of the muscle in which it occurs. It was not activated as a result of a trigger point in another muscle.

- **Satellite:** A satellite trigger point (sometimes called a secondary or "baby" trigger point) is activated because of key trigger points in a referral zone or in an overloaded synergist muscle compensating for the muscle in which the key trigger point is located.

Formation of Trigger Points

Exactly how trigger points form is unknown. A number of researchers have advanced theories about why they occur. Many believe they form as a result of contracted **sarcomeres** caused by a chemical imbalance at the point where a nerve and a muscle communicate with one another. Muscle tissue is made up of specialized contractile cells called muscle fibers. Muscle fibers are composed of hundreds of myofibrils, which

are themselves composed of specialized proteins called myofilaments. Myofilaments are submicroscopic, slender, stringy structures. There are two types. Thick myofilaments are composed of myosin, and thin myofilaments are composed of actin. Thick and thin myofilaments lie parallel to one another and overlap, creating the dark and light striations that are visible when muscle is viewed under a microscope. Units of myofilaments are separated by protein fibers called Z-lines. Z-lines run at right angles to the myofilaments and hold the thin (actin) myofilaments in place. A sarcomere is the length of a myofibril between two Z-lines (Fig. 21-3). Sarcomeres are the functional unit (the smallest structures of an organ that can perform the function) of muscle, and the activity of the sarcomeres is what causes the muscle to contract (millions of sarcomeres must be activated to make even the smallest movement).

The sliding filament model explains the contraction of a muscle at a molecular level. When the muscle is stimulated to contract by the axon of a communicating nerve, the thick and thin myofilaments attach to one another to form "bridges." The bridges behave as levers that pull the myofilaments past each other. Calcium and adenosine triphosphate must be present for the bridges to form correctly and for the muscle contraction to occur.

Trigger points develop when a group of sarcomeres enter a state of prolonged contracture. Prolonged contracture of sarcomeres occurs without stimulation from the nerve axon that innervates the muscle fiber. Researchers believe contracture is caused by dysfunctional motor endplate activity due to a chemical imbalance. Chemical imbalances are most likely caused by some level of mechanical overload (acute trauma, overuse, repetitive use, etc.) to the muscle, but other factors might also play a role (explained in the next section). The pain produced by trigger points may cause muscles in the area to enter a protective spasm to splint the region. This results in decreased circulation, leading to an oxygen and nutrient deficit that further complicates the condition.

Concept Brief 21-4
Contracted Sarcomere Theory

The theory that trigger points are formed as a result of contracted sarcomeres caused by a chemical imbalance at the point where a nerve and muscle communicate.

Factors that Contribute to the Formation of Trigger Points

Travell and Simons note that myofascial trigger points are very common in all sectors of the population. For example, trigger points don't just affect people as they grow older. In a study of 200 young adults, latent trigger points were identified in the shoulder girdle muscles of 54% of females and 45% of males.[7] A number of factors likely contribute to the formation of trigger points:

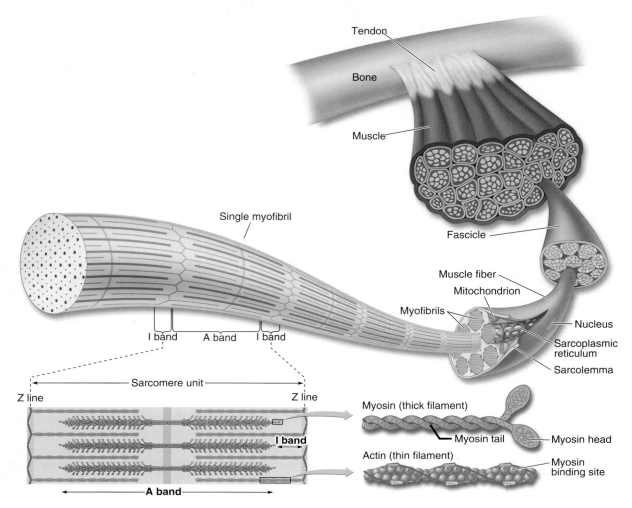

Figure 21-3 A sarcomere is the length of a myofibril between two Z-lines as shown in this image. Sarcomeres are the functional unit (the smallest structures of an organ that can perform the function) of muscle, and the activity of the sarcomeres is what causes the muscle to contract (millions of sarcomeres must be activated to make even the smallest movement).

- **Muscle overload:** Poor posture, repetitive work activities, a sudden increase in physical activity, hard physical training in athletes, or abnormalities in anatomical structure can overload muscles and increase the likelihood of trigger point formation.

- **Muscle trauma:** Soft-tissue injuries such as sprains, strains, or contusions may activate the formation of trigger points. This may be due to the changes in circulation to the region that occur as part of the inflammatory process and pain-spasm-pain cycle.

- **Vitamin and mineral deficiency:** Travell and Simons noticed a correlation between chronic myofascial pain and vitamin deficiency. Almost half of the patients treated for chronic pain lacked vitamins B_1, B_6, B_{12}, C, and folic acid. Calcium, iron, magnesium, and potassium levels were also low.

- **Metabolic disorders:** Metabolic disorders including low thyroid function, hypoglycemia, anemia, and uricemia (high levels of uric acid in the blood) may contribute to the formation and persistence of trigger points.[8]

- **Mental and emotional stress:** Stress impacts every system of the body and often causes increased muscular tension that decreases circulation in regional muscle tissue. Stress also causes metabolic changes in the body that may contribute to the formation and persistence of trigger points.

- **Other factors:** Exposure to cold, the onset of a virus or bacterial infection, or conditions like fibromyalgia may contribute to the formation of trigger points.

To treat trigger points effectively, we must alert our clients to factors that may contribute to their formation and persistence. These factors must be resolved, eliminated, or reduced for trigger points to remain deactivated after treatment.

The Locations of Trigger Points

A trigger point can form in any muscle, but postural muscles of the neck, shoulder, and pelvic girdles, and the upper trapezius, scalenes, sternocleidomastoid, levator scapulae, and quadratus lumborum muscles commonly produce active trigger points. Later in this chapter, you will learn how to identify the regions where trigger points are likely to be located in the muscles of individual clients based on subjective and objective data gathered during client assessment.

Symptoms of Trigger Points

People experience a variety of symptoms due to trigger points in muscles. Some of these symptoms, like pain, they recognize and report, while others, like watery eyes, they don't associate with muscular issues and often don't report. Specific questions related to the autonomic and general motor disturbances caused by trigger points can be added to your health intake form to help you better capture the subjective experiences of your clients during the intake process. Common symptoms of trigger points include:

- **Pain:** Active trigger points produce pain that the patient recognizes, even at rest.
- **Paresthesia:** An active trigger point may cause the sensation of numbness rather than pain in a referral zone (the predictable pain pattern associated with common trigger points in specific muscles).
- **Muscle tension:** Latent trigger points may cause increased muscular tension in the region of the trigger point and shortened muscles.
- **Reduced range of motion:** Both active and latent trigger points cause muscles to be shortened, reducing the range of motion at an affected joint.
- **General motor function disturbances:** As a result of trigger points in a region, other muscles might go into spasm, there may be increased weakness of muscles in the region, coordination may be reduced, and muscles in the area may be less able to recover after fatigue and be more susceptible to mechanical stress.
- **Autonomic disturbances:** Travell and Simons found that symptoms related to autonomic nervous system disturbances caused by trigger points include abnormal sweating, eye redness and irritation, watering of the eyes, blurry vision, persistent runny nose, increased salivation, and goose bumps.
- **Sleep disturbances:** The pain and other symptoms caused by trigger points may cause sleep disturbances. Active trigger points may become more painful when the sleeper's body position places muscles where they are located in shortened positions. In addition, some active and latent trigger points might be compressed by sleep positions, increasing pain in certain muscles.

Guidelines for the Application of Neuromuscular Therapy

The goal of NMT is to locate and treat trigger points that are causing pain, muscle shortness, and muscle weakness. The treatment of trigger points can lead to pain reduction and help prevent chronic pain conditions.

Locating Trigger Points

Regular assessment methods such as a health intake form and interview, posture assessment, and range-of-motion assessment help you locate broad regions where trigger points are often most irritable. For example, during the health intake process, clients usually identify areas where they feel pain. These areas are likely to be places where active trigger points are located. You may also notice postural holding patterns that cause postural distortions during a posture analysis. Any misaligned body position causes increased stress to joints and muscles in a region, and this stress is likely to lead to the formation of trigger points. Range-of-motion testing will reveal a reduced range of motion in joints affected by muscles with trigger points, and particular muscles may be noticeably weakened during resisted range-of-motion testing. During palpation or general massage of a region, the body may respond to the pressure of your stroke with signs that indicate the presence of trigger points. These signs include:

- **The presence of taut bands:** The taut bands that form around trigger points have a ropey, cable-like (larger muscles) or stringy, wire-like consistency when the muscle is palpated. This tissue feels decidedly unlike the pliable, springy texture of healthy tissue.
- **The presence of tender nodules:** The contracted sarcomeres that make up the tender nodules that are trigger points feel like a small pea, knot, or mass of tissue. Be careful not to confuse trigger points with lymph nodes in lymph node–rich areas like the neck and armpit.
- **General pain in a region:** The soft tissue in a region where trigger points are located is likely to be tender and hypertonic. Active trigger points become more active when tender nodules are compressed.
- **Pain with compression of a tender nodule:** Latent trigger points produce pain when the trigger point is compressed. Usually, clients are unaware of latent trigger points and may suddenly wince or jump when the point is touched.
- **Referred pain:** Active trigger points or compressed latent trigger points may produce pain that radiates out from the trigger point and is felt at an area distant to the trigger point.
- **Numbness:** Active or latent trigger points may create a sensation of numbness that radiates out from the trigger point to areas distant to the trigger point when the point is compressed.

Once you have identified trigger points in a region, your goal is to improve the health of the muscle tissue around the points and deactivate specific points.

Deactivation of Trigger Points

The deactivation of trigger points is an uncomfortable process for the client. Remind clients throughout treatment to focus on long, slow, deep belly breathing. Because of the stress caused to the nervous system (trigger point work stimulates the sympathetic nervous system response) during deactivation of trigger points, treat no more than five muscles in a given session. Spend the remainder of sessions applying soothing strokes that stimulate the parasympathetic nervous system response to aid the body in rest and recovery. Follow these general guidelines when deactivating trigger points:

- **Clusters:** Identify areas that contain clusters of trigger points, and focus on these areas first in your treatment.

- **Identify the most irritable point:** Treat the most irritable trigger points first because this trigger point is often a key point. Sometimes, the deactivation of one key point will deactivate a number of satellite points.
- **Medial and superior points:** Treat trigger points that are medial and superior before points that are distal and lateral.
- **Superficial first:** Often, trigger points occur in muscles that are stacked in layers. Treat the trigger points in superficial muscles before those in deeper layers.
- **Muscle bellies:** When treating a specific muscle with multiple trigger points, deactivate the points in the muscle belly before points occurring at attachment sites.
- **Place the muscle in a lengthened position:** Place the muscle with trigger points in a lengthened position for treatment. Trigger points are more likely to deactivate when the muscle is not contracted during the application of static compression.
- **Warm the tissue:** Warm the tissue that surrounds the trigger point with hydrocollator packs and with massage strokes such as skin rolling and friction. The goal is to increase circulation to improve the overall metabolic health of the muscles where trigger points occur.
- **Apply static compression to the point:** Apply static compression to the point for 8 to 12 seconds as described in Technique 84 (Static Compression).

- **Stretch the muscle:** Immediately after deactivating a trigger point, passively lengthen and stretch the muscle to reset the muscle's resting length. Encourage clients to regularly stretch muscles where trigger points form, as part of their self-care routine. The more regularly a muscle is stretched, the less likely it is to form trigger points.[9]

Document the location where you identified trigger points, and chart the trigger points you deactivated and your results. Share with clients the factors that contribute to trigger point formation, and encourage self-care activities such as stretching, regular exercise, and reducing repetitive activities to improve the treatment's success. Use subsequent treatments to continue to locate and deactivate trigger points.

Techniques for Trigger Point Deactivation

In previous chapters, you learned how to apply hot packs and warm the muscle tissue with strokes like skin rolling and friction. Review Chapters 13 and 16 if you need a refresher in these techniques. The primary techniques used in trigger point deactivation are static compression (also called ischemic compression) and pincer compression. These methods are taught in Techniques 84 and 85.

Because trigger point deactivation usually causes the client discomfort, constant communication is required with the client during NMT. Before you deactivate trigger points, work out a pain scale with clients so that they can keep you

| **Technique 84** | **Static Compression (Ischemic Compression)** |

Using your thumbs, elbow, or fingers, apply direct downward pressure over the top of the tender nodule that forms a trigger point for 8 to 12 seconds or longer if pressure continues to cause the pain produced by the point to decrease. Every other second, ask the client to report his or her sensation of pain using the scale described in the text. Adjust your pressure based on the client's feedback. If the treatment is successful, the client will report a lessening of the pain each time you ask her to rate the experience.

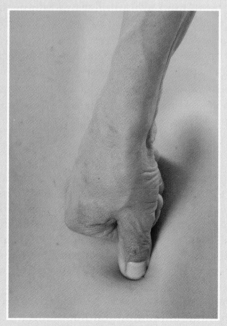

1. Placement of thumbs for the application of static pressure.

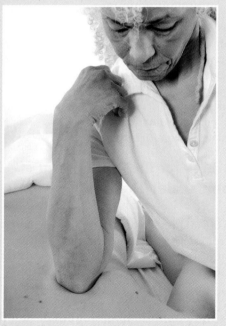

2. Placement of the elbow for the application of static pressure.

| **Technique 84** | **Static Compression (Ischemic Compression) (Continued)** |

3. Placement of reinforced fingers for the application of static pressure.

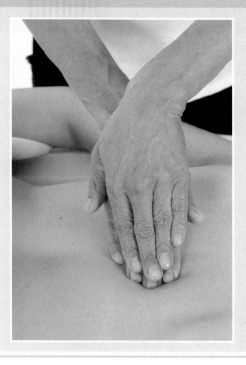

apprised of their experience and you can adjust the technique as suggested by their feedback. Explain to the client that deactivation of a point can increase the pain they feel in a particular area and cause the pain to travel down a referral pathway. Encourage them to breathe deeply during deactivation and to rate their experience on a scale of 1 to 3:

- 1: Very little pain and too little pressure
- 2: Tolerable pain with the right amount of pressure
- 3: Too much pain and too much pressure

If the deactivation of the point is successful, the client should initially feel an increase of pain and referred pain followed by a gradual reduction of pain as the point is deactivated. If the pain does not diminish, make sure that you have correctly lengthened the muscle and warmed the tissue and that another point in the same muscle is not the most active of the points. You can try to reduce a point two times. If the point still does not diminish, move on to another muscle and try again at the next session.

| **Technique 85** | **Pincer Compression** |

Grasp the belly of the muscle in which the trigger point is located, and "pinch" the muscle between the fingers and thumb. Hold the pincer compression for 8 to 12 seconds or longer if pressure continues to decrease the pain produced by the point. Every other second, ask the client to report his or her sensation of pain using the scale described in the text. Adjust your pressure based on the client's feedback. If the treatment is successful, the client will report a lessening of the pain each time you ask her to rate the experience.

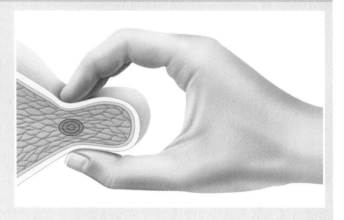

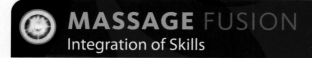

MASSAGE FUSION
Integration of Skills

STUDY TIP: The Any Page Game

When students learn techniques like postisometric relaxation, they often watch the instructor demonstrate the technique on one muscle but then have difficulty applying the technique to other muscles. Think of each technique as a "formula" that can be applied to many different muscles, and then explore the techniques fearlessly with the "Any Page Game." Open a kinesiology book at any page. Pick the muscle on that page, and apply origin and insertion technique to the muscle. Turn to a new page and apply postisometric relaxation to the new muscle. Do this with each of the techniques in this chapter at the end of each of your massage sessions. Soon, you will be applying these techniques effortlessly to a variety of muscles.

GOOD TO KNOW: Resources for Neuromuscular Therapy

If you want to learn more about NMT, begin with a few good books. Here are some helpful titles:

- Hendrickson T. *Massage for Orthopedic Conditions*. Lippincott Williams & Wilkins.
- Travell J, Simons D. *Myofascial Pain and Dysfunction: The Trigger Point Manual*. . Lippincott Williams & Wilkins. *Upper Half of the Body;* vol 1. *Lower Half of the Body;* vol 1.
- Scheumann D. *The Balanced Body: A Guide to Deep Tissue and Neuromuscular Therapy*. 3rd ed. Lippincott Williams & Wilkins.
- Sharkey J. *The Concise Book of Neuromuscular Therapy: A Trigger Point Manual*. North Atlantic Books.

MASSAGE INSPIRATION: Trigger Point Body Map

One way to better understand the trigger point patterns of clients is to create a trigger point body map. You can do this on a practice body with grease pencils and then transfer the information to a SOAP chart. To make your map, locate trigger points on the posterior of your practice body, and indicate the position of each point with a dot made with a grease pencil. Now press on the point, and if it refers to another area, lightly color in the areas where the practice body feels pain or numbness. As you contemplate the trigger points and referral patterns on your practice body, think about the long-term treatment program you might adopt to benefit the client. Also think about the different types of trigger points and see if you can differentiate those that are active, associated, attachment, central, key, latent, primary, or satellite.

CHAPTER WRAP-UP

By this point in your massage therapy training, you have developed a fairly extensive number of "tools" in your toolbox. Not only can you assess a client using a variety of methods, but you can also plan a meaningful treatment and document your results. You might already notice that your healthcare massages follow certain patterns. If you found myofascial release effective, you might apply these techniques to a body region first to address fascial restrictions while the skin is free of massage lubricants. Next, you might apply general Swedish massage for its benefits and because it allows the client to relax into the session, breathe deeply, and focus on body sensations. General Swedish techniques can be followed by deep tissue techniques and then by the techniques you have learned in this chapter, such as neuromuscular work or proprioceptive techniques. Finally, you return to Swedish techniques to help flush the tissue of metabolic wastes and to finish the body area in a relaxing manner.

Take a moment to appreciate how far you have come as a massage therapist. You really know a lot! In the final chapters of this textbook, you will use all of the methods and techniques you have learned to develop treatment plans for clients with chronic pain conditions and selected pathologies and for special populations such as athletes, the elderly, and obese clients. You are well on way to becoming a knowledgeable and highly skilled professional.

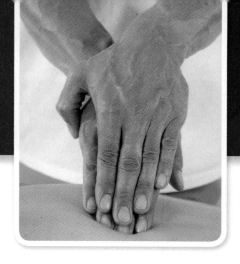

Musculoskeletal Injury and Massage

KEY TERMS

acute stage

acute traumatic injury

chronic inflammation

compensation patterns

deformation

delayed-onset muscle soreness

forces

inflammatory response

injury

load

maturation stage

mechanical strength

overexertion injury

overuse injury

repair stage

tissue failure

tissue load

tissue strain

tissue stress

LEARNING OBJECTIVES

Having read the chapter and used the related student learning tools, the student will be able to:

1 Define *musculoskeletal injury* and outline classifications of injury types affecting structures in the musculoskeletal system.

2 Identify at least three forces that load soft-tissue structures.

3 Define the terms *stress, strain,* and *deformation* as they apply to tissue load.

4 Describe four risk factors that increase the potential for injury.

5 Explain the term *compensation pattern* and describe one method a massage therapist would use to treat a compensation pattern.

6 State the signs and symptoms of acute inflammation, and explain the causes of each.

7 Distinguish among the massage treatment goals and techniques for the acute stage, repair stage, and maturation stage of the inflammatory response.

8 Explain two reasons why an injury site might enter a chronic inflammatory process.

9 Describe the similarities between the massage treatments for carpal tunnel syndrome and thoracic outlet syndrome.

10 List three massage techniques that could be used with a muscle strain in the maturation phase of the inflammatory response.

11 Outline a treatment plan for an ankle sprain in the acute stage of the inflammatory process.

In simple terms, **injury** is tissue damage. This chapter focuses on damage involving muscle tissue, connective tissue, veins, arteries, and nervous tissue caused by physical trauma. Topic 22-1 examines the forces and mechanisms that lead to musculoskeletal injuries, while Topic 22-2 describes the stages and physiological changes that occur as tissue repairs itself. Topic 22-3 defines specific injuries, explains their causes, and provides treatment goals and treatment techniques appropriate for rehabilitative sessions. A number of related topics in other chapters support and round out this discussion. This chapter together with Chapters 19 23, provide a foundation for therapists who wish to offer healthcare massage, work in medically oriented settings, work with athletes, or make injury and rehabilitation a cornerstone of their private practices.

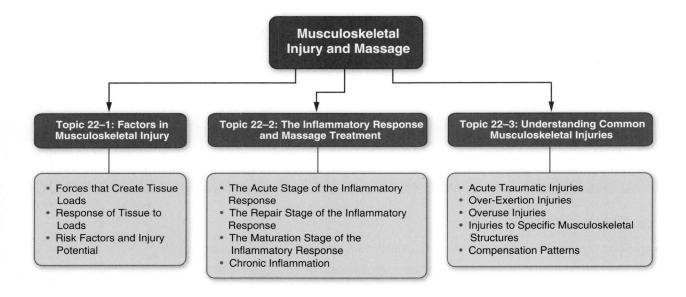

Musculoskeletal Injury and Massage

Topic 22–1: Factors in Musculoskeletal Injury
- Forces that Create Tissue Loads
- Response of Tissue to Loads
- Risk Factors and Injury Potential

Topic 22–2: The Inflammatory Response and Massage Treatment
- The Acute Stage of the Inflammatory Response
- The Repair Stage of the Inflammatory Response
- The Maturation Stage of the Inflammatory Response
- Chronic Inflammation

Topic 22–3: Understanding Common Musculoskeletal Injuries
- Acute Traumatic Injuries
- Over-Exertion Injuries
- Overuse Injuries
- Injuries to Specific Musculoskeletal Structures
- Compensation Patterns

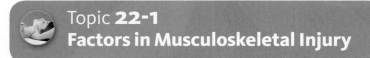

Topic **22-1**
Factors in Musculoskeletal Injury

Musculoskeletal injury involves damage to muscles, tendons, ligaments, joints, nerves, blood vessels, or other related soft-tissue structures that causes discomfort, pain, or loss of function. This section examines factors that contribute to musculoskeletal injury including tissue loads, the forces that act on soft-tissue structures, how forces might overload tissue leading to injury, and risks that increase the potential for injury.

Forces that Create Tissue Loads

Understanding **tissue load** and how forces act on soft-tissue structures helps massage therapists better understand movement, evaluate an injury, and choose effective techniques for supporting rehabilitation. The term **load** refers to the amount of stress soft-tissue structures are under due to **forces**.

In biomechanics (the study of the movement of living things using the science of mechanics), a force is something that internally or externally causes the movement of the body to change or body structures to deform. Forces create loads by pushing or pulling on the body in a variety of ways. Forces include gravity; the primary axial forces (when a force is applied along a single line or a primary axis of a structure) of compression, tension, and shear; and combined forces (two forces acting at the same time) such as torsion and bending. Friction is a low-magnitude force in which opposing structure surfaces resist movement across one another (Fig. 22-1).

Gravity

Gravity's constant downward pull has a profound influence on the body. Each person's posture and movement patterns are an expression of how he or she negotiates with gravity to stand and move. Certain skeletal muscles, often called postural muscles (Box 22-1), sustain a semicontracted state for long periods of time to hold the body upright against the forces of gravity; otherwise, we would end up in a heap of bones on the ground. Each person has a center of gravity, the imaginary point around which body weight is evenly distributed. The center of gravity of the human body can move because joints allow body segments to move. Some body positions are more stable than others because of the position of the center of gravity, and so the body is able to interact with gravity and remain balanced with the least possible amount of energy and effort. When a person's posture is distorted, the center of gravity becomes displaced and the body cannot stand and move efficiently against Earth's gravitational pull. Postural muscles become hypertonic by bracing misaligned joints, and myofascia becomes thick and contracted over time.

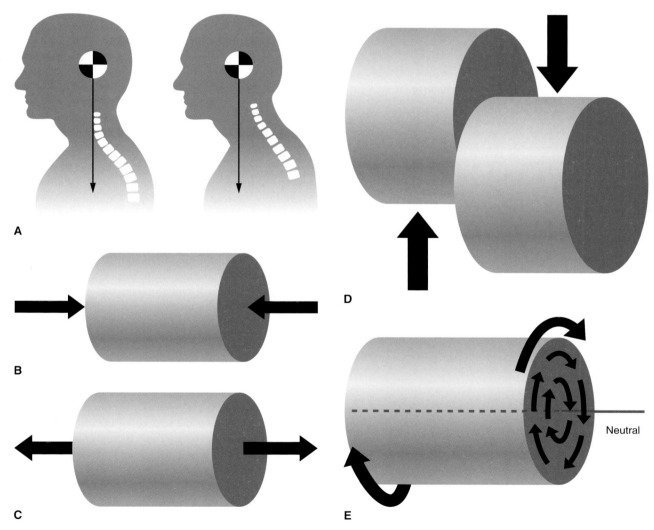

Figure 22-1 Forces that create tissue loads. The term load refers to the amount of stress soft-tissue structures are under due to *forces*. **A. Gravity's** constant downward pull has a profound influence on the body. **B. Compression** is a force in which the tissue is loaded when structures are pressed together. **C. Tension,** sometimes referred to as tensile force, loads the tissue by pulling two ends of a structure apart. **D. Shear forces,** or shearing forces, are parallel forces that act perpendicular to a structure and load the tissue by creating tensions that pull in opposite directions. **E. Torsion,** also called torque, is a twisting force that occurs along a shaft or an axis.

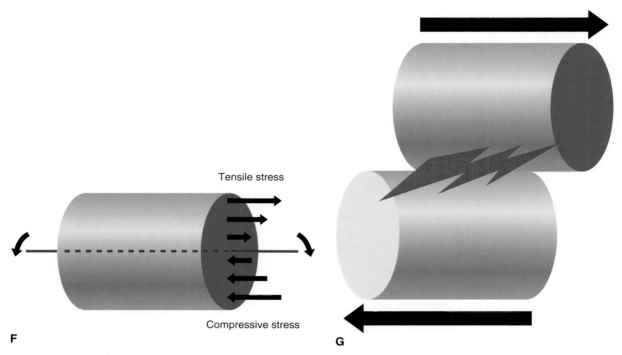

F

G

Figure 22-1 *(Continued)* **F.** In a **bending force** the inner surface experiences compressive force, while the outer surface experiences tensile force. **G. Friction** is defined here as a low-magnitude force in which resistance is created when one structure of the body contacts another as the structures move in opposite directions.

Compression

Compression is a force in which the tissue is loaded when structures are pressed together. Numerous types of compressive forces might cause injury. In a simple example, a tight muscle or tendon can compress a nerve and cause pain and dysfunction. Sudden compressive forces occur when

BOX 22-1 Postural Muscles

Postural muscles remain in partially contracted states for long periods of time to maintain the body's posture against the force of gravity. Postural muscles include:

- Adductor longus
- Adductor magnus
- Erector spinae group
- Gastrocnemius
- Hamstrings
- Iliopsoas
- Levator scapula
- Pectoralis major
- Piriformis
- Quadratus lumborum
- Rectus femoris
- Soleus
- Sternocleidomastoid
- Upper trapezius

two football players collide in a headfirst tackle; contact occurring at the crown of the head causes the cervical spine to be compressed between the head and the torso. When this compressive force exceeds the spine's absorption capabilities, the soft-tissue structures fail and injury results.[1,2] In a whiplash injury, often caused when one car hits another from behind, the hips and trunk move forward and upward.[3] The upward and forward thrust of the trunk cause the head to move backward into extension and then forward into flexion, placing the facet joints under extreme compression and sometimes causing minor fractures to the inferior facet joints.[4–6]

Tension

Tension, sometimes called tensile force, loads the tissue by pulling two ends of a structure apart. Soft tissues like muscle, tendon, and ligaments can absorb tensile forces and stretch. If the tensile force exceeds the strength of the soft-tissue structure and its ability to elongate, tears or ruptures result in the structure. Nerve injuries can occur due to tensile forces when a nerve is rapidly stretched.

Shear

Shear forces, or shearing forces, are parallel forces that act perpendicular to a structure and load the tissue by creating tensions that pull in opposite directions. For example, shear forces place the knee under pressure while running. The momentum of the body's mass above the knee joint causes the femur to slide over the tibial plateau, placing shear stresses on the hyaline cartilage of the knee joint and menisci.[7] A head-forward position causes shear stress in the lower cervical vertebrae.

Torsion

Torsion, also called torque, is a twisting force that occurs along a shaft or an axis. The larger the radius of the shaft, or the stiffer the material being twisted, the more resistance it has to torsion, and the greater potential for tissue damage. For example, asymmetrical contractures of the muscles on either side of the spine can cause torsion in the spine in which vertebrae rotate slightly in opposite directions. Twisting your knee or ankle torques the joints placing soft-tissue structures under compressive, tensile, and shearing forces leading to damage in muscles, ligaments, cartilage, and tendons.

Bending

Structures that are long and slender like long bones and the spine are susceptible to bending forces. In a bending force, the inner surface experiences compressive force while the outer surface experiences tensile force. This combination of stresses causes the structure to bend. For example, in skiing accidents, the ski boot can place compressive forces on the front of the tibia that can fracture the bone if the skier hits a pile of ice or falls while at a high speed.[8] Spinal deformities like scoliosis displace the vertebral discs in a way that subjects the body to constant bending forces. The muscles must assume distorted positions in an attempt to absorb and support the weight of the body.

Friction

Friction is not usually classified as a primary or combined force but is a factor in injuries such as tendinitis. In repetitive stress injuries like tendinitis, friction could be understood as a low-magnitude force with which resistance is created when one structure of the body contacts another as the structures move in opposite directions. If the opposing surfaces of the structures have irregularities, they create greater resistance and may begin to stick to each other. Over time, the repeated resistance causes stress to the tissue of both structures, eventually leading to inflammation, pain, and dysfunction.

Concept Brief 22-1
Forces

Gravity: A force that compresses structures downward

Compression: A force that pushes structures together

Tension: A force that pulls the ends of a structure apart

Shear: Parallel forces that act perpendicular to a structure and pull in opposite directions

Torsion: A twisting force that occurs along a shaft or axis

Bending: A force that causes a structure to bend

Friction: A low-magnitude force in which contacting structures move in opposite directions and resist one another

Response of Tissue to Loads

When loaded, musculoskeletal tissues resist the load. The amount of resistance the tissue exhibits to a load is called **tissue stress**. For example, the resistance of tissue to being pushed together is called compressive stress, while the resistance of tissue to being pulled apart is called tensile stress. Whenever a tissue is subjected to a load (e.g., lifting a heavy object, being elongated), the tissue changes shape, sometimes imperceptibly. This change of shape is called **deformation. Tissue strain** is the amount of deformation experienced by the tissue. If the tissue is elongated due to a tensile load, it is referred to as tensile strain, while deformation of the tissue due to a compressive load is compressive strain. Stress and strain are closely related and play a role in a tissue's susceptibility to injury. Compressively loaded bone is highly stressed because it is highly resistant to compressive forces. It deforms very little when compressed. If the compressive load is heavy enough, the bone will resist until it fails and develops stress fractures or breaks.

The mechanical strength of the tissue (not to be confused with muscular strength) affects its response to loads. **Mechanical strength** can be described as the amount of force a tissue can absorb or resist before failure. As discussed in Chapter 20, musculoskeletal tissue is *viscoelastic*; that term comes from the words *viscous* (thick, sticky, gummy) and *elastic* (stretchy, expandable, flexible). If a substance is viscous, it will become deformed when an outside force manipulates it and will remain deformed. Imagine compressing your fist into a piece of clay. The clay will flatten and remain flattened. If a substance is elastic, it will deform when manipulated by an outside force but will then snap back into its original shape when the outside force is removed (think of pulling and releasing a rubber band). Obviously, some tissue is more viscoelastic than others. Bone has very little viscoelasticity and can break when a strong compressive or bending force is applied to it. Muscles, tendons, and ligaments have greater degrees of viscoelasticity and so can withstand compressive forces more easily than bone. When tissue is deformed (strained) by loads (forces acting on tissue) past the point where it can absorb or resist the load (stress), it fails, and tissue damage results. A number of factors influence the nature and severity of loads that are great enough to cause injury:

- **Location:** Where on the body or on the structure is the force applied? As previously noted, a compressive load on a bone can cause the bone to fracture. A compressive load on a muscle might cause only bruising.

- **Magnitude:** How much force is applied? A tensile load, such as might be experienced when a muscle is stretched, may or may not cause tissue damage depending on how much force is applied. If the stretch (load) is applied gently, the tissue is less likely to tear (fail) than if the stretch (load) is applied forcefully.

- **Rate:** How quickly is the force applied? A tissue may be able to absorb greater loads if the load is applied slowly. Previously we discussed the application of a stretch (tensile force) to a muscle. If the muscle is stretched slowly, it is more likely to stretch further without tearing (failure). If the muscle is stretched rapidly, muscle spindles (proprioceptors that monitor rate and degree of muscle lengthening) may react to cause a reflexive contracture, which may lead to tearing of muscle fibers as the application of the stretch continues.

- **Direction and position:** Where is the force directed and what position is the body in when it experiences tissue loading? For example, when a joint is exposed to torsion forces, such as could occur with a twisted ankle (the force is directed in two opposing directions while the body is traveling along a straight line), ligaments commonly fail (tear or rupture) due to the tensile stress they experience as they try to stabilize the joint and keep it from twisting while the body's momentum continues to carry it on its original straight-ahead path. Forces loading the tissue of an arm that is hyperextended and externally rotated will cause a different injury pattern than forces loading the tissue of an arm that is flexed and internally rotated.

- **Duration:** Over what period of time is the force applied? Earlier, we discussed friction and explained that resistance experienced over a long period of time leads to inflammation and damage to the tissue. If the issues causing friction are resolved quickly, the friction is less likely to cause tissue damage.

- **Frequency:** How often is the force applied? If a particular tissue is repeatedly loaded, an injury is more likely to develop than if the body area has time to rest and recover between the applications of forces that load the tissue. For example, carpal tunnel syndrome (CTS) often results from frequently working on a computer keyboard. The body is repeatedly exposed to the compressive and tensile forces at play while typing and does not have time to heal minor irritations and tissue damage. Over time, tissue damage becomes pronounced, and pain and dysfunction result.

Concept Brief 22-2
Tissue Loads

Load: A normal or an abnormal internal or external force applied to a tissue that causes the tissue to experience normal or abnormal mechanical stress and strain

Stress: The amount of resistance a tissue experiences when loaded

Strain: The amount of deformation experienced by the tissue in response to a load

Deformation: The way in which a tissue changes shape in response to a load

Mechanical strength: The amount of force a tissue can absorb or resist before failure

Tissue failure: The point at which structures are damaged by loads and lose their mechanical integrity, usually resulting in injury

Risk Factors and Injury Potential

Risk factors are particular internal and external conditions that increase the potential for an injury to occur. Risk factors influence the mechanical strength of the tissue and its ability to resist a load without failure, and the frequency with which the body is exposed to loads that could cause tissue damage.

- **Age:** In younger people, tissues are growing and developing and tend to regenerate more quickly. The body can withstand greater frequency of loads without injury. As we age, repetitive stress and chronic injury may result as the body's tissues begin to degenerate and lose their optimal strength and density.

- **Gender:** Men and women demonstrate statistical differences in injury and disease patterns of the musculoskeletal system based on the circumstances. For example, men are more likely to fall off ladders and scaffolding (29:1), be injured on machinery (22:1), or be injured by electric current (19:1), while women are more likely than men to develop osteoporosis. Gender-specific differences are related to hormones, sociology, and activity patterns.[9]

- **Genetics:** Genetic factors influence tissue composition and its predisposition toward certain types of injury like intervertebral disk degeneration, tendon ruptures, CTS, and rotator cuff degeneration.[10]

- **Physical condition:** A person's lifestyle can predispose the individual to injury. Poor diet, a sedentary lifestyle, and the use of tobacco can cause tissue to degenerate and become thickened, hypertonic, or weakened. The fitter a person is, the less likely he or she is to sustain an injury. If an injury occurs, healthy tissue is likely to repair itself more rapidly than unhealthy tissue. However, athletes, who are often very fit, may sustain injury due to the repetitive loads applied to body tissue that occurs during training to maintain or increase fitness.

- **Psychological condition:** A person's psychological condition can predispose the individual to injury. Influencing factors include stress levels, depression, anxiety, inattention and human error, personality, and the ability to cope under pressure.

- **Fatigue:** Fatigue from physical and mental exertion increases the potential for injury because muscle strength, coordination, and postural control as well as mental attention are compromised. For example, ski accidents are more frequent after multiple runs down the mountain, and risk of injuries in athletes increases during the latter stages of an event or game.[11]

- **Environment:** Weather conditions, lighting, terrain, altitude, and the type of activity performed in a given environmental condition can predispose a person to injury. In addition, the type of equipment used in a sport or type of work may increase the potential for injury.

- **Previous injury:** If a person has sustained tissue damage in a particular structure, it is likely that the repaired tissues are not fully returned to their preinjury condition and are more susceptible to re-injury. An injury may cause a compensation pattern that, over time, leads to a secondary injury.

Now, we can turn to examine how tissues respond when they are injured and the massage techniques that support the return of tissue to full function following injury.

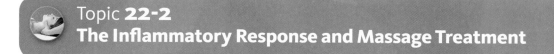

Topic **22-2**
The Inflammatory Response and Massage Treatment

As discussed earlier, when tissue is loaded beyond its mechanical strength, or when tissue is repeatedly loaded without sufficient time for rest and recovery, **tissue failure** and injury result. To repair the damage done to tissue, the body rapidly reacts to any injury with a series of specific vascular, chemical, and cellular events referred to as the **inflammatory response.** This healing process aims to remove damaged tissue, provide the necessary materials to repair the tissue, and support the new tissue as it grows and matures (Fig. 22-2).

The inflammatory response has three stages (acute, repair, and maturation) in which specialized events lead to tissue healing and a return to full function. Different terms are used to describe inflammation and tissue healing. These terms are listed in Box 22-2; you may see these used in various massage therapy textbooks. While it is possible to assign a loose time frame to each stage of healing, the stages tend to overlap and are influenced by the location of the injury and the type of tissue that is damaged, the severity of the damage, and the state of health of the person who is injured. The inflammatory response occurs as a reaction to any type of tissue damage including that caused by infection, autoimmune diseases, exposure to chemicals, sensitivity to irritants, and illnesses. This section focuses on the repair of soft tissue injured by acute traumatic events, overexertion, or overuse of musculoskeletal structures.

Chapter 19 discussed signs, symptoms, and treatment goals. You learned how to assess clients by observing their posture, gait, and range of motion and through their feedback about pain and decreased ability to participate in activities of daily living. Chapter 19 described how to develop a treatment plan based on a general rehabilitation process. The massage treatment of most musculoskeletal injuries depends on the current stage of the inflammatory response of the healing tissue. Treatment goals and techniques tend to be very similar despite the different structures or regions where the injury is located. This section now examines specific treatment goals and techniques, and the following Topic 22-3 discusses massage treatment considerations for particular structures and locations.

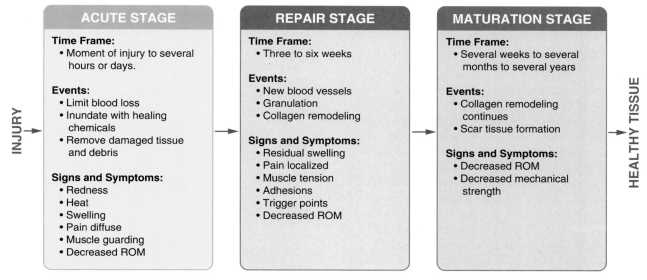

Figure 22-2 The inflammatory response. The body's healing process, which aims to remove damaged tissue, provides the necessary materials to repair the tissue, and supports the new tissue as it grows and matures.

BOX 22-2 Use of Terms Associated with the Healing Process

Term used in this textbook	Other terms commonly used to describe the same thing
Inflammatory response	Stages of inflammation, inflammatory process, inflammation
Repair stage of the inflammatory response	Subacute inflammation, regeneration phase
Maturation stage of the inflammatory response	Chronic inflammation, resolution phase
Collagen remodeling to form scar tissue	Fibrosis

The Acute Stage of the Inflammatory Response

The **acute stage** of the inflammatory response begins seconds after tissue damage has occurred and lasts from several hours to several days depending on the severity of the injury. The events of the acute stage of the inflammatory response are initiated and managed by over 180 different chemicals released from cells or activated plasma proteins.[12] Redness, swelling, heat, pain, and loss of function are often noticeable in the local area.

Physiological Events of the Acute Stage of the Inflammatory Response

In the acute stage of the inflammatory response the body attempts to limit blood loss, inundate the injured area with healing components, and remove damaged tissue and debris so that the body can enter the repair stage. Acute inflammation is a very complex process, and it is not possible or practical to describe every detail here. The key events will be outlined. Although this description may seem to imply that inflammation follows a neat, orderly progression, in fact many of these events are occurring simultaneously or in overlapping sequences.

Limit Blood Loss and Inundate the Area with Healing Components

Immediately after the injury occurs, surrounding blood vessels briefly constrict to limit possible blood loss and quickly repair any damage to the vessels. Within minutes, minor blood loss is controlled, and the body instigates vascular changes that allow the injured area to be flooded with cells that prevent infection and remove damaged tissue. Chemical mediators including histamine, serotonin, prostaglandin E2, and bradykinin trigger vasodilation and an increase in the permeability of blood vessels. Components normally contained in the blood vessels are allowed to leak out into the tissue spaces of the damaged area.

SWELLING, REDNESS, AND HEAT
When soft tissue is damaged, blood and fluids spill out of the damaged tissue into the surrounding area causing primary edema (swelling), often referred to as exudates. In some injuries the damage is extensive, and primary edema is pronounced. In other cases the damage is limited, and primary edema is minimal. The vasodilation and permeability of blood vessels caused as part of the acute inflammatory response cause the redness and heat in the injured region. These vascular changes ensure that relevant leukocytes and plasma proteins can gain entry to the damaged area. Normally, the capillary membranes retain plasma proteins, but when they slip into tissue spaces they exert an osmotic (water attracting) force that draws additional interstitial fluids toward the injury site, causing secondary edema for a period after the initial trauma occurred. It is believed that edema caused by the inflammatory response disrupts nearby capillaries, causing congestion in the injured region. This congestion prevents nearby undamaged tissue from receiving the nutrient-rich blood (referred to as ischemia) and oxygen (referred to as hypoxia) it needs for normal cellular activity, causing cell death in otherwise healthy tissue and thereby increasing the zone of injury. Cold applications are used to decrease the swelling, redness, heat, and pain associated with inflammation. Cooling the region lowers the metabolic activity of the tissue, reducing the demand for oxygen and allowing cells to survive a period of hypoxia. The more cells that survive, the less total tissue loss occurs, ensuring that the resolution of acute inflammation happens more rapidly.

PAIN
The initial pain felt at an injury site is caused by tissue damage and chemicals released by the tissue to mediate the inflammatory response. Shortly thereafter, pain is also caused by pressure placed on surrounding structures by edema. The primary chemicals that contribute to the sensation of pain experienced with acute inflammation are prostaglandin E2 and bradykinin. Bradykinin is a plasma protein that increases capillary membrane permeability and interacts with prostaglandins to stimulate free nerve endings, causing pain. The sensation of pain at the injury site causes the muscles surrounding the area to involuntarily contract (spasm), splinting the region and holding it immobile. This splinting action is called muscle guarding and early in the healing process it provides a useful function. Usually, muscle guarding subsides as the injury moves out of the acute stage and into the repair stage. In many cases, muscle guarding decreases circulation to the area, causing the region to enter a pain-spasm-pain cycle

(discussed in detail in Chapter 4) that can inhibit the healing process if it is not disrupted and resolved.

Removal of Damaged Tissue and Debris

During the process that synthesizes prostaglandins to mediate vascular changes, free radicals are released into the tissue. The free radicals activate proteases (enzymes that break down proteins) causing the destruction of nearby cell membranes. This provides a necessary function in that damaged cell membranes are broken down for removal from the area. Unfortunately, healthy cells may also be damaged in this process, resulting in an increased zone of injury.[13]

Many of the chemical mediators of the inflammatory response are *chemotaxins*. Chemotaxins cause a process called *chemotaxis* in which circulating leukocytes (white blood cells) are attracted to the area of injury. The first types of leukocytes drawn to the injured area are neutrophils, which fight infection by attacking bacteria. Neutrophils begin to stick to the inner surface of capillaries and venules near the injury site. Because of increased blood vessel permeability, the neutrophils are able to migrate through the capillary and venule walls into the interstitial spaces of the damaged tissue. Neutrophils are soon followed by monocytes that are transformed into macrophages, a larger leukocyte that has the ability to engulf and remove damaged tissue through phagocytosis. Leukocytes continue to migrate to the injury site until the removal of damaged tissue is completed and then exit the area through general blood and lymph circulation. If the area becomes infected with bacteria or if a foreign body is present, leukocytes persist in the area, and the body may enter a chronic inflammatory process (discussed below).

Treatment during the Acute Stage of the Inflammatory Response

If you have ever watched a sporting event in which an athlete is injured during the game, you may have seen the athletic trainer or the coach instantly apply ice to the injury or immerse the injured area in ice water. This first aid is applied to limit the inflammatory response and keep swelling to a minimum in order to prevent damage to surrounding healthy tissue through ischemia and hypoxia, as discussed above. If you practice sports massage or onsite work, you may be the person who applies first aid to an acute injury. Usually, clients visit a massage therapist after an injury has received first aid (sometimes clients don't receive first aid for an acute injury and the zone of injury is increased because swelling, ischemia, and hypoxia go unchecked). Treatment involves assessing the injury by observing the signs and symptoms demonstrated or described by the client and then targeting specific treatment goals to ensure proper tissue healing in the acute stage.

Signs and Symptoms of the Acute Stage of the Inflammatory Response

In general, the acute stage of the inflammatory response lasts for 3 to 4 days after the injury. You may observe redness, swelling, and heat at the injury site. If the tissue is bruised, it tends to be dark red, black, and blue. The client is likely to report feeling pain at the site that radiates out into the surrounding region. Muscles in the local area may splint the region, with protective spasms causing visible muscle tension and client discomfort. The client may be reluctant to move joints related to the injury site and report a loss of function and increased pain with movement.

Treatment Goals and Massage Techniques for the Acute Stage of the Inflammatory Response

The treatment goals for a massage therapy session used to address an acute injury are usually the same regardless of the region where the injury occurs or the type of tissue affected. A wide range of massage techniques may be applied to meet treatment goals. The techniques suggested here provide a starting place from which to work. You can add more techniques as you develop additional skills and learn new massage modalities. Treatment goals and massage techniques include:

- **Reduce tissue swelling:** One of the most effective ways to reduce tissue swelling is to apply cold hydrotherapy and elevate the area with pillows (if possible). You might place an ice pack or a cold compress on the area, or submerge the area in ice water (see Chapter 16 for details). Manual lymphatic drainage (MLD) techniques help move excess fluid out of the tissue and back into normal circulation. While MLD is an advanced bodywork system, a few basic application methods are easy to learn and prove useful. These basics are demonstrated in Technique 86. In some cases, a compression bandage might be used to limit swelling during the first 3 days after an injury. Compression bandages are often misused and actually increase pain and swelling if they are wrapped too tightly or incorrectly and thus disrupt circulation too much. Don't use compression bandages in combination with elevation or when the client is lying down. Ensure that the bandage is applied so that it is not tighter at the proximal end than at the distal end. The bandage should give some comfort to the client and provide mild pain relief. If the bandage feels uncomfortable, it should be removed. Clients can usually wrap injuries on the extremities themselves and can use compression bandages for self-care. In some states, the use of compression bandages by massage therapists is prohibited, so check your state regulations before you use them.

- **Reduce muscle spasms:** Muscle spasms in the acute stages of inflammation protect the injury site by splinting it and preventing movements that might cause increased injury or re-injury to healing tissue. You don't want to completely eliminate muscle spasms that splint injury, but you want to reduce their intensity to ensure proper circulation in the area and to decrease client discomfort. General Swedish massage provides full body relaxation and decreases sympathetic nervous system firing. Usually, you can apply massage to all body areas that are not injured. If the injury site is located in one extremity, massage applied to the uninjured

Technique 86   Manual Lymphatic Drainage Basics

Emil and Estrid Vodder, Danish physical therapists, developed MLD in the 1930s. Using light, rhythmic strokes applied in a specific order and manner, MLD stimulates lymph flow and fluid movement. It is used for conditions in which fluid collects in the tissue, including inflammatory conditions, lymphedema, and circulatory disturbances. MLD is an advanced bodywork skill, and the training for foundational certification is 40 hours. The skills described here are very basic but useful for working with the acute and early repair stage of the inflammatory response that occurs with musculoskeletal injury.

These techniques are not recommended for use with other conditions that cause fluid accumulation without specific training in MLD (because there is not room in this chapter to explain the important contraindications that may exist or to adequately describe all the specific pathologies that might cause edema). Review your anatomy and physiology textbook for a description of the lymphatic system and its functions to better understand the use of this technique.

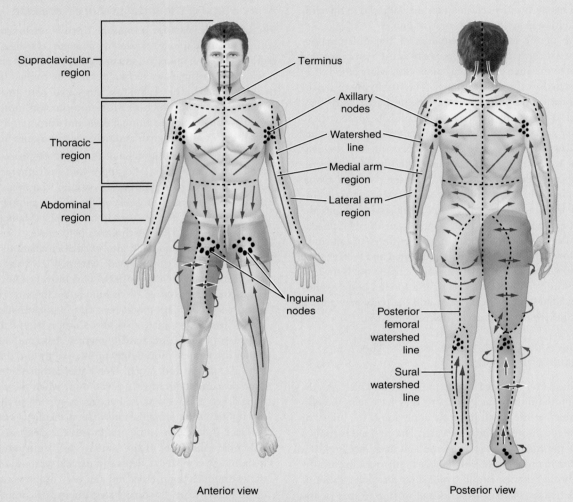

Anterior view   Posterior view

1. Review Lymph Drainage Patterns. Superficial lymphatic vessels form an interconnected and overlapping network of specific drainage patterns. The lymph from the right arm, right shoulder, and right side of the head drain through the right lymphatic duct. All other areas of the body drain through the thoracic duct. When encouraging the flow of lymph from an area of congestion, such as the swelling around an injury site, you stimulate flow at the main drainage points first (the terminus and axillary nodes for the upper body, and the inguinal nodes for the lower body) and then work backward (proximal to distal) toward the swelling. In the final application, you work distal (from the proximal edge of the swelling) to proximal. Never work distal to the injury or on the site of the injury in the acute or early repair stage of the inflammatory response because you don't want to exacerbate the congestion already present in the tissue. For example, if the swelling is on the wrist, you might perform nodal pumping (described below) at the terminus first. Next you would stimulate the lymph nodes in the axillary region, and then in the cubital fossa. Then, you might use stationary circles to treat the areas between lymph nodes at the terminus, axillary, and cubital fossa regions. Finally, "webbing" and effleurage strokes are used to move fluid just proximal to the swelling of the injury toward the cubital fossa, axillary nodes, and finally the terminus. Diaphragmatic breathing (described in Technique 14), cool hydrotherapy applications, and passive range of motion within the client's pain tolerance to nearby joints support the benefits and effects of MLD techniques.

| **Technique 86** | **Manual Lymphatic Drainage Basics** (Continued) |

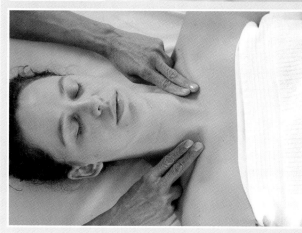

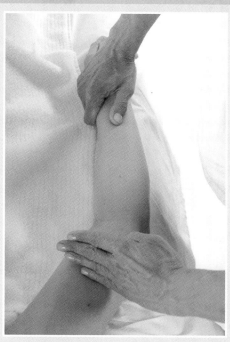

2. Nodal Pumping with the Fingers. Nodal pumping is the first technique applied to an area to stimulate the flow of lymph and to move excess fluid from tissue. It is performed on primary drainage points (the terminus, axillary lymph nodes, nodes in the cubital fossa, and nodes in the inguinal area) with two fingers or the palm of the hand in a wavelike motion. The fingers are placed just distal to the nodes and then rolled from distal to proximal with very light pressure (anything other than very light pressure collapses lymphatic vessels). Repeat the rolling finger motion lightly five to seven times to move fluid into the node, and then repeat the process on the next set of nodes.

3. Nodal Pumping with the Palm. Place the palm of the hand distal to the nodes and roll the palmar surface of the hand lightly from the heel of the hand to the fingers in a wavelike motion so that fluid distal to the node is pushed into the node (your palm moves in a distal-to-proximal motion).

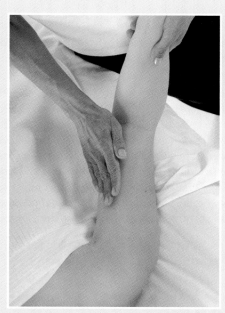

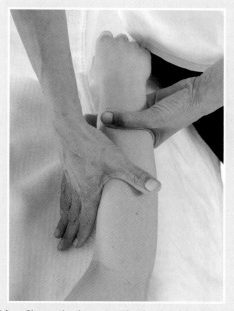

4. Stationary Circles. After each of the primary drainage points is stimulated with nodal pumping, use stationary circles to push lymph from the distal regions of the extremity to the proximal regions of the extremity between primary drainage points. To perform stationary circles, apply the palm of one hand or both hands lightly in a circular motion rotating the palm and fingers toward the next proximal drainage sight. Stimulate one region and then move the circles up to the next region. Remember to keep the strokes light to avoid collapsing lymph vessels.

5. Webbing. Place one hand just proximal to the edge of the swelling (remember that you don't want to work distal to swelling or over the top of the swollen region), and use the "web" between the thumb and index finger to lightly stroke the tissue in a proximal direction. The ulnar border of the hand or the edge of the thumb might also be used. Effleurage strokes applied from just proximal to the swelling toward the heart are also useful.

extremity may cause a consensual response and help reduce spasms in the injured extremity. Apply massage within the client's tolerance proximal to the injury site, but not distal to the injury site.

- **Decrease pain:** Massage techniques like Swedish massage and myofascial release can be applied to uninjured areas to decrease pain through the gating mechanism of the spinal column. (Review the section on the Gate Theory of Pain Management in Chapter 4 for details.)
- **Decrease sympathetic nervous system firing (flight-or-fight response):** Swedish massage, energetic bodywork, or other gentle techniques might be used to elicit a parasympathetic nervous system response and relax the body to decrease sympathetic activity that may add to a client's perception of pain or increase muscle spasms.
- **Maintain available pain-free range of motion:** If movement causes pain, then don't move the injured area. If the client can tolerate some movement, use passive range of motion or gentle active range of motion to maintain any available movement. For example, a client with a deltoid tear might be able to gently circle his or her arm by hanging the arm off the massage table while prone.
- **Prevent re-injury:** To ensure that you do not exacerbate the injury or cause re-injury, work gently and avoid any techniques that increase the client's pain or discomfort. Encourage the client to rest the injured site and to participate in self-care activities.
- **Encourage client self-care:** Encourage the client to rest the area, keep it elevated if possible (but not in combination with compression bandages), and ice it regularly. The range of motion in uninjured joints should be maintained. If active movement in the joints surrounding the injury site does not cause increased pain, it is encouraged. Any movements that cause increased pain are restricted.

The Repair Stage of the Inflammatory Response

As the acute stage of the inflammatory response concludes, muscle guarding subsides; heat, redness, swelling, and pain diminish; and the area regains some limited function as it enters the repair stage of the healing process. Depending on the severity of the injury, and on the types of tissues to be repaired, this stage of healing can take 3 to 6 weeks.[14]

Physiological Events in the Repair Stage of the Inflammatory Response

In the first phases of the **repair stage**, new blood vessels develop from venules located at the edge of the injury site to provide blood, oxygen, nutrients, and waste removal to the regenerating tissue. Granulation begins when fibroblasts (collagen-producing cells) lay down a weak, delicate form of collagen in a web-like matrix across the area where tissue was

lost. This connective tissue matrix, called granulation tissue, is very fragile, allowing for the possibility of re-injury if the region is subjected to mechanical stress and strain before it has matured.

As the repair stage continues, thicker and stronger collagen strands replace the frail granulation tissue in a process called collagen remodeling to produce scar tissue (Box 22-3). Scar tissue is distributed in such a way as to build strength in the tissue with the formation of crosslinks among collagen fibers. Collagen fibers are not necessarily distributed along the lines of mechanical stress in the tissue (i.e., muscle fiber direction), and this can lead to the formation of adhesions that cause the new tissue to be shorter and thicker than the original tissue. In some cases, abnormal amounts of connective tissue fibers are distributed in disorganized patterns and dense scar tissue forms, reducing range of motion and increasing the potential for re-injury and chronic inflammation (described later). Massage therapists play an essential role in reducing the occurrence of disorganized collagen fibers, adhesions, and thick patches of scar tissue through a variety of techniques like crossfiber friction, pétrissage, passive movement, and gentle stretching.

Treatment during the Repair Stage of the Inflammatory Response

In the early period of the repair stage, the tissue is delicate and the treatment goals of a massage session remain the same as in the acute stage. In the later repair stage, your treatment options increase and the goals of the session expand.

Signs and Symptoms of the Late Repair Stage of the Inflammatory Response

You may observe mild residual swelling at the injury site, but swelling, redness, and heat have likely vanished. If the tissue is bruised, it has changed from black and blue to yellow, brown, and green coloring. If the tissue is healing properly, muscle guarding has disappeared, but the client's range of motion and overall function are still inhibited. You may palpate muscle tension and imbalances, adhesions, and trigger points in the surrounding tissue, and stress to compensating structures may cause secondary injury or dysfunction to appear in related structures. Pain has localized to the injury site.

Treatment Goals and Massage Techniques for the Late Repair Stage of the Inflammatory Response

As mentioned previously, the treatment goals and techniques for the early repair stage remain the same as for the acute stage. As healing progresses into the late repair stage, treatment goals and massage techniques expand to include those described here:

- **Increase circulation for improved tissue health:** Chapter 16 described the effects of contrasting hot and cold applications. For example, a hot pack may be applied to the injury site to cause vasodilation and bring fresh, nutrient-rich blood to the area for 3 minutes. Next, an ice pack is applied

BOX 22-3 Scar Tissue

Scar tissue is a permanent mass of connective tissue that replaces normal tissue after tissue damage has occurred. It can be found on any tissue of the body including skin, muscle, tendon, and internal organs. The formation of scar tissue is part of the normal collagen remodeling process and occurs with every type of wound or injury (musculoskeletal failure, laceration, surgery, etc.). Scar tissue is mechanically weaker and less functional than the original tissue it replaces. For example, scars in the skin do not have sweat glands and hair follicles and are less resistant to ultraviolet light. Scars in muscle tissue are usually shorter and less flexible than normal muscle tissue and may pull on the fibers of surrounding tissue, placing them under abnormal stresses. Collagen fibers are produced randomly in a disorganized format during collagen remodeling. If the area of injury enters a chronic inflammatory process, an extended healing process, if it is not rehabilitated appropriately to align fibers down the lines of mechanical stress, or if the structure or the region remains immobilized for a prolonged period after the injury, unhealthy scar tissue may result in a bulky mass of stiff, brittle tissue that remains weak, painful, and prone to re-injury. Types of scar tissue often seen by massage therapists include:

- **Soft-tissue contracture**: Scar tissue that occurs in the tissues (muscle, tendon, ligament, fascia, joint capsule) around a joint, causing a shortening of tissue that prevents the joint from moving fully through its range of motion.
- **Adhesions:** Scar tissue that forms between surfaces (muscle fibers, tendons, fascia, etc.) that should slide over one another. Instead, the fibers pack together, form abnormal crosslinks, and cause the tissue to become thicker, shorter, and less elastic, decreasing local circulation and range of motion.
- **Hypertrophic scarring:** An overgrowth of dermal tissue that remains within the boundaries of the wound, which is caused by second- and third-degree burns or with skin grafting.
- **Keloid:** A tumor-like growth of scar tissue past the boundaries of the original wound that occurs in the skin.

to cause vasoconstriction for 1 minute, and the sequence is repeated three times ending with the cold application. This creates a *vascular flush,* in which the tissues are "pumped" free of metabolic waste buildup due to the alternating vasoconstriction and vasodilatation of the peripheral blood vessels. As a result, tissue health is improved. Contrast hydrotherapy applications can be used at the beginning of the session or after other techniques have been applied to the region.

- **Reduce trigger points:** Chapter 21 explained the physiology of trigger points. Tissue trauma can cause the formation of trigger points around the area of injury and in compensating structures. Techniques described in Chapter 21 to reduce trigger points are applied proximal to the injury site within the client's pain tolerance.
- **Reduce adhesions:** Myofascial techniques, pétrissage, and friction are applied to the injured region and to compensating structures within the client's pain tolerance to reduce adhesions and restricted tissue.
- **Promote proper collagen alignment:** Use techniques like myofascial release, pétrissage, and gentle friction in the region of the injury and to the injury site as long as they do not cause pain and discomfort to the client. After myofascial and friction techniques are applied to the tissue, gently stretch the tissue at affected joints to promote proper collagen alignment.
- **Increase range of motion:** Passive and active range-of-motion techniques are used, as long as they do not cause pain, to increase the range of motion and function in affected joints.
- **Encourage client self-care:** As they start to feel better, clients often re-injure themselves by returning to full activity before the tissue has progressed significantly into the maturation stage of the inflammatory response. Encourage clients to use contrast hydrotherapy applications at home, to participate in stress-reduction activities, to pay attention to their activity levels, and to rest if pain or symptoms related to their injury increase.

The Maturation Stage of the Inflammatory Response

As tissue enters the final stage of healing, all evidence of edema is gone, but the area has not regained full range of motion or mechanical strength. This **maturation stage** can last from several weeks to several months to a year or longer, depending on the severity and location of the injury, the health and self-care practices of the injured person, the types of techniques used for rehabilitation, and the regularity with which those techniques are applied. The collagen remodeling process produces scar tissue (the type of tissue that replaces normal tissue after damage has occurred, as described in Box 22-3) and continues rapidly in the early maturation stage and then slows. In the healthy formation of scar tissue, the alignment of fibers down the lines of mechanical stress improves and the links between fibers become stronger. The tissue is gradually able to withstand greater and greater mechanical loads but is likely to only achieve 70% to 80% of the strength of the original tissue when the healing process concludes.[15]

Treatment during the Maturation Stage of the Inflammatory Response

Proper treatment during the maturation stage of the inflammatory response is important to prevent the tissue from entering a recurrent inflammatory process as described in the later section on chronic inflammation. As the client feels better, he or she may begin to pay less attention to the healing process and re-injure the area through overuse or may fail to continue massage and other treatment because of a lack of perceived need.

Signs and Symptoms of the Maturation Stage of the Inflammatory Response

While swelling, redness, and heat have completely disappeared, the injured region has not returned to full function. The client may have difficulty performing full range of motion of affected joints, and some muscles are likely to be weakened, leading to muscular imbalances and compensation patterns. Symptoms like pain, stiffness, and tissue heat may reappear after activities that stress the tissue.

Treatment Goals and Massage Techniques for the Maturation Stage of the Inflammatory Response

The treatment goals for massage sessions addressing the maturation stage of an injury are similar to those of the late repair stage; you continue to reduce trigger points and adhesions while increasing range of motion in affected joints. Additional treatment goals and techniques include

- **Balance muscular tension:** The muscles involved in an injury or in the region of an injury commonly become unbalanced. Some muscles went into a protective guarding function during the acute stage and may be hypertonic as a result, while others were held immobilized and lost strength. Think carefully about the balance of the muscles around joints and lengthen chronically shortened muscles, decrease tension in hypertonic muscles, and build strength in weakened muscles. Hot packs are often applied to increase circulation in hypertonic muscles and as part of the process to reduce trigger points. Techniques such as myofascial release, deep-tissue massage, active isolated stretching, postisometric relaxation, active, passive, and resisted range of motion, and many others are effective for returning the muscles around the joint to balanced function.

- **Reduce scar tissue:** Techniques used to reduce adhesions are now applied more vigorously to areas of scar tissue. Any techniques that use friction to break down tissue usually cause the region to reenter a brief inflammatory cycle. Always stretch the area after treating it and then cool the tissue with an ice pack or other cold hydrotherapy application. Cyriax crossfiber friction is an effective method for reducing areas of dense scar tissue, as shown in Technique 87.

- **Treat compensating structures:** When one area of the body is injured, other areas compensate by bracing the body to balance it in new ways or by overworking to take the stress off the injured region. Often, the client will adopt dysfunctional postural positions that don't disappear, even when the injury has healed. It is important to address the needs of compensating structures by ensuring the tissue is healthy, maintains proper circulation, and is not hypertonic or not weakened.

Technique 87 — Cyriax Crossfiber Friction

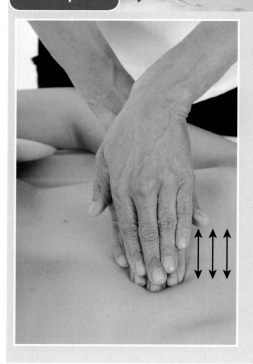

Cyriax crossfiber friction is a specific technique developed by James Cyriax in the 1930s as a means to break down scar tissue and adhesions. The technique is applied across the fibers of the muscle, tendon, or ligament instead of following the muscle, tendon, or ligament fiber direction with rapid and transverse rubbing at the deepest level tolerated by the client. This technique creates inflammation in the tissue, which stimulates tissue repair mechanisms and helps to reorganize connective tissues along the lines of mechanical stretch. The application of Cyriax crossfiber friction follows a specific set of steps:

1. Warm the tissue over and around the adhesion or scar tissue with myofascial and Swedish strokes, and then remove the massage lubricant from the skin with a wet wipe or alcohol so that you don't slip over the structures and can engage the tissue effectively.

2. Place the structure with the adhesion or scar tissue under the appropriate tension. Muscles are placed in a shortened position. Tendons without a synovial sheath are placed in a shortened position. Tendons with a synovial sheath are placed in a lengthened position.

3. Use reinforced fingers or thumbs to compress the tissue directly over scar tissue (make sure you are right on the lesion site), and move the reinforced fingers or thumbs transversely and rapidly across the tissue fibers with enough pressure to penetrate the scar tissue but at a level still tolerable to the client. Apply the technique continually for 2 to 5 minutes.

4. Perform passive range of motion to all of the joints associated with the muscle, tendon, or ligament within the client's pain tolerance. As long as the client can tolerate it, stretch the structures to help collagen align properly.

5. Apply an ice pack or a cold hydrotherapy application to the area to limit the inflammatory response of the tissue.

Chronic Inflammation

In many cases, the injury site does not progress normally through the maturation stage and the conclusion of the healing process. Instead, the tissue enters a recurrent inflammatory process that leads to excessive scar tissue formation, prolonged pain, and additional loss of function.

Chronic inflammation has many different causes depending on the type of tissue damage sustained by the body. For example, inflammation may recur or persist because of the presence of a foreign body or bacteria in the area of injury. In diseases like rheumatoid arthritis, an autoimmune response ignites repeated bouts of acute inflammation. Constant exposure to chemical irritants may cause a chronic inflammatory process in tissues of the body like the lungs or skin. In musculoskeletal injuries, chronic inflammation is most often caused by a misdiagnosis of the injury leading to a flawed treatment plan, the return to full activity without sufficient healing time, overly aggressive treatment, failure to correct faulty body mechanics, and poor self-care.

Misdiagnosis and a Faulty Care Plan

In many cases, the client visits a massage therapist with a referral from a physician, chiropractor, or physical therapist with a diagnosed injury (e.g., CTS, thoracic outlet syndrome [TOS], plantar fasciitis). The diagnosis informs the types of treatment choices you make in terms of massage techniques and the areas of the body where you focus your work. A misdiagnosis could lead to a faulty care plan that causes everyone on the healthcare team to provide ineffective treatment. In one case, a female athlete was diagnosed by a physician with bilateral plantar fasciitis and received daily massage treatments including active and passive stretching. The pain from the injury failed to improve, and treatment seemed to exacerbate the condition. The massage therapist encouraged the client to visit an orthopedic physician and request further diagnostic testing. An MRI revealed that the client did not have plantar fasciitis but had stress fractures in the navicular bones of her feet. While massage therapists cannot diagnose a treatment, it is appropriate to refer clients to healthcare professionals who can. Alternately, the therapist can share the results of sessions and SOAP notes with the diagnosing physician, which may lead to re-evaluation of the original findings.

Re-Injury

As discussed previously, collagen slowly becomes stronger as it progresses through the maturation phase. The signs of inflammation, including redness, swelling, heat, pain, and pronounced loss of function, have long disappeared. The injured person may feel fully functional and jump back into his normal level of activities or work tasks before the tissue is ready. Re-injury may occur, sending the tissue back to the acute stage of the inflammatory process. This cycle is often witnessed with professional athletes who feel pressure to return to competition. Reconditioning requires the athlete to carefully control exercise intensity, frequency, and duration. Workers with repetitive stress injuries may also feel pressure to return to work. If the conditions that caused the injury are not resolved before the worker resumes the job, re-injury is probable. A good rule of thumb for both athletes and workers is that activity that was possible yesterday should be possible today. What this means is that if a workout or day on the job caused soreness, pain, or an increase of symptoms that prevents the same level of activity today, the intensity of activity was too high yesterday and needs further modification.

Overly Aggressive Treatment

Massage therapists use techniques like crossfiber friction, deep-tissue massage, and passive, active, and resisted range of motion when working with injuries in the maturation stage. If these techniques are applied too forcefully before the tissue has regained adequate mechanical strength and pliability, the tissue may experience microtrauma and re-enter the inflammatory process, prolonging healing. While clients often report minor increases in symptoms the day after a massage treatment (e.g., some soreness, some stiffness, etc.), by the following day the symptoms should be reduced and improvement experienced. If the client does not respond to treatment in a positive way, assess the intensity of the techniques and work more gently to see if you get a better result. This is why a phone call or an e-mail to the client the day following a massage is so important. It helps you capture and record the results of the session so that you can best adapt the next session for the client's benefit.

Failure to Correct Faulty Body Mechanics

Evaluation of an injured person's body mechanics as healing progresses is important. Faulty body mechanics are often the cause of the initial injury and can lead to re-injury if new habits are not adopted. Poor body mechanics or compensation patterns may be at the root of a persistent chronic condition because misalignment in one area can cause dysfunction in another. As a massage therapist, you work with the degree of balance between muscles to promote better posture and movement patterns. Referral of the client to a chiropractor, physical therapist, or movement specialist (e.g., Feldenkrais or Alexander Movement Therapist), if he or she is not already working with one, can help the client correct faulty body mechanics and learn more efficient and supported movement patterns.

Poor Self-Care

Throughout the healing process, clients need to practice good self-care to ensure a complete return to function. In the acute stage, the client might apply ice packs at home, maintain any available pain-free movement, and limit activity. When the tissue enters the repair stage, the client can apply hot or cold applications and participate in gentle stretching regimens that help collagen organize down the lines of mechanical stress.

As the tissue enters the maturation stage, the client can stretch and undergo exercises that strengthen the muscles and promote muscular balance. Attention to posture and work tasks is likely important. If the client fails to take part in self-care activities and continues to practice poor posture or work tasks that cause repetitive stress, he or she is likely to cause microtrauma to tissue and set off another bout of acute inflammation.

Chronic inflammation causes excessive amounts of collagen fibers to be laid down across the injury site, forming a dense, hard mesh of ropy or sticky sheet-like tissue. Muscle, tendon, fascia, ligaments, and joint capsules "glue down" and lose the ability to contract or elongate fully. If the situation is not resolved, chronic inflammation can last for several years.

Concept Brief 22-3
Chronic Inflammation

Definition: When the injury site does not progress normally through the maturation stage and enters a recurrent inflammatory process.

Causes related to musculoskeletal injuries include misdiagnosis leading to a flawed treatment plan, a return to full activity without sufficient healing time, overly aggressive treatment, failure to correct faulty body mechanics, and poor self-care

Topic 22-3
Understanding Common Musculoskeletal Injuries

Musculoskeletal injuries can be categorized in numerous ways. This topic explores injuries based on occurrence patterns such as acute traumatic injuries, overexertion injuries, and overuse injuries. Musculoskeletal injuries are also categorized by structure as muscle injuries, tendon injuries, joint injuries, bone injuries, or nerve injuries. Note that the conditions described here are injuries and not diseases like rheumatoid arthritis, fibromyalgia, or cancer, which also affect the musculoskeletal system but are outside the scope of this chapter. Massage treatment for these conditions is discussed in Chapter 23. Chapter 19 explains methods for assessing injuries and outlines the rehabilitation process, and provides important supplemental materials to increase your understanding of these topics.

As noted earlier, every injury is unique to the person experiencing it, and massage therapists must often adjust treatment goals and techniques to ensure the comfort of the individual client. Injuries are complex, and a novice therapist can be overwhelmed by all the factors that create a client's particular injury pattern. Therefore, it is important to start slowly, rely on experienced people around you, refer often to reference books, and trust yourself and your instincts. If you feel an injury requires a physician's release before you treat the client, hold your ground, even when clients insist that they just need a relaxation massage to feel better. If you are uncertain where to begin, return to your foundation by determining the stage of inflammation first and use the treatment goals associated with each inflammatory stage as a guideline. Whenever possible, consult with other members of the client's healthcare team to coordinate treatment. It's okay to explain that you have never worked with a particular injury type before and to get input on your treatment plan from more experienced professionals.

Acute Traumatic Injuries

An **acute traumatic injury** is an injury or a wound to the physical body caused by the application of extreme external force or violence. This type of force or violence might occur in many different situations, such as a mugging, a blow sustained during a sporting event (e.g., crossbody block in football), or blows, compression, rapid speed acceleration, and rapid speed deceleration as might occur in a work or car accident. Acute traumatic injuries often affect structures outside the musculoskeletal system (e.g., brain injury, internal bleeding, gunshot wound, kidney, or liver damage caused in a car accident, etc.). Examples of acute traumatic injuries in the musculoskeletal system include bone fractures (crack, break, or shattering of bones), contusions (blows to the body that cause damage to vascular tissue and bleeding into surrounding tissue), high-grade strains (serious tears or ruptures of muscle and tendon tissue) and sprains (tears or ruptures of ligaments), and lacerations (cuts that penetrate through the skin and are deep enough to require stitches).

Overexertion Injuries

Overexertion injuries usually occur suddenly when you push your body too hard or try to lift, lower, push, pull, or carry something that is too heavy. Overexertion injuries often occur because of an abrupt increase in activity. For example, a weekend athlete might not run regularly for 2 weeks and then strain a hamstring muscle because of running too far without the proper preparation and fitness level. In the workplace, 25% of overexertion injuries occur to the low back because of lifting, pushing, or pulling objects.[16] Movements of the body associated with overexertion injuries include repeated bending at the waist while picking up and moving an object, bending at the waist and twisting, long-term bending at the waist, reaching for an object, sitting or standing for long periods of time with poor posture, or absorbing vibration through the body during activities like using a jack hammer or driving a truck. Overexertion injuries often occur when people are moving too quickly to perform a particular task or perform the task while positioned in an awkward and unsupported posture.

Overuse Injuries

Overuse injuries (often called repetitive stress injuries, cumulative stress injuries, occupational overuse syndrome, and other similar names) occur when you repeatedly do the same task or movement without sufficient recovery time. They are generally caused by repetitive movements and repetitive movements performed from awkward and unsupported postures. Overuse breaks down structures like muscle and tendon, such that they weaken, fatigue, and eventually fail. In a study of injuries in middle-aged, fit athletes, 80% of the overexertion injuries occurred in runners who had been training regularly for more than 1 year and trained between three and five times per week. The level of preparation of these athletes suggests that the overexertion injury occurred because the structures involved were overused and failed when they hit a certain level of fatigue. Approximately 30% of these injuries took place in the knee, 24% in the ankle, heel or foot, 17% in the muscles of the leg, and 9% in the Achilles tendon.[17] You only have to imagine the number of times a weight-lifter lifts a weight or a foot hits the ground on a 5-mi run to understand how overuse injuries occur in athletes. In the workplace, overuse injuries are caused by repetitive movements like typing at a keyboard, filing, process work on assembly lines, packing boxes, tasks like sewing or moving automated machinery, or manual work like bricklaying, carpentry, or dry wall installation. The potential for injury is increased when furniture, tools, or equipment don't conform comfortably to the individual worker or when workplace design requires repeated bending, twisting, or reaching. Tight deadlines might prevent workers from taking sufficient breaks, or machinery might operate at a pace too fast for worker comfort requiring the worker to rush to move objects from conveyer belts. In many cases, poor worker posture and bad habits like lifting boxes incorrectly increase the potential for injury.

Concept Brief 22-4
Occurrence Pattern Injury Types

Acute traumatic injury: An injury or a wound to the body caused by the application of extreme external force

Overexertion injury: An injury that occurs from an abrupt increase in activity without proper preparation

Overuse injury: An injury that occurs from performing a movement repeatedly without sufficient recovery time

---

Injuries to Specific Musculoskeletal Structures

This section considers musculoskeletal injuries in categories based on the primary structure involved in the injury such as muscles, tendons, nerves, and joints. While this helps us to grasp injury basics, we must not forget that injuries affect the entire body, regardless of where they are located (review Chapter 20 for a detailed discussion of this concept). Furthermore, many common injuries such as whiplash, TOS, and CTS affect multiple structures in various ways. What you are likely to notice is that your treatment choices are often based largely on the stage of the inflammatory response the tissue is in as it progresses through the healing process. For example, if the injury is acute, despite the structures that are involved, you should use techniques to reduce tissue swelling, reduce but not eliminate muscle spasms, decrease pain, decrease sympathetic nervous system firing, maintain available pain-free range of motion, prevent re-injury, and encourage client self-care. These treatment goals and techniques were described in the earlier Topic 22-2. Instead of repeating that information for each individual structure, this section first describes the injury is defined and the reasons for its occurrence. Special considerations based on the particular injury and unique treatment goals and massage techniques are explained. In addition, apply the earlier concepts about the stages of the inflammatory response and the treatment goals and techniques used for those stages.

Muscle Injuries

Skeletal muscles have the capacity to contract forcefully without sustaining injury. But if too much force is transmitted through the muscle, if the muscle is compelled to elongate past its mechanical capacity, if the muscle suffers a direct blow, or if metabolic wastes build up from sustained anaerobic work, injury may result. Common muscle injuries include contusions or hematomas, muscle stiffness, acute muscle soreness, delayed-onset muscle soreness, muscle spasm, muscle guarding, strains, and whiplash.

Contusion or Hematoma

A contusion is an injury to a muscle caused by a blow or an impact to the tissue. With a contusion, there is damage to muscle fibers and bleeding into the subcutaneous tissue and skin. Contusions are classified as mild with little or no loss of function, moderate with some loss of function, and severe with significant loss of function. A hematoma is extensive bleeding and pooling of blood in muscle tissue and tissue surrounding muscle. The pooling blood causes the tissue to swell rapidly and places pressure on nearby nerve endings. Contusions and hematomas cause local swelling, pain at the location of the impact and in the surrounding tissue, bruising, decreased range of motion, and muscle spasms depending on the severity of the injury. Assess the injured area and refer the client for a medical evaluation if the contusion is severe with pronounced bruising, swelling, and loss of function. If you decide that you can continue with massage treatment, apply the treatment goals and techniques based on the stage of inflammation. One exception is the maintenance of available range of motion in the acute stage, because movement at this stage can increase the bleeding into the tissue and exacerbate the situation. Encourage the client to keep the area quiet and don't apply any range-of-motion techniques until the tissue has entered the late repair stage.

Muscle Stiffness and Soreness

Muscle stiffness is restricted mobility due to decreased muscle length. Often, stiffness and soreness occur together because of overuse, but not always. Sometimes, stiffness in muscle is not accompanied by pain and is not caused by overuse. For example, a sedentary lifestyle causes connective tissue to thicken and set, while poor posture causes muscular imbalances where certain muscles are chronically shortened as others are chronically lengthened. There is increasing evidence that intramuscular connective tissue, in particular the fascial layer known as the perimysium, is capable of active contraction and is likely to influence passive muscle stiffness, especially in tonic muscles.[18] Some diseases and drug side effects can cause muscle stiffness.

Muscle soreness usually occurs during or immediately after physical activity and is caused by lack of oxygen in the muscles and the buildup of lactate from anaerobic work. This type of injury tends to be mild and resolves within a few minutes to a few hours of rest.

Delayed-onset muscle soreness is a type of muscle soreness experienced from 12 to 48 hours after a vigorous workout or after a period of inactivity followed by unaccustomed strenuous physical activity. Symptoms include diffuse muscle tenderness, stiffness, swelling, and pronounced soreness. Researchers are not completely sure of the exact cause of delayed-onset muscle soreness. One idea is that exercise involving eccentric or isometric contractions causes increased tension in muscle tissues and disrupts the muscle fibers themselves or the connective tissue that binds muscle fibers together.[19] Muscles analyzed with a high-power microscope after intense exercise show evidence of microscopic muscle tissue damage.[20] This damage leads to an inflammatory response that causes the accumulation of fluid in the tissue. The fluid places pressure on surrounding structures leading to pain, while white blood cells activated by the inflammatory process secrete chemicals that trigger pain receptors.[21] Blood samples from runners the day after a marathon exhibit high levels of the enzyme creatine kinase. This is a marker of muscle damage because this particular enzyme "leaks" from damaged muscle.[22]

If the stiffness or soreness in one region is pronounced, assess the client to ensure that an injury is not present. If the tissue is hot or noticeably inflamed, apply cold hydrotherapy applications and general Swedish massage to the client's tolerance level. With mild stiffness and soreness, aim to increase circulation and the pliability of muscle fibers by using contrast hydrotherapy applications and a variety of massage techniques including myofascial release, Swedish massage,

and range of motion with gentle stretches. If stiffness and soreness are from inactivity, use warm to hot hydrotherapy applications and a range of techniques to reduce muscle tension and increase the pliability of the muscle and fascia.

Muscle Spasm and Muscle Guarding

A muscle spasm (in lay terms, a cramp) is a sustained, painful, involuntary contraction of a muscle or muscle group. A spasm can occur for many reasons, such as a response to pain, inflammation, infection, cold, increased sympathetic nervous system activity, dehydration, and electrolyte deficiencies (e.g., athletes in competition who get dehydrated), emotional stress, muscle fatigue, or vitamin deficiencies (associated with vitamin E and B vitamins), and as a symptom of pregnancy.

Muscle guarding is an involuntary reaction of muscles surrounding an injury site to protect an area of pain, as discussed previously. Muscle spasms that occur to guard and splint an injury site should never be completely eliminated. They provide an important function for ensuring the area remains immobile. Usually, muscle guarding resolves on its own as the local injury site heals and pain decreases. In some cases, muscle guarding may not fully resolve and problems may arise because other structures start to compensate for the dysfunctional region, creating the potential for secondary injury.

Firm, direct pressure or reciprocal inhibition helps to reduce an active muscle spasm that is causing acute pain and discomfort, such as an athlete might feel at the end of a sporting event. Proper rest and hydration are also important. Both hot and cold hydrotherapy applications help to reduce acute and chronically recurring muscle spasms, but hot hydrotherapy should not be used if the spasm occurs in relation to an acute or an early repair stage injury. For chronically spastic muscles or to break the pain-spasm-pain cycle around an injury site that has entered the maturation phase of healing, use hot hydrotherapy applications and a variety of massage techniques that reduce hypertonicities, adhesions, and fascial restrictions. The goal is to ensure that nutrient-rich blood can circulate freely and that metabolic wastes are effectively removed from the tissue. Never passively stretch a muscle in spasm because you might tear its fibers and injure the client.

Torticollis (also called wryneck) is caused by a severe spasm, usually of the sternocleidomastoid muscle, on one side (Fig. 22-3). This unilateral spasm locks the head in a painful rotated and flexed position. Trigger points in the sternocleidomastoid muscle may cause tinnitus (ringing in the ears) and watering of the eyes on the affected side. Simply sleeping in the wrong position or poor body mechanics may cause it, as may congenital abnormalities or central nervous system problems. If the condition is recurrent or severe, the client should be referred for medical assessment and diagnosis before proceeding with massage. In most cases, massage is an effective intervention with the client positioned supine so that slow and gentle Swedish massage is applied to relax the muscles on both sides of the neck and decrease sympathetic nervous system firing. Warm hydrotherapy applications increase local circulation and feel comforting. A variety of techniques may be used to reposition the head.

Work within the client's pain tolerance, and avoid passive stretching until the muscle spasm is diminished and even muscle tone has been established, to protect against unintended muscle tears.

Strain

A strain is a tear in the fibers of a muscle's belly, where the muscle and tendon interweave, in the fascia that wraps the muscle, or where the tendon attaches to the bone. Strains most often occur because the muscle-tendon unit is suddenly overstretched or because the muscle is asked to perform an extreme contraction against a heavy load. Overuse, fatigue, muscular imbalances, muscle stiffness, or inadequate warm-up before physical activity may contribute to tissue failure leading to a strain. Muscles prone to strains are the hamstring muscles, the deltoids, rotator cuff muscles, and the spinalis group of the back.

Strains are categorized in grades based on their level of severity. Grade 1 is a mild or first-degree strain where tearing occurs in individual muscle fibers (<5% of fibers show damage) and physical activity is slightly uncomfortable. In a grade 2 strain, also called a moderate or second-degree strain, tearing of muscle fibers and connective tissue is more extensive, but the muscle or tendon has not completely ruptured. Pain and muscle weakness are pronounced and prevent normal activity. Grade 3 strains, or severe or third-degree strains, involve a complete rupture of the muscle and tendon or an avulsion fracture where the bony attachment of the tendon is torn off while the muscle-tendon unit remains intact. The muscle may bunch up and a palpable gap may appear. Often, surgery is required to repair the damage. First assess the severity of the strain and refer the client for medical attention if the signs and symptoms of the injury are moderate to severe. In severe cases, the massage is contraindicated until the client has received an evaluation by a physician and a physician's release. If massage can proceed, apply treatment based on the stage of inflammation of the healing region.

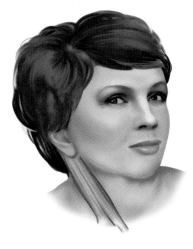

Figure 22-3 Torticollis (also called wryneck) is caused by a severe spasm, usually of the sternocleidomastoid muscle, on one side.

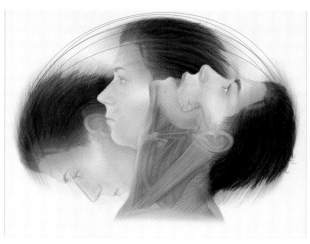

Figure 22-4 Whiplash is an injury to the head and neck from a rapid acceleration–deceleration of the head and neck during a motor vehicle collision or because of high-speed or contact sports.

Whiplash

Whiplash is an injury to the head and neck because of rapid acceleration–deceleration of the head and neck during a motor vehicle collision or high-speed or contact sports (Fig. 22-4). Massage therapists often see whiplash caused by rear-impact car accidents. When a person's car is struck from behind, the body undergoes an intricate series of movements in which the acceleration rate of the head is greater than that of the vehicle. On impact, the torso is pushed into the back of the seat and then thrown rapidly upward, compressing the cervical spine and causing possible injury to the cervical discs. The head and neck first stay in place as the torso moves forward, forcing the neck into hyperextension, causing shearing forces to the cervical and thoracic spine, and overstretching the anterior muscles and ligaments of the neck. Facet joints can experience damage during this movement. The head and torso then rapidly decelerate when the shoulder portion of the seatbelt prevents the torso from falling forward. The head and the neck are pushed into forceful hyperflexion, overstretching the posterior muscles and ligaments of the neck and causing injury to the lower cervical and upper thoracic spine.

The head position at the time of impact can influence the pattern of injury. For example, if a person's head is turned to look into the rearview mirror during the impact, the cervical spine is less able to extend, placing greater compressive stress on the ipsilateral facet joints and the splenius cervicis muscles. A headrest position that is too low can allow the head to hyperextend over the top of the headrest and increase the severity of the injury. An improperly fitted seatbelt allows the torso and shoulders to rotate asymmetrically, causing low back spinal injuries.

Whiplash injuries potentially involve all of the structures of the head, neck, and spine, and in some cases are severe enough to require surgical intervention or medical stabilization of the head. If the head hits the dashboard, windshield, or another object in the car, head trauma, loss of consciousness, and postconcussion headache are possible. The vertebrae, intervertebral discs, facet joints, joint capsules, ligaments, temporomandibular joints, muscle, fascia, blood vessels, and nerves could all suffer injury. Often, the client has few symptoms in the first 24 hours after injury and so does not seek medical assistance. Over the following 72 hours, symptoms of acute inflammation develop and may be accompanied by some hearing loss, headache, dizziness, memory loss, nausea, jaw pain, thoracic outlet symptoms (see below), tinnitus, and difficulty swallowing. Any client having undergone a rear, side, or front impact accident (even at low speeds) should receive medical analysis and a physician's release prior to massage therapy treatment. If possible, consult with the client's other caregivers to determine treatment protocol and to outline self-care activities for the client to use at home. Otherwise, if the client is released for massage, apply techniques based on the stage of inflammation while remaining attentive to the client's response to treatment. Any treatment that increases symptoms or pain, either during or following the massage, should be adjusted.

Tendon Injuries

Tendons are bands of fibrous connective tissue that attach muscles to bones. When a muscle contracts, the tendon and its corresponding bone are pulled toward the contracting muscle, producing movement. Certain tendons, like those of the wrist and ankle, are enclosed by a tendon sheath, which can be thought of as a fibrous tube. Between the layers of the tendon sheath and the tendon is a cavity that contains synovial fluid. This allows tendons to slide back and forth more easily. Tendons are exposed to high levels of tensile stress. When a load is placed on a tendon, the collagen fibers deform and temporarily straighten. So long as the load does not exceed the tissue's mechanical strength (4% increased length), the tendon can return to its normal length and shape. The collagen links in tendons begin to fail when the tendon length exceeds 8%.[22] A tendon injury may happen suddenly such as in a sports injury that causes tendon tissue to tear or completely rupture. This type of injury and its treatment are described in the previous "Muscle Injuries" section. Commonly, tendon injuries are the result of overuse from repetitive movements on the job or regular participation in a particular sport or activity. Factors that contribute to tendon injuries include muscle imbalances, poor posture, chronic degeneration of the tendon, poor circulation to the tendon, lack of flexibility, and the use of poorly designed or poorly fitting equipment on the job or in an activity.

Tendinitis

Tendinitis is a general term for a group of related tendon pathologies that may occur simultaneously in the same tendon. These pathologies include tendinitis, paratendinitis, tenosynovitis, tenovaginitis, tendinosis, and fasciitis.

- **Tendinitis** is inflammation of a tendon that occurs because of microscopic tearing of the tendon fascicles from repetitive movements that overload the tendon (Fig. 22-5).
- **Paratendinitis** (paratendon is another word for tendon sheath) is caused when the tendon sheath becomes irritated from rubbing over a bony prominence. In some cases, the terms paratendinitis, tenosynovitis, or tenovaginitis are used interchangeably. In other contexts, the terms differentiate among conditions (see tenosynovitis and tenovaginitis).
- **Tenosynovitis** is a term used to indicate irritation and inflammation of the inner surface of the tendon sheath because of friction with the tendon itself.
- **Tenovaginitis** is a term used to indicate that repeated irritation has led to a thickening of the tendon sheath.
- **Tendinosis** is the term used to describe degenerative changes that occur in the tendon at the cellular level without inflammation. With overuse, tendons may be subjected to repeated microtrauma (tiny tears or damage to structures that triggers an inflammatory response). When the tendon is not allowed to heal properly, fibroblasts begin to produce abnormal collagen. First, the total amount of collagen is decreased, and the ratio of different types of collagen normally found in tendons is out of balance. The normal parallel bundled fiber structure is disturbed, and many of the collagen fibers are thin, fragile, and separated from each other. Vascularity of the tissue is increased, and the size and shape of mitochondria (structures in cells concerned with chemical processes that make energy available to cells) in the nuclei of the tenocytes (tendon cells) is altered.

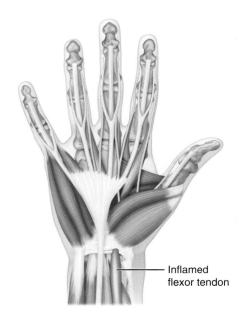

Inflamed flexor tendon

Figure 22-5 Tendinitis is the general term for a group of related tendon pathologies that may occur simultaneously in the same tendon.

- **Fasciitis** means inflammation of the fascia. The most common type is plantar fasciitis, in which the plantar fascia on the bottom of the foot becomes inflamed due to overuse, often from sporting activities.

LOCATIONS WHERE TENDINITIS IS COMMON

While there are many tendons in the body that can be injured, the tendons of the rotator cuff muscles and the Achilles and patellar tendons are particularly vulnerable to repetitive stress injury.

The rotator cuff tendons include the tendons for the supraspinatus, infraspinatus, subscapularis, and teres minor muscles (Fig. 22-6). Sports like swimming, baseball, tennis, golf, or other sports with throwing motions, and jobs that require workers to hold their arms over their heads for extended periods, like dry wall hangers or painters, cause stress to these tendons because they may become regularly impinged under the arch of the acromion where they are subjected to mechanical stress. Pain may be particularly noticeable when the humerus is abducted, trapping the tendons, particularly the tendon of the supraspinatus, against the acromion. This type of impingement, normal aging, or tissue degeneration for other reasons can lead to tears in the rotator cuff tendons. In some cases, surgery is required to remove portions of the acromion and re-attach the tendons to the humerus.

Achilles tendinitis causes painful sensations along the Achilles tendon during normal activity and is usually caused by tight gastrocnemius and soleus muscles and activities like running while overpronating or wearing poor-quality shoes that don't properly support and cushion the feet.

Patellar tendinitis is caused by activities that include running or jumping, such as track and field sports, professional cheerleading, and dancing. Pain is felt in the tendon below the patella and where it attaches to the tibia. During activity, the pain is sharp and shooting and then dulls to a persistent ache with rest.

Tendon injuries are classified into four grades depending on patterns of pain. Grade 1 injuries are mild, and discomfort occurs only after a particular activity. In grade 2 injuries, pain is felt at the beginning of the activity; the pain disappears during the activity as the tissue warms up but returns shortly after the conclusion of the activity. People with grade 3 injuries experience moderate pain at the beginning of the activity, throughout the activity, and after the activity. Grade 4 injuries are painful before, during, and after activities and with unrelated activities. In all cases, the pain is likely to worsen if the client does not seek treatment and modify repetitive patterns.

Treat tendinitis according to the stage of inflammation in the healing tissue, and discuss with the client the repetitive activities he or she is doing that lead to the issue. In many cases, the client will need to decrease the amount of the exacerbating activity and rest for healing to progress normally.

Joint Injuries

Joints are intricate structures that function with complex mechanical loading patterns occurring in multiple tissues. Forces applied to a joint may tear or rupture the ligaments that strap the joint together, or the fibrous joint capsule may be damaged or irritated. If sufficient force is applied

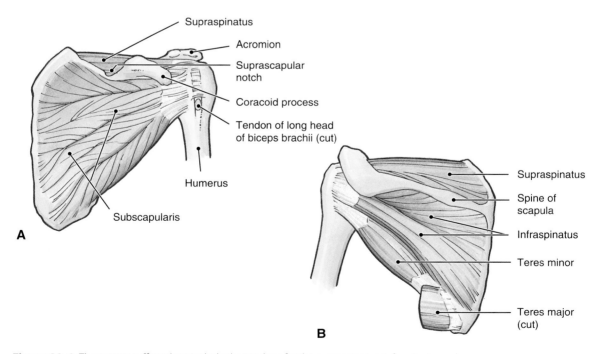

Figure 22-6 The rotator cuff tendons include the tendons for the supraspinatus, infraspinatus, subscapularis, and teres minor muscles. Sports like swimming, baseball, tennis, golf, or other sports with throwing motions cause stress to these tendons and may lead to injury **A.** Anterior view. **B.** Posterior view.

to structures of a joint, the articulating bones may become displaced (pulled from their normal structural relationship). Common injuries that affect joints include sprains, synovitis, subluxations, dislocations, capsulitis, bursitis, and meniscal injuries.

Sprains

When serious tensile forces are applied to a ligament, the tissue elongates past its mechanical capacity and is overstretched, torn, or ruptured. Depending on the severity of the damage, the ligament may no longer maintain the integrity of the joint's structure to prevent abnormal movements. Sprains often result when the joint is twisted beyond its normal range of motion (twisted ankle) while playing sports, stepping onto a surface that is irregular, or awkwardly placing the foot when running or walking. Three levels of severity are used to describe sprains (Fig. 22-7). In grade 1 (or a mild or first-degree sprain), the ligament experiences a minor stretch or minor tearing but the structure of the joint and regular movement is preserved, and activities can continue with only minor discomfort. Grade 2 sprains (or moderate or second-degree) involve tearing of ligament fibers, causing joint instability, pain, and dysfunction. In a grade 3 sprain (severe or third-degree), there is a rupture of the ligament or an avulsion fracture where the bony attachment of the ligament is torn away as the ligament remains intact. Significant joint instability, pain, and dysfunction are experienced in a grade 3 sprain, which usually requires surgery.

With sprains you apply massage techniques based on the inflammatory stage with some minor adaptations. First, assess the severity of the injury and refer the client to a physician if the sprain is moderate or severe. Passive joint movement to maintain range of motion is applied only to the joints proximal to the injured joint and not to the injured joint itself or to distal joints in the acute stage and early repair stage. In the late repair stage, passive joint movements are applied to proximal and distal joints and to the injured joint according to the client's tolerance. If the extremity was immobilized because of surgery, focus on balancing and strengthening muscles that cross the joint, and be careful not to overmobilize the joint after the casting is removed.

Synovitis

Synovitis occurs when the synovial membrane of a synovial joint becomes inflamed. It is caused when conditions like sprains, arthritis, lupus, gout, or other pathologies irritate the synovial membrane such that it produces increased levels of synovial fluid, causing the joint capsule to swell. It is a regular symptom of rheumatoid arthritis and is also associated with rheumatic fever and tuberculosis. The joint appears swollen and hot and feels boggy when touched. Pain and dysfunction result from the pressure placed on joint structures by fluid accumulation. Clients with synovitis should see a physician for proper diagnosis. Physicians may perform a synovial fluid analysis to determine the cause of the condition. This test is useful in the diagnosis of rheumatoid arthritis, arthritis caused by infection, gout, and pseudogout. Consult with the client's physician or healthcare team about the best way to proceed with the particular client based on the diagnosis.

Subluxation

A subluxation occurs when the articulating surfaces of the bones that form joints move out of their proper positions but remain in partial contact with one another. For example, the vertebrae in the spine may move out of place due to a traumatic event like a car accident or because of pressure

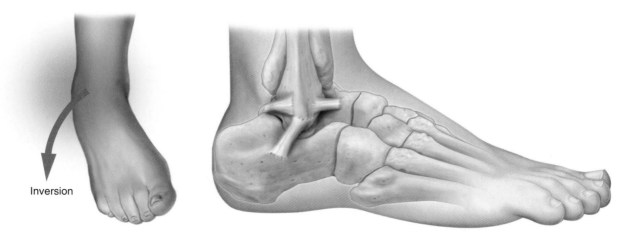

Inversion

Figure 22-7 Sprains occur when serious tensile forces are applied to a ligament, and the tissue elongates past its mechanical capacity and is overstretched, torn, or ruptured.

from muscular imbalances. When the vertebrae move out of their proper alignment, they place mechanical stresses on surrounding tissues such as muscles, ligaments, discs, and nerves that can accelerate degeneration of tissues and cause pain and loss of function. It is out of the massage scope of practice to manipulate bone. Massage promotes muscular balance so that uneven tension does not pull bones out of their proper orientation. In many cases, massage can create an environment where bone can naturally fall back into place. Treat tissue surrounding bone according to the stage of inflammation, and refer clients to chiropractors or other healthcare providers for diagnoses and treatment if you suspect a subluxation.

Dislocation

A dislocation occurs when the articulating surfaces of bones that make up a joint completely separate from one another. The anatomical structure of certain joints makes them more susceptible to dislocation than others. For example, the glenohumeral joint is unstable because the humeral head articulates only with a shallow glenoid fossa. This joint relies on ligaments and muscles for stabilization. Compare this to the deep ball-and-socket configuration of the hip joint. When a traumatic force separates the bones of a joint, surrounding ligaments, muscles, tendons, cartilage, blood vessels, and nerves are also damaged, requiring immediate medical attention. Medical personnel treat a dislocation by tractioning the bones that make up a joint back into their proper configuration (referred to as joint reduction). In some cases, surgery is required to repair the joint capsule and related structures. Often, the limb is immobilized for several weeks to allow the joint capsule and ligaments to heal. Massage is an important part of the rehabilitation process following joint reduction by a physician, and you are encouraged to communicate with the client's healthcare team to coordinate treatment goals. In general, you follow the treatment protocols for the stages of inflammation. Gentle passive joint movements are applied to the proximal joints (not the injured joint) within the client's pain tolerance during the early repair stage. As healing progresses, active and passive joint movements are used to increase range of motion within the injured joint's midrange of movement. Avoid overmobilizing the joint, especially in the direction of movement that caused the dislocation. In the maturation phase, strengthening the muscles that cross the joint becomes an important focus.

Capsulitis

Capsulitis is a chronic inflammatory condition that results from prolonged inflammation, scarring, thickening, and shrinkage of the joint capsule, leading to restricted movement and pain. It most often occurs in the glenohumeral joint (usually called frozen shoulder or adhesive capsulitis), and its causes are not completely understood. It could result

as a complication of tendinitis, bursitis, rotator cuff injuries, diabetes, and trigger points in the subscapularis muscle; trauma to muscles of the shoulder; head-forward postures; or shoulder surgery. One theory suggests that hyperkyphosis changes the alignment of the scapula, causing it to inferiorly rotate as it protracts over the thorax. This places the glenoid fossa in a downward-facing position and forces the head of the humerus to slightly abduct when the arm hangs freely. The rotator cuff muscles are positioned under increased tension as they attempt to maintain the head of the humerus in the glenoid fossa. The improper position of the joint causes collagen formation and capsular fibrosis. Treat the condition according to the stage of inflammation in the healing tissue. Pay special attention to the condition of the myofascia (Chapter 20), the reduction of trigger points (Chapter 21), and joint movement techniques that maintain or increase range of motion. Working with the healthcare team on the client's treatment goals is important. Exercises prescribed by a physical therapist may be the client's best chance to meet treatment goals effectively.

Bursitis

Bursae are small, fluid-filled sacs that cushion places where pressure or friction occurs between structures such as tendons, muscles, ligaments, and bones at joints (Fig. 22-8). When repetitive movements, muscle imbalances, poor posture, or muscle tension places bursae under prolonged or repetitive pressure, they become irritated and inflamed. Bursitis can also be caused by acute trauma, infections, or pathologies like gout, osteoarthritis, or rheumatoid arthritis, which are less common. When inflammation occurs, movement becomes painful. In some cases, calcific bursitis develops in which calcium deposits degenerate the internal lining of the bursa, leading to further pain and loss of function. Bursitis might occur in several places:

- Greater trochanteric bursa: There are two bursae at the greater trochanter that might become inflamed. The first is situated between the gluteus maximus tendon and the greater trochanter. The second is between the gluteus medius tendon and the greater trochanter.
- Iliopectineal bursa: Situated between the iliopsoas muscle and the iliofemoral ligament.
- Infrapatellar bursa: Situated between the tibia and the patellar ligament.
- Ischial bursa: Situated between the ischial tuberosity and the gluteus maximus.
- Olecranon bursa: Situated between the olecranon and the subcutaneous fascia.
- Pes anserine bursa: Situated between the tendons of the sartorius, gracilis, and semitendinosus muscles and the medial tibia.
- Prepatellar bursa: Situated between the inferior half of the patella and the patellar ligament.

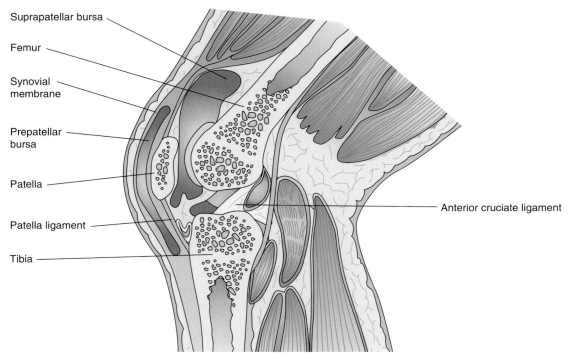

Suprapatellar bursa
Femur
Synovial membrane
Prepatellar bursa
Patella
Patella ligament
Tibia
Anterior cruciate ligament

Figure 22-8 Bursae are small, fluid-filled sacs that cushion places where pressure or friction occurs between structures such as tendons, muscles, ligaments, and bones at joints. Repetitive stress can cause bursae to become irritated and inflamed, a condition called bursitis.

- Retrocalcaneal bursa: Situated between the calcaneus and the Achilles tendon.
- Subacromial bursa: Situated between the acromion and the supraspinatus tendon with a section of the bursa between the deltoid muscle and the humerus.
- Subscapular bursa: Situated between the scapula and the subscapularis muscle.

Massage treatment follows the stage of inflammation of the tissue. Use caution with ice packs in the acute stage to avoid the weight of the pack placing pressure on the inflamed bursa. Bags of frozen peas make a good substitute for a heavy ice pack. As the inflammation in the bursa subsides, focus on reducing muscular imbalances surrounding the affected joint, reducing trigger points, and reducing restrictions or adhesions in myofascia.

Meniscal Injuries

The two menisci (medial and lateral) located between the femur and the tibia in the knee provide shock absorption for compressive and shear forces incurred with normal movement (Fig. 22-9). During a twisting injury in which the foot is weight bearing, the menisci may tear under the strain of torsion forces, leading to inflammation, pain, and loss of function. The posterior portion of the medial meniscus is the most commonly injured because it is less mobile than the lateral meniscus. Meniscal injuries are located deep in the knee and are not directly accessible to the massage therapist. If the injury is mild, rest, physical therapy, and a supportive brace

might be prescribed. In more serious cases, the client may require surgery. Massage therapists support rehabilitation efforts by limiting inflammation, maintaining available range

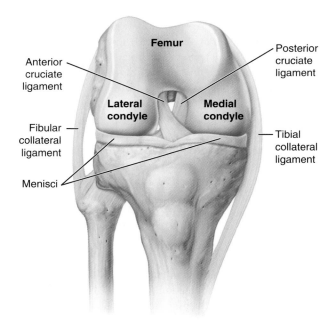

Femur
Anterior cruciate ligament
Posterior cruciate ligament
Lateral condyle
Medial condyle
Fibular collateral ligament
Tibial collateral ligament
Menisci

Flexed knee, anterior view

Figure 22-9 Meniscal injuries. During a twisting injury in which the foot is weight bearing, the menisci may tear under the strain of torsion forces, leading to inflammation, pain, and loss of function.

of motion, treating compensating structures, reducing pain, and reducing adhesions in surrounding tissue.

Temporomandibular Joint Dysfunction

Temporomandibular joint dysfunction (also called temporomandibular disorder, temporomandibular joint pain dysfunction syndrome, and temporomandibular joint syndrome, or commonly just as TMJD) is a condition that affects the temporomandibular joints, the muscles of mastication, and associated structures, causing jaw, head, and ear pain (Fig. 22-10). It is a complicated condition that can have many causes. For example, if the cranial bones are improperly aligned, especially the temporal bone, or if there is a postural dysfunction such as hyperkyphosis or scoliosis that causes imbalances in the neck and shoulder muscles, this could lead to faulty joint mechanics placing stress on jaw structures, leading to TMJD. The muscles of mastication might become unbalanced due to tension, spasm, trigger points, or overuse and alter joint mechanics. Habits like chewing gum, chewing only on one side of the mouth, pipe smoking, or wearing a mouthpiece or guard for long periods can cause these types of imbalances. Tooth extraction of the molars, tooth loss, or an improper bite can lead to imbalances, as can stress, which could cause a person to clench the jaw or grind the teach during sleep (bruxism). Joint pathologies, sinus infection, or prolonged sinus blockage or acute trauma to the face and jaw might all lead to TMJD. Clients presenting with the symptoms of TMJD should be referred to a physician for diagnosis and to rule out other pathologies such as sinusitis, trigeminal neuralgia, and pain caused by tooth decay. Relaxation massage helps to release tension in surrounding and compensating structures of the neck and shoulders. Reduce hypertonicities and trigger points

in these muscles. Apply myofascial techniques to the face and neck and focus moderate pressure on the muscles of mastication outside the mouth. These muscles are the temporalis and masseter. If you have specialized training and work in a state that allows interoral massage, you are likely to also massage the medial pterygoid, lateral pterygoid, and digastric muscles.

Bone Injuries

The ability of bone to absorb forces without failure depends on the bone's cellular health and the way in which the bone is loaded. For example, osteoporosis is a condition in which the bone becomes more porous and brittle, leading to a loss of bone strength and an increased risk of fractures. Alternately, the bone might be strong and healthy but subjected to a single, large-magnitude load imposed by an external violent force as might occur in a car accident. Repeated applications of lower-magnitude compressive forces, such as might occur with repeated running or jumping, may cause fatigue to structures and eventual injury. While massage therapists don't treat bone, they do address the effects of bone injuries on surrounding structures (apply techniques based on the level of inflammation in soft-tissue structures) and help the body deal with compensation patterns.

Peripheral Nerve Injuries

While nerve tissue is not part of the musculoskeletal system, it has a pronounced effect on musculoskeletal function and is often damaged in musculoskeletal injuries. Severe injuries of the central nervous system like brain concussions and spinal cord injuries require immediate medical intervention and are not discussed here. Massage therapists are most often concerned with injuries that affect the peripheral nervous system when compressive, tensile, or shear forces damage nerve tissue causing pain and loss of function.

Nerve injuries are often referred to as nerve lesions to describe the effect of the injury on the fibers of the nerve. In a complete nerve lesion, all of the fibers of the nerve are affected, while in a partial nerve lesion only some of the fibers are affected. Remember that different nerve fibers provide different functions. Some carry information to the central nervous system (afferent fibers), while others carry information from the central nervous system (efferent fibers). Some convey sensory information (sensory fibers), while others convey impulses for motor function (e.g., motor nerves responsible for stimulating muscles to contract). The type of fibers affected by the injury influences the level and type of function that is lost. In many cases, the nerve lesion can regenerate and the nerve heals. In others, the nerve is unable to repair itself and the damage is permanent. The severity of peripheral nerve lesions is classified in three grades[24]:

- **Neuropraxia (grade 1):** Neuropraxia is the mildest form of nerve injury, in which there is a reduction or block to the conduction of the nerve signal across one segment of the nerve due to demyelination of local nerve fibers. The conduction both proximal and distal to the lesion is

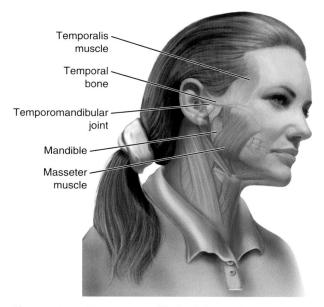

Figure 22-10 Temporomandibular joint syndrome is a condition that affects the temporomandibular joints, the muscles of mastication, and associated structures, causing jaw, head, and ear pain.

Temporalis muscle

Temporal bone

Temporomandibular joint

Mandible

Masseter muscle

maintained, and full recovery of nerve function is expected as the myelin is repaired.

- **Axonotmesis (grade 2):** Axonotmesis is more severe than neuropraxia because prolonged compression of the nerve results in a lesion at the site of compression and degeneration of the axons of the nerves distal to the compression site. Healing takes place over weeks or months, but usually full regeneration of the axons is expected.

- **Neurotmesis (grade 3):** Neurotmesis is the most severe grade of peripheral nerve injury because the nerve trunk is completely or partially severed, causing the nerve to degenerate. In some cases surgery can repair the damage, but in others the entire nerve is lost and function does not return to the area.

Nerve lesions are caused by a number of different forces, which might be applied to the tissue suddenly and violently or repetitively over time. Internal compressive forces overload a nerve by placing prolonged pressure on the nerve fibers, which eventually leads to nerve tissue failure. Examples of internal compressive forces include chronically tight muscles, the subluxation of bones, the buildup of fluid, or the growth of a tumor. Alternatively, external compressive forces such as the strap of a backpack slung over the shoulder, crutches used to support body weight, or the weight of a body region placed on an unprotected nerve during a movement performed repetitively at work might cause damage. Trauma from a blow to a body region, a gunshot or knife wound, or impact during a car accident can cause compressive damage to nerves. Nerves can be damaged due to tensile forces that compel the tissue to elongate past its mechanical capacity, leading to lesions or to shear forces that cause friction and irritation. Nerve damage also occurs because of systemic conditions like hypothyroidism, diabetes, kidney conditions, heart conditions, and pregnancy.

Peripheral nerve pain is often experienced as a result of peripheral nerve lesions. Neuritis refers to the inflammation of a nerve in which the sheath and local connective tissue are affected, but the nerve axon is unaffected. The condition causes dull pain and is often the result of a pathology, trauma to the nerve, or exposure to a toxic substance, drugs, or alcohol. Neuralgia, or nerve pain, is most often caused by regional compression of a nerve, subluxation of a bone, or prolonged exposure to cold. TOS, CTS, and piriformis syndrome are conditions massage therapists work with regularly.

Thoracic Outlet Syndrome

The brachial plexus is a bundle of nerves arising from the cervical spine that supplies the arm with sensation. The subclavian vein and the subclavian artery run parallel to the brachial plexus as it travels under the clavicle and pectoralis minor muscle to supply the arm with blood. (Vein and artery names change as these structures travel down the arm; in the axillary region as the structures pass under the pectoralis minor, they are called the axillary vein and artery.) TOS is a collective name for a number of conditions caused by the compression of these structures anywhere between the base of the neck and the axilla (Fig. 22-11). Three primary areas of compression are possible:

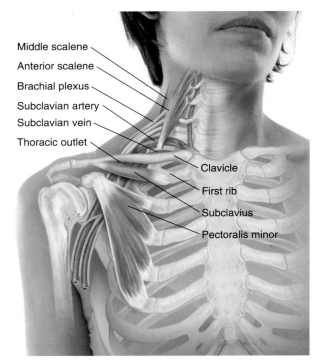

Figure 22-11 TOS is a collective name for a number of conditions caused by the compression of the brachial plexus, subclavian vein, and/or subclavian artery anywhere between the base of the neck and the axilla.

- **Anterior scalene syndrome:** The brachial plexus and the subclavian artery are compressed between the anterior scalene muscle and the middle scalene muscle, usually because these muscles become hypertonic and develop trigger points in reaction to stress or heavy lifting or through respiratory dysfunction like extreme coughing from bronchitis or heavy breathing because of asthma or emphysema. In rare cases, a client may have an anatomical anomaly such as an additional rib that forms at C7, or the insertion of the anterior scalene may be overly large. The subclavian vein is not compressed in anterior scalene syndrome because it passes in front of the anterior scalene muscle at this level.

- **Costoclavicular syndrome:** The brachial plexus, subclavian artery, and subclavian vein are compressed as they travel through the space between the clavicle anteriorly and the first rib posteriorly. The size of the space can change because of posture (e.g., rounded or dropping shoulders), trauma or anomalies of the clavicle or first rib (e.g., fracture or the development of a bony callus), chronic respiratory disorders that cause disordered breathing (emphysema, asthma), and hypertonicity and trigger points in the subclavius muscle. Costoclavicular syndrome often leads to edema in the extremity because of impaired venous return due to the compression of the subclavian vein.

- **Pectoralis minor syndrome:** The brachial plexus, axillary artery, and axillary vein (as the subclavian artery and vein enter the axillary region their names change to the axillary artery and axillary vein) are compressed as they pass through the subpectoral space created by the clavicle and the insertion of the pectoralis minor muscle. This compression is most often due to the position of the arm when it is elevated over the head for prolonged periods of time as with jobs like painting or drywall installation or by sleeping with the arm positioned over the head. People who regularly carry a heavy backpack that places weight on the shoulders or who use crutches can also develop pectoralis minor syndrome.

Arm symptoms can be confusing and suggest a variety of conditions in addition to TOS. CTS, ulnar nerve compression, tendinitis, osteoarthritis in the glenohumeral joint, and cervical spine spondylosis can share similar symptoms to TOS, so it is important to refer the client for a physician's diagnosis before treatment begins.

The goal of massage treatment for TOS is to eliminate the compression of the brachial plexus and subclavian vein and arteries caused by soft-tissue structures. Seek to reduce hypertonicities, fascial restrictions, and trigger points in the entire area including the upper back, shoulders, neck, and upper chest. Use joint movements to improve range of motion to the cervical spine and shoulder joint.

Carpal Tunnel Syndrome

In CTS (Fig. 22-12), the median nerve is pinched by surrounding structures as it passes through the tunnel created by the carpal bones and the flexor retinaculum (also called the transverse carpal ligament). The flexor retinaculum is a strong fibrous band that spans the carpal bones forming a tunnel through which the flexor tendons and median nerve

pass (the flexor tendons attach muscles originating around the elbow and forearm to the fingers). Usually the carpal tunnel provides enough space for the median nerve to pass through unhampered, but when the area is under stress, the flexor tendons thicken, the flexor retinaculum thickens, irritation causes inflammation, inflammation causes edema, and this puts pressure on the nerve. The median nerve provides sensation for the thumb, index finger, middle finger, and half of the ring finger. When squeezed, numbness, weakness, burning sensations, shooting pain, or tingling results. Without proper attention, permanent nerve damage can occur. CTS is sometimes caused by factors other than repetitive stress. For example, edema caused by pregnancy, menopause, or obesity can fill up the space of the carpal tunnel, as can a subluxation (when a bone loses its proper juxtaposition with neighboring bones) of the capitate bone (a centrally placed carpal bone). Other conditions occurring in the neck, shoulder, arm, wrist, and hand can cause symptoms mimicking those of CTS.

While a massage therapist can't always address the underlying cause of CTS, you can reduce edema, fascial restrictions, hypertonicity in muscles, and trigger points that contribute to the condition. Follow the protocol for the appropriate stage of inflammation, and focus on reducing tension in any soft-tissue structures that compress the median nerve.

Piriformis Syndrome

The piriformis is a muscle that originates on the anterior sacrum and inserts on the greater trochanter of the femur to laterally rotate the thigh (it abducts and medially rotates the thigh if the thigh is flexed). The sciatic nerve, the largest nerve in the body, supplies sensation to the leg and foot. It originates in the lower back at L5-S2 and travels between the piriformis and the superior gemellus (another muscle that laterally rotates the thigh) before branching into the tibial nerve and common peroneal nerve at the popliteal fossa. When the piriformis is tight, it may compress the sciatic nerve, resulting in numbness, a burning sensation, a sharp and shooting pain, tingling, and loss of function (Fig. 22-13). In some individuals, the sciatic nerve travels directly through the fibers of the

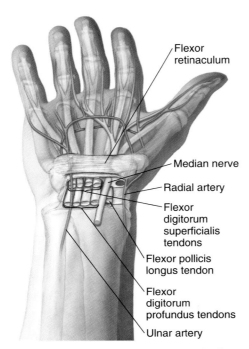

Figure 22-12 In **CTS,** the median nerve gets pinched by surrounding structures as it passes through the tunnel created by the carpal bones and the flexor retinaculum (also called the transverse carpal ligament).

Flexor retinaculum
Median nerve
Radial artery
Flexor digitorum superficialis tendons
Flexor pollicis longus tendon
Flexor digitorum profundus tendons
Ulnar artery

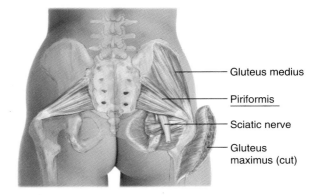

Figure 22-13 **Piriformis syndrome.** When the piriformis is tight, it may compress the sciatic nerve, resulting in numbness, a burning sensation, sharp, shooting pain, tingling, and loss of function.

Gluteus medius
Piriformis
Sciatic nerve
Gluteus maximus (cut)

piriformis, which might cause a person to be predisposed to piriformis syndrome. Clients with persistent piriformis syndrome symptoms should be referred to a physician to rule out other causes of radiating gluteal pain.

Massage treatment for piriformis syndrome involves reducing facial restrictions, hypertonicities, adhesions, and trigger points in muscles related to the lumbar spine and pelvic girdle because postural compensation often contributes to the condition.

Compensation Patterns

Compensation patterns refer to new behaviors that offset a weakness. When the body is injured, it adopts new movement patterns as a means to protect the weakened areas and to manage the resulting loss of function. For example, if you sprain an ankle, you limp. If you break one hand, you use the other. If you suffer a shoulder injury, you contract muscles to keep it immobile and use the other arm and hand in an effort to allow the injury to heal. Whenever an injured person adjusts his or her movement patterns in response to weakness, pain, or loss of function, the altered pattern redistributes loads to other joints, muscles, tendons, ligaments, nerves, and bones of the body. The compensating body tissues are often unaccustomed to these new loads, and the tissue becomes fatigued and a new injury may result. Sometimes compensation patterns disappear as the primary injury heals, and sometimes the compensation pattern becomes a subconscious habit that persists long after the original injury has healed. An injury caused by a long-held compensation pattern may be more severe than the original injury that triggered the pattern. Massage therapists may recognize compensation from old injuries in postural holding patterns,

hypertonic or hypotonic muscles, restricted fascial regions, disordered movement, limited range of motion, and pain.

Concept Brief 25-3
Injury to Structures

- Common muscle injuries include contusions or hematomas, muscle stiffness, acute muscle soreness, delayed-onset muscle soreness, muscle spasm, muscle guarding, strains, and whiplash.
- Tendinitis is the general term for a group of related tendon pathologies that may occur simultaneously in the same tendon. These pathologies include tendinitis, paratendinitis, tenosynovitis, tenovaginitis, tendinosis, and fasciitis.
- Common injuries that affect joints include sprains, synovitis, subluxations, dislocations, capsulitis, bursitis, and meniscal injuries.
- Neuritis refers to the inflammation of a nerve in which the sheath and local connective tissue are affected, but the nerve axon is unaffected.
- Neuralgia, or nerve pain, is most often caused by regional compression of a nerve, subluxation of a bone, or prolonged exposure to cold.
- Compensation patterns refer to new behaviors that offset a weakness. When the body is injured, it adopts new movement patterns as a means to protect the weakened areas and to manage the resulting loss of function.

MASSAGE FUSION
Integration of Skills

STUDY TIP: Catchwords

Catchwords, catch phrases, and acronyms, like SHARP, used to remember the signs and symptoms of acute inflammation, useful memory devices. When you are trying to remember something, write out its aspects in brief notes and see if they don't suggest a catchword or catch phrase. Come test time, you will be glad you made the extra effort. Here are examples:

- You can remember the signs and symptoms of acute inflammation by using the catchword SHARP:

  S = Swelling
  H = Heat
  A = A loss of function

R = Redness
P = Pain

- RICE, the first aid for acute inflammation:

  R = Rest
  I = Ice
  C = Compression
  E = Elevation

CHAPTER WRAP-UP

Professional massage therapists tell many stories about their experiences with injury rehabilitation and the sense of fulfillment they have when people heal and return to full function through massage and other treatments. Therapists might also describe the emotional difficulties of working

MASSAGE FUSION (*Continued*)
Integration of Skills

with clients whose conditions fail to progress normally to the maturation stage of healing. In some instances, massage is the key that changes the progression of pain and helps the client live with higher levels of function and greater ease. But for some clients, massage provides a brief period of some relief but no lasting change. Injury affects each person differently. Each person copes with the pain and loss of function in his or her own way. If you plan to work with athletes or with other medical professionals in a hospital, hospice, wellness center, clinic, chiropractic office, or sports medicine clinic, understanding how the musculoskeletal system may sustain an injury and how soft tissue repairs itself is crucial to your work. This chapter provides you with this essential knowledge. In other chapters, you

learn additional components of working with injury and chronic pain conditions. In previous chapters, you have already learned assessment tools and massage techniques that provide proven effects and benefits.

While you learn all of these things, keep in mind the psychological aspects of injury and pain. It is out of your scope of practice to counsel clients, but it is within your scope of practice to listen. Take the time to understand how an injury affects the client's life. What has the client lost that is important to him or her? Can a grandfather still pick up his grandkids? Can a wife take a walk with her husband? Can a teenager go to the prom? The information you learn will help you focus your techniques to better address activities of daily living that are particularly important to the client.

Chapter
23

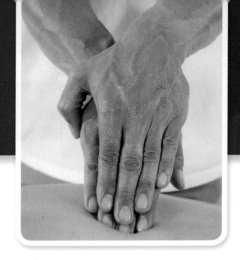

Massage for Chronic Pain Conditions and Selected Pathologies

KEY TERMS

cancer
chemical headache
chronic pain
cluster headache
fibromyalgia
inflammatory headache
migraine headache

nociceptor
osteoarthritis
pain
rheumatoid arthritis
tension headache
traction headache
vascular headache

LEARNING OBJECTIVES

Having read the chapter and used the related student learning tools, the student will be able to:

1 Define the terms *pain*, *suffering*, and *chronic pain*.

2 Outline the anatomy and mechanisms of pain.

3 Describe two ways in which chronic pain affects the quality of a person's life.

4 Discuss four ways that massage can assist in the process of pain management.

5 Define the term *fibromyalgia*, identify one cause, and choose two treatment goals

and techniques to use in a session for fibromyalgia.

6 Define the term *rheumatoid arthritis (RA)*, identify one cause, and choose two treatment goals and techniques to use in a session for RA.

7 Define the term *osteoarthritis*, identify one cause, and choose two treatment goals and techniques to use in a session for osteoarthritis.

8 Compare and contrast tension headaches with migraine headaches.

9 Define the term *cancer*, identify one cause, and choose two treatment goals and techniques to use in a session for cancer with a client in a weakened state undergoing treatment.

10 Define the term *AIDS*, identify its cause, and choose two treatment goals and techniques to use in a session for AIDS with a client in a weakened condition.

In your massage practice, regardless of the setting (e.g., clinic, spa, cruise ship, home office), you will encounter clients with pathologies, many of which cause chronic pain. Some of these clients seek massage purely as a luxury, while others are looking to massage to help them manage their conditions. In any case, you must have a strong understanding of how the body works, how massage techniques affect systems of the body, and how to use critical thinking skills to determine if massage is safe or contraindicated for each client's particular condition. This chapter discusses pain in detail before introducing common pathologies you are likely to work with during your massage career. Because it is almost impossible to know everything about every pathology you might encounter in your massage career, you should have a detailed pathology textbook for reference in your massage practice and know how to gather information and apply it in treatment planning. Ruth Werner's *A Massage Therapist's Guide to Pathology* is highly recommended.

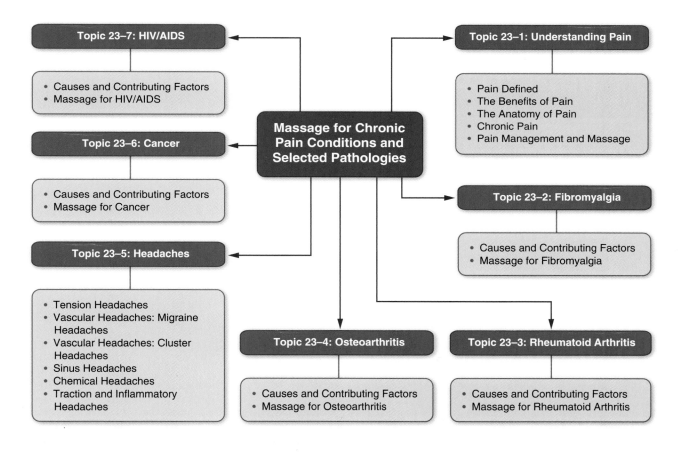

Topic 23–7: HIV/AIDS
- Causes and Contributing Factors
- Massage for HIV/AIDS

Topic 23–6: Cancer
- Causes and Contributing Factors
- Massage for Cancer

Topic 23–5: Headaches
- Tension Headaches
- Vascular Headaches: Migraine Headaches
- Vascular Headaches: Cluster Headaches
- Sinus Headaches
- Chemical Headaches
- Traction and Inflammatory Headaches

Massage for Chronic Pain Conditions and Selected Pathologies

Topic 23–1: Understanding Pain
- Pain Defined
- The Benefits of Pain
- The Anatomy of Pain
- Chronic Pain
- Pain Management and Massage

Topic 23–2: Fibromyalgia
- Causes and Contributing Factors
- Massage for Fibromyalgia

Topic 23–4: Osteoarthritis
- Causes and Contributing Factors
- Massage for Osteoarthritis

Topic 23–3: Rheumatoid Arthritis
- Causes and Contributing Factors
- Massage for Rheumatoid Arthritis

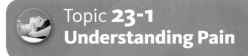

Topic **23-1**
Understanding Pain

A 1999 national pain survey found that approximately 50 million Americans live with chronic pain caused by accidents or disease, while an additional 25 million suffer acute pain resulting from surgery or an accident. Two thirds of the people surveyed had been living with pain for more than 5 years.[1] Researchers in 2000 found that 36 million Americans had missed work in 1999 due to pain and that 83 million reported that pain affected their participation in activities of daily living.[2] Similar research conducted in 2006 indicates that the number of people affected by pain is increasing.[3]

Regardless of where you choose to practice massage, you will encounter clients living with pain. If you focus your career on healthcare massage, you will regularly work with clients living with pain. The judgments you make about the validity of the client's pain story, your knowledge of pain and its causes, your personal experience of pain, and your personal beliefs about how people should respond to pain are likely to influence how you interact with these clients and the quality of the care you provide. This section will define pain, explain the anatomy of pain sensations, discuss the impact of chronic pain on activity levels and quality of life, and identify reliable massage techniques that reduce pain.

Pain Defined

Pain is an unpleasant physical and emotional sensation associated with tissue damage or the immediate potential for tissue damage. This definition describes pain associated with physical trauma and not pain in the broader sense (often differentiated from physical pain with the term *suffering*), which occurs mentally and emotionally and without tissue damage in response to life's challenges.

The intensity and quality of pain due to physical trauma vary among individuals because of genetics, ethnicity, gender, past experiences, present expectations, cultural background, situation and context, and a variety of other psychological and physiological factors. An individual's personality, emotional reaction patterns, and mental state can play a role in his or her reaction to and experience of pain. For example, in a study conducted on depressed patients of the same age and sex, patients with more severe types of depression reported greater occurrence and sensations of physical pain than patients with less severe types of depression.[4] Note that the pain perceived by a client may not always seem proportional to the degree and severity of tissue damage observed by the therapist. Pain is a highly subjective and personal experience; this fact has prompted the nursing profession to widely adopt the following definition of pain: "Pain is whatever the experiencing person says it is, existing whenever the experiencing person says it does."[5] Pain is classified and further described according to time, its location, tissue type, and how it is generated, as shown in Table 23-1.

TABLE 23-1 Classification of Pain

	Term	Defined	Example
Time	Acute pain	Pain that comes on quickly, can be severe, but lasts only as long as the reason for the pain is present.	Stubbed toe, burn, scrapped knee, etc.
	Recurrent acute pain	Acute pain that occurs regularly or irregularly.	Menstrual pain, migraine headaches.
	Chronic pain	Pain that persists for a long period of time past the point of typical injury recovery or in relationship to a medical condition.	Old musculoskeletal injury, cancer, fibromyalgia, arthritis.
	Intractable pain	Chronic pain that persists despite treatment.	Not associated with a particular disease or injury.
Location	Focal pain	Pain restricted to one local region of the body. The pain is felt in only one place.	Stubbed toe, scrapped knee, broken bone.
	Multifocal pain	Pain sensations are broadly distributed. Pain is felt in more than one place.	Stomachache, toothache.
	Radiating pain	Pain that extends out from the injured area along specific spinal nerve root distributions (dermatomes).	Sciatica, thoracic outlet syndrome, trigger points.
	Referred pain	Pain experienced at a site different from the injured or diseased organ or body part, with a nerve supply different from that of the source of pain, often with recognized referral patterns.	Heart attack causes referred pain in the arm and jaw. Gallbladder injury causes referred pain in the scapula area.
Tissue type	Somatic pain	Pain associated with structures of the body wall.	Broken limbs, burns, cuts.
	Visceral pain	Pain associated with internal organs of the body.	Damage to liver, spleen, intestines, lungs, or other internal organs.
	Nociceptive pain	Pain caused by tissue injury or the potential for tissue injury detected by nociceptors. This type of pain diminishes as tissues heal.	Musculoskeletal injury, injury to the skin.
	Neuropathic pain	Pain resulting from injury or malfunction in the peripheral or central nervous system. Pain is often triggered by an injury but then persists for months or years beyond the healing of damaged tissues.	Nerve trauma, neuropathy caused by diabetes, alcohol abuse, exposure to chemicals, vitamin deficiencies, or others.
	Allodynia	A type of neuropathic pain in which stimuli that are not usually experienced as painful cause pain.	Cutaneous allodynia (pain from nonpainful touch stimuli)
How the pain is generated	Psychogenic pain	Pain associated with psychological factors such as depression or anxiety.	Headaches, muscle pain, back pain, stomach pains associated with depression.
	Idiopathic pain	Pain with an unknown cause that cannot be categorized or diagnosed.	Can present as many painful conditions like fibromyalgia or persistent back pain.
	Phantom pain	Pain experienced in a limb that has been amputated. Believed to be caused by spontaneous nerve impulses generated due to damage from the amputation.	Amputated limbs
	Malingering	Pain fabricated for the purposes of achieving personal reward or satisfaction.	Pain that is fabricated to ensure an insurance payout

The Benefits of Pain

Acute physical pain, an important part of the body's defense system, alerts a person that something is wrong. It causes changes in behavior and promotes learning. A person takes action to end a painful experience (e.g., removes a hand from a hot surface) and learns from the experience to avoid activities that cause pain and potential injury in the future (never touch hot surfaces again). People seek medical help when they experience abnormal painful sensations; their descriptions of their pain often help pinpoint the cause of the underlying problem. As part of the healing process, pain encourages an injured person to protect the damaged area and decrease normal activity in an attempt to avoid further pain, thereby allowing the area to heal. These benefits do not relate to chronic pain, however.

> ### Concept Brief 23-1
> **Pain**
>
> - **Defined:** Pain is an unpleasant physical and emotional sensation associated with tissue damage or the immediate potential for tissue damage.
> - **Variations:** Variations in the experience of pain are caused by genetics, ethnicity, gender, past experiences, present expectations, cultural background, and the situation and context.
> - **Benefits:** Pain is part of the body's alert system to promote changes in behavior and learning to ensure survival.

The Anatomy of Pain

This brief discussion of the anatomy of pain is intended only as an introduction (Fig. 23-1). For more in-depth information about the conduction of nerve impulses and pathways to the brain, review your anatomy and physiology textbook.

Nerves in the peripheral nervous system transmit signals between the central nervous system and all other parts of the body. **Nociceptors** are the sensory receptors that transmit sensations of pain. They are found at the ends of small unmyelinated or myelinated afferent neurons and are activated by mechanical stimuli (e.g., bending, twisting, compression), thermal stimuli (e.g., hot or cold), and chemical stimuli (e.g., prostaglandin and bradykinin).

Pain stimuli are conveyed to brain centers via two types of axons. Alpha-beta axons are myelinated and convey information rapidly from precise locations, while C-fiber axons do not possess myelin and convey less-defined information more slowly. Alpha-beta axons are responsible for immediate, sharp, intense pain like that of a stubbed toe. C-fibers carry the secondary diffuse and throbbing pain that follows.

Myelin is a fatty, membranous sheath formed by supporting Schwann cells that wrap around areas of the axon. Spaces between myelin wraps are called nodes of Ranvier, which expose the axon's membrane to extracellular fluid. The nodes of Ranvier are the "excitable" areas of the axon. Nerve signals (action potentials) travel the length of the axon quickly by jumping from one node of Ranvier to the next (Fig. 23-2). If myelin is disturbed when nerves are injured, large areas of excitable axons may be uncovered. Nerve impulses can be spontaneously produced at these injury sites, resulting in numerous pain signals being conducted to the brain and intensifying the experience of pain.

The cell bodies of peripheral neurons having similar functions are clustered together in groups called ganglia. The afferent fibers carrying pain and other sensory information from the body to the brain are called the dorsal root ganglia because they enter the spinal cord via the dorsal root on the backside of the cord. The axons then ascend toward the brain along complex pathways, after passing through the gray matter of the spinal cord at an area called the dorsal horn.

The thalamus receives sensory information from the body and relays it to the cerebral cortex. In the cerebral cortex, all sensory stimuli including pain are examined and compared with memories, expectations, and emotional states to inform any required modifications of behavior. It is during this process that pain information can be interpreted and its experience modified based on cultural beliefs, past experiences, attitudes, and viewpoints.[6]

> ### Concept Brief 23-2
> **Anatomy of Pain**
>
> - **Nociceptors:** Sensory receptors that detect pain
> - **Alpha-beta axons:** Myelinated afferent neurons that convey sharp, precise, acute pain quickly to the brain.
> - **C-fiber axons:** Unmyelinated afferent neurons that convey diffuse, throbbing pain more slowly to the brain.
> - **Thalamus:** Receives sensory information from the body and relays it to the cerebral cortex.
> - **Cerebral cortex:** Compares sensory information including pain to memories, expectations, and emotional states to inform behavioral changes.

Chronic Pain

Chronic pain is pain that persists for a period of time past the point of typical injury recovery. Chapter 22 described how a musculoskeletal injury triggers an inflammatory response and the body begins to progress through the stages of healing. Most people respond well to treatment and return to full strength and function within a predictable time frame. In some cases, the tissue does not progress normally through the stages of healing and enters a recurrent inflammatory process that leads

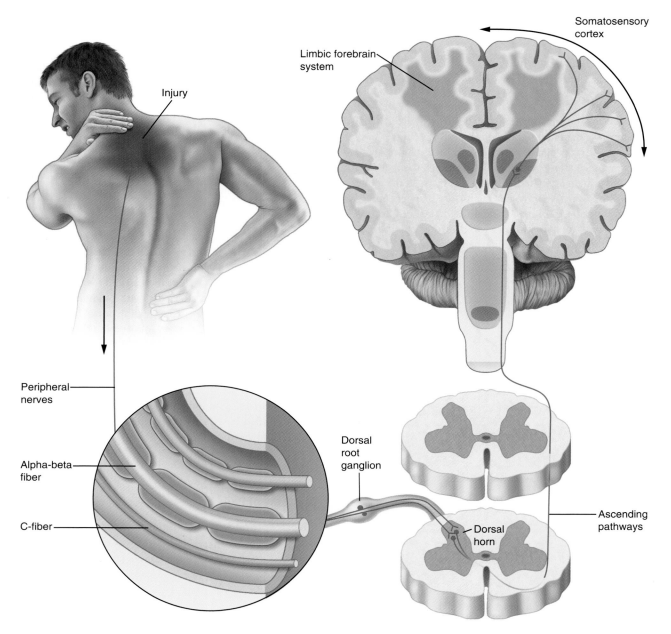

Figure 23-1 Pain stimuli are conveyed to brain centers via two types of axons. Alpha-beta axons are myelinated and convey information rapidly from precise locations, while C-fiber axons do not possess myelin and convey less-defined information more slowly. *Nociceptors* are pain receptors found at the ends of small unmyelinated or myelinated afferent neurons and are activated by mechanical, thermal, and chemical stimuli.

to a prolonged experience of pain. Chronic pain can also be a persistent symptom of a medical condition such as fibromyalgia, rheumatoid arthritis (RA), cancer, or lupus (Box 23-1).

The Impact of Chronic Pain on Quality of Life

Chronic pain impacts people physically, psychologically, socially, and economically. Each person's experience of chronic pain is different. You will work with many clients whose mild pain does not significantly limit their activities of daily life but still impacts their quality of life. It is important to honor each person's experience of pain and not compare it

to another's. Following are some of the impacts that chronic pain can have on a person's quality of life:

- **Loss of mobility:** People suffering from chronic pain often lose the ability to move around comfortably and perform tasks that are usually taken for granted. For example, daily tasks like hair brushing, showering, getting dressed, driving, grocery shopping, laundry, and housework may be difficult or impossible. Other family members may have to assume responsibilities for the person living with chronic pain, and this can lead to feelings of lost self-worth.

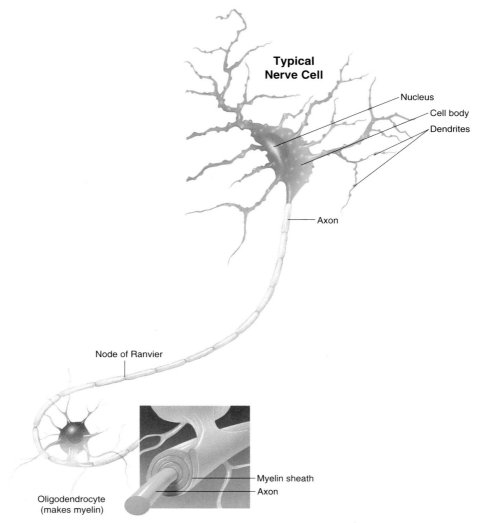

Figure 23-2 Myelin is a fatty, membranous sheath formed by supporting Schwann cells that wrap around areas of the axon. Spaces between myelin wraps, called nodes of Ranvier, expose the axon's membrane to extracellular fluid.

BOX 23-1 Conditions Commonly Associated with Chronic Pain

AIDS	Irritable bowel syndrome
Cancer and cancer treatment	Migraines
Chronic fatigue syndrome	Myofascial pain syndrome
Cluster headaches	Osteoarthritis
Complex regional pain syndrome	Persistent low back pain
Crohn's disease	RA
Depression	Sickle cell disease
Diabetic neuropathy	Tension headache
Fibromyalgia	Whiplash-induced neck pain
Heart disease	

- **Pain avoidance:** People living with chronic pain may begin to focus on their pain to the extent that they avoid any activity that might increase pain. This leads to pronounced inactivity and higher levels of disability as the body gradually loses overall condition and remains immobile. Over time, the intense focus on pain causes more and more sensations, which would otherwise not be unpleasant, to be perceived as painful.

- **Medication issues:** Medications may decrease the amount of pain a person feels but can also produce side effects like gastrointestinal problems, drowsiness, fogginess, or aggressive behavior. Over time, the drug may lose its effectiveness and breakthrough pain might occur, or a person could develop a physical addiction to or psychological dependence on the drug. Drugs may cause other physical problems such as liver toxicity when they are used for extended periods of time.

- **Sleep disturbances:** Persistent pain makes normal sleep difficult, and people living with chronic pain usually experience pronounced sleep disturbances that leave them feeling lethargic, moody, foggy, and inattentive.

- **Loss of relationships:** Chronic pain places a huge strain on relationships with family and friends. A person constantly restrained by pain often cannot enjoy normal sexual relations with his or her partner. It may be impossible to pick up and carry young children or place them into and out of car seats, highchairs, strollers, and bathtubs without a risk of increased pain. Activities that once promoted bonding and connection with friends and family may be impossible for a person in pain. For example, sitting through a movie, sports event, or lunch date may increase pain. Going for a walk with a loved one, playing a golf game, gardening, or preparing to host a dinner might increase pain. As time passes, friends and family stop asking the person living with chronic pain to participate in activities, and so he or she becomes more and more isolated from other people.

- **Loss of income:** A person living with chronic pain may have to quit a job or cut back significantly in the number of hours worked in a week. If the injury happened on the job, failure to heal from the injury may lead to a conflict with an employer or a disability manager over an injury settlement. The loss of income or conflict leads to increased stress, which may exacerbate the pain.

- **Loss of credibility:** The friends and family members of people living with chronic pain often doubt the validity of pain levels reported by a person in pain. At first, friends and family are supportive. Gradually, as the person with pain fails to respond to treatment and show improvement, frustration and helplessness set in. Their feelings of frustration and helplessness due to being unable to help their loved one transform into doubt that their loved one is really in pain. The person in pain loses his or her credibility and retreats further into isolation.

- **Anxiety, stress, and depression:** It is easy to understand why people living with chronic pain experience high levels of anxiety and stress. They may feel that they are no longer who they once were, or want to be, and can no longer participate in activities that give life meaning. They may feel that they are a burden on spouses, children, other family members, and friends. As they become more and more isolated from people they love and from activities that hold value, they may slip into depression. In fact, research suggests that people living with chronic pain are four times more likely to attempt suicide than people without pain.[7]

Research demonstrates that when people are encouraged to talk about their pain and set goals for pain reduction with their healthcare providers, the quality of pain management improves and they find greater relief from pain.[8] As a professional massage therapist, you can discuss pain with clients and ask them the right questions that will help you choose effective techniques and methods, while providing a baseline from which to judge the effectiveness of sessions over time. Chapter 19 described specific methods for gathering and documenting pain data. Remember that some factors increase pain levels while others decrease pain levels (Box 23-2). Develop a resource list for people living with chronic pain that includes books, pain clinics, local support groups, and referrals to other healthcare

---

BOX 23-2 Factors that Increase or Decrease Pain Levels

Factors That Decrease Pain Levels

- Counseling from a mental health specialist
- Positive internal dialogue
- Program of strengthening and conditioning based on a physical therapist's recommendations to maintain available activity levels
- Relaxation techniques (e.g., meditation, hypnosis, massage, etc.)
- Self-care with thermal therapies (e.g., application of ice, use of hot packs, hot baths, etc.)
- Distraction methods to remove focus from pain

Factors That Increase Pain Levels

- Conflict
- Depression
- Faulty body mechanics or poor posture
- Inactivity
- Increased focus on pain
- Increased stress levels
- Negative internal dialogue
- Pain avoidance behaviors
- Progression of a pain-causing disease
- Overactivity
- Sleep disturbances

providers like orthopedic surgeons, chiropractors, naturopathic physicians, acupuncturists, physical therapists, and mental health professionals who may provide useful services.

Concept Brief 23-3
Chronic Pain

- **Defined:** Chronic pain persists for a period of time past the point of typical injury recovery or is a persistent symptom of a medical condition.
- **Impact:** Loss of mobility, pain avoidance behaviors, drug issues, sleep disturbances, loss of relationships, loss of income, loss of credibility, anxiety, stress, and depression.

Pain Management and Massage

Research demonstrates that massage effectively reduces pain. Although the mechanism by which pain is reduced is not always clear, certain techniques have proven reliable.

- **Promote relaxation:** Any type of pain information received by the brain signals a threat to survival and so triggers the fight-or-flight response of the sympathetic nervous system. The increase in blood pressure, heart rate, breathing rate, and blood flow to voluntary muscles, the heart, and lungs is often accompanied by mental and emotional anxiety, anger, and fear. Norepinephrine, one of the neurotransmitters that mediate the fight-or-flight response, enhances transmission of nerve impulses, increasing the intensity of the experience of pain. Stress increases the sensation of pain, and pain increases stress. Therefore, the reduction of stress brought about by the parasympathetic nervous system response to massage is one way that massage helps in the management of pain.
- **Break the pain-spasm-pain cycle:** As described in previous chapters, the pain-spasm-pain cycle refers to a persistent cycle in which pain triggers muscle spasms, muscle spasms cause decreased blood flow and a buildup of metabolic wastes in the tissue leading to pain, which then triggers more muscle spasms and a recurrence of the dysfunctional cycle. Massage breaks the pain-spasm-pain cycle by reducing muscle spasms, triggering the parasympathetic nervous system response to reduce sympathetic firing, and increasing circulation to the local area, which removes metabolic wastes, thereby reducing pain.
- **Use the gating mechanism of the spinal cord to reduce pain:** Chapter 4 described Melzack and Wall's gate control theory of pain management. To briefly review, because the spinal cord has a limited ability to attend to multiple sources of sensory stimuli at one time, pain stimuli traveling on the slower C-fiber axons can be locked out when lots of sensory stimuli (such as caused by massage) are traveling to the brain. Dull, aching or throbbing pain, the type often associated with chronic conditions, can be blocked by somatic stimuli like massage.
- **Apply thermal applications:** Cold applications like ice packs or ice massage are most appropriate for acute pain because they cause vasoconstriction of blood vessels and slow the metabolic process of cells allowing them to survive a period of hypoxia, reducing the zone of secondary injury as discussed in previous chapters. Cold applications have a numbing effect on the tissue and reduce the velocity of pain stimuli transmissions. Heat is most often used for chronic conditions because it increases circulation to the local tissue, improving the condition of the tissue through enhanced oxygen, nutrient, and waste exchange to decrease muscle spasm. Heat lowers pain perception because it slows the conduction of pain stimuli to the brain and sedates the central nervous system to aid relaxation.
- **Reduce trigger points:** Trigger points are hypersensitive spots that usually occur within a taut band of muscle or fascia and cause the affected muscle to be shortened. Trigger points have a predictable pain referral pattern. They are related to tissue ischemia (vasoconstriction and decreased circulation) and increased metabolic processes in the local tissue brought on by many factors including stress, injury, a sedentary lifestyle, poor posture, and repetitive stress. Reducing trigger points is an important treatment goal in the rehabilitation of clients with many different conditions, as discussed in Chapter 21.

The compassion and understanding you demonstrate toward clients living with chronic pain enhances the therapeutic relationship, builds trust, and provides psychological comfort. The therapeutic value of this increased awareness and level of empathy cannot be quantified but will help you provide the best possible care to clients.

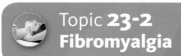

Topic 23-2
Fibromyalgia

Fibromyalgia affects 3% of the U.S. population (women comprise 85% of those affected) and causes diverse symptoms that include the distribution of tender points all over the body, chronic pain in soft tissues, fatigue, and sleep disturbances.[9] The tender points that develop with fibromyalgia seem to be distributed in nine pairs over all the regions of the body but

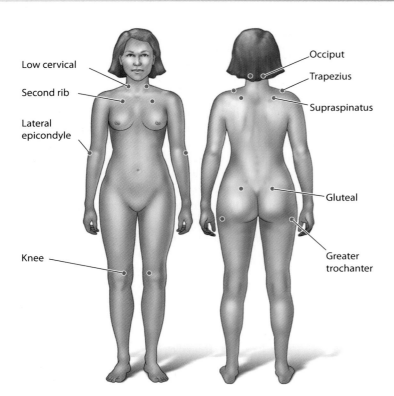

Low cervical

Second rib

Lateral
epicondyle

Knee

Occiput

Trapezius

Supraspinatus

Gluteal

Greater
trochanter

Figure 23-3 The tender points that develop with fibromyalgia seem to be distributed in nine pairs over all the regions of the body but are particularly concentrated in the neck and shoulder area.

are particularly concentrated in the neck and shoulder area (Fig. 23-3). Additional tender points seem to form when the condition is triggered by soft-tissue trauma. The pain felt by people living with fibromyalgia varies widely. Pain can change locations without explanation, might be experienced as mild to severe, and may change dramatically from day to day. Many people develop sensitivity to any stimulus that is perceived as potentially painful and thus avoid exposure to bright light, noise, cold, and pressure. Fibromyalgia is often associated with other chronic conditions such as chronic fatigue syndrome, irritable bowel syndrome, and psychological issues.

Causes and Contributing Factors

Researchers report that fibromyalgia could be triggered by a wide array of factors that might include soft-tissue trauma, neuroendocrine disturbances, abnormal nociception (a term for the perception of pain), and many others.[10] The cerebrospinal fluid of fibromyalgia patients demonstrates higher than normal levels of the neurotransmitters substance P and nerve growth factor. These neurotransmitters increase tissue vasodilation, stimulate nerve activity, and increase the sensation of pain. In addition, sleep studies indicate that people with fibromyalgia rarely reach the deepest level of Stage IV sleep. As a result, growth hormone levels and serotonin levels are lower than normal. Growth hormone helps the body heal tissue damage and recover. Serotonin is an important neurotransmitter that moderates pain sensations.[11]

Medical diagnosis is difficult because the symptoms of fibromyalgia share common characteristics with other conditions such as chronic fatigue syndrome, myofascial pain syndrome, hypothyroidism, and sleep disorders. Treatment focuses on management of pain and encouraging a person living with fibromyalgia to stay healthy with good nutrition, adequate sleep and exercise, and stress-reduction strategies.

Massage for Fibromyalgia

Massage is an effective support strategy for people living with fibromyalgia. Remember to carefully assess a client with fibromyalgia before each session and customize the massage to how he or she feels at that moment. Clients often vary widely in their needs based on how they are feeling on a particular day, and also often have very different responses to massage. Deep work or techniques that overstretch muscles might cause flare-ups and persistent pain for days after a session. Therefore, the techniques you choose should be applied with light-to-moderate pressure. Many therapists report that session length is important. Clients seem to do better with shorter sessions that last 30 minutes to 1 hour than with longer sessions of 90 minutes to 2 hours. Treatment goals might include:

● **Increase relaxation and decrease stress:** A wide variety of techniques can be applied that increase relaxation and reduce stress, including general Swedish massage and energetic bodywork techniques. Researchers point to a link between psychological stress and fibromyalgia because chronic stress causes abnormalities in neuroendocrine function that show up in fibromyalgia cases.[12] Decreasing stress can be a powerful intervention to decrease pain and improve quality of life.

- **Warm the tissue:** Hot, moist hydrotherapy might be applied before massage techniques to warm the tissue and increase local circulation to the area.

- **Decrease pain:** A wide variety of techniques can be applied that activate the gating mechanism of the spinal column and break the pain-spasm-pain cycle if present. Review the first part of this chapter and try general Swedish massage and energetic bodywork techniques.

- **Deactivate trigger points:** People living with fibromyalgia often develop trigger points. Provide trigger point work as long as it is tolerable to the client and proves effective after a session. If the client has an adverse reaction to trigger point work, deactivate fewer points in a session or lighten the depth of treatment.

- **Work with what you find in the tissue:** Each client's experience of fibromyalgia is unique. Work with what you find in the tissue using techniques that feel good to the client.

For example, if you palpate and find fascial restrictions or adhesions, apply myofascial techniques.

Call the client 24 hours after the session and ask for feedback about his or her response to treatment. If the client reports that muscles feel overly tender or that pain increased, this indicates the tissue was overworked. Adjust your treatment depth and evaluate the appropriateness of the techniques you used during the session. Document your findings in the client's chart. Fibromyalgia can be tricky, and it may take you a few sessions to figure out what works best for each client.

Concept Brief 23-4
Fibromyalgia

- A condition characterized by tender points distributed over the body, chronic pain, fatigue, and sleep disturbances.
- Massage techniques that reduce stress, decrease pain, deactivate trigger points, and feel good to the client are indicated within the client's tolerance level.

Topic **23-3**
Rheumatoid Arthritis

Rheumatoid arthritis is an autoimmune disorder that affects primarily the synovial membranes of joints but may also affect other tissues including blood vessels, the lungs, and fascia. A variety of symptoms might be experienced at the onset of RA. Often, people feel as if they have a low-grade illness like a cold or the flu and experience fatigue with a low fever, loss of appetite, and general muscle pain. Gradually, the condition becomes specific to joints (particularly the joints of the hands, feet, wrists, and ankles), and joints become hot, swollen, stiff, and painful. RA usually occurs bilaterally but may affect one side of the body more severely than the other. The condition is characterized by flare-ups followed by periods of remission, but each person's flare-remission cycle is unique. Some people have few lifetime flare-ups and experience low levels of life impact. Others have a number of flare-ups each year, and some experience regular flare-ups that never completely subside.

Concept Brief 23-5
Arthritis

Arthritis (from the Greek, *arthron* meaning joint + *itis* meaning inflammation) is something of a catch-all term that might be applied to over 100 disorders that affect joints. Many of these conditions are noninflammatory, prompting some authors to use the term arthrosis as well.

Causes and Contributing Factors

Autoimmune diseases like RA occur when the immune system malfunctions and starts to treat normal body cells and tissues as if they were an infectious agent. A person who is exposed to some types of streptococcus bacteria, some retroviruses, or the bacteria that causes Lyme's disease may develop RA as a result of exposure. A protein found in synovial membranes is structured in a similar fashion to these invading pathogens and causes immune system confusion. The immune system attacks synovial membrane proteins, causing inflammation in the joint and the release of chemicals that break down cartilage. Joints are painful, hot, swollen and may become deformed over time due to cartilage erosion and the development of fibrous scar tissue. Muscles associated with the affected joint often become hypertonic and develop trigger points, leading to muscle spasms and further constriction of the joint. The impact on a person's quality of life and ability to perform activities of daily living is determined by the severity of the flare-up and the number of flare-ups experienced in a year.

Medical treatments for RA aim to reduce inflammation and pain and to limit damage to the joint's structure through the use of nonsteroidal anti-inflammatory drugs. Other drugs like steroidal anti-inflammatory medications and immune suppressants might be used to interrupt the diseases process, but many of these drugs have serious side effects and cannot be used for long periods of time. In some cases, joint replacement surgery is an option.

Massage for Rheumatoid Arthritis

When a client with RA is experiencing a flare-up in which joints are red, hot, swollen, and painful, massage is contraindicated. If the client is in a period of remission, the joints may be stiff but will not be swollen, hot, and red. During this phase, massage can help maintain available range of motion and decrease stress, which may decrease the occurrence of flare-ups. Each client is unique. One may like deep work, while another finds deep work increases symptoms or flare-ups. Communicate with clients about what they experience from sessions. Work moderately at first to get a feel for the client's tissue and tolerance level. Work deeper if the client indicates that she or he feels it will be beneficial. Avoid hot hydrotherapy, which may cause a flare-up. Focus on these treatment goals:

- **Increase relaxation and decrease stress:** A wide variety of techniques can be applied that increase relaxation and reduce stress, including general Swedish massage and energetic bodywork techniques.
- **Reduce fascial restrictions:** Use myofascial techniques to reduce fascial restrictions around affected joints and compensating areas.
- **Focus on muscles at affected joints:** Reduce hypertonicities and trigger points in muscles around affected joints with proprioceptive and neuromuscular techniques.

- **Maintain range of motion:** Joint movements and gentle stretches within the client's comfort tolerance help to maintain or even improve range of motion.
- **Cool the tissue:** Use cold applications at the conclusion of the session or at the conclusion of a particular body area to cool the tissue and decrease the chances that the body might enter an inflammatory cycle.

Call the client 24 hours after the session and ask for feedback about his or her response to treatment. If the client reports that muscles felt overly tender or that joints responded with increased stiffness, this indicates that the tissue was overworked. Adjust your treatment depth and evaluate the appropriateness of the techniques you used during the session. Document your findings in the client's chart.

> ### Concept Brief 23-6
> **Rheumatoid Arthritis**
>
> - **Defined:** RA is an autoimmune disorder that primarily affects the synovial membranes of joints.
> - **Massage:** Massage is contraindicated in flare-ups but used during periods of remission to decrease stress, reduce fascial restrictions, hypertonicities, and trigger points around affected joints, maintain range of motion, and provide comfort.

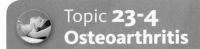

Topic 23-4
Osteoarthritis

Osteoarthritis (also called degenerative joint disease) is a condition related to wear and tear of a synovial joint's structures that causes the joint to become painful and inflamed (Fig. 23-4). It is especially prevalent in weight-bearing joints like the hips and knees. If the symptoms are acute, the joint is hot, swollen, and painful. In chronic osteoarthritis, the joint tends to be stiff, tight, and mildly painful and to feel better as it warms up with mild activity. Overuse can cause a flare-up of a chronic condition back into an acute stage of inflammation.

Causes and Contributing Factors

Osteoarthritis is most often caused by wear and tear due to repetitive stress, muscular imbalances that place additional stress on joints, a ligament laxity that causes joint instability, overweight that increases the stress on joints, hormonal imbalances, nutritional insufficiencies, and aging. For example, a recurring physical activity like running places cumulative stress on particular joints like the hips and knees that are exposed to repeated compressive forces. Over time, the smooth

cartilage of articulating bones starts to roughen. Instead of gliding smoothly over each other, the articulating bones start to irritate each other and inflammation develops. Chemicals related to the inflammatory process further break down and damage the cartilage. Bones start to adapt to the situation by thickening at the condyles. This often results in the formation of small bone spurs that increase irritation and pain, leading to further inflammation. Muscles related to the damaged joint become hypertonic and develop trigger points, leading to muscle spasms and further constriction of the joint. Soon, a person with osteoarthritis starts to decrease his or her use of the joint or stop moving in ways that cause increased pain. This lack of use causes muscles and joint structures to weaken and become atrophied, leading to increased dysfunction and even disability.

Medical treatment for osteoarthritis aims to reduce pain and inflammation and reduce the damage occurring to articulating cartilage. Depending on the severity of the condition, a physician might recommend anti-inflammatory medications, injections of hyaluronic acid into the joint to increase joint lubrication, the use of nutritional supplements like glucosamine and chondroitin that improve joint function, or joint replacement surgery.

Right knee

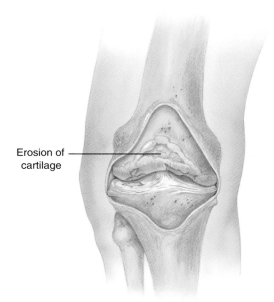

Erosion of cartilage

Figure 23-4 Osteoarthritis (also called degenerative joint disease) is a condition related to wear and tear of a synovial joint's structures that causes the joint to become painful and inflamed.

Massage for Osteoarthritis

Chronic osteoarthritis usually does not cause joints to be hot, red, and swollen. If mild inflammation is present, treat the affected joints with ice and apply techniques with caution proximal to the inflamed area. Following are common treatment techniques when working with osteoarthritis:

- **Warm the tissue:** Hot, moist hydrotherapy might be applied before massage techniques to warm the tissue and increase local circulation to the area. Avoid the use of heat if the tissue appears inflamed.
- **Decrease pain:** A wide variety of techniques can be applied that increase relaxation, activate the gating mechanism of

the spinal column, and break the pain-spasm-pain cycle if present. Try general Swedish massage and energetic bodywork techniques.

- **Reduce fascial restrictions:** Use myofascial techniques to reduce fascial restrictions around affected joints and compensating areas.
- **Focus on muscles at affected joints:** Reduce adhesions, hypertonicities, and trigger points in muscles around affected joints with Swedish massage, myofascial techniques, proprioceptive techniques, and neuromuscular techniques.
- **Maintain range of motion:** Joint movements and gentle stretches within the client's comfort tolerance help maintain or improve range of motion. Apply joint movements to the cervical region and hips with extreme caution depending on the overall condition of the client and the progression of osteoarthritis. In severe cases, these joint movements might be omitted from the treatment plan.

Call the client 24 hours after the session and ask for feedback about his or her response to treatment. If the client reports that muscles felt overly tender or that joints responded with increased stiffness or pain, this indicates that the tissue was overworked. Adjust your treatment depth and evaluate the appropriateness of the techniques used during the session. Document your findings in the client's chart.

Concept Brief 23-7
Osteoarthritis

- **Defined:** Osteoarthritis (also called degenerative joint disease) is a condition involving wear and tear of a synovial joint's structures, causing the joint to become painful and inflamed.
- **Massage:** Massage aims to decrease pain, fascial restrictions, adhesions, hypertonicities, and trigger points around affected joints, and maintain or improve range of motion.

Topic **23-5**
Headaches

Headache can generally be defined as pain experienced in the region of the head that can be caused by many different situations. Headaches are currently classified as tension, vascular, chemical, or traction-inflammatory types. Tension and vascular headaches are the most common types experienced regularly (Fig. 23-5). The following sections consider each type's symptoms, causes, and contributing factors, and massage techniques that are helpful.

Tension Headaches

Tension headaches are the most common type of headache, causing mild-to-moderate pain that is often described as a diffuse tight band around the head. The soft tissue of the scalp, neck, and shoulders often feels tender. Some people experience tension headaches occasionally (episodic pattern), while others experience tension headaches regularly (chronic pattern).

Headaches

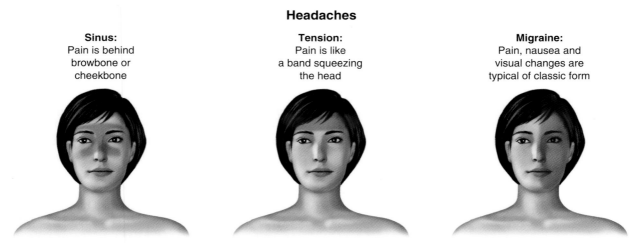

Sinus:	Tension:	Migraine:
Pain is behind browbone or cheekbone	Pain is like a band squeezing the head	Pain, nausea and visual changes are typical of classic form

Figure 23-5 Headache types and their pain patterns.

Causes and Contributing Factors

The exact causes of tension headaches are unknown. At one time, experts believed that the pain of tension headaches was caused by hypertonic muscles of the face, neck, and scalp, brought about by stress or heightened emotions (hence the name tension headache). Current research indicates that changes in numerous brain chemicals stimulate pain pathways to the brain and interfere with the brain's ability to stifle pain. For example, lower-than-normal serotonin levels may cause the trigeminal nerve (the main sensory nerve for the head and face) to release neuropeptides that dilate blood vessels in the brain's periphery, leading to increased pressure and pain sensations.

Factors that increase the occurrence of tension headaches include stress, depression, and anxiety, poor posture, working in awkward positions, and clenching the jaw for prolonged periods. Women have a higher occurrence of tension headaches than men, and middle-aged people (40 to 50 years) experience more tension headaches than other age groups. Injuries to the head and neck such as that caused in whiplash, subluxation of cervical vertebrae, or muscle tension in the muscles of the head, neck, and jaw flexors may contribute to the occurrence of tension headache. Medical treatment is not generally necessary for tension headaches, and over-the-counter analgesics are often the first choice of treatment by clients.

Massage for Tension Headaches

Massage for tension headaches focuses on the region of the head, neck, shoulders, and back. If the client is actively experiencing a headache, you may need to use alternative positions to ensure his or her comfort. For example, pressure from the face cradle may increase pain, so you might adjust by performing the massage with the client in the side-lying position. General treatment goals include

- **Increase relaxation and decrease stress:** A wide variety of techniques can be applied that increase relaxation and reduce stress, including general Swedish massage and energetic bodywork techniques. Simply reducing stress can ease the pain of a tension headache and decrease the number of headache episodes experienced by the client.
- **Decrease pain:** A wide variety of techniques can be applied that activate the gating mechanism of the spinal column and break the pain-spasm-pain cycle if present. Try general Swedish massage and energetic bodywork techniques.
- **Decrease muscle tension and spasm:** Warm or hot packs might be applied to the posterior neck, shoulders, and upper back at the start of the session to warm the tissue, increase local circulation and reduce pain. A variety of techniques might then be used to reduce adhesions, hypertonicities, and fascial restrictions.
- **Deactivate trigger points:** Trigger points are likely a factor in tension headaches. Reduce trigger points in the trapezius (which refer to the eye, ear, and lateral neck), splenius capitis (refer to the top of the head), splenius cervicis (refer to the temporal region and posterior neck), suboccipitals (refer around the ears), sternocleidomastoid (refer to the occiput, around the eye, into the ear, and across the forehead), masseter (refer to the eye, ear, jaw, and teeth), and temporalis (refer to the temporal region).

Vascular Headaches: Migraine Headaches

Migraines and cluster headaches are considered **vascular headaches** because these types of headaches are related to irregularities in blood flow in the brain. The pain from these types of headaches tends to pulsate or throb along with the body's pulse.

Migraine headaches are chronic vascular headaches that cause significant pain for hours or days. Symptoms often begin in childhood, adolescence, or early adulthood and can be severe. The pain might be confined to one side of the head or may affect both sides, and is likely to interfere with activities of daily living. The pain tends to worsen with physical activity and exposure to light or sound. Nausea and vomiting may accompany migraine pain.

People sometimes experience warning symptoms hours or even days before the onset of a migraine. These symptoms can include flashes of light, blind spots, tingling in the arms or legs, feelings of elation or increased energy, heightened thirst, sweet cravings, fatigue, irritability, and depression.

Causes and Contributing Factors

Like tension headaches, migraines are accompanied by a drop in serotonin levels. This drop in serotonin likely activates the trigeminal nerve to release neuropeptides that place pressure on the meninges, resulting in pain. Researchers also believe that fluctuations in estrogen trigger migraines in women and that food sensitivities to alcohol (especially beer and wine), cheese, chocolate, aspartame, caffeine, many Asian foods, salt, and chemicals found in processed foods are also factors. Increased stress levels, overly bright lights or sun glare, loud sounds, strong smells, changes in wake-sleep patterns such as missing sleep, physical exertion, changes in barometric pressure from weather patterns, or certain medications may trigger migraines in some people.

Medical treatment for migraines includes the use of selective serotonin reuptake inhibitors (commonly used for treating depression) both as a preventive and to shorten the migraine once it begins. Other medications such as ergot compounds, beta-blockers, and calcium channel blockers might also be prescribed by a physician.

Massage for Migraine Headaches

Many clients experiencing migraine headaches cannot tolerate any massage work during the actual attack. If the client can tolerate massage, a few adaptations in the treatment room and session are helpful. You may need to limit treatment time to 30 minutes to avoid exhausting the client. Darken the room, turn off the sound system, and don't use any products, even if they are natural, which contain fragrances. Clients with migraines often cannot tolerate the prone position, so the side-lying and supine positions are recommended. In general, sessions during an attack will strive to attain these treatment goals:

- **Increase relaxation and decrease stress:** Diaphragmatic breathing is helpful to open the session and start the relaxation process. If the client can't tolerate direct work such as slow, soothing Swedish strokes, try some of the energetic techniques explained in Chapter 18.
- **Cool the tissue:** Apply cold packs to the back of the head and neck at the beginning and end of the session.

- **Decrease pain:** The most effective pain relief will likely come from cold hydrotherapy, as above, and gentle Swedish massage. Sometimes the head, shoulders, neck, and back cannot tolerate work, but the gating mechanism of the spinal column can be activated by gently massaging the hands and feet.

Between migraine attacks the client can likely handle much deeper work, with the focus on the prevention or decrease of attacks. In this case, treatment goals might include:

- **Deactivation of trigger points:** Explore the regions of the head, neck, shoulders, and upper back. Focus on deactivating trigger points in these regions to support prevention of migraine attacks.
- **Work with what you find in the tissue:** Each client's tissue will be unique. Work with what you find in the tissue, using techniques that feel good to the client. For example, if you palpate and find fascial restrictions or adhesions, apply hot hydrotherapy packs, myofascial techniques, and deep-tissue work to the client's tolerance.
- **Stretching:** Demonstrate some neck and shoulder stretches the client can use at home for self-care.

Vascular Headaches: Cluster Headaches

Cluster headaches are rare vascular headaches that cause debilitating pain, which is usually located around one eye but may spread out to other areas of the face, head, neck, and shoulders. The pain is more likely located on the side of the affected eye. This eye is red and swollen, may have a drooping eyelid and reduced pupil size, and tear. Nasal passages may be runny or stuffy in the nostril on the affected side of the face. People experiencing a cluster headache are often restless and rock or pace because lying down increases the pain. Migraine-like symptoms including nausea and sensitivity to light and sound might also occur with a cluster attack.

Cluster headaches get their name because the headaches often come in groups. Attacks, known as cluster periods, may last from weeks to months followed by a remission period in which the person is headache free. During a cluster period, the person is likely to get a headache everyday or numerous times a day. Each headache can last from 15 minutes to 3 hours and is likely to occur at the same time in each 24-hour period. The pain usually begins and ends suddenly. Often, cluster periods are seasonal. For example, a person gets a cluster period every fall.

Causes and Contributing Factors

While the exact cause of cluster headaches is unknown, the seasonal and hourly regularity of cluster headaches suggests that the hypothalamus and the body's biological clock are involved. Research shows that the hypothalamus becomes more active during a cluster period. Other factors that are likely to play a role in cluster headaches include abnormal levels of the hormones melatonin and cortisol, as well as low serotonin as described earlier for migraines and tension headaches. Cluster headaches are different from migraines in that foods, stress levels, and physical activity do not act as triggers. However, once a cluster period begins, alcohol tends to trigger more frequent and longer headaches.

Medical treatment for cluster headaches includes the use of a daily cortisone-like medication that may prevent a cluster period in some instances. Calcium channel blockers, lithium carbonate, and anticonvulsant medications may also prevent cluster headaches. Once a cluster period starts, oxygen inhalation and triptan-type medications might be used.

Massage for Cluster Headaches

Like migraine headaches, cluster headaches are usually so painful that clients avoid massage or other stimuli that may exacerbate their condition. If a client does seek massage during a cluster period, follow the recommendations earlier for migraine headaches. Between cluster periods, you can provide massage based on the client's goals and to the client's level of comfort.

Sinus Headaches

Sinus headaches are caused by sinus pressure that leads to pain and pressure around the eyes, cheeks, and forehead. The pain increases when the person bends forward or lies down. It is usually accompanied by the symptoms of sinusitis (described in the next section), which include yellow, greenish, or blood-tinged nasal discharge, sore throat, fever, cough, fatigue, and achy teeth.

Causes and Contributing Factors

Sinus headaches are caused by sinusitis, a condition that often accompanies colds, bacterial or fungal infections, low immunity, or structural disorders in the nasal cavity. Asthma, allergies, and exposure to cigarette smoke can also cause or worsen sinusitis. The condition leads to swollen, inflamed sinus membranes that can cause pressure resulting in headache pain. Medical treatment involves the use of antibiotics to clear up the infection, corticosteroid nasal sprays to reduce inflammation, surgical correction in the event of structural problems, and the use of over-the-counter medications.

Massage for Sinus Headaches

Massage is contraindicated for acute sinus headaches because of the inflammation accompanying this condition. In chronic or noninfectious cases, massage can proceed based on the client's goals for the session. In some cases, even when inflammation is not present, the client may be uncomfortable in the face cradle, so the prone position is avoided.

Chemical Headaches

Chemical headaches are triggered by chemical imbalances in the body. Symptoms vary and may resemble tension headaches or might lead to a migraine.

Causes and Contributing Factors

Chemical headaches occur with some type of chemical imbalance in the body, such as low blood sugar suggesting that a person needs to eat, dehydration from physical exertion such as running long distances without drinking more water or alcohol consumption (the headache experienced as part of a hangover), hormonal changes accompanying the menstrual cycle, pregnancy, or childbirth, or imbalances caused by some medications. Medical treatment is not always needed and depends on the nature of the chemical imbalance.

Massage for Chemical Headaches

Massage should be postponed until the imbalance causing the headache has been remedied.

Traction and Inflammatory Headaches

Traction and **inflammatory headaches** are symptoms of other disorders that may be serious and that require immediate medical intervention. Headaches of this type often have a sudden onset and are severe. They may occur in association with a stiff neck, fever, convulsions, confusion, slurred speech, loss of consciousness, numbness in any area of the body, difficulties with motor control, severe pain in the eye or ear, or following a blow to the head. With a persistent headache in someone who was previously headache free, especially over the age of 50, or occurring with a gradual onset but no remission, medical assistance is necessary.

Causes and Contributing Factors

The term "traction" refers to pulling on tissues, as might be experienced in the head when a tumor is present or there is bleeding in the brain. Traction headaches can be caused by a head injury, brain tumor, stroke, diseases of the head or neck, subdural hematoma, subarachnoid hemorrhage, subdural hemorrhage, or spinal tap, among other causes. With inflammatory headache, inflammation may be occurring because of an infection like severe sinusitis, meningitis, encephalitis, dental problems, trigeminal neuralgia, shingles, ear infection, nose infection, or brain abscess, among other causes.

Massage for Traction and Inflammatory Headaches

Because traction and inflammatory headaches are often symptoms of serious underlying medical conditions, massage is contraindicated. If a client presents with these symptoms, he or she should be referred immediately to a medical provider.

Concept Brief 23-8
Headaches

- **Tension headaches** present as a tight band around the head and are the most common type of headache.
- **Migraine headaches** are chronic vascular headaches that cause significant pain for hours or days.
- **Cluster headaches** are rare vascular headaches that cause debilitating pain in clustered attacks.

- **Sinus headaches** are headaches caused by sinus pressure, often due to infection, that results in pain and pressure around the eyes, cheeks, and forehead.
- **Chemical headaches** are headaches triggered by a chemical imbalance in the body.
- **Traction and inflammatory headaches** are symptoms of other disorders that may be serious and that require immediate medical intervention.

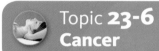

Topic 23-6
Cancer

Cancer is the general term for a large number of diseases typified by the growth of abnormal cells that replicate uncontrollably. These cells may permeate and destroy normal body tissue, form masses called tumors, and travel to other areas of the body to infiltrate new tissue. The signs and symptoms of cancer vary depending on the system or structure of the body affected and the type of cancer. In general, a person may experience fatigue, a lump or thickening of tissue felt under the skin, changes in skin color such as yellowing, darkening, or redness, sores that won't heal or changes to moles, changes in normal weight (sudden weight gain or weight loss), changes in bowel or bladder patterns, persistent coughing, difficulty swallowing, indigestion or discomfort after eating, continual or unexplained muscle or joint pain.

Causes and Contributing Factors

Cancer originates when the DNA in cells mutates causing the cells grow and divide incorrectly. An oncogene is a gene that directs a cell to grow and divide rapidly. Triggers that may activate oncogenes are not always clear but may include environmental toxins, some viruses, genetic predisposition, lifestyle choices that increase exposure to carcinogens such as smoking or repeated overexposure to the sun, or consumption of carcinogenic substances. DNA repair genes identify and attempt to correct DNA mutations. If the DNA repair gene has a mutation, it is likely to miss DNA errors, allowing more DNA mutations to occur. Cells contain genes known as tumor suppressor genes that identify abnormally rapid growth and work to stop it. Mutations in tumor suppressor genes may cause them to turn off or lose their effectiveness. Mutated cells are free to grow and divide. These are just some of the gene mutations that cause cancer.

Common medical treatments for cancer include surgery (to remove malignant tumors or affected lymph nodes),

chemotherapy (drugs that kill fast-growing cells), radio-frequency thermal ablation (the use of an electrical current to attack tumors), bone marrow transplants (to replace lost immune system cells), radiation (the use of high-energy rays to attack tumors), hormonal therapy, and hypothermia (freezing malignant cells).

Massage for Cancer

Massage provides a meaningful way to decrease stress, pain, muscle tension, and improve sleep patterns, appetite, and quality of life for people living with cancer.[13] Each person's cancer is unique, and each person's overall condition is different. In some cases while a person is undergoing medical treatment, only gentle stroking, energetic techniques, or massage of the hands and feet is tolerable. After medical treatment, depending on the client's overall condition, massage to reduce adhesions, scar tissue, fascial restrictions, and trigger points might be appropriate. It is imperative for the massage therapist to work with the client's physician and healthcare team to develop an effective and safe massage treatment plan at each stage of the client's medical treatment and recovery. Adaptations to treatment will likely be required based on the type of cancer treatment the client is undergoing.

- **Surgery:** Surgery is used to remove tumors or affected lymph nodes and may cause nerve damage and lymphedema. Obviously, massage is contraindicated over a recent surgery scar and distal or local to areas of inflammation. Therapists trained in manual lymphatic drainage may use these techniques with lymphedema under the supervision of a physician. Lymphedema contraindicates the use of warm or hot hydrotherapy.
- **Radiation:** External radiation can cause burns on the skin, lowered immunity, lymphedema, and fatigue. Massage is

contraindicated over damaged skin. In addition, be careful to ensure the highest possible standards of sanitation and hygiene to prevent the spread of pathogens to a client in a weakened condition.

- **Chemotherapy:** Chemotherapy causes a number of various side effects including severely impaired immunity, fatigue, nausea, ulcers in mucus membranes, and an overall weakened condition. Again, the highest standards of sanitation and hygiene are important to prevent the spread of pathogens to the client.

Massage treatment goals while a client is undergoing medical treatment are determined based on the type of treatment and the client's condition. People living with cancer often seek massage to reduce stress, decrease pain, and provide nurturing touch and comfort. In some cases, you may simply massage the client's hands and feet and provide slow, gentle effleurage down the spine or on the limbs. In other situations, the client may tolerate and appreciate a full-body Swedish massage with firm pressure. As the client recovers from medical treatment, you may start to apply deeper work with the intent to decrease fascial restrictions, reduce trigger points, improve range of motion, and rebalance muscles. Maintain good communication with both the client and healthcare team to plan safe and effective sessions.

Concept Brief 23-9
Cancer

- **Defined:** Cancer is the general term for a large number of diseases typified by a growth of abnormal cells that replicate uncontrollably.
- **Massage:** Massage treatment for clients living with cancer depends on the type of medical treatment the client is receiving and the client's overall condition. Communication with the client and physician is imperative.

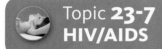

Topic 23-7
HIV/AIDS

As discussed in Chapter 3, the human immunodeficiency virus (HIV) causes AIDS. HIV is a retrovirus that can live in an infected individual for long periods of time before causing symptoms. The National Institute for Allergies and Infectious Diseases reports that people infected with HIV generally develop a flu-like illness 1 to 2 months after initial exposure to HIV. The symptoms are often mistaken for another viral infection and clear up within a week or 2. Severe symptoms may not appear for 10 years or more (Children born with HIV develop symptoms around the age of 2.) During this period, the HIV virus is slowly multiplying and killing immune system cells. Gradually, infected people experience periodic symptoms such as swollen glands, decreased energy, weight loss, fevers and night sweats, persistent yeast infections, short-term memory loss, persistent pelvic inflammatory disease, frequent and severe herpes outbreaks, and shingles.

Causes and Contributing Factors

AIDS is caused by the HIV virus, which is transmitted through body fluids including semen, vaginal secretions, and blood, and during pregnancy from a mother to her baby or through breast milk. HIV can be spread through needle sharing between drug users, from accidental needle pricks, and from infected blood in a blood transfusion (rare in developed countries). There is no evidence that HIV is transmitted through saliva, sweat, tears, urine, or feces except when blood is present. There is no evidence that HIV is spread through casual contact such as sharing towels, food utensils, or telephones or using swimming pools. HIV is not believed to be spread by biting insects like mosquitoes or fleas.

Acquired immunodeficiency syndrome (AIDS) occurs when the HIV-infected person has fewer than 200 CD4+ T cells (the immune system's primary infection-fighting blood cells). Uninfected adults usually have CD4+T cells numbering 1,000 or more. The immune system, gradually destroyed by the HIV virus, loses its ability to fight off common pathogens that generally don't cause illness in healthy individuals. In people with AIDS, these opportunistic infections are severe and often fatal. People with AIDS are also prone to developing various cancers, especially those caused by viruses and cancers of the immune system called lymphomas.

Massage and HIV/AIDS

Research on the benefits of massage for clients living with HIV has shown that massage improves immune function in children and adults infected with HIV by increasing natural killer cell numbers, CD4 cells, and the ratio of CD4/CD8 cells. It also decreases anxiety, decreases stress, and improves coping skills for people living with HIV.[14,15] For clients who are HIV-positive but asymptomatic, massage is absolutely indicated and delivered based on the client's overall treatment goals.

Clients with AIDS require greater caution but benefit from stress reduction, increased immunity, and the sense of comfort provided by massage. As with cancer patients, the massage treatment you provide is based on the client's overall condition and conversations with the client and the healthcare team. In some cases, you might provide only gentle stroking techniques for 30-minute sessions. In other cases, the client can handle more vigorous techniques. Following are some key factors to consider when providing massage to clients with HIV/AIDS:

- **Medications:** The client is likely to be on medications that may be impacted by massage. Use a current drug reference guide and stay abreast of medication changes in the client's treatment plan. Discuss medications and massage with the client's treating physician. Similarly, the client may have side effects from medications such as nausea or dizziness. These side effects may require an adaptation in the application of strokes or session length. For example, you want to avoid fast strokes or rocking strokes if the client experiences nausea as a drug side effect.

- **Secondary diseases:** The client may have secondary diseases such as shingles, tuberculosis, and lymphoma. Check that any secondary diseases do not contraindicate massage, and adapt the massage to such diseases as appropriate.

- **Site contraindications:** The client may have lesions or enlarged lymph nodes as a result of AIDS. Treat these areas as site contraindications and work around them.

- **Massage in a hospital:** If the client is hospitalized, you will likely have to work around medical equipment such as tubes, catheters, needles, and monitors.

- **Universal precautions:** Universal precautions to prevent disease transmission are discussed in depth in Chapter 3. Review that information and practice universal precautions and the highest possible sanitation and hygiene standards when providing massage to clients with HIV/AIDS.

Concept Brief 23-10
HIV/AIDS

- **Defined:** The HIV causes AIDS.
- HIV is a retrovirus that can live in the infected individual for long periods of time before causing symptoms.
- AIDS occurs when the HIV-infected person has fewer than 200 CD4+T cells (the immune system's primary infection-fighting blood cells).
- **Massage:** Massage is indicated for clients living with HIV/AIDS, depending on the client's overall condition.

MASSAGE FUSION
Integration of Skills

STUDY TIP: Internet-Work!

The Internet provides people with fast access to information, which can be very helpful when you want to learn more about an unfamiliar chronic pain condition. Some information on the Internet comes from questionable sources, however, necessitating having to sort through advertising, false claims, and misleading information. One way to surpass this sorting process is to use a teaching and research-oriented search engine like Google Scholar (at www.google.scholar.com) when looking for more reputable information. If you want to see visual examples of massage techniques being applied to clients, look for videos supplied by massage teachers on TeacherTube (www.teachertube.com). Finally, ask other massage professionals for information on www.massageprofessionals.com. This social networking site created for the massage profession by Associated Bodywork & Massage Professionals lets you connect with massage people across the country. If you're having difficulty making progress with a client who has fibromyalgia, for example, you can simply ask other people for advice in one of the forums. Make sure to keep identifying factors about your client out of the conversation to protect his or her privacy.

IT'S TRUE: Massage for Pain Management

Numerous research studies have demonstrated that massage is an effective treatment for pain management in clients with various chronic pain conditions. In Germany, massage was compared to standard medical treatment (e.g., prescription analgesics) for chronic pain affecting the back, neck, shoulders, and limbs. Patients rated their pain and feelings including depression, anxiety, mood, and body concept before and after treatments. Both the test group (massage) and the control group (standard medical treatment) improved, but the massage group rated their pain lower and their feelings more positive than the group receiving standard medical treatment. Three months after the final treatments, the massage group had maintained their benefits while the standard medical group had not.[16]

In a study to determine whether one session of nurse-delivered massage could reduce the severity of chronic pain in a hospitable setting, patients were placed in a test group to receive 15 minutes of massage or in a control group to talk about their pain for 15 minutes. Pain and anxiety levels were

(Continued)

⊕MASSAGE FUSION *(Continued)*
Integration of Skills

tested before and immediately after the sessions. Patients in the massage group had significantly lower pain and anxiety scores after the treatment than the control group.[17]

GOOD TO KNOW: The American Pain Society

The American Pain Society (www.ampainsoc.org) and the American Pain Foundation (www.painfoundation.org) are two national organizations that conduct pain research and seek to improve the quality of life for people living with pain. Their websites include research, the latest interventions for pain management, and other resources that you or your future clients may find useful.

CHAPTER WRAP-UP

You may be noticing that everything you have been learning in your massage training is becoming integrated. Pieces of the massage practice puzzle are forming into larger conceptual frameworks filled in with meaningful detail. Using the information in this chapter fully involves much of what you have already learned. For example, you use your knowledge of cautions and contraindications (learned in Chapter 5) to determine if massage is safe for a client with a particular pathology. Your assessment and documentation skills (learned in Chapters 12 and 19) are essential to ensure that you can assess the client's condition. Virtually every massage technique you have learned so far can be applied to help achieve the treatment goals for clients with the pathologies described in this chapter. Through it all you are applying good ethics (Chapter 6), building therapeutic relationships (Chapter 7), and communicating effectively (Chapter 8). Congratulations! This is an exciting time because everything is coming together and you are very close to achieving your goal of being a knowledgeable and skilled massage therapist. Just one more chapter to go!

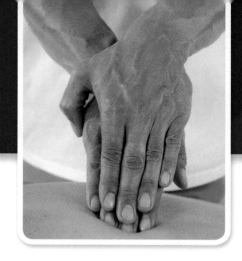

Chapter 24

Massage for Special Populations

KEY TERMS

assertive technology

disability

end-of-life care

event massage

first trimester

high-risk pregnancy

hyperthermia

hypothermia

intraevent massage

maintenance massage

obesity

older adult

people-first language

post-event massage

postpartum massage

pre-event massage

special population

terminal illness

LEARNING OBJECTIVES

Having read the chapter and used the related student learning tools, the student will be able to:

1 Describe the three primary categories of sports massage, and list three benefits of massage for athletes.

2 Organize the logistics for delivering massage at a sporting event.

3 Deliver appropriate techniques at the appropriate pace for pre-event and post-event massages.

4 List three benefits of massage for mothers and infants.

5 Identify signs and symptoms of high-risk pregnancy.

6 Outline three important considerations including correct positioning for the application of massage in the first, second, and third trimesters.

7 List three benefits of massage for older adults.

8 Describe two cautions for working with older adults in a weakened condition.

9   Outline three important considerations for the application of massage to older adults.

10 List three benefits of massage for obese clients.

11 Describe two important considerations for the application of massage to obese clients.

12 Explain the purpose of people-first language, and identify personal responses to disability.

13 List two physical disabilities and describe the massage adaptations for each.

14 List one consideration for the application of massage to a person living with a mental health issue.

15 Define end-of-life care and describe techniques useful for supporting the dying process.

Special populations are groups of people who may require specific considerations and adaptations during a massage session. While massage is most often always customized to some degree for the individual client, special populations require an in-depth understanding of the client's particular circumstances, physical and psychological needs, and possible cautions or contraindications. When you work with special populations, you apply everything you know about ethics, communication, building a positive therapeutic relationship, assessment, cautions and contraindications, session adaptations, and proper techniques. Special populations discussed in this chapter include athletes, mothers and infants, older adults, obese clients, clients with disabilities, and people at the end of life.

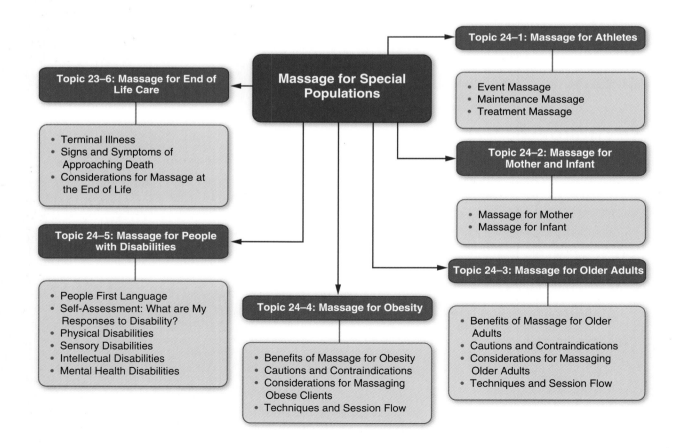

Topic **24-1**
Massage for Athletes

Athletes are people who are physically active and train to participate in sports. Sports require mental commitment, physical strength, speed, endurance, flexibility, coordination, or a combination of these abilities. Athletes include professionals who make their living in sports and amateurs who take part in sports for fitness and enjoyment.

Massage for athletes is commonly called sports massage (Fig. 24-1). Sports massage uses the same techniques as many other massage systems but is differentiated by an emphasis on particular muscle groups related to the sport, by the location where massage is delivered (massage often takes place onsite at a sporting event), and by timing (techniques are adapted based on when the massage is provided: before, during, or after the event).

This section introduces the categories of sports massage and explains the focus, benefits, considerations, and techniques of each. All of the techniques described in previous chapters are useful in sports massage, assuming they are applied at the proper time to appropriate muscle groups with specific pacing adaptations. Other chapters support your working with athletes, especially Chapters 19 and 22.

Categories of Sports Massage

The categories of sports massage recognize the particular focus of the massage for the specialized needs of an athlete at different stages of training, participation in a sporting event, recovery from training sessions or a sporting event, or rehabilitation from an injury. The primary categories of sports massage are event massage, maintenance massage, and treatment massage.

Event Massage

Event massage is a category of sports massage in which the massage is applied on the day of a sporting event at the location of the sporting event. It is used to help the athlete prepare for optimal performance, prevent injury, and recover effectively from strenuous physical effort. Environmental conditions, muscles in focus, and logistics are key issues.

Environmental Conditions

Weather, the topography (surface features or geography) at the event, altitude, time changes, travel to out-of-town events, and factors like pollution, traffic, and noise all influence the athlete's ability to perform, avoid injury, and recover optimally from the event. Ideally, athletes have trained to expect and manage the environmental conditions they might face at an event. Massage therapists administering massage to athletes at events must also anticipate and plan for environmental conditions to ensure their own safety, comfort, and efficacy. They should be able to recognize the signs and symptoms of hyperthermia (overheating), hypothermia (loss of heat), and frostbite (freezing of tissues) in athletes and know how to respond and obtain help when these conditions occur.

HYPERTHERMIA

Hyperthermia is a general term for a number of heat-related characteristics associated with illnesses. The human body maintains a relatively steady core temperature of 98.6°F. When the weather is hot or when a person performs vigorous activity, the body perspires. Perspiration evaporates from the

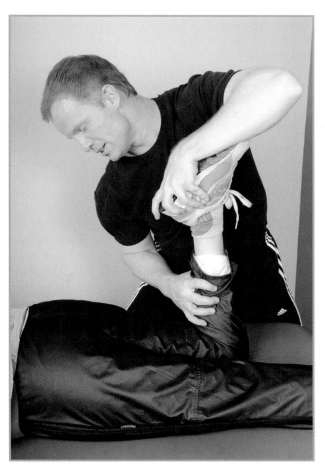

Figure 24-1 Massage for athletes is commonly referred to as sports massage. Image provided by Associated Bodywork & Massage Professionals.

skin to cool the body. If exposure to heat is prolonged or if there is inadequate replacement of fluids causing dehydration and limiting perspiration, hyperthermia may result. The two most common forms of hyperthermia are heat exhaustion and heatstroke.

- **Heat exhaustion** is characterized by pale or splotchy skin that may feel cool and clammy to touch, heavy sweating, shallow and rapid breathing, weakness, fatigue, and possible fainting. The athlete might complain of headache, lightheadedness or dizziness, nausea, muscle cramping, chills, and fatigue. If the athlete exhibits signs of heat exhaustion, move him or her to a cool place (inside into air conditioning if possible) or shaded location and have him or her sit down. Sitting is preferable to lying down because it helps prevent blood pressure from dropping too rapidly. Heat exhaustion is a medical condition requiring first aid skills. If you do not have sufficient training in first aid, try to find a medical professional who can manage the athlete's care. If no medical support is available, help the athlete cool off by removing excess clothing such as a hat or a headband, shoes and socks, and outerwear. Pour cool water over the athlete or use cool wet towels to cover the body. The athlete may shiver, complain of chills, or have goose bumps while cooling off. Dry the skin with a towel if this occurs but don't cover the athlete or attempt to warm him or her; keep cooling. Encourage the athlete to sip an electrolyte drink or water, but avoid sodas, juice, coffee, or alcoholic beverages. Monitor the athlete carefully and don't leave him or her alone. The athlete's condition should improve as he or she cools down. If the athlete's condition fails to improve or worsens, call emergency services because he or she may have heatstroke.

- **Heatstroke** is characterized by red, flushed skin that is hot to touch and dry. Completely dry skin indicates that the tissue is dehydrated and perspiration has shut down. In some cases the athlete may feel a little moist, but body temperature is elevated and the skin is hot. The person may have a strong, rapid heartbeat and rapid and shallow or deep breathing. You may see irritability or confusion and hear complaints of headache, dizziness, lightheadedness, and nausea. The person may faint or become unconscious. Heatstroke is a life-threatening condition and requires immediate cooling and medical attention. Call emergency services and then take rapid action to cool the athlete by removing excess clothing, immersing him or her in cold water, pouring cold water over the body, or draping the body with cold, wet towels until help arrives. If the athlete can safely take in fluids, offer cool water.

HYPOTHERMIA

Hypothermia is the opposite condition of hyperthermia. It occurs when the core temperature of the body falls below 96°F. Hypothermia may occur during sporting events where the body is exposed to cold or wet weather for prolonged periods of time. Risk factors include:

- Low air temperatures.
- Wind on the body (wind chill).
- Skin exposure to the elements caused by inadequate clothing or protection.
- Moisture due to wetness from water spray, immersion in water (rowers, paddlers), rain, or excess perspiration in cold conditions, which magnify the effects of wind chill.
- Inactivity in low air temperatures or in persistent rain as might happen between events after the athlete has perspired. For example, crosscountry runners waiting for the start of an event or football players standing on the sidelines.
- Consumption of caffeine or other diuretics, which reduce fluid volumes in the body.
- Consumption of alcohol, which stimulates blood flow to the periphery contributing to heat loss.

Signs and symptoms of hypothermia include pronounced shivering, numbness, and a feeling of cold throughout the body. A person with hypothermia may exhibit an inability to move quickly, dizziness, and confusion. In advanced hypothermia, shivering stops and the athlete may experience rigidity in his or her muscles followed by a lapse into a coma. Organ damage, organ failure, and death can result.

Hypothermia is a medical condition requiring first aid skills. If you do not have sufficient training in first aid, attempt to find a medical professional who can manage the athlete's care. If no medical support is available, the goal is to safely warm the athlete as quickly as possible without inducing perspiration, which further reduces body fluid levels. Remove the athlete from the cold environment if it is possible, or place him or her in an area that is protected from wind and moisture. For example, is a warm car available? Remove any wet clothing from his or her body and replace it with dry clothing. Cover the athlete with blankets or other protective layers such as coats, mittens, hats, and scarves. Make sure to cover the head and neck because this area of the body rapidly dissipates heat. Only if help will be delayed, use an external heat source like a hot water bottle, electric blanket, electric heating pad, or space heater to continue to warm the athlete if such an option is available. Resist the temptation to rub the extremities or skin to stimulate the athlete because this may direct cold blood from the limbs to the heart and cause a shock-like reaction. If the athlete can take in fluids, give him or her warm water to sip and as the athlete recovers support him or her while walking around. If the athlete's condition does not improve or if it worsens, immediately contact emergency services once you have administered first aid to ensure he or she is covered in dry layers.

Frostnip and Frostbite

Mountaineers, winter runners, skiers, ice skaters, and other cold-weather outdoor enthusiasts are prone to cold-related skin injuries. Frostnip and frostbite are the most common and are conditions in which the temperature in the skin and superficial muscles dramatically decreases while the core body temperature remains normal. While hypothermia and frostbite are different, they can occur simultaneously in athletes.

- **Frostnip** develops slowly and painlessly and may affect the tips of the ears, nose, cheeks, chin, fingers, and toes. Signs and symptoms include blanching or whiteness of the skin and the formation of ice crystals on the skin's surface. The skin may feel numb, tingly, or itchy. There is usually no permanent tissue damage with frostnip, and it is easily treated by warming the area with air blown through cupped hands, covering the tissue (e.g., cover the tips of the ears with a hat), holding warm hands against the affected region, or holding the affected body area against a warmer body area (e.g., placing cold hands under the armpits).

- **Frostbite** refers to freezing of the tissue and usually affects the hands, feet, nose, cheeks, and ears. It can be classified as superficial or deep. Superficial frostbite causes sensations of burning, numbness, tingling, itching, and cold. The affected area appears white and frozen, but if you press on the tissue it retains some tone. Deep frostbite causes a loss of sensation in the affected area, tissue swelling, and blistering. Blisters appear blood-filled over the top of white or yellowish skin. The area is hard and may even appear blackened or dead.

If you suspect that an athlete has frostbite, assess him or her to rule out hypothermia. If he or she does demonstrate the signs and symptoms of hypothermia, respond as described above. Frostbite is a medical condition requiring first aid skills. If you do not have sufficient training in first aid, attempt to find a medical professional who can manage the athlete's care. If no medical support is available, keep the affected body area elevated to reduce tissue swelling, and avoid asking the athlete to walk on frostbitten feet, which could increase tissue damage. Cover the affected area in dry, sterile bandages or place cotton between the fingers or toes to prevent rubbing, and contact emergency services for transport to a medical facility. If emergency services are not available and you must rewarm the tissue yourself, do so in lukewarm (not hot) water. Rewarming the tissue if it is likely to freeze again can lead to increased tissue damage. Do not rub the area with snow (an old folk remedy that causes increased tissue damage) or with anything else including the hands. Avoid rubbing, friction or heating the area with an external heat source like a heating pad. Instead, warm the tissue rapidly in a water bath (the affected area should be placed in a lukewarm water bath that is large enough so that the tissue does not touch the sides of the container) heated to 104 to 107°F. The process of rewarming the tissue is painful and usually lasts 15 to 30 minutes. The injured athlete should receive medical attention as quickly as possible.

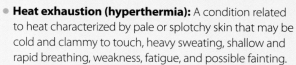

Concept Brief 24-1
Environment-Related Medical Conditions in Athletes

- **Heat exhaustion (hyperthermia):** A condition related to heat characterized by pale or splotchy skin that may be cold and clammy to touch, heavy sweating, shallow and rapid breathing, weakness, fatigue, and possible fainting.

- **Heat stroke (hyperthermia):** A life-threatening condition related to heat characterized by red, flushed skin that is hot to touch and dry, a strong, rapid heartbeat, and rapid and shallow or rapid and deep breathing with irritability, confusion, headache, dizziness, lightheadedness, and nausea. Fainting and unconsciousness are possible.

- **Hypothermia:** A life-threatening condition in which the core temperature of the body falls below 96°F characterized by pronounced shivering, numbness, and a feeling of cold throughout the body, dizziness, and confusion. Rigidity of muscles followed by a lapse into a coma is possible.

- **Frostnip:** A condition related to cold temperatures characterized by blanching or whiteness of the skin and the formation of ice crystals on the skin's surface. The skin may feel numb, tingly, or itchy.

- **Frostbite:** A condition related to cold temperatures characterized by freezing of the tissue affecting the hands, feet, nose, cheeks, and ears. It can be superficial or deep.

Muscles in Focus

At sporting events, your focus is often on large muscle groups associated with the particular activity in which the athlete is competing. Think about the main regions of the body the athlete will stress during the event. For example:

- **Baseball and softball:** Focus on the muscles of the neck, shoulders, upper and lower back, and abdominal muscles.
- **Basketball:** Focus on the muscles of the lower extremities and the shoulders.
- **Cycling:** Focus on the lower extremities and the muscles of the neck, upper back, and forearms.
- **Equestrian sports:** Focus on the muscles of the back, neck, hips, and abdominal region.
- **Football:** Focus on the lower extremities, low back, and shoulders.
- **Golf:** Focus on the upper extremities, neck, back, shoulders, chest, and knees.
- **Racquet sports:** Focus on the lower extremities, upper extremities, and back.
- **Rock climbing:** Focus on the upper extremities, especially the shoulders, forearms and hands, and feet.
- **Rowing and paddling:** Focus on the upper extremities and back.

- **Runners:** Focus on the lower extremities.
- **Skiing:** Downhill skiing particularly stresses the lower extremities, while crosscountry skiing stresses both the lower and upper extremities and back.
- **Soccer:** Focus on the lower extremities, neck, and back.
- **Swimming:** The focus may depend on the particular stroke used by the swimmer, but both the upper and lower extremity and the back and neck are likely to need attention.
- **Volleyball:** Focus on the lower extremities and shoulders.

While you focus on these main muscle groups, you must also take into consideration the needs of the individual athlete. For example, a runner may experience back stiffness as a result of running and want particular focus on the back during the event. A rock climber may notice that tight gluteal muscles and hamstrings make it difficult to tuck the hips into the rock wall or high step onto a hold and want focused attention on these areas. Always consult the athlete about his or her particular wants and needs and customize the massage with this feedback.

Logistics and Planning

Because massage is performed onsite, often outside at the sporting event location, it requires careful planning and organization. First, consider your own health and safety. Dress in layers to ensure you are protected from the elements should the weather change. Bring water and snacks to guarantee you stay hydrated and fueled. If you plan to do a lot of sports massage, it may be worth investing in a mobile structure like a tent that protects you and athletes from sun, wind, and moisture. Bring your massage table, but the use of linens is not usually necessary. Athletes dress for their event, and massage is provided over or around this clothing. If you work on multiple athletes, bring wipes or a spray bottle of disinfectant and paper towels to sanitize the massage table surface, an alcohol-based hand sanitizer, a container for trash, and a first aid kit. As discussed above, it's a good idea to bring a warm blanket for cooler or rainy days and some towels that can be drenched in cold water and used to cool an athlete on hot days.

Types of Event Massage

Three types of massage are performed at sporting events. Each of these massage types is characterized by specific timing of the massage, pacing of the strokes, technique considerations, and duration of the treatment.

PRE-EVENT MASSAGE

Pre-event massage refers to the massage given to the athlete before participating in the sporting event. In some cases this type of massage may be given 1 to 2 days before the event, but most often it is used within 2 hours of the start of the event to support the athlete's warm-up preparations. The benefits of pre-event massage include increased circulation to the primary muscles used for the particular sport, decreased muscle tension, warming of muscles and connective tissue,

increased flexibility, and an improved mental attitude and concentration.

Pre-event massage is performed at a brisk pace and for a short duration (sessions last 10 to 20 minutes) to maintain the athlete's readiness to perform optimally. Avoid the use of slow, overly relaxing techniques that might sedate the athlete and send the body into rest and recovery mode; pick an upbeat, fast-tempo song and practice massaging at that speed to understand the proper pacing for pre-event massage. Lubricants may or may not be used depending on the situation. For example, you wouldn't want to cover a runners arms and legs with oil or cream. This would prevent the runner from perspiring freely and may impact his or her performance. Athletes are usually dressed in their event clothing or warm-up clothing (e.g., a sweats over the top of a sports top and shorts) and so strokes are often applied over clothing without lubricants.

Common techniques used in pre-event massage include rhythmic compression, pétrissage, superficial friction, brisk effleurage, joint movement, gentle stretching, and tapotement (often used to end the pre-event session). The depth of the strokes is light to moderate, and techniques that change proprioception or address imbalances or compensation patterns are avoided. For example, the athlete may have a tight hamstring in one leg for which he or she has developed compensation patterns during training. The pre-event massage is not the time to address such patterns, because substantive changes to muscle length, balance, or proprioception may throw off the athlete's sense of his or her body and negatively impact performance. For the same reason, avoid comments that may affect mental readiness. The comment, "Wow, your right hamstring is really tight" could distract the athlete and cause him or her anxiety before the race.

INTRA-EVENT MASSAGE

Intra-event massage refers to a massage provided between heats or innings, at half time, or between different events at a match or meet. It is provided anytime after the first athletic effort and up to 10 minutes before the second athletic effort in a 10- to 20-minute session. The goal is to decrease any areas of muscular tension that have resulted from the first athletic effort and to help the muscles recover for better performance in the second athletic effort. As in pre-event massage, the pace is brisk and the techniques are delivered with light-to-moderate pressure. Common techniques are the same as for pre-event massage.

POST-EVENT MASSAGE

Post-event massage is the massage performed after all athletic efforts have concluded and usually within 2 hours of the last effort. The goal is to aid muscle recovery through improved circulation, reduce muscular tension resulting from the effort exerted during the event, decrease the occurrence of delayed-onset muscle soreness (DOMS) (Box 24-1), maintain range of motion and flexibility, decrease muscle cramping, and provide first aid for injury or weather exposure if required.

BOX 24-1 Delayed-Onset Muscle Soreness

The term "delayed-onset muscle soreness" (DOMS) refers to muscle pain, soreness, and stiffness felt 12 to 48 hours after exercise. DOMS is different from acute muscle soreness felt during or directly after an activity. Acute muscle soreness is associated with an increase in hydrogen ions due to lactic acid accumulation in the tissues. Several theories have been proposed to explain the cause of DOMS, but none is universally accepted. Many believe that DOMS is the result of muscle tissue breakdown, because muscle biopsies performed on marathon runners after competition have shown considerable cell damage in muscles.[1] The sarcolemma (cell membrane) may be ruptured, allowing the contents of the cell to seep between other muscle fibers.[2] Damage to the contractile filaments actin and myosin has also been reported.[1] In addition, this damage triggers an inflammatory response that causes the accumulation of chemicals that stimulate nerve endings and increase sensations of pain.[3,4] A number of studies demonstrate that massage reduces the discomfort associated with DOMS, but these results vary depending on the time of the massage application.[5–7]

Unlike pre-event and intra-event massage, the pace of the post-event massage is soothing and relaxing. The duration may be shorter (10 to 25 minutes) or longer depending on the needs of the athlete. Lubricant, which may be unadvised during pre- or intra-event massage, can now be used with traditional strokes like effleurage, pétrissage, light-to-moderate friction, passive joint movement, and gentle stretching. Avoid tapotement, which can be too stimulating and cause muscle cramping during a post-event massage. Finish the treatment with effleurage delivered toward the heart to support muscle recovery.

PROMOTIONAL EVENT MASSAGE

Promotional event massage is massage delivered at a sporting event where the athletes are not currently your clients. The goal is to promote the benefits of massage for athletes and to support athletes in achieving their full potential at the event. Provide pre-event, intra-event, and post-event massage as described in the previous sessions, but also include a verbal description of the benefits of massage as a support to a healthy lifestyle and pass out your cards and informational brochures. Encourage athletes to seek you to receive all the benefits related to event, maintenance, and treatment massage.

Maintenance Massage

Maintenance massage refers to the regular massage the athlete receives between sporting events while in training. It is often performed on the athlete's less strenuous training days because its primary goal is to aid in the recovery process.

Sessions vary in length from 30 to 90 minutes and might be delivered once a week to twice a month. The benefits of maintenance massage include regular evaluation of muscular balance, compensation patterns, and minor injuries, decreased muscle tension, increased flexibility, enhanced range of motion, decreased occurrence of DOMS, improved recovery from strenuous workouts, and better mental attitude.

Maintenance massage is a form of healthcare massage. You are assessing the athlete, discussing his or her fitness goals, and planning sessions to meet the athlete's needs and support his or her training program. You are likely to use a wide range of techniques including Swedish massage, deep-tissue work, myofascial release, neuromuscular therapy, and many others. If the athlete has a coach or trainer, it can be very helpful to include him or her in the treatment planning process as long as the athlete has given his or her informed consent.

Treatment Massage

Treatment massage refers to the massage given to an athlete when he or she sustains an injury and massage is part of the rehabilitation process. You learned about the forces that create tissue loads and the response of soft tissue to loads in Chapter 22. Athletes often maintain rigorous training schedules that expose their soft tissue to repeated heavy loading. An athlete is at higher risk for injury if he or she fails to warm up carefully, lacks overall flexibility, is using faulty or poorly fitted equipment, overtrains without taking enough recovery time, is undernourished or dehydrated, is training or competing in adverse weather conditions, or performs exercises with poor body mechanics. Chapter 22 describes the stages of inflammation, the treatment goals for each stage, and the types of techniques you might use to promote soft-tissue healing. Use the information in Chapter 22 to provide the foundation for developing treatment plans for athletes with injuries.

Concept Brief 24-2
Categories of Sports Massage

- **Event massage:** Massage performed at a sporting event.
  - **Pre-event:** Massage performed before the athlete's event.
  - **Intra-event:** Massage performed after the first athletic effort and before a second or third athletic effort.
  - **Post-event:** Massage performed after the athlete's events.
  - **Promotional event:** Massage performed at a sporting event to promote a massage practice.
- **Maintenance massage:** Regular massage provided to athletes while in training.
- **Treatment massage:** Massage provided to athletes as part of recovery from an injury.

Topic **24-2**
Massage for Mother and Infant

In one study, 26 pregnant women were assigned to a massage therapy group or a relaxation therapy group for 5 weeks. Both groups reported feeling a reduction in anxiety and leg pain, but only the massage therapy group reported improved mood, better quality of sleep, and less back pain by the conclusion of the study.[8]

Another study showed that women who received massage therapy demonstrated decreased cortisol levels and lower premature birth occurrences. During labor and delivery, women who received massage therapy reported significantly less pain, and their labors were on average 3 hours shorter with less need for medication than the nonmassage control group.[9]

Premature infants given massage therapy averaged a 21% greater weight gain per day, were discharged from the hospital 5 days earlier, and were more active during stimulation sessions than infants in the control group who did not receive massage.[10]

There is little doubt that massage is beneficial for healthy women with pregnancies that are progressing normally, during the birthing process, and after the baby is born, or that regular structured touch supports infant development and health. However, massage during high-risk pregnancy and for unhealthy infants may be contraindicated depending on the situation. This section provides only introductory information to students of massage and entry-level therapists working with healthy women with low-risk pregnancies and healthy infants. Work with high-risk pregnancy and infants who have complicating conditions requires additional specialized training. In all cases, obtain a physician's release before providing massage to mothers and babies.

Massage for Mother

A woman's body undergoes many changes during pregnancy (Table 24-1). These changes can lead to increased emotional, mental, and physical stress and physical discomfort (Box 24-2). Massage provides an effective means to decrease

TABLE 24-1 Select Changes in a Pregnant Woman's Body

First Trimester (first 13 wk)	Second Trimester (wk 14–28)	Third Trimester (wk 28–40)
• Blood volume increases	• Baby movement felt toward end of trimester	• Baby continues to grow
• Body temperature increases	• Back pain occurs	• Carpal tunnel syndrome may develop
• Heart rate increases	• Breasts are tender and swollen	• Discomforts like varicose veins, hemorrhoids, heartburn, and insomnia may be present
• Hormonal changes cause headache, fatigue, nausea, constipation, mood swings, smell and taste sensitivity, and possible vomiting	• Breathing becomes more shallow as diaphragm moves upward	• Edema may be present in the legs, ankles, and feet
• Metabolism increases	• Edema may be present in the legs, ankles, and feet	• Pregnancy posture increases, causing tension to muscles and joints and difficulty walking and bending over
• Relaxin present at wk 10	• Linea alba begins to separate	• Shortness of breath occurs as the uterus moves up into the ribcage
• Urination frequency increases	• Muscle cramping may occur	• Growing baby presses on nerves, blood vessels, and internal organs, causing a variety of symptoms
• Uterus size increases	• Organs may be pushed aside to accommodate the growing fetus • Pelvis expands • Posture changes cause muscular stresses • Relaxin affects ligaments • Ribs expand up and out • Stretch marks appear • Weight increases	

BOX 24-2 **Discomforts of Pregnancy**

- Carpal tunnel syndrome
- Constipation
- Difficulty walking or bending over
- Dizziness
- Fatigue
- Frequent urination
- Headache
- Heartburn
- Hemorrhoids
- Indigestion
- Insomnia
- Leg cramps
- Low back pain
- Nasal congestion
- Nausea
- Neck and shoulder pain
- Postural changes
- Shortness of breath
- Stretch marks
- Swollen and tender breasts
- Swollen legs, ankles, and feet
- Varicose veins
- Vomiting
- Weight gain

many of the discomforts of pregnancy, reduce stress, and provide nurturing and social contact to pregnant women (Fig. 24-2).

Benefits of Massage for Mothers

The advantages of massage for mothers during pregnancies, during birthing processes, and after childbirth have been well researched by Tiffany Field and her team at the Touch Research Institute at the University of Miami School of Medicine. Field's research has documented these benefits:

- Anxiety decreased
- Blood and lymph circulation improved
- Blood pressure control increased
- Depression reduced
- Fatigue decreased
- Headache pain reduced
- Immunity improved
- Insomnia reduced
- Joint pain and stiffness reduced
- Leg cramps reduced
- Marital adjustment to newborn improved
- Muscle pain reduced
- Muscle spasms decreased

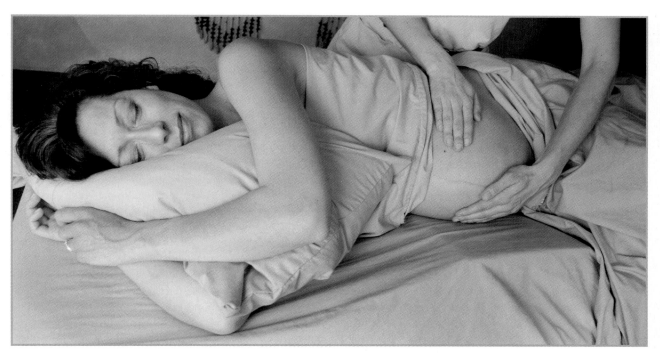

Figure 24-2 Massage provides an effective means to decrease many of the discomforts of pregnancy, reduce stress, and provide nurturing and social contact to pregnant women. Image provided by Associated Bodywork & Massage Professionals.

- Muscle tension decreased in preparation for labor and delivery
- Postpartum (after the baby is born) stress and depression reduced
- Premature birth rates decreased
- Self-image improved
- Skin elasticity and condition improved
- Sleep quality improved
- Stress decreased
- Stretch marks decreased

In addition, perineum massage applied by the woman to herself or by her partner or birth coach during the last 6 weeks of pregnancy and during labor decreases the likelihood of tearing the perineum during delivery. Because the perineum is located in the genital region, massage therapists are not permitted to apply perineum massage techniques. Advanced training courses in massage for mothers and babies often guides massage therapists on how to instruct clients in perineum massage techniques.

Cautions and Contraindications

Every woman's experience of pregnancy, labor, and delivery is unique. Because complications related to pregnancy can occur for a variety of reasons, it is important to obtain a physician's release before providing massage even when the pregnancy seems to be progressing normally. In all cases, be vigilant and pay attention to the changes in the body and signs or symptoms that signify caution or contraindicate massage. Cautions include:

- **Abdominal massage:** Light nurturing strokes or gentle holding strokes on the abdominal area are usually acceptable. Moderate-to-deep abdominal work can cause damage or trauma to the uterus or the fetus and is contraindicated.
- **Acupoints:** Traditional Chinese medicine cautions that the use of some acupressure points might encourage uterine and cervical activity and should be avoided during pregnancy. These points include those of the gallbladder channel, spleen 6, and large intestine 4.
- **Aromatherapy:** While many essential oils are safe for use during pregnancy and can support the relaxation process, aromatherapy should be avoided during pregnancy without specific training in this area. Many essential oils that are sold as "natural" are in fact synthetic and can cause nausea, headache, and emotional irritation. While unlikely, essential oils applied incorrectly could possibly complicate an existing condition or be unsafe for the mother and baby.
- **First-trimester massage:** Massage during the **first trimester** (the first 3 months of pregnancy) is controversial. Some advise avoiding massage because of the major changes occurring in the embryo that lead to the development of a fetus during this period. However, some women are unaware of an early pregnancy or don't disclose their pregnancies until they begin to show signs. It is likely that many

women have received massage during this stage without complications. It is during the first trimester that women often experience systems like nausea, vomiting, fatigue, smell hypersensitivity, and emotional swings that might contraindicate massage. According to Associated Bodywork & Massage Professionals, the largest massage membership organization in the United States, no liability claims have been reported for therapists providing massage during the first trimester of pregnancy in the most recent time period reported.[11] Ask your massage instructor to provide insight about working with pregnant women in the first trimester, and work with caution until you gain more experience or have had an advanced pregnancy massage course.

- **Lower leg massage:** There is a widely held belief that the use of reflexology or massage on the medial lower leg and ankle can cause premature birth. While there is some evidence that reflexology in these areas can stimulate labor and delivery, there is little or no documentation that it causes complications in normally progressing pregnancies.[12] In research studies that demonstrated that reflexology can promote labor, therapists applied techniques with significant pressure and focus. General moderate massage or reflexology should not be problematic. However, if the client has poor circulation in her legs, is on bed rest, or has severe or pitting edema, massage of the lower extremity is contraindicated, and these symptoms may indicate a condition that completely contraindicates all massage treatment.
- **Medial thigh massage:** Use caution when massaging the medial thigh because the iliac, great saphenous, and femoral veins accessible in the medial thigh are more prone to develop blood clots during pregnancy. Techniques that use an open and flat hand and gentle pressure are recommended.
- **Modalities:** Modalities like myofascial release or connective tissue work should be avoided during pregnancy because of the presence of relaxin. Relaxin is a hormone produced during pregnancy that causes the cervix and pubic symphysis to soften and lengthen to facilitate delivery. Its presence causes the production of collagen to decrease and promotes collagen breakdown. It also plays a role in the timing of delivery by inhibiting contractions of the uterus until labor.
- **Positioning:** Pay attention to the positioning recommendations in the later section here. Proper positioning not only ensures the mother's comfort but also the health and safety of mother and baby. For example, when a pregnant woman in the late second or third trimester is positioned supine, the weight of the fetus could impinge on the abdominal aorta and inferior vena cava, reducing the flow of blood and oxygen to the woman's lower extremities and also to the fetus.
- **Postpartum massage:** After childbirth, **postpartum massage** is a useful support as the mother recuperates and adjusts to her new responsibilities. If the mother received an epidural for pain relief during delivery, avoid the injection area for 72 hours or longer depending on the sensitivity experienced by the client. If the client had a normal vaginal

birth, vaginal bleeding is normal for 2 weeks after delivery and is not a contraindication. C-section births indicate the use of side-lying and supine positions for 8 weeks after delivery. Obtain a physician's release before providing massage to a woman who recently had a C-section.

- **Range-of-motion techniques:** Apply range-of-motion techniques gently and slowly because the presence of relaxin (described previously) may cause increased ligament laxity and instability in the joints.
- **Varicose veins:** As the uterus grows during pregnancy, it puts pressure on the inferior vena cava, increasing pressure in the veins of the legs. For this reason, many women develop varicose veins during pregnancy or find that existing varicose veins become worse. Massage over varicose veins should be avoided to prevent further damage to the veins.

Some signs and symptoms that usually contraindicate massage, such as the nausea and vomiting associated with morning sickness, are normal in pregnancy. Others signs and symptoms indicate that a serious underlying condition may be present and medical intervention necessary. If your client has vaginal bleeding, a fever, decreased fetal movement for 24 hours, abdominal pain, abdominal cramping, excessive swelling in the extremities, or uterine contractions, advise her to contact her physician immediately. If signs and symptoms are severe, contact emergency services. Signs, symptoms, or conditions that contraindicate massage include:

- Abdominal cramps
- Abdominal pain
- Any condition that normally contraindicates massage
- Back pain with vaginal bleeding, abdominal cramps, or pain
- Decreased fetal movement over a 24-hour period
- Diarrhea
- High-risk pregnancy (see Box 24-3)
- Morning sickness including nausea and vomiting
- Severe swelling or pitting edema in the extremities
- Severe pain anywhere in the body
- Uterine contractions
- Vaginal bleeding

Considerations for Pregnancy Massage

As a therapist working with pregnant clients, you can increase a woman's safety, comfort, and enjoyment of massage by paying attention to:

- **Assistance getting on and off the massage table:** In the late second and third trimesters, a woman may need assistance getting on and off the massage table, as discussed in Chapter 10. Put a hydraulic table in the lowered position until the woman is situated and the massage begins, and then again at the end of the session. Manually adjustable tables can be set a little lower in the later stages of pregnancy to facilitate the application of strokes in the side-lying position and to adjust for the larger body size of the client.

BOX 24-3 High-Risk Pregnancy

Every pregnancy involves a risk that problems will develop or that pre-existing conditions will be complicated by the changes happening in a woman's body during pregnancy. A high-risk pregnancy is a pregnancy that puts the mother or the developing fetus at higher than normal risk for complications. Factors that lead to high risk include:

- Young or old maternal age
- Overweight
- Underweight
- History of problems with other pregnancies, such as miscarriage or preterm labor and delivery
- Multiple fetuses (twins, triplets, etc.)
- Pre-existing health conditions including HIV/AIDS, heart disease, high blood pressure, kidney disorders, autoimmune disorders, sexually transmitted diseases, diabetes, or cancer
- Conditions that may occur during pregnancy such as pre-eclampsia, eclampsia, gestational diabetes, or results of prenatal tests indicating that the fetus is abnormal.

- **Emotional release:** Mood swings and emotional release are more common during massage of pregnant clients due to the increased hormonal activity that facilitates a normal pregnancy. Follow the process for management of emotional release described in Chapter 7, if your client demonstrates the signs of emotional release during the session.
- **Frequency of sessions:** Massage can be applied during pregnancy in the second and the third trimesters as frequently as twice a week. Sessions every other week or once a month are also helpful.
- **Health intake questions:** Use your regular health history form and ask additional questions during the health intake process (thoroughly document the client's answers to your questions) or adapt your current health history form to include questions for a pregnant woman. Ask questions that help you rule out a **high-risk pregnancy** or the development of symptoms that require medical intervention. Ask about the current symptoms she is experiencing that may require to session adaptations (e.g., breast tenderness) and about symptoms that indicate high risk or a contraindication (e.g., vaginal bleeding and abdominal cramping in the last 24 hours, etc.).
- **Massage during labor and delivery:** Massage during labor and delivery might be applied by a doula, midwife, childbirth assistant, massage therapist, partner, or friend. Massage applied during this period helps the mother to deal with the demands placed on her physically, mentally, and emotionally. Because massage therapists interested in participating in the labor and delivery process would gain from advanced training in techniques for the delivery room, this topic is not covered here. Available texts detail this in theory and practice.

- **Massage postpartum:** Postpartum massage refers to massage applied in the weeks after the baby is born. It can help the mother adjust to exhaustion experienced with the care of new babies and the muscular tension and pain from the physical exertion of labor and delivery, Cesarean section delivery, or learning to breastfeed. If the client had a normal vaginal birth, she can receive massage without a physician's release. If she had a C-section, obtain a physician's release before providing massage for 8 weeks after delivery.

- **Positioning:** Positioning clients, the use of bolsters, and draping techniques were described in Chapter 10. Review that chapter for specific instructions and details for placing clients in the prone, supine, semireclined, side-lying, and seated positions. If you perform massage in the first trimester of pregnancy, the woman's body is not yet undergoing significant outward changes that prevent the use of any of the common massage positions. As the fetus grows and the mother's abdomen starts to expand, certain positions are more comfortable and safer for the mother and baby. In the early months of the second trimester, the side-lying position allows access to the back and hips without the woman having to be placed face down on tender breasts and her larger abdomen. Rather than having her lie flat in the supine position, which puts pressure on the abdominal aorta and inferior vena cava, use the semireclined position instead. Toward the end of the second trimester and into the third trimester, even the semireclined position may put too much pressure on blood vessels, and only the side-lying position is used. Alternatively, a seated position might be used, depending on the woman's comfort level. Fill in any spaces with bolsters, pillows, or rolled towels so that the woman's body is completely supported by soft surfaces. Communicate openly with your client to get feedback on her comfort level, and remind her to alert you if a particular position starts to cause discomfort. Postpartum clients who had vaginal births can safely receive massage in any position that feels comfortable. Breasts tender from breast feeding may make the side-lying position more comfortable than the prone position. Clients who had a C-section birth usually receive massage with a physician's release in the side-lying position for up to 8 weeks after delivery.

- **Restroom use:** Frequent urination is a common symptom of pregnancy. In the first trimester, it is caused by an increased amount of blood in the body, which must be processed through the kidneys. In the second and third trimesters, the growing uterus places pressure on the bladder. Suggest that a pregnant client use the restroom immediately before a session. Let her know that you can pause the session at any time so that she can use the restroom if needed. Provide a robe and slippers for pregnant clients so they can move back and forth to the restroom without dressing if there is not a private restroom attached to the treatment room.

- **Room temperature:** Increased hormonal levels raise a pregnant woman's body temperature, and she may feel hot if you do not lower the treatment room's temperature. Communicate with the client and cool the room if necessary to ensure her body temperature feels comfortable.

- **Room ventilation:** Women experience smell and taste hypersensitivities during pregnancy, especially in the first trimester. Make sure your treatment room is well ventilated, and avoid the use of scented detergents, room fresheners, fragranced massage lubricants, or other aromas during the session.

- **Session length:** Massage sessions can last from 15 to 60 minutes depending on the client's tolerance level. Longer sessions can sometimes be fatiguing and require multiple stops for restroom use.

- **Use of heat packs:** Do not use heat because of the pregnant client's increased body temperature.

Concept Brief 24-3
Positioning of Pregnant Clients

- **First trimester:** Supine, prone, side-lying, and semireclined
- **Early second trimester:** Supine, side-lying, and semireclined
- **Late second trimester:** Side-lying and semireclined
- **Third trimester:** Side-lying and semireclined

Techniques and Session Flow

Techniques and pressure during the massage of an expectant mother depend on the individual client's preferences and comfort as long as they are not contraindicated (review the earlier section on contraindications). A wide variety of techniques might be applied with special attention on the neck, shoulders, low back, sacral area, and feet. These areas require more focused work because the body assumes a particular posture to compensate for the expanding uterus and weight gain. Pregnant women often exhibit a head-forward position that causes hypertonicities in the muscles of the neck and shoulders. The chest may sink slightly and the pelvis tilt forward, causing low back pain and pain in the hips and around the sacrum. As the pregnancy progresses, the client's knees are likely to remain in a hyperextended position when she stands, and her feet may rotate laterally. Foot and knee pain may result. Aim to enhance relaxation and provide relief from muscle tension and pain. Structure the session to prevent turning the client repeatedly from one side to the other in the side-lying position, and offer a restroom break halfway through the massage.

Massage for Infants

Chapter 7 discussed the fact that in the early years of the 20th century, children in orphanages died in alarming numbers from touch deprivation. Those who did survive were permanently damaged. They experienced retarded bone growth, low weight, suppressed immunity, poor coordination, general apathy, and decreased mental function. Touch is essential for life, proper development, and good health. Infant massage provides a structured way for babies to receive the tactile stimulation and touch bonding they need to thrive.

Benefits of Massage for Infants

Tiffany Field's extensive research on the benefits of massage for preterm infants demonstrated that massage stimulates growth, aids digestion, positively affects sympathetic and adrenocortical function, aids sleep, and decreases fussing, crying, and behaviors related to stress such as hiccupping.[13–18] In general, infant massage educators note that when infants receive massage:

- Bonding between parents and baby is increased
- Circulation is increased, supporting the baby's developing tissues
- Digestion is improved
- Digestive discomforts like teething and gas are decreased
- Neurological development is supported
- Respiration slows and deepens
- Sensory and motor nerves are stimulated
- Sensory awareness is increased
- Sleep quality improved
- Stress indicators are decreased
- Vocalization is increased, which may assist speech and language development

In addition, parents benefit because they develop self-confidence in their ability to bond with and support their new baby. Spouses and partners sometimes find it challenging to identify their roles in the process of pregnancy, labor, and delivery. Infant massage gives them a means to be an active part in the child's development. Parents also "tune in" to their children and learn how to read their behavioral cues and understand their moment-by-moment needs. Women feel more supported by their partners when they share responsibility for the child's development.

Cautions and Contraindications

Infant massage is very different from adult massage, and therapists and parents must learn to read the baby's behavioral cues to avoid overstimulation. Certain signs indicate that the baby is engaged and ready to receive massage, while other signs indicate that the baby is disengaged and that massage is not appropriate at the time. If the baby has bright eyes and is making eye contact, smiling, making happy vocalizations, and reaching toward the parent, these signal receptiveness to massage. If the baby is breaking eye contact and looking away from the parent, arching the back, kicking or jerking the arms and legs, and flaring the fingers and toes, he or she may not be receptive to massage. Crying and pulling away can be strong cues to decrease the stimulation (e.g., turn off music, dim lights, use quiet voices, and wait to proceed).

Wait 30 to 45 minutes after the baby has been fed to provide massage. If the baby has signs of nausea, is vomiting, or has diarrhea, or if the parents report that the baby is sick, massage is contraindicated. Use only cold-pressed natural food oils for a massage lubricant. Babies often place their hands in their mouths and could get sick from exposure to the synthetic dyes, fragrances, and chemicals in many massage lubricants. Working with preterm infants, babies with injuries or medical conditions, or special needs children requires advanced training and is not discussed here.

Considerations for Infant Massage

As a therapist working with parents and infants, you can increase the family's comfort and enjoyment of a massage session in these ways:

- **Advanced training:** The strokes used to massage infants are not difficult to learn. However, understanding behavioral cues of babies and interacting effectively with parents who are often sleep-deprived and overwhelmed can be more challenging. If infant massage is an area of special interest, you are encouraged to take an advanced continuing education course and earn credentials as an infant massage instructor. This will give you the skills you need to work effectively with parents and their infants.
- **Baby determines the massage:** With signs of stress and engagement cues, the baby will let you know if this is a good time for massage or if massage would be overstimulating. Let the baby determine how the session should progress, and be ready to adapt. For example, if the baby is deeply asleep, it is not the right time for massage.
- **Crawlers and toddlers:** Crawlers and toddlers are mobile. As the infant grows into these stages, massage has to be mobile and flexible. It works well to turn the massage into play. Sing a song along with the strokes, and use rhymes and facial expressions to keep the child engaged while receiving massage.
- **Duration:** Infant massage sessions last from 5 to 15 minutes depending on the engagement level of the baby. The overall session may last longer as you work with the parents to determine their infant's behavioral cues and needs.
- **Environment for massage:** The environment for infant massage varies. It can be delivered on the parent's lap, on the floor, on a couch, on a bed, or in the baby's cradle. The room should be warmer than usual to prevent the baby from becoming chilled. Cover any areas of the baby's body that are not receiving massage. The lights should be soft but not dark, and eliminate noise distractions. Often, music is not played so that the baby can focus on the sound of his or her parent's voice.
- **Frequency:** Parents can apply massage strokes to their babies everyday as long as the baby demonstrates receptiveness to massage.
- **Health intake questions:** Keep chart notes for babies just as you do with adults so that there is a written record of

Technique 88   Infant Massage Strokes

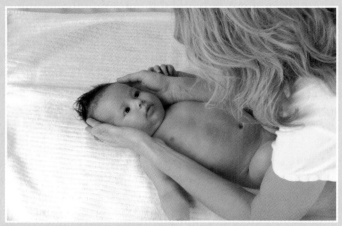

Image provided by Associated Bodywork and Massage Professionals

1. Make eye contact with the infant while using gentle effleurage strokes to the abdominal area in clockwise circles. Use only cold-pressed (edible) oil on infants.
2. Make eye contact with the infant while applying strokes that run diagonally from the abdomen to the shoulder.
3. Apply circular fingertips to the forehead, top, and sides of the infant's head.
4. Apply gentle arm and leg movements that bring the arms or legs into the centerline of the body and then open the arms or legs outward. The infant's legs can also be gently mobilized so that the knees come towards the belly and then are straightened.
5. Apply diagonal thumb strokes to the infant's palms and feet.
6. With a flat, soft palm apply long effleurage strokes to the arms and the legs from the feet or the hands toward the heart.
7. With a flat, soft palm apply long strokes over the back and legs with the infant in the prone position.
8. Apply diagonal thumb strokes to the infant's palms and feet, up the legs toward the heart, and from the hands up the arms toward the heart.
9. Gently squeeze and twist the tissue on the arms and legs. Perform it lightly so that you can work down the legs toward the feet and back again. The intent is to move the superficial tissue.
10. Begin and end sessions and body areas with holding strokes that warm the tissue and relax the baby.

what occurred during the session. You want to find out and record the expectations of the parents for session outcomes and also learn about what the baby likes in regards to touch. For example, the parents might report that the baby enjoys having his or her feet stroked. Another baby might dislike having his or her feet touched.

- **Therapist role:** In an infant massage session, your role is often to educate parents about the benefits of massage for their babies, about behavioral cues that signal the baby is receptive to receiving massage, and about the types of strokes for the session. Some therapists teach parents massage using a doll until they develop some basic skills that they can transfer to their infant.

Techniques and Session Flow

The techniques used to massage infants are gentle but firm, often with the baby situated between the giver's legs on the floor or even across the giver's lap. As mentioned above, part of the session is dedicated to learning the parents' expectations and needs and responding with information and resources. The infant determines the way in which the massage progresses, but sessions usually begin with the baby supine so that touch is combined with eye contact, soothing vocalizations, and facial expressions. Technique 88 provides direction for basic strokes that are effective for infants. It may work well to demonstrate the strokes on a doll as the parents perform the strokes on their baby, and give your verbal guidance on their technique.

Topic 24-3
Massage for Older Adults

The word elderly generally refers to people in the later stages of life. The term geriatric" refers specifically to people who are 70 years old or older, and the phrase senior citizen is generally used for people who are 60 or 65 years of age or older. Most healthcare professionals now use the phrase **older adult** to minimize any negative connotations related to the phrase "senior citizen." The number of older adults in the United States is rapidly increasing because people are living longer. By 2030, about one in every five Americans, or 20% of the population, will be an older adult.[19] Massage provides many benefits for this special population and promotes life-long health and healthy aging (Fig. 24-3).

Figure 24-3 Massage provides many benefits for older adults and promotes lifelong health and healthy aging. Image courtesy of Mary Kathleen Rose.

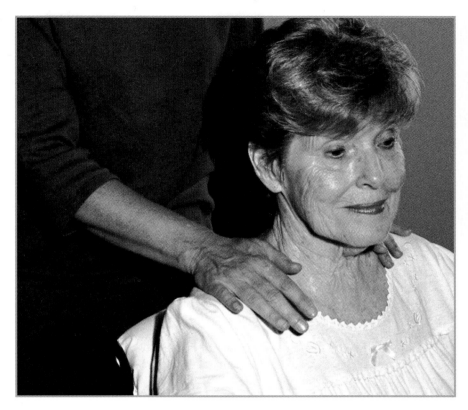

Benefits of Massage for Older Adults

As people age, every organ system in the body is affected. The epidermis of the skin atrophies and becomes thinner, and changes in collagen and elastin production lead to less skin elasticity and tone. Cardiac output decreases and blood pressure increases as arteriosclerosis often develops. Lean body mass and strength decline with age due to loss and atrophy of muscle cells and often a decrease in general mobility. The body experiences slower nerve conduction, decreased circulation and lymph flow, decreased immunity, and loss of flexibility. Degenerative changes occur in many joints as bone mass decreases, and osteoporosis may develop. The lungs often have impaired gas exchange and a decrease in vital capacity, while functional changes in the gastrointestinal system may lead to digestive and elimination issues.[20] While massage can't prevent these changes, it can help the body to adapt to aging more effectively and lead to improved quality of life. In addition, massage provides a means of social contact for individuals who are often coping with the loss of life-long friends or a spouse and feelings of isolation resulting from decreased mobility. The benefits of massage for older adults include:

- Agitated behaviors in Alzheimer's patients decreased[21]
- Appetite increased
- Circulation increased
- Digestion and elimination improved
- Flexibility increased
- Immune function improved
- Lymph flow improved
- Muscle tension decreased
- Pain decreased
- Skin condition improved
- Sleep quality improved
- Social contact gained
- Stress decreased

Cautions and Contraindications

Every older adult is unique, and the age span of this population ranges from 60 to over 100. Some clients look far younger than their years and are healthy, physically active, energetic, and mentally sharp. Many people continue to live independently and manage all of the normal activities of daily life. Others look their chronological age, have decreased physiological functioning, and may show early signs of mental deterioration. They may live independently with some outside assistance or may live in assisted care facilities. Some older adults could be characterized as extremely frail and need continuous assistance with routine activities of daily living or may be confined to a hospice bed. Healthy, robust older adults should receive the same type of massage as any healthy middle-aged client. Proceed with your normal massage unless your health intake process uncovers a condition that requires caution.

Use a thorough health history process to gather information about the client's medications and health conditions, such as the use of blood thinners, a history of blood clots, a heart condition, diabetes, and other reasons for caution. Watch for bedsores, arthritic joints, varicose veins, and recent surgeries. Obtain a physician's release for older adults who demonstrate decreased physiological or psychological function due to aging, and adapt your session as described below.

Considerations for Massaging Older Adults

As with any massage, use critical thinking skills and a thorough health history process to determine treatment goals and appropriate techniques. Remember that each older adult is unique and may fall anywhere on a broad spectrum from very healthy to very frail. Following are considerations when working with older adults:

- **Communication and interaction:** When interacting with an older adult, remember to speak clearly and look directly at the person. If the client has hearing loss, this provides the best opportunity for the person to understand your questions. In some situations, attending family members may also be able to help during the health intake process and may fill in important health information that ensures the client's safety. Speak directly to the client even if family members are giving input during the health intake process.

- **Condition of the feet:** As people age, it becomes more difficult for them to bend over and care for their feet. The condition of an older adult's feet may be quite poor. As long as a condition like advanced diabetes does not contraindicate foot massage, this is an important region for focus to ensure good circulation and lymphatic flow. The client's feet can be placed on a bath towel and cleansed with warm water and liquid soap. Remove the soap with warm, moist hand towels, and proceed with the massage. This use of a simple spa-like treatment can enhance the session and aid relaxation.

- **Condition of the skin:** An older adult's skin may be quite delicate. Assess the condition of the skin before providing massage, and work at a depth that is comfortable to the client. If the skin is delicate, avoid techniques like myofascial release that stretch the skin and could cause tearing.

- **Environment:** Massage of older adults can take place in a number of settings. Clients might come to your office, or you might provide massage at their homes when travel is difficult. Massage might take place in an assisted care facility, in a family member's home, a hospice, or a hospital room. Remain flexible and adaptable in these environments, and pay special attention to sanitation and hygiene issues.

- **Level of dress:** Some older adults may be shy about removing clothing, or they may demonstrate what seems to be immodesty and undress while you are still in the treatment room. In other cases, older clients may have difficulty dressing and undressing and need assistance. Remain flexible and helpful while being sensitive to the client's boundaries and your own level of comfort. Family members or attendants may help the client dress or undress. You can also simply work around some clothing or directly over clothing.

- **Memory loss:** Some clients have some memory loss and may miss appointments. Be proactive and enlist the help of family members or caregivers to remind clients of appointment times. Often, a reminder call on the day of the appointment is appreciated.

- **Orthostatic hypotension:** Orthostatic hypotension is the clinical term for the sudden drop in blood pressure an older person might experience upon moving from a reclining position to a seated or standing position. Assist an older person to a seated position toward the end of the session, and finish the session with the client upright before asking him or her to move off the massage table and stand up.

- **Physical assistance:** Be ready to assist an older client at all times before, during, and after the session. Assistance may include helping the client exit or enter a car, walk into the office through heavy entrance doors, walk to the restroom, undress, get onto the massage table, get off of the massage table, and get dressed.

- **Positioning:** Position clients based on their level of health and communication about what feels comfortable. For example, a robust client may feel comfortable in both the prone and supine positions, while a frail client may need to be in a semireclined position the entire session. Pressure from the face cradle may cause sinus issues that could be prevented by using the side-lying position. Medical equipment (e.g., an IV drip) may restrict how a client can be positioned in a hospice or hospital setting, or the client may want to keep his or her clothing on and remain seated. Again, be flexible and do your best to accommodate the client's particular needs and wants.

- **Session length:** Typically, frail clients cannot tolerate long sessions and do better with 30-minute sessions. Healthy and robust clients enjoy 60- to 90-minute sessions. Base the session length on the overall health of the client, and communicate with the client or the caregivers about what the client is likely to enjoy and tolerate.

Techniques and Session Flow

The techniques you choose, the session's length, and the flow of the session all depend on a number of factors reviewed during the health intake process. As previously noted, healthy older adults who are functioning well, active, and mentally sharp may appreciate a variety of techniques and respond well to firm pressure. However, if you determine that the client is in a weakened condition or frail, use only Swedish techniques with light pressure, even rhythm and pace, and slow strokes. Gentle face massage, foot massage, and abdominal massage are often beneficial. Position the client for comfort, and insulate with extra blankets. Five minutes before the end of the session, have the client sit up slowly, and perform the remainder of the massage with the client upright. This is a good time to work on the client's hands and arms. Having the client upright the last 5 minutes helps ensure that he or she won't experience a sudden drop in blood pressure.

Topic **24-4**
Massage for Obesity

Obesity is an excessive amount of body fat in relation to lean body mass. Extra calories not used to fuel body functions are stored as body fat. Lean body mass is the mass of the body without fat. Body composition, involving the ratio of fat to lean body mass, is calculated based on the weight and height of an individual and is commonly determined as body mass index (BMI). A BMI chart can be used to determine one's BMI (Fig. 24-4).

People are considered overweight with a BMI from 25 to 29.9. A person with a BMI of 30 or higher is considered obese. In 2007 to 2008, the prevalence of obesity in the United States was 32.2% of adult men and 35.5% of adult women.[22] The prevalence of obesity in children 2 to 19 years of age is 16.1%.[23] Obesity contributes to serious health conditions including diabetes, heart disease, hypertension, metabolic syndrome, stroke, and other conditions, currently resulting in an estimated 400,000 deaths a year in the United States. Obesity impacts lifestyle and can lead to lowered self-esteem, depression, and significantly diminished quality of life.[24] It is caused by a number of factors including genetic predisposition, lifestyle choices, environmental factors such as access to safe places to walk or be active, access to healthy foods, social factors, cultural factors, pre-existing conditions like hypothyroidism, and some prescription drugs.

Overweight and obese adults generally use CAM therapies including massage less than normal-weight adults.[25] This may be so because they are reluctant to expose themselves and feel vulnerable to prejudice and criticism. Compassionate massage free of judgment can be a valuable means of supporting the physiological and psychological concerns of people who are obese. This section discusses the benefits of massage for obesity, cautions and contraindications for working with this population, special considerations, and techniques and session flow.

Benefits of Massage for Obesity

Massage can benefit people living with obesity by helping them overcome common challenges related to the physical and psychological stresses that accompany this condition. Muscle fatigue, soreness, and joint pain are common in people who are overweight or obese because of the constant stress that extra weight places on the skeletal and muscular systems. In addition, fascial restrictions and hypertonicities develop because range of motion is decreased, and postural shifts occur due to extra body mass. Conditions like sleep apnea, asthma, and labored breathing, common with obesity, disrupt sleep patterns and make full relaxation difficult.

Circulation is decreased due to the pressure of adipose tissue on blood and lymph vessels. Psychologically, people who are obese often feel disconnected from their bodies and may feel negative emotions such as shame that lead to depression and social isolation.

Massage can benefit people who are obese through increased relaxation, improved circulation, better breathing, decreased muscle tension, and reduced pain. Clients benefit psychologically from the social contact provided by massage and from improved self-image, increased sense of connection to the body, and a sense of acceptance that are made possible through safe, nurturing touch.

Cautions and Contraindications

Obesity is often a contributing factor to many other health conditions that may make specific adaptations to the massage necessary or may completely contraindicate massage. Conduct a thorough health history and intake process to best understand the client's overall health. Look up in a massage pathology reference book any pathology or medication with which you are unfamiliar, and adjust the massage as necessary based on your research. If you are uncertain about to the safety of massage for a particular client, contact the client's physician and ask for recommendations or obtain a physician's release.

Be cautious when working with areas where adipose deposits are particularly excessive because this tissue tends to be highly vascular and may be prone to bruising. Adipose tissue may make it difficult to access muscle tissue. In some cases, it is possible to gently draw back the adipose tissue to better access the muscle. Don't make an effort to push through adipose tissue to the underlying muscle because this is likely to damage the adipose tissue. Also avoid deep work over any folds of excess skin that may occur if a client has lost a significant amount of weight.

Considerations for Massage of Obese Clients

When working with overweight and obese clients, consider the client's psychological state and comfort with level of undress, draping, positioning, table condition, and your body mechanics and attitudes and beliefs about obesity.

- **Client's psychological state:** In American society, an attractive physical appearance is often associated with slimness. Overweight and obese people may feel unattractive. They

Body Mass Index (BMI) Table

To determine your BMI, look down the left column to find your height and then look across that row and find the weight that is nearest your own. Now look to the top of the column to find the number that is your BMI.

BMI	Normal						Overweight					Obese										Extreme Obesity														
	19	20	21	22	23	24	25	26	27	28	29	30	31	32	33	34	35	36	37	38	39	40	41	42	43	44	45	46	47	48	49	50	51	52	53	54
Height (feet & inches)	Body Weight (pounds)																																			
4'10" (58")	91	96	100	105	110	115	119	124	129	134	138	143	148	153	158	162	167	172	177	181	186	191	196	201	205	210	215	220	224	229	234	239	244	248	253	258
4'11" (59")	94	99	104	109	114	119	124	128	133	138	143	148	153	158	163	168	173	178	183	188	193	198	203	208	212	217	222	227	232	237	242	247	252	257	262	267
5'0" (60")	97	102	107	112	118	123	128	133	138	143	148	153	158	163	168	174	179	184	189	194	199	204	209	215	220	225	230	235	240	245	250	255	261	266	271	276
5'1" (61")	100	106	111	116	122	127	132	137	143	148	153	158	164	169	174	180	185	190	195	201	206	211	217	222	227	232	238	243	248	254	259	264	269	275	280	285
5'2" (62")	104	109	115	120	126	131	136	142	147	153	158	164	169	175	180	186	191	196	202	207	213	218	224	229	235	240	246	251	256	262	267	273	278	284	289	295
5'3" (63")	107	113	118	124	130	135	141	146	152	158	163	169	175	180	186	191	197	203	208	214	220	225	231	237	242	248	254	259	265	270	278	282	287	293	299	304
5'4" (64")	110	116	122	128	134	140	145	151	157	163	169	174	180	186	192	197	204	209	215	221	227	232	238	244	250	256	262	267	273	279	285	291	296	302	308	314
5'5" (65")	114	120	126	132	138	144	150	156	162	168	174	180	186	192	198	204	210	216	222	228	234	240	246	252	258	264	270	276	282	288	294	300	306	312	318	324
5'6" (66")	118	124	130	136	142	148	155	161	167	173	179	186	192	198	204	210	216	223	229	235	241	247	253	260	266	272	278	284	291	297	303	309	315	322	328	334
5'7" (67")	121	127	134	140	146	153	159	166	172	178	185	191	198	204	211	217	223	230	236	242	249	255	261	268	274	280	287	293	299	306	312	319	325	331	338	344
5'8" (68")	125	131	138	144	151	158	164	171	177	184	190	197	203	210	216	223	230	236	243	249	256	262	269	276	282	289	295	302	308	315	322	328	335	341	348	354
5'9" (69")	128	135	142	149	155	162	169	176	182	189	196	203	209	216	223	230	236	243	250	257	263	270	277	284	291	297	304	311	318	324	331	338	345	351	358	365
5'10" (70")	132	139	146	153	160	167	174	181	188	195	202	209	216	222	229	236	243	250	257	264	271	278	285	292	299	306	313	320	327	334	341	348	355	362	369	376
5'11" (71")	136	143	150	157	165	172	179	186	193	200	208	215	222	229	236	243	250	257	265	272	279	286	293	301	308	315	322	329	338	343	351	358	365	372	379	386
6'0" (72")	140	147	154	162	169	177	184	191	199	206	213	221	228	235	242	250	258	265	272	279	287	294	302	309	316	324	331	338	346	353	361	368	375	383	390	397
6'1" (73")	144	151	159	166	174	182	189	197	204	212	219	227	235	242	250	257	265	272	280	288	295	302	310	318	325	333	340	348	355	363	371	378	386	393	401	408
6'2" (74")	148	155	163	171	179	186	194	202	210	218	225	233	241	249	256	264	272	280	287	295	303	311	319	326	334	342	350	358	365	373	381	389	396	404	412	420
6'3" (75")	152	160	168	176	184	192	200	208	216	224	232	240	248	256	264	272	279	287	295	303	311	319	327	335	343	351	359	367	375	383	391	399	407	415	423	431
6'4" (76")	156	164	172	180	189	197	205	213	221	230	238	246	254	263	271	279	287	295	304	312	320	328	336	344	353	361	369	377	385	394	402	410	418	426	435	443

Source: National Heart, Lung, and Blood Institute.

Figure 24-4 BMI chart.

may cope regularly with prejudice and discrimination at their jobs, while in school, or in social situations. Many people think that obesity is caused by laziness and gluttony and project their judgments onto obese people, causing feelings of shame, rejection, and even self-loathing. Recognize that it may take bravery and a leap of faith for people living with obesity to seek massage. They risk exposing themselves to a therapist who may be prejudiced and judgmental. Sensitivity, compassion, and professionalism are especially important when working with this special population.

- **Clothing:** Overweight and obese clients may prefer to leave some or all of their clothing on while receiving massage. Make sure clients understand that they can disrobe to their level of comfort and that you can work through clothing if they prefer.
- **Draping:** Make sure that your top massage sheet and other draping materials like towels and blankets are large enough to provide good coverage for overweight or obese clients.
- **Positioning:** Overweight or obese clients may experience discomfort or difficulty breathing when supine or prone for long periods of time. Remain flexible and ask the client for input about their most comfortable sleep positions. Side-lying may be an option, as is the semireclined position.
- **Table size and strength:** Make sure that your massage table is in good condition, that leg bolts are screwed on tightly, and that the table is fully open before the client arrives. While this is important with every client, it is especially important with a client weighing more than 300 lb. For a large person a regular massage table may be too narrow, and the client may harbor valid fears that the table will collapse. Many tables have side pieces that can be adjusted to increase the width of the table. It may also be difficult for a large client to get on and off the massage table. With a hydraulic table, set it in the lowered position before the client arrives, and raise it to a comfortable height after the client is on the table. A step stool is helpful if a hydraulic table is not available. You might also consider working with the client situated on a floor mat like the type used for some Asian bodywork therapies.

- **Therapist's body mechanics:** Lower the massage table before the client arrives in order to gain height leverage, and maintain proper body mechanics while working on obese clients. Pay attention to bending at the waist, and do your best to reach all the areas of the client's body without undue stress on your own body. Again, you may consider working with the client situated on a floor mat in order to better leverage height and body position.
- **Therapist's psychological state:** Take time to assess your beliefs and feelings about obesity. Do you harbor judgments or prejudices about this condition? Be honest with yourself, and if you find you do have some prejudices or discomfort about working with obese clients, make an effort to develop a better understanding of the causes of obesity and the needs of people living with obesity. Your client deserves a massage that is accepting and free of judgment. Powerful transformations can happen in an environment that is nurturing, supportive, sensitive, and caring.

Techniques and Session Flow

You can use a wide variety of massage techniques depending on the client's overall physical condition and session goals. Because larger clients often have breathing issues, it can be very beneficial to include the diaphragmatic breathing or pursed-lipped breathing exercises described in Chapter 10 to open the session. Remember that the client may not be able to lay prone or supine for prolonged periods of time, so a number of different positions might work best, from prone to side-lying to supine or semireclined. Another concern is the space required to maneuver from one position to another. Give your client good directions when it comes time to turn over, and be sure to position your body so that you can prevent a client from rolling off the table as he or she turns.

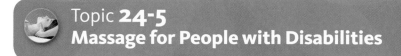

Topic **24-5**
Massage for People with Disabilities

Governmental, political activist, aid, and international organizations use the terms disability and impairment in different ways. Disability theorists are still debating the proper use of these terms. In this section, the term **disability** is used in a medical sense to mean a functional impairment. It is a condition caused by an accident, trauma, genetics, or disease that may limit a person's mobility, hearing, vision, speech, or mental function. The term **impairment** is used to imply a problem in body structure or function that impacts the person's ability to execute a task or an action. This section discusses the use of people-first language, explores the personal responses we need to assess as massage therapists before we work with people with disabilities, and then describes considerations for improving the massage experience of clients with disabilities.

People-First Language

People-first language is a form of disability etiquette that aims to diminish the subconscious dehumanization that can occur when discussing people with disabilities. It puts the person before the disability and helps to decrease the discrimination people with disabilities experience in society by raising awareness and understanding. It describes *what a person has*, not *who a person is* (Table 24-2). It seeks to focus on abilities and not limitations and avoid terminology that generates pity, negativity, discrimination, or fear.

Assertive technology and adaptive technology are accepted generic terms for devices and societal or personal modifications that help people with disabilities overcome impairments and broaden the accessibility of places and things. Examples of assertive technology devices include wheelchairs, prosthetics, accessible keyboards, large-print publications, and speech recognition software. Societal modifications include curb cuts to make sidewalks more accessible to wheelchairs, accessible parking spaces, and accessible restrooms and hotel rooms.

Remember that assertive technology is something a person with a disability uses to better access the world—not something that limits him or her in some way. For example, avoid phrases like "He is confined to a wheelchair," which conveys a sense of the person imprisoned in a wheelchair when in fact the wheelchair provides access to the world that might otherwise be impossible. The correct language is to say, "He uses a wheelchair" or "She uses sign language" or "He uses a prosthetic" in the same way we would say, "She uses reading glasses."

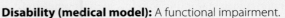

Concept Brief 24-4
Key Terminology in Disability

Disability (medical model): A functional impairment.

Impairment: A problem in body structure or body function that impacts the ability to execute a task.

People-first language: A form of disability etiquette used when discussing people with disabilities.

Assertive (or adaptive) technology: Devices and societal or personal modifications that help people with disabilities overcome impairments and broaden the accessibility of places and things.

TABLE 24-2 People-First Language Preferred Expressions

Preferred	Avoided
Child with a disability	Handicapped or disabled
Individual with cerebral palsy	Palsied, CP, or spastic
Person who has….	Person afflicted with or suffering with, victim of
Nonverbal	Mute or dumb
Child with autism	Autistic
Child with developmental delay	Slow, special-needs child, retarded
Person with a mental illness	Crazy, insane
Person with a hearing impairment, (deaf or hard of hearing is sometimes preferred)	Dumb
Communicates with sign language	Signer
Uses a wheelchair	Confined to a wheelchair
Child with a cognitive impairment	Retarded
Has epilepsy	Epileptic
Adult with Down's syndrome	Mongoloid, suffers from Down's syndrome
Has a learning disability	Is learning disabled
Has a physical disability	Is physically disabled, crippled
A person with a congenital disability	Birth defect, birth defective
Has seizures	Has fits
Has a cleft lip	Has a hare lip
Has a mobility impairment	Is lame or crippled
Is paralyzed	Paralytic
Has quadriplegia	Quadriplegic
Accessible parking, accessible hotel room	Handicapped parking, handicapped hotel room
Needs or uses	Has a problem with, has special needs

Self-Assessment: What Are My Responses to Disability?

If you do not have a disability or have not often interacted with people with disabilities, you may not understand disabilities in a way that supports effective care during massage. If you are uncomfortable or lack awareness, your behaviors may be subtly patronizing, discriminatory, or dehumanizing even without an intention to offend. For example, you might overcompensate and be too helpful by rushing to open a door for a person using a wheelchair who is perfectly capable of opening the door independently. When a companion is present at the health intake interview, you may feel more comfortable asking health-related questions to him or her instead of to the person with the disability who is about to receive massage. You might act as if the disability didn't exist and thus fail to provide useful support to improve massage access. Uneasiness, reluctance, or fear might be noticeable in your facial expressions, quality of touch, or communication.

Because our attitudes, beliefs, and knowledge influence our responses to people, self-assessment helps to increase one's personal awareness and to formulate a plan to develop any needed improved communication, understanding, or other skill sets. Write down your thoughts about the following questions in your journal:

- Imagine a person with a disability, and notice responses in your body. How do you feel? Do your palms perspire? Do you feel tightness in your chest or stomach? Do you feel relaxed, nervous, shy, confident, or other emotions? Write about your feelings.

- Imagine a different person with a different disability, and notice your thoughts. What would you say to him or her if you met for the first time on a street corner? Write down your thoughts.

- For each of the following disabilities, write down your initial body sensations and thoughts: amputation, visual impairment, hearing impairment, intellectual disability, and mental health disability.

- Picture yourself with a disability, and imagine how you would interact with the world. What concerns do you have? How do your family members and friends respond to you? How do you navigate through the tasks related to your job? What kind of support would be most useful for you? What do you wish others understood about your disability? Write about these ideas.

- Imagine that one of your family members has a disability. How does this affect each member of your family? What sorts of family activities are difficult to continue? How do people respond to your family member? How does this make you feel?

- Imagine a person with a disability coming for a massage, and notice your thoughts and feelings. What concerns do you have about providing the person with effective care?

Note that the self-assessment above makes some assumptions that may not be helpful. First, it assumes that you feel some level of discomfort (as many people do), which may not be true. It also puts you in a position of viewing disabilities as something like pathologies, implying that a functional limitation is the source of a problem. It is more helpful to view disabilities as "normal"—and in fact, it is the normal reality for the person with the disability. A person who walks normally gets around by walking. A person who uses a wheelchair normally gets around by using a wheelchair. Now we can see that our ideas about disability should focus not on limitation (a patient or client in need of help) but rather on how we as a society can organize our environment to remove barriers to participation. As massage therapists, we must analyze the environment in which we offer care and remove any barriers that limit the use of massage by a particular person seeking care. In this approach, a person with a disability is an expert about himself or herself and uses massage as a way to enhance his or her experience of life, just like every other client. Think about these things to remove barriers in your own massage practice:

- **The massage environment:** When you design the environment for your practice, or when you work as an employee at a massage business, think about how the environment might be enhanced to remove barriers to access. Are the hallways and doorways wide enough to accommodate a wheelchair? Are Braille placards present to identify areas like restrooms, the lobby, and session rooms? Do you have a hydraulic massage table that can be placed in a lowered position to reduce the challenge of getting on and off the table? Do you have an accessible parking space with a curb cut and a smooth sidewalk surface?

- **Communication:** Ask clients to explain and needs they may have. What assistance, if any, would be useful, and how would they like that assistance to be provided? Don't try to act as if a disability is not present. Instead, cultivate an attitude that disabilities create different normal ways of navigating through the environment. Your goal is to make the environment as hospitable as possible to every person. If a companion is present, address all health and session questions to the person who will receive the massage, even if it is necessary for the companion to respond or to translate your message. For example, a companion might use sign language to convey your question to a person with a hearing impairment. In some cases, the companion may answer your questions (e.g., a person with a cognitive impairment or brain injury may not be able to respond to your question), but even in these cases you should avoid talking about the person instead of talking to the person. If you are concerned that you may not be able to meet needs of a person with a disability and provide appropriate support, discuss this concern openly and arrive at a solution in collaboration with the person.

- **Professional limitations:** Sometimes, people are not ready to shift their thinking and continue to feel uncomfortable when with people with disabilities. If so, recognize this professional limitation and refer clients to other massage therapists who can provide appropriate and meaningful care when necessary.

Physical Disabilities

Physical disability or impairment refers to a number of disabilities that affect the muscular, skeletal, nervous, respiratory, and cardiovascular system. Physical disabilities related to sensory organs are discussed separately.

Physical disabilities may result from congenital causes, an injury, amputation, or a disease such as muscular dystrophy, multiple sclerosis, cerebral palsy, heart disease, pulmonary disease or others. Some physical disabilities may not be noticed through usual observation or interaction but may still create lifestyle challenges. Such disabilities include pulmonary disease, respiratory disorders, epilepsy, and others. People with physical disabilities may use assertive devices like wheelchairs, artificial limbs, braces, crutches, or canes for mobility. Considerations for working with physical disabilities include

- **Access challenges:** Access challenges related to the massage environment such as accessible parking and restrooms were described earlier. Impairments in eye-hand coordination, verbal communication, mobility, and decreased physical stamina and endurance may also require consideration. Discuss the client's needs openly, and work together to decrease access challenges. For example, if the client is easily fatigued, limit the session to 30 minutes to avoid overtaxing the client. If a verbal impairment makes understanding the client difficult, ask him or her to repeat a question or statement. In some cases the client may need to text, write, or have a translator convey information.

- **Balance disorders:** A client may experience a balance disorder, which causes feelings of unsteadiness, sensations like spinning or floating, or feelings of wooziness. The eyes, ears (vestibular system), and proprioception need to work together for the body to feel balanced when standing and walking. If asked, be ready to offer assistance, and structure the session to ensure the client can sit up for a period of time before being asked to stand from the table.

- **Body space:** Wheelchairs and other mobility devices are part of a person's body space. Don't hang or lean on a wheelchair, push a wheelchair without assistance having been requested, or move a mobility device that was set aside without the consent of the person with the disability.

- **Contraindications:** As with any client, conduct a thorough health history intake, and pay attention to cautions or contraindications related to diseases and conditions that cause physical disabilities. Research any medications the client is taking to determine whether there may be a related caution. (Cautions related to sensory impairments are discussed later.)

- **Eye level:** During the health intake interview, try to be on the same eye level as the person with the disability. For example, sit down or squat at the same eye level as a person using a wheelchair.

- **Medical equipment:** If the client is using medical equipment such as a catheter or a breathing apparatus, ask the client about the best way to help him or her stay comfortable and provide good massage without disrupting the equipment. He or she can instruct you what methods work best.

- **Paralysis:** Paralysis is the loss of muscle function in one or more muscles. Often caused by damage to the nervous system, usually the spinal cord, it may be accompanied by a loss of feeling in the area. Causes include spinal cord injury, stroke, other nerve injury, multiple sclerosis, Guillain-Barre syndrome, and others. Paraplegia is an impairment of motor or sensory function of the lower extremities. Quadriplegia is the partial or total loss of function in both the upper and lower extremities and the torso. If your client has an area that is paralyzed, learn whether sensory as well as motor function is lost. If sensory function is diminished, the client will not be able to give feedback about your pressure or temperature, so you must adjust your strokes accordingly.

- **Prosthesis:** People with a limb amputation may or may not want a prosthetic removed for the session and may or may not want the remainder of the limb massaged. It is usually safe and beneficial to massage the entire length of a limb as long as the client gives permission. Ask clients about their wishes and follow their recommendations.

- **Requests for assistance:** If a person seems to need assistance, ask if you can help. Most people will ask for assistance if they need it. If the client declines your assistance, accept their wishes graciously and do not take it personally.

- **Speech impairments:** Speech impairments can occur for a variety of reasons including hearing loss, neurological disorders, brain injuries, cognition impairments, or a cleft lip and palate. If a person has a speech impairment, communicate by listening attentively and encouragingly. Avoid interrupting or attempting to complete the person's sentences, and demonstrate patience. If you are having difficulty understanding, ask the person to repeat what you don't understand. It can be helpful to ask questions with yes or no answers or short answers. Don't raise your voice, because a person with a speech impairment may hear and understand perfectly.

- **Techniques and session flow:** The techniques you use and how you structure the session depend on the individual client, his or her overall physical condition, the treatment goals, and the feedback he or she gives during the massage about techniques that feel effective. Discuss the client's needs and wants openly to plan the session.

- **Transfer to a massage table:** When transferring a client from a wheelchair to the massage table, ask the client to direct how he or she wishes to be transferred. You may need to lower the table and adjust your body mechanics during the session. Lower a hydraulic table for the transfer and then adjust it to your comfortable working height.

Sensory Disabilities

A sensory disability can involve any of the five senses, although the inability to smell or taste is often not considered a disability. Visual impairments and hearing impairments are the main disabilities that limit access or create life challenges.

Visual Impairment

Visual impairment refers to a loss of visual capacity. In the United States, the terms "blind," "legally blind," "low vision," and "partially sighted" are used by educational and governmental organizations to describe degrees of visual impairment. The causes of visual impairment include disease, trauma, congenital, or degenerative conditions that cannot be corrected by glasses or contact lenses, medication, or surgery. Following are considerations for working with people who have visual impairments:

- **Access issues:** Think about ways you can improve your space to increase access to massage care. For example, is the lobby crowded and difficult to navigate from the doorway to the session room using a cane or service dog? Are Braille placards present to identify the restrooms, lobby, and session rooms? You might also consider printing your brochure and informed consent documents in Braille.

- **Assumptions:** Avoid making assumptions about any client's degree of visual impairment. Ask the client directly and respectfully what type of assistance he or she might need. Do not behave in a way that suggests you think the person has total blindness. Try to provide the right level of assistance for the individual client.

- **Physical guidance:** Do not take hold of a person with a visual impairment and pull in an attempt to physically guide him or her. Ask clients if they would like assistance, and offer your right elbow while standing slightly in front of the client on the left. The client can grasp your elbow and use it as a directional guide.

- **Communication:** Use the name of a person with a visual impairment so that he or she knows you are addressing him or her rather than someone else. Use a normal tone of voice unless the person also has a hearing impairment. Give very specific location information when introducing the person to your session room. If the person is legally blind or totally blind, you might give directions such as, "The massage table is on your left about three steps from this doorway. You can place your clothing on the chair to your right about four steps from the doorway and two steps from the massage table. Here is the massage table. You want to position yourself underneath this sheet." Some clients may want a kinesthetic feel for the position of objects; provide guidance by walking the client to each object and by placing the edge of the sheet in his or her hand so that the client is properly oriented to the space. When you re-enter the room, speak to the client to identify yourself and let the client know what you are doing if you move around the room to adjust the temperature or music.

- **Placement of personal items:** Don't move a personal item belonging to a person with a visual impairment unless necessary. Ask for permission and then describe where it is now placed in relationship to the client's position.

- **Service dogs:** Don't pet, feed, or play with a service dog. The service dog is working, and these activities only distract the dog from its job.

Hearing Impairment

Hearing impairment refers to a loss of the ability to detect or perceive some or all sound frequencies. The clear perception of sound may also be diminished. Some people can hear sound but not be able to understand speech due to diminished clarity. Hearing impairments may be mild, moderate, severe, or profound depending on the loudness a sound must be before the individual detects it. Language skills are often influenced by the age at which hearing loss occurred. Prelingual deafness is hearing loss that occurred before the person learned to speak. Postlingual deafness is hearing loss that occurred after the acquisition of language. The causes of hearing loss include trauma, genetics, disease, long-term exposure to noisy environments, the use of some medications, and exposure to some types of chemicals. Considerations for working with people who have hearing impairments include:

- **Background noise:** Reduce or eliminate background noise, which can create difficulties for people using hearing aids because it muddies sound.

- **Communication:** People with hearing impairments have different communication skills. Some can speech read (lip read), some use hearing aids, and some use interpreters. When communicating with a person with a hearing impairment, get his or her attention by touching the client on the shoulder or waving your hand. Look at the client directly, and speak clearly at a comfortable pace. Do not exaggerate your volume, lip movement, body language, facial expressions, or gestures in an attempt to aid understanding. Written notes can be used as needed to aid communication. If an interpreter is present, do not consult that person about health issues of the person for whom he or she is interpreting. Direct all questions to the person with the hearing impairment who will receive massage.

- **Hearing aids:** Avoid massaging too closely to hearing aids, as this can cause squeaking sounds.

Intellectual Disability

An intellectual or a cognitive disability is broadly defined as any disability that affects mental processes. Cognitive disabilities range from mild to severe and may be present from birth or may have developed later in life. Many organizations have their own definitions of cognitive disabilities related to certain challenges to access. There are a number of terms in use. For example, the term *developmental disability* describes lifelong disabilities caused by mental or physical impairments that manifested before age 18. Developmental delay, in contrast occurs temporarily as the result of illness or trauma during childhood. Developmental disabilities include mental retardation, cerebral palsy, autism, and fetal alcohol spectrum disorders. They may be classified as mild, moderate, severe, or profound.

Autism

Autism is a general term describing a group of complex developmental cognitive disorders, including Asperger's syndrome,

Rett's syndrome, and childhood disintegrative disorder. Many healthcare professionals now refer to these conditions as autism spectrum disorders. Currently 1 in 110 children is diagnosed with autism, and the incidence of autism is increasing 10% to 17% annually. No one knows what causes autism, but various combinations of factors may play a role, including genetic components (e.g., fragile X syndrome, tuberous sclerosis, and Angelman's syndrome) and exposure to environmental factors (e.g., maternal rubella while pregnant). Symptoms of autism vary but typically include impaired social functions such as a resistance to make eye contact, failure to develop peer relationships, lack of spontaneous seeking to share interests, achievements, or enjoyment with other people, delay in spoken language, repetitive or stereotypic patterns of behavior such as hand or finger twisting, and others.

Massage seems to provide useful support for children with autism. In one study, 20 children 3 to 6 years old with autism were assigned to a massage therapy or a reading attention (control) group. A massage therapist trained the parents of the massage therapy group to provide massage for 15 minutes prior to bedtime every night for a month. The parents of the control group read Dr. Seuss stories to their children for 15 minutes a night. After 1 month the children were assessed, and the massage group exhibited less stereotypic behavior, experienced fewer sleep problems, and showed more on-task and positive social-relating behavior during play observations at school than the control group.[27] Additional studies indicate that massage decreases anxiety, increases attention span, and reduces the autistic behaviors of inattentiveness, touch aversion, and withdrawal.[28]

Michael Regina-Whitely provides massage session recommendations.[29] He suggests that therapists use firm strokes instead of light pressure, keep sessions brief, and watch out for immune sensitivities related to environmental issues such as synthetic fragrances in massage lubricants or allergies to laundry detergent used with sheets. Caregivers should remain in the treatment room to provide feedback based on their better understanding of the child's behavior patterns and tolerance.

Mental Retardation

The term mental retardation is still in use, although some now refer to this condition as mild, moderate, severe, or profound intellectual disability. Mental retardation affects 1% to 3% of the population and may be caused by a broad spectrum of conditions and diseases.[30] Causes include infections at birth or after birth, chromosomal abnormalities, environmental conditions leading to deprivation syndrome, genetic abnormalities, inherited metabolic disorders, malnutrition, exposure to toxic substances like alcohol, cocaine, amphetamines, lead, or methylmercury, trauma during birth (lack of oxygen, or intracranial hemorrhage before or during birth), or severe head injury. Symptoms may be mild or severe. In mild cases, a child might demonstrate quiet behavior and a lack of curiosity. In severe cases, the child might demonstrate infant-like behavior that continues throughout life. Complications can include an inability to care for oneself, the inability to interact with others effectively, or complete social isolation.

Although there is not a wide body of research on massage for mental retardation, based on limited information we can speculate that massage therapy is beneficial. For example, in one study 21 moderate- to high-function children (median age: 2 years) with Down's syndrome received two 30-minute massage therapy or reading sessions (control group) per week. Children in the massage therapy group demonstrated less severe hypotonicity in their limbs and improved motor and muscle function than those in the reading group.[31] General recommendations for providing massage to people with mental retardation include:

- **Communication:** How you interact with the client depends on his or her level of function and cognitive ability. In some cases, you will interact directly with a caregiver. Speak and interact as directly as possible with the person who will receive massage.

- **Contraindications:** Research complicating physical conditions or medications to rule out contraindications and to provide a safe massage. Conduct a thorough health intake process and develop a session plan to best meet the person's needs. In many cases, you will develop session goals with the caregiver and the client's healthcare team instead of directly with the client.

- **Response to massage:** The client's responses to massage sessions are likely to be very specific to the individual client and may take fine tuning over a number of sessions. This includes the techniques used, session length, and environmental variables such as lighting, music, and temperature. It is often helpful to have the caregiver present to provide feedback based on his or her better knowledge of the client's behavioral cues. Often, it is appropriate to require the caregiver to be present to ensure the comfort of the client and your own safety (e.g., to prevent liability issues such as accusations of physical or sexual abuse). Start with firm pressure and avoid either light or overly deep work until you learn the client's preferences. Start with 30-minute sessions and progress to longer sessions if appropriate. Demonstrate patience and flexibility while watching and listening to the cues from the client. Adapt your techniques and the session goals moment by moment as needed.

Learning Disabilities

Learning disabilities are neurological impairments that affect the brain's ability to receive, process, store, and respond to information. They include difficulties with reading, writing, spelling, math, listening, and using language. They can be mild to severe. In moderate-to-severe cases, continued academic struggles often take a toll on the person's emotional and psychological health and his or her ability to participate in strong peer relationships. Massage benefits children and adults with learning disabilities through a reduction of stress and improved self-image. Though research is limited, massage improved the cognitive performance of preschoolers in one study of massage for early child development.[32] Massage is customized for the individual client and his or her needs.

Brain Injury

A brain injury occurs with trauma to the brain, such as a skull fracture, concussion, a lack of oxygen to the brain (anoxic injury), bleeding inside the brain (hemorrhage), swelling of brain tissues (edema), and others. A mild injury may cause a brief loss of consciousness, loss of memory before and after the injury, nausea, dizziness, headache, fatigue, temporary changes in cognition, and temporary behavioral changes. Moderate-to-severe brain injuries can include loss of consciousness for hours, confusion, agitation, slurred speech, weakness in the extremities, loss of coordination and bladder control, convulsions or seizures, and persistent cognitive, behavioral and mobility disorders. In severe cases, a person could enter a prolonged comatose or vegetative state. Massage following a recent head injury is contraindicated. As the client heals and with permission from the treating physician, massage can be very beneficial and serve as part of the rehabilitative process. For those in a comatose or vegetative state, massage can help preserve the heath of the tissues as long as techniques are moderate and do not overtax the fragile client. Because each case is unique, you are advised to consult with the client's healthcare team for specific session recommendations.

Mental Health Disabilities

Mental health disabilities are functional impairments caused by mental health disorders that interfere with or limit one or more major life activities.[33] Mental health disorders are mental, behavioral, or emotional patterns associated with subjective distress that are not part of normal development or culture. The National Institute of Mental Health estimates that tens of millions of people each year are impacted by mental health issues.[34] The World Health Organization notes that mental health disorders comprise 5 of the 10 leading causes of disability worldwide.[35]

The causes of mental health disorders are still being explored. Most are thought to arise from many causative factors, including:

- **Biological**: Brain chemistry may be disordered, such as with the abnormal functioning of neurotransmitters, or there may be a brain pathology or a structural abnormality that causes dysfunction. Biological factors can also involve genetic vulnerabilities triggered by environmental stress.
- **Psychological**: Psychological factors include cognitive function and reasoning, emotional processes, personality, temperament, and coping style.
- **Social**: Social factors include gender-specific influences (e.g., female-specific indicators of mental illness may be linked to rape, domestic violence, or high progesterone oral contraceptive use, etc.), a history of abuse or bullying, negative or highly stressful life experiences (e.g., post-traumatic stress in soldiers who served in combat areas), which may or may not be associated with cultural influences or socioeconomic inequality.

Mental health disorders include anxiety disorders (general anxiety disorder, obsessive-compulsive disorder, panic disorder, post-traumatic stress disorder, and social anxiety disorder), eating disorders (anorexia nervosa, bulimia nervosa, binge-eating disorder), mood disorders (bipolar disorder, depression), personality disorders (antisocial personality disorder, avoidant personality disorder, borderline personality disorder), schizophrenia, and substance abuse (alcohol and drug abuse). People who survive physical, mental, or emotional abuse often develop survival behaviors that are associated with some mental health disorders, but surviving abuse is not in itself a mental health disorder (discussed separately in Box 24-4).

BOX 24-4 **Massage for Survivors of Abuse**

The word "abuse" is defined in a number of ways, including treating someone with cruelty or violence or to cause damage or harm, especially regularly or repeatedly. Abuse exists in many forms, including child abuse, child sexual abuse, dating violence, domestic abuse or domestic violence, elder abuse, emotional abuse, group psychological abuse, hate crimes, intimidation, rape, school bullying, self-abuse, sexual abuse, and many others.

Abuse crosses all cultural, gender, and generational boarders but is most often perpetrated by family members or people intimate with the family, such as extended family or friends of the family. There are no clear answers about why some people abuse other people or why adults in abusive situations choose to stay in those situations. Patterns of abuse are often learned while growing up. People who were abused as children become abusers or subconsciously seek abusive relationships as adults. In many cases, abusive behavior is linked to mental health disorders.

During your professional practice, you will likely work with clients who are survivors of abuse. In some cases you won't know that your client is a survivor of abuse, while other clients may seek massage as a support strategy for coping with present or past abuse. Survivors of abuse may experience feelings of unease or emotional release because massage sessions may trigger associations with circumstances in which abuse occurred. Common triggers in a massage session include low light levels, certain colors, particular types of music, certain aromas, and touch on specific areas of the body. If you practice ethically, are competent in setting good boundaries, understand bodymind factors in therapeutic relationships, and can manage emotional processes of clients as discussed in Chapters 6 and 7, and if you understand core concepts in communication (Chapter 8), then you have a solid foundation for working with survivors of abuse. However, you are encouraged to obtain advanced training in continuing education classes after you graduate to provide the very best care to this group.

Mental health disorders range from mild to severe, and each person's physical condition, medications, and response to massage is unique. As described in depth in Chapter 4, relaxation-oriented massage is beneficial as a support strategy for people living with many mental health disorders. For example, a Swedish study found that people with general anxiety disorder who received massage reported sensations of being relaxed in their bodies and increased self-confidence. Massage in this case seemed to allow patients to "rediscover their own capacity during the massage session."[36] In an Australian study, massage delivered over a 7-week period to young adults hospitalized as psychiatric patients decreased levels of cortisol, self-reported anxiety, and the frequency and severity of aggressive incidents.[37] Massage has a positive effect on biochemistry related to anxiety and depression, such as decreased levels of cortisol and increased levels of serotonin and dopamine.[38] Anorexic women who received massage as compared to standard treatment reported lower stress and anxiety levels and had lower cortisol (stress) hormone levels following massage. Over the 5-week treatment period, they also reported decreases in body dissatisfaction on an eating disorder inventory (a rating of patient perception about a condition) and showed increased dopamine and norepinephrine levels.[39]

People with mental health disorders are often under the care of a mental health professional. Consult with the mental health professional (with the client's consent) about appropriate treatment goals and techniques. Have a referral list of mental health professionals available for clients not under professional care. As with other special populations, conduct a thorough health history intake process, rule out cautions or contraindications from medications, and work with the client to determine session goals and techniques.

Clients withdrawing from alcohol or drug addictions are likely to find the stress-reducing effects of massage beneficial, but avoid deep work during a withdrawal period to avoid accelerated detoxification symptoms as the body eliminates toxic substances related to addictions. Massage is contraindicated for anyone who is actively abusing substances or who shows signs of inebriation.

Use caution also if the client demonstrates behavior that indicates he or she has failed to take medication for a mental health disorder. If you feel that you or the client is in any danger, don't hesitate to contact the client's treating mental healthcare provider or emergency services for assistance. In one example, a massage therapist had worked successfully with a client with severe bipolar disorder over a number of sessions. During one particular session, the client's behavior rapidly deteriorated and the client tried to kick and bite the therapist. The therapist ended the session and called emergency services. The client's mental healthcare provider informed the therapist that the client had failed to take her medication. After the client had resumed taking her medication, she was able to proceed with massage therapy sessions.

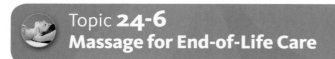

Topic 24-6
Massage for End-of-Life Care

End-of-life care is broadly defined as any care provided to a person nearing death due to natural causes or terminal illness. In medicine, end-of-life care refers to medical care provided in the final days or hours of a person's life or to care provided in the final months of a terminal illness. For example, when a person's doctors determine that cancer can no longer be controlled, medical testing and cancer treatment usually stop. The goal now is to make the person as comfortable as possible. Medications to control pain and symptoms like constipation, nausea, and shortness of breath are provided, but drugs once used to fight the cancer are discontinued. This section discusses terminal illness, the signs and symptoms of approaching death, and considerations for massage at the end of life.

Terminal Illness

A **terminal illness** is a disease that is considered ultimately incurable and likely to cause death within a short period of time (typically a life expectancy of 6 months or less, although people often outlive their life expectancy). An illness is considered terminal when there are no standard therapies to eliminate it from the body or cure it. In some cases, a disease allow for a relatively long life span, such as AIDS and neurological diseases like Alzheimer's and Parkinson's.

When people are diagnosed with a terminal illness, they often go through defined stages of acceptance. In the first stage, people often experience disbelief or shock progressing to anger or guilt that they have done something to deserve the diagnosis. In the second stage, depression sets and can last for several weeks. Eventually, depression fades as many people move into the final stage of acceptance.

Symptoms experienced during terminal illness include pain, nausea, difficulty breathing, difficult urination and constipation, depression, and refusal of food and water. Medical care seeks to reduce these symptoms with medications. Many people with terminal illnesses turn to complementary and alternative medicine modalities like massage to ease their symptoms.

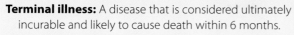

Concept Brief 24-5
Terminal Illness and End-of-Life Care

Terminal illness: A disease that is considered ultimately incurable and likely to cause death within 6 months.

End-of-life care: Care provided to manage symptoms and provide comfort after treatment to cure or fight a disease ends.

Signs and Symptoms of Approaching Death

The Hospice Patients Alliance describes two phases of approaching death.[40] The first phase is called the preactive phase of dying, which begins approximately 2 weeks before death. In this phase, a person demonstrates increased restlessness and confusion. He or she finds it difficult to remain in one position and changes positions frequently. The person withdraws from social activities and experiences increased periods of sleep and lethargy and reduced food or liquid intake. The person may demonstrate periods of breathing pauses (apnea) when awake or during sleep and may have difficulty healing from wounds or infections. Edema often occurs in the extremities or entire body. During this period, the person often requests to see family members and wants to settle unfinished business or actively say goodbye. The person is likely to state that he or she is dying and may report seeing persons who have already died.

The second phase of dying, called the active phase, is characterized by an unresponsive state. He or she may be difficult to arouse or may fall into a semicoma or coma. In some cases, a person exhibits severe agitation, including hallucinations or pronounced personality changes. Abnormal breathing patterns including long pauses in breathing, rapid chest breathing, or shallow breathing are common. The person may not be able to speak but holds the mouth open for breathing. Inability to swallow food or liquids occurs, and urine output is decreased and often darker in color or abnormally colored. Urinary or bowel incontinence may occur. Blood pressure drops, and the person's extremities may feel very cold or turn bluish or purple, and the body is held in a rigid and unchanging position. The jaw drops or is held in a sideways position. Although the person seems unresponsive, he or she can hear the words of loved ones up until passing.

Considerations for Massage at the End of Life

There is limited research on the benefits of massage specifically for end-of-life care. It is likely that massage reduces pain, increases relaxation, improves mood, supports better sleep patterns, reduces anxiety, and provides a sense of comfort for people at the end of life. One study shows that massage reduced anxiety and evoked feelings of calmness in 30 hospice patients in the final stages of life.[41] Another noted that aromatherapy massage demonstrated short-term effects to decrease pain and depression and over a longer term improved sleep patterns.[42] A study at the University of Colorado showed that massage provided immediate and noticeable relief of pain and anxiety in cancer patients at the end of life.[43] Massage considerations when working with clients at the end of life include the following:

- **Therapist's response to dying process:** Each of us responds to the dying process in different ways, and it is important to assess your personal level of comfort with this process before you work with clients and their families. You must be ready to make a personal commitment to remain present throughout the dying process to ensure that the client and loved ones do not feel abandoned. It is normal to feel attachment to a client who is dying and to grieve the loss of the client along with family members. A wide variety of useful books and audio CDs are available with information about the stages of grief and the dying process. Some of these resources are listed in the Massage Fusion section of this chapter.

- **Pathology knowledge:** Research the particular disease for the person to whom you provide massage, and learn about the ways the disease progresses.

- While this knowledge is unlikely to change the way you deliver massage, it will help you understand the bodymind histories of both the client and his or her loved ones. This understanding leads to greater empathy, compassion, and sensitivity in your work.

- **Environments:** Massage is typically provided in the client's home, a family member's home, hospice, or hospital room. Remain flexible and adaptable in these new environments while still practicing the best possible body mechanics and self-care.

- **Techniques:** Techniques should be very gentle and calming. Slow strokes on the arms and hands, holding at the base of the neck, and energetic bodywork techniques are indicated. Your goal is to promote calm and offer support.

- **Massage as a support for family:** Family members, especially family members who are primary caregivers during a time of transition, can benefit from massage delivered in the home, hospice, or hospital. Massage provides the person with the opportunity to regroup and rest from the ongoing stress of a loved one's approaching death. You may choose to offer 15-minute sessions that can be conducted in a massage chair or in a regular chair for caregivers.

MASSAGE FUSION
Integration of Skills

STUDY TIP: Plan to Learn Forever

Continuing education is training that takes place after you graduate from your primary massage program and obtain your initial credentials. Continuing education is widely available as live training and online courses. You can usually find listings of courses through your professional massage therapy association (Associated Bodywork & Massage Professionals or American Massage Therapy Association) or through the National Certification Board of Therapeutic Massage & Bodywork. As noted throughout this chapter, therapists who wish to specialize in massage for special populations should consider advanced training through continuing education. You can also take courses in advanced assessment and techniques. Continuing education allows you to explore your interests and stay inspired with a life-long passion for learning.

GOOD TO KNOW: Resources for Understanding Death and the Grief Process

1. *On Death and Dying* by Elisabeth Kubler-Ross
2. *Death and Dying: Life and Living* by Charles Corr, Clyde Nabe, and Donna Corr
3. *Final Gifts: Understanding the Special Awareness, Needs, and Communications of the Dying* by Maggie Callanan and Patricia Kelley
4. *Questions and Answers on Death and Dying* by Elisabeth Kubler-Ross

5. *A Healing Touch: True Stories of Life, Death, and Hospice* by Richard Russo
6. *Facing Death: Images, Insights, and Interventions: A Handbook for Educators, Healthcare Professionals, and Counselors* by Sandra L. Bertman.

CHAPTER WRAP-UP

Massage for special populations requires a complete integration of everything you have learned in your massage training program. You must know the sciences including anatomy, physiology, and pathology to understand the benefits and effects of massage for specific groups of people. You must also be able to evaluate a client's current level of health and rule out contraindications or make adaptations for the changing bodies of pregnant women, older people, clients with a disability, people at the end of life, or athletes at a particular stage of training. You must practice a wide variety of techniques while using good body mechanics and proper self-care. If this isn't enough, you must also maintain strong professional boundaries, manage the emotional processes of your clients, communicate actively and effectively, and navigate gray ethical issues. Reading this chapter now, you are likely close to finishing your foundation training and are looking forward to graduation. Congratulations! You are a massage therapist—and it is a wonderful and rewarding profession. I hope that you will continue to grow and develop your skills. Good luck as you prepare to take your massage boards and obtain your credentials. Welcome to your new career!

Appendix A: Healthcare Terminology

Every profession has developed its own language so that its professionals can communicate more efficiently and effectively. Lawyers must understand legal terms, plumbers must know the names of different types of pipes, and landscape designers must learn all the botanical names of plants. Similarly, massage therapists must learn the names of body areas and muscles as well as medical and healthcare-related terms.

There are many benefits to learning healthcare terminology (often called medical terminology). First, it helps you better understand written information in textbooks and verbal information conveyed during lectures and demonstrations. Your improved understanding leads to greater enjoyment of your massage training program (and better grades). In addition, massage therapists who are proficient in the use of healthcare terminology can convey the benefits of massage more successfully to other healthcare providers. This leads not only to clearer communication but also to more respect. Other healthcare professionals are more likely to refer their clients or patients to a massage therapist who understands the human body and can convey that knowledge using the correct terms. Knowing and using a healthcare vocabulary can literally improve your ability to increase your income and attract new clients. A good vocabulary helps you feel confident when interacting with other healthcare providers and understand your role in an integrated healthcare team.

The ability to reason clinically and rule out massage contraindications is important for a knowledgeable massage therapist. Understanding healthcare terminology supports clinical reasoning and helps a therapist when researching specific conditions and medications. It also improves the quality of the written documentation of the session.

This appendix aims to provide a resource to learn word elements and general healthcare terms, as well as the correct terms for body positions, regions, surface anatomy, planes, and directions and important terms associated with the musculoskeletal system. It is unlikely that you will learn every term you will encounter during your massage career, however. For this reason, it is essential to keep a medical dictionary on hand as a reference, both as a student and later when you become a professional. Since everyone usually makes pronunciation mistakes when learning new and sometimes complicated terms, you should proceed fearlessly and not be embarrassed by such mistakes. Note that the terms used in Eastern bodywork are discussed in Chapter 17, Eastern Approaches.

Word Elements

Most medical and healthcare terms are built from Greek and Latin words elements. Chapter 1 discussed how the Greeks moved medicine out of the magical realm and into a more logical and objective science. Hippocrates sought to describe the body and human physiological conditions precisely. The ancient Greek language was flexible, and Greeks tended to join two or more words to form a new word. This still happens in modern times. For example, the word telephone is a combination of two Greek words: tele meaning "distant" and phone meaning "voice." When the Romans conquered Greece in 146 BCE, they adopted many elements of Greek society. Greek physicians became teachers and central figures in Roman society, and soon Roman physicians trained by the Greeks were adding their own Latinized version of words to medical writings.

During the Renaissance (14 to 16th centuries), there was a surge of interest in classical learning, and Latin became the preferred language of scholars and the educated elite. In addition, educated men wrote to each other in Latin so that scholars from many different countries could share their ideas and scientific advances. Today, healthcare providers around the world still use the same vocabulary to describe medical conditions. This is one of the values of having a consistent and standardized healthcare terminology. Healthcare professionals, regardless of their nationality, can thus understand each other.

Medical terms are composed of individual components called word elements. Word elements are prefixes, roots, and suffixes. Prefixes are often written with a dash at the end, while roots are written with no dash and suffixes are written with a dash at the beginning. When you review Tables A-1, A-2, and A-3, you may notice that some word elements are both a prefix and a suffix or both a prefix and a root. Notice also that sometimes multiple word elements mean the same thing, or that very similar word elements mean different things. This can seem confusing at first, but as you develop

(706 MASSAGE MASTERY: FROM STUDENT TO PROFESSIONAL)

TABLE A-1   Prefixes

Prefix	Meaning	Origin
A-, an-	Without, not	Greek, *a-, an-*
Ab-, abs-	Off, motion away	Latin, *ab* meaning "from"
Ad-	Towards, increase	Latin, *ad* meaning "towards"
Allo-	Other, different	Greek, *allos*
Ambi-	Both, both sides, around	Greek, *amphi*, corresponds to Latin *ambo* meaning "both"
Ana-	Up, towards, apart	Greek, *ana* meaning "up"
Ante-	Before	Latin, *ante*
Antero-	Anterior	Latin, *anterior*
Anthropo-	Human	Greek, *anthropos*
Anti-	Against, opposing	Greek, *anti*
Apico-	Apex	Latin, *apex, apicis* meaning "summit" or "tip"
Atreto-	Lack of an opening	Greek, *atretos* meaning "imperforate" (no perforation or no hole)
Auto-, aut-	Self, same	Greek, *autos*
Axio-, axo-	Axis	Latin, *axis* corresponding to the Greek, *axon*
Baro-	Weight, pressure	Greek, *baros*
Bi-	Twice, double, dual actions	Latin, *bi*
Blasto-	Budding by cells or tissue	Greek, *blastos* meaning "germ"
Carcino-, carcin-	Cancer	Greek, *karkinos* meaning "crab" or "cancer"
Cerebello-, cerebro-, cerebri	Cerebellum	Latin, *cerebrum* meaning "brain"
Cervico-	Neck (may also relate to the uterine cervix)	Latin, *cervix*
Cheilo-, cheil-	Lip	Greek, *cheilos*
Cheiro-, Cheir-	Hand	Greek, *cheir*
Chyl-, chyli-, chylo-	Chyle	Greek, *chylos* meaning "juice"
Cili(o)-	Cilia, ciliary	Latin, *cilium* meaning "eyelash"
Con-	Together	Latin, *cum* meaning "with" or "together"
Crym(o)-, cry(o)-	Cold	Greek, *kryos*
Cyan(o)-	Blue	Greek, *kyanos* meaning "a dark blue substance"
Cyt(o)-	Cell	Greek, *kytos*
Dacry(o)-	Tears	Greek, *dakryon*
Dactyl(o)-	Fingers, sometimes toes	Greek, *daktylos*
De-	Away from	Latin, *de*
Dent(i), dent(o)	Teeth	Latin, *dens* meaning "tooth"
Derm-, derma-, dermat-	Skin	Greek, *derma* corresponds to the Latin *cut-*
Dis-	Apart, not	Latin, *dis* meaning "separation"
Dys-	Bad, difficult, opposite	Greek, *dis*
Ec-	Out of, away from	Greek, ek meaning "out"
Embro-	Embryo	Greek, *embryo* meaning "a young one"
Encephalo-, encephal-	Brain	Greek, *enkephalo*

TABLE A-1   Prefixes *(Continued)*

Prefix	Meaning	Origin
Endo-, end	Within, inner, absorbing	Greek *endon* meaning "within"
Epi-	On, following, subsequent	Greek, *epi*
Ethmo-	Ethmoid	Greek, *ethmos* meaning "sieve"
Ex-	Out of, away from	Latin, *ex*
Exo-	Exterior, external, outward	Greek, *exo*
Extra-	Without, outside	Latin, *extra*
Fascio-	Fascia	Latin, *fascia* meaning "a band"
Gen-	Birth	Greek, *genos*
Gyn-, gyne-, gyneco-, gyno	Female	Greek, gyne
Holo-	Whole, entire, complete	Greek, *holos*
Hyper-	Excessive, above normal	Greek, *hyper*
Hypo-	Deficient, below normal	Greek, *hypo*
Ideo-	Idea	Greek, *idea*
Idio-	Distinctive, peculiar	Greek, *idios* meaning "one's own"
In-	Not	Greek, *a-, an-* synonymous with un-
Infra-	Below	Latin, *infra*
Inter-	Between	Latin, *inter*
Intra-	Inside, within	Latin, synonymous with endo-, ento-
Iso-	Equal	Greek, *isos*
Jejuno-	Jejunum	Latin, *jejunus* meaning "empty"
Laparo-	Loins	Greek, *lapara* meaning "flank"
Mal-	Ill, bad	Latin, *malus* meaning "bad"
Meti, medio	Middle, median	Latin, *medius*
Mega-, megalo-	Large	Greek, *megas*
Meta-	After, subsequent to	Greek, *meta*
Micro-	Small	Greek, *mikros*
Mis-	Not, opposite, incorrect	Greek, *miseo* meaning "to hate"
Mono-	Single, single part	Greek, *monos*
Multi-	Many	Latin, *multus* meaning "much"
Narco-	Narcosis, deaden	Greek, *narkoo* meaning "to benumb"
Necro-	Death	Greek, *nekros* meaning "corpse"
Neo-	New	Greek, *neos*
Organo-	Organ	Greek, *organon*
Oro-	Mouth	Latin, *os, oris*
Osmo-	Osmosis	Greek, *osme*
Para-	Departure from the normal	Greek, *para-* meaning "alongside" or "near"
Para-	Meaning two like parts or a pair	Greek, *para-* meaning "alongside" or "near"
Ped-, pedi-, pedo-	Foot, feet	Latin, *Pes* meaning "foot"
Per-	Through	Latin, *per* meaning "through," "extremely"

(Continued)

TABLE A-1 Prefixes *(Continued)*

Prefix	Meaning	Origin
Peri-	Around, about, near	Greek, *peri-* meaning "around"
Petro-	Hard, stone-like	Latin, *petra*, Greek, *petros* meaning "stone"
Phago-	Eating, devouring	Greek, *phago* meaning "to eat"
Physio-, physi-	Physical, natural	Greek, *physis* meaning "nature"
Plano-, plan-, plani-	Plane, flat, level	
Pleur-, Pleuro-	Rib, side or pleura	Greek, *pleura* meaning "a rib" or "the side"
Poly-	Many	Greek, *polys*
Post-	After, behind	Latin, *post*
Pre-	Before, anterior	Latin, *prae*
Pro-	Before or forward	Greek, *pro*
Proto-	The first in a series	Greek, *protos* meaning "first"
Proxi-, prox-	Proximal	Latin, *proximus* meaning "nearest"
Quadri-	Four	Latin, *quattuor*
Semi-	One-half	Latin, *semis*
Spino-, spin	Spine, spinous process	Latin, *spina*
Super-, supra-	Excess, above, superior	Latin, *supra*
Syn-	Together, joined	Greek, *syn* corresponds to Latin, *con-*
Trans-	Across, through, beyond	Latin, *trans*
Tri-	Three	Latin and Greek, *tri*
Ultra-	Excess, exaggeration, beyond	Latin, *ultra*
Un-	Not, a reversal	Relates to Latin, *in-* and Greek *a-* and *an-*
Uni-	One, single, not paired	Latin, *unus* corresponds to Greek, *mono-*
Xipho-	Xiphoid process	Greek, *xipho* meaning "sword"

TABLE A-2 Roots

Root	Meaning	Origin
Abdomin(o),	Abdomen	Latin, *abdominis*
Acr(o)	Extremity, tip, end	Greek, *akron*
Aden(o)	Gland	Greek, *aden* and Latin, *glandul* or *glandi*
Adip(o)	Fat	Latin, *adeps, adipis* "lard or grease" corresponds to Greek, *lip* or *lipo*
Adren(o), adren	Adrenal gland	Latin, *ad* "toward" and *renes* "the kidney"
Are(o)	Air	Greek, *are*
Alge, algesi, algio, algo	Pain	Greek, *algos* corresponds to Latin *dolor*
Ambly	Dull, dim	Greek, *amblys*
Andr(o)	Male	Greek, *aner* or *andros* meaning "a male human"
Angi(o)	Blood or lymph vessels	Greek, *angeion* meaning "vessel" corresponds to Latin, *vas-* or *vaso-* or *vasculo-*

TABLE A-2 Roots *(Continued)*

Root	Meaning	Origin
Anis(o)	Unequal, unlike, dissimilar	Greek, *anisos*
Ankyl(o)	Bent, crooked, stiff, fixed	Greek, *ankylos* meaning "bent" and *ankylosis* meaning "stiffening of the joints"
Ap(o)	Derived from	Greek, *apo* or *ap*
Appendic(o)	Appendix	Latin, *appendix*, *appendicis* meaning "appendage"
Arch(o), arche, archi	Primordial, ancestral, first	Greek, *arche* meaning "origin" or "beginning"
Arteri(o)	Artery	Latin, *arteria*
Arthr(o)	Joint, articulation	Greek, *anthron* corresponds to the Latin, *articul-*
Ather(o)	Soft, pasty	Greek, *athere* meaning "gruel" which is a type of porridge that has a soft, pasty appearance
Atlant(o), atlo	Atlas (bone that supports the head)	Greek, Atlas, *Atlantos* - named for the Greek god who supported the universe on his shoulders
Audi(o)	Sense of hearing	Latin, *audio* meaning "to hear"
Aur(i), aur(o)	Ear	Latin, *auris*
Bacteri(o)	Bacteria	Greek, *baktron* meaning "staff" referring to the shape of bacteria when viewed under a microscope (named in the 1800s by Robert Koch)
Bath(o), bathy	Depth, deep	Greek, *bathos*
Bili	Bile	Latin, *bilis*
Bio	Life	Greek, *bios*
Brachi(o)	Arm	Latin, *brachium*
Brady	Slow	Greek, *bradys*
Bronch(i), bronch(o)	Bronchus	Greek, *bronchos* meaning "windpipe"
Bucc(o)	Cheek	Latin, *bucca*
Calcane(o)	The heel	Latin, *calcaneum*
Cardi(o)	Heart	Greek, *kardia*
Carp(o), carpal, carpus	Wrist	Greek, *karpos*
Cata	Down	Greek, *kata*
Caud(o)	Tail, lower part of the body	Latin, *caudalis*
Cec(o)	Cecum	Latin, *cecum* meaning "blind"
Celi(o)	Abdomen	Greek, *koilia* meaning "belly"
Centr(o)	Center	Greek, *kentron*
Cephal(o)	Head	Greek, *kephale*
Chem(o)	Chemistry	Greek, *chemeia* meaning "alchemy"
Chir(o)	Hand	Greek, *cheir*
Chole, chol(o)	Bile	Greek, *chole*
Chondr(o), chondri(o)	Cartilage	Greek, *chondrion* or *chondros* which was a type of course grain
Chrom(o), chromat(o)	Color	Greek, *chroma*
Circum	Circular movement	Latin, *circum* meaning "around"
Cleid(o), clid(o)	Clavicle	Greek, *kleis* meaning "bar"
Coen(o)	Shared in common	Greek, *Koinos* meaning "common"

TABLE A-2 Roots *(Continued)*

Root	Meaning	Origin
Contra, counter	opposite, opposed	Latin, *contra* meaning "against"
Core(o), cor(o)	Pupil of the eye	Greek, *kore* meaning "pupil"
Dermat(o)	Skin	Greek, *derma*
Duoden(o)	Duodenum	Latin, *duodenum*
Dynam(o)	Force, energy	Greek, *dynamis* meaning "power"
Enter(o)	Intestines	Greek, *enteron*
Erg(o)	Work	Greek, *ergon*
Erythr(o)	Red, red blood cell	Greek, *erythros* meaning "red"
Eu	Good, well	Greek, *eu*
Fibr(o)	Fiber	Latin, *fibra*
Hemangi(o)	Blood vessel	Greek, *haima* meaning "blood" and *angeion* meaning "vessel"
Hemat(o), hem, hemo	Blood	Greek, *haima*
Hepat(o), hepatic(o)	Liver	Greek, *hepar*
Hidr(o)	Sweat, sweat glands	Greek, *hidros*
Hist(o)	Tissue	Greek, *histos*
Histi(o)	Connective tissue	Greek, *histion* meaning "web"
Hyster(o)	The uterus	Greek, *hystera* meaning "womb"
Ili(o)	Ilium	Latin, *ilium*
Kinesi(o), kines(o), kino	Motion	Greek, *kinesis* meaning "motion," *kineo* meaning "to move"
Laryng(o)	Larynx	Greek, *larynx*
Later(o)	Lateral	Latin, *lateralis*
Lecu(o), leuk(o)	White or white blood cell	Greek, *leukos*
Lingu(o)	Tongue	Latin, *lingua*
Lip(o)	Fatty	Greek, *Lipos* meaning "fat"
Lymphaden(o)	Lymph node	Latin, *lympha* meaning "spring water" and Greek, *aden* meaning "gland"
Lymphangi(o)	Lymphatic vessel	Latin, *lympha* meaning "spring water" and Greek, *angeion* meaning "vessel"
Lymph(o)	Lymph	Latin, *lympha*, meaning "spring water"
Macr(o)	Large	Greek, *makros* corresponds with *mega-*, *megalo-*
Meat(o)	Meatus	Latin, *meatus* meaning "passage"
Morph(o)	Shape, form	Greek, *morphe*
Muci, muc(o)	Mucous	Latin, *mucus*
My(o)	Muscle	Greek, *mys*
Nas(o)	Nose	Latin, *Nasus*
Nephr(o)	Kidney	Greek, *nephros* corresponds with Latin, *reno*
Neur(o), neuri	Nerve, nerve tissue, nervous system	Greek, *neuron*
Occipit(o)	Occiput	Latin, *occiput*
Ocul(o)	Eye	Latin, *oculus*
Ole(o)	Oil	Latin, *oleum*

TABLE A-2   Roots *(Continued)*

Root	Meaning	Origin
Onc(o)	Tumor	Greek *onkos* meaning "mass"
Osse(o), ossi, ost(o)	Bone, bony	Latin, *osseus*
Ot(o)	Ear	Greek, *ous*
Pancreat(o)	Pancreas	Greek, *pankreas*
Path(o), pathic	Disease	Greek, *pathos,* meaning "feeling," "suffering"
Pelvi(o), pelvo	Pelvis	Latin, *pelvis* meaning "basin"
Perioste(o)	Periosteum	Modern Latin
Pharyng(o)	Pharynx	Greek, *pharynx*
Phleb(o)	Veins	Greek, *phleps*
Plasma, Plasmat(o)	Plasma	Greek, *plasma* meaning "something formed"
Pne(o)	Breath, respiration	Greek, *pneo* meaning "to breath"
Pseud(o)	False, deceptive	Greek, *pseudes*
Psych(o), psyche	Mind	Greek, *psyche* meaning "soul" or "mind"
Pulm(o)	Lungs	Latin, *pulmo*
Ren(o), reni	Kidney	Latin, *ren*
Scapul(o)	Scapula	Latin, *scapulae* meaning "shoulder blade"
Seb(o), sebi	Sebum	Latin, *sebum* meaning "tallow"
Sensori	Sensory	Latin, *sensorius*
Somat(o)	Body	Greek, *soma*
Splen(o)	Spleen	Greek, *splen*
Spondyl(o)	Vertebrae	Greek, *spondylos*
Stern(o)	Sternum, sternal	Greek, *sternon* meaning "chest"
Syndesm(o)	Ligament	Greek, *syndesmos* meaning "fastening"
Tal(o)	Talus	Latin, *talus*
Tars(o)	Tarsal bones	Greek, *tarsos* meaning "flat surface"
Tempor(o)	Temporal bone, temple	Latin, *temporalis*
Tend(o), ten(o), tenont	Tendon	Latin, *tendo*
Therm(o)	Heat	Greek, *therme*
Thromb(o)	Blood clot	Greek, *thrombos* meaning "clot"
Tibi(o)	Tibia	Latin, *tibia*
Ton(o)	Tone, tension	Greek, *tonos*
Tixi(o), tox, toxo	Toxin, poison	Greek, *toxikon* meaning "bow" referring to an arrow tipped with poison
Trachel(o)	Neck	Greek, *trachelos*
Vas(o), vascul(o)	Blood vessel	Latin, *vas* and *vasculum* meaning "a small vessel"
Vene-, veno, veni	Veins or venous	Latin, *vena*
Vertebro	Vertebra or vertebral	Latin, *vertebra*
Viscer(o)	Viscera	Latin, *viscus* or *viscera* meaning "internal organs"
Vivi	Living	Latin *vivus* meaning "alive"

TABLE A-3   Suffixes

Suffix	Meaning	Origin
-Acouousis, -acusis	Refers to hearing	German, *akoustikos*
-Agog, -agogue	Promoting, stimulating	Greek, *agogos* meaning to "lead forth"
-Al, -ar, -ary	Pertaining to	
-Algia, -algio, -algo	Pain, or a painful condition	Greek, *algos*
-Blast	Precursor cell	Greek, *blastos* meaning "germ"
-Cele	Hernia, swelling	Greek, kele meaning "tumor"
-Chrome	Relationship to color	Greek, *chroma*
-Cide, -cido	To kill	Latin, *-cida, -cidium*
-Cleisis	Closure	Greek, *kleisis* meaning "a closing"
-Cyte	Cell	Greek, *kyton*
-Ectasia, -ectasis	Dilation, expansion	Greek, *ektasis* meaning "stretching"
-Emia	Blood	Greek, from *haima* meaning "blood"
-Form	Shape of, form	Latin, *formis*
-Fugal	Movement away	Latin, *fugio* meaning "to flee"
-Genic	Producing, forming	Greek, *genos* meaning "birth"
-Ia, -iasis	Condition (usually unhealthy)	Greek, *ia*
-Ism	medical condition	Greek, *isma*
-Ismus	Spasm	Latin from Greek, *ishos*
-Itis	Inflammation	Greek, *itis*
-Logia, -logy	Study of	Greek, logos meaning "discourse," "treatise"
-Megaly	Large	Greek, *megas*
-Odes, -oid	Resemblance of form	Greek, *eidos*
-Oma	Tumor, neoplasm	Greek, *oma*
-Osis	Abnormal state	Greek, *osis*
-Penia	Deficiency	Greek, *penia* meaning "poverty"
-Phage, phagia, phagy	Eating, devouring	Greek, *phago* meaning "to eat"
-Phi, phile, philic, philia	Affinity for, craving	Greek, *philos* meaning "fond" or "loving"
-Phrenia	Diaphragm	Greek, *phren* "seat of emotions"
-Plegia	Paralysis	Greek, *plege* meaning "stroke"
-Stat	An agent to keep something from changing or moving	Greek, *states* meaning "stationary"
-Tome	Cutting, segment	Greek, *tomos* meaning "a cutting," "section" or "segment"

your understanding of roots, prefixes, and suffixes, your comprehension of healthcare terminology will dramatically improve. When you encounter new words in your reading, you will often be able to break them down and figure them out for greater comprehension.

Prefixes

A prefix is not an independent word. It is a word element attached to the beginning of a root to modify its meaning. For

example, the prefix sub- is often used to modify Latin roots. It means "under," "beneath," or "less than" what is normal. For example:

- Subcartilaginous: partly cartilaginous or beneath the cartilage
- Subclavian: below the clavicle
- Subconscious: not completely conscious, or an idea or impression present in the mind that the person is not consciously aware of

- Subcutaneous: beneath the skin (cutaneous is Latin for skin)

The prefix epi-, on the other hand, usually means "over" or "on top." It might also mean "following" or "subsequent" to something else. For example:

- Epicranium: refers to the muscle, aponeurosis (a sheet-like tendon), and skin covering the cranium (skull).
- Epidermis: refers to the superficial (top) layer of the skin. The word dermis refers to the layer of the skin under the epidermis.
- Epicondyle: a projection from a long bone above or on a condyle. A condyle is a rounded articular bony projection. The word articular refers to a joint.

A prefix may also modify the number of the root word. Bi-, for example, means "two," "twice," or "double." It might refer to the number of structures, as in the word biceps, which refers to a muscle (structure) with two origins (an origin is the place where a muscle starts on the bone), or bicuspid, which refers to two points (cusp is from cuspis, Latin for point) as in bicuspid tooth, a premolar tooth that has two points. Bi- can also refer to dual actions, as in the term biaxial joint, which refers to a joint that moves in two main directions (axes). Tri- means "three," and knowing that biceps means a muscle with two origins, we can assume that triceps is a muscle with three origins.

A prefix often modifies the amount of the root word. The prefix a- or an- means "not" or "without," as in the term *acellular*, which means devoid of cells, or *achromatic*, which means colorless (the Greek word for color is *chroma*), or *anemia*, which refers to a condition in which a person has too few red blood cells (*haima* is the Greek word for blood and is seen as *hem-*, *hemat-*, and *hemato-*).

Prefixes that describe directions, positions, and sizes are also common in medical terminology. *Ad-* means "towards," while *ab-* means "away from." When you adduct the arm you bring it toward the body, but when you abduct the arm you move it away from the body. *Macro-* (also *macr-*, *mega-*, and *megalo-*) means "large," while *micro-* means "small." *Infra-* means "below," while *supra-* (also *super*) means above. Thus, it is not difficult to surmise that a muscle called the infraspinatus is likely to be situated below a muscle called the supraspinatus.

Roots

Roots are word elements that provide the core meaning of the word. They are usually combined with prefixes and suffixes to create medical terms. Roots often refer to an anatomical structure such as an organ or body region. They might also refer to a disease or condition. When one word element ends with a consonant and the word element that follows begins with a consonant, a combining vowel is added for smooth pronunciation. Usually the combining vowel is o, but sometimes it is i. This is why root words are often written with (o) after them.

The root word *cardi(o)* refers to the heart. It can be combined with a wide variety of prefixes and suffixes to indicate different meanings relating to the heart. For example:

- Cardiology is the medical specialty that is concerned with the diagnosis and treatment of the heart (-logy comes from the Greek logos meaning "study").

- Cardioplegia is the paralysis of the heart, which is sometimes induced with chemicals as part of heart surgery (-plegia comes from the Greek plege meaning "stroke").
- A cardiograph is an instrument for recording the movements of the heart (-graph comes from the Greek grapho meaning "to write").
- The term cardiovascular relates to the heart and blood vessels or circulation (vascular comes from the Latin vasculum meaning "vessel").

Whenever you see the root *cardi(o)*, regardless of prefixes or suffixes, you know the term relates in some way to the heart. This is true of other root words such as *hepat(o)*, which refers to the liver, or *my(o)*, which refers to muscle, or *pulm(o)* or *plumon(o)*, which refers to the lung.

Suffixes

A suffix is not an independent word. It is a word element attached to the end of a root to modify its meaning. When encountering a difficult term, it is helpful to first define the suffix because it tells you how the word is used and if it is a noun or adjective. The suffix *-algia* means "characterized by pain," so you know that *neuralgia* means some type of pain. When you know that the root *neur(o)* means nerve, it is easy to deduce that *neuralgia* means a condition involving nerve pain. Other words using the suffix *-algia* include:

- Arthralgia: arthr(o) is a root from the Greek that means "joint." When combined with -algia, it means "joint pain."
- Cephalalgia: cephal(o) is a Greek root that means "head." When combined with -algia, it means "headache."
- Fibromyalgia: fibro- is a prefix meaning "fiber," derived from the Latin fibra. My(o) is a root that means "muscle," derived from the Greek mys. When combined with -algia, it means a condition in which the fibers (tendons, ligaments, and fascia) and muscle are painful.
- Mastalgia: mast(o) is Greek for breast, and mamma (mamme plural) from the Latin is also used. When combined with -algia it means "breast pain" or "painful breasts."
- Myalgia: my is Greek for "muscle," so this word means "muscle pain."

Breaking Terms Apart

In the sections above, we have already begun the process of breaking down terms to determine their meaning. By knowing common prefixes, roots, and suffixes, we can easily understand the separate word elements that comprise terms and then break words down and put them back together. Notice that many terms have only two word elements, not all three. As you read your textbooks, take note of medical terms, and get in the habit of breaking words down to help you understand them. (Some students write the breakdown in the margin of the textbook to help them remember the word during review for an exam.)

While the tables included here contain common prefixes, roots, and suffixes, they cannot replace the information included in a medical dictionary. The information from these tables was prepared using Stedman's Medical Dictionary for the Health Professions and Nursing.

Must-Know Terminology

Anatomy and physiology are closely related biological sciences. Anatomy is the study of the structures that make up an organism, and physiology is the study of the way in which the organism functions. Kinesiology is the science and study of movement and the active and passive structures (joints, muscles, tendons, ligaments, and fascia) involved in facilitating that movement. A solid understanding of anatomy, physiology, and kinesiology is essential for building informed massage and bodywork skills. This textbook focuses primarily on the theory and practice of massage and leaves the in-depth study of anatomy, physiology, and kinesiology to textbooks dedicated to those subjects. Therefore, the focus here is on terminology related directly to the practice of massage. Additional terms and terms related to more in-depth anatomy and physiology can be found in the glossary.

The Basics of the Musculoskeletal System

You can't get very far in massage training without running into terms for the muscular and skeletal system, called collectively the musculoskeletal system. While all body systems are important, these two are prominent in a massage therapist's knowledge base, and it is helpful for the massage students to have some basic knowledge right from the start. Basic terms related to these systems are described before the terms for positions, directions, body regions, planes of the body, and movements.

The Basics of the Skeletal System

The skeletal system is the body's frame. It supports and protects other body systems while allowing movement. The skeletal system is composed of 206 bones and is divided into the axial skeleton and the appendicular skeleton. The axial skeleton is composed of the bones of the skull and the vertebral column. *Axial* comes from the Greek *axon* meaning "axis." An axis is an imaginary straight line about which an object rotates. In this case, the body is said to rotate around a straight line represented by the vertebral column.

The appendicular skeleton consists of the shoulder girdle and arms, and the pelvic girdle and legs. The clavicle and the scapula form the shoulder girdle, and the arms are attached to the shoulder girdle at the glenohumeral joint where the glenoid fossa of the scapula articulates with the head of the humerus (the upper arm bone). The pelvic girdle is formed by the ilium, ischium, and pubis. The legs are attached to the pelvic girdle at the coxal joint (hip joint) formed by the articulation of the head of the femur with the acetabulum formed by the bones of the pelvis. The term *appendicular* comes from

---

BOX A-1 Word Breakdown and Origins for Important Musculoskeletal Term

- **Cartilage:** The word cartilage comes from the Latin cartilago meaning "gristle," referring to the gristle-like consistency of cartilage, which is in fact gristle.

- **Articulate:** The word articulate comes from the Latin articul meaning "to join" or "fit together."

- **Synovial:** The term synovial refers to synovial fluid, the clear liquid that lubricates this type of joint; the term is from the Greek syn meaning "together" and Latin ovum meaning "egg" because the fluid resembles egg whites.

- **Ligaments:** This word comes from the Latin ligamentum meaning "a band" or "bandage."

- **Endomysium:** This word is a combination of the Greek prefix endo- meaning "within," "inner," or "containing," and mys meaning "muscle."

- **Fascicle:** This word comes from the Latin fascis meaning "a bundle." The term perimysium is a combination of the Greek prefix peri- meaning "around" and mys meaning "muscle."

- **Epimysium:** This word is a combination of the Greek prefix epi- meaning "on" and mys meaning "muscle."

- **Fascia:** This word is from the Latin meaning "a band" or "fillet."

- **Hypertonicity:** This term comes from the Greek prefix hyper- meaning "excessive" or "above normal" and tonus meaning "tension."

- **Hypotonicity:** This term comes from the Greek prefix hypo- meaning "deficient" or "below normal" and tonus.

- **Contraction:** The term comes from the Latin word contractus meaning "draw together."

- **Isotonic contraction:** Iso- is a Greek prefix meaning "equal," so this term literally means "equal tone."

- **Isometric contraction:** Metron is Greek for "measure," so this term means "equal measure" referring to the fact that the muscle does not change measurement (length).

- **Agonist:** The word comes from the Greek agon meaning "a contest," referring to the fact that some muscles must lengthen (give way) while others contract.

- **Antagonist:** This term comes from the Greek antagonisma meaning "to fight," derived from anti-meaning "against" and agon meaning "contest."

- **Synergist:** This term comes from the Greek prefix syn-meaning "together" and ergon meaning "work."

the Latin root *appendic(o)*, meaning "appendage" (attached to the main structure). So the limbs are often called appendages or extremities.

BONE SHAPES AND MARKINGS

Bones have different shapes to serve specific purposes. They are covered by a fibrous, white membrane called the periosteum, except over areas of articular cartilage. The term *periosteum* is modified Latin from the Greek *peri*, meaning "around," and *osteon*, meaning "bone." It functions in bone growth, repair, and nutrition. It also serves as a point of attachment for ligaments and tendons. Bone shapes include long bones, short bones, flat bones, irregular bones, and sesamoid bones.

Bones also have surface markings that serve specific functions. Roughened areas on a bone might serve as attachment points for tendons or ligaments. Some bones have grooves where blood vessels pass through. A bone might have a hole in it to allow for the passage of nerves or vessels. Long bones have large, rounded ends that form strong joints.

Following are some important terms related to bones:

- Condyle: A rounded articular surface at the end of a bone. An epicondyle is a small projection above a condyle (from the Greek kondylos meaning "knuckle").
- Crest: A bony ridge or distinct border on a bone (from the Latin crista meaning "crest").
- Foramen: An opening in a bone through which blood vessels, ligaments, or nerves pass (from the Latin aperture meaning "a small narrow opening").
- Fossa: A depression in or on a bone (from the Latin term for "a trench or ditch").
- Facet: A small, smooth area on a bone like the facets on each vertebra that articulate with the vertebrae above and below.
- Head: The rounded articular ends at the top of some long bones. The top portion of the femur is called "the head of the femur," while the top portion of the humerus is called "the head of the humerus."
- Meatus: A passageway shaped like a tube that runs within a bone (from the Latin for "passage").
- Process: Any prominent projection on a bone, like the mastoid process of the temporal bone or the spinus processes of the vertebrae (from the Latin processus meaning "an advance, progress, or process").
- Tuberosity: A large, rough, rounded process, like the ischial tuberosity of the pelvis.
- Trochanter: The greater and lesser trochanters are found only on the femur and serve as attachment sites for some of the muscles of the thigh and gluteals. The word trochanter is Greek meaning "a runner" and originally referred to horses that have three trochanters (tro meaning three and canter referring to a horse's running gait), whereas humans have only two.

CARTILAGE

Cartilage is an important connective tissue that provides structure and absorbs shock. Hyaline cartilage occurs over the ends of long bones (where it is also called articular cartilage) and forms the nose, larynx, trachea, bronchi, and anterior ends of the ribs (called costal cartilage). Fibrocartilage is tough and flexible, acting often as a shock absorber in joints like the knees (medial and lateral meniscus) and between the vertebrae (intervertebral discs).

JOINTS

Muscles attach to the bones and contract to move bones where they articulate (meet) at the joints. The varieties of joint types in the body are classified by how the joint is structured and how the joint functions. Some joints move freely, while others move very little, depending on their structure. Some joints have a capsule enclosing the joint, and some don't. Synovial joints are freely movable joints, like the joints at the shoulder and hips. These types of joints have a joint capsule and a synovial membrane that encloses the joint and nourishes the articular cartilage.

Bones in freely movable joints, like synovial joints, are held together by bands of connective tissue called ligaments. Some ligaments are called extracapsular ligaments because they reside outside of the joint capsule. Others are called intracapsular ligaments because they occur within the joint capsule. Sometimes these ligaments are called accessory ligaments to note that they act as an accessory to the joint capsule. For more information on the structure of synovial joints, see Chapter 13, Topic 13-6 (Joint Movements). Following are other important terms related to joints:

- Fibrous joint: A structural classification that refers to joints that have no joint capsule and are held together by fibrous connective tissue like the sutures that hold together the bones of the skull.
- Cartilaginous joint: A structural classification that refers to joints that have no joint capsule and are held together by cartilage. Sometimes the joint is held together by hyaline cartilage that slowly ossifies (hardens) as the individual matures (e.g., the first rib and the sternum). These joints are referred to as synchondroses joints and are immovable. The joints held together by tough, flat discs of fibrocartilage are called symphyses joints and are slightly moveable, like the intravertebral discs.
- Synarthrosis joint: A functional classification that refers to joints that are immovable, like the fibrous suture joints between the bones of the skull.
- Amphiarthrosis joint: A functional classification that refers to joints that are slightly movable, like the cartilaginous discs found between the vertebrae.
- Diarthrosis joint: A functional classification that refers to joints that are freely movable like synovial joints. The name refers to the fact that synovial diarthrotic joints move in paired directions, such as flexion and extension, and adduction and abduction.

The Basics of the Muscular System

The muscular system includes the skeletal muscles that attach to the bones and initiate movement, the cardiac muscle that makes up the walls of the heart, and the smooth muscle present in the walls of organs.

The involuntary muscle that forms most of the heart wall and automatically beats an average of 75 times a minute is called the cardiac muscle. Involuntary muscle contracts as needed automatically, and the contractions cannot be controlled voluntarily through conscious thought. Cardiac muscle is striated (meaning "furrowed"), referring to alternating band-like structures that give the tissue its particular appearance when viewed under a microscope. Smooth muscle is nonstriated involuntary muscle tissue. It is found in the walls of hollow internal structures like blood vessels and the intestines. Smooth muscle tissue has its own integral rhythm, influenced by certain hormones and involuntary nerves. For example, food is moved through the intestines automatically by the wave-like contractions of smooth muscle.

Skeletal muscle is striated muscle that is termed voluntary because it can be deliberately made to contract or relax. It is attached mainly to the bones and moves the skeleton, produces heat to maintain body temperature, helps the body maintain an erect posture, and protects organs from injury. Each muscle is formed from individual muscle fibers wrapped in fibrous connective tissue (fascia) called the endomysium. Individual muscle fibers are formed into bundles called fascicles and wrapped by a fascial perimysium. Multiple groups of fascicles are wrapped by an epimysium to complete the muscle. The meatiest section of a muscle is called the muscle belly. The epimysium is a fibrous connective tissue covering that is continuous with the deep fascia.

FASCIA

Fascia is a sheet-like connective tissue that envelopes the body just below the skin and encloses muscles, groups of muscles, and organs. Superficial fascia (also called the subcutaneous layer) lies just beneath the skin and surrounds the entire body. It varies in thickness from very thin (over the top of the hand) to thick (over the inferior abdominal wall). Superficial fascia is composed of an inner and outer layer filled with adipose (fat) tissue, blood and lymph vessels, and nerves. Deep fascia surrounds individual muscle bellies, penetrates into muscle bellies to surround each muscle fiber, and encloses groups of muscles and organs. It lines the body wall and extremities and carries blood vessels, lymph vessels, and nerves. Continuous with the epimysium, deep fascia provides the point of attachment to the bones for some muscles and fills in the spaces between muscles.

TENDONS

The connective tissue (epimysium) enclosing a muscle merges at each end of the muscle's belly with a tendon. Tendons are a form of connective tissue composed of parallel collagen fibers that connect muscles to the periosteum (the connective tissue that surrounds the bone, as described earlier). In the simplest terms, tendons connect the muscle to the bone. The term *aponeurosis* refers to a very broad, flat tendon.

MUSCLE CHARACTERISTICS

Skeletal muscle has four important characteristics. It responds to stimuli, contracts, extends, and is elastic.

- Muscles responds to stimuli: The characteristic of muscle tissue (also of nerve tissue) that allows it to receive and respond to stimuli is called excitability. The nervous system keeps the muscles in a constant state of readiness, partially contracted. The term tone means the tension present in resting muscle. Hypertonic muscle or hypertonicity refers to a muscle with too much resting tension. Hypotonicity refers to a muscle with too little resting tension.

- Muscles contract: Contractility is the characteristic of muscle tissue that allows it to contract (shorten and thicken) to produce movement at the joints.

- Muscles extend: Opposing muscles usually lengthen during a contraction. The characteristic of muscle tissue that allows it to extend (lengthen) when opposing muscles contract is called extensibility.

- Muscle is elastic: Elasticity is the characteristic of muscle tissue that allows it to return to its original shape after contracting or extending.

MUSCLE CONTRACTIONS

The word "contraction" is a general term indicating that a muscle is either shortening or increasing in tension in response to an effort. The place where a muscle starts on the bone is called its origin. The place where a muscle ends on a bone is called its insertion. The origin and insertion are both called attachment sites, so sometimes the origin is referred to as the proximal attachment and the insertion as the distal attachment. When a muscle shortens, the insertion moves toward the origin; put in another way, the origin and insertion are drawn together. The term *fire* is slang for contraction (e.g., "fire your deltoid muscle"). The muscle might also be "shortened," which refers to an isotonic contraction, a specific type of muscle contraction. Muscle contractions are further defined as follows:

- Isometric contraction: In an isometric contraction, tension is generated but the joint angle and muscle length do not change. Isometric contractions are important because they are used to stabilize joints such as when an object is held in a fixed position. For example, pushing the hands against a wall causes an isometric contraction because the tension increases in the arm muscles but their length stays the same.

- Isotonic contraction: This is a muscle contraction where the muscle length and joint angle are changed in response to the tension generated in the muscle. Eccentric and concentric contractions are the two different types of isotonic contractions.

- Concentric contraction: In a concentric contraction, tension shortens the muscle and the joint angle decreases to initiate or accelerate movement.

- Eccentric contraction: In an eccentric contraction tension is generated while the muscle lengthens and the joint angle increases. These types of contractions are often used to control movement such as lowering yourself into a chair.

Isotonic contractions produce movements like walking, running, and bending over, but isometric contractions are also occurring. Most movements involve a combination of both types of contractions from different muscle groups. For example, when walking, certain muscles must contract isotonically to move the body forward, while other muscles contract isometrically to stabilize the body so it can remain upright.

Muscle Roles in Movement

During movement, different sets of muscles play different roles and muscles must work together to create movement, assist with a movement, or perform opposite actions.

- Agonists, also called prime movers, are muscles that contract to carry out a specific action (movement). They are the main muscles involved in performing the movement.
- Antagonists are muscles that have the opposite action to the agonist; they must extend when the prime mover contracts.
- A synergist is a muscle that aids the action of another. Synergistic muscles have similar actions and thus support each other in movements.

Terms for Body Positions

During a massage session, the client's body takes a number of different body positions, which are identified by specific names. Instructors usually use these positional terms when giving directions. Massage therapists use these terms to document a session, describe certain steps of a session to another therapist, or discuss the client's condition with another healthcare provider. For example, an instructor might say, "Please have your client get on the massage table in the prone position."; in this case the student will be working on the client's posterior body because in a prone position the client

BOX A-2 Terms to Know for the Musculoskeletal System

Agonists (prime movers)	Fascia	Muscle tone
Antagonists	Fascicle	Nonstriated
Appendicular skeleton	Hyaline cartilage	Perimysium
Articulation	Hypertonic	Periosteum
Axial skeleton	Hypotonic	Skeletal muscle
Cartilage	Involuntary muscle	Smooth muscle
Contractility	Isometric contraction	Striated
Deep fascia	Isotonic contraction	Superficial fascia
Elasticity	Joint	Synergists
Endomysium	Ligament	Synovial fluid
Epimysium	Muscle belly	Tendon
Excitability	Muscle insertion	Vertebral column
Extensibility	Muscle origin	Voluntary muscle

is lying face down. Following are commonly used position terms:

- Anatomical position: In this position, a person stands with both feet facing forward, a shoulders-width apart. The arms are at the sides with the palms facing forward. In the following section on directional terms, the planes of the body and body regions are described in terms of the anatomical position. When the location of body structures is described, it is assumed that the body is in the anatomical position because otherwise descriptions could be confusing. For example, the liver is located superior to (above) the transverse colon on the right side of the body with the body in the anatomical position. If the person were doing a handstand, however, the liver would seem to be inferior to (below) the transverse colon.
- Supine position: In this position, a person is lying on the back face up. With the client in a supine position, the therapist can massage the anterior legs, feet, abdominal muscles, upper chest, arms, neck, and face. In some techniques, certain areas of the back can also be massaged while in the supine position, with the therapist using the client's body weight to facilitate the stroke.
- Prone position: In this position, a person is lying face down, usually with the face in a cradle so the cervical vertebrae are aligned with the rest of the spinal column. With the client in a prone position, the therapist can massage the posterior legs, feet, gluteal muscles, back, posterior neck, and arms.
- Side-lying position: In this position, the client lies on the side with one leg positioned on a bolster and a pillow in front of the chest to support the upper body. This position is most often used for pregnant women or for clients who feel uncomfortable lying prone or supine. All body areas are accessible in this position, although appropriate draping and good body mechanics during techniques require some practice. The side-lying position is also called the lateral recumbent position.
- Semi-reclined position: In this position, a client lies supine but pillows elevate the upper body so that the client is half-sitting. This position is most often used for pregnant women or clients whose sinuses have become congested during the first part of the treatment (usually from lying in the prone position).
- Seated position: In this position, a client is seated in a regular chair or a massage chair for the massage or for assessment (e.g., range of motion assessment).
- Erect position: In this position, the client stands in a relaxed posture with the arms hanging naturally at the sides. This position is used during posture assessments and is different from the anatomical position in that the client assumes their normal standing position so that the therapist can determine muscular holding patterns.

Although these terms are used with other healthcare providers, they should not be used to give the client directions. A client who is asked to "please situate yourself in the supine position under the sheet" is likely to feel confused. Instead, use layman's terms to explain directions to clients, such as saying, "Please lie down face up and under the sheet when you finish undressing."

Directional Terms

Directional terms provide a precise way to indicate where a structure is located or to indicate the relationship of one structure to another structure. For example, an instructor might say, "I want everyone to focus on the anterior of the body today during massage exchanges." This means students will likely place their client in the supine position and massage the front of the body. When documenting the massage session, the therapist also uses directional terms to indicate where a client reported pain or another sensation; where a muscle felt especially tight, or the location of a spasm, tender point, or other condition. Massage therapists use a number of different terms to indicate location and direction, as follows.

- Anterior (ventral): Refers to the front of the body or to structures toward the front of the body. The term ventral is used less often than anterior. This term is from the Latin venter meaning "belly."
- Posterior (dorsal): Refers to the back of the body or to structures toward the back of the body. The term dorsal is also widely used and is Latin for "back." It might also refer to the top of the foot or the back of the hand.
- Proximal: Refers to being nearest the trunk or, when a specific structure is being referred to, the part nearest the structure's point of origin. A massage therapist massaging the client's leg is working nearest the trunk (proximal) when working on the thigh.
- Distal: Refers to being furthest away from the trunk or, when a specific structure is being referred to, the area of the structure that is furthest from the point of origin.
- Medial: Refers to the middle or centerline of the body. A therapist wanting to explain the position of the heart in relationship to the lungs might note that the heart is medial and the lungs are lateral. Or a therapist might say, "The client experiences mild pain on the medial wrist." In this case, the anatomical position becomes important: if the client is in a completely relaxed position, the medial wrist could be confused with the lateral wrist depending on how the client's hand is positioned. Therapists should describe the wrist as if the client were in the anatomical position, such that the medial wrist is on the ulnar side (on the side of the little finger, also known as the fifth phalange).
- Lateral: Refers to the structures that are on the sides of the body and out from the body's center. The lateral cartilage of the nose is located in the outside walls of the nose rather than the center. In the anterior thigh, there are four muscles known collectively as the quadriceps. They are the quadriceps femoris, rectus femoris, vastus lateralis, and vastus medialis. From the muscle names, it is easy to figure out

that vastus lateralis is on the outside of the leg and the vastus medialis on the inside of the leg.
- Unilateral: Refers to something on one side only. A client with unilateral neck pain is experiencing pain only on one side of the neck.
- Bilateral: Refers to both sides. A client with bilateral neck pain is experiencing pain on both sides of the neck.
- Superior: Refers to being situated above something or closer to the head.
- Inferior: Refers to being situated below something or closer to the feet. You can deduce that the inferior angle of the scapula (as opposed to the superior angle) is the curved section of the scapula that lies closest to the feet.
- Palmar/dorsal: The term palmar is used only for the palm of the hand. The term dorsal refers to the back of the hand (away from the palm). An instructor might say, "Make sure you massage both the palmar and dorsal surfaces of the hand" (e.g., the front and back).
- Plantar/dorsal: The term plantar is used only when referring to the sole, bottom, or plantar surface of the foot. The term dorsal refers to the top of the foot. For example, when the foot is plantar flexed, the foot is pointed down (the foot moves toward the plantar surface). When the foot is dorsiflexed, the toes move up toward the knee (the foot moves away from the plantar surface).
- Internal: The word internal is from the Latin internus meaning "inside." In anatomy, the term is used to refer to anything situated away from the surface of the body, such as organs like the liver and spleen.
- External: From the Latin externus meaning "outside," this term refers to the outer surface of the body.
- Superficial: Structures that are superficial lie closer to the surface. For example, if you are told the trapezius is superficial to the rhomboid muscles, you know the rhomboids are underneath the trapezius.
- Deep: Structures that are deep lie away from the surface of the body. It is important to consider the anatomical position when using the terms superficial and deep. In the anatomical position facing the front of the body, the kidneys are deep to the lungs, liver, and heart. When describing the position of the kidneys in relationship to these other structures, this anatomical position is assumed, even though when the massage therapist is working on a client's back, the kidneys are actually above the lungs, liver, and heart.
- Valgus: Valgus is the modified Latin meaning "turned outward." The term refers to any of the paired joints in the extremities such as the elbow or knees. Valgus is a deformity where the bone distal to the joint deviates laterally from the proximal bone causing an outward angulation of the distal bone. In a valgus deformity of the lower extremity, the knees look as if they are knocking together and one or both lower legs jut outward at a distinct angle.
- Varus: Varus is the modified Latin meaning "bent inward." Like valgus, varus refers to the paired joints of the

extremities. In this case, the bone distal to the joint deviates medially from the proximal bone causing an inward angulation of the distal bone. In a varus deformity of the lower extremity, the knees look as if they are rounded out (bowlegged) and one or both lower legs jut inward at a distinct angle.

- Radial: Refers to the radius, a bone in the forearm, or to the structures that lie close to it (e.g., radial artery, radial nerve). In the anatomical position, the radius is situated lateral to the ulna; therefore the term radial is equivalent to the term lateral when discussing the upper extremity.

- Ulnar: Refers to the ulna, a bone in the forearm, or to the structures that lie close to it (e.g., ulnar nerve, ulnar vein). In the anatomical position, the ulna is situated medial to the radius; therefore the term ulnar is equivalent to the term medial when discussing the upper extremity.

- Peripheral: Refers to the periphery of the body or parts that lie away from the center. It is used in anatomical terms such as the peripheral nervous system (as opposed to the central nervous system).

- Central: Refers to the middle of the body, the internal core of the body, or the middle of specific structures or systems. The central nervous system consists of the brain and spinal cord and is the processing center for everything that happens in the body.

Terms for Body Planes

Body planes are imaginary planes that divide the body into different sections. Because joint movements occur within these imaginary planes, they help us to explain and understand movement. Motion at the body's joints occur parallel to the imaginary planes. Front to back movements occur in the sagittal plane. Side to side movements occur in the frontal (also called the coronal) plane and rotational movements occur in the transverse plane.

- The sagittal plane divides the body into left and right parts with a straight vertical line (also referred to as a longitudinal line). The sagittal plane runs through the midline of the body and is also called the midsagittal plane or the median plane when the left and right parts are equal. A parasagittal plane is a straight vertical line that divides the body into unequal left and right parts. The word sagittal is from the Latin sagitta meaning "arrow." The movements of flexion and extension (front to back movements) occur in the sagittal plane.

- The frontal plane, also called the coronal plane, divides the body into anterior and posterior parts with a straight vertical line that is at right angles to the sagittal plane. The movements of adduction and abduction (side-to-side movements) occur in the frontal plane.

- The transverse plane divides the body into superior and inferior parts with a straight horizontal line. Rotation occurs in the transverse plane.

Terms for Body Movements

Body movement terms referring to the appendicular skeleton usually refer to joints and not to general structures like "legs" or "arms." For example, the triceps brachii muscle extends the elbow joint (not the forearm) and extends the shoulder joint (not the arm). The semitendinosus muscle flexes the knee joint (not the lower leg) and extends the hip joint (not the thigh). When referring to the axial skeleton, the general structures are often referred to, and sometimes the specific joints also. For example, the scalenes rotate the head and neck (general structure) to the opposite side. The erector spinae group produces lateral flexion of the vertebral column (specific joints), although one can also correctly say trunk (general structure). Massage therapists use a number of different terms to indicate movement, as described below.

- Flexion takes place in the sagittal plane with the body part moving anteriorly (with the exception of the knee). The knee flexes posterior in the sagittal plane. It is the opposite movement to extension.

- Extension takes place in the sagittal plane with the body part moving posteriorly (with the exception of the knee). The knee extends in an anterior movement in the sagittal plane. It is the opposite movement to flexion.

- Abduction takes place in the coronal plane with the body part moving laterally away from the body. Abduction happens only in the appendicular skeleton as the limbs move out from the midline of the body. The fingers and toes are abducted when they are spread apart. Abduction is an opposite movement to adduction.

- Adduction takes place in the coronal plane with the body part moving medially toward the body. Like abduction, adduction happens only in the limbs, which move in toward the midline of the body. The fingers and toes are adducted when they are brought together. Adduction is an opposite movement to abduction.

- Lateral rotation takes place in the transverse plane when a limb (anterior surface) turns away from the midline to face laterally. Lateral rotation only occurs in the appendicular skeleton (hip joint and shoulder joint). Lateral rotation is an opposite movement to medial rotation.

BOX A-3 Terms to Know for Positions and Directions

Anatomical position	Internal	Semi-reclined
Anterior	Lateral	Side lying
Bilateral	Medial	Superficial
Central	Palmar	Superior
Deep	Peripheral	Supine
Distal	Plantar	Ulnar
Dorsal	Posterior	Unilateral
Erect	Prone	Valgus
External	Proximal	Varus
Inferior	Radial	

- Medial rotation takes place in the transverse plane when a limb (anterior surface) turns in to face the midline. Medial rotation only occurs in the appendicular skeleton (hip joint and shoulder joint). Medial rotation is an opposite movement to lateral rotation.

- Rotation (right or left) takes place in the transverse plane when the anterior surface of the body part rotates right or left. Rotation refers only to the axial body (head and vertebral column). For example, stand with your face forward and turn your chin toward your right shoulder. Your head and neck have just performed the right rotation. Now, stand in the anatomical position and turn your trunk to the left without moving your feet. This is left rotation of the trunk (or vertebral column).

- Ipsilateral rotation refers to a movement that may occur in the axial skeleton. The term ipsilateral means on the same side with reference to a given point; the term is from the Latin ipsi meaning "same" and latus meaning "side." For example, the levator scapulae are muscles located on either side of the posterior neck. One of the actions of the individual levator muscles is ipsilateral rotation of the neck. This means that the muscle turns the head to the same side on which the muscle is located. The right levator scapula rotates the head to the right. The left levator scapula rotates the head to the left.

- Contralateral rotation refers to a movement that may occur in the axial skeleton. The term means on or to the opposite side with reference to a given point. It may refer to muscle movements or to a situation in which pain or another sensation is felt on the side opposite an injury or condition. The trapezius is a large, diamond-shaped muscle on the posterior neck and back that has upper, middle, and lower sections. It also has left and right sections. The actions of the upper sections include contralateral rotation of the neck and head. The left upper section of the trapezius turns the head to the right, and the right upper section turns the head left. The superior portions of the muscles cross the cervical spine and so can turn the head in the opposite direction to the side where the muscle is located.

- Lateral flexion (right or left) takes place in the coronal plane when the axial body part bends either to the right or to the left. Stand in the anatomical position and move your right ear toward your right shoulder without rotating your head and neck and without lifting your shoulder—this is right lateral flexion of the head and neck. Now place your hands on your waist and bend your trunk to the left to perform left lateral flexion of the trunk, head, and neck.

- Supination is a movement where the forearm rotates so that the palm is facing upward and the radius and ulna are parallel to each other. Supination is an opposite movement to pronation.

- Pronation is a movement where the forearm rotates so that the palm is facing downward and the radius crosses over the ulna. Pronation is an opposite movement to supination.

- Elevation is a movement that can occur at the mandible, scapula, clavicle, pelvis, and hyoid bone where the body part moves superiorly (up). When the mouth is closed, the mandible is elevated. When you shrug your shoulders, the scapula is elevated. Elevation is an opposite movement to depression.

- Depression is a movement that can occur at the mandible, scapula, clavicle, pelvis, and hyoid bone where the body part moves inferiorly (down). When the mouth is open, the mandible is depressed. Depression is an opposite movement to elevation.

- Protraction is a movement that can occur at the mandible, scapula, and clavicle where the body part moves anteriorly. When the jaw is jutted forward, the mandible is protracted. Protraction is an opposite movement to retraction.

- Retraction is a movement that can occur at the mandible, scapula, and clavicle where the body part moves posteriorly. When the jaw is pulled back, the mandible is retracted. Retraction is an opposite movement to protraction.

- Upward rotation is a movement when the scapula rotates so that the glenoid fossa moves superiorly. Upward rotation is an opposite movement to downward rotation.

- Downward rotation is a movement when the scapula rotates so that the glenoid fossa moves inferiorly. Downward rotation is an opposite movement to upward rotation.

- Inversion is a movement that occurs in the tarsal joints of the foot when the plantar surface of the foot pivots to face the midline of the body. Inversion is an opposite movement to eversion.

- Eversion is a movement that occurs in the tarsal joints of the foot when the plantar surface of the foot pivots to face laterally. Eversion is an opposite movement to inversion.

- Dorsiflexion is a movement that occurs in the joints of the foot when the dorsal surface of the foot moves superiorly so that the toes point up to the sky and slightly back toward the knee. Dorsiflexion is an opposite movement to plantarflexion.

- Plantarflexion is a movement that occurs in the joints of the foot when the plantar surface of the foot moves inferiorly so that the toes are pointed downward. Plantarflexion is an opposite movement to dorsiflexion.

- Opposition is a series of movements that occur at the thumb allowing the thumb to flex, adduct, and medially rotate to cross the palm and touch the fifth finger (little finger).

- Circumduction is a series of movements that occur at the shoulder and hip joints when these body areas flex, abduct, extend, and then adduct in an arching motion such as when swimming the backstroke.

Muscle Names

A massage student who recognizes muscle names can more easily find the muscle in the body, palpate the muscle, and understand how the muscle works.

Muscles are named by the fiber direction of the muscle, the location of the muscle or its location in relationship to other muscles, its size and structure or shape of the muscle, where

BOX A-4 **Terms to Know for Planes and Movements**

Abduction	Flexion	Plantarflexion
Adduction	Frontal (coronal) plane	Pronation
Circumduction	Inversion	Protraction
Contralateral rotation	Ipsilateral rotation	Retraction
Depression	Lateral flexion	Rotation
Dorsiflexion	Lateral rotation	Sagittal plane
Downward rotation	Medial rotation	Supination
Elevation	Opposition	Transverse plane
Eversion	Planes of the body	Upward rotation
Extension		

the muscle originates or inserts, or what types of actions (movements) the muscle performs.

The term *rectus* means "straight" and refers to the organization of muscle fibers along the sagittal axis of the body (running in a vertical line). Several muscles in the body have the name rectus, including the rectus abdominus (abdominal area) and rectus femoris (thigh area). You should therefore know that the muscle fibers run straight up and down. Other muscle names that refer to fiber direction are transversus (running along the coronal/frontal plane) and oblique. Oblique muscles run at an oblique angle across the sagittal axis of the body. A muscle called a "flexor" is likely to flex a body part while a muscle called an "extensor" is likely to extend the body part. Adductors adduct and abductors abduct. The gluteus maximus is likely to be larger than the gluteus medius or gluteus minimus. Table A-4 describes word components in muscle names to help you better understand muscles and their actions.

Terms Related to Pathology

Pathology is the medical science concerned with disease or abnormal function. *Path(o)* is from the Greek word *pathos* meaning "suffering" and is part of words like *pathogen* (an agent that causes disease), *pathological* (the nature of a disease), and *pathologist* (a physician who specializes in understanding disease). Pharmacology is the science of drugs and their sources. *Pharmacology* is from the Greek word *pharmakon* meaning "medicine." Pharmacology terms and medications that may affect a client's response to massage

TABLE A-4   **Muscle Name Components**

Word Component	Meaning	Word Component	Meaning
Abdominal, abdominis	Abdominal region	Middle	Middle
Abductor	Abducts the part	Minimi, minimus	Least
Anconeus	Refers to the elbow	Minor	Smaller
Anguli	Angle	Multi	Many
Anterior	Front	Nasalis, nasi	Nose
Articularis	Refers to a joint	Oblique, obliquus	Running at an oblique angle
Auricularis	Ear	Obturator	To stop or obstruct
Biceps	Two heads (origins)	Occipitals, occipito	Refers to the occiput
Brachialis, brachii	Refers to the arm	Oculi	Refers to the eye
Brevis	Brief, short	Opponens	Opposing
Buccinator	Refers to the cheek	Orbicularis	A small circle
Capitis	Head	Oris	Mouth
Carpi	Carpal bones	Ossei	Bone
Cervicis	Cervical vertebrae	Palmar, palmaris	Refers to the palm
Clavius, cleido	Clavicle	Pectineus	Means "comb"
Colli	Neck	Pectoralis	Refers to the chest
Coraco	Relating to the coracoid process of the scapula	Pedis	Refers to the foot
Costarum, costal, costales, costalis	Ribs	Piriformis	Means "pear shaped"
Deltoid	Shaped like the Greek letter delta	Plantae, plantar, plantaris	Refers to the plantar surface of the foot
Depressor	Flattens or lowers the part	Platysma	Broad, referring to the shape of the muscle

(Continued)

TABLE A-4   Muscle Name Components *(Continued)*

Word Component	Meaning	Word Component	Meaning
Diaphragm	Means "partition"	Pollicis	Refers to the thumb
Digastric	Muscle with two bellies	Popliteus	Means "ham of the knee" the back of the knee
Digiti, digitorum	Finger or toe	Posterior	Behind, toward the back
Dorsal, dorsi	Back, backside	Profundus	Deep
Erector	Muscles that raise or erect the vertebral column	Pronator	Turns the part so that it faces downward
Extensor	Extends the part	Proparietalis	Refers to the parietal bone
External, externus	Outside, outer	Psoas	Loin
Fasciae	Means "bandage"	Pterygoid	Wing shaped
Femoris	Relating to the femur or thigh	Quadratus	Squared
Fibularis	Relating to the fibula	Qudriceps	Four heads
Fidus	To split	Radialis	Refers to the radius
Flexor	Muscle that flexes a part	Rectus	Straight
Frontalis	Refers to the frontal bone	Rhomboids	Referring to a geometric shape
Gastrocnemius	Refers to the calf	Rotatores	To turn
Gemellus	Means "twin"	Sartorius	Means "tailor"
Genu	Refers to the knee	Scalene	Uneven or a ladder referring to the way the muscles attach up the cervical vertebrae
Gluteus	Relating to the buttocks	Scapulae, scapularis	Scapula
Gracilis	Means "slender," "graceful"	Semi	Half
Hallucis	Refers to the big toe	Semimembranosus	Name refers to its tendon that resembles a flat membrane
Hyoid	Refers to the hyoid bone	Semitendinosus	Name refers to the muscles long tendon
Iliacus, ilio	Refers to the ilium	Septi	Refers to the nasal septum
Indicis	Refers to the index finger	Serratus	A "notching" referring to the way the muscles attach to the ribs
Inferior, inferioris, infra	Below	Soleus	Sole of the foot
Inter	Between	Spinae	A thorn, referring to the spine
Internal, internus	Inside, inner	Spinalis	Refers to the spinus processes
Interossei	Between the bones	Spinatus	Spine
Intertransversarii	Between the transverse processes	Splenius	Means "bandage"
Labii	Refers to the lip	Sterno	Refers to the sternum
Latae	Refers to lateral (the side)	Sub	Under
Lateral, lateralis	To the side	Superficialis	Superficial
Latissimus	Wide	Superior, superioris	Upper, higher than
Levator	Muscle that lifts a part	Supinator	Turns the part so that it faces upward
Longissimus	Very long	Supra	Above
Longus	Long	Tempo, temporalis	Refers to the temporal bone
Lubricals	Means "earthworm"	Tensor	Means "stretcher"

TABLE A-4   Muscle Name Components *(Continued)*

Word Component	Meaning	Word Component	Meaning
Lumborum, lumbricals	Low back, lumbar region	Teres	Round
Magnus	Great, large	Tertius	Third, referring to where the muscle occurs on the bone
Major	Larger	Thoracis	Referring to the thorax
Manus	Refers to the hand	Tibialis	Refers to the tibia
Masseter	Means "chewer"	Transverso	Refers to the transverse processes
Mastoid	Refers to the mastoid process	Transversus	Running transversely (horizontally)
Maximus	Greatest	Trapezius	Name refers to the shape of a muscle, like a trapezoid
Medial, medius	Medial	Triceps	Three heads
Membranosus	Shape of a membrane	Ulnaris	Refers to the ulna or ulnar side
Mentalis	Chin	Vastus	Vast
		Zygomaticus	Refers to the zygomatic bone

are discussed in depth in Chapter 5, Massage Cautions and Contraindications.

- Indication: When a therapeutic treatment is likely to benefit a client and have no adverse reactions, it is indicated (from the Latin in-dico, meaning "to point out"). In medicine, the term refers more specifically to the rationale behind the use of a treatment based on signs, symptoms, or a diagnosis.

- Contraindication: When a therapeutic treatment might harm a client or cause an adverse reaction, it is contraindicated (Latin prefix contra- meaning "opposed" or "against").

- Idiopathic: A disease or condition that develops spontaneously or without a known cause is referred to as an idiopathic disease.

- Etiology: The study of the cause of a disease, or the theory of the origin of a disease. This term might also be used to describe the set of factors that contributes to the occurrence of a disease.

- Inflammation: Inflammation is the response of living tissue to injury, infection, or irritation. Heat, redness, swelling, and pain are present at the site and in surrounding tissue.

- Acute: A disease may be classified as acute, subacute, or chronic, based on the severity of the symptoms and the duration of the disease. These terms also apply to the healing process of soft-tissue injuries. Acute diseases are severe but only last a short time. A soft-tissue injury like a sprained ankle is considered to be acute while it is red, hot, swollen, and very painful. As the sprain begins to heal, it moves into the subacute stage and then into the chronic stage.

- Subacute: A patient or client with a condition that has entered the subacute stage still has symptoms, but they are less severe than in an acute stage. Normal function is slowly returning, but the body or body area is not yet at full strength.

- Chronic: The term chronic has two related but different meanings. Sometimes a condition or disease persists for a very long time or regularly recurs. This is called a chronic condition, such as chronic hepatitis. In the case of a soft-tissue injury, the term chronic indicates the last stage of healing. In the chronic stage of healing, the therapist aims to help the client return to full function and build strength to avoid re-injury. Diagnose: Before treating a patient, the doctor must first identify the disease or condition. The naming of a set of signs and symptoms is called diagnosis. Massage therapists never diagnose conditions or diseases because this activity is out of our scope of practice.

- Signs: Signs are defined as objective physical manifestations that the doctor or therapist can observe. For example, if a therapist is performing a posture analysis of a client and observes that one shoulder is elevated higher than the other, this is a sign of likely muscle tension in the region.

- Symptoms: Symptoms are defined as subjective abnormal physical manifestations that the patient or client reports. For example, if the client reports pain on both sides of the neck, this is a symptom.

- Prognosis: A prognosis (from the Greek pro- meaning "before" and gignosko "to know") is a prediction of the probable course and outcome of the disease based on the condition of the patient and the doctor's knowledge of the disease.

Abbreviations

Abbreviations are used in written communication such as SOAP charting, a form of charting often used to document massage sessions and by healthcare providers or the public during verbal communication. For example, people regularly

BOX A-5 Terms to Know for Pathology

Acute	Idiopathic	Prognosis
Chronic	Indication	Signs
Contraindication	Inflammation	Subacute
Diagnose	Pathology	Symptoms
Etiology	Pharmacology	

say AIDS and MS rather than acquired immune deficiency syndrome or multiple sclerosis. Abbreviations for words or phrases take up less space on the page and allow the therapist to write more quickly. Most common medical abbreviations can be found in a medical dictionary, but some abbreviations specific to massage may not be included. Therapists may also develop their own abbreviations when they do not already exist for common massage terms. This is fine, so long as a key is provided in the event another person must read the chart notes. Common abbreviations related to appropriate terms are listed in Tables A-5, A-6, and A-7. Students are encouraged

TABLE A-5 Common Abbreviations for Position and Directions

Anterior	Ant
Bilateral	BL
Caudal	Cd
Cephalic	ceph
Deep	dp
Distal	dist
External	ext
Inferior	inf
Internal	int
Lateral	lat
Left	L
Medial	med
Midline	ML
Posterior	post
Prone	pr
Proximal	prox
Right	R
Side-lying	sl
Superficial	super
Superior	sup
Supine	sup
Unilateral	unilat

TABLE A-6 Common Abbreviations for Body Planes and Movements

Abduction	abd
Adduction	add
Articulation	art
Circumduction	circ
Depression	dep
Dorsiflexion	DF
Elevation	ele
Eversion	ever
Extension	extn
External	ext
Flexion	flex
Frontal/coronal plane	front
Inversion	inv
Lateral flexion	lat flex
Opposition	opp
Planter flexion	PF
Pronation	pro
Protraction	ptx
Retraction	rtx
Rotation	rot
Sagittal plane	sag
Supination	sup
Transverse plane	trans

to use abbreviations when taking notes in class to build and integrate this important skill.

In any massage textbook or class, and in any conversation with other healthcare providers, healthcare terminology factor is prominent in communication. Examine the following paragraph from this chapter and consider the medical terms you need to know in order to understand what you are reading:

Small oval- or bean-shaped structures that reside along the length of lymphatic vessels are called lymph nodes. On its way back to the cardiovascular system, lymph enters a lymph node and circulates through the node's sinuses where foreign substances are filtered out of the lymph and destroyed by white blood cells and phagocytic cells. Lymph nodes usually occur in groups (named for the region in which they reside as in axillary nodes or inguinal nodes) and are arranged in superficial and deep layers.

Wow, just one paragraph requires you to know a lot of information about the body! Too often, students rush through reading assignments or fail to completely understand an instructor's lecture. Students who take the time to learn

TABLE A-7　Common Abbreviations for Anatomy and Body Regions

Abdominal muscles/region	abs
Bone	os
Central nervous system	CNS
Cervical region	C, C1-C7
Chest	ch
Cranium	Cr
Diaphragm	dia
Elbow	elb
Femur	FE
Gluteal muscles/region	gluts
Greater trochanter	GT
Head	hd
Head and neck	H&N
Heart	he
Humerus	hum
Intervertebral disc	IVD
Joint	J, jt
Large intestine	LI
Lower extremity	LE
Lumbar region	L, L1-5

TABLE A-7　Common Abbreviations for Anatomy and Body Regions (*Continued*)

Lymph node	LN
Lymph vessel	LV
Muscle	mm
Musculoskeletal	ms
Nerves	nn
Nervous system	ns
Occiput or occipital region	occ
Parasympathetic nervous system	PNS
Rib cage	RC
Shoulder	sh
Soft tissue	ST
Sternum	st
Subcutaneous	sc
Thoracic region	T, T1-12
Throat	th
Tibia	tib
Upper extremity	UE
Vertebrae	vert
Viscera	visc

healthcare terminology, look up unknown words, and ask the instructor questions are most likely to achieve academic and professional success. At the end of a reading assignment, lecture, or class discussion ask yourself:

- Did I have the vocabulary I needed to understand the text?
- Did I understand the vocabulary the instructor used?
- Did I have the vocabulary I needed to express my ideas about the human body clearly?

If the answer to any of these is "no," start by making flash cards of terms and their definitions and begin to build your vocabulary now. If you work hard, you will have the words you need to convey your ideas and thoughts about the human body. You are also more likely to pass your licensure or certification examination and build a better client base through referrals from other healthcare providers.

Appendix B: References

CHAPTER 1

1. Calvert RN. *The History of Massage: An Illustrated Survey from Around the World*. Rochester, VA: Healing Arts Press; 2002.
2. Berndt CH, Berndt RM. *The Aboriginal Australians: The First Pioneers*. Carlton, Australia: Pitman Publishing Pty Ltd.; 1978.
3. Devanesen D. Traditional aboriginal medicine practice in the Northern Territory. Paper presented at the International Symposium on Traditional Medicine. World Health Organization Center for Development. Kobe, Japan, 2000.
4. Elkin AP. *Aboriginal Men of High Degree*. 2nd ed. Brisbane, Australia: University of Queensland Press; 1977.
5. Lhuillier AR. *The Ancient Maya*. http://www.mayacalendar.com/theancientmaya.html. Viewed August 16, 2006.
6. Rombough J. *Aztec Medicine*. http://lark.cc.ku.edu/family/julia/hiscover.htm. Viewed August 16, 2006.
7. Ortiz de Montellano B. *Aztec Medicine, Health, and Nutrition*. New Brunswick, NJ: Rutgers University Press; 1990.
8. Smith ME. *The Aztecs*. London, UK: Blackwell Publishers Ltd.; 1996.
9. Alba HR. *Sweat Lodge: Temazcal—The Traditional Mexican Sweat Bath*. Instituto Mexicano de Medicinas Tradicionales Tlahuilli A.C. http://www.experiencefestival.com/a/Sweat_Lodge/id/1014. Viewed August 16, 2006.
10. Garrett JT, Garrett M. *Medicine of the Cherokee: The Way of Right Relationships*. Rochester, VA: Bear and Company Publishing; 1996.
11. Moon C. *A Medicine Woman Speaks. An Exploration of Native American Spirituality*. Franklin, NJ: New Page Books; 2001.
12. Graham D. *Manual Therapeutics: A Treatise on Massage: Its History, Mode of Application and Effects*. 3rd ed. Philadelphia, PA: J.B. Lippincott; 1902.
13. Page J. *In the Hands of the Great Spirit: The 20,000 Year History of the American Indians*. New York, NY: Free Press; 2003.
14. Kerenyi C. *The Gods of the Greeks*. London, UK: Thames & Hudson; 1951.
15. Burckhardt J. *A History of Greek Culture*. Mineola, NY: Dover Publication Inc.; 2002.
16. Guthrie D. *A History of Medicine*. 2nd ed. London, UK: Nelson and Sons; 1958.
17. Osler W. *The Evolution of Modern Medicine*. Whitefish, MT: Kessinger Publishing; 2004.
18. Kellogg JH. *The Art of Massage: A Practical Manual for the Nurse, the Student, and the Practitioner*. Whitefish, MT: Kessinger Publishing; 2004.
19. Green RM. *A Translation of Galen's Hygiene*. Springfield, IL: Charles C. Thomas Publishing; 1951.
20. Roberts JM. *The New Penguin History of the World*. London, UK: Penguin Books; 2002.
21. Mochizuki JS. *Anma: The Art of Japanese Massage*. Saint Paul, MN: Kotobuki Publications; 1995.
22. Amaro J. *Historical Perspectives of Accurpuncture*. http://www.iama.edu/articles/historicalperspectiveofacu.htm. Viewed August 15, 2006.
23. Somma C. Shiatsu. Princeton, NJ: Pearson Education, Inc,. 2007.
24. Wujastyk D. *The Roots of Ayurveda: Selections from Sanskrit Medical Writings*. London, UK: Penguin Books; 2003.
25. Warrier G, Gunawant D. *The Complete Illustrated Guide to Ayurveda: The Ancient Indian Healing Tradition*. Shaftesbury, Dorset, UK: Element Books Inc.; 1997.
26. Frawley D, Ranade S. *Ayurveda, Nature's Medicine*. Twin Lakes, WI: Lotus Press; 2001.
27. Apfelbaum A. *Thai Massage, Sacred Bodywork*. New York: Avery (Penguin Group); 2004.
28. Chow KT, Moody E. *Thai Yoga Therapy, An Ayurvedic Tradition*. Rochester, VA: Healing Arts Press; 2006.
29. Introduction to Tibetan Medicine by Bonnie Pasqualoni. http://www.dharma-haven.org/tibetan/tibetan-art-of-healing.htm#Tibetan%20Art%20of%20Healing. Viewed August 2006.
30. Tibetan Medicine Foundation. http://www.amfoundation.org/tibetanmedicine.htm. Viewed August 2006.
31. The Timeless Wisdom of the Tibetans, by Craig Hamilton-Parker: http://www.tibetan-buddhism.com/tibetanmedicine.html. Viewed August 2006.
32. Traditional Tibetan Medicine. http://www.ctibet.org.cn/en/tm.htm. Viewed August 2006.
33. Medicine Buddha and Tibetan Medicine: http://www.tibetan-medicine.org/medicinebuddha.asp Tibetan Medical and Astro. Institute of H. H. Dalai Lama. Viewed August 2006.
34. Freeman C. *Egypt, Greece and Rome: Civilizations of the Ancient Mediterranean*. 2nd ed. New York, NY: Oxford University Press; 2004.
35. Behringer W. *Witches and Witch Hunts, A Global History*. Cambridge, UK: Polity Press; 2004.
36. Burns WE. *Witch Hunts in Europe and America: An Encyclopedia*. Westport, CT: Greenwood Press; 2003.
37. Medieval Medicine. http://www.wikipedia.org/wiki/medieval_medicine. Viewed August 2006.
38. Cantor N. *In the Wake of the Plague: The Black Death and the World it Made*. New York, NY: Perennial Books; 2001.
39. Porter R. *Cambridge Illustrated History of Medicine*. Cambridge, UK: Cambridge University Press; 1996.
40. Da Vinci L, Brown JW. *A Treatise on Painting: With a Life of Leonardo and an Account of His Works*. Adament Media Company, Elibron Classics Series; 2006.
41. Vesilius A, Jackson I, Park K. De *Humani Corporis fabrica (CD-ROM)*. Italy: Octavo, Bilingual Edition; 1998.
42. Arcangeli A. *Recreation in the Renaissance. Attitudes towards Leisure and Pastimes in European Culture*. New York, NY: Palgrave Macmillan; 2003.
43. Dossey B. *Florence Nightingale: Mystic, Visionary, Healer*. Baltimore, MD: Lippincott Williams & Wilkins; 2000.
44. Reich W, Carfagno V. *Character Analysis*. 3rd ed. New York: Farrar, Straus and Giroux; 1980.
45. Anderson WT. *The Upstart Spring: Esalen and the Human Potential Movement: The first 20 years*. Backinprint.com. 2004.
46. Harvard School of Medicine. Spirituality and Healing in Medicine Conference available at http://cme.med.harvard.edu/cmeups/pdf/00261464.pdf. Viewed March 2007.

47. 2006 Massage Therapy Fast Facts. Associated Bodywork & Massage Professionals available at http://www.abmp.com. Viewed February 10, 2007.

48. Monteson P, Singer J. *What Today's Spa Client Seeks*. ISHC Lodging Hospitality; 1998 (November).

49. 2005 Massage Therapy Industry Fact Sheet. American Massage Therapy Association available at http://www.amtamassage.org. Viewed February 10, 2007.

50. 2006 Massage Therapy Fast Facts. Associated Bodywork & Massage Professionals available at http://www.abmp.com. Viewed February 10, 2007.

51. Key Findings of the 2003 ISPA Spa Goer Survey. Available at http://www.discoverspas.com. Viewed September 2006.

52. American Pain Foundation. Fast facts about pain. Available at: http://www.painfoundation.org/page.asp?file=Library/FastFacts.htm. Viewed September 14, 2006.

53. Vickers A, Ohlsson A, Lacy JB, et al. Massage therapy for premature and/or low birth-weight infants to improve weight gain and / or to decrease hospital length of stay. In *Cochrane Collaboration*. Issue 3. Oxford, UK: The Cochrane Library; 1998.

54. Associated Bodywork & Massage Professionals Web site available at http://www.abmp.com. Viewed December 10, 2007.

55. Caplan RL, Scarpaci JL. The consequences of increased competition on alternative health care practitioners in the United States. *Holistic Med*. 1989;4:125–135.

56. Einsenberg DM, Davis RB, Ettner SL, et al. Unconventional medicine in the United States. *N Engl J Med*. 1993;328:246–252.

57. Wetzel MS, Eisenberg DM, Kaptchuk TJ. Courses involving complementary and alternative medicine at U.S. medical schools. *J Am Med Assoc*. 1998;280:784–787.

58. *The Landmark Repost on Public Perceptions of Alternative Care*. Sacramento, CA: Landmark Healthcare, Inc.; 1998.

59. International Spa Association Spa-goer Study for 2006. Compiled by the Hartman Group and available from the International Spa Association at http://www.experienceispa.com/ISPA/.

60. Miraval Resort. Life in Balance Program available at http://www.miravalresort.com. Viewed November 2, 2007.

61. Chopra Center for Wellbeing. Perfect Health Program available at http:www.chopra.com. Viewed November 2, 2007.

62. http://www.canyonranch.com/tucson/index.asp. The Canyon Ranch Health Resort in Tucson, Arizona. Accessed March 2, 2005.

63. National Centers for Complementary and Alternative Medicine Web site. *Reducing End-of-Life Symptoms with Touch*. Available at http://www.clinicaltrials.gov/ct/show/NCT00065195?order=1. Viewed October 2, 2007.

64. National Centers for Complementary and Alternative Medicine Web site. Treatment of Depression With Massage in HIV. Available at http://www.clinicaltrials.gov/ct/show/NCT00033852?order=1. Viewed October 2, 2007.

65. Field T, Hernandez-Reif M, Hart S, et al. Pregnant women benefit from massage therapy. *J Psychosomat Obstetr Gynecol*. 1999;20:31–38.

66. Field T, Hernandez-Reif M, LaGreca A, et al. Massage therapy lowers blood glucose levels in children with diabetes mellitus. *Diabetes Spectrum*. 1997;10:237-239.

67. Hernandez-Reif M, Field T, Dieter J, et al. Migraine headaches are reduced by massage therapy. *Int J Neurosci*. 1998;96:1–11.

68. Field T, Quintino O, Hernandez-Reif M et al. Adolescents with attention deficit hyperactivity disorder benefit from massage therapy. *Adolescence*. 1998;33:103–108.

69. Massage Therapy Foundation Web site available at http://www.massagetherapyfoundation.org. Viewed October 12, 2007.

CHAPTER 2

1. Friedman Z, Shochat SJ, Maisels MJ, et al. Correction of essential fatty acid deficiency in newborn infants by cutaneous application of sunflower-seed oil. *Pediatrics*. 1976;58(5):650–654.

2. Bohles H, Bieber MA, Heird WC. Reversal of experimental essential fatty acid deficiency by cutaneous administration of safflower oil. *Am J Clin Nutr*. 1976;29(4):398–401.

3. Michalun N, Michalun MV. *Skin Care and Cosmetics Ingredients Dictionary*. 2nd ed. Albany, NY: Thomson Learning, Milady Publishing; 2001.

4. Begoun P. *The Cosmetic Cop, Myth Busters*. Available at http://www.cosmeticcop.com. Viewed July 5, 2004.

5. Tan E. *Light and Color Therapy—Psychological, Biological and Spiritual Effects*. Available at http://mindreality.com/light-and-color-therapy-psychological-biological. Viewed September 14, 2006.

6. Color Psychology. Available at http://library.thinkquest.org/27066/psychology/nlcolorpsych.html. Viewed September 14, 2006.

7. Johnson D. Psychology of Color: Do Colors Affect Mood? Available at http://www.infoplease.com/spot/colorsl.html. Viewed September 6, 2006.

8. Color Psychology. Available at http://www.wikipedia.org/wiki/color-psychology. Viewed September 8, 2006.

9. Knight WE, Rickard NS. Relaxing music prevents stress-induced increases in subjective anxiety, systolic blood pressure and heart rate in healthy males and females. *J Music Ther*. 2001;38(4):254–272.

10. Zakharova NN, Avdeev VM. Functional changes in the central nervous system during music perception (study of positive emotions). Available as an abstract at http://www.pubmed.com. Viewed September 11, 2006.

11. Krout RE. the effects of single-session music therapy interventions on the observed and self-reported levels of pain control, physical comfort, and relaxation of hospice patients. *Am J Hosp Palliat Care*. 2001;18(6):383–390.

12. Thorgaard B, Henriksen BB, Pedersbaek G, et al. Specially selected music in the cardiac laboratory—an important tool for improvement of the wellbeing of patients. *Eur J Cardiovasc Nurs*. 2004;3(1):21–26.

13. Uhlig T, Kallus KW. The brain: a psychoneuroimmunological approach. *Curr Opin Anesthesiol*. 2005;18(2):147–150.

14. Julkunen J, Ahlstrom R. Hostility, anger, and sense of coherence as predictors of health-related quality of life. *J Psychosom Res*. 2006;6(1):33–39.

15. Parasuraman R. Effects of fragrances on behavior, mood and physiology. Paper presented at the annual meeting of the American Association for the Advancement of Science, Washington, DC, 1991.

16. Fox K. The Smell Report. The Social Issues Research Center. Available at http://www.sirc.org/publik/smell_contents.html.

CHAPTER 3

1. Medline Plus Medical Encyclopedia Web site. Causes of Autoimmune Disorders available at http://www.nlm.nih.gov/medlineplus/ency/article/000816.htm#Causes,%20incidence,%20and%20risk%20factors. Viewed September 23, 2006.

2. American Association for Clinical Chemistry Web site. Autoimmune Disorders. http://www.labtestsonline.org/understanding/conditions/autoimmune.html. Viewed September 23, 2006.

3. Autoimmune Book. The Autoimmune Report available at http://www.autoimmunebook.com. Viewed September 23, 2006.

4. National Cancer Institute. Cancer Causes and Risk Factors available at http://www.nci.nih.gov/cancertopics/prevention-genetics-causes/causes. Viewed September 23, 2006.

5. United States Department of Energy and the National Institute of Health, Human Genome Project. Medicine and the New Genetics available at http://www.ornl.gov/sci/techresources/Human_Genome/medicine/medicine.shtml. Viewed September 23, 2006.

6. Kenneth Todar. University of Wisconsin-Madison Department of Bacteriology. Online Textbook of Bacteriology for *Streptococcus pyogenes* available at http://textbookofbacteriology.net/streptococcus.html. Viewed September 23, 2006.

7. The Centers for Disease Control: Guidelines for Hand Hygiene in Health-Care Settings. Recommendations of the Healthcare Infection Control Practices Advisory Committee and the HICPAC/SHEA/APIC/IDSA Hand Hygiene Task force. Available at htpp://www.cdc.gov. Viewed September 23, 2006.

8. Abram S. Benenson, eds. *The Control of Communicable Diseases Manual*. 16th ed. (1995). Washington, DC: The American Public Health Association; 2005.

9. The Centers for Disease Control and Prevention. Available at http://www.cdc.gov. Viewed September 23, 2006.

10. Journal of the American Medical Association (JAMA). HIV: The Basics. Available at http://jama.ama-assn.org/cgi/content/full/296/7/892. Viewed September 23, 2006.

11. National Institute of Diabetes and Digestive and Kidney Diseases. Viral Hepatitis: A Through E and Beyond. Available at http://digestive.niddk.nih.gov/ddiseases/pubs/viralhepatitis/. September 23, 2006.

12. Werner R. *A Massage Therapist's Guide to Pathology*. 3rd ed. Baltimore, MD: Lippincott Williams & Wilkins; 2005.

13. Hernandez-Reif M, Ironson G, Field T, et al. Breast cancer patients have improved immune and neuroendocrine functions following massage therapy. *J Psychosom Res*. 2003;57(1):35–52.

14. Hernandez-Reif M, Field T, Ironson G, et al. Natural killer cells and lymphocytes increase in woman with breast cancer following massage therapy. *Int J Neurosci*. 2005;115(3):395–510.

15. Diego MA, Field T, Hernandez-Reif M, et al. HIV adolescents show improved immune function following massage therapy. *Int J Neurosci*. 2001;106(1–2):35–35.

CHAPTER 4

1. Dieter JN, Field T, Hernandez-Reif M, et al. Stable preterm infants gain more weight and sleep less after five days of massage therapy. *J Pediatr Psychol*. 2003;28(6):403–411.

2. Mitchell J. How We Know What We Know. A Different Way to Heal. PBS Scientific American Frontiers available at www.pbs.org/saf/1210/features/know.htm. Viewed December 24, 2007.

3. Rennard BO, Ertl RF, Gossman GL, et al. Chicken soup inhibits neutrophil chemotaxis in vitro. *Chest*. 2000;118(4):1150–1157.

4. Cassidy C. Methodological issues in investigations of massage/bodywork therapy. Massage Therapy Foundation. 2002. Available at http://www.massagetherapyfoundation.org/pdf/Cassidy1.pdf. Viewed December 24, 2007.

5. Brown M, Pitch C. Research Literacy: Levels of Evidence. Massage Therapy Foundation available at http://www.amtamassage.org/journal/spring06_journal/pdf/ResearchLiteracy.pdf. Viewed December 24, 2007.

6. Juhan D. *Job's Body: A Handbook for Bodywork*. Expanded ed. Barrytown, NY: Barrytown, Ltd.; 1998.

7. Premkumar K. *The Massage Connection: Anatomy and Physiology*. 2nd ed. Baltimore, MD: Lippincott Williams & Wilkins; 2004.

8. Bardot J. Cutaneous cicatrix: natural course, anomalies and prevention. *Rev Prat*. 1994;44(13):1763–1768.

9. Roh YS, Cho H, Oh Jo, et al. Effects of skin rehabilitation massage therapy on pruritus, skin status, and depression in burn survivors. *Taehan Kanho Hakhoe Chi*. 2007;37(2):221–226.

10. Field T, Peck M, Hernandez-Reif M, et al. Postburn itching, pain, and psychological symptoms are reduced with massage therapy. *J Burn Care Rehabil*. 21(3):189–193.

11. Hakkinen A, Salo P, Tarvainen U, et al. Effects of manual therapy and stretching on neck muscle strength and mobility in chronic neck pain. *J Rehabil Med*. 2007;39(7):575–579.

12. Hopper D, Deacon S, Das S, et al. Dynamic soft tissue mobilization increases hamstring flexibility in healthy male subjects. *Br J Sports Med*. 2005;39(9):594–598.

13. Van den Dolder PA, Roberts DL. A trial into the effectiveness of soft tissue massage in the treatment of shoulder pain. *Aust J Physiother*. 2003;49(4):275.

14. Robertson A, Watt JM, Galloway SD. Effects of leg massage on recovery from high intensity cycling exercise. *Br J Sports Med*. 2004;4:173–176.

15. Zainuddin Z, Newton M, Sacco P, et al. Effects of massage on delayed-onset muscle soreness, swelling, and recovery of muscle function. *J Athl Train*. 2005;40:174–180.

16. Brooks CP, Woodruff LD, Wright LL, et al. The immediate effects of manual massage on power-grip performance after maximal exercise in healthy adults. *J Altern Complement Med*. 2005;11:1093–1101.

17. Hilbert JE, Sforzo GA, Swensen T. The effects of massage on delayed onset muscle soreness. *Br J Sports Med*. 2003;37:72–75.

18. Rinder AN, Sutherland CJ. An investigation of the effects of massage on quadriceps performance after exercise fatigue. *Complement Ther Nurs Midwifery*. 1995;1:99–102.

19. Weiss JM. Treatment of leg edema and wounds in a patient with severe musculoskeletal injuries. *Phys Ther*. 1998;78(12):1338–1339.

20. Melham TJ, Sevier TL, Malnofski MJ, et al. Chronic ankle pain and fibrosis successfully treated with a new noninvasive augmented soft tissue mobilization technique (ASTM): a case report. *Med Sci Sports Exerc*. 1998;30(6):801–804.

21. Field T, Diego M, Cullen C, et al. Carpal tunnel syndrome symptoms are lessened following massage therapy. *J Bodywork Movement Ther*. 2004;8:9–14.

22. Pettitt R, Dolski A. Corrective neuromuscular approach to the treatment of iliotibial band friction syndrome: a case report. *J Athl Train*. 2000;35(1):96–99.

23. Wu LD, Xiong Y, Yan SG, et al. Total knee replacement for post-traumatic degenerative arthritis of the knee. *Clin J Traumatol*. 2005;8(4):195–199.

24. Pellino TA, Grodon DB, Engelke ZK, et al. Use of nonpharmacologic interventions for pain and anxiety after total hip and total knee arthroplasty. *Orthop Nurs*. 2005;24(3):182–190.

25. Bost N, Wallis M. The effectiveness of a 15 minute weekly massage in reducing physical and psychological stress in nurses. *Aust J Adv Nurs*. 2006;23(4):28–33.

26. Fogaca MC, Carvalho WB, Peres CA, et al. Salivary cortisol as an indicator of adrenocortical function in healthy infants, using massage therapy. *Sao Paulo Med J*. 2005;123(5):215–218.

27. Field T, Hernandez-Reif M, Diego M, et al. Cortisol decreases and serotonin and dopamine increase following massage therapy. *Int J Neurosci*. 2005;115(10):1397–1413.

28. Field T, Diego MA, Hernandez-Reif M, et al. Massage therapy effects on depressed pregnant women. *J Psychosom Obstet Gynaecol*. 2004;25(2):115–122.

29. Field T, Schanberg S, Kuhn C, et al. Bulimic adolescents benefit from massage therapy. *Adolescence*. 1998;33(131):555–563.

30. Field T. Violence and touch deprivation in adolescents. *Adolescence*. 2002;37(148):735–749.

31. Bender T, Nagy G, Barna I, et al. The effects of physical therapy on beta-endorphin levels. *Eur J Appl Physiol*. 2007;100(4):371–382.

32. Kaada B, Torsteinbo O. Increase of plasma beta-endorphins in connective tissue massage. *Gen Pharmacol*. 1989;20(4):487–489.

33. Kim MS, Cho KS, Woo H, et al. Effects of hand massage on anxiety in cataract surgery using local anesthesia. *J Cataract Refract Surg*. 2001;27(6):884–890.

34. Field T, Pickens J, Prodromidis M, et al. Targeting adolescent mothers with depressive symptoms for early intervention. *Adolescence*. 2000;35(138):381–414.

35. Juhan D. *Job's Body: A Handbook for Bodywork*. Expanded ed. Barrytown, NY: Barrytown, Ltd.; 1998.

36. Field T. Violence and touch deprivation in adolescents. *Adolescence*. 2002;37(148):735–749.

37. Turner RA, Altemus M, Enos T, et al. Preliminary research on plasma oxytocin in normal cycling women: investigating emotion and interpersonal distress. California School of Professional Psychology, San Francisco, CA. 1999. Available at http://www.oxytocin.org/oxy/oxywomen.html. Viewed December 7, 2007.

38. Field T, Hernandez-Reif M, Deigo M, et al. Cortisol decreases and serotonin and dopamine increase following massage therapy. *Int J Neurosci.* 2005;115(10):1397–1413.

39. DeVane LC. Substance P: a new era, a new role. *Pharmacotherapy.* 2001;21(9):1061–1069.

40. Field T, Deigo M, Cullen C, et al. Fibromyalgia pain and substance P decrease and sleep improves after massage therapy. *J Clin Rheumatol.* 2002;8(2):72–76.

41. Ebner M. *Connective Tissue Massage.* Huntington, IN: Robert Krieger; 1980.

42. Yates J. *A Physician's Guide to Therapeutic Massage: Its Physiological Effects and Their Application to Treatment.* Vancouver, BC: Massage Therapist's Association of British Columbia; 1990.

43. Liu Y, Xu S, Yan J, et al. Capillary blood flow with dynamic change of tissue pressure caused by exterior force. *Sheng Wu Yi Xue Gong Cheng Xue Za Zhi.* Translation from the Chinese. 2004;21(5): 699–703.

44. Premkumar K. *The Massage Connection Anatomy and Physiology.* 2nd ed. Baltimore, MD: Lippincott Williams & Wilkins; 2004.

45. Ernst E, Matrai A, Magyarosy I, et al. Massage causes changes in blood fluidity. *Physiotherapy.* 1992;73:43–45.

46. Mein EA, Richards DG, McMillin DL, et al. Physiological regulation through manual therapy. Physical Medicine and Rehabilitation. A state-of-the-art review. *Psy Med Rehab.* 2000;14(1):27–42.

47. Hernandez-Reif M, Field T, Krasnegor J, et al. High blood pressure and associated symptoms were reduced by massage therapy. *J Bodywork Mov Ther.* 2000;4:31–38.

48. McNamara NE, Burnham DC, Smith C, et al. The effects of back massage before diagnostic cardiac catheterization. *Altern Ther.* 2003;9:50–57.

49. Mondry TE, Riffenburgh RH, Johnstone PA. Prospective trial of complete decongestive therapy for upper extremity lymphedema after breast cancer therapy. *Cancer J.* 2004;10(1):42–48.

50. Hamner JB, Fleming MD. Lymphedema therapy reduces the volume of edema and pain in patients with breast cancer. *Ann Surg Oncol.* 2007;14(6):1904–1908.

51. Vignes S, Porcher R, Arrault M, et al. Long-term management of breast cancer-related lymphedema after intensive decongestive physiotherapy. *Breast Cancer Res Treat.* 2007;101(3):285–290.

52. Hernandez Reif M, Field T, Ironside G, et al. Natural killer cells and lymphocytes increase in women with breast cancer following massage therapy. *Int J Neurosci.* 2005;115:495–510.

53. Ironson G, Field T, Scafidi F, et al. Massage therapy is associated with enhancement of the immune system's cytotoxic capacity. *Int J Neurosci.* 1996;84:205–217.

54. McCool FD, Rosen MJ. Nonpharmacologic airway clearance therapies. ACCP evidence-based clinical practice guidelines. *Chest.* 2006;129(1):250S–259S.

55. Faling LJ. Pulmonary rehabilitation physical modalities. *Clin Chest Med.* 1986;7(4):599–618.

56. Wu HS, Lin LC, Wu SC, et al. The psychologic consequences of chronic dyspnea in chronic pulmonary obstruction disease: the effects of acupressure on depression. *J Altern Complement Med.* 2007;13(2):253–261.

57. Beeken JE, Parks D, Cory J, et al. The effectiveness of neuromuscular release massage therapy in five individuals with chronic obstructive lung disease. *Clin Nurs Res.* 1998;7(3):309–325.

58. Roy N, Leeper HA. Effects of the manual laryngeal musculoskeletal tension reduction technique as a treatment for functional voice disorders: perceptual and acoustic measures. *J Voice.* 1993;7(3):242–249.

59. Ayas S, Leblebici B, Sozay S, et al. The effect of abdominal massage on bowel function in patients with spinal cord injury. *Am J Phys Med Rehabil.* 2006;85(12):951–955.

60. Field T, Hernandez-Reif M, Hart S, et al. Pregnant women benefit from massage. *J Phychosomatic Obstetr Gynecol.* 1999;20: 31–38.

61. Chang, MY, Chen, CH, Huang, KF. A comparison of massage effects on labor pain using the McGill Pain Questionnaire. *J Nurs Res.* 2006;14(3):190–197.

62. Cullen C, Field T, Escalona A, et al. Father-infant interactions are enhanced by massage therapy. *Early Child Develop Care.* 2000;164:41–47.

63. Field T. Review—massage therapy facilitates weight gain in preterm infants. *Curr Direct Psychologic Sci.* 2001;10:51–54.

64. Field T, Schanberg SM. Massage alters growth and catecholamine production in preterm newborns. *Advances in Touch.* Skillman, NJ: 1990.

65. Field T, Hernandez-Reif M. Sleep problems in infants decrease following massage therapy. *Early Child Develop Care.* 2001;168:95–104.

66. Shulman KP, Jones GE. The effectiveness of massage therapy intervention on reducing anxiety in the work place. *J Appl Behav Sci.* 1996;32:160–173.

67. Field T, Morrow C, Valdeon C, et al. Massage reduces anxiety in child and adolescent phychiatric patients. *J Am Acad Child Adolesc Psychiatry.* 1992;31:125–131.

68. Cooke M, Holzhauser K, Jones M, et al. The effect of aromatherapy massage with music on the stress and anxiety levels of emergency nurses: comparison between summer and winter. *J Clin Nurs.* 2007;16(9):1695–1703.

69. Anderson PG, Cutshall SM. Massage therapy: a comfort intervention for cardiac surgery patients. *Clin Nurse Spec.* 2007;21(3):161–165.

70. Wilkinson SM, Love SB, Westcombe AM, et al. Effectiveness of aromatherapy massage in the management of anxiety and depression in patients with cancer: a multicenter randomized controlled trial. *J Clin Oncol.* 2007;25(5):532–539.

71. Collinge W, Wentworth R, Sabo S. Integrating complementary therapies into community mental health practice: an exploration. *J Altern Complement Med.* 2005;11(3):569–574.

72. Diego MA, Field T, Hernandez-Reif M, et al. Aggressive adolescents benefit from massage therapy. *Adolescence.* 2002;37:597–607.

73. Field T, Quintino O, Hernandez-Reif M, et al. Adolescents with attention deficit hyperactivity disorder benefit from massage therapy. *Adolescence.* 1998;33:103–108.

74. Khilnani S, Field T, Hernandez-Reif M, et al. Massage therapy improves mood and behavior of students with attention deficit hyperactivity disorder. *Adolescence.* 2003;38:623–638.

75. Escalona A, Field T, Cullen C, et al. Behavior problem preschool children benefit from massage therapy. *Early Child Develop Care.* 2001;161:1–5.

76. Field T, Kilmer T, Hernandez-Reif M, et al. Preschool children's sleep and wake behavior: effects of massage therapy. *Early Child Develop Care*; 120:39–44.

77. Song RH, Kim DH. The effects of foot reflexology massage on sleep disturbance, depression disorder and the physiological index of the elderly. *Taehan Kanho Hakhoe Chi.* Translated from the Korean. 2006;36(1):15–24. 2006.

78. Richards KC. Effect of back massage and relaxation intervention on sleep in critically ill patients. *Am J Crit Care.* 1998;7:288–299.

79. Diego MA, Field T, Sanders C, et al. Massage therapy of moderate and light pressure and vibrator effects on EEG and heart rate. *Int J Neurosci.* 2004;114(1):31–44.

80. Jones NA, Field T. Massage and music therapies attenuate frontal EEG asymmetry in depressed adolescents. *Adolescence.* 1999;34(135):529–534.

81. Energy Medicine: An Overview by the National Center for Complementary and Alternative Medicine. http://nccam.nih.gov/health/backgrounds/energymed.htm. Viewed December 8, 2007.

82. Gallob R. Reiki: a supportive therapy in nursing practice and self-care for nurses. *J N Y State Nurses' Assoc.* 2003;34(1):9–13.

83. Lawler SP, Cameron LD. A randomized, controlled trial of massage therapy as a treatment for migraine. *Ann Behav Med.* 2006;32(1):50–59.

84. Price. C. Body-oriented therapy in recovery from child sexual abuse: an efficacy study. *Altern Ther Health Med*. 2005;11(5):46–57.

85. Lindera KB, Stainton MC. A case study of infant massage outcomes. *MCN AM J Matern Child Nurs*. 2000;25(2):95–99.

86. Rowe M, Alfred D. The effectiveness of slow-stroke massage in diffusing agitated behaviors in individuals with Alzheimer's disease. *J Gerontol Nurs*. 1999;25(6):22–34.

87. Kim EJ, Buschmann MT. The effect of expressive physical touch on patients with dementia. *Int J Nurs Stud*. 1999;26(3):235–243.

88. Malaquin-Pavan E. Therapeutic benefit of touch-massage in the overall management of demented elderly. *Rech Soins Infirm*. 1997;(49):11–66.

89. Chen Z. 48 cases of anxiety syndrome treated by massage. *J Tradit Chin Med*. 1998;18(4):282–284.

90. Field T, Morrow C, Valdeon C, et al. Massage reduces anxiety in child and adolescent psychiatric patients. *J Am Acad Child Adolesc Psychiatry*. 1992;31(1):125–131.

91. McKechnie AA, Wilson F, Watson N, et al. Anxiety states: a preliminary report on the value of connective tissue massage. *J Psychosom Res*. 1983;27(2):125–129.

92. Brooks CP, Woodruff LD, Write LL, et al. The immediate effects of manual massage on power-grip performance after maximal exercise in healthy adults. *J Altern Complement Med*. 2005;11(6):1093–1101.

93. Hilbert JE, Sforzo GA, Swensen T. The effects of massage on delayed onset muscle soreness. *Br J Sports Med*. 2003;37(1):72–75.

94. Rinder AN, Sutherland CJ. An investigation of the effects of massage on quadriceps performance after exercise fatigue. *Complement Ther Nurs Midwifery*. 1995;1(4):99–102.

95. Escalona A, Field T, Singer-Strunck R, et al. Brief report: improvements in the behavior of children with autism following massage therapy. *J Autism Dev Disord*. 2001;31(5):513–516.

96. Cullen-Powell LA, Barlow JH, Cushway D. Exploring a massage intervention for parents and their children with autism: the implications for bonding and attachment. *J Child Health Care*. 2005;9(4):245–255.

97. Field T, Quintino O, Hernandez-Reif M, et al. Adolescents with attention deficit hyperactivity disorder benefit from massage therapy. *Adolescence*. 1998;33:103–108.

98. Khilnani S, Field T, Hernandez-Reif M, et al. Massage therapy improves mood and behavior of students with attention-deficit/hyperactivity disorder. *Adolescence*. 2003;38:623–638.

99. Escalona A, Field T, Cullen C, et al. Behavior problem preschool children benefit from massage therapy. *Early Child Develop Care*. 2001;161:1–5.

100. Roh YS, Cho H, Oh JO, et al. Effects of skin rehabilitation massage therapy on pruritus, skin status, and depression in burn survivors. *Taehan Kanho Hakhoe Chi*. 2007;37(2):221–226. 2007.

101. Gallager G, Rae CP, Kinsella J. Treatment of pain in severe burns. *Am J Clin Dermatol*. 2000;1(6):329–335.

102. Gatlin CG, Schulmeister L. When medication is not enough: nonpharmacologic management of pain. *Clin J Oncol Nurs*. 2007;11(5):699–704.

103. Dibble SL, Luce J, Cooper BA, et al. Acupressure for chemotherapy-induced nausea and vomiting: a randomized clinical trial. *Oncol Nurs Forum*. 2007;34(4):813–820.

104. Warren AG, Brorson H, Borud LJ, et al. Lymphedema: a comprehensive review. *Ann Plast Surg*. 2007;59(4):464–472.

105. Sagar SM, Dryden T, Wong RK. Massage therapy for cancer patients: a reciprocal relationship between body and mind. *Curr Oncol*. 2007;14(2):45–56.

106. Mehling WE, Jacobs B, Acree M, et al. Symptom management with massage and acupuncture in postoperative cancer patients: a randomized controlled trial. *J Pain Symptom Manage*. 2007;33(3):258–266.

107. Hernandez-Reif M, Ironson G, Field T, et al. Breast cancer patients have improved immune functions following massage therapy. *J Psychosomat Res*. 2003;57:45–52.

108. Hernandez-Reif M, Field T, Largie S, et al. Cerebral Palsy symptoms in children decreased following massage therapy. *J Early Child Develop Care*. 2005;175:445–456.

109. Powell L, Barlow J, Cheshire A. The Training and Support Program for parents of children with cerebral palsy: a process evaluation. *Complement Ther Clin Pract*. 2006;12(3):192–199.

110. Barlow J, Cullen L. Increasing touch between parents and children with disabilities: preliminary results from a new program. *J Fam Health Care*. 2002;12(1):7–9.

111. Jones JF, Maloney EM, Boneva RS, et al. Complementary and alternative medical therapy utilization by people with chronic fatiguing illnesses in the United States. *BCM Complement Altern Med*. 2007;7:12.

112. Field T, Sunshine W, Hernandez-Reif et al. Chronic fatigue syndrome: massage therapy effects on depression and somatic symptoms in chronic fatigue syndrome. *J Chronic Fatigue Synd*. 1997;3:43–51.

113. Wu HS, Lin LC, Wu SC, et al. The psychologic consequences of chronic dyspnea in chronic pulmonary obstruction disease: the effects of acupressure on depression. *J Altern Complement Med*. 2007;13(2):253–261.

114. Beeken JE, Parks D, Cory J, et al. The effectiveness of neuromuscular release massage therapy in five individuals with chronic obstructive lung disease. *Clin Nurs Res*. 1998;7(3):309–325.

115. Mehl-Madrona L, Kilgler B, Silverman S, et al. The impact of acupuncture and craniosacral therapy interventions on clinical outcomes in adults with asthma. *Explore*. 2007;3(1):28–36.

116. Field T, Henteleff T, Hernandez-Reif M, et al. Children with asthma have improved pulmonary functions after massage therapy. *J Pediatr*. 1998;132:854–858.

117. Inoue M, Ohtsu I, Tomioka S, et al. Effects of pulmonary rehabilitation on vital capacity in patients with chronic pulmonary emphysema. *Nihon Kyobu Shikkan Gakkai Zasshi*. 1996;34(11):1182–1188.

118. Ernst E. Abdominal massage therapy for chronic constipation: a systematic review of controlled clinical trials. *Forsch Komplementarmed*. 1999;6(3):149–151.

119. Coggrave M, Burrows D, Durand MA. Progressive protocol in the bowel management of spinal cord injuries. *Br J Nurs*. 2006;15(20):1108–1113.

120. Harrington KL, Haskvitz EM. Managing a patient's constipation with physical therapy. *Phys Ther*. 2006;86(11):1511–1519.

121. Preece J. Introducing abdominal massage in palliative care for the relief of constipation. *Complement Ther Nurs Midwifery*. 2002;8(2):101–105.

122. Hart S, Field T, Hernandez-Reif M, et al. Anorexia nervosa symptoms are reduced by massage therapy. *Eat Disord*. 2001;9(4):289–299.

123. Field T, Schanberg S, Kuhn C, et al. Bulimic adolescents benefit from massage therapy. *Adolescence*. 1998;33(131):555–563.

124. Filed T. Massage therapy for infants and children. *J Dev Behav Pediatr*. 1995;16(2):105–111.

125. Field T, Diego M, Cullen C, et al. Fibromyalgia pain and substance P decrease and sleep improves after massage therapy. *J Clin Rheumatol*. 2002;8(2):72–76.

126. Gordon C, Emiliozzi C, Zartarian M. Use of a mechanical massage technique in the treatment of fibromyalgia: a preliminary study. *Arch Phys Med Rehabil*. 2006;87(1):145–147.

127. Goffaux-Dogniez C, Vanfraechem-Raway R, Verbanck P. Appraisal of treatment of trigger points associated with relaxation to treat chronic headache in the adult. Relationship with anxiety and stress adaptation strategies. *Encephale*. 2003;29(5):377–390.

128. Quinn C, Chandler C, Moraska A. Massage therapy and frequency of chronic tension headaches. *Am J Public Health*. 2002;92(10):1657–1661.

129. Lawler SP, Cameron LD. A randomized, controlled trial of massage therapy as a treatment for migraine. *Ann Behav Med*. 2006;32(1):50–59.

130. Aourell M, Skoog M, Carleson J. Effects of Swedish massage on blood pressure. *Complement Ther Clin Pract*. 2005;11(4):242–246.

131. Olney CM. The effects of therapeutic back massage in hypertensive persons: a preliminary study. *Biol Res Nurs*. 2005;7(2):98–105.

132. Shor-Posner G, Hernandez-Reif M, Miguez MJ, et al. Impact of a massage therapy clinical trial on immune status in young Dominican children infected with HIV-1. *J Altern Complement Med*. 2006;12(6):511–516.

133. Diego MA, Field T, Hernandez-Reif M, et al. HIV adolescents show improved immune function following massage therapy. *Int J Neurosci*. 2001;106(1–2):35–45.

134. Anderson PG, Cutshall SM. Massage therapy: a comfort intervention for cardiac surgery patients. *Clin Nurse Spec*. 2007;21(3): 161–165.

135. McRee LD, Noble S, Pasvogel A. Using massage and music therapy to improve postoperative outcomes. *Aorn J*. 2003;78(3):433–442.

136. Milligan M, Fanning M, Hunter S, et al. Reflexology audit: patient satisfaction, impact on quality of life and availability in Scottish hospices. *Int J Palliat Nurs*. 2002;8(10):489–496.

137. MacDonald G. Massage as a respite intervention for primary caregivers. *Am J Hosp Palliat Care*. 1998;15(1):43–47.

138. Cullen C, Field T, Escalona A, et al. Father-infant interactions are enhanced by massage therapy. *Early Child Develop Care*. 2000;164:41–47.

139. Field T. Review—massage therapy facilitates weight gain in preterm infants. *Curr Direct Psychologic Sci*. 2001;10:51–54.

140. Field T, Hernandez-Reif M. Sleep problems in infants decrease following massage therapy. *Early Child Develop Care*. 2001;168: 95–104.

141. Field T, Grizzle N, Scafidi F, et al. Massage therapy for infants of depressed mothers. *Infant Behav Develop*. 1996;19:109–114.

142. Field T. Massage therapy for infants and children. *J Develop Behav Pediatr*. 1995;16:105–111.

143. Field T, Kilmer T, Hernandez-Reif M, et al. Preschool children's sleep and wake behavior: effects of massage therapy. *Early Child Develop Care*. 1998;120:39–44.

144. Schiff A. Literature review of back massage and similar techniques to promote sleep in elderly people. *Pflege*. 2006;19(3):163–173.

145. Richards K, Nagel C, Markie M, et al. Use of complementary and alternative therapies to promote sleep in critically ill patients. *Crit Care Nurs Clin North Am*. 2003;15(3):329–340.

146. National Digestive Diseases Information from the National Institute of Diabetes and Digestive and Kidney Diseases. Irritable Bowel Syndrome. Available at http://digestive.niddk.nih.gov/ddiseases/pubs/ibs/. Viewed December 15, 2007.

147. Huang ZD, Liang LA, Zhang WX. Acupuncture combined with massage for the treatment of irritable bowel syndrome. *Zhongguo Zhen Jiu*. 2006;26(10):717–718.

148. Bosseckert H. Irritable colon syndrome. *Dtsch Z Verdau Stoffwechselkr*. 1982;42(4):161–168.

149. Hernandez-Reif M, Field T, Theakston H. Multiple sclerosis patients benefit from massage therapy. *J Bodywork Movement Ther*. 1998;2:168–174.

150. Siev-Ner I, Gamus D, Lerner-Geva L, et al. Reflexology treatment relieves symptoms of multiple sclerosis: a randomized controlled study. *Mult Scler*. 2003;9:356–361.

151. Werner R. *A Massage Therapists Guide to Pathology*. 3rd ed. Baltimore, MD: Lippincott, Williams & Wilkins; 2005.

152. Buonocore M, Manstretta C, Mazzucchi G, et al. The clinical evaluation of conservative treatment in patients with thoracic outlet syndrome. *G Ital Med Lav Ergon*. 1998;20(4):249–254.

153. Field, T, Diego, M, Cullen, C, et al. Carpal tunnel syndrome symptoms are lessened following massage therapy. *J Bodywork Movement Ther*. 2004;8:9–14.

154. Perlman AI, Sabina A, Williams AL, et al. Massage therapy for osteoarthritis of the knee. A randomized controlled trial. *Arch Intern Med*. 2006;166(22):2533–2538.

155. Cherkin DC, Eisenberg D, Sherman KJ, et al. Randomized trial comparing traditional Chinese medical acupuncture, therapeutic massage, and self-care education for chronic low back pain. *Arch Intern Med*. 2001;161:1081–1088.

156. Foster KA, Liskin J, Cen S, et al. The Trager approach in the treatment of chronic headache: A pilot study. *Altern Ther Health Med*. 2004;10:40–46.

157. Nixon M, Teschendorff J, Finney J, et al. Expanding the nursing repertoire: the effect of massage on post-operative pain. *Aust J Adv Nurs*. 1997;14(3):21–26.

158. Field T, Hernandez-Reif M, Taylor S, et al. Labor pain is reduced by massage therapy. *J Psychosom Obstet Gynecol*. 1997;18:286–291.

159. Field T, Diego M, Hernandez-Reif M. Prenatal depression effects on the fetus and newborn. A review. *Infant Behav Dev*. 2006;29(3):445–455.

160. Hernandez-Reif M, Martinez A, Field T, et al. Premenstrual symptoms are relieved by massage therapy. *J Psychosom Obstet Gynaecol*. 2000;21(1):9–15.

161. Oleson T, Flocco W. Randomized controlled study of premenstrual symptoms treated with ear, hand, and foot reflexology. *Obstet Gynecol*. 1993;82(6):906–911.

162. Anderson C, Lis-Balchin M, Kirk-Smith M. Evaluation of massage with essential oils on childhood atopic eczema. *Phytother Res*. 2000;14:452–456.

163. Schachner L, Field T, Hernandez-Reif M, et al. Atopic dermatitis symptoms decreased in children following massage therapy. *Pediatr Dermatol*. 1998;15:390–395.

164. Cook M, Holzhauser K, Jones M, et al. The effect of aromatherapy massage with music on the stress and anxiety levels of emergency nurses: comparison between summer and winter. *J Clin Nurs*. 2007;16(9):1695–1703.

165. Cady SH, Jones GE. Massage as a workplace intervention for reduction of stress. *Perceptual Motor Skills*. 1997;84:157–158.

166. Field T, Seligman S, Scafidi F, et al. Alleviating posttraumatic stress in children following Hurricane Andrew. *J Appl Develop Psychol*. 1996;17:37–50.

167. Tian X, Krishnan S. Efficacy of auricular acupressure as an adjuvant therapy in substance abuse treatment: a pilot study. *Altern Ther Health Med*. 2006;12(1):66–69.

168. Reader M, Young R, Connor JP. Massage therapy improves the management of alcohol withdrawal syndrome. *J Altern Complement Med*. 2005;11(2):311–313.

169. Hernandez-Reif M, Field T, Hart S. Smoking cravings are reduced by self-massage. *Prevent Med*. 1999;28:28–32.

170. De Laat A, Stappaerts K, Papy S. Counseling and physical therapy as treatment for myofascial pain of the masticatory system. *J Orofac Pain*. 2003;17(1):42–49.

171. Vander AJ, Sherman JH, Luciano D. *Human Physiology. The Mechanisms of Body Function*. International Edition. 5th ed. New York, NY: McGraw-Hill; 1990.

172. Nuernberger P. *Freedom from Stress: A Holistic Approach*. Honesdale, PA: The Himalayan Institute Press; 1981.

173. Mollica RF. *Healing Invisible Wounds: Paths to Hope and Recovery in a Violent World*. Orlando, FL: Harcourt Books; 2006.

174. Holmes and Rahe Stress Scale. Available at http://www.ta-tutor.com/webpdf/ram015.pdf. Viewed May 14, 2008.

175. Brown BB. *Stress and the Art of Biofeedback*. New York, NY: Bantam Books; 1982.

176. Reduce Stress with a Strong Social Support Network. Available at http://www.mayoclinic.com/health/social-support/SR00033.Viewed May 14, 2008.

177. Bost N, Wallis M. The effectiveness of a 15 minute weekly massage in reducing physical and psychological stress in nurses. *Aust J Adv Nurs*. 2006;23(4):28–33.

178. Fogaca MC, Carvalho WB, Peres CA, et al. Salivary cortisol as an indicator of adrenocortical function in healthy infants, using massage therapy. *Sao Paulo Med J*. 2005;123(5):215–218.

179. Kim MS, Cho KS, Woo H, et al. Effects of hand massage on anxiety in cataract surgery using local anesthesia. *J Cataract Refract Surg.* 2001;27(6):884–890.

180. Field T, Pickens J, Prodromidis M, et al. Targeting adolescent mothers with depressive symptoms for early intervention. *Adolescence.* 2000;35(138):381–414.

CHAPTER 5

1. Billhult A, Bergbom I, Stener-Victorin E. Massage relieves nausea in women with breast cancer who are undergoing chemotherapy. *J Altern Complement Med.* 2007;13(1):53–57.

2. Molassiotis A, Helin AM, Dabbour R, et al. The effects of P6 acupressure in the prophylaxis of chemotherapy-related nausea and vomiting in breast cancer patients. *Complement Ther Med.* 2007;15(1):3–12.

3. Helm S. Shiel WC. Peripheral Neuropathy. Available at www.medicinenet.com/peripheral_neuropathy/article.htm. Viewed December 25, 2007.

4. Hitti M, Nazario B. Older Adults Have More Adverse Events from Common Drugs. Available at www.medicinenet.com/script/main/art.asp?articlekey=46374. Viewed December 25, 2007.

5. *Nursing 2008 Drug Handbook.* Baltimore MD: Lippincott, Williams & Wilkins; 2007.

6. American Diabetes Association. All About Diabetes. Available at http://www.diabetes.org/about-diabetes.jsp. Viewed December 29, 2007.

7. Wible JM. *Pharmacology for Massage Therapy.* Baltimore, MD: Lippincott Williams & Wilkins; 2005.

CHAPTER 6

1. Irwin T. *The Development of Ethics: From Socrates to the Reformation.* Vol. 1. New York, NY: Oxford University Press; 2007

2. Plato Ferrari GRF, Plato GT. *The Republic: Cambridge Texts in the History of Political Thought.* Cambridge, UK: Cambridge University Press; 2000.

3. Aristotle CR. *Nicomachean Ethics: Cambridge Texts in the History of Philosophy.* Cambridge, UK: Cambridge University Press; 2000.

4. Blondell R. *The Play of Character in Plato's Dialogues.* Cambridge, UK: Cambridge University Press; 2002.

5. Sherman, N. *The Fabric of Character: Aristotle's Theory of Virtue.* New York, NY: Oxford University Press; 1991.

6. Allport GW. *The Nature of Prejudice: 25th Anniversary Edition.* New York: Perseus Books Group; 1979.

CHAPTER 7

1. Whiston S, Sexton T. An overview of psychotherapy outcome research: implications for practice. *Profess Psychol Res Pract.* 1993;24(1):43–51.

2. West W, Client's experience of bodywork psychotherapy. *Counsel Psychol Quart.* 1994;7(3)287–303.

3. Forman S, Marmar C. Therapist actions that address initially poor therapeutic alliances in psychotherapy. *Am J Psychiatry.* 142:922–926.

4. Chapin HD, Pisek GR. *Diseases of Infants and Children.* New York, NY: William Wood Publishers; 1919.

5. Cullen C, Field T, Escalona A, et al. Father-infant interactions are enhanced by massage therapy. *Early Child Develop Care.* 2000;164:41–47.

6. Field T. Review—massage therapy facilitates weight gain in preterm infants. *Curr Direct Psychol Sci.* 2001;10:51–54.

7. Field T, Hernandez-Reif M. Sleep problems in infants decrease following massage therapy. *Early Child Develop Care.* 2001;168:95–104.

8. Field T, Grizzle N, Scafidi F, et al. Massage therapy for infants of depressed mothers. *Infant Behav Develop.* 1996;19:109–114.

9. Field T. Massage therapy for infants and children. *J Develop Behav Pediatr.* 1995;16:105–111.

10. Reich W. *Character Analysis.* 3rd ed. New York, NY: Farrar, Straus and Giroux; 1972.

11. University of California (2000). Comparison of anger expression in men and women reveals surprising differences. *ScienceDaily.* Available at http://www.sciencedaily.com/releases/2000/01/000131075609.htm. Viewed April 2, 2008.

12. Gottschalk LA, Serota HM, Shapiro LB. Psychologic conflict and neuromuscular tension. I. preliminary report on a method, as applied to rheumatoid arthritis. *Psychosom Med.* 1950;12:315–319.

13. Reich W. *Character Analysis.* 3rd ed. Translated by Vincent Carfagno. New York, NY: Farrar, Straus and Giroux; 1945.

14. Weinberger DA. *The Construct Validity of the Repressive Coping Style. Repression and Dissociation.* Chicago, IL: University of Chicago Press; 1990.

15. Gottlieb A. *The Dream of Reason: A History of Philosophy from the Greeks to the Renaissance.* New York, NY: W.W. Norton & Company; 2002.

16. Pert C. *Molecules of Emotion: The Science Behind Mind-Body Medicine.* New York, NY: Scribner; 1997.

17. Freeman H, Elmadjian F. The relationship between blood sugar and lymphocyte levels in normal and psychotic subjects. *Psychosom Med.* 1947;9:226–233.

18. Phillips L, Elmadjian F. A Rorschach tension score and the diurnal lymphocyte curve in psychotic subjects. *Psychosom Med.* 1947;9:364–371.

19. Vaughan WTJ, Sullivan JC, Elmadjian F: Immunity and schizophrenia. *Psychosom Med.* 1947;11:327–333.

20. Rosch PJ. *Future Directions in Psychoneuroimmunology: Psycho-electroneuroimmunology?* New York, NY: American Institute of Stress. Available at http://www.stress.org/archives/SISandP.pdf?AIS=2ad4f0814d4d64867b7bb6500e41ea. Viewed April 2, 2008.

21. Ader R, Lee J, Cohen N. Conditioning phenomena and immune function. *Ann N Y Acad Sci Neuroimmune Interact.* 1987;496–532. 1987.

22. Ader R. *Psychoneuroimmunology.* Burlington, MA: Elsevier Academic Press; 2007.

23. Temoshok L. *The Type C Connection: The Behavioral Links to Cancer and Your Health.* New York, NY: Random House; 1992.

24. Spiegel D, Butler LD, Giese-Davis J, et al. Effects of supportive-expressive group therapy on survival of patients with metastatic breast cancer: a randomized prospective trial. *Cancer.* 2007;12:112(2):443–444.

25. Temoshok L. Clinical Psychoneuroimmunology in AIDS. Proceedings from the annual meeting of the Society of Behavioral Medicine, San Francisco, 1986.

26. Wilkinson RG. *Unhealthy Societies: The Afflictions of Inequality.* New York, NY: Routledge Publishers; 1996.

27. Williams RB, Haney TL, Lee KL, et al. Type A behavior, hostility, and coronary atherosclerosis. *Psychosom Med.* 1980;42(6):539–549.

28. O'Regan B. *Positive Emotions: The Emerging Science of Feelings.* New York, NY: Institute for the Advancement of Health; 1985.

29. Zajonc RB. Emotion and facial efference. A theory reclaimed. *Science.* 1985;22(4695):15–21.

30. Alder N, Matthews K. Health psychology: why do some people get sick and some stay well? *Annu Rev Psychol.* 1994;45:229–254.

31. Williams RB. Neurobiology, cellular and molecular biology, and psychosomatic medicine. *Psychosom Med.* 1994;56:308–315.

32. Borysenko J. Psychoneuroimmunology: behavioral factors and the immune response. *Revision.* 1984;7(1):56–65.

33. Nordenberg T. The healing power of placebos. *FDA Consumer Magazine.* January-February 2000 available at http://www.fda.gov/fdac/features/2000/100_heal.html. Viewed May 29, 2008.

34. Dubos R. *Self-Healing. From the Healing Brain Series Recording number 15.* Los Altos, CA: Institute for the Study of Human Knowledge; 1981.

35. Grabe S, Ward LM, Hyde JS. The role of the media in body image concerns among women: a meta-analysis of experimental and correlational studies. *Psychol Bull.* 2008;134(3):460–476.

36. Hill AJ. Motivation for eating behavior in adolescent girls: The Body Beautiful. *Proc Nutr Soc*. 2006;65(4):376–384.

37. Ricciardelli LA, McCabe MP, Williams RJ, et al. The role of ethnicity and culture in body image and disordered eating among males. *Clin Psychol Rev*. 2007;27(5):582–606.

38. Spring B. Possible mechanisms underlying diet-behavior effects. Report from the presentations at the annual meeting of the Society of Behavioral Medicine. San Francisco, 1986. Available at http://repositories.cdlib.org/cgi/viewcontent.cgi?article=1000&context=sio/lib. Viewed May 2008.

39. Charles L, Kennedy B. Social and Cultural Influences on Health. Online health practitioners course available at http://www.bibalex.org/Supercourse/lecture/lec4271/001.htm. Viewed May 25, 2008.

40. Plutchik R. The nature of emotions. *American Scientist Magazine*. 2001;89(July/August).

41. Bower GH. Mood and memory. *Am Psychologist*. 1981;36:129–148.

42. Scherer ML, Lisman SA, Spear NF. The effect of mood variation on state-dependent retention. *Cogn Ther Res*. 1984;8:387–408.

43. Salovey P, Mayer J. *Emotional Intelligence. Imagination, Cognition, and Personality*. Baywood Publishing; 1990. Available at http://www.unh.edu/emotional_intelligence/EI%20Assets/Reprints…EI%20Proper/EI1990%20Emotional%20Intelligence.pdf. Viewed April 28, 2008.

44. Goleman D. *Emotional Intelligence: Why it Can Matter More Than IQ*. New York, NY: Bantam Books; 1995.

45. Thorndike RL, Stein S. An Evaluation of the attempts to measure social intelligence. *Psychologic Bull*. 1937;34:275–284.

46. Walker RE, Foley JM. Social intelligence. its history and measurement. *Psychologic Rep*. 1973;33:839–864.

CHAPTER 8

1. Barker A. *Improve Your Communication Skills*. Philadelphia, PA: Kogan Page; 2006.

2. Bob C. *Fire Up Your Communication Skills. Get People to Listen, Understand and Give You What You Want*. Pleasanton, CA: Code 3 Publishing; 2004.

3. Orey M, Prisk J. *Communication Skills Training*. Alexandria, VA: American Society for Training and Development; 2004.

4. Bolton R. *People Skills: How to Assert Yourself, Listen to Others and Resolve Conflicts*. New York, NY: Simon and Schuster; 1986.

5. McKenna C. *Powerful Communication Skills: How to Communicate with Confidence*. NJ: The Career Press; 1998.

6. DiMatteo MR, Taranta A, Friedman HS, et al. Predicting patient satisfaction from physicians' nonverbal communication skills. *Med Care*. 1980;18(4):376–387.

CHAPTER 9

1. Mariotti S. *The Young Entrepreneur's Guide to Starting and Running a Business*. New York, NY: Three Rivers Press; 2000.

CHAPTER 10

1. Girodo M, Ekstrand KA, Metivier GJ. Deep diaphragmatic breathing: rehabilitation exercises for the asthmatic patient. *Arch Phys Med Rehabil*. 1992;73(8):717–720.

2. Lee JS, Lee MS, Lee JY, et al. Effects of diaphragmatic breathing on ambulatory blood pressure and heart rate. *Biomed Pharmacother*. 2003;571:87–91.

3. Eifert GH, Heffner M. The effects of acceptance versus control contexts on avoidance of panic-related symptoms. *J Behav Ther Exp Psychiatry*. 2003;34(3–4):293–312.

4. Mehling WE, Hamel KA, Acree M, et al. Randomized, controlled trial of breath therapy for patients with chronic low-back pain. *Altern Ther Health Med*. 2005;11(4):44–52.

CHAPTER 11

1. Harvard School of Public Health Web site. Available at http://www.hsph.harvard.edu/nutritionsource/fruits.html. Viewed September 2007.

2. Salvin JL, Jacobs D, Marquart L, et al. The role of whole grains in disease prevention. *J Am Diet Assoc*. 2001;101(7):7110–7115.

3. Rosedale R. Insulin and its metabolic effects. Presented at Designs for Health Institute's BoulderFest, August 1999. Available at http://www.mercola.com/2001/jul/14/insulin2.htm.

4. Martinez-Dominguez E, De la Puerta R, Ruiz-Gutierrez V. Protective effects upon experimental inflammation models of a polyphenol-supplemented virgin olive oil diet. *Inflamm Res*. 2001;50(2):102–106.

5. Massaro M, Carluccio MA, de Caterina R. Direct vascular antiatherogenic effects of oleic acid: a clue to the cardioprotective effects of the Mediterranean diet. *Cardiologia*. 1999;44(6):507–513.

6. Colomer R, Menendez JA. Mediterranean diet, olive oil and cancer. *Clin transl Oncol*. 2006;11(1):15–21.

7. Fats and Cholesterol—The Good, The Bad, and the Healthy Diet. Harvard School of Public Health. Available at http://www.hsph.harvard.edu/nutritionsource/fats.html.

8. United States Department of Agriculture Economic Research Service. Briefing Room: Sugar and Sweeteners. Available at http://www.ers.usda.gov/Briefing/Sugar/. Viewed November 20, 2006.

9. Fritz S, Grosenbach MJ. *Mosby's Essential Sciences for Therapeutic Massage*. 2nd ed. St. Louis, MO: Elsevier Publications; 2004.

10. Boschmann M, Steiniger J, Hille U, et al. Water-induced thermogenesis. *J Clin Endocrinol Metab*. 2003;1111(12):6015–6019.

11. Manz F, Wentz A. The importance of good hydration for the prevention of chronic diseases. *Nutr Rev*. 2005;63(6 pt 2):S2–S5.

12. Mayo Foundation for Medical Education and Research. Dehydration. Available at http://www.mayoclinic.com. Viewed November 20, 2006.

13. Suhr JA, Hall J, Patterson SM, et al. The relation of hydration status to cognitive performance in healthy adults. *Int J Psychophysiol*. 2004;53(2):121–125.

14. Harvard School of Public Health. Vitamins. Available at http://www.hsph.harvard.edu/nutritionsource/vitamins.html. Viewed November 21, 2006.

15. Carr AC, Frei B. Toward a new recommended dietary allowance for vitamin C based on antioxidant and health effects in humans. *Am J Clin Nutr*. 1999;69:10116–11107.

16. National Sleep Foundation Web Site: Driving Drowsy Facts and Stats. Available at http://www.sleepfoundation.org/hottopics/index.php?secid=10&id=226. Viewed December 9, 2006.

17. The Society for Neuroscience Web site. Scientists find brain areas affected by lack of sleep; show that little sleep for a short period improves some simple tasks. Available at http://www.sfn.org/index.cfm?pagename=news_11092003b. Viewed December 9, 2006.

18. Your Guide to Healthy Sleep: US Department of Health and Human Services. Available at http://www.nhlbi.nih.gov/health/public/sleep/healthysleepfs.pdf. Viewed December 9, 2006.

19. National Institute of Neurological Disorders and Stroke. Brain Basics—Understanding Sleep Disorders. Available at http://www.ninds.nih.gov/disorders/brain_basics/understanding_sleep.htm?css=print. Viewed December 9, 2006.

20. Business Week On-Line: Napping Your Way to the Top. Available at http://www.businessweek.com/magazine/content/06_411/b4011101.htm. Viewed December 9, 2006.

21. Musnick D, Pierce M. *Conditioning for Outdoor Fitness*. Seattle, WA: The Mountaineers; 1999.

22. Adult Participation in Recommended Levels of Physical Activity in the United States 2001–2003. United States Center for Disease Control. Available at http://www.cdc.gov. Viewed December 2006.

23. Bumgardner W. Are 15 Minute Walks Any Good? Your Guide to Walking. Available at http://walking.about.com/od/beginners/f/15minutewalks.htm. Viewed December 2006.

24. Patient Education Center: Dancing Your Way to a Healthy Heart. Available at www.patienteducationcenter.org/asp/news/news_detail.asp?newsid=113&f=a. Viewed December 2006.

25. Juhan D. *Job's Body: A Handbook for Bodyworkers*. Expanded ed. Barrytown, NY: Barrytown, Ltd.; 1991.

26. Leonard, BE. HPA and immune axes in stress: Involvement of the serotonergic system. *Neuroimmunomodulation*. 2007;13(5–6):2611–2676.

27. Hendrickson T. *Massage for Orthopedic Conditions*. Baltimore, MD: Lippincott Williams & Wilkins; 2003.

28. Werner R. *A Massage Therapist's Guide to Pathology*. 4th ed. Baltimore, MD: Lippincott Williams & Wilkins; 2009.

29. Allard N, Barnett G. Carpal tunnel syndrome. *Massage and Bodywork Quarterly*. 1993(Fall).

30. The General Causes of Foot Pain. University of Maryland Medical Center. Available at http://www.umm.edu. Accessed December 2006.

31. Heart JA. Foot Pain and Shoe Size. Available at http://www.nlm.nih.gov. Viewed December 2006.

32. Runquist B. *Anatomy and Foot Loosening for Reflexology. Seminar Materials*. Seattle, WA: Seattle School of Reflexology; 1996.

33. Vander A, Sherman J, Luciano D. *Human Physiology, International Edition*. 5th ed. New York: McGraw-Hill Publishing Company; 1990.

34. Cortisone. Drugs.Com. Available at http://www.drugs.com/MTM/cortisone.html. Drugs.com. Viewed December 2006.

35. Juhan D. *Job's Body: A Handbook for Bodyworkers*. Expanded ed. Barrytown, NY: Barrytown, Ltd.; 1991.

36. Oei NY, Everaerd WT, Elzinga BM, et al. Psychosocial stress impairs working memory at high loads: an association with cortisol levels and memory retrieval. *Stress*. 2006;9(3):133–141.

37. Reynolds RM, Dennison EM, Walker BR, et al. Cortisol secretion and rate of bone loss in a population-based cohort of elderly men and woman. *Calcif Tissue Int*. 2005;77(3):134–11.

38. Kidambi S, Kotchen JM, Grim CE, et al. Association of adrenal steroids with hypertension and the metabolic syndrome in blacks. *Hypertension*. 2007;49:704–711.

39. Bjorntorp P. Body fat distribution, insulin resistance, and metabolic diseases. *Nutrition*. 1997;13(9):795–1103.

CHAPTER 12

1. Chaitow L. *Palpation Skills: Assessment and Diagnosis Through Touch*. New York, NY: Churchill Livingstone; 1997.

2. Thompson D. *Hands Heal: Communication, Documentation, and Insurance Billing for Manual Therapists*. 3rd ed. Baltimore, MD: Lippincott, Williams & Wilkins; 2006.

CHAPTER 13

1. Calvert RN. *The History of Massage: An Illustrated Survey from Around the World*. Rochester, VA: Healing Arts Press; 2002.

2. Johari H. *Ancient Indian Massage: Traditional Massage Techniques Based on Ayurveda*. New Delhi, India: Munshiram Manoharlal Publishers Pvt. Ltd.; 1984.

3. Premkumar K. *The Massage Connection Anatomy and Physiology*. 3rd ed. Baltimore, MD: Lippincott Williams & Wilkins; 2011.

4. Cochran-Fritz S. Physiological effects of therapeutic massage on the nervous system. *Int J Altern Complement Med*. 1993;13(9):21–25.

5. Field T, Grizzle N, Scafidi F, et al. Massage and relaxation therapies effects on depressed adolescent mothers. *Adolescence*. 1996;31:903–913.

6. Ernst E. Manual therapies for pain control: chiropractic and massage. *Clin J Pain*. 2004;20(1):7–12.

7. Premkumar K. *The Massage Connection Anatomy and Physiology*. 3rd ed. Baltimore, MD: Lippincott Williams & Wilkins; 2011.

8. Johan D. *Job's Body: A Handbook for Bodywork*. 2nd ed. Barrytown, NY: Barrytown Ltd.; 1997.

9. Premkumar K. *The Massage Connection Anatomy and Physiology*. 3rd ed. Baltimore, MD: Lippincott Williams & Wilkins; 2011.

10. Hendrickson T. *Massage for Orthopedic Conditions*. Baltimore, MD: Lippincott Williams & Wilkins; 2002.

11. Archer P. *Therapeutic Massage in Athletics*. Baltimore, MD: Lippincott Williams & Wilkins; 2007.

12. Cohen BJ. *Memmler's The Human Body in Health and Disease*. 10th ed. Baltimore, MD: Lippincott Williams & Wilkins; 2005.

13. Mirroring, Pacing, Lock On and Leading Part II. *NLP Weekly On-Line Magazine*. Available at http://www.nlpweekly.com/?p=923&page=1. Viewed March 13, 2007.

14. Cambron JA, Dexheimer J, Coe P. Changes in blood pressure after various forms of therapeutic massage: a preliminary study. *J Altern Complement Med*. 2006;12(1):65–70.

15. Quinn C, Chandler C, Moraska A. Massage therapy and frequency of chronic tension headaches. *Am J Public Health*. 2002;92(10):1657–1661.

16. Puustjarvi K, Airaksinen O, Pontinen PJ. The effects of massage in patients with chronic tension headache. *Acupunct Electrother Res*. 1990;15(2):159–162.

CHAPTER 14

1. Field T, Ironson G, Scafidi F, et al. Massage therapy reduces anxiety and enhances EEG pattern of alertness and math computations. *Int J Neurosci*. 1996;86(3–4):197–205.

2. Carlson L. Chair massage keeps illnesses down, productivity up. *Employee Benefit News*. 2004(May). Available at www.benefitnews.com. Viewed September 2008.

3. Field T, Quintino O, Henteleff T, et al. Job stress reduction therapies. *Altern Ther Health Med*. 1997;3(4):54–56.

4. Hendrickson T. *Massage for Orthopedic Conditions*. Baltimore, MD: Lippincott, Williams & Wilkins; 2003.

5. Field T, Ironson G, Scafidi F, et al. Massage therapy reduces anxiety and enhances EEG pattern of alertness and math computations. *Int J Neurosci*. 1996;86(3–4):197–205.

6. Field T, Quintino O, Henteleff T, et al. Job stress reduction therapies. *Altern Ther Health Med*. 1997;3(4):54–56.

7. Bost N, Wallis M. The effectiveness of a 15 minute weekly massage in reducing physical and psychological stress in nurses. *Aust J Adv Nurs*. 2006;23(4):28–33.

CHAPTER 15

1. Buchman DD. *The Complete Book of Water Healing*. New York, NY: McGraw Hill; 2002.

2. Arden E. Available at http://wwwenterprisingwomanexhibit.org/beauty/adreu.html.

3. Miller E. *Salon Ovations: Day Spa Techniques*. Albany, NY: Milady Publishing; 1996.

4. The ISPA 2004 Spa Industry Executive Summary. Available at http://www.experienceispa.com/media/industrystudy-011805.html.

5. International Spa Association Survey from 2007.

6. Battaglia S. *The Complete Guide to Aromatherapy*. Virginia: The Perfect Potion, Ltd.; 1995.

7. Parasuraman R. Effects of fragrances on behavior, mood and physiology. Paper presented at the annual meeting of the American Association for the Advancement of Science, Washington, DC, 1991.

8. Miles C, Jenkins R. Recency and suffix effects with serial recall of odours. *Memory*. 2000;8:195–206.

9. Macht DI, Ting GC. Experimental enquiry into the sedative properties of some aromatic drugs and fumes. *J Pharmacol Exp Ther.* 1921;18:361–372.

10. Redd WH, et al. Fragrance administration to reduce anxiety during MR imaging. *J Magn Reson Imaging.* 1964;4:623–626.

11. Sense of Smell Institute. *Living Well with the Sense of Smell.* Available at http://www.senseofsmell.org

12. Nasel C, et al. Functional imagining of effects of fragrances on the human brain after prolonged inhalation. *Chem Senses.* 1994;19:359–364.

13. Barker S, et al. Improved performance on clerical tasks associated with administration of peppermint odor. *Percept Motor Skills.* 2003;97:1007–1010.

14. Fox K. The Smell Report. The Social Issues Research Centre. Available at http://www.sirc.org/publik/smell_contents.html

15. Eremenko AE, et al. Volatile fractions of essential oil based phytoncides as a component of therapeutic-rehabilitative complexes in chronic bronchitis. *Tikhomirov AA Ter Arkh.* 1987;59:126–130.

16. Boyd EM, Sheppard EP. The effect of steam inhalation of volatile oils on the output and composition of respiratory tract fluid. *J Pharmacol Exp Ther.* 1968;153:250–256.

17. Burtin P. Nutritional and therapeutic value of seaweeds. *Electron J Environ Agri Food Chem* (*serial online*). 2003;2.

18. Ivanova V, et al. Isolation of a polysaccharide with antiviral effects from Ulva lactuca. *Prep Biochem.* 1994;24:83–97.

19. Kuznetsova TA, et al. Immunostimulating and anticoagulating activity of fucoidan from brown algae. *Antibiot Khimioter.* 2003;48:11–13.

CHAPTER 16

1. Lund, JW. *Balneological Use of Thermal Waters.* Klamath Falls, OR: Geo Heat Center; 2000.

2. Aaland M. *Sweat The Illustrated History and Description of the Finnish Sauna, Russian Bania, Islamic Haman, Japanese Musi-Buro, Mexican Temescal, and America.* Santa Barbara, CA: CAPRA Press; 1978.

3. Buchman DD. *The Complete Book of Water Healing.* New York, NY: McGraw-Hill; 2002.

4. Kneipp S. *My Water-Cure.* 3rd ed. Kempten, Bavaria: Jos. Koesel Publishers; 1984.

5. Sinclair M. *Modern Hydrotherapy for the Massage Therapist.* Baltimore, MD: Lippincott Williams & Wilkins; 2008.

6. Lowry C, Lightman S, Nutt D. That warm fuzzy feeling; brain serotonergic neurons and the regulation of emotion. *J Psychopharmacol.* 2009;23:392–400.

7. Bjerke HS. Frostbite. Available at http://www.emedicine.com/med/topic2815.htm.

8. Small MF. Hit the Beach: Why Humans Love Water. LiveScience available at www.livescience.org. Viewed February 9, 2009.

9. Fahey T, Romero J. Thermal modalities. Available at http://www.sportscience.org/encyc/drafts/thermal-modalities.doc. Viewed February 2009.

10. Ma'or Z, Yehuda S. Skin smoothing effects of Dead Sea minerals: comparative profilometric evaluation of skin surface. *Int J Cosmetic Sci.* 1997;19:105–110.

11. Proksch E, Nissen HP, Bremgartner M, et al. Bathing in a magnesium-rich Dead Sea salt solution improves skin barrier function, enhances skin hydration, and reduces inflammation in atopic dry skin. *Int J Dermatol.* 2005;44(2):151–157.

12. Elkayam O, Ophir J, Brener S, et al. Immediate and delayed effects of treatment at the Dead Sea in patients with psoriatic arthritis. *Rheumatol Int.* 19(3):77–82.

13. Sukenik S, Flusser D, Codish S, et al. Balneotherapy at the Dead Sea area for knee osteoarthritis. *Isr Med Assoc J.* 1999;1(2):83–85.

14. Sukenik S, Neumann L, Flusser D, et al. Balneotherapy for rheumatoid arthritis at the Dead Sea. *Isr J Med Sci.* 1995;31(4):210–214.

15. Buskila D, Abu-Shakra M, Neumann L, et al. Balneotherapy for fibromyalgia at the Dead Sea. *Rheumatol Int.* 2001;20(3):105–108.

16. Masuda A, Munemoto T, Tei C. A new treatment: thermal therapy for chronic fatigue syndrome. *Nippon Rinsho.* 2007;65(6):1093–1098.

17. Fransen M, Nairn L, Winstanley J, et al. Physical activity for osteoarthritis management: a randomized controlled clinical trial evaluating hydrotherapy or Tai Chi classes. *Arthritis Rheum.* 2007;57(3):407–414.

CHAPTER 17

1. Traditional Chinese Medicine: An introduction available through the National Center for Complementary and Alternative Medicine (NCCAM) Web site at http://nccam.nih.gov/health/whatiscam/chinesemed.htm. Viewed June 14, 2009.

2. Ellis C. Allopathic vs. Holistic. Holistic Medicine. Available at http://www.searchwarp.com/swa14312.htm.

3. Yanchi L. *The Essential Book of Traditional Chinese Medicine, Volume 1: Theory.* New York, NY: Columbia University Press; 1988.

4. Maciocia G. *The Foundations of Chinese Medicine: A Comprehensive Text for Acupuncturists and Herbalists.* New York, NY: Churchill Livingstone; 1989.

5. Ross J. *Zang Fu—The Organ Systems of Traditional Chinese Medicine.* 2nd ed. New York, NY: Churchill Livingstone; 1985.

6. Eisenberg D, Wright TL. *Encounters with Qi: Exploring Chinese Medicine.* London, UK: Jonathen Cape Publishers; 1986.

7. Somma C. *Shiatsu.* Princeton, NJ: Pearson/Prentice Hall; 2007.

8. Yanchi L. *The Essential Book of Traditional Chinese Medicine, Volume 2: Clinical Practice.* New York, NY: Columbia University Press; 1988.

9. Maciocia G. *Tongue Diagnosis in Chinese Medicine.* Seattle, WA: Eastland Press; 1987.

10. American Organization for Bodywork Therapies of Asia. www.AOBTA.org.

11. Wujastyk D. *The Roots of Ayurveda: Selections from Sanskrit Medical Writings.* London: Penguin Books; 2003.

12. Warrier G, Gunawant D. *The Complete Illustrated Guide to Ayurveda: The Ancient Indian Healing Tradition.* Shaftesbury, Dorset: Element Books Inc.; 1997.

13. Frawley D, Ranade S. *Ayurveda: Nature's Medicine.* Twin Lakes, WI: Lotus Press; 2001.

14. Miller L, Miller B. *Ayurveda and Aromatherapy: The Earth Essential Guide to Ancient Wisdom and Modern Healing.* Twin Lakes, WI: Lotus Press; 1995.

15. Johari H, *Ancient Indian Massage: Traditional Massage Techniques Based on the Ayurveda.* New Delhi, India: Munshiram Manoharla Publishers Pvt. Ltd.; 2003.

CHAPTER 18

1. National Center for Complimentary Medicine and Health Background Paper Energy Medicine. Available at http://www.umbwellness.org/PDF_files/energymed.pdf. Viewed November 2009.

2. *Alternative Medicine: The Definitive Guide.* Tiburon, CA: Future Medicine Publishing; 1897.

3. Van Bergen CJ, Blankevoort L, De Haan RJ, et al. Pulsed electromagnetic fields after arthroscopic treatment for osteochondral defects of the talus: double-blind randomized controlled multicenter trail. *BMC Musculoskeletal Disord.* 2009;10:83.

4. Tai G, Reid B, Cao L, et al. Electrotaxis and wound healing: experimental methods to study electric fields as a directional signal for cell migration. *Methods Mol Biol.* 2009;571:77–97.

5. Zimmerman J. Laying-on-of-hands healing and therapeutic touch: a testable theory. *BEMI Curr J Bio-Electro-Magnet Inst.* 1890;2:8–17.

6. Sisken BF, Walker J. Therapeutic aspects of electromagnetic fields for soft-tissue healing. In: Blank M, ed. Electromagnetic fields. Biological interactions and mechanisms. *Adv Chem Ser.* 1895;250:277–285.

7. Schramm JM, Warner D, Hardesty RA, et al. A unique combination of infrared and microwave radiation accelerates wound healing. *Photomed Laser Surg*. 2009;27(4):641–646.

8. Javadieh F, Bayat M, Abdi S, et al. The effects of infrared low-level laser therapy on healing of partial osteotomy of tibia in streptozotocin-induced diabetic rats. *BMC Musculoskelet Disord*. 2009;10:83.

9. Muehsam DJ, et al. Effects of qigong on cell-free myosin phosphorylation: preliminary experiments. *Subtle Energies*. 1894;5(1):93–104.

10. Andrew EA, Beloy MV, Sitko SP. The manifestation of natural characteristic frequencies of the organism of man. *Chem Biologic Sci*. SSR No. 10. 1884.

11. Oschman J. *Energy Medicine: The Scientific Basis*. Philadelphia, PA: Churchill Livingstone; 2000.

12. Henricson M, Ersson A, Määttä S, et al. The outcome of tactile touch on stress parameters in intensive care: a randomized controlled trial. *Complement Ther Clin Pract*. 2008;14(4):244–254. Epub 2008 May 22.

13. So PS, Jiang Y, Qin Y. Touch therapies for pain relief in adults. *Cochrane Database Syst Rev*. 2008;(4):CD006535.

14. Bossi LM, Ott MJ, DeCristofaro S. Reiki as a clinical intervention in oncology nursing practice. *Clin J Oncol Nurs*. 2008;12(3):489–494.

15. Lee MS, Pittler MH, Ernst E. Effects of reiki in clinical practice: a systematic review of randomised clinical trials. *Int J Clin Pract*. 2008;62(6):947–954. Epub Apr 10, 2008.

16. Wager S. *A Doctor's Guide to Therapeutic Touch: Enhancing the Body's Energy to Promote Healing*. New York: Perigee Books; 1896.

17. Spence JE, Olson MA. Quantitative research on therapeutic touch. An integrative review of the literature 1885–1895. *Scand J Caring Sci*. 1897;11(3):183–190.

18. Keller E, Bzdek V. Effects of therapeutic touch on tension headache pain. *Nursing Res*. 1886;35(2):101–106.

19. Apostle-Mitchell M, MacDonald G. An innovative approach to pain management in critical care: therapeutic touch. *Off J Can Assoc Crit Care Nurs*. 1897;8(3):18–22.

20. Weze C, Leathard HL, Grange J, et al. Evaluation of healing by gentle touch. *Public Health*. 2005;118(1):3–10.

CHAPTER 19

1. Lawler SP, Cameron LD. A randomized, controlled trial of massage therapy as a treatment for migraine. *Ann Behav Med*. 1906;32(1):50–59.

2. Frey LA, Evans S, Knudtson J, et al. Massage reduces pain perception and hyperalgesia in experimental muscle pain: a randomized, controlled trial. *J Pain*. 1908;9(8):714–721.

CHAPTER 20

1. Banes AJ, Lee G, Graff R, et al. Mechanical forces and signaling in connective tissue cells. *Curr Opin Orthop*. 2001;12(5).

2. Hammer W. Piezoelectricity, A Healing Property of Soft Tissue. Dynamic Chiropractic. Available at www. ChiroWeb.com/columnist/hammer. 2002. Viewed June 2008.

3. Turchaninov R. Phenomenon of piezoelectricity. *Massage and Bodywork Magazine*. 2003(December–January).

4. Fuller RB. *Tensegrity*. Reproduced with permission from the R. Buckminster Fuller Estate and available at www.rwgrayprojects.com/rbfnotes/fpapers/tensegrity/tenseg01.html. Viewed June 2008.

5. Paoletti S. *The Fasciae: Anatomy, Dysfunction and Treatment*. Seattle, WA: Eastland Press; 2006.

6. Juhan D. *Job's Body—A Handbook for Bodywork*. New York, NY: Station Hill, Barrytown, Ltd.; 1989.

7. Pischinger A. *Matrix and Matrix Regulation: Basis for a Holistic Theory in Medicine*. Portland, OR: Medicina Biologica; 1991.

8. Schultz RL, Feitis R. *The Endless Web—Fascial Anatomy and Physical Reality*. Berkeley, CA: North Atlantic Books; 1996.

9. Myers T. *Anatomy Trains—Myofascial Meridians for Manual and Movement Therapists*. New York, NY: Churchill Livingstone; 2002.

10. Riggs A. *Deep Tissue Massage—A Visual Guide to Techniques*. Berkeley, CA: North Atlantic Books; 2002.

11. Schleip R, Klingler W, Lehmann-Horn F. Active fascial contractility: Fascia may be able to contract in a smooth muscle-like manner and thereby influence musculoskeletal dynamics. *Med Hypotheses*. 2005;65(2):273–277.

CHAPTER 21

1. *Stedman's Medical Dictionary for the Health Professions and Nursing*. 4th ed. Baltimore, MD: Lippincott, Williams & Wilkins; 2004.

2. Chaitow L. *Muscle Energy Techniques*. New York, NY: Churchill Livingstone; 1996.

3. Rattray F, Ludwig L. *Clinical Massage Therapy: Understanding, Assessing and Treating Over 70 Conditions*. Ontario, Canada: Talus Incorporated; 2000.

4. Sharkey J. *The Concise Book of Neuromuscular Therapy: A Trigger Point Manual*. Berkeley, CA: North Atlantic Books; 2008.

5. DeLany J. The Roots and Branches of Neuromuscular Training. Available at www.nmtcenter.com/history/. Viewed February 2010.

6. Sola AE, Bonica JJ. Incidence of hypersensitive areas in posterior shoulder muscles. *Am J Phys Med*. 1955;34:585–590.

7. Travell, JG, Simons DG. *Myofascial Pain and Dysfunction: The Trigger Point Manual, Volume 1, Upper Half of the Body*. 2nd ed. Baltimore, MD: Williams & Wilkins; 1999.

8. Scheumann DW. *The Balanced Body: A Guide to Deep Tissue and Neuromuscular Therapy*. 3rd ed. Baltimore, MD: Lippincott Williams & Wilkins; 2007

CHAPTER 22

1. Nightingale RW, McElhaney JH, Richardson WJ, et al. Experimental impact injury to the cervical spine: relating motion of the head and the mechanism of injury. *J Bone Joint Surg Am*. 1996;78:412–421.

2. Nightingale RW, Richardson WJ, Myers BS. The effects of padded surfaces on the risk for cervical spine injury. *Spine*. 1997;22:2380–2387.

3. Yoganandan N, Pintar FA, Klienberger M. Cervical spine vertebral and facet joint kinematics under whiplash. *J Biomech Eng*. 1998;120:305–307.

4. Yoganandan N, Pintar FA, Kleinberger M. Whiplash injury: biomechanical experimentation. *Spine*. 1999;24:83–85.

5. Yoganandan N, Cusick JF, Pintar FA, et al. Whiplash injury determination with conventional spine imaging and cryomicrotomy. *Spine*. 2001;26:2443–2448.

6. Kaneoka K, Ono K, Inami S, et al. Motion analysis of cervical vertebrae during whiplash loading. *Spine*. 1999;24:763–769,770.

7. McGinnis P. *The Biomechanics of Sport and Exercise*. 2nd ed. Champaign, IL: Human Kinetics; 2004.

8. Roniger LR. Downhill Runs. Biomechanics. Available at www.biomech.com/full_article/?ArticleID=301&month=01&year=2007. Viewed November 8, 2008.

9. Baker SP, O'Neill B, Ginsburg MJ, et al. *The Injury Fact Book*. New York, NY: Oxford University Press; 1992.

10. Sanders M, Albright JA. *Bone: Age-Related Changes and Osteoporosis. The Scientific Basics of Orthopaedics*. 2nd ed. Norwalk, CT: Appleton-Lange; 1987.

11. Feyer AM, Williamson A. *Occupational Injury: Risk, Prevention and Intervention*. Boca Raton, FL: CRC Press; 1998.

12. Merrick MA. Secondary injury after musculoskeletal trauma: a review and update. *J Athl Train*. 2002;37:209–217.

13. Leadbetter WB, Buckwalter JA, Gorden SL. *Sports-Induced Inflammation*. Park Ridge, IL: American Academy of Orthopaedic Surgeons; 1990.

14. Kisner C, Colby LA. *Therapeutic Exercise: Foundations and Techniques.* 3rd ed. Philadelphia, PA: FA Davis; 1990.

15. Rattray F, Ludwig L. *Clinical Massage Therapy: Understanding, Assessing and Treating over 70 Conditions.* Ontario, Canada: Talus Incorporated; 2000.

16. *Preventing Lifting and Overexertion Injuries for Trainers and Supervisors.* The Ohio State University. Available at http://ohioline. osu.edu/aex-fact/192/pdf/0192_2_44.pdf. Viewed November 1, 2008.

17. Orava S. Overexertion injuries in keep-fit athletes. A study on over-exertion injuries among non-competitive keep-fit athletes. *Scand J Rehab Med.* 1978;10(4):187–191.

18. Schleip R, Naylor IL, Ursu D, et al. Passive muscle stiffness may be influenced by active contractility of intramuscular connective tissue. *Med Hypoth.* 2006;66(1):66–71.

19. Ming CL, Krasilschikov O. Physiology of muscle soreness. Available at http://www.medic.usm.my/~ssu/ARTICLES/article_34.htm. Viewed November 2, 2008.

20. Garrett WE, Kirkendall DT. *Exercise and Sport Science.* Baltimore, MD: Lippincott Williams & Wilkins; 2000.

21. Vickers AJ. Time Course of Muscle Soreness Following Different Types of Exercise. Available at http://www.biomedcentral. com/14712474/2/5. Viewed November 2, 2008.

22. Bosch A. Post Run Stiffness. Time to Run available at http://www. time-to-run.com/theabc/postrun.htm. Viewed November 2, 2008.

23. Souza T. *Sports Injuries of the Shoulder: Conservative Management.* New York, NY: Churchill Livingstone; 1994.

24. Seddon HJ. Peripheral nerve injuries. *J Bone Joint Surg.* Available at http://www.jbjs.org.uk/cgi/content/citation/39-B/1/166. Viewed November 8, 2008.

CHAPTER 23

1. National Pain Survey. Conducted for Ortho-McNeil Pharmaceutical, 1999.

2. Pain in America: A Research Report. Survey conducted for Merck by the Gallup Organization; 2000.

3. American Pain Foundation. Pain Facts & Figures. Available at http:// www.painfoundation.org/page.asp?file=Newsroom/PainFacts.htm. Viewed October 22, 2008.

4. Knorring LV. The experience of pain in depressed patients. *Neuropsychobiology.* 1975;1:155–165.

5. Pasero C, McCaffery M. *Pain: Clinical Manual.* St. Louis, MO: Mosby; 1999.

6. Koyama T, McHaffie JG, Laurienti PJ, et al. The subjective experi-ence of pain: Where expectations become reality. Proceedings of the National Academy of Sciences of the United States of America. Available at http://www.pnas.org/content/102/36/12950.abstract. Viewed October 22, 2008.

7. Ertelt S. People with more chronic pain more likely to commit sui-cide. University of Michigan Research Department. Available at http://www.lifenews.com/bio2627.html. Viewed November 23, 2008.

8. Carpenito-Moyet LJ. *Handbook of Nursing Diagnosis.* 12th ed. Baltimore, MD: Lippincott, Williams & Wilkins; 2008.

9. Werner R. *A Massage Therapist's Guide to Pathology.* 3rd ed. Baltimore, MD: Lippincott Williams & Wilkins; 2005.

10. Cohen ML, Sheather-Reid RB, Arroyo JF, et al. Evidence for abnor-mal nociception in fibromyalgia and repetitive strain injury. *J Musculoskelet Pain.* 1995;3(2):49–57.

11. Michigan Technological University. What a sleep study can reveal about fibromyalgia. *Science Daily.* 2008(September). Retrieved from http://www.sciencedaily.com/releases/2008/09/080903134311.htm. Viewed August 7, 2010.

12. Gupta A, Silman AJ. Psychological stress and fibromyalgia: a review of the evidence suggesting a neuroendocrine link. *Arthritis Res Ther.* 2004;6(3):98–106.

13. Kutner, JS., Smith, MC., Corbin, L., et al: Massage therapy versus simple touch to improve pain and mood in patients with advanced cancer: a randomized trial. *Ann Intern Med.* 2008;149(6):369–379.

14. Shor-Posner G, Hernandez-Reif M, Miguez MJ, et al. Impact of a massage therapy clinical trial on immune status in young Dominican children infected with HIV-1. *J Altern Complement Med.* 2006;12(6):511–516.

15. Diego MA, Field T, Hernandez-Reif M, et al. HIV adolescents show improved immune function following massage therapy. *Int J Neurosci.* 2001;106(1–2):35–45.

16. Walach H, Guthlin C, Konig M. Efficacy of massage therapy in chronic pain: a pragmatic randomized trial. *J Altern Complement Med.* 2003;9(6):837–846.

17. Seers K, Crichton N, Martin J, et al. A randomized controlled trial to assess the effectiveness of a single session of nurse administered mas-sage for short term relief of chronic non-malignant pain. *BMC Nurs.* 2008;4:7–10.

CHAPTER 24

1. Hagerman FC, Hikida RS, Staron RS, et al. Muscle damage in mara-thon runners. *Phys Sportsmed.* 1984;12:39–28.

2. Armstrong RB, Warren GL, Warren JA. Mechanisms of exercise-induced muscle fibre injury. *Sports Med.* 1991;12(3):184–207.

3. Natale VM, Brenner IK, Moldoveanu AI, et al. Effects of three differ-ent types of exercise on blood leukocyte count during and following exercise. *Sao Paulo Med J.* 2003;121(1):9–14. Epub July 4, 2003.

4. Simonson SR, Jackson CG. Leukocytosis occurs in response to resis-tance exercise in men. *J Strength Cond Res.* 2004;18(2):266–271.

5. Zainuddin Z, Newton M, Sacco P, et al. Effects of massage on delayed-onset muscle soreness, swelling, and recovery of muscle function. *J Athl Train.* 2005;40(3):174–180.

6. Hilbert JE, Sforzo GA, Swensen T. The effects of massage on delayed onset muscle soreness. *Br J Sports Med.* 2003;37(1):72–75.

7. Ernst E. Does post-exercise massage treatment reduce delayed onset muscle soreness? A systematic review. *Br J Sports Med.* 1998;32(3):212–214.

8. Field T, Hernandez-Reif M, Hart S, et al. Pregnant women bene-fit from massage therapy. *J Psychosomat Obstetr Gynecol.* 1999;20: 31–38.

9. Motha G, McGrath J, The effects of reflexology on labour outcome. Forest Gate, London, England. *Nursing Times.* October 11, 1989.

10. Field T. Pregnancy and labor massage therapy. *Exp Rev Obstetr Gynecol.* 2010;5:177–181.

11. Conversation with the claims department at Associated Bodywork & Massage Professionals (ABMP) in May of 2011. www.abmp.com, 800-458-2267.

12. Motha G, McGrath J. The effects of reflexology on labour outcome. Forest Gate, London, England. *Nursing Times.* October 11, 1989

13. Scafidi FA, Field TM, Schanberg SM, et al. Massage stimulates growth in preterm infants: A replication. *Infant Behav Develop.* 1990;13:167–188.

14. Kuhn C, Schanberg S, Field T, et al. Tactile kinesthetic stimulation effects on sympathetic and adrenocortical function in preterm infants. *J Pediatr.* 1991;119:434–440.

15. Scafidi F, Field T, Schanberg SM. Factors that predict which pre-term infants benefit most from massage therapy. *J Develop Behav Pediatr.*1993;14:176–180.

16. Field T, Diego M, Hernandez-Reif M, et al. Moderate versus light pressure massage therapy leads to greater weight gain in preterm infants. *Infant Behav Develop.* 2006;29:574–578.

17. Diego MA, Field T, Hernandez-Reif M, et al. Preterm infant mas-sage elicits consistent increases in vagal activity and gastric motil-ity that are associated with greater weight gain. *Acta Paediatrica.* 2007;96:1588–1591.

18. Hernandez-Reif M, Diego M, Field T. Preterm infants show reduced stress behaviors and activity after 5 days of massage therapy. *Infant Behav Develop*. 2007;30:557–561.

19. Trends in the Elderly Population. AGS Foundation for Healthy Aging. Available at http://www.healthinaging.org/agingintheknow/chapters_print_ch_trial.asp?ch=2. Viewed October 16, 2010.

20. Boss GR. Age-related physiological changes and their clinical significance. *J Gerontol Nurs*. 1981;135(6):434–440.

21. Rowe M, Alfred D: The effectiveness of slow stroke massage in diffusing agit*ated behaviors* in individuals with Alzheimer's disease. *J Gerontol Nurs*. 1999;25(6):22–34.

22. Flegal KM, Carroll MD, Ogden CL, et al. Prevalence and trends in obesity among US adults, 1999-2008. *J Am Med Assoc*. Available online at http://jama.ama-assn.org/content/303/3/235.full?ijkey=ijKHq6YbJn3Oo&keytype=ref&siteid=amajnls

23. Ogden C, Carroll M. Prevalence of obesity among children and adolescents: United States, trends 1963-1965 through 2007-2008. Division of Health Nutrition Examination Survey. Available at http://www.cdc.gov/nchs/data/hestat/obesity_child_07_08/obesity_child_07_08.htm

24. Understanding Obesity: Obesity in America Web site. http://www.obesityinamerica.org.

25. Bertisch SM, Wee CC, McCarthy EP. Use of complementary and alternative therapies by overweight and obese adults. *Obesity*. 2008;16(7):1610–1615.

26. Hernandez-Reif M, Field T, Bornstein J, et al. Children with Down Syndrome improved in motor function a*nd* muscle tone following massage therapy. *J Early Child Develop Care*. 2006;176:395–410.

27. Bernard R, Baker, S. Brief report: alternative approaches to the development of effective treatments for autism. *J Autism Develop Disord*. 1996;26(2):237–238.

28. Field, T, Lasko, D, Mundy, P, et al. Brief report: autistic children's attentiveness and responsivity improve after touch therapy. *J Autism Develop Disord*. 1997;27(3):333.

29. Regina-Whitely M. Autism and Treatment with Massage Therapy. Massage Today Magazine available at http://www.massagetoday.com/mpacms/mt/article.php?id=13157. Viewed December 12, 2010.

30. Mental Retardation. MedlinePlus (A service of the U.S. National Library of Medicine and National Institutes of Health) available at http://www.nlm.nih.gov/medlineplus/ency/article/001523.htm. Viewed May 2011.

31. Hernandez-Reif M, Field T, Bornstein J, et al. Children with Down syndrome improved in motor function and muscle tone following massage therapy. *J Early Child Develop Care*. 2006;176:395–410.

32. Hart S, Field T, Hernandez-Reif M, et al. Preschoolers' cognitive performance improves following massage. *Early Child Develop Care*. 1998;143:59–64.

33. Mental Health Information. National Institute of Mental Health Web site available at http://www.nimh.nih.gov/index.shtml. Viewed May 2011.

34. Statistics Resources. National Institute of Mental Health Web site available at http://www.nimh.nih.gov/statistics/index.shtml. Viewed May 2011.

35. World Health Organization. Mental Health and Work: Impact, issues and good practices available at http://www.who.int/mental_health/media/en/712.pdf. Viewed May 2011.

36. Billhult A, Maatta S. Light pressure massage for patients with severe anxiety. *Complement Ther Clin Pract*. 2009;15(2):96–101.

37. Garner B, Phillips LS, Schmidt H, *et al*. Pilot study evaluating the effect of massage therapy on stress, anxiety and aggression in a young adult psychiatric inpatient unit. *Aust N Z J Psychatry*. 2008;42(5):414–422.

38. Field T, Hernandez-Reif M, Diego M, et al. Cortisol decreases and serotonin and dopamine increase following massage therapy. *Int J Neurosci*. 2005;115(10):1397–1413.

39. Hart S, Field T, Hernandez-Reif M, *et al*. Anorexia nervosa symptoms are reduced by massage therapy. *Eat Disord*. 2001;9(4):289–299.

40. Hospice Patience Alliance directory available at http://www.hospicepatients.org/maintopics.html. Viewed May 2011.

41. Meek SS. Effects of slow stroke back massage on relaxation in hospice clients. *Image J Nurs Sch*. 1993;25(1):17–21.

42. Soden K, Vincent K, Craske S, et al. A randomized controlled trial of aromatherapy massage in a hospice setting. *Palliat Med*. 2004;18(2):87–92.

43. Kutner JS, Smith MC, Corbin L, et al. Massage therapy versus simple touch to improve pain and mood in patients with advanced cancer: a randomized trial. *Ann Intern Med*. 2008;149(6):369–379.

Glossary

Abbreviations: Symbols and shortened words used in health-care documentation because they take up less space on the page and are faster to write.

Abdominal cavity: The abdominal cavity contains the spleen, liver, stomach, gallbladder, pancreas, small intestine, and most of the large intestine.

Abdominal region: The abdominal region is the area of the trunk inferior to the thorax (separated by the diaphragm) and superior to the pelvic region. The abdominal region is broken into four quadrants.

Abdominopelvic cavity: The abdominopelvic cavity is separated from the thoracic cavity by the diaphragm. It is divided into the abdominal cavity (superior) and the pelvic cavity (inferior).

Abduction: Takes place in the coronal plane with the body part moving laterally away from the body.

Abhyanga: The Sanskrit word for oil massage.

Accessibility: Refers to ease of access and user-friendliness of a massage business.

Acromial region: The region related to the acromion, a bony protrusion on the scapula, which articulates with the clavicle to form the highest point of the shoulder.

Active communication: A form of communication that requires awareness, active listening, and the ability to communicate a message honestly.

Active treatment group: Part of a clinical trial group who receive the treatment being researched.

Acupoints: Places along channels where qi can be accessed and manipulated to improve qi flow (also known as Qi Xue meaning "energy cavities" in Chinese, qi points in Tuina massage, or Tsubo, meaning "body points" in Japanese).

Acute stage: The acute stage of the inflammatory response begins seconds after tissue damage has occurred and lasts from several hours to several days depending on the severity of the injury. Signs and symptoms may include redness, swelling, and pain at the injury site.

Acute traumatic injury: An injury or wound to the body caused by the application of extreme external force.

Acute: A disease with a rapid onset and severe symptoms that only lasts a short time (less than 6 months).

Adaptive measures: Modifications made by a therapist during the massage session in response to the overall health and condition of the client.

Adduction: Takes place in the coronal plane with the body part moving medially toward the body.

Adrenal glands: Situated above the kidneys, each adrenal (from the Latin prefix *ad-* meaning "toward" or "on" and *ren* meaning "kidneys") gland has two parts. The inner area (medulla) secretes epinephrine (adrenaline) and norepinephrine (noradrenaline), the flight-or-fight hormones that ready the body for maximum action in times of danger or high stress. The outer area (cortex) secretes hormones that regulate carbohydrate reserves, suppress inflammatory responses, and regulate the balance of electrolytes.

Adverse reaction: An undesirable response to treatment in which current symptoms are exacerbated or new symptoms occur.

Afferent nerves: A type of neuron that conducts impulses to the spinal cord and brain (from the Latin *afferens* meaning "to bring to"; opposite of *efferent* and synonymous with *centripetal*).

Agonists: Also called prime movers, these are muscles that contract to carry out a specific action (movement). They are the main muscles involved in performing the movement.

Amphiarthrosis joint: A functional classification that refers to joints that are slightly movable, like the cartilaginous discs found between the vertebrae.

Anatomical position: In this position, a person stands with both feet facing forward shoulders-width apart. The arms are at the sides with the palms facing forward.

Andreas Vesalius: A Flemish anatomist (1514–1564 CE) who wrote *On the Workings of the Human Body* in 1543, which became one of the most influential books on human anatomy during that period.

Antagonists: Muscles that have the opposite action to the agonist; they must extend when the prime mover contracts.

Antebrachial region: *Ante-* is the Latin prefix meaning "before" and *brachial* means "arm." The antebrachial region refers to the forearm.

Anterior (ventral): Refers to the front of the body or to structures toward the front of the body. The term *ventral* is used less often than anterior. This term is from the Latin *venter* meaning "belly."

Anterior triangle: An area of caution defined by the trachea, mandible, and sternocleidomastoid muscles on each side of the neck.

Antiseptic: Cleaning products that are safe for use on the skin and create an unfavorable environment for pathogen reproduction. Hand soap, iodine, hydrogen peroxide, and rubbing alcohol are commonly used antiseptics.

Aorta: The aorta (from Latin from the Greek aeiro meaning "to lift up") is the largest artery in the body and receives blood from the left ventricle. It moves downward and then branches to other arteries to supply the body's tissues with oxygenated blood.

Approach: Different systems that share many similar characteristics are collectively called an "approach" (which might also be referred to as a modality, form, or style).

Area of caution: Any region of the body where delicate structures are superficial and unprotected, requiring caution from the massage therapist.

Armoring: A concept introduced by Wilhelm Reich to explain the use of physical tension to support psychological defenses.

Aromatherapy: The use of essential oils (aromatic plant extracts) for health and wellness.

Arteries: Blood vessels that transport blood from the heart to the body's tissues.

Asian bodywork therapy: A general term used to describe a number of different forms of bodywork that have developed over the centuries in Asian countries, and more recently in the West.

Assertive relating: A style of relating to other people in which one remains open, listening, and responsive in order to collaborate with others toward a common goal or cause.

Assertive technology: Devices and societal or personal modifications that help people with disabilities overcome impairments and broaden the accessibility of places and things.

Assessment: A judgment based on an understanding of the situation.

Autonomic nervous system (ANS): The section of the nervous system that regulates smooth muscle, cardiac muscle, and certain glands without conscious control.

Axilla area: The area of the armpit.

Axillary region: In lay terms, the axillary region is called the armpit. It lies inferior to the shoulder joint and contains the axillary artery, axillary vein, part of the brachial plexus, and the axillary lymph nodes.

Ayurveda: The traditional medical system of India.

Basalt: Main type of stones used in hot stone massage because they hold heat well.

Benefit: A good effect that promotes well-being, even if a specific pathology, postural dysfunction, or muscular tension pattern is not an issue.

Bilateral: Refers to both sides.

Biomagnetic field: The electromagnetic field produced as a result of the body's electrical activity that is projected into the space around the body.

Blood vessels: Blood flows in a closed system of five groups of vessels: arteries, arterioles, capillaries, venules, and veins.

Blood: A connective tissue composed of formed elements and plasma. Formed elements include erythrocytes (from the Greek *erythros* meaning "red"), which are red blood cells, leukocytes (from the Greek *leukos* meaning "white"), which are white blood cells, and platelets (from the Greek *platys* meaning "flat" or "broad" referring to the shape of the platelet), also referred to as thrombocytes, which function in blood clotting. Plasma is the fluid portion of blood, comprising 55% of blood volume and made up mainly of water and proteins.

Board of massage: Appointed in states that regulate massage to supervise the practice of massage through reviews of therapist applications, investigations of complaints, and overseeing licensees who practice in the state.

Body mechanics: Refers to the proper way to stand, sit, bend, and lift to avoid movements that lead to injury or burnout.

Body planes: Imaginary planes that divide the body into different sections.

Bodymind connection: The recognition that the body and mind mirror each other and are intimately connected.

Bodymind split: The unconscious belief that the body and mind do not reflect each other.

Bolster: One of many specially shaped pillows that are used to support the client's body so that she or he can relax completely without undo pressure on joints while receiving massage.

Boney landmarks: Boney prominences, such as irregularly shaped bones with knobs, grooves, holes, depressions, and angles; these help therapists find their way around the body.

Boundary: An imaginary border that marks the limits of an individual's personal space.

Brachial plexus: The collection of nerves that innervate the upper extremity. Three large trunks of the brachial plexus pass under the clavicle and divide into five major nerves.

Brachial region: *Brachial* is the Latin word for "arm," modified from the Greek word *brachion*. In anatomy, the arm is considered the area superior to the elbow and inferior to the shoulder both anteriorly and posteriorly.

Bronchi: The trachea branches into the right main bronchus (which goes to the right lung) and the left main bronchus (which goes to the left lung). When they enter the lungs, the bronchi branch into three smaller lobar bronchi, then into smaller bronchioles, then into smaller terminal bronchioles, which divide into microscopic branches called respiratory bronchioles. *Bronch(o)* is the Greek root meaning "windpipe."

Buccal region: *Bucca* is the Latin root that means "cheek." The buccal region follows the outline of the zygomatic bones, called the cheekbones in lay terms.

Buoyancy: Refers to floating in water.

Business plan: A written guide to starting and running a business.

Calcaneal region: The calcaneus is the tarsal bone that forms the heel. This region relates to the heel.

CAM therapies: Complementary and Alternative Medicine (CAM) include such diverse forms of practice as acupuncture, Tai Chi, biofeedback, chiropractic medicine, meditation, dance therapy, aromatherapy, art therapy, ayurvedic medicine, Traditional Chinese Medicine, hypnosis, and many others. The term "complementary medicine" describes alternative healing practices used in conjunction with conventional medicine.

Cancer: General term for a large number of diseases typified by the growth of abnormal cells that replicate uncontrollably.

Capillaries: These tiny vessels have thin walls that allow substances to move between tissue cells and capillary blood in exchanges. Capillaries (from the Latin *capillaris* relates to "hair," referring to their shape and size) link arterioles and venules.

Carpal region: *Carpal* is Latin modified from the Greek *karpos* meaning "wrist." Eight small bones (the carpal bones) articulate directly with the radius and indirectly with the ulna to form the wrist. The carpal region refers to the anterior and posterior wrist.

Cartilaginous joint: A structural classification that refers to joints that have no joint capsule and are held together by cartilage. Sometimes the joint is held together by hyaline cartilage that slowly ossifies (hardens) as the individual matures (e.g., the first rib and the sternum). These joints are referred to as synchondrosis joints and are immovable. Joints held together by tough, flat discs of fibrocartilage are called symphysis joints and are slightly moveable, like the intravertebral discs.

Cellular level: Cells (from the Latin *cella* meaning "storeroom") are the smallest units of living structure and are highly specialized (e.g., blood cell, nerve cell, muscle cell). They are the basic units of structure and function in the human body. Cells make up tissues.

Centered: Refers to a person's ability to find an emotional, mental, and physical center.

Central nervous system (CNS): The CNS includes the brain and spinal cord. It receives input from the body's nerves, processes the information, and responds in a coordinated manner.

Central: Refers to the middle of the body, the internal core of the body, or the middle of specific structures or systems.

Cervical region: *Cervix* is the Latin word for "neck," and the cervical vertebrae form the top seven vertebrae of the vertebral column. This region most often refers to the posterior area of the neck where the cervical vertebrae might be palpated.

Channels: A term used in some Asian therapies to refer to pathways or routes where qi flows.

Chemical headache: Headache triggered by chemical imbalances in the body.

Chemical level: The chemicals (from the Greek *chemeia* meaning "alchemy") of the human body are composed of atoms such as hydrogen, carbon, oxygen, nitrogen, calcium, sodium, and potassium. These atoms combine to form molecules such as proteins and carbohydrates. Chemicals combine to form cells.

Chinese four pillars of examination: A primary assessment method in some Asian therapies that promote observation, listening, asking, and touching as key methods of determining treatment choices.

Chronic: The term *chronic* has two related but different meanings. Sometimes a condition or disease persists for a very long time or regularly recurs. This is called a chronic condition, such as chronic hepatitis. In the case of a soft-tissue injury, the term *chronic* indicates the last stage of healing. In the chronic stage of healing, the therapist aims to help the client return to full function and build strength to avoid re-injury.

Chronic inflammation: When the injury site does not progress normally through the maturation stage and enters a recurrent inflammatory process.

Chronic pain: Pain that persists for a period of time past the point of typical injury recovery.

Circumduction: A series of movements that occur at the shoulder and hip joints when these body areas flex, abduct, extend, and then adduct in an arching motion such as when swimming the backstroke.

Client self-care: Actions the client performs that aid in recovering from an injury or in managing a condition or disease.

Clinical trial: A type of research study that compares a treatment to a placebo (inactive treatment), to another treatment, or to standard treatment to establish safety and efficacy, using randomization and controls in study design.

Cluster headache: A rarely occurring vascular headache that causes debilitating pain that is usually located around one eye but may spread out to other areas of the face, head, neck, and shoulders.

Cocoon: A type of body wrap where treatment product is applied directly to the client before the client is wrapped in plastic and blankets in order to absorb the product into the skin.

Code of ethics: A professional group's ethical principles.

Collagen fibers: Collagen is a protein that forms the tough rope-like strands that make up the fibrous content of skin, fascia, tendons, ligaments, cartilage, bone, blood vessels, and organs.

Compensation patterns: Refers to new behaviors that offset a weakness. When the body is injured, it adopts new movement patterns as a means to protect the weakened areas and to manage the resulting loss of function.

Compress: A cloth that is dipped in hot, warm, neutral, cool, or cold water, wrung out, and placed on the body.

Compression: A massage technique in which the therapist pushes the muscle belly directly toward the bone beneath it with a rhythmic pumping action.

Condyle: A rounded articular surface at the end of a bone. An epicondyle is a small projection above a condyle (from the Greek *kondylos* meaning "knuckle").

Confidentiality: The therapist's obligation to ensure the client's privacy by not discussing the client's information with anyone but the client or other healthcare professionals, and then only with the client's permission.

Conflict resolution: A process used to resolve a conflict through conversation or mediation.

Connective tissue: Connective tissue includes bone, cartilage, ligaments, tendons, joint capsules, adipose tissue (fat), blood, and lymph. Connective tissue is widely distributed throughout the body and shapes the body's form with an interweaving network that binds various body parts together, while separating certain structures so that they can move freely over one another.

Contraindication: When a therapeutic treatment might harm a client or cause an adverse reaction, it is *contraindicated* (Latin prefix *contra-* meaning "opposed" or "against").

Control group: Part of the clinical trial group who receive the standard treatment (if there is one), no treatment, a placebo treatment, or a second treatment being researched as a comparison.

Counter-transference: When a therapist personalizes the therapeutic relationship.

Cover letter: A letter used by someone seeking a job that provides an introduction to an employer.

Cranial cavity: The space within the skull that contains the brain and cerebrospinal fluid. It is sometimes referred to as the intracranial cavity.

Cranial nerves: The 12 pairs of cranial nerves handle impulses for the special senses (smell, vision, taste, hearing), general senses (pain, touch, temperature, pressure, and vibrations), motor impulses resulting in control of skeletal muscles, and visceral motor impulses for the involuntary control of cardiac muscle, smooth muscle, and glands.

Cranial region: *Cranio-* is a prefix from the Greek *kranion* meaning "skull" and is synonymous with the term *cephalic* from the Greek *kephale* meaning "head." The skull is divided into two portions, the cranium and the facial area.

Crest: A bony ridge or distinct border on a bone (from the Latin *crista* meaning "crest").

Crural region: The term *crural* can relate to both the thigh and the leg. It is most often used to denote the region distal to the knee on the anterior leg.

Cubital region: The area of the elbow.

Décor: What the client sees when entering a massage space.

Deep tissue: An approach to soft-tissue structures where the therapist works slowly while applying more pressure to deeper muscular structures, creating greater length and pliability in soft tissue.

Deep: Refers to structures that are positioned away from the surface of the body.

Deformation: A term used to describe the change in shape that occurs to soft-tissue structures in response to the application of a massage stroke.

Delayed-onset muscle soreness: A type of muscle soreness that is experienced from 12 to 48 hours after a vigorous workout or after a period of inactivity followed by unaccustomed strenuous physical activity. Symptoms include diffuse muscle tenderness, stiffness, swelling, and pronounced soreness.

Deltoid region: The deltoid is a muscle that "caps" the shoulder and flexes, extends, and laterally or medially rotates the shoulder joint. The surface area over any of these structures is called the shoulder or deltoid region.

Depression: Movement that can occur at the mandible, scapula, clavicle, pelvis, and hyoid bone where the body part moves inferiorly (down).

Dermis: The dermis (from the Greek *derma* meaning "skin") is the skin layer below the epidermis. Components of the dermis are responsible for the strength, elasticity, and extensibility of the skin (collagen and elastin fibers), blood supply to the skin, and nerve endings sensitive to touch.

Diarthrosis joint: A functional classification that refers to joints that are freely movable like synovial joints. The name refers to the fact that synovial diarthrotic joints move in paired directions, such as flexion and extension, and adduction and abduction.

Disability: A medical condition or functional impairment that impacts the ability to perform particular activities.

Disease transmission: Disease is caused by pathogens which are transmitted by direct contact, indirect contact, vehicle transmission, or vector transmission.

Disinfectants: Cleaning products that are stronger than antiseptics and should not be used on the skin. They kill or are effective against most bacteria and viruses.

Distal: Refers to being farthest away from the trunk or, when a specific structure is being referred to, the area of the structure that is furthest from the point of origin.

Documentation: The records kept by a therapist to record the particular techniques used during a session and the results they achieved. A health history form and SOAP notes are standard forms used to document massage sessions.

Dorsiflexion: Movement that occurs in the joints of the foot when the dorsal surface of the foot moves superiorly so that the toes point up to the sky and slightly back toward the knee.

Dosha: A concept in Ayurvedic medicine that explains the nature of the universe. The three doshas (vata, pitta, and kapha) govern the qualities of different times of the day or night, different seasons or climates, the characteristics of the physical body, and a person's mental and emotional tendencies.

Downward rotation: When the scapula rotates so that the glenoid fossa moves inferiorly.

Draping: The use of a sheet, bath towel, or blanket to establish professional boundaries, preserves the modesty of both the client and therapist, and ensure that the client stays warm during the massage.

Drug: A synthesized chemical that may be prescribed by a physician to treat a particular condition, purchased over-the-counter without a prescription (e.g., cold medication, pain reliever, etc.), or categorized as illegal substances (e.g., cocaine, heroin, etc.).

Dry room: A tiled room with drains in the floor that allows services using water to be applied efficiently.

Dry skin brushing: A technique in which natural bristle brushes, rough hand mitts, or textured cloths are used to stimulate the sebaceous glands, increase local circulation, remove dead skin cells, and invigorate the nervous system to revitalize the body.

Dual relationships: A situation in which more than one relationship with a client is present.

Ebers papyrus: A lengthy scroll written around 1,550 BCE that contains around 700 formulae and remedies demonstrating ancient Egypt's advanced understanding of human anatomy and the use of herbal medicine.

Efferent nerves: A type of neuron that conducts impulses from the central nervous system to the muscles and glands (from the Latin *efferens* meaning "to bring out"; opposite of *afferent* and synonymous with *centrifugal*).

Effleurage: The French word for the gliding strokes used in Swedish massage.

Elevation: Movement that can occur at the mandible, scapula, clavicle, pelvis, and hyoid bone, in which the body part moves superiorly (up).

Embodiment: Refers to the subjective sensation of having and using a body.

Emotion: A state of psychological arousal accompanied by detectable physiological responses and feelings of tenderness or vulnerability.

Emotional intelligence: The ability to monitor one's own and other's feelings and emotions, to discriminate among them and to use this information to guide one's thinking and actions.

Emotional release: A natural process that may occur during a massage session in which a client relaxes his or her defenses and experiences emotions such as sadness, happiness, or other emotions.

Employee: A person who is hired by another person to perform particular duties for a determined fee.

End feel: During passive range of motion, it is the point at which the therapist feels the structures of the joint and surrounding the joint "push back." There are three different types of normal end feel: hard, soft, and firm.

Endocrine gland: Endocrine glands secrete hormones into the space around them. The hormones pass into capillaries and are conveyed through the blood to target cells.

Energy medicine: One of five domains of Complementary and Alternative Medicine therapy identified by the National Center for Complementary and Alternative Medicine (NCCAM).

Energy: The exertion of power; the capacity to do work, taking the forms of kinetic energy, potential energy, chemical energy, electrical energy, and others.

Epidermis: The epidermis (from the Greek epi- meaning "on" and dermis meaning "skin") is the outer layer of the skin, which has four sublayers. Components in the epidermis are responsible for waterproofing the skin (keratin), some of the color of the skin (melanin), protection from UV radiation, and some immune function (Langerhans' cells and Granstein cells).

Erect position: In this position, the client stands in a relaxed posture with the arms hanging naturally at the sides.

Esophagus: The esophagus (from the Greek *oisophagos* meaning "gullet") secretes mucus and transports food to the stomach. Food is pushed through the esophagus by involuntary muscular contractions called peristalsis (from the Greek *peri* meaning "around" and *stalsis* meaning constriction), which also occurs in the gastrointestinal tract.

Essential oil: Pleasant-smelling substances that come from specific species of aromatic plants.

Ethics: A major branch of philosophy exploring values, morals, right and wrong, good and evil, and responsibility. Also called moral philosophy.

Etiology: The study of the cause of a disease, or the theory of the origin of a disease.

Event massage: A category of sports massage where the massage is applied on the day of a sporting event at the location of the sporting event.

Eversion: Movement that occurs in the tarsal joints of the foot when the plantar surface of the foot pivots to face the midline of the body.

Exfoliation: A coarse-textured product or hand-held cloth, brush, or mitt is applied to the skin to brighten it by removing the dull top layer of dead cells.

Exocrine gland: Exocrine glands secrete their products into ducts where they are carried to certain organs (digestive glands) or the body's surface (sudoriferous and sebaceous glands of the integumentary system).

Expenses: All of the monies that go out of a business related to startup or operational costs.

Extension: Takes place in the sagittal plane with the body part moving posteriorly (with the exception of the knee). The knee extends in an anterior movement in the sagittal plane. It is the opposite movement to flexion.

External: From the Latin *externus* meaning "outside," this term refers to the outer surface of the body.

Facet: A small, smooth area on a bone, such as the facets on each vertebra, that articulate with the vertebrae above and below.

Facial region: The facial region of the head includes the area of the eyes, nose, mouth, and cheeks. It can be broken down into smaller areas.

Fascia: A type of connective tissue that forms a fibrous membrane covering that supports and separates muscles and other structures in the body.

Fees: A monetary cost paid by a client to a professional for a desired service.

Femoral region: The word *femoral* means "relating to the femur," the long bone in the thigh. This region refers to the thigh.

Femoral triangle: An area of caution defined by the inguinal ligament, sartorius, and adductor longus in the thigh.

Fibromyalgia: A condition characterized by the distribution of tender points over the body, chronic pain, fatigue, and sleep disturbances.

Fibrous joint: A structural classification that refers to joints that have no joint capsule and are held together by fibrous connective tissue, such as the sutures that hold together the bones of the skull.

Filter: The concept that all people have individual needs, values, beliefs, attitudes, assumptions, and experiences that become a "filter" for how we view the world, listen to others, communicate ideas, or feel in certain situations.

First trimester: The first three months of pregnancy.

Flexibility: The range of motion available at a given joint or series of joints.

Flexion: A movement that takes place in the sagittal plane with the body part moving anteriorly (with the exception of the knee). The knee flexes posterior in the sagittal plane. It is the opposite movement to extension.

Flight-or-fight response: The body's response to a perceived threat (run away or stay and fight) mediated by the sympathetic nervous system.

Foramen: An opening in a bone through which blood vessels, ligaments, or nerves pass (from the Latin *aperture* meaning "a small narrow opening").

Forces: Something that internally or externally causes the movement of the body to change or body structures to deform.

Fossa: A depression in or on a bone (from the Latin term for "a trench or ditch").

Friction treatments: A classification of spa treatments such as salt glows, dry or wet skin brushing, cold mitt friction, and loofah scrubs that stimulate the skin, blood circulation, and lymph flow when applied to one body area or the entire body.

Friction: A heat-producing, chafing stroke or a stroke applied with deeper pressure to outline particular muscle structures and break up adhered tissue. One of the traditional strokes used in Swedish massage.

Frontal plane: Also called the coronal plane, divides the body into anterior and posterior parts with a straight vertical line that is at right angles to the sagittal plane.

Frontal region: The frontal bone of the skull forms the forehead and the superior portion of the eye socket. The frontal region of the head follows the outline of the frontal bone.

Functional goals: Goals developed with clients that define the particular activities the client would most like to accomplish in daily life without a significant increase in symptoms.

Functional limitations: Activities of daily living that are limited by a condition or by soft-tissue injury.

Functional outcomes reporting: A form of writing SOAP or chart notes that focus on the client's ability to function in activities of daily life.

Gait: The client's walking patterns.

Galen: Claudius Galenus of Pergamum (129-200 CE), known in English as Galen, was a Greek physician who built on the theories of Hippocrates. Eventually Galen moved to Rome where he lectured, conducted experiments on animals to develop his understanding of anatomy, and wrote twenty-two volumes. He wrote *The Elements According to Hippocrates* to expand on the idea of the four humors.

Gallbladder: A small sac located on the surface of the liver that stores bile until it is needed in the small intestine.

Gate theory: In 1965 psychologist Ronald Melzack and physiologist Patrick Wall introduced the gate control theory of pain management in a paper published in *Science* magazine. Melzack and Wall believed that the spinal cord had a gating mechanism whereby nerve fibers carrying somatic stimuli relating to touch, temperature, pressure, or movement can "close the gate" to dull aching pain information traveling to the brain.

Gluteal region: The gluteal muscles form the buttocks. This region lies on either side of the sacral region.

Golgi tendon organs: Propriocepters that monitor muscle tension and tendon strain.

Ground substance: A fluid produced by fibroblasts that looks like egg whites and surrounds all the cells in the body to support cellular metabolism.

Grounded: Refers to a person's ability to find a relaxed and connected state of being.

Growth: Refers to the body's ability to develop and increase in size to reach maturity.

Head-forward position: An abnormal posture in which the head is positioned forward of its correct alignment.

Health intake form: A document the client completes before his first session that provides contact details, current health conditions, medications, past health conditions, and health-related goals.

Health intake interview: A conversation that occurs between the therapist and client to rule out contraindications and plan the treatment.

Heart: An organ located between the lungs that pumps blood throughout the body. The two upper chambers, called the right atrium and left atrium (plural atria, from the Latin meaning "entrance hall"), receive blood. The two lower chambers (right and left side), called the ventricles (from the Latin *ventriculus* from *venter* meaning "belly" and referring to a cavity), pump blood. The right side of the heart pumps blood through the pulmonary circuit, where the blood is oxygenated by the lungs. The left side of the heart pumps blood through all other parts of the body.

High-risk pregnancy: A pregnancy that puts the mother or developing fetus at higher than normal risk for complications.

Hippocrates: A Greek physician (460–377 BCE) widely regarded as the "Father of Western Medicine" because he based his medical practice on observation and an extensive study of anatomy.

HIV/AIDS: The human immunodeficiency virus (HIV) is the virus that causes acquired immunodeficiency syndrome (AIDS).

Homeostasis: The relative constancy of the body's internal environment maintained by adaptive responses in spite of changing environmental conditions.

Hot sheet wrap: A common spa and massage treatment in which the treatment product (herbs, coffee, milk, honey, seaweed, mud, etc.) is dissolved in hot water. Two muslin sheets (or a sheet and a bath towel) are steeped in the dissolved product and then wrapped around the client.

Hydrostatic pressure: Refers to the amount of pressure exerted by a liquid, in this case water, when the liquid is at rest.

Hydrotherapy: The use of water for health and wellness.

Hyperkyphosis: An abnormal increase in the thoracic curve of the spine (also called kyphosis).

Hyperlordosis: An abnormal increase in the lumbar curve of the spine (also called lordosis).

Hyperthermia: General term used to describe a number of heat-related characteristics that are associated with illnesses.

Hypothermia: A condition that occurs when the core temperature of the body falls below 96 degrees Fahrenheit.

Ida Rolf: An American biochemist working in the 1940s, who extensively researched musculoskeletal components and founded structural integration (also "Rolfing"). Her methods continue to profoundly influence massage today.

Idiopathic: A disease or condition that develops spontaneously or without a known cause is referred to as an idiopathic disease.

Independent contractor: A person or business that performs services for another person or business under an agreement.

Indication: When a therapeutic treatment is likely to benefit a client and have no adverse reactions, it is *indicated* (from the Latin *in-dico*, meaning "to point out").

Infectious agents: Pathogens that cause infections like bacteria, viruses, fungi, and protozoa.

Infectious diseases: Diseases (also known as communicable diseases) caused by an infectious agent referred to as a pathogen. Infectious diseases are spread by contact with another person or an animal, or to an infant from its mother.

Inferior: Refers to being situated below something or closer to the feet.

Inflammation: Inflammation is the response of living tissue to injury, infection, or irritation. Heat, redness, swelling, and pain are present at the site and in surrounding tissue.

Inflammatory response: The response of living tissue to injury. To repair the damage done to tissue, the body rapidly reacts to any injury with a series of specific vascular, chemical, and cellular events.

Informed consent: A process by which a fully informed client consents to participate in the massage treatment.

Infrared radiation: Electromagnetic radiation of a wavelength longer than that of visible light, but shorter than that of radio waves.

Injury: Damage to the body's tissues caused by physical trauma or repetitive stress.

Internal: The word *internal* is from the Latin *internus* meaning "inside." In anatomy, the term is used to refer to anything situated away from the surface of the body.

Inversion: Movement that occurs in the tarsal joints of the foot when the plantar surface of the foot pivots to face the midline of the body.

Ipsilateral rotation: Refers to a movement that may occur in the axial skeleton. The term *ipsilateral* means on the same side with reference to a given point; the term is from the Latin *ipsi* meaning "same" and *latus* meaning "side."

Isometric contraction: In an isometric contraction tension is generated, but the joint angle and muscle length do not change. Isometric contractions are important because they are used to stabilize joints such as when an object is held in a fixed position. For example, pushing the hands against a wall causes an isometric contraction because the tension increases in the arm muscles but their length stays the same.

Isotonic contraction: This is a muscle contraction in which the muscle length and joint angle are changed in response to the tension generated in the muscle. Eccentric and concentric contractions are the two different types of isotonic contractions.

Jurisprudence exam: Basic law exams required by some states to obtain massage credentials, that ensures knowledge of the laws relating to massage in the particular state, general massage ethics, and continuing education requirements.

Kickback: Any money, fee, commission, credit, gift, gratuity, thing of value, or compensation of any kind, provided for referrals of clients.

Lateral flexion: A movement that takes place in the coronal plane when the axial body part bends either to the right or left.

Lateral rotation: A movement that takes place in the transverse plane when a limb (anterior surface) turns away from the midline to face laterally.

Lateral: Refers to the structures that are on the sides of the body and out from the body's center.

Laws: Rules, recognized by a community as binding and enforceable by authority.

License: A printed, state-issued document that gives a person official permission to practice massage within the limits of a scope of practice. Allows qualifying therapists to use a protected title and list their massage credentials after their names.

Liver: The liver (from the Greek *hepato*) conducts many vital functions needed for normal digestion, metabolism, blood production, and the elimination of wastes. Activities of the liver include carbohydrate, fat, and protein metabolism; removal of drugs and hormones from the body; production of bile to process fats; synthesis of bile salts; storage of vitamins, minerals, and glycogen; phagocytosis of worn-out red and white blood cells and some bacteria; and the activation of vitamin D.

Load: Refers to the amount of stress soft-tissue structures are under due to *forces*.

Local contraindication: One area of the body is contraindicated for massage.

Lubricant: A product such as oil, lotion, gel, or cream that is used with many massage techniques to prevent undue friction between the therapist's hands and the client's skin.

Lumbar region: The lumbar region refers to the low back in relationship to the five lumbar vertebrae.

Lymph nodes: Small oval or bean-shaped structures that reside along the length of lymphatic vessels and filter lymph.

Lymph: A clear fluid that is collected from tissue spaces throughout the body by the lymph capillaries and channeled into lymphatic vessels to be filtered by lymph nodes.

Marketing: All the activities a massage therapist undertakes to attract and retain clients.

Mastoid region: The mastoid process is a bony projection of the temporal bone that serves as a place for muscles to attach. It is located directly behind the inferior portion of the ear lobe, and this region is comprised of the area behind the ear.

Mechanical effect: A response of the body to massage that occurs as a direct result of the manual manipulation of the client's soft tissue.

Mechanical strength: The amount of force a tissue can absorb or resist before failure.

Medial rotation: A movement that takes place in the transverse plane when a limb (anterior surface) turns in to face the midline.

Medial: Refers to the middle or centerline of the body.

Meridian system: A concept in many Asian therapies that describes an energy network composed of channels, collaterals, and their associated zang fu organs, sense organs, and tissues.

Metabolism: Metabolism (from the Greek *metabole* meaning "change") refers to all of the chemical reactions that occur in the body to break down food, release energy, and make up substances that form the body's structural and functional components.

Migraine headache: Chronic vascular headaches that cause significant pain for hours or days.

Movement: Movement (from the Latin *moveo* meaning "to move") refers to the body's ability to move from one place to another or to move one part in relation to another. It also refers to the cells and organs that must move in order to carry out the body's essential processes.

Elasticity: Elasticity is the characteristic of muscle tissue that allows it to return to its original shape after contracting or extending.

Muscle spindles: A propriocepter that helps control muscle movement by detecting the amount of stretch placed on a muscle.

Muscle tissue: Muscle tissue is formed by fibers that are highly specialized to contract, thereby generating heat and movement. Muscle tissue is classified as skeletal (the type that creates body movements), cardiac (the type that forms the heart wall and produces regular heart contractions), and smooth (the type that forms the walls of hollow organs and causes movements like the wavelike contractions of digestion).

Contractility: Contractility is the characteristic of muscle tissue that allows it to contract (shorten and thicken) to produce movement at joints.

Extensibility: The characteristic of muscle tissue that allows it to extend (lengthen) when opposing muscles contract.

Excitability: The characteristic of muscle tissue (also of nerve tissue) that allows it to receive and respond to stimuli.

Neuromuscular therapy: A form of bodywork that aims to locate, treat, and prevent chronic pain associated with myofascial trigger points.

Neuron: The functional unit of the nervous system. It consists of a cell body, dendrites, and axons. Dendrites conduct impulses to the cell body, while axons conduct impulses away from the cell body.

Nociceptor: Sensory receptors that transmit sensations of pain.

Obesity: An excessive amount of body fat in relation to lean body mass for an individual of a given height.

Objective data: Information the therapist gathers through observation and palpation.

Occipital region: The occipital bone forms the posterior and base section of the skull. The occipital region of the head follows the outline of the occipital bone.

Older adult: People who are 60 years of age or older.

Onsite massage: Refers to massage taken to clients at their businesses, homes, or events they attend, or situated close to businesses they frequent.

Opposition: A series of movements that occur at the thumb allowing the thumb to flex, adduct, and medially rotate to cross the palm and touch the fifth finger (little finger).

Osteoarthritis: A condition (also called degenerative joint disease) related to wear and tear of a synovial joint's structures that cause the joint to become painful and inflamed.

Otic region: The otic region is the area directly around the ear.

Over-exertion injury: An injury that occurs from an abrupt increase in activity without proper preparation.

Overuse injury: An injury that occurs from performing a movement repeatedly without sufficient recovery time.

Pack: A hot, warm, cool, or cold application that causes changes in soft-tissue structures when it is placed on the body.

Pain assessment: Involves a number of methods that might be used to capture a client's experience of pain at a given point in time.

Pain: An unpleasant physical and emotional sensation associated with tissue damage or the immediate potential for tissue damage.

Pain-spasm-pain cycle: A persistent cycle in which pain triggers muscle spasms, which then lead to more pain.

Palpation: Data obtained through touch based on the client's tissue textures, tone, temperature, and hydration.

Paraffin: A waxy substance obtained from the distillates of wood, coal, petroleum, or shale oil that is heated and applied to body areas to produce changes in soft-tissue structures.

Parasympathetic nervous system response: The rest and recovery response of the body mediated by the parasympathetic nervous system that is often trigged by the relaxation brought about through massage.

Parasympathetic nervous system: The division of the autonomic nervous system associated with the body's ability to rest and recover (from the Greek prefix *para-* meaning "alongside").

Pathology: The medical science concerned with disease or abnormal function.

Pelvic cavity: The pelvic cavity contains the urinary bladder, portions of the large intestine, and the internal reproductive organs.

People First Language: A form of politically correct disability etiquette that aims to diminish the subconscious dehumanization that occurs when discussing people with disabilities.

Per Henrik Ling: An Austrian (1776–1839) credited with creating medical gymnastics, he built on the work of many other people to develop a structured movement system called Swedish massage.

Peripheral: Refers to the periphery of the body or parts that lie away from the center.

Peripheral nervous system (PNS): This part of the nervous system is made up of all nerves outside the CNS. It includes the cranial nerves, which transmit impulses to and from the brain, and the spinal nerves, which transmit impulses to and from the spinal cord.

Personal space: The physical, emotional, mental, and spiritual space people hold around themselves.

Petrissage: A rhythmic massage technique utilized in Swedish massage that seeks to lift tissue away from the bone to increase tissue pliability and decrease adhesions.

Physical history: The past physical state of the client, which influences the present physical state of the client. It includes genetics, nutrition, age, fitness level, past diseases, conditions, or injuries, and current diseases, conditions, or injuries.

Physician's release: A document that notes that a physician approves the use of massage for a client.

Physiological effect: The physical changes the body undergoes in response to massage treatment.

Piezo-electricity: The ability of tissue to generate electrical potentials in response to mechanical deformation such as the deformation that occurs with massage treatment.

Pin and stretch: Refers to a technique in which a muscle is first shortened passively or actively (placed in a shortened position through passive range of motion by the therapist or placed in a shortened position by an active movement performed by the client), then "pinned" by the therapist's hand at its origin, insertion, or muscle belly, before it is lengthened passively or actively.

Pineal gland: Located posterior to the midbrain, the pineal gland produces melatonin, which regulates waking and sleeping cycles (from the Latin *pineus* meaning "pine tree," relating to the shape of the gland).

Plantarflexion: Movement that occurs in the joints of the foot when the plantar surface of the foot moves inferiorly so that the toes are pointed downward.

Plaster: The application of an herbal paste (herbs mixed with either water or oil) to a body region.

Plexus: A network of nerves that occurs on both the right and left sides of the body.

Polarity therapy: An energy-based system that aims to address the body, mind, and spirit of the client through energetic bodywork, diet, exercise, and improved self-awareness.

Popliteal region: The muscles of the posterior leg form a diamond-shaped surface where they converge at the posterior knee to form what is called the popliteal fossa. The popliteal fossa and the popliteal region are the same area.

Positioning: Refers to the different positions a client takes while on the massage table or massage chair to allow access to specific areas of the body.

Posterior (dorsal): Refers to the back of the body or to structures toward the back of the body. The term *dorsal* is also widely used and is Latin for "back." It might also refer to the top of the foot or the back of the hand.

Posterior triangle: An area of caution defined by the clavicles, sternocleidomastoid muscles, and trapezius muscles on either sides of the neck.

Post-event massage: Massage performed after an athlete's sporting event.

Postpartum massage: Massage applied in the weeks after the baby is born.

Postural dysfunction: Any position of the body that exerts undue strain on body structures including joints, ligaments, fascia, muscle, nerves, blood vessels, and bones.

Posture assessment: The assessment of the client's posture in order to determine where structures are experiencing undue strain.

Posture: The arrangement of the body's parts in space, in other words, the body's position. The way in which a client holds his or her body while standing and moving.

Power differential: The power advantage that a therapist naturally holds over a client due to his or her knowledge of the body and massage skills.

Practical exam: In some states an applicant performs massage techniques in front of a panel to demonstrate competency in the application of techniques, sanitation and hygienic practices, communication with clients, and overall professionalism.

Prana: In the ayurvedic medical system of India, prana is defined as spiritual, physical, and mental energy. This vital energy is the fundamental life force of the body and the source of all knowledge.

Pre-event massage: Massage performed before an athlete's event.

Process: Any prominent projection on a bone, like the mastoid process of the temporal bone or the spinus processes of the vertebrae (from the Latin *processus* meaning "an advance, progress, or process").

Prognosis: A prediction of the probable course and outcome of the disease based on the condition of the patient and the doctor's knowledge of the disease.

Promotion: Marketing activities that increase a massage therapist's business visibility and attract the attention of potential clients.

Pronation: Movement in which the forearm rotates so that the palm is facing downward and the radius crosses over the ulna.

Prone position: In this position, a person is lying face down, usually with the face in a cradle so the cervical vertebrae are aligned with the rest of the spinal column.

Proprioception: Comes from the Latin *proprius*, meaning "one's own," and the word perception. It refers to the position of the body in space and the relationship of body parts to one another and to the environment around them.

Protraction: Movement that can occur at the mandible, scapula, and clavicle where the body part moves anteriorly.

Proximal: Refers to being nearest the trunk or, when a specific structure is being referred to, the part nearest the structure's point of origin.

Psychological defenses: Mental processes that enable the mind to deal with conflicts it can't resolve.

Psychological effect: Responses to massage that occur in the mind and emotions of clients.

Psychological history: Refers to the client's attitudes, beliefs, expectations, and cultural influences and how these influences might determine the outcome of a massage session.

Publicity: Media exposure arising from an event related to the massage business.

Pursed-lip breathing: A breathing technique that aims to tone and strengthen the diaphragm and help to re-educate the client's kinesthetic sense of breath.

Qi: A concept in Chinese medicine that seeks to explain the energy that underlies everything in the universe.

Radial: Refers to the radius, a bone in the forearm, or to the structures that lie close to it (e.g., radial artery, radial nerve).

Range of motion assessment: An assessment procedure that aims to evaluate the client's ability to move and to identify if there are any pathological restrictions present in a particular joint.

Range of motion: Refers to the amount of movement that is possible at a joint based on its structure and condition.

Reciprocal inhibition: Refers to a reflex mechanism in the body that ensures coordinated movement between groups of opposing muscles.

Reflecting: A listening skill with which the listener gathers information conveyed by the speaker and then summarizes the information in a brief phrase back to the speaker.

Reflexive effect: An involuntary and rapid response of the nervous system to stimuli that result in changes to the structural or systemic condition of the body.

Reflexology: A therapy based on the belief that there are points on the feet, hands, and ears that stimulate the function of different parts of the body including the glands and organs.

Reiki: An energetic approach to health and healing wherein a reiki practitioner places his or her hands on a recipient or above the recipient, or heals from a distance.

Resting and holding strokes: A technique in which the hands are placed, without lubricant, on the client with the intent to greet the client and allow the client time to become accustomed to the unfamiliar touch.

Resume: A summary of a person's background, experience, education, training, and skills used by employers to determine if you have the experience necessary to fill an open position.

Retraction: Movement that can occur at the mandible, scapula, and clavicle where the body part moves posteriorly.

Revenue: All of the monies that come into a business through payment on services by clients.

Rheumatoid arthritis: An autoimmune disorder that primarily affects the synovial membranes of joints, but may also affect other tissues including blood vessels, the lungs, and fascia.

Rotation: A movement that takes place in the transverse plane when the anterior surface of the body part rotates right or left.

Routines: A series of massage strokes that are planned in advance, delivered to body areas in a pre-set order, and practiced until they flow smoothly together.

Sacral region: This region lies over the sacrum and between the gluteal muscles. The sacrum is formed by the fusion of five vertebrae that lie inferior to the lumbar vertebrae.

Sagittal plane: Divides the body into left and right parts with a straight vertical line (also referred to as a longitudinal line). The sagittal plane runs through the midline of the body and is also called the midsagittal plane, or the median plane when the left and right parts are equal.

Salt glow: A spa treatment in which different types of mineral salts (Dead Sea salt, Bearn salt, sea salt, Epson salt, etc.) are rubbed across the surface of the skin with gentle massage strokes.

Sarcomeres: The functional unit of muscle that causes the muscle to contract (millions of sarcomeres must be activated to make even the smallest movement).

Scapular region: The scapula is a flat, triangular bone that lies over the ribs on the posterior trunk and articulates with the humerus to form the shoulder joint. The scapular region is the area directly over and around the scapula.

Scientific method: A process that scientists use to develop an accurate representation of the world, investigate phenomena, acquire new knowledge, integrate established knowledge with new knowledge, and correct existing knowledge.

Scoliosis: An abnormal lateral curve of the spine.

Scope of practice: The methods and techniques a professional can utilize in practice.

Seated massage: A massage applied to a fully clothed client sitting in a specialized chair.

Seated position: In this position, a client is seated in a regular chair or a massage chair for the massage or for assessment (e.g., range of motion assessment).

Sebaceous (oil) glands: Sebaceous glands (from the Latin *sebum* meaning "tallow" like animal fat used for candles) are located in the dermis and secrete an oily product called sebum into hair follicles to lubricate the hair and skin and prevent dryness.

Self-care: Attention to one's own health and wellness.

Semi-reclined position: In this position, a client lies supine but pillows elevate the upper body so that the client is half-sitting.

Sequencing: Refers both to the sequence of strokes (the order in which strokes are applied to a given body area) and to the overall sequence of the massage (the order in which body areas are massaged).

Session planning: The use of information gathered during an assessment to determine goals and techniques that will be used during the session.

Shiatsu: A bodywork form from Japan based on principles of traditional Chinese medicine. Composed of the Japanese words *shi* meaning "finger" and *atsu* meaning "pressure", and so translates literally to finger-pressure.

Shoulder region: The shoulder region refers to the shoulder girdle composed of the clavicle and the scapula. The shoulder joint (glenohumeral joint) is formed by the humerus and the glenoid fossa of the scapula.

Side effect: A secondary effect of a medication or therapy that goes beyond the desired effect or causes unwanted responses in addition to the therapeutic effect.

Side-lying position: Also called the lateral recumbent position. In this position, the client lies on the side with one leg positioned on a bolster and a pillow in front of the chest to support the upper body.

Signs: Objective physical manifestations that the doctor or therapist can observe.

Somatic nervous system: A division of the autonomic nervous system that involves the skeletal muscles under voluntary control (from the Greek root *soma* meaning "the body"). It consists of peripheral nerves that send sensory information to the central nervous system and motor nerves that send impulses to the skeletal muscles.

Special populations: Groups of people who require specific considerations and adaptations during a massage session.

Spinal cavity or canal: The spinal cavity or canal is a boney cavity formed by the vertebrae of the spine that encloses the spinal cord and the roots of the spinal nerves. It is sometimes referred to as the vertebral canal.

Spinal cord: The spinal cord is positioned in the spinal canal of the vertebral column. The function of the spinal cord is to transport sensory impulses from the periphery to the brain and motor impulses from the brain to the periphery.

Spinal nerves: The 31 pairs of spinal nerves connect the central nervous system to sensory receptors, muscles, glands, and the somatic part of the peripheral nervous system.

Spleen: The spleen is the largest mass of lymphatic tissue in the body, but it does not have sinuses like a lymph node and does not filter lymph. It functions in the production of B cells, which develop into antibody-producing cells and aid in immunity. Bacteria, worn-out or damaged red blood cells, and old platelets are removed from circulation by phagocytic cells in the spleen. The spleen serves as a blood reservoir for the body and releases blood in the event of an emergency involving blood loss.

Standards of practice: Professional guidelines based on ethical principles.

State-approved exam: The written examination chosen by the state to test entry-level knowledge. Massage therapists must pass this test in order to obtain massage credentials in most states.

Sternal region: The sternum is a long, flat bone that articulates with the first seven ribs and with the clavicle forming the middle section of the anterior wall of the thorax. The sternal region resides between the two mammary regions.

Stone massage: The use of heated or cooled stones to apply massage techniques.

Stress: Any event that threatens homeostasis and causes the body to adapt.

Stressor: Any stimulus that produces stress.

Stretch reflex: A somatic reflex mediated by proprioceptors called muscle spindles that are located in the muscle belly and monitor the muscle's length.

Subacute: A patient or client with a condition that has entered the subacute stage still has symptoms but they are less severe than in an acute stage. Normal function is slowly returning, but the body or body area is not yet at full strength.

Subcutaneous layer: The subcutaneous layer (from the Latin *sub-* meaning "under" and Latin *cutis* meaning "skin") is located directly beneath the dermis and is composed of loose connective tissue and adipose (fat) tissue (from the Greek *adip(o)* meaning "lipid" or Latin *adipis* meaning "lard" or "fat"). It is sometimes called the hypodermis or the superficial fascia and connects the skin to the underlying muscles while insulating the body and protecting underlying structures.

Subjective data: Information the client tells the therapist about his or her condition based on what he or she feels and his or her opinions. Gathered through the health intake form and interview.

Sudoriferous (sweat) glands: Sudoriferous glands (from the Latin *sudor* meaning "perspiration" and *fero* meaning "to bear") are located in the subcutaneous layer and dermis.

They cool the body and eliminate a small amount of waste through perspiration.

Superficial: Structures that are superficial lie closer to the surface.

Superior: Refers to structures situated above something or closer to the head.

Supination: Movement where the forearm rotates so that the palm is facing upward and the radius and ulna are parallel to each other.

Supine position: In this position a person is lying on the back face up.

Sympathetic nervous system: A division of the autonomic nervous system that controls the flight-or-fight response, fear responses, and responses to feelings (from the Greek *sympathetikos* meaning "to feel with").

Symptoms: Subjective abnormal physical manifestations that the patient or client reports.

Synarthrosis joint: A functional classification that refers to joints that are immovable, like the fibrous suture joints between the bones of the skull.

Synergist: A muscle that aids the action of another. Synergistic muscles have similar actions and thus support each other in movements.

Synovial joints: Freely moveable (diarthrosis) joints where the bones do not touch each other.

Taila: Oils infused with herbs that are believed to have a medicinal effect. They are used in ayurvedic medicine and bodywork.

Tapotement: A rhythmic percussion stroke used in Swedish massage.

Target market: The group of specific clients that a business aims to attract.

Tarsal region: Seven bones make up the ankle and instep of the foot, called tarsal bones. The region of the ankle is referred to as the tarsal region.

Temporal region: The two temporal bones of the skull form the sides and part of the base of the skull. The temporal region of the head follows the outline of the temporal bone and includes the otic region and mastoid region.

Tendon reflex: A somatic reflex mediated by proprioceptors called Golgi tendon organs that monitor muscle tension and tendon strain. Golgi tendon organs are located in tendons near where the tendon joins muscles (Fig. 4-5).

Tensegrity: A term coined by an architect and designer named Buckminster Fuller that has been adopted by massage therapists and bodyworkers. Fuller's architecture was based on a geometrical model where structures maintain their integrity because of a balance of continuous tensile forces through the building. Tensile forces refer to stretching forces (tension) pulling at both ends of a structure.

Tension headache: Most common type of headache with mild to moderate pain that is often described as a diffuse, tight band around the head.

Terminal illness: A disease that is considered ultimately incurable and likely to cause death within six months.

Therapeutic edge: The particular pace and depth of deep tissue manipulation that allows the greatest possibility of therapeutic change to occur in the tissue. The client experiences some pain, but the pain feels right, appropriate, and good.

Therapeutic relationship: A professional partnership between a massage therapist and client in which safe, structured touch is used to help the client achieve reasonable and clearly defined treatment goals.

Therapeutic Touch: An energetic healing method that aims to balance and increase the body's energy as a way to support health and wellness.

Thixotropy: The phenomenon by which gels become more fluid or more solid.

Thoracic region: The thoracic region encircles the upper trunk and includes the area directly inferior to the neck and directly superior to the abdominal region. Structures in the thoracic region include the thoracic vertebrae, ribs, and sternum.

Thymus gland: Located in the lower part of the neck, the thymus gland plays an important role in the maturation of T cells (a type of white blood cell), which are necessary for immune function.

Thyroid gland: *Thyroid* is from the Greek *thyreoides* meaning "an oblong shield," referring to the shield-like shape of the gland, which sits in front and to the sides of the upper part of the trachea. The thyroid gland secretes hormones that regulate metabolism.

Tissue failure: The point at which structures are damaged by loads and lose their mechanical integrity, usually resulting in injury.

Tissue level: Tissues (from the Latin *texo* meaning "to weave") are groups of similar cells that perform special functions. There are four basic tissues in the body: epithelium, connective tissue, muscle, and nerve tissue. Specialized tissues make up organs.

Tissue load: A normal or abnormal internal or external force applied to a tissue.

Tissue strain: The amount of deformation experienced by the tissue.

Tissue stress: The amount of resistance the tissue exhibits to a load.

Tonsils: These large lymphatic nodes are fixed in the mucus membranes and located in a circle at the intersection of the oral cavity and pharynx. They protect against foreign substances that are inhaled or ingested. *Tonsil* comes from the Latin *tonsilla* meaning "a stake."

Transference: When a client personalizes the therapeutic relationship.

Transverse plane: Divides the body into superior and inferior parts with a straight horizontal line.

Trigger point: Hyperirritable spot in skeletal muscle that is associated with a hypersensitive palpable nodule in a taut band.

Trochanter: The greater and lesser trochanters are found only on the femur and serve as attachment sites for some of the muscles of the thigh and gluteals. The word *trochanter* is Greek meaning "a runner" and originally referred to horses that have three trochanters (*tro* meaning three and *canter* referring to a horse's running gait), whereas humans have only two.

Tuberosity: A large, rough, rounded process, such as the ischial tuberosity of the pelvis.

Tuina: A bodywork form practiced as part of traditional Chinese medicine for over 4000 years and based on principles of Chinese medicine. Tui means "push" and Na means "grasp" in Chinese, conveying the vigorous and firm quality of this massage system in which squeezing, compression, kneading, and joint movements are used to positively manipulate qi.

Ulnar: Refers to the ulna, a bone in the forearm, or to the structures that lie close to it (e.g., ulnar nerve, ulnar vein).

Unilateral: Refers to something on one side only.

Universal precautions: Guidelines for dealing with broken skin and mucus membranes, blood and other body fluids, and the clean-up of body fluids. Important components of universal precautions include: correctly using gloves, properly linens soiled in blood or body fluids, and properly cleaning surfaces contaminated with blood or bodily fluids.

Upward rotation: Movement when the scapula rotates so that the glenoid fossa moves superiorly.

Valgus: Valgus is modified Latin meaning "turned outward." The term refers to any of the paired joints in the extremities such as the elbow or knees. Valgus is a deformity in which the bone distal to the joint deviates laterally from the proximal bone, causing an outward angulation of the distal bone.

Varus: Varus is modified Latin meaning "bent inward." Like valgus, varus refers to the paired joints of the extremities.

Vasoconstriction: A decrease in a blood vessel's diameter resulting in decreased blood flow to an area (from the Latin root *vas(o)* meaning "blood vessel").

Vasodilation: An increase in a blood vessel's diameter allowing for more blood to an area.

Veins: Veins (from the Latin *vena*) receive deoxygenated blood from venules and form larger vessels that drain into the venae cavae. Veins have one-way valves that allow blood to flow in only one direction, toward the heart.

Vena cava (plural, venae cavae): The superior vena cava and the inferior vena cava are two large veins that receive deoxygenated blood from the veins and deposit the blood in the heart's right atrium.

Vibration: A pulsating, tremor-like, oscillating stroke practiced as part of Swedish massage.

Wellness chart: A simple form used to document wellness sessions when the client is healthy, a condition is not the reason for the visit, sessions are standardized or sessions are provided purely for relaxation and enjoyment.

Wellness massage: Used by the public to decrease stress, promote relaxation, support the body's natural restorative mechanisms, and have an enjoyable experience that leaves the body feeling refreshed and revitalized.

Index

(Note: Page numbers in italics indicates figure and those followed by "t" indicates tables and those followed "B" indicates boxes.)